Interventional Cardiology

1133 Questions: An Interventional Cardiology Board Review

THIRD EDITION

Interventional Cardiology

1133 Questions: An Interventional Cardiology Board Review

THIRD EDITION

Editors

Debabrata Mukherjee, MD

Chairman and Professor
Department of Internal Medicine
Paul L. Foster School of Medicine
Texas Tech University Health Sciences Center El Paso
El Paso, Texas

Richard A. Lange, MD, MBA

President and Dean
Paul L. Foster School of Medicine
Texas Tech University Health Sciences Center El Paso
El Paso, Texas

Saurav Chatterjee, MD

Fellow, Interventional Cardiology
Temple University Hospital
Philadelphia, Pennsylvania

Leslie Cho, MD

Director, Women's Cardiovascular Center
Preventive Cardiology & Rehabilitation
Cleveland Clinic Foundation
Cleveland, Ohio

David J. Moliterno, MD

Chairman and Professor
Department of Internal Medicine
Gill Heart and Vascular Institute
University of Kentucky
Lexington, Kentucky

Managing Editor

Nadia M. Whitehead

Texas Tech University Health Sciences Center El Paso
El Paso, Texas

Wolters Kluwer

Philadelphia • Baltimore • New York • London
Buenos Aires • Hong Kong • Sydney • Tokyo

Acquisitions Editor: Sharon Zinner
Development Editor: Mary Woodman
Editorial Coordinator: Mary Woodman/Annette Ferran
Editorial Assistant: Virginia Podgurski
Marketing Manager: Rachel Mante Leung
Production Project Manager: Bridgett Dougherty
Design Coordinator: Stephen Druding
Manufacturing Coordinator: Beth Welsh
Prepress Vendor: SPi Global

Third edition

9 8 7 6 5 4 3 2 1

Printed in China

Library of Congress Cataloging-in-Publication Data
Names: Mukherjee, Debabrata, editor.
Title: 1133 questions : an interventional cardiology board review / [edited by] Debarata Mukherjee.
Other titles: 1001 questions | Interventional cardiology board review
Description: Third edition. | Philadelphia : Wolters Kluwer, [2019] | Preceded by 1001 questions / editors, Debabrata Mukherjee, Leslie Cho, David J. Moliterno. c2012. | Includes index.
Identifiers: LCCN 2018015044 | ISBN 9781496386199
Subjects: | MESH: Cardiovascular Diseases—diagnosis | Cardiovascular Diseases—therapy | Examination Questions
Classification: LCC RC669.2 | NLM WG 18.2 | DDC 616.10076—dc23 LC record available at https://lccn.loc.gov/2018015044

LWW.com

CCS0618

"To interventional fellows and colleagues everywhere for their hard work and dedication to patient care; to my parents for their infinite patience, love, and understanding; and to Suchandra, for her love and support."

—Debabrata Mukherjee

"To interventional fellows worldwide who will use this text to expand their knowledge and advance our field … and to my parents, wife and sons who've taught me more about issues of the heart than any cardiology text."

—Richard A. Lange

"To my parents, my wife and my daughter–who inspire me to keep learning–and to my innumerable mentors over the years."

—Saurav Chatterjee

"With gratitude to the interventional fellows at Cleveland Clinic past, present, and future for their dedication and hard work."

—Leslie Cho

"To our chapter authors and interventional cardiology teachers worldwide; thoughtful questions and thorough answers will continue to advance the field and guide us all in contemporary medical practice."

—David J. Moliterno

PREFACE

Insightful questions have been used throughout the ages as a metric to assess one's knowledge, but when coupled with carefully delivered answers, they can become a powerful teaching tool. This book of questions and annotated answers covering the field of interventional cardiology is meant to serve as a helpful resource for individuals preparing for the interventional cardiovascular medicine board exam, as well as for clinicians who wish to perform an in-depth self-assessment on individual topics or the full spectrum of cardiovascular medicine. The book has many key features, which we believe will make the reader successful in passing the boards and improving clinical practice.

Of foremost importance, the areas covered are relevant not only to the day-to-day practice of interventional cardiology but have also been modified to fit the scope and content of the actual board examination. The book begins with several chapters dedicated to the anatomy and physiology associated with interventional cardiology and the pathobiology of atherosclerosis and inflammation. This corresponds to the 15% of the board examination, which targets material in the basic sciences. The subsequent chapters focus on the essential interventional pharmacotherapy of antiplatelets, anticoagulants, and other commonly used medications in the catheterization laboratory and outpatient setting for patients with atherosclerosis. These chapters correspond to the next 15% of the boards centering on pharmacology. A similar-sized 15% of the board examination is directed toward imaging; this book includes specific chapters on radiation safety, catheterization laboratory equipment and technique, contrast agents, and intravascular ultrasound. The two largest areas of the examination, each covering 25% of the content, include case selection management and procedural techniques. This review book dedicates several chapters to comprehensively cover these areas as well. Finally, we have included chapters for the miscellaneous remaining areas covered by the board examination, including peripheral vascular disease, cerebrovascular and structural heart interventions, ethics, statistics, and epidemiology, as well as a chapter directed at improving test-taking skills.

Also essential to the quality and appropriateness of the questions and annotated answers is the expertise of the chapter authors. We are fortunate to have assembled the "who's who" of academic interventional cardiology. The contributing authors from leading medical centers around the world have over 8,000 articles cited in PubMed. We are greatly indebted to these authors who are recognized both for their interventional expertise and for their teaching skills. In the end, the true value of this textbook is not only the relevance of the questions and the outstanding quality of the authors but also the value of the annotated answers. The text includes more than 1,000 questions and over 400 figures and tables. The corresponding answers have been appropriately detailed to provide relevant facts, information, and up-to-date journal citations.

The practice of interventional cardiology is exciting, rewarding, and a privilege each of us enjoys. Likewise, it has been our privilege to work with the superb contributors, our colleagues in interventional cardiology, and Ms. Nadia Whitehead at Texas Tech University Health Sciences Center El Paso and Ms. Mary Goodman at Wolters Kluwer for their editorial assistance. It is our personal hope that you will enjoy this book and that it will be a valuable resource to you in passing the board examination and providing the highest quality care possible to your patients

Debabrata Mukherjee, MD
Richard A. Lange, MD, MBA
Saurav Chatterjee, MD
Leslie Cho, MD
David J. Moliterno, MD

CONTRIBUTORS

Harsh Agrawal, MD
Division of Cardiology
Paul L. Foster School of Medicine
Texas Tech University Health Sciences Center El Paso
El Paso, Texas

Robert J. Applegate, MD
Cardiovascular Medicine
Wake Forest School of Medicine
Medical Center Boulevard
Winston-Salem, North Carolina

Subhash Banerjee, MD
University of Texas Southwestern Medical Center
Division of Cardiology
Veterans Affairs North Texas Health Care System
Dallas, Texas

Olivier F. Bertrand, MD, PhD
Québec Heart-Lung Institute
Laval University
Department of Mechanical Engineering
McGill University
Québec City, Québec, Canada

Sorin J. Brener, MD
Cardiac Catheterization Laboratory
New York—Presbyterian Brooklyn Methodist Hospital
Weill Cornell Medical College
Brooklyn, New York

Saurav Chatterjee, MD
Fellow, Interventional Cardiology
Temple University Hospital
Philadelphia, Pennsylvania

Adnan K. Chhatriwalla, MD
University of Missouri—Kansas City
Saint Luke's Mid America Heart Institute
Kansas City, Missouri

Leslie Cho, MD
Director, Women's Cardiovascular Center
Preventive Cardiology & Rehabilitation
Cleveland Clinic Foundation
Cleveland, Ohio

Joaquin E. Cigarroa, MD
Knight Cardiovascular Institute
Oregon Health & Science University
Portland, Oregon

Antonio Colombo, MD
Interventional Cardiology Unit
San Raffaele Scientific Institute
EMO-GVM Centro Columbus Hospital
Milan, Italy

Harold L. Dauerman, MD
University of Vermont College of Medicine
Burlington, Vermont

Ali Denktas, MD
Division of Cardiology
Department of Medicine
Baylor College of Medicine
Houston, Texas

Steven P. Dunn, PharmD
Heart and Vascular Center
University of Virginia Health System
University of Virginia School of Medicine
Charlottesville, Virginia

Mouhammad Fathallah, MD
Department of Cardiovascular Medicine
Duke University Medical Center
Durham, North Carolina

Stephan D. Fihn, MD, MPH
Departments of Medicine and Health Services
University of Washington
Seattle, Washington

Giuseppe Gargiulo, MD
Department of Cardiology, Inselspital
Bern University Hospital
Bern, Switzerland

Jay Giri, MD, MPH
Interventional Cardiology & Vascular Medicine
Division of Cardiovascular Medicine
Perelman School of Medicine
University of Pennsylvania
Philadelphia, Pennsylvania

Kashish Goel, MBBS
Department of Cardiovascular Diseases
Mayo Clinic
Rochester, Minnesota

Ziyad M. Hijazi, MD, MPH
Weill Cornell Medical College
Cornell University
Department of Pediatrics
Sidra Medical and Research Center
Doha, Qatar

Terence Hill, MD
Department of Cardiovascular Medicine
Heart and Vascular Institute
Cleveland Clinic Foundation
Cleveland, Ohio

Elizabeth M. Holper, MD, MPH
Interventional Cardiology
Interventional Cardiology Research
The Heart Hospital Baylor Plano
Plano, Texas

Samuel E. Horr, MD
Department of Cardiovascular Medicine
Heart and Vascular Institute
Cleveland Clinic
Cleveland, Ohio

Sei Iwai, MD
Westchester Medical Center
New York Medical College
Hawthorne, New York

Alice K. Jacobs, MD
Cardiac Catheterization Laboratory
Boston University School of Medicine
Boston, Massachusetts

Hani Jneid, MD
Interventional Cardiology Research
Michael E. DeBakey VA Medical Center
Baylor College of Medicine
Houston, Texas

Ankur Kalra, MD
Division of Cardiovascular Medicine
Department of Medicine
Case Western Reserve University School of Medicine
Harrington Heart & Vascular Institute
University Hospitals Cleveland Medical Center
Cleveland, Ohio

David E. Kandzari, MD
Piedmont Heart Institute
Piedmont Healthcare
Atlanta, Georgia

Ryan Kaple, MD
Interventional Cardiology
Westchester Medical Center
New York Medical College
Valhalla, New York

Dimitri Karmpaliotis, MD, PhD
Columbia University Medical Center
New York Presbyterian Hospital
New York, New York

Waleed Kayani, MD
Division of Cardiology
Department of Medicine
Baylor College of Medicine
Houston, Texas

Morton J. Kern, MD
Division of Cardiology
Veterans Affairs Long Beach HealthCare System
Long Beach, California
University of California Irvine Medical Center
Orange, California

Richard A. Krasuski, MD
Adult Congenital Heart Disease Center
Duke University Medical Center
Durham, North Carolina

Richard A. Lange, MD, MBA
President and Dean
Paul L. Foster School of Medicine
Texas Tech University Health Sciences Center El Paso
El Paso, Texas

Azeem Latib, MD
Interventional Cardiology Unit
San Raffaele Scientific Institute
EMO-GVM Centro Columbus Hospital
Milan, Italy

John J. Lazarus, MD
Department of Internal Medicine
University of Michigan Medical School
Ann Arbor, Michigan

Glenn N. Levine, MD
Cardiac Care Unit
Michael E. DeBakey VA Medical Center
Baylor College of Medicine
Houston, Texas

Tracy E. Macaulay, PharmD
College of Pharmacy
University of Kentucky
Lexington, Kentucky

Rajendra H. Mehta, MD, MS
Duke Clinical Research Institute
Duke University Medical Center
Durham, North Carolina

Timothy A. Mixon, MD
Interventional Cardiology, Division of Cardiology
Texas A&M College of Medicine
Scott & White Medical Center
Temple, Texas

David J. Moliterno, MD
Gill Heart and Vascular Institute
University of Kentucky
Lexington, Kentucky

Pedro R. Moreno, MD
Mount Sinai Health System
New York, New York

Debabrata Mukherjee, MD
Chairman and Professor
Department of Internal Medicine
Paul L. Foster School of Medicine
Texas Tech University Health Sciences Center El Paso
El Paso, Texas

Srihari S. Naidu, MD
Hypertrophic Cardiomyopathy Program
Interventional Cardiology
Westchester Medical Center
New York Medical College
Long Island, New York

Brahmajee K. Nallamothu, MD
Department of Internal Medicine
University of Michigan
Ann Arbor, Michigan

Craig R. Narins, MD
Divisions of Cardiology and Vascular Surgery
University of Rochester School of Medicine
Rochester, New York

Stephane Noble, MD
Division of Cardiology
University Hospital of Geneva
Geneva, Switzerland

Hussein Othman, MD
Central Michigan University College of Medicine
Detroit, Michigan

Devin Patel, MD
Division of Cardiovascular Medicine
Vanderbilt University Medical Center
Nashville, Tennessee

Timir K. Paul, MD, PhD
Department of Internal Medicine
Quillen College of Medicine
East Tennessee State University
Johnson City, Tennessee

Guillaume Plourde, MD, PhD
Québec Heart-Lung Institute
Université Laval
Québec, Canada

Abhiram Prasad, MD
Department of Cardiovascular Diseases
Mayo Clinic
Rochester, Minnesota

Mark Robbins, MD
Division of Cardiovascular Medicine
Vanderbilt University Medical Center
Nashville, Tennessee

Marco Roffi, MD
Division of Cardiology
University Hospital of Geneva
Geneva, Switzerland

Sonia Samtani, MD
Division of Cardiology
Irvine School of Medicine
University of California
Memorial Care Heart & Vascular Institute
Long Beach, California

Jacqueline Saw, MD
Interventional Cardiology
Vancouver General Hospital
University of British Columbia
Vancouver, Canada

Karen Segerson, MD
Department of Medicine
University of Washington
Seattle, Washington

Arnold H. Seto, MD
Division of Cardiology
Veterans Affairs Long Beach Health Care System
Long Beach, California
University of California Irvine Medical Center
Orange, California

Madhan Shanmugasundaram, MD
Sarver Heart Center
University of Arizona College of Medicine
Southern Arizona Veterans Affairs Health Care System
Tucson, Arizona

Mehdi Shishehbor, DO, PhD, MPH
Director, Cardiovascular Interventional Center
Co-Director, Vascular Center
University Hospitals Harrington Heart & Vascular Institute
Cleveland, Ohio

Michael H. Sketch Jr., MD
Department of Medicine
Duke University
Durham, North Carolina

Paul Sorajja, MD

Center for Valve and Structural Heart Disease
Minneapolis Heart Institute
Abbott Northwestern Hospital
Minneapolis, Minnesota

Hussam S. Suradi, MD

Rush Center for Structural Heart Disease
Rush University Medical Center
Structural Heart & Valve Center
St. Mary Medical Center
Munster, Indiana

Rajesh V. Swaminathan, MD

Duke University Medical Center
Duke Clinical Research Institute
Durham, North Carolina

Jay Thakkar, MD

Vancouver General Hospital
University of British Columbia
Vancouver, Canada

Marco Valgimigli, MD, PhD

Bern University Hospital
University of Bern
Bern, Switzerland

Amit N. Vora, MD, MPH

Department of Medicine
Duke University
Durham, North Carolina

Frederick G.P. Welt, MD

Division of Cardiovascular Medicine
Department of Medicine
Cardiac Catheterization Laboratory
University of Utah Health Sciences Center
Salt Lake City, Utah

Katherine Yu, MD

Olive View-UCLA Medical Center
University of California, Irvine
Long Beach, California

Khaled M. Ziada, MD

Interventional Cardiology
Gill Heart and Vascular Institute
University of Kentucky
Lexington, Kentucky

CONTENTS

ABBREVIATIONS

AAA	abdominal aortic aneurysm
ABI	ankle–brachial index
ABIM	American Board of Internal Medicine
ACAS	Asymptomatic Carotid Atherosclerosis Study
ACC	American College of Cardiology
ACCF	American College of Cardiology Foundation
ACE	angiotensin-converting enzyme
ACEI	angiotensin-converting enzyme inhibitor
ACGME	Accredited Council for Graduate Medical Education
ACLS	Advanced Cardiac Life Support
ACP	American College of Physicians
ACS	acute coronary syndrome
ACT	Acetylcysteine for Contrast-induced Nephropathy Trial
ACT	activated clotting time
ACUITY	Acute Catheterization and Urgent Intervention Triage strategy
AD	advance directive
ADP	adenosine diphosphate
AHA	American Heart Association
AIVR	accelerated idioventricular rhythm
AL	Amplatz left
ALARA	as low as reasonably achievable
ALI	acute limb ischemia
AMI	acute myocardial infarction
ANA	antinuclear antibody
ApoE	apolipoprotein E
aPTT	activated partial thromboplastin time
APV	average peak velocity
AR	Amplatz right
ARC	Academic Research Consortium
ARFD	acute renal failure requiring dialysis
ART	allRight™
AS	aortic stenosis
ASA	acetylsalicylic acid
ASD	atrial septal defect
ATP III	Adult Treatment Panel III
AV	atrioventricular
AVM	arteriovenous malformation
AVR	aortic valve replacement
AYMYDA	atorvastatin for reduction of myocardial damage during angioplasty
BARI	bypass versus angioplasty revascularization investigation
BE	balloon expandable
BMI	body mass index
BMS	bare-metal stent
BNP	brain natriuretic peptide
BP	blood pressure
BSA	body surface area
BVS	bioresorbable vascular scaffold
CABG	coronary artery bypass graft
CAD	coronary artery disease
cAMP	cyclic adenosine monophosphate
CAS	carotid artery stenting
CBC	complete blood count
CCA	common carotid artery
CCD	charge-coupled device
CCS	Canadian Cardiovascular Society
CCU	coronary care unit
CEA	carotid endarterectomy
CFR	coronary flow reserve
CHD	coronary heart disease
CHF	congestive heart failure
CI	confidence interval
CKD	chronic kidney disease
CK-MB	creatine kinase-MB
CME	continuing medical education
CMR	cardiovascular magnetic resonance
CNS	central nervous system
CO	cardiac output
COPD	chronic obstructive pulmonary disease

COX	cyclooxygenase
CPO	cardiac power output
CREDO	clopidogrel for the reduction of events during observation
CREST	Carotid Revascularization Endarterectomy versus Stenting Trial
CRP	C-reactive protein
CSA	cross-sectional area
CT	computed tomography
CTA	computed tomography angiography
cTFC	corrected TIMI frame count
CTO	chronic total occlusion
CVA	cerebrovascular accident
CVD	comorbid cardiovascular disease
2D	two-dimensional
D2B	door-to-balloon
DAP	dose area product
DAPT	dual antiplatelet therapy
DCA	directional coronary atherectomy
DES	drug-eluting stent
DM	diabetes mellitus
DNA	deoxyribonucleic acid
DNR	do not resuscitate
DREAM	Dutch Endovascular Aneurysm Management
DSA	digital subtraction angiography
DVT	deep vein thrombosis
EAST	Emory Angioplasty versus Surgery Trial
EBU	extra back-up
ECA	external carotid artery
ECG	electrocardiogram
ECST	European Carotid Surgery Trial
ED	emergency department
EDRF	endothelial-derived relaxing factor
EEM	external elastic media
EEOC	Equal Employment Opportunity Commission
EES	everolimus-eluting stent
EF	ejection fraction
EKG	electrocardiogram
EMERALD	enhanced myocardial efficacy and recovery by aspiration of liberated debris
EMS	emergency medical services
EP	electrophysiologic
EPC	endothelial progenitor cell
EPD	emboli protection device
ER	emergency room
ERBAC	excimer laser, rotational atherectomy, and balloon angioplasty comparison
ESSENCE	efficacy and safety of subcutaneous enoxaparin in non-q-wave coronary events
EVAR	endovascular aneurysm repair
FDA	Food and Drug Administration
FFR	fractional flow reserve
FIRE	FilterWire EX Randomized Evaluation
FMD	fibromuscular dysplasia
FPS	frames per second
Fr	French
GERD	gastroesophageal reflux disease
GFR	glomerular filtration rate
GIK	glucose–insulin–potassium
GP	glycoprotein
GPI	glycoprotein IIb/IIIa inhibitor
GRACE	Global Registry of Acute Coronary Events
Gy	gray
HCM	hypertrophic cardiomyopathy
HDL	high-density lipoprotein
HF	heart failure
HIT	heparin-induced thrombocytopenia
HMG-CoA	hydroxymethylglutaryl coenzyme A
HORIZONS	Harmonizing Outcomes with Revascularization and Stents in Acute Myocardial Infarction
HPS	Heart Protection Study
HR	hazard ratio
HR	heart rate
HS	hockey stick
HTN	hypertension
IABP	intra-aortic balloon pump
IC	intracoronary
ICA	internal carotid artery
ICAM	intercellular cell adhesion molecule
ICD	implantable cardioverter defibrillator
ICE	intracardiac echocardiography
ICU	intensive care unit
IgE	immunoglobulin E
IL	interleukin
IM	internal mammary
IMA	inferior mesenteric artery
IMA	internal mammary artery
IPA	inhibition of platelet aggregation
IRA	infarct-related artery

IRB	Institutional Review Board
ITT	intention-to-treat
IV	intravenous
IVC	inferior vena cava
IVUS	intravascular ultrasound
J	joule
JL	Judkins left
JR	Judkins right
KERMA	kinetic energy released to matter
keV	kiloelectron volt
kg	kilogram
kVp	peak kilovoltage
LA	left atrium
LAD	left anterior descending
LAD	leukocyte adhesion deficiency
LAO	left anterior oblique
LBBB	left bundle-branch block
LCB	left coronary bypass or left graft seeker
LCx	left circumflex
LDH	lactate dehydrogenase
LDL	low-density lipoprotein
LDL-C	low-density lipoprotein cholesterol
LIMA	left internal mammary artery
LM	left main
LMCA	left main coronary artery
LMT	left main trunk
LSVC	left-sided vena cava
LTA	light transmission aggregometry
LV	Left ventricular
LVEDP	left ventricular end-diastolic pressure
LVEF	left ventricular ejection fraction
LVH	left ventricular hypertrophy
LVOT	left ventricular outflow tract
mA	milliampere
MA	malignant arrhythmias
MACE	major adverse cardiac events
MAP	mean arterial pressure
MBG	myocardial blush grade
MCA	middle cerebral artery
MCE	myocardial contrast echocardiography
MDR	multidrug resistance
MERLIN	Middlesbrough Early Revascularization to Limit Infarction
mg	milligram
mGy	milligray
MI	myocardial infarction
mL	milliliter
MLA	minimum lumen area
MLD	minimal lumen diameter
mm	millimeter
MONA	morphine, oxygen, nitroglycerin, and aspirin
MP	multipurpose
MPA	maximal platelet aggregation
MR	mitral regurgitation
MRA	magnetic resonance angiography
MS	mitral stenosis
mSv	millisievert
MVD	multivessel disease
MVP	mitral valve leaflet prolapse
NASCET	North American Symptomatic Carotid Endarterectomy Trial
NCEP	National Cholesterol Education Program
ng	nanogram
NNT	number needed to treat
NO	nitric oxide
NPH	neutral protamine Hagedorn
NSAID	nonsteroidal anti-inflammatory drug
NSTEMI	non–ST-segment elevation myocardial infarction
NSVT	nonsustained ventricular tachycardia
NTG	nitroglycerine
NTR	no-torque right
NYHA	New York Heart Association
OCT	optical coherence tomography
OM	obtuse marginal
OR	odds ratio
PA	plasminogen activator
PA	pulmonary arterial
PA	pulmonary artery
PAD	peripheral arterial disease
PAF	paroxysmal atrial fibrillation
PAI-1	plasminogen activator inhibitor-1
PAR-1	protease activator receptor-1
PAV	percent atheroma volume
PB	plaque burden
PBMA	poly n-butyl methacrylate
PCI	percutaneous coronary intervention
PCL	poly(e-caprolactone)
PCW	pulmonary capillary wedge
PCWP	pulmonary capillary wedge pressure
PD	pharmacodynamic

PDA	patent ductus arteriosus
PDA	posterior descending artery
PE	pulmonary embolism
PES	paclitaxel-eluting stent
PEVA	polyethylene-co-vinyl acetate
PFO	patent foramen ovale
PFT	pulmonary function test
PGA	poly(glycolic acid)
PK	pharmacokinetics
PKC	protein kinase C
PLC	phospholipase C
PLE	protein-losing enteropathy
PLLA	poly-L-lactic acid
PPI	proton pump inhibitor
PT	prothrombin time
PTA	percutaneous transluminal angioplasty
PTCA	percutaneous transluminal coronary angioplasty
PTSMA	percutaneous transluminal septal myocardial ablation
PV	peripheral vascular
PV	pulmonary vein
Q	Q curve catheter
QCA	quantitative coronary angiography
R	roentgen
RA	right atrial
RAGE	receptor for advanced glycation end products
RAO	right anterior oblique
RAS	renin–angiotensin system
RBC	red blood cell
RCA	right coronary artery
RCB	right coronary bypass
rCFR	relative coronary flow reserve
RCT	randomized clinical trial
RD	reference diameter
RI	ramus intermedius
RIMA	right internal mammary artery
RN	registered nurse
RP	retroperitoneal
RPH	retroperitoneal hematoma
RV	right ventricular
RVSP	right ventricular systolic pressure
SA	stable angina
SAFER	saphenous vein graft angioplasty free of emboli randomized
SBP	systolic blood pressure
SCAI	Society of Coronary Angiography and Interventions
sCD40L	soluble CD40 ligand
SCI	spinal cord ischemia
SD	sudden death
SE	self-expanding
SES	sirolimus-eluting stent
SFA	superficial femoral artery
SI	silent ischemia
SMA	superior mesenteric artery
SOB	shortness of breath
SS	spot stenting
STEMI	ST-segment elevation myocardial infarction
STR	segment resolution
Sv	sievert
SVC	superior vena cava
SVG	saphenous vein graft
SYC	syncope
TAA	thoracic aortic aneurysm
TAPAS	Thrombus Aspiration During Percutaneous Coronary Intervention in Acute Myocardial Infarction Study
TAV	total atheroma volume
TAVI	transcatheter aortic valve replacement
TCFA	thin-cap fibroatheromas
TEE	transesophageal echocardiogram
TFC	TIMI frame count
TFPI	tissue factor pathway inhibitor
TG	triglycerides
ThCFA	thick-cap fibroatheroma
TIA	transient ischemic attack
TIMI	thrombolysis in myocardial infarction
TLR	target lesion revascularization
TMP	TIMI myocardial perfusion
TMPG	TIMI myocardial perfusion grade
TNF	tumor necrosis factor
TnI	troponin I
TnT	troponin T
TOF	tetralogy of Fallot
TOPAS	Thrombolysis or Peripheral Arterial Surgery trial

TOSCA	Total Occlusion Study of Canada
tPA	tissue plasminogen activator
TS	traditional stenting
TVR	target vessel revascularization
UA	unstable angina
UFH	unfractionated heparin
VASP	vasodilator-stimulated phosphoprotein
VCAM	vascular cell adhesion molecule
VF	ventricular fibrillation
VH	virtual histology
VKOR	vitamin K epoxide reductase
VL	Voda left
VLDL	very-low-density lipoprotein
VSD	ventricular septal defect
VSR	ventricular septal rupture
ZES	zotarolimus-eluting stent

1 Vascular Biology

Frederick G.P. Welt and Pedro R. Moreno

QUESTIONS

1.1 A 64-year-old female with diabetes, hypertension, and an active smoking history undergoes cardiac catheterization and stent implantation in a 90% obstructive lesion found in her left anterior descending (LAD) artery. In addition to the stented lesion, she is found to have an additional nonobstructive lesion in her proximal right coronary artery (RCA). You suspect that the nonobstructive lesion has a large necrotic lipid core, as shown in Figure Q1-1. The following statements are TRUE regarding this plaque containing a lipid core, EXCEPT:

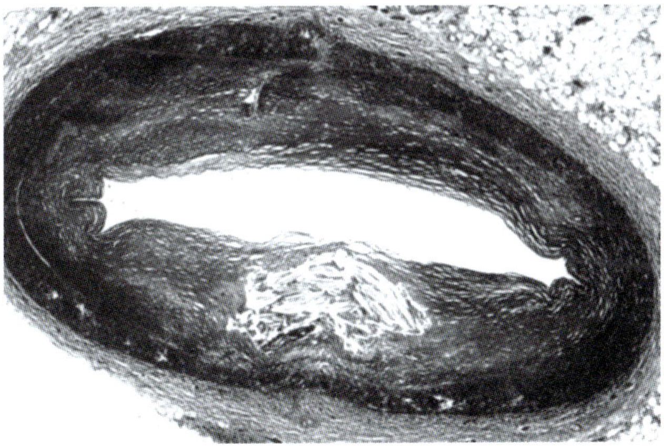

Figure Q1-1

(A) It is composed of cholesterol crystals and collagen
(B) The predominant cell is the smooth muscle cell
(C) It is reflected as a green structure on polarized microscopy using the Picrosirius red stain
(D) It may be suitable for imaging using percutaneous techniques

1.2 You are evaluating a 59-year-old male patient with a history of diabetes, hypertension, peripheral vascular disease, hypercholesterolemia, and coronary artery disease (CAD). He has previously undergone coronary artery bypass grafting (CABG), drug-eluting stent (DES) implantation twice, and bilateral below the knee amputation. His laboratory results showed an elevated high-sensitivity C-reactive protein (hs-CRP). Which of the following statements is FALSE regarding the pathophysiology of the atheroma of this patient?

(A) Given this advanced atherosclerosis burden, this patient has a defective resolution of inflammation
(B) The complex atherosclerotic plaques in this patient are rich in neovascularization, which is promoted by inflammation
(C) Macrophages are the main source of metalloproteinases in the plaque
(D) Plaque stabilization is characterized by defective efferocytosis

1.3 A 49-year-old male who is an active smoker is rushed into the catheterization laboratory after presenting to the emergency department with a 20-minute history of excruciating, pressure-like substernal chest pain radiating to his left arm and associated with nausea and diaphoresis, which occurred while rapidly climbing upstairs. The initial coronary angiogram is shown in Figure Q1-3. A successful thrombectomy was performed. Which of the following best describes the coronary substrate that led to the clinical presentation of the patient?

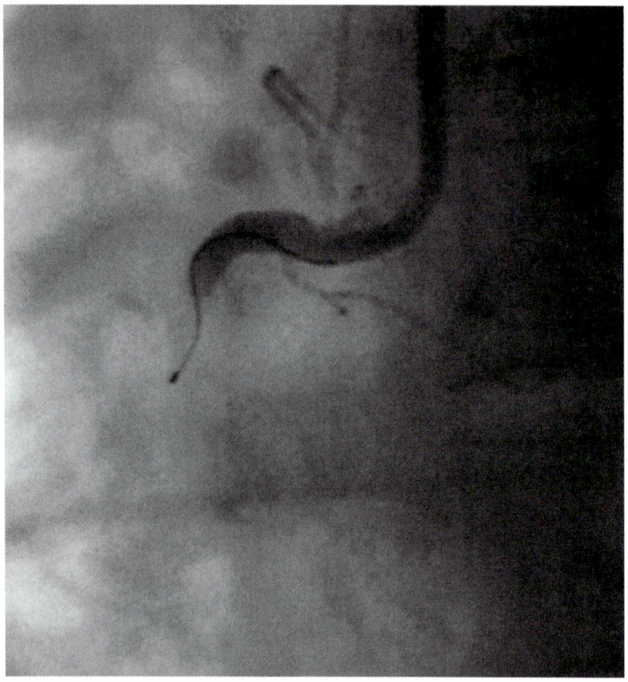

Figure Q1-3

(A) A ruptured atherosclerotic plaque with increased collagen content
(B) A ruptured atherosclerotic plaque with decreased lipid content
(C) A ruptured atherosclerotic plaque with increased proteoglycan content
(D) A ruptured atherosclerotic plaque with increased matrix metalloproteinase expression

1.4 Consider the patient in Question 1.3. The atherosclerotic plaque responsible for his clinical event would most likely be characterized by which of the following?

(A) A rupture at the shoulder region of the plaque
(B) A rupture at the center of the cap
(C) A rupture at the thickest portion of the cap
(D) No rupture, but superficial erosion

1.5 A 55-year-old male presents with stuttering chest pain at rest and electrocardiogram (ECG) changes of T-wave inversion in the inferior leads. His troponin is elevated. Just 1 month prior to this event, he had a catheterization revealing only mild obstructive disease in the RCA. Repeat catheterization reveals a hazy irregular lesion in the RCA at the site of the prior plaque but with normal-appearing flow. What is the most likely explanation for his elevated troponin?

(A) Rapid progression of the lesion resulting in myocardial oxygen supply demand mismatch at rest
(B) Microemboli from a ruptured plaque leading to downstream microvascular obstruction
(C) Intermittent complete occlusion of the vessel with endogenous lysis
(D) Intermittent severe vasospasm
(E) False-positive elevation of troponin

1.6 In the patient above, angioscopy is utilized to evaluate and characterize the lesion. What would you expect to find?

(A) A white lesion secondary to abundant fibrin and red cell deposition
(B) A red lesion secondary to abundant fibrin and red cell deposition
(C) A white lesion secondary to abundant platelet deposition
(D) A red lesion secondary to abundant platelet deposition
(E) A glistening yellow lesion secondary to abundant cholesterol deposition

1.7 A 72-year-old patient develops sudden-onset excruciating substernal chest pain associated with severe shortness of breath. He is rapidly taken to the cardiac catheterization laboratory where a DES implantation is successfully performed, as shown in Figure Q1-7. Based on previous evidence, you consider the most likely histopathologic event leading to this patient's clinical presentation is plaque rupture. All of the following statements are TRUE, EXCEPT

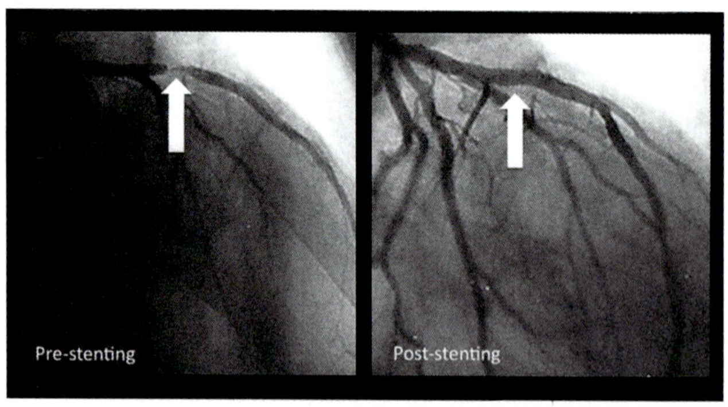

Figure Q1-7

(A) Plaque rupture may occur simultaneously in two different arteries
(B) Plaque healing after rupture is mediated by smooth muscle cell production of collagen type III
(C) Smooth muscle cells are responsible for weakening the fibrous cap
(D) T lymphocytes increase proteolytic activity and decrease collagen synthesis

1.8 A 62-year-old male without prior cardiac history, but with history of diabetes mellitus, hypertension, and tobacco use, presents with crushing substernal chest pain and ST-segment elevation in leads V2 through V4. He is taken immediately to the catheterization laboratory where he is found to have an occluded LAD and a high-grade ulcerated-appearing left circumflex (LCx) lesion with what appears to be thrombus. What is the best explanation for these findings?

(A) Embolization to the coronary arteries from a noncoronary source
(B) Embolization of a left main thrombus to both the LAD and LCx
(C) Evidence of an inherited hypercoagulable state
(D) Simultaneous plaque rupture in two separate arteries

1.9 A 67-year-old male is referred to you for evaluation after a positive stress test. His laboratory evaluation included an elevated low-density lipoprotein (LDL) level, low levels of high-density lipoprotein (HDL), and elevated CRP levels. Regarding CRP, all of the following statements are TRUE, EXCEPT

(A) CRP is an acute phase reactant that binds to phosphocholine in dying cells or bacteria
(B) CRP is produced in the liver as a proinflammatory response to interleukin (IL)-4
(C) CRP has been found within the plaque at the lipid core
(D) CRP has intrinsic atherogenic properties stimulating foam cell formation

1.10 Cardiac catheterization performed in a 58-year-old demonstrates nonobstructive lesions in the proximal RCA. You confirm these findings with quantitative coronary angiography (QCA) and intravascular ultrasound (IVUS) (Fig. Q1-10) and suspect that these lesions could represent thin cap fibroatheromas (TCFA). All of the following statements about TCFA are TRUE, EXCEPT:

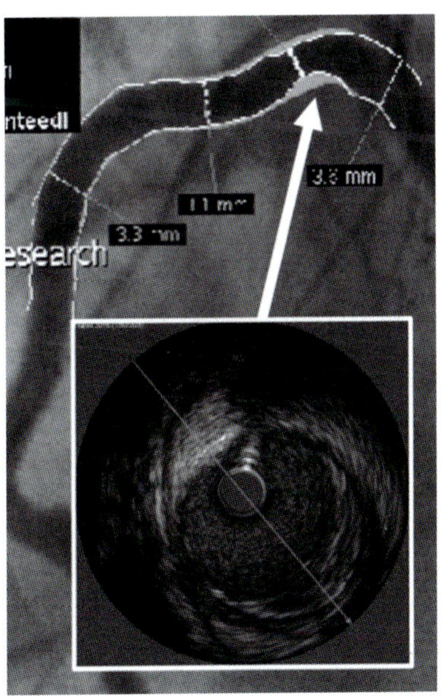

Figure Q1-10

(A) The nonthrombosed lesion that most resembles the acute plaque rupture is the TCFA
(B) TCFA is characterized by a necrotic core with an overlying fibrous cap measuring <65 μm, containing rare smooth muscle cells but numerous macrophages
(C) TCFAs are most frequently observed in patients dying with acute myocardial infarction (MI) and are least common in plaque erosion
(D) TCFAs have a greater degree of calcification than other advanced plaques

1.11 You are evaluating a 64-year-old with a history of multiple MIs, who is visiting your office for the first time. You notice that the patient has high levels of inflammatory markers including hs-CRP and leukocytosis. Which of the following is the most accurate regarding the diagnostic benefit of biomarkers?

(A) LDL levels are more accurate for determining prognosis than hs-CRP
(B) Methotrexate has been proven to reduce cardiovascular events in clinical trials
(C) Leukocytosis is not an independent predictor for future events
(D) The beneficial effects of aspirin in primary prevention are dependent on the degree of inflammation, measured as plasma hs-CRP levels

1.12 A 69-year-old male patient with a history of hypertension, uncontrolled diabetes, and smoking undergoes cardiac catheterization and IVUS imaging that reveal numerous atherosclerotic plaques with positive remodeling as seen in Figure Q1-12. All of the following statements are true, EXCEPT:

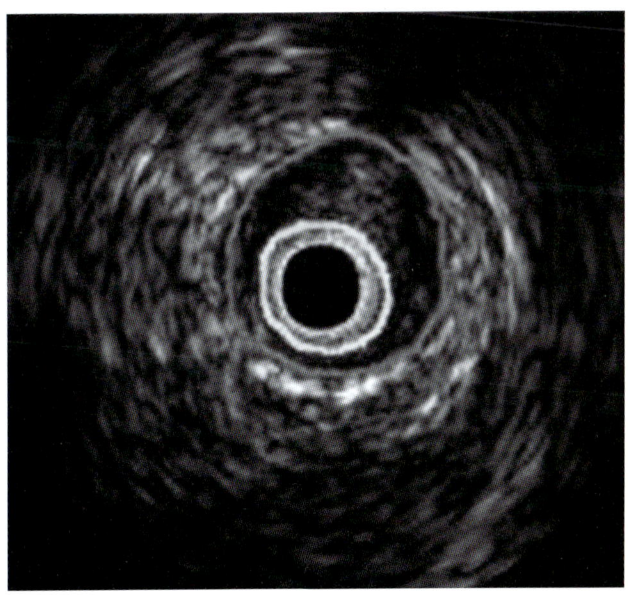

Figure Q1-12

(A) Remodeling preserves the lumen and protects against heart attacks
(B) Positive remodeling is most frequently seen in unstable syndromes
(C) Positive remodeled plaques have more macrophages
(D) Plaques can grow up to 40% area of stenosis without obstructing the lumen

1.13 In the patient from Question 1.12, you are concerned that most of the nonobstructive lesions observed during his coronary angiogram are vulnerable plaques. Which of the following statements is most accurate regarding vulnerable plaques?

(A) Neoangiogenesis is associated with vessels predominantly entering from the luminal surface of the lesion
(B) Vulnerable plaques have been shown to be less rupture prone when treated with antiangiogenic factors in clinical trials
(C) Density of neovascularization is not associated with plaque vulnerability
(D) Intraplaque hemorrhage is related to increased plaque vulnerability

1.14 The cardiac catheterization laboratory at your institution is part of a multicenter prospective study that evaluates the use of optical coherence tomography (OCT) in coronary plaque characterization. One of your patients, a 61-year-old female, is enrolled in the study. During OCT pullback, you observe a dense layer of tissue covering an atherosclerotic lesion as showed in Figure Q1-14. This plaque can be classified as:

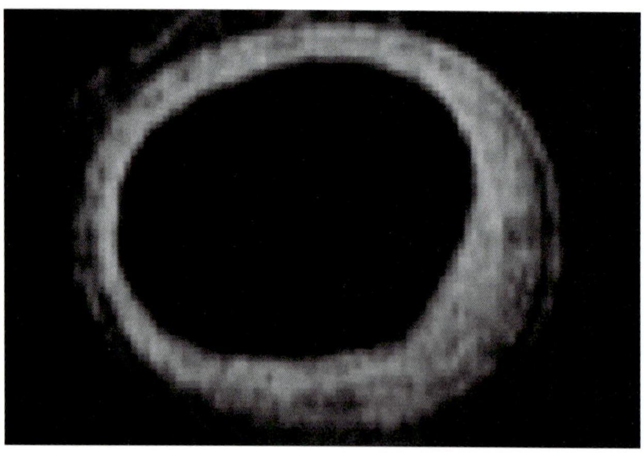

Figure Q1-14

(A) Plaque rupture
(B) Thin cap fibroatheroma
(C) Thick cap fibroatheroma
(D) Plaque erosion

1.15 The angiogram of a 49-year-old male with atypical chest pain is presented in Figure Q1-15. After 100 mcg of intracoronary nitroglycerin, the angiogram dramatically improves. The following statements are all TRUE, EXCEPT:

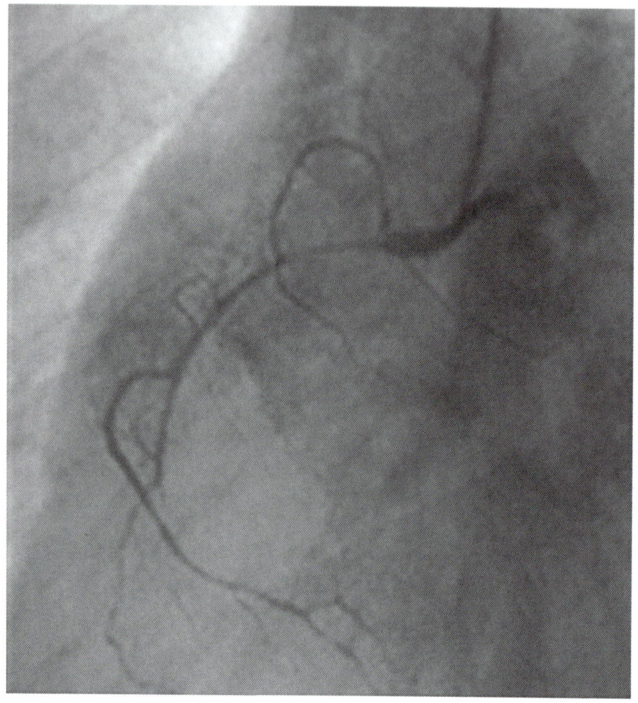

Figure Q1-15

(A) The improvement is related to increased endothelial-dependent relaxation
(B) The improvement is related to increased endothelial-independent relaxation
(C) This patient will benefit from long-acting calcium channel blockers (CCBs)
(D) Coronary stenting is associated with repeat spasm in nonstented areas

1.16 In the above patient, normal function of the endothelium utilizes the enzyme endothelial nitric oxide synthase to catalyze which of the following intracellular reactions?

(A) Arginine to citrulline releasing NO
(B) Arginine to citrulline releasing NO_2
(C) Thiamine to arginine releasing NO
(D) Thiamine to arginine releasing NO_2

1.17 Regarding the patient presented in Question 1.15, which of the following statements best describes the role of nitric oxide in the vascular tissue?

(A) Blocks endothelial-dependent vasodilation
(B) Activates thrombin
(C) Induces smooth muscle cell proliferation
(D) Activates cyclic guanosine monophosphate (cGMP)

1.18 A 58-year-old male patient with a history of smoking and early CAD in both parents is undergoing a diagnostic cardiac catheterization. OCT is performed and demonstrates areas of high-intensity signal with stripe pattern shadow suggestive of macrophage infiltration (Fig. Q1-18). This increased macrophage activity in vulnerable plaques can lead to:

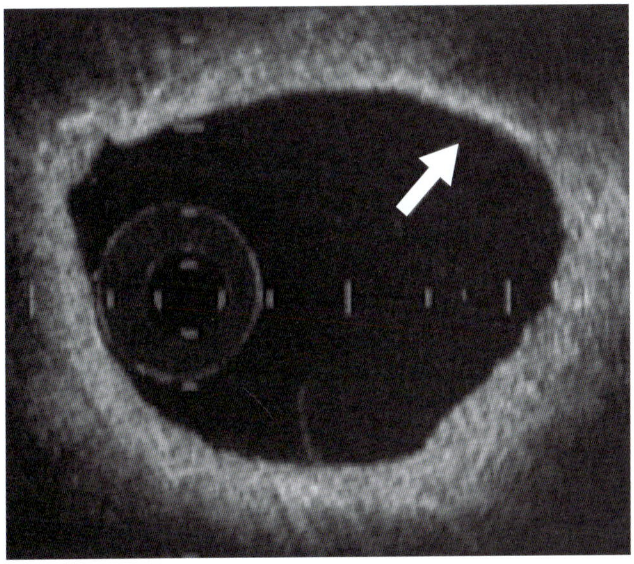

Figure Q1-18

(A) Expression of matrix metalloproteinases
(B) Antiapoptotic cell survival
(C) Production of NO
(D) Expression of antithrombin III

1.19 You are doing rounds evaluating patients after cardiac catheterization. One of your patients, a 65-year-old female, with advanced diabetes and history of multiple coronary events, CABG, and stent implantation, asks you to explain why she has had multiple cardiovascular complications. Which one of the following is TRUE about diabetic atherosclerosis?

(A) It is associated with decreased atherosclerotic burden
(B) It is characterized by decreased plaque macrophage infiltration
(C) It is associated with lower levels of hs-CRP
(D) It is associated with upregulation of macrophage receptor for advanced end-glycation (RAGE) products

1.20 IVUS imaging performed in a 62-year-old diabetic female patient reveals positive remodeling in several vascular segments as shown in Figure Q1-20. Which of the following is not an independent predictor of positive remodeling?

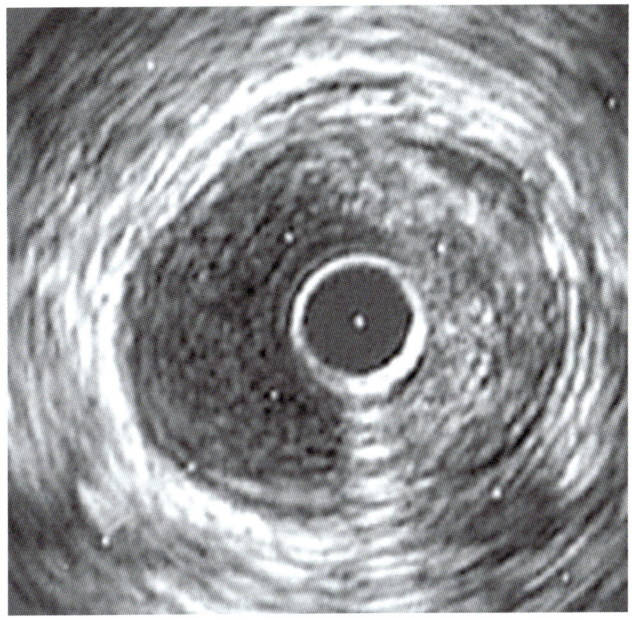

Figure Q1-20

(A) Inflammation
(B) Calcification
(C) Medial atrophy
(D) Cigarette smoking

1.21 A 71-year-old female diabetic patient undergoes bare metal stent (BMS) implantation in a 78% lesion in her mid-RCA after a positive nuclear stress test. The patient undergoes a follow-up coronary angiogram with OCT imaging as part of a clinical trial in which she was enrolled at the time of the stenting.

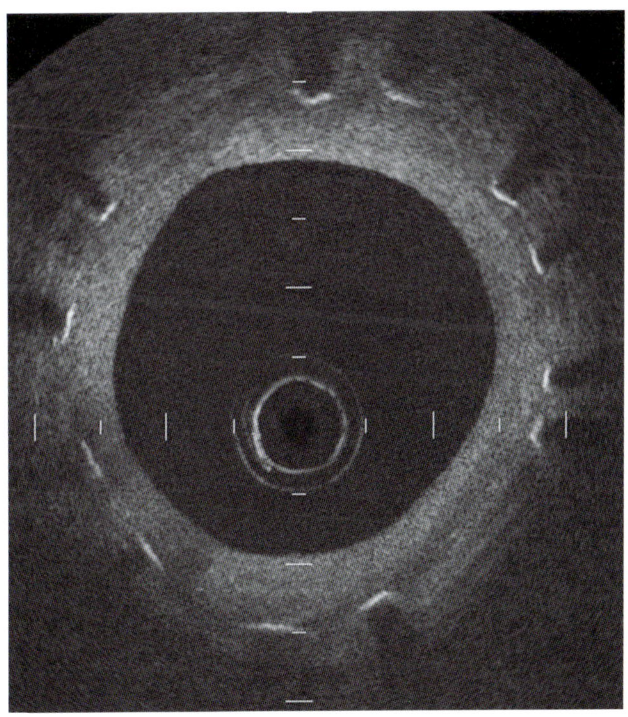

Figure Q1-21

OCT reveals neointimal coverage over the implanted stent struts as shown in Figure Q1-21. Which of the following statements is FALSE regarding smooth muscle cell proliferation after stent deployment?

(A) Is increased in diabetic lesions after BMS
(B) Is characterized by increased production of collagen I
(C) Is associated with inflammation
(D) Is reduced after complete endothelialization
(E) Is associated with increased cell apoptosis

1.22 A 64-year-old male patient with history of hypertension, hypercholesterolemia, and previous cigarette smoking presents to the emergency room with chest pain in the midchest radiating to his back and left shoulder. An ECG taken upon arrival is displayed in Figure Q1-22. His pain starts to improve after two sublingual nitroglycerin tablets. His initial troponin-I level is 3.5 ng/mL. He is taken to the cardiac care unit at your institution for medical management. Which of the following statements is FALSE regarding coronary thrombosis in unstable angina and non–ST-segment elevation myocardial infarction (NSTEMI)?

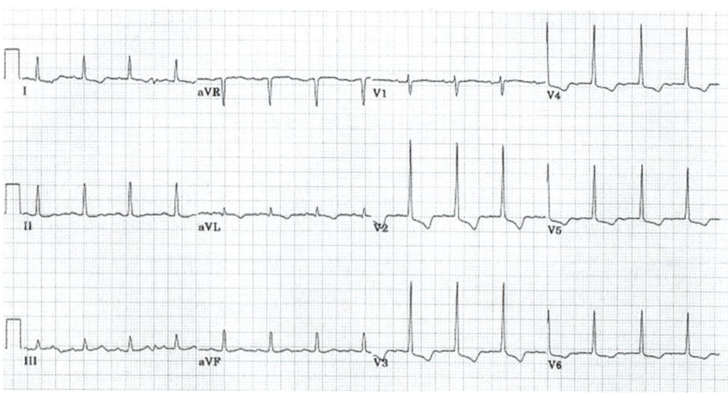

Figure Q1-22

(A) Is more frequently mediated by plaque rupture rather than erosion
(B) Can induce distal emboli, predominately composed of cholesterol crystals and necrotic debris
(C) Thrombolysis reduces embolization and facilitates intervention
(D) Is associated with increased circulating tissue factor particles and cell apoptosis

1.23 A 78-year-old female patient is admitted to the medical service with a 6-hour history of weakness and paresthesias in the left upper and lower extremities. On physical exam, besides her motor and sensory deficits in the left limbs, she also presents right mouth droop and a right carotid bruit. You order a carotid ultrasound that shows an 80% atherosclerotic plaque in the right internal carotid artery (Fig. Q1-23), so you call for a neurosurgery consult. Studies of carotid endarterectomy have shown all of the following, EXCEPT:

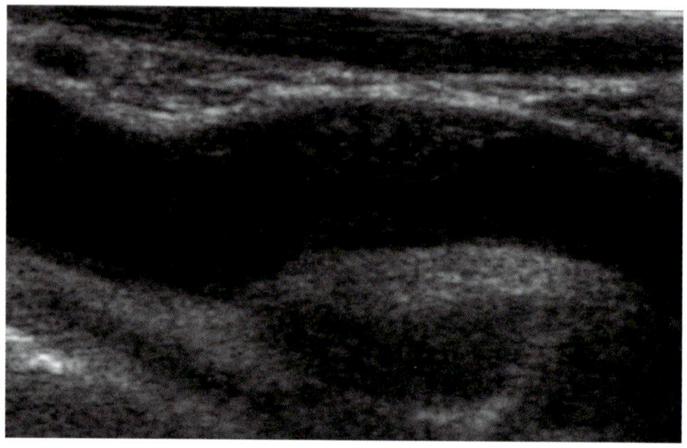

Figure Q1-23

(A) Thrombotic plaques are more frequently observed in patients with stroke as compared to transient ischemic attack (TIA)
(B) Asymptomatic patients can have thrombotic carotid plaques in up to 27% of individuals
(C) Hypertension and low HDL cholesterol are associated with vulnerable and thrombotic carotid plaques
(D) Low HDL cholesterol does not correlate with macrophage infiltration

1.24 A 67-year-old male patient and active smoker with a history of dyslipidemia, obesity, and hypertension undergoes a coronary computed tomography (CT) angiogram as recommended by his primary care physician. The report of the test reveals extensive coronary calcification and a high coronary calcium score (Fig. Q1-24). The following statements about coronary calcification are all TRUE, EXCEPT:

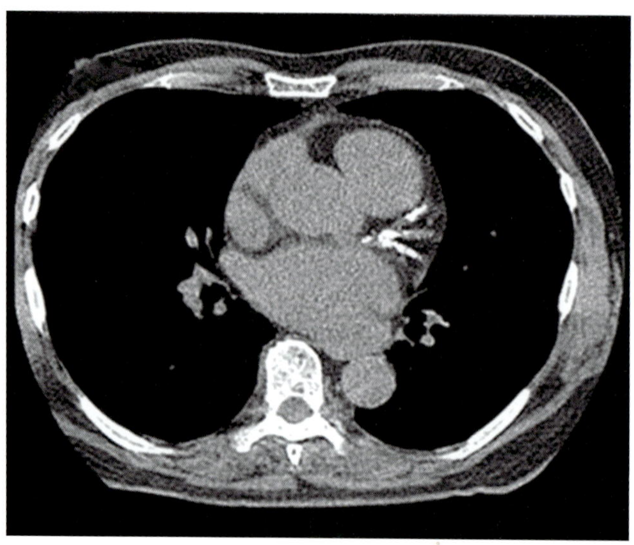

Figure Q1-24

(A) Coronary calcification is a predictor for future coronary events
(B) Coronary calcification typically reflects advanced disease by histologic criteria
(C) Plaque erosion is more frequently seen in smokers
(D) Chronic stable angina lesions may be healed ruptured plaques
(E) Plaque rupture more frequently occurs at the center of the fibrous cap

1.25 A 52-year-old diabetic female with a history of two episodes of pulmonary thromboembolism and several third trimester miscarriages is referred to you for follow-up after being discharged for an NSTEMI. Given her high incidence of thrombotic events, you decide to perform a workup for hypercoagulable state. In regard to vascular thrombosis, all of the following statements are TRUE, EXCEPT:

(A) Her coronary thrombus is predominately platelet-rich
(B) Her deep vein thrombosis (DVT) and pulmonary embolism (PE) are mostly fibrin-rich
(C) Her natural anticoagulants to be evaluated include protein C, protein S, and tissue factor pathway inhibitor (TFPI)
(D) Her plasminogen-activator inhibitor (PAI)-1 level will be low

1.26 While talking to a pathologist who has performed an autopsy on a 70-year-old male who experienced sudden cardiac death, he describes to you that the immunostaining analysis of the specimens revealed abundant matrix metalloproteinases as observed in the following image (Fig. Q1-26). The role of these matrix metalloproteinases is relevant for all of the following, EXCEPT:

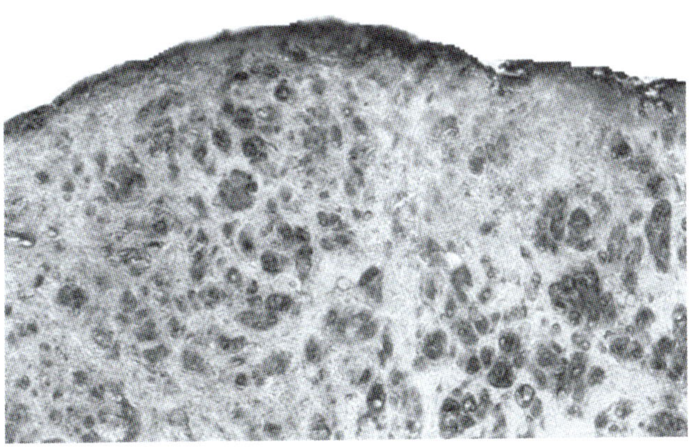

Figure Q1-26

(A) Positive remodeling by digesting the internal elastic lamina
(B) Plaque angiogenesis by mediating tunnelization of neovessels
(C) Plaque rupture by digesting the collagen of the fibrous cap
(D) Myocardial salvage preventing expansion and remodeling

1.27 In further evaluation of the specimen from the patient in Question 1.26, the pathologist describes significant amounts of monocyte-derived macrophages infiltrating the atheroma (Fig. Q1-27). The role of these monocyte-derived macrophages in atherosclerosis can be described by all of the following, EXCEPT:

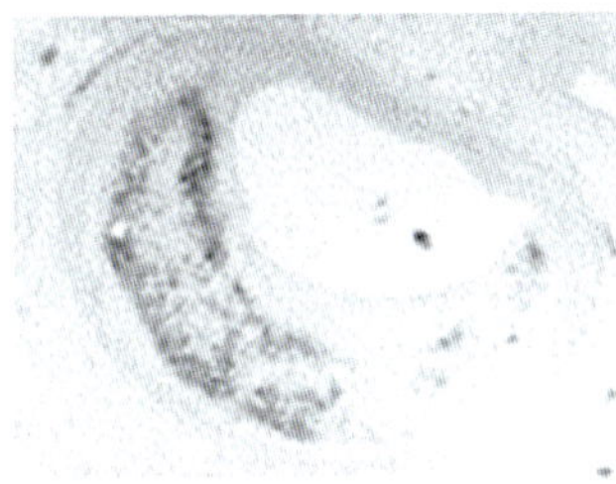

Figure Q1-27

(A) Removal of oxidized LDL by the scavenger receptor CD-36
(B) Transfer of free cholesterol to HDL by the ABC1 and ABCG transporters
(C) Removal of apoptotic bodies from the plaque
(D) Antithrombogenic effects during apoptosis by the expression of protein C

1.28 You are asked to bring a patient with end-stage renal disease (ESRD) to the catheterization laboratory to evaluate his coronary anatomy prior to possible renal transplant. Your angiogram reveals dense calcification and a moderate lesion in the left main artery. IVUS is performed showing what appears to be a 50% lesion with predominantly intimal calcification. In addition to circulating osteoblast progenitor cells, which resident cells of the plaque likely contribute to the cellular mechanisms of atherosclerotic calcification?

(A) Vascular smooth muscle cells
(B) Fibroblasts
(C) Macrophages
(D) T cells

1.29 A 75-year-old male presents with stable angina and is referred for catheterization. He has a history of DES placement in the LAD approximately 3 years ago. Angiography reveals a 50% narrowing in the prior placed stent. OCT is performed and shows a lesion (Fig. Q1-29). Which of the following is TRUE about this lesion?

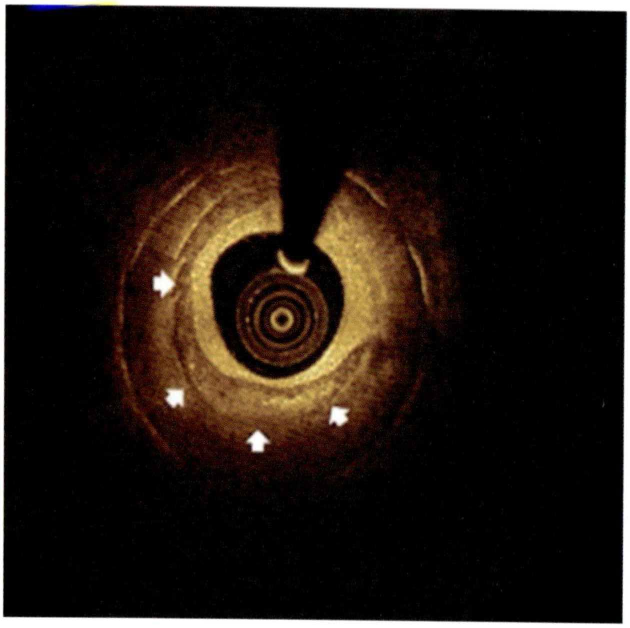

Figure Q1-29 (Adapted from Lee SY, et al. *Circ Cardiovasc Interv* 2015;8(2):e001878, with permission.)

(A) It is likely an extension of the underlying atherosclerotic plaque, which has grown through the stent struts
(B) It forms by virtue of stent thrombosis with subsequent remodeling of the plaque
(C) It more commonly occurs in the first year after stent implantation
(D) It more commonly occurs after DES placement than BMS placement

1.30 A 82-year-old patients is admitted to the hospital with gastrointestinal (GI) bleeding and syncope. You are asked to consult regarding a murmur. The patient has no prior history of cardiac issues but complains of progressive shortness of breath with exertion. On exam, you hear a harsh systolic murmur at the right upper sternal border radiating to the carotids. The patient has gone through upper and lower endoscopy without an obvious source of bleed. What is the likely bleeding diathesis affecting this patient?

(A) Thrombocytopenia
(B) Factor V deficiency
(C) Acquired von Willebrand's disease
(D) Bernard–Soulier syndrome

1.31 A 32-year-old female with a history of cardiac transplantation 1 year prior is brought to the cardiac catheterization laboratory for her annual evaluation, including right heart catheterization, coronary angiography, and myocardial biopsy. On angiography, you see diffuse "pruning" of the vessels without focal disease. If you were able to study cross-sections of the arteries with histologic staining, what might help you differentiate the lesions evident in this patient vs. one with native atherosclerosis?

(A) More abundant levels of collagen in this patient
(B) More abundant levels of proteoglycans in this patient
(C) Lack of foam cells in this patient
(D) More abundant platelet deposition in this patient

1.32 You are performing a catheterization on a 55-year-old male with angina and a positive stress test. You observe a lesion at the bifurcation of the LAD and a large diagonal artery (Medina classification 1,0,1). A cardiology fellow asks you whether lesions are more common at bifurcations. What is the most accurate statement to tell her?

(A) No, lesions are less common at bifurcations
(B) Yes, they typically occur at the carina between the two vessels
(C) Yes, they typically occur opposite the carina in both vessels
(D) Yes, they typically occur in the main branch

ANSWERS AND EXPLANATIONS

1.1 Answer B. A necrotic core characterizes plaque rupture with an overlying thin-ruptured cap infiltrated by macrophages and lymphocytes. There are few or no smooth muscle cells within the cap. With polarized microscopy, collagen fibers will be bright yellow or orange and the thinner fibers will be green.The lipid core is suitable for imaging using radiofrequency analysis of IVUS (virtual histology) or near infrared spectroscopy. More recently, intracoronary OCT, a technique that measures backscattered light, or optical echoes, and is derived from an infrared light source directed at the arterial wall, has been proposed as a high-resolution analogue of IVUS (Finn AV, et al. *Arterioscler Thromb Vasc Biol* 2010;30(7):1282–1292).

1.2 Answer D. Plaque stabilization is characterized by *effective*, not defective, efferocytosis, which relates to the ability of macrophages to remove apoptotic bodies from the core of atherosclerotic plaques (Tabas I. *Nat Rev Immunol* 2010;10(1):36–46). All other statements are true.

1.3 Answer D. Ruptured plaques are characterized by decreased collagen content, increased lipid content, and increased metalloproteinase expression (Finn AV, et al. *Arterioscler Thromb Vasc Biol* 2010;30(7):1282–1292).

1.4 Answer A. Plaque ruptures typically occur at the shoulder regions where circumferential stress is highest (Arroyo LH, et al. *Cardiovasc Res* 1999;41(2):369–375).

1.5 Answer B. It is unlikely that there has been rapid progression of a stable plaque in the timeframe of a month. It is also unlikely that in the face of EKG changes and symptoms that this is a false elevation of troponin. It is more likely that this represents a ruptured plaque with thrombus and the troponin rise is due to downstream emboli. Vasospasm and intermittent total occlusion can be causes of troponin rise, and these mechanisms are not mutually exclusive but less likely (Braunwald E. *Am J Respir Crit Care Med* 2012;185(9):924–932).

1.6 Answer C. Angioscopy of plaques in patients with acute coronary syndromes (ACS) has revealed that plaques associated with NSTEMI typically are predominantly platelet-based and white to gray. In contrast, plaques associated with STEMI typically are more red due to fibrin and red cell deposition often overlying a platelet-based lesion (Mizuno K, et al. *N Engl J Med* 1992;326(5):287–291).

1.7 Answer C. Smooth muscle cells are responsible for strengthening, not weakening, of the fibrous cap. All other statements are correct.

1.8 Answer D. Multiple complex plaques are common and provide evidence of contribution of systemic inflammation to the process of plaque rupture. Such patients are typically found to have higher levels of inflammatory markers such as hs-CRP compared to normal controls or patients with a single complex plaque (Goldstein JA, et al. *N Engl J Med* 2000;343(13):915–922).

1.9 Answer B. CRP is produced in the liver as a proinflammatory response to IL-6, not IL-4.

1.10 Answer D. TCFAs have a lesser degree of calcification than other advanced plaques (Virmani R, et al. *J Am Coll Cardiol* 2006;47(8 Suppl):C13–C18). The other statements are correct.

1.11 Answer D. The beneficial effects of aspirin in primary prevention are closely related to CRP levels (Ridker PM, et al. *N Engl J Med* 1997;336(14):973–979). In patients with the lowest quintile of CRP, acetylsalicylic acid (ASA) does not prevent cardiovascular events (13% reduction when compared to placebo; p = NS). However, in patients with the highest quintile of CRP, aspirin prevents cardiovascular events (53% reduction when compared to placebo; $p < 0.0001$). Leukocytosis is a predictor of future cardiac events. Compared to LDL, hs-CRP is at least as predictive for future cardiac events. Methotrexate is currently being studied as a protective strategy in patients, but the results are not known as of yet.

1.12 Answer A. Remodeling preserves the lumen but does not protect from heart attacks. It is actually more frequent in plaques from patients with acute coronary events (Schoenhagen P, et al. *Circulation* 2000;101(6):598–603).

1.13 Answer D. Intraplaque neovascularization occurs mainly from the vasa vasorum and is associated with plaque growth, hemorrhage, and vulnerability. In vivo studies have suggested that antiangiogenic strategies can retard plaque growth but have been associated with worse outcomes in clinical trials to date (Camaré C, et al. *Redox Biol* 2017;12:18–34).

1.14 Answer C. A plaque with a dense layer of tissue covering the lipid core is considered a thick cap fibroatheroma.

1.15 Answer A. Nitroglycerin acts directly on the smooth muscle cell of the tunica media, classically known as endothelial-independent relaxation. Coronary stenting is associated with repeat spasm in nonstented areas and is not indicated.

1.16 Answer A. Arginine to citrulline releasing NO. NO_2 is nitrous, not nitric, oxide and is a common mistake.

1.17 Answer D. The mechanism of action of NO is related to the activation of cGMP.

1.18 Answer A. Increased macrophage activity in vulnerable plaques can lead to the expression of matrix metalloproteinases.

1.19 Answer D. Diabetes atherosclerosis is characterized by increased atherosclerotic burden, higher levels of CRP plaque macrophage infiltration, and upregulation of RAGE (Wendt T, et al. *Atherosclerosis* 2006;185(1):70–77).

1.20 Answer D. The independent predictors of positive remodeling include inflammation, calcification, and medial atrophy (Burke AP, et al. *Circulation* 2002;105(3):297–303). Cigarette smoking is associated with plaque erosion but not positive remodeling.

1.21 Answer B. Smooth muscle cell proliferation after stent deployment is characterized by increased production of collagen III, not collagen I. All other statements are correct.

1.22 Answer C. Coronary thrombosis in unstable angina and NSTEMI is mediated by platelet-rich thrombus (Fuster V, et al. *J Am Coll Cardiol* 2005;46(6):937–954). Thrombolysis activates platelets and may be harmful in ACS and should not be used. Other statements are correct.

1.23 Answer D. Low HDL cholesterol is an independent predictor for macrophage infiltration in carotid endarterectomy studies in humans. In addition, asymptomatic patients can have thrombotic carotid plaques in up to 27% of the cases (Mauriello A, et al. *Atherosclerosis* 2010;208(2):572–580).

1.24 Answer E. Plaque rupture more frequently occurs at the shoulders, not the center of the fibrous cap (Richardson PD, et al. *Lancet* 1989;2(8669):941–944). The other statements are correct.

1.25 Answer D. PAI-1 is increased in diabetic plaques not lowered (Jax TW, et al. *Cardiovasc Diabetol* 2009;8:48). All other statements are true.

1.26 Answer D. Metalloproteinases do not salve myocardium. On the contrary, metalloproteinase is associated with expansion and remodeling of the ventricle after MI (Lindsey ML, et al. *Circulation* 2002;105(6):753–758). All other statements are correct.

1.27 Answer D. Macrophages are associated with thrombogenic effects during apoptosis by the expression of tissue factor. All other statements are correct.

1.28 Answer A. The main body of evidence points toward transformation of vascular smooth muscle cells and to some degree arterial pericytes into osteoblast cells that contribute to calcification (Johnson RC, et al. *Circ Res* 2006;99(10):1044–1059).

1.29 Answer D. The lesion shows an eccentric plaque with a cap overlying a less dense core. This is consistent with neoatherosclerosis, a process resembling native atherosclerosis that has been found to occur more often following DES (first generation > newer DES) than BMS. It is typically a late process and does not appear to be structurally associated with the underlying lesion although it may be more common when implanted in patients with an initial presentation of ACS (Otsuka F, et al. *Eur Heart J* 2015;36(32):2147–2159).

1.30 Answer C. The likely diagnosis is Heyde's syndrome or acquired von Willebrand's deficiency with associated arteriovenous malformations, usually in the small intestine. This is a syndrome associated with severe aortic stenosis, which may be caused by deformation of the von Willebrand's protein due to turbulent flow across the aortic valve (Loscalzo J. *N Engl J Med* 2013;368(6):579–580).

1.31 Answer B. Acquired vasculopathy in the transplanted heart has many distinct differences when compared to native atherosclerosis, most notably the presence of abundant proteoglycan and less collagen deposition. Platelet deposition tends to be more prominent in native atherosclerosis while foam cells are present in both conditions (Rahmani M, et al. *Circ Res* 2006;99(8):801-815).

1.32 **Answer C.** Statistically, lesions more often occur at bifurcations, specifically at the walls opposite the carina where shear stress is lower. This leads to both biologic and mass transport conditions favoring lesion growth (Ku DN, et al. *Arteriosclerosis* 1985;5(3):293-302).

2 Anatomy and Physiology

Richard A. Lange and Joaquin E. Cigarroa

QUESTIONS

2.1 An 80-year-old man is referred for coronary angiography for evaluation of retrosternal pain at rest. Pressure recordings from the coronary catheter tip during its engagement in the right coronary artery (RCA) ostium and withdrawal (see *arrow*, Fig. Q2-1) into the aorta indicate:

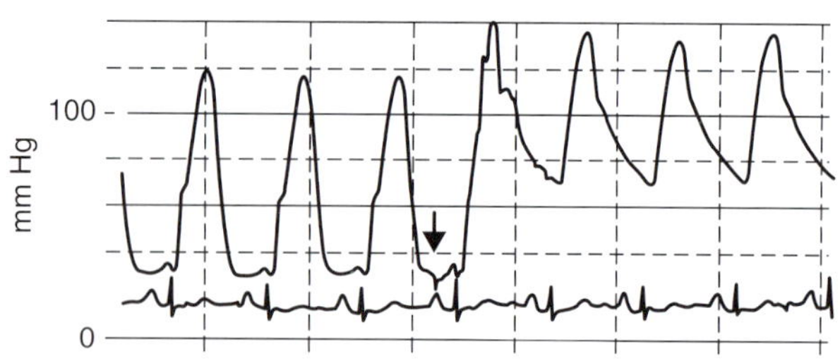

Figure Q2-1

(A) Collateral coronary flow
(B) Severe aortic stenosis
(C) Anomalous origin of a coronary artery
(D) Obstruction of antegrade coronary flow by the catheter

2.2 Which of the following projections allows the operator to visualize a proximal left circumflex (LCx) stenosis optimally?

(A) 30-degree right anterior oblique (RAO)
(B) 30-degree RAO, 30-degree cranial
(C) 60-degree left anterior oblique (LAO), 30-degree cranial
(D) 30-degree RAO, 30-degree caudal

2.3 A 45-year-old man with a bicuspid aortic valve is found to have a left dominant coronary circulation at cardiac catheterization. What is the incidence of this?

(A) 90%
(B) 50%
(C) 30%
(D) 10%

2.4 A 55-year-old man undergoes coronary angiography for evaluation of nonexertional chest pain. The left lateral view of the left anterior descending (LAD) artery obtained during diastole (panel A) and systole (panel B) is displayed in Figure Q2-4. He has:

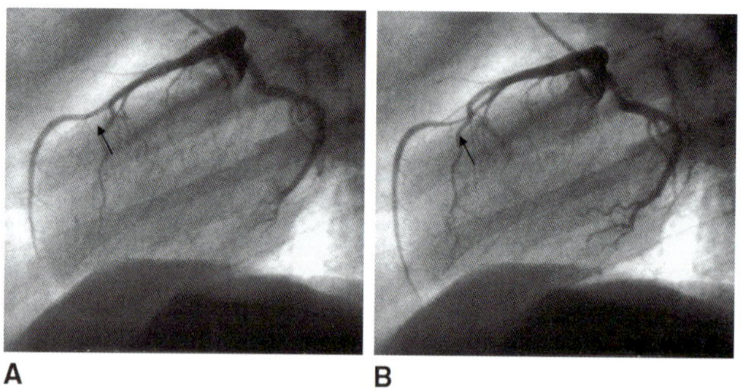

Figure Q2-4 (With permission from Bauters C, et al. *Circulation* 2002;105(1):130.)

(A) An eccentric atherosclerotic stenosis
(B) Myocardial bridging
(C) Prinzmetal's angina
(D) Coronary dissection

2.5 In order to obtain a "spider view" to visualize the left main (LM) coronary artery as well as the proximal LAD and LCx arteries optimally, the image intensifier should be positioned:

(A) 50 degrees LAO, 20 degrees caudal
(B) 30 degrees RAO, 30 degrees caudal
(C) 50 degrees LAO, 35 degrees cranial
(D) 15 degrees RAO, 30 degrees cranial

2.6 In a 30-year-old survivor of sudden cardiac death, left ventriculography in the 30-degree RAO projection shows a "button" projecting from the aortic root (Fig. Q2-6). This suggests that the patient has:

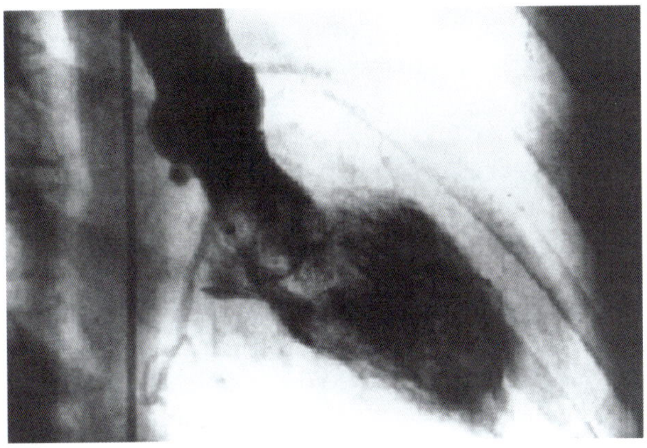

Figure Q2-6

(A) Occlusion of the proximal RCA
(B) Anomalous origin of the LCx artery
(C) Pseudoaneurysm of the proximal ascending aorta
(D) Coronary ectasia from Kawasaki's disease

2.7 In routine clinical practice, the severity of coronary stenosis is estimated from visual inspection of the coronary angiogram. Compared with quantitative coronary angiography, such a visual estimation of coronary stenoses usually:

(A) Provides similar results
(B) Underestimates the severity of the stenosis by 35%
(C) Underestimates the severity of the stenosis by 20%
(D) Overestimates the severity of the stenosis by 20%

2.8 Impaired vasodilator reserve is first noted when the coronary luminal diameter narrowing (i.e., stenosis) is:

(A) 50%
(B) 60%
(C) 75%
(D) 90%

2.9 What is a Kugel's artery?

(A) Anomalous origin of the LAD coronary artery from the pulmonary artery
(B) Coronary arteriovenous fistula (AVF)
(C) Conus artery branch
(D) Right-to-right collateral (from proximal to distal RCA through the atrioventricular [AV] node branch)

2.10 A 55-year-old woman with exertional chest pain and an abnormal myocardial perfusion scan has a coronary angiogram that demonstrates a 50% stenosis of the mid-RCA. This corresponds to a cross-sectional area narrowing of:

(A) 50%
(B) 60%
(C) 75%
(D) 90%

2.11 Which is TRUE of coronary blood flow?

(A) Phasic coronary blood flow is more pronounced for diastolic compared to systolic flow
(B) The diastolic predominance is greater in the left than the RCA
(C) With an epicardial stenosis, translesional pressure loss (i.e., the aortic coronary gradient) will initially be evident in diastole
(D) All of the above

2.12 In what percentage of individuals does the LCx coronary artery provide the blood flow to the sinoatrial node?

(A) 10%
(B) 40%
(C) 60%
(D) 90%

2.13 Which of the statements regarding coronary blood flow autoregulation is TRUE?

(A) During exercise, the resistance of the coronary microvasculature increases
(B) An epicardial stenosis increases epicardial resistance, which is compensated by an equivalent increase in microvascular resistance to maintain coronary autoregulation
(C) When a coronary stenosis becomes "critical," the compensation capacity of the microvasculature is exhausted
(D) The Bayliss phenomenon (i.e., increased perfusion pressure causes reflex coronary vasodilation) helps to maintain coronary autoregulation
(E) A low coronary flow reserve (CFR) (<2 in adults) is diagnostic for abnormal microvascular resistance

2.14 Which of the following is TRUE of the coronary venous system?

(A) Veins and venules are innervated by sympathetic nerves
(B) Venous volume increases with sympathetic stimulation
(C) Veins dilate in response to local metabolic factors
(D) Veins are constricted in the basal state

2.15 All the following are TRUE regarding coronary vascular resistance, EXCEPT:

(A) Left ventricular (LV) hypertrophy can impair microcirculatory (R3) resistance
(B) In the absence of stenosis, R1 (epicardial vessel) resistance is trivial
(C) The R2 (prearteriolar) vessels are responsible for most of the total coronary resistance
(D) The R3 (arteriolar and intramyocardial) vessels are regulated neurogenically and locally

2.16 Which of the following are limitations of using CFR to assess the presence of a significant epicardial stenosis?

(A) Hyperemic flow is directly dependent on systemic blood pressure
(B) Tachycardia decreases hyperemic flow, thus reducing CFR
(C) The hyperemic and resting measurements are not performed simultaneously
(D) CFR is not specific for epicardial stenosis
(E) All of the above

2.17 Before placement of a catheter in the coronary sinus, a venogram is performed (Fig. Q2-17). What does the *arrow* denote?

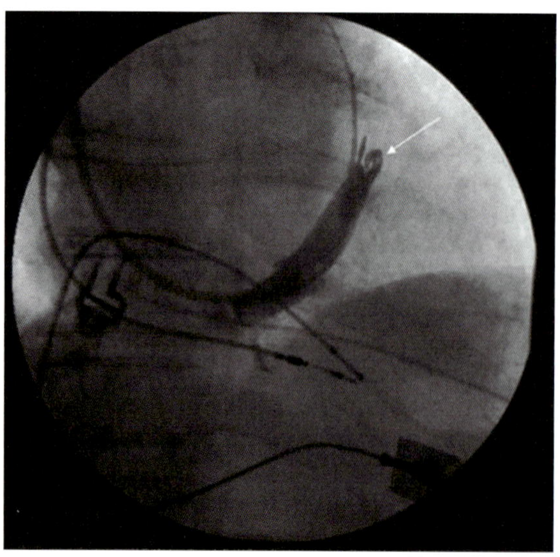

Figure Q2-17 (With permission from Habib A, et al. *Europace* 2009;11:15–21.)

(A) A prominent Vieussens valve is visualized
(B) The proximal coronary sinus has a thrombotic occlusion
(C) The middle cardiac vein is seen coursing superiorly after emptying into the coronary sinus
(D) A persistent left superior vena cava (SVC) is visualized

2.18 The CORRECT formula for determining myocardial oxygen consumption (MVO_2) from the coronary arterial or venous flow (Q), arterial oxygen content (AoO_2), and coronary sinus oxygen content (CSO_2) is:

(A) $MVO_2 = Q/(AoO_2 - CSO_2)$
(B) $MVO_2 = (AoO_2 - CSO_2)/Q$
(C) $MVO_2 = Q \times (AoO_2 - CSO_2)$
(D) Cannot calculate with the data provided

2.19 The "abbreviated" form of the Gorlin formula (so-called Hakki equation: valve area (cm^2) = flow (L/min)/$\sqrt{\text{peak-to-peak pressure gradient}}$) is often used to estimate valve area in patients with valvular stenosis referred for catheterization. It may be inaccurate in which of the following circumstances?

(A) Valve area < 1.0 cm^2
(B) High cardiac output
(C) Low transvalvular gradient
(D) Bradycardia (heart rate < 60 beats per minute [bpm]) or tachycardia (heart rate > 100 bpm)

2.20 In which of the following circumstances may the use of an LV–Ao pullback pressure recording to assess aortic valve area yield inaccurate results?

(A) Low (<35 mm Hg) transvalvular gradient
(B) Atrial fibrillation
(C) Immediately after left ventriculography
(D) All of the above

2.21 A 50-year-old gentleman with a left bundle-branch block (LBBB) is referred for cardiac catheterization to evaluate "atypical" chest pain because his noninvasive testing was nondiagnostic. Coronary angiography demonstrates a 65% mid-LAD stenosis. You decide to assess his instantaneous wave-free ratio (iFR) to determine the hemodynamic significance of his stenosis. Which of the following best characterizes this assessment?

(A) For measurement of iFR, adenosine intravenous (IV) (140 mcg/kg/min) or intracoronary (IC) (100 mcg bolus) is preferable to regadenoson for achieving maximal hyperemia
(B) Aortic and distal coronary artery pressures are compared during early diastole to obtain iFR
(C) An iFR of 0.85 is an indication for revascularization
(D) An iFR of 0.90 is a contraindication to revascularization, as medical therapy is effective in patients with this measurement

2.22 Coronary venous oxygen saturation is typically:

(A) 30%
(B) 50%
(C) 65%
(D) 80%

2.23 A 66-year-old woman presents to the emergency department with acute shortness of breath and dizziness. She is noted to have a blood pressure of 90/60 mm Hg, a heart rate of 35 bpm, elevated neck veins, and rales to the midlung fields. Her electrocardiogram (ECG) shows an inferior ST-segment elevation myocardial infarction (STEMI) and third-degree heart block. An echo shows a markedly decreased left ventricular ejection fraction (LVEF) with inferior akinesis and anterior hypokinesis. She is brought to the cardiac catheterization laboratory where a temporary transvenous pacing is placed in the right ventricle and dobutamine is initiated prior to angiography. Catheterization revealed a 100% occlusion of the RCA and 60% proximal LAD stenosis. Primary percutaneous coronary intervention (PCI) of the RCA is successful with placement of a 3.0- × 20-mm drug-eluting stent (DES). To evaluate the "intermediate" LAD stenosis, you decide to:

(A) Assess FFR after the dobutamine infusion is stopped because the increased contractility alters FFR reliability
(B) Assess FFR after the temporary pacing wire is discontinued, as changes in heart rate by pacing may affect the accuracy of FFR measurement
(C) Proceed with FFR without changing dobutamine infusion or pacing therapy, as neither affects this measurement
(D) Defer FFR and proceed directly to PCI of the proximal LAD stenosis, as FFR is unreliable in the setting of an acute myocardial infarction (MI) due to microvascular dysfunction

2.24 Which of these coronary anomalies is commonly associated with ischemic complications?

(A) An RCA arising from the left sinus of Valsalva
(B) Origin of the LCx from the right coronary sinus
(C) A left main coronary artery arising from the noncoronary sinus
(D) An RCA originating from the noncoronary sinus
(E) All of the above

2.25 Which is TRUE of the normal endothelial layer of coronary arteries?

(A) Endothelial cells produce and secrete von Willebrand factor
(B) Endothelial cells secrete nitric oxide
(C) Endothelial cells secrete matrix metalloproteinases
(D) Endothelial cells secrete extracellular matrix components, such as elastin and fibronectin
(E) All of the above

2.26 Which is TRUE of the capillary vessels?

(A) They consist of a single layer of endothelial cells
(B) They lack the ability to change their diameter actively because they have no smooth muscle cells
(C) They have the largest cross-sectional and surface area of the vessels in the vasculature
(D) All of the above

2.27 Coronary blood flow velocity is directly:

(A) Proportional to cross-sectional area of the artery
(B) Proportional to vascular resistance
(C) Proportional to blood flow
(D) All of the above

2.28 Which of the following induces coronary arterial vasodilation?

(A) Angiotensin II
(B) Vasopressin
(C) Alpha-1 adrenergic receptor stimulation
(D) Beta-2 adrenergic receptor stimulation
(E) All of the above

2.29 Which of the following statements regarding the structure of coronary arteries is CORRECT?

(A) The media of all arteries is contained within a connective tissue layer called the internal elastic lamina
(B) At the point the epicardial arteries turn into the myocardium, they become more muscular arteries with few if any elastic fibers
(C) The media contains a network of small blood vessels (vasa vasorum), which is responsible for the nutrition of the inner third of the artery
(D) The internal elastic lamina contains nerves, which control the tone of the artery

2.30 In a normal subject at rest, coronary blood flow is what percentage of cardiac output?

(A) 40%
(B) 20%
(C) 10%
(D) 5%

2.31 Which of the following statements regarding the left main coronary artery is correct?

(A) The left main ostium lacks adventitia and has a greater portion of elastic tissue than other segments of the coronary tree
(B) Since the left main ostium has fewer elastic fibers, it is not subject to diseases affecting the aortic wall, such as syphilitic aortitis, radiation-induced aortitis, and Takayasu's arteritis
(C) Trifurcation of the left main, with the third artery called the ramus intermedius, occurs in 10% to 20% of the population
(D) A high takeoff in the left main is associated with an increased risk of left main stenosis and ischemia
(E) Origin of the left main from the noncoronary cusp is associated with sudden cardiac death

2.32 A 45-year-old woman developed acute-onset, severe substernal chest pain and anterior ST elevation on her ECG following an intense argument with her son (Fig. Q2-32A and B). Arteriography demonstrated no significant coronary stenoses, and her left ventriculogram is shown in Figure Q2-32C. She most likely has:

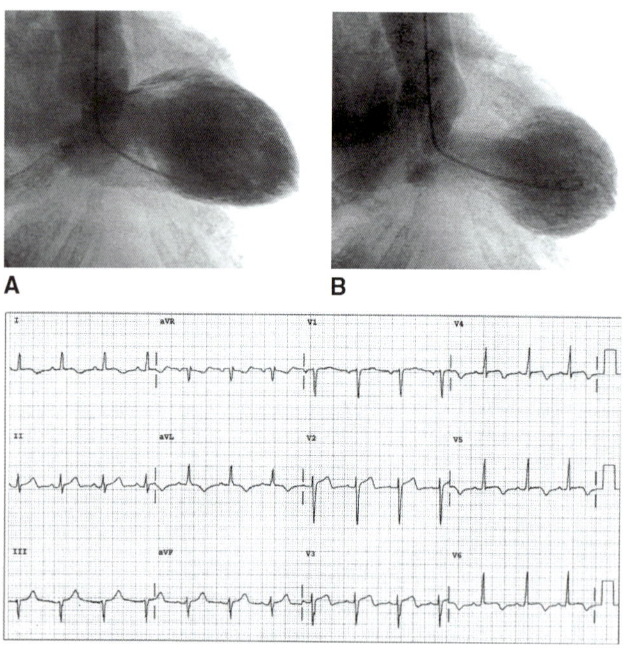

Figure Q2-32 (With permission from Witzke C, et al. *Circulation* 2003;108(16):2014.)

(A) Prinzmetal's angina
(B) Myopericarditis
(C) Dilated cardiomyopathy
(D) Takotsubo cardiomyopathy

2.33 A 70-year-old woman presents with an acute inferior MI. Following primary PCI of an occluded RCA, coronary angiography shows persistent staining of the inferior myocardium, with the blush persisting at the time of the next coronary injection (Fig. Q2-33). Using the thrombolysis in myocardial infarction (TIMI) myocardial perfusion grade (TMPG) system, you would classify this as:

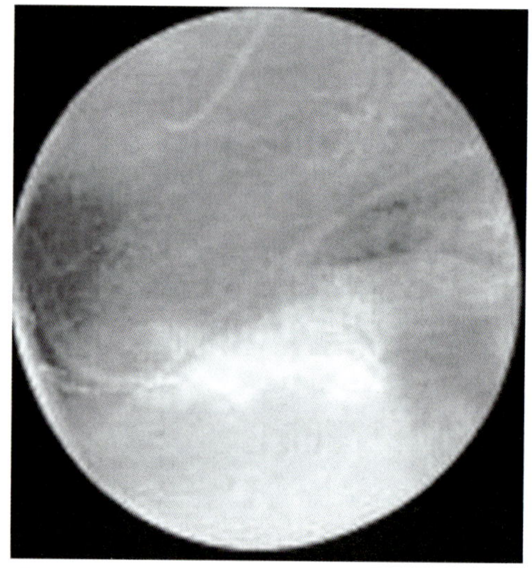

Figure Q2-33 (Adapted from Gibson CM, et al. *Circulation* 2004;109(25);3096–3105.)

(A) TMPG 0
(B) TMPG 1
(C) TMPG 2
(D) TMPG 3

2.34 A 71-year-old male smoker presents with chest pain. Coronary angiography reveals a normal left coronary artery and severe stenoses in the proximal and mid-RCA (Fig. Q2-34A). Immediately following successful stenting of the RCA (Fig. Q2-34B), the patient developed severe chest pain and marked anterior ST-segment elevation (Fig. Q2-34C). The most likely cause is:

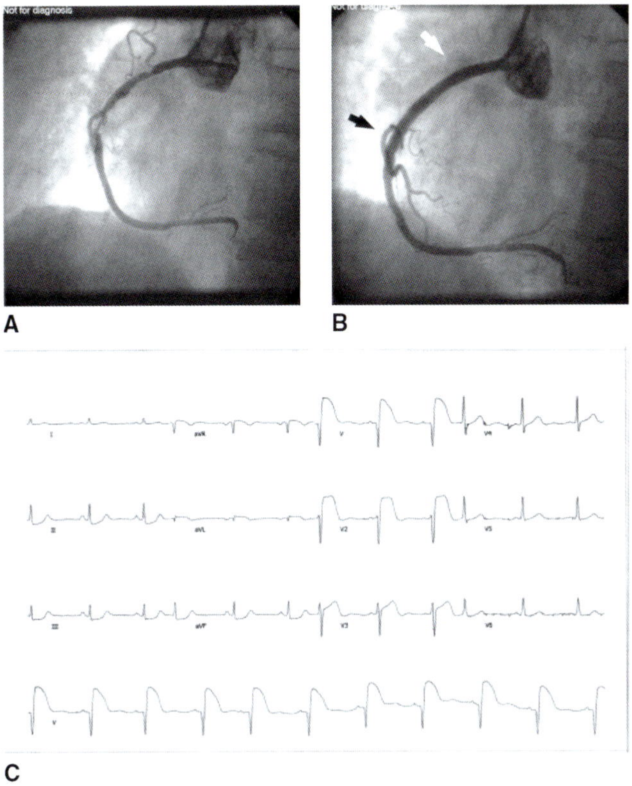

Figure Q2-34 (With permission from Eichhöfer J, et al. *Circulation* 2005;111(9);e113–e114.)

(A) Microvascular obstruction
(B) Occlusion of sinoatrial branch of the RCA
(C) Transient occlusion of right ventricular branch of the RCA
(D) Transient occlusion of the conus branch of the RCA

2.35 A 60-year-old man with previous coronary artery bypass surgery for LM disease undergoes coronary angiography for the evaluation of angina with minimal exertion (Fig. Q2-35), which demonstrates occlusion of the LM and a patent RCA. The LAD, LCx, and ramus intermedius arteries are perfused via collaterals (*solid black arrow*), the source (*open arrow*) of which is:

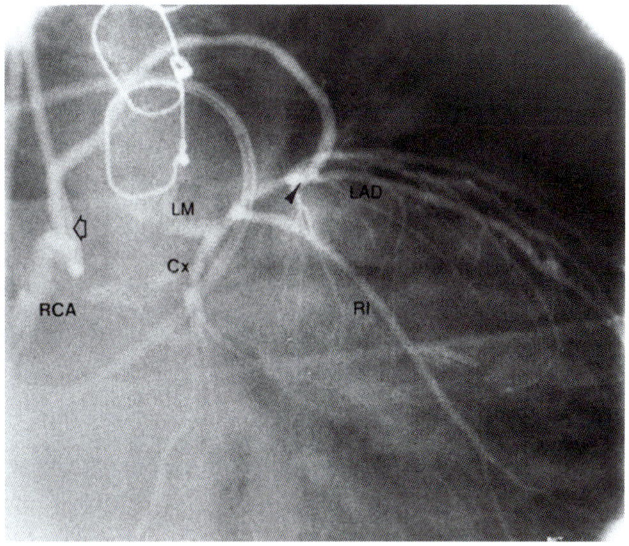

Figure Q2-35 (With permission from O'Leary EL, et al. Vieussens' ring. *Circulation* 1998;98(5):487–488.)

(A) Kugel's artery
(B) Aorta-coronary fistula
(C) Anomalous origin of the LAD from the pulmonary artery (Bland-Garland-White syndrome)
(D) Large conus branch from RCA

ANSWERS AND EXPLANATIONS

2.1 Answer D. The pressure recording shows "ventricularization," in which diastolic pressure is reduced but systolic pressure is preserved. Normally, the catheter tip pressure and the peripheral arterial pressure are similar. If an ostial coronary stenosis is present, engagement of the catheter may obstruct antegrade blood flow and cause ventricularization of the catheter pressure waveform (Pacold I, et al. *Am Heart J* 1989;118(6):1160–1166).

2.2 Answer D. In the 30-degree RAO projection, one is looking down the AV plane, in which the LCx artery resides. Because the proximal portion of the vessel is foreshortened in this view, caudal angulation must be employed to unforeshorten it. With the other angles listed, the proximal LCx is foreshortened or overlapped by other vessels.

2.3 Answer C. In the general population, only 10% of individuals are left dominant (i.e., the posterior descending artery [PDA] arises from the distal LCx artery), but 30% of subjects with a bicuspid valve are left dominant (Hutchins GM, et al. *Am J Cardiol* 1978;42(1):57–59).

2.4 Answer B. Not infrequently, the LAD will course beneath a muscle bundle on the epicardial surface of the heart, resulting in its compression during ventricular systole; this is known as myocardial bridging. It is usually an incidental finding of no consequence, but rarely, it has been associated with myocardial ischemia (Bauters C, et al. *Circulation* 2002;105(1);130).

2.5 Answer A. The LAO caudal view projects the LAD upward from the LM in the appearance of a spider and permits improved visualization of the LM and the bifurcation.

2.6 Answer B. The most common coronary anomaly is origin of the LCx artery from the right sinus of Valsalva. This can often be visualized during left ventriculography (30-degree RAO projection) as a "dot" or "button" projecting from the aortic root as the LCx courses posterior to the aorta (Page HL, et al. *Circulation* 1974;50(4):768–773; Ueyama K, et al. *Ann Thorac Surg* 1997;63(2):377–381).

2.7 Answer D. Visual estimation of coronary stenoses is subject to substantial operator variability and a systematic form of "stenosis inflation," in which the operator's estimate of diameter stenosis is approximately 20% greater than that measured by quantitative coronary angiography (Stadius ML, et al. *Circulation* 1990;82(6):2231–2234). Therefore, a stenosis that measures 50% by quantitative angiography is typically called 70% by visual estimation.

2.8 Answer A. A 50% reduction in luminal diameter (hence, a 75% reduction in cross-sectional area) is "hemodynamically significant," in that it impairs CFR (i.e., the three- to fourfold augmentation in coronary flow in response to increased myocardial oxygen demands). The ability to increase flow during vasodilator stimulus is first impaired when luminal diameter is reduced 50% and abolished when it is reduced >70% (Uren NG, et al. *N Engl J Med* 1994;330(25):1782–1788).

2.9 Answer D. A Kugel's artery passes from either the proximal right or left coronary artery along the anterior margin of the atrial septum to anastomose with the AV nodal branch of the distal RCA to provide blood supply to the posterior circulation (Fig. A2-9) (Nerantzis CE, et al. *Tex Heart Inst* 2004;31(3):267–270; Riseman JE, et al. *Am Heart J* 1950;40(2):260–270).

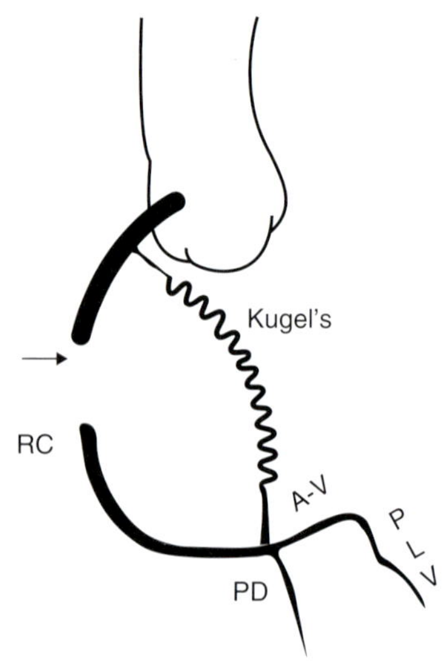

Figure A2-9

2.10 Answer C. A 50% stenosis represents a 75% narrowing in cross-sectional area (Fig. A2-10).

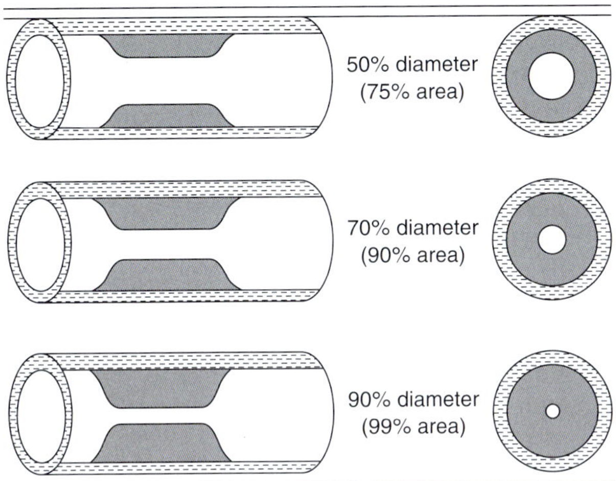

Figure A2-10

2.11 Answer D. Because of ventricular contraction, coronary blood flow occurs mainly during diastole. Accordingly, phasic coronary blood flow is more pronounced for diastolic compared to systolic flow. Flow in the left coronary artery has a greater diastolic predominance than the RCA because the compressive forces of the right ventricle are less than those of the left ventricle. The diastolic predominance is greater in the left than the RCA. At least 85% of coronary flow in the LAD occurs during diastole, whereas the RCA blood flow is more or less equal in systole and diastole. With an epicardial stenosis, the aortic-coronary gradient is initially evident in diastole.

2.12 Answer B. The sinus node artery originates from the LCx artery in 40% of individuals and from the proximal RCA in 60%, regardless of whether the patient is right or left dominant.

2.13 Answer C. During exercise or any other form of increased oxygen demand, the resistance of the microvasculature decreases, allowing for an increased blood flow. Similarly, an epicardial stenosis increases epicardial resistance, which is compensated by an equivalent decrease in microvascular resistance. This results in a maintained total resistance to blood flow and a preserved resting flow, with residual—albeit reduced—CFR. When the stenosis becomes "critical," the compensation capacity of the microvasculature (i.e., CFR) is exhausted. Hence, a lower CFR (<2 in adults) suggests that either the epicardial resistance is very high (i.e., a critical epicardial stenosis is present) or the microvascular resistance is abnormal, but it does not indicate which is affected. The maintenance of constant resting coronary blood flow is referred to as autoregulation. An example of an autoregulatory mechanism is the Bayliss phenomenon, in which increased perfusion pressure causes reflex vasoconstriction.

2.14 Answer A. Like arterioles, veins and venules are innervated by sympathetic nerves, with increased sympathetic tone resulting in venoconstriction and a decrease in venous volume. Unlike arteries, the venous system is not regulated by local metabolic factors and has little basal tone. Therefore, veins are generally in a dilated state.

2.15 Answer C. In the absence of stenoses, the R3 vessels (arteriolar and intramyocardial) are responsible for 40% to 50% of total coronary resistance, the R2 vessels (prearteriolar) are responsible for 25% to 35%, and the R1 (epicardial) vessels contribute little to coronary resistance.

2.16 Answer E. CFR—the ratio of maximal hyperemic blood flow to resting myocardial blood flow—is obtained from successive (i.e., nonsimultaneous) flow measurements. CFR can be altered by changes in basal and hyperemic flows, both of which are influenced by hemodynamics, loading conditions, hypertrophy, and contractility. Additionally, tachycardia increases basal flow and decreases hyperemic flow, thus reducing CFR by 10% for each 15-beat increase in heart rate. A low CFR (<2 in adults) suggests that either the epicardial resistance is very high (i.e., a critical epicardial stenosis is present) or the microvascular resistance is abnormal, but it does not indicate which is affected. In clinical terms, CFR is best used to assess the microcirculation in the absence of epicardial artery narrowing.

2.17 Answer A. The valve of Vieussens lies at the junction of the great cardiac vein and the coronary sinus. Its position is marked by the vein of Marshall, which can be seen coursing superiorly after emptying into the coronary sinus. In this particular patient, the valve of Vieussens is preventing reflux of contrast material from the coronary sinus into the great cardiac vein.

2.18 Answer C. According to the Fick principle, the uptake of a substance (e.g., oxygen or MVO_2) is the product of flow (Q) and the AV concentration difference of the substance ($AoO_2 - CSO_2$). Therefore, $MVO_2 = Q \times (AoO_2 - CSO_2)$.

2.19 Answer D. At extremes of heart rate (<60 bpm or >100 bpm), the Hakki equation should not be used to estimate valve area, as it may be inaccurate (Grishkin IuN. *Kardiologiia* 1991;31(5):40–44).

2.20 Answer D. Assessment of the transvalvular aortic gradient with nonsimultaneous measurement of LV and aortic pressures may be inaccurate when the transvalvular gradient is low, if the systolic pressure is fluctuating (e.g., with atrial fibrillation), or if contrast material administered during left ventriculography causes depression of ventricular systolic function and systemic vasodilation (Brogan WC III, et al. *Am Heart J* 1992;123(4 Pt 1):948–953).

2.21 Answer C. Instantaneous wave-free ratio (iFR) is a measurement of the hemodynamic significance of a coronary artery stenosis that relies on comparison of pressures during diastole in the absence of hyperemia. It is measured during the wave-free period of mid to late diastole, when flow during the cardiac cycle is the highest and the microcirculatory resistance is the lowest. During this period, pressure and flow are linearly related, allowing pressure ratios to be used to determine whether a flow-limiting lesion is present. Unlike in FFR assessment, hyperemia is not required.

An iFR threshold of <0.9 has been proposed for revascularization based on the RESOLVE study. The ADVISE studies took a different approach and proposed a hybrid iFR-FFR approach, which involves performing revascularization for iFR < 0.86, deferral for iFR > 0.93, and using FFR to guide revascularization if iFR is between 0.86 and 0.93. This approach allowed a 95% classification agreement between the hybrid strategy and FFR, while sparing 60% of patients from adenosine.

2.22 Answer A. At rest, transmyocardial oxygen extraction is nearly maximal, with typical coronary venous oxygen saturations of 25% to 35%.

2.23 Answer C. Because each myocardial territory and its resistance bed serves as its own control, FFR is a lesion-specific index. Unlike most other physiologic indexes, FFR has a normal value of 1 for every patient and every coronary artery. FFR has high reproducibility and low intraindividual variability. Furthermore, because FFR is measured only at maximal hyperemia, it is independent of microcirculation, heart rate, blood pressure, and other hemodynamic variables. De Bruyne and associates demonstrated that in humans, FFR is independent of hemodynamic conditions (De Bruyne B, et al. *Circulation* 1996;94(8):1842–1849); changes in heart rate by pacing, contractility by dobutamine infusion, and blood pressure by nitroprusside infusion did not alter FFR. In an acute STEMI, FFR of most nonculprit lesions at a distance from the infarct-related artery has been shown to be accurate (Ntalianis A, et al. *JACC Cardiovasc Interv* 2010;3(12):1274–1281). Hence, FFR measurement in the LAD can proceed reliably without changing therapy.

2.24 Answer A. The course of an anomalous coronary artery, rather than the actual location of the coronary ostium, is a major discriminating factor for the anomaly being benign or associated with clinical complications such as angina, ventricular arrhythmias, syncope, or sudden death. Adverse outcomes occur more frequently when the anomalous coronary artery has a course that passes between the aorta and the pulmonary artery, or less commonly via a septal pathway. The mechanism of ischemia, infarction, or sudden death in this situation appears related to the shape of the coronary ostium of the anomalous vessel rather than compression related to the interarterial course. An RCA arising from the left sinus of Valsalva or the proximal left main almost invariably (>99%) will pass between the aorta and pulmonary artery. The clinical course in these patients is variable with some having no symptoms or evidence of cardiac dysfunction and others having complications including angina, MI, syncope, and sudden death. Anomalous coronary origins of the LCx from the right coronary sinus, the left main from the noncoronary sinus, and the right coronary from the noncoronary sinus do not typically result in passage of a coronary artery between the aorta and pulmonary artery (Fig. A2-24).

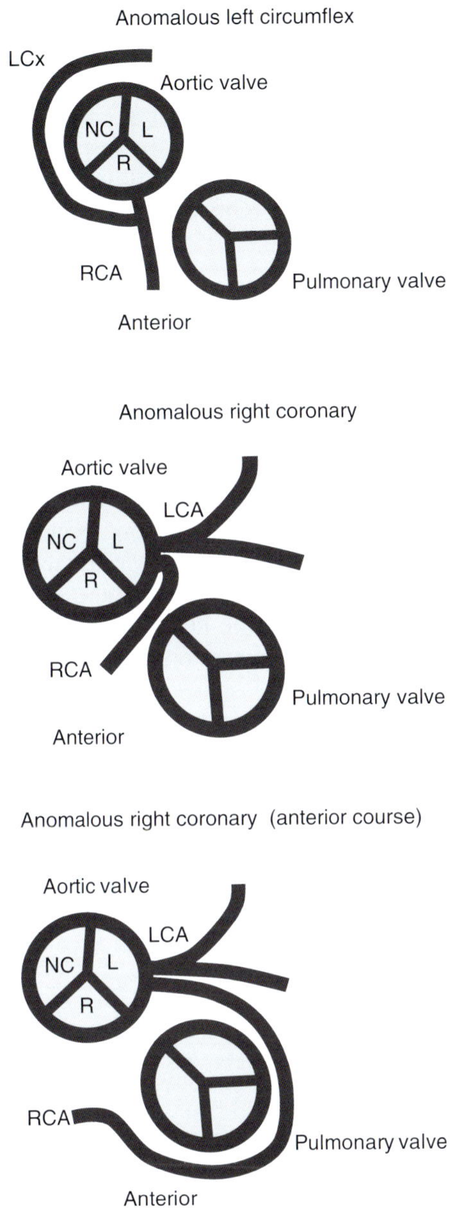

Figure A2-24

2.25 Answer E. The endothelium is a metabolically active secretory tissue. Endothelial cells secrete both vasodilator substances such as prostacyclin, nitric oxide and endothelial-derived hyperpolarizing factors, and vasoconstrictor substances (endothelin and vasoconstrictor prostanoids). Endothelial cells also produce and secrete von Willebrand factor, factor VIII antigen, tissue factor, and tissue plasminogen activator, which have important roles in coagulation and fibrinolysis. Moreover, endothelial cells secrete certain structural components of the extracellular matrix, such as elastin, glycosaminoglycans, and fibronectin and, along with smooth muscle cells, matrix metalloproteinases, which are critical in arterial remodeling.

2.26 Answer D. Capillaries are the smallest vessels in the vasculature with the largest cross-sectional and surface area. The capillary wall consists of a single layer of endothelial cells, thereby allowing the capillaries to act as the exchange vessels of the cardiovascular system. Because they contain no smooth muscle cells, they lack the ability to change their diameters.

2.27 Answer C. Velocity (V) is proportional to blood flow (Q) and inversely proportional to the cross-sectional area (A) of the artery and vascular resistance (R). This can be expressed as $V = Q/A$. Since flow (Q) is proportional to the pressure gradient (ΔP) and inversely proportional to resistance ($Q = \Delta P/R$), then velocity (V) = $\Delta P/(A \times R)$. Thus, blood flow velocity (V) increases when flow (Q) increases and decreases if the cross-sectional area of the artery (A) or vascular resistance increases.

2.28 Answer D. Stimulation of vascular beta-2 adrenergic receptors causes vasodilation, whereas stimulation of alpha-1 adrenergic receptors causes vasoconstriction. Since beta-2 receptors are more sensitive to epinephrine, moderately elevated levels of circulating epinephrine typically cause vasodilation, whereas higher levels cause alpha-1 receptor–mediated vasoconstriction. Angiotensin II and vasopressin are potent vasoconstrictors.

2.29 Answer B. Large arteries have additional circumferential layers of elastic tissue within the media and are thus referred to as elastic arteries. The epicardial coronary arteries are elastic arteries as are the carotids, cerebral arteries, and the aorta. However, at the point the epicardial arteries turn into the myocardium, usually at a right angle from the parent vessel, they become more muscular arteries with few if any elastic fibers. The media of all arteries is contained within a connective tissue layer called the tunica adventitia, or simply adventitia. The adventitia contains a network of small blood vessels (vasa vasorum), which is responsible for the nutrition of the outer two-thirds of the artery. The inner third of the artery derives nutrition by diffusion through the endothelium. The adventitia also contains nerves, which control the tone of the artery.

2.30 Answer D. Coronary blood flow is approximately 250 mL/min, which represents 4% to 5% of cardiac output.

2.31 Answer A. The left main ostium lacks adventitia and has a greater portion of elastic tissue than other segments of the coronary tree. This may account for some of the differences in response to coronary interventions involving this segment of the LM. Since the LM ostium technically lies within the wall of the aorta, it is subject to diseases affecting the aortic wall, such as syphilitic aortitis, radiation-induced aortitis, and Takayasu's arteritis. Trifurcation of the LM has been reported in 37% of the general population (Levin DC, et al. *Invest Radiol* 1982;17(5):458–462). A high takeoff of the LM is not generally felt to have any clinical significance. The origin of the left coronary has been rarely observed from the noncoronary cusp but has never been associated with symptoms or complications in this location.

2.32 Answer D. Takotsubo cardiomyopathy is characterized by systolic apical ballooning of the ventricle with preservation of basal contraction. Excessive amounts of epinephrine (endogenous or exogenous) are thought to cause it. The ventricular regional wall motion abnormalities do not follow any particular coronary anatomic pattern and probably are not a result of transient coronary arterial occlusion. The acute onset of severe chest pain following emotional stress and the pattern of ventricular involvement are not characteristic of myopericarditis.

2.33 Answer B. In the TMPG system, TMPG 0 represents minimal or no myocardial blush; in TMPG 1, contrast material stains the myocardium, and the stain persists on the subsequent injection; in TMPG 2, contrast material reaches the distal vessel lumen but dissipates slowly; and in TMPG 3, normal vessel perfusion is noted (Gibson CM, et al. *Circulation* 2004;109(25);3096–3105).

2.34 Answer D. The post-PCI angiogram shows occlusion of the conus branch of the RCA, whereas the right ventricular branch is patent. Anterior ST-segment elevation due to occlusion of a right ventricular RCA branch has been reported previously and is thought to be a mirror image of right ventricular ischemia. This is a profound example of this phenomenon, caused by acute conus branch occlusion. Occlusion of the sinoatrial branch of the RCA may cause dysrhythmias but not anterior ST-segment elevation, and microvascular obstruction of the RCA would typically cause inferior, rather than anterior, ST-segment alterations.

2.35 Answer D. The patient has a large (3.3-mm) conus branch off the RCA that passes upward and over the right ventricular outflow tract to provide collateral flow to the LAD and subsequently the other vessels of the left coronary artery system. This type of collateral system is known as Vieussens' ring.

3 Principles of Radiation Use, Protection, and Basic Physics Concepts

Guillaume Plourde and Olivier F. Bertrand

QUESTIONS

3.1 Recent data from large-scale randomized trials comparing radial and femoral access support radial artery adoption as the default access site, especially since a mortality reduction has been observed with radial access in patients undergoing primary percutaneous coronary intervention (PCI) for ST-elevation myocardial infarction (STEMI). Despite this advantage, radial access has been associated with higher patient radiation exposure. According to a recent meta-analysis, however, this relative increase has declined consistently for the past 20 years. In contemporary practice, radial access is associated with:

(A) An average 2-minute increase in fluoroscopy time per procedure
(B) A radiation excess dose equivalent to 25 to 50 x-rays per procedure
(C) An overall 10% absolute increase in radiation-induced cancer risk
(D) An overall 10% relative increase in total radiation dose per procedure

3.2 The arteriogram shown in Figure Q3-2 was obtained with digital subtraction technique, which eliminates background structures and enhances the visibility of contrast-filled vessels. Which of the following statements about digital subtraction angiography and radiation is TRUE?

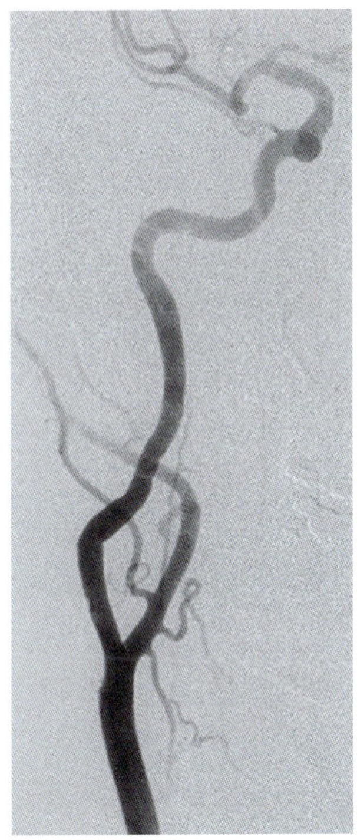

Figure Q3-2

(A) Compared to cardiac "cine" acquisitions, each frame of a subtraction study delivers a much larger dose of radiation to the patient
(B) A principal advantage of the digital subtraction technique is that each frame delivers a reduced dose of radiation to the patient
(C) Digital subtraction is a form of postprocessing that does not influence patient dose
(D) Subtraction technique can enhance low-quality images obtained with very low x-ray exposure settings

3.3 Which of the following statements regarding fluoroscopy in the modern cardiac catheterization laboratory is TRUE?

(A) The x-ray exposure for fluoroscopy is much lower than the exposure for diagnostic cineangiography
(B) Most reports of radiation skin injury due to fluoroscopy occurred before 1996 and were linked to improperly calibrated analog imaging equipment
(C) The federal government limits the maximum allowable fluoroscopic exposure rate to 88 mGy per minute (10 R per minute)
(D) Modern catheterization laboratories have reduced the potential for x-ray exposure to patients and operators

3.4 The interventional cardiologist shown in Figure Q3-4 wishes to minimize his own radiation exposure during a procedure that will require imaging in a lateral projection. Which of the following statements is TRUE?

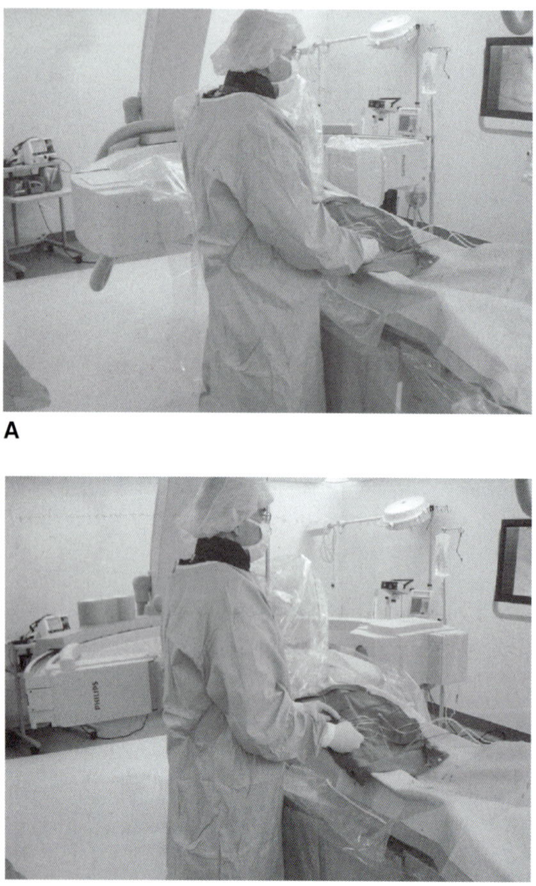

Figure Q3-4

(A) Panel B is preferred because the principal source of scatter radiation is positioned farthest from the operator
(B) Panel A is preferred because the x-ray beam is directed away from the operator
(C) There is no difference as long as the distances between the x-ray tube, patient, and image receptor are held constant
(D) There is no difference because the x-ray beam penetrates the same thickness of tissue

3.5 The images in Figure Q3-5 were obtained from the same patient using the same radiographic equipment. Panel A has a grainy appearance, whereas Panel B is smoother and sharper. Which of the statements best explains the difference?

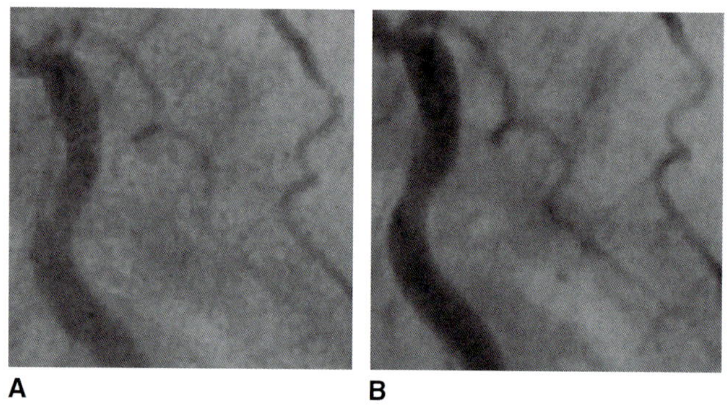

Figure Q3-5

(A) Panel A was acquired with an excessively high milliampere (mA) setting
(B) Panel B has been electronically processed with an edge enhancement filter
(C) The speckled appearance of Panel A could have been improved by decreasing the pulse width
(D) Panel B is visually superior because it was made with a larger dose of x-rays
(E) Panel A indicates that the charge-coupled device (CCD) camera is out of focus and should be recalibrated by the service technician

3.6 The three plots in Figure Q3-6 depict the energy spectra of x-rays produced by a typical cardiac fluoroscopy unit. In each case, the dashed line represents a change that has been made to the settings. Which of the following statements is TRUE?

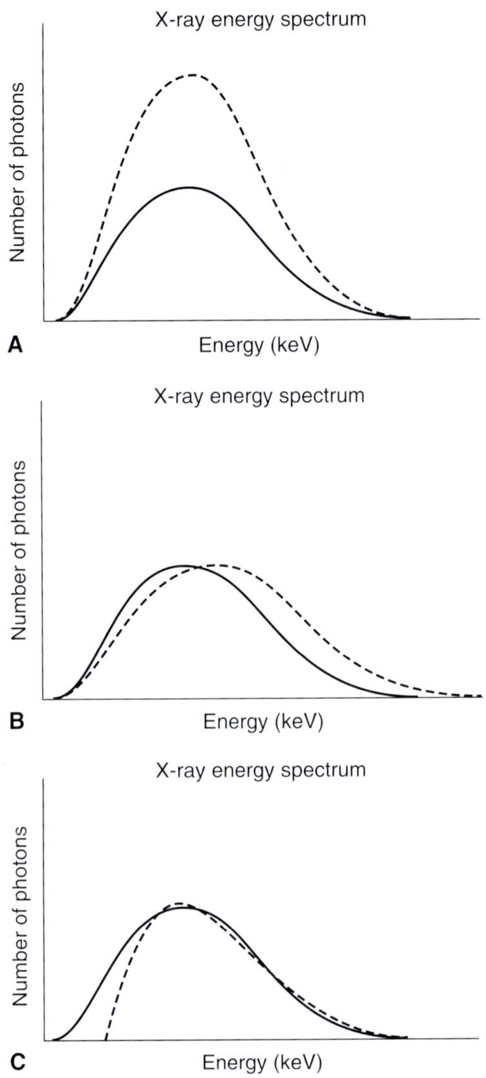

Figure Q3-6

(A) The dashed line in Panel A indicates that peak kilovoltage (kVp) has been increased
(B) The dashed line in Panel B indicates that mA has been increased
(C) The dashed line in Panel B indicates that the pulse width has been increased
(D) The dashed line in Panel C indicates that the beam has been hardened by placing copper or aluminum filters over the output port of the x-ray tube

3.7 Which of the following statements about tube filament current (mA) is CORRECT?

(A) Doubling the mA will decrease the patient dose rate by 50%
(B) Doubling the mA will increase the patient dose rate by 50%
(C) Doubling the mA will double the patient dose rate
(D) Doubling the mA will quadruple the patient dose rate

3.8 A patient is to receive 10 mSv of radiation during a routine cardiac catheterization and PCI procedure. What is the equivalent number of chest radiographs this exposure would represent and how long would it take for such an exposure to occur from natural background radiation?

(A) 50 chest radiographs, 1 year
(B) 500 chest radiographs, 4 years
(C) 50 chest radiographs, 10 years
(D) 500 chest radiographs, 30 years

3.9 Figure Q3-9 illustrates the use of collimation during coronary arteriography. Which of the following statements about collimation is FALSE?

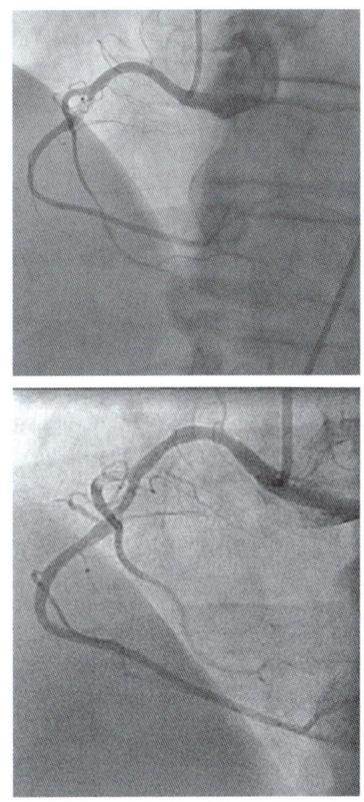

Figure Q3-9

(A) Collimation reduces the skin entrance dose
(B) Collimation reduces x-ray exposure everywhere in the room
(C) Collimation improves image quality
(D) As a means of reducing x-ray exposure, collimation is superior to selecting a smaller field of view (higher magnification) that just encompasses the area of interest

3.10 In Figure Q3-10, a dotted line has been superimposed on the plot of photon energies produced by a typical cardiac fluoroscopy unit. Which of the following statements about this dotted line is TRUE?

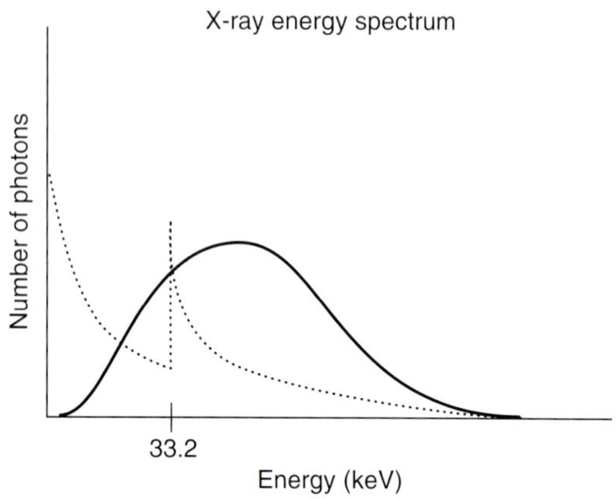

Figure Q3-10

(A) The spike in the dotted line depicts Compton scatter, which peaks at 33.2 keV
(B) The dotted line illustrates how copper beam filters reduce skin dose by eliminating x-rays with energies above 33.2 keV
(C) The spike in the dotted line depicts characteristic x-rays originating from the K shell of the tungsten atom
(D) The spike in the dotted line depicts the bremsstrahlung effect
(E) The dotted line depicts the absorption spectrum of iodine, which has an absorption peak at 33.2 keV

3.11 Time, distance, and shielding are the three general guidelines for controlling exposure to ionizing radiation during catheterization procedures. Which of the following statements about shielding is FALSE?

(A) Lead aprons typically provide the equivalent of 0.5 mm lead thickness and block >90% of scatter radiation
(B) Lead eyeglasses reduce radiation exposure to the lens by a factor between 1 and 3, depending on the model and the operator's position
(C) Operators who find lead glasses uncomfortable can utilize a transparent, movable leaded acrylic shield to provide equivalent eye protection
(D) A transparent, movable shield should be placed between the operator and the face of the image intensifier or flat-panel detector
(E) Assistants can reduce their exposure to scatter radiation by standing directly behind the primary operator

3.12 Which of the following is TRUE about radiation exposure-associated risks?

(A) A single 5 mGy exposure comprises a greater stochastic risk compared to five repeated 1 mGy exposures over a 6-month period
(B) There is actually no evidence of deterministic effects (tissue reactions) for operators at exposures below 0.5 mSv
(C) National Cancer Institute (NCI) grade 2 radiation-induced dermatitis tends to resolve completely with supportive care in 2 to 3 months
(D) Since radiation-induced cancer is extremely rare, it should not be routinely discussed with patients when obtaining consent

3.13 Ionizing radiation interacts with organic matter in several ways. Concerning the biologic effects of ionizing radiation, which of the following is TRUE?

(A) Most of molecular interactions between x-rays and DNA are direct in nature (DNA structural alterations)
(B) Radiation-induced carcinogenesis is a process that affects a particular tissue regardless of its metabolic activity or replication rate
(C) Women tend to be more radiosensitive than men during PCI procedures, which entails fluoroscopy because of their breast tissue
(D) Circulating lymphocyte anomalies is now recognized as a valid prognostic tool for long-term radiation-induced carcinogenesis

3.14 Modern cardiac fluoroscopy systems display values for air kinetic energy released per unit mass (KERMA) and dose area product (DAP). Interventional cardiologists should understand what these metrics mean. Which of the following statements is TRUE?

(A) Air KERMA estimates the skin dose and can be used to predict the risk of radiation skin injury
(B) DAP is a valuable measure of total x-ray exposure because it cannot be manipulated by collimation or any other operator-controlled variable
(C) Air KERMA is a measure of scatter radiation in the air surrounding the image receptor (intensifier or flat detector)
(D) Air KERMA and DAP are instantaneous values that should never be used to infer the skin dose or the total absorbed dose

3.15 PCI constitutes one of many cardiovascular imaging modalities. Concerning radiation exposure, which of the following best compares PCI to other imaging modalities?

(A) Single-isotope, rest-stress single-photon emission computed tomography (SPECT) is associated with greater exposure, on average, than standard coronary angiography
(B) Radiation exposure associated with a cardiac calcium-score computed tomography (CT) is equivalent to a natural background exposure of about 3 years (which is the same as a standard coronary angiography)
(C) A dual-isotope SPECT study exposes the patient to less radiation than a cardiac ^{82}Rubidium positron emission tomography (PET) scan
(D) Radiation exposure associated with a standard percutaneous coronary angioplasty (15 mSv) is equivalent to a natural background exposure of about 1 to 2 years

3.16 To optimize radiation exposure to the patient, the operator and the catheterization laboratory staff should be familiar with variants of arterial anatomy. Which of the following variants of the aortic arch vessels is the most common?

(A) Right common carotid originating from the innominate artery
(B) Right common carotid originating from the aortic arch
(C) Common origin of the left carotid and the innominate artery
(D) Common origin of the right carotid and the innominate artery

3.17 The operator controls several technical factors that significantly influence radiation exposure and image quality. Among these are table height, tube position, and image detector position. Figure Q3-17 shows that the image detector (*arrow*) is positioned well above the patient's chest. Which of the following statements is TRUE?

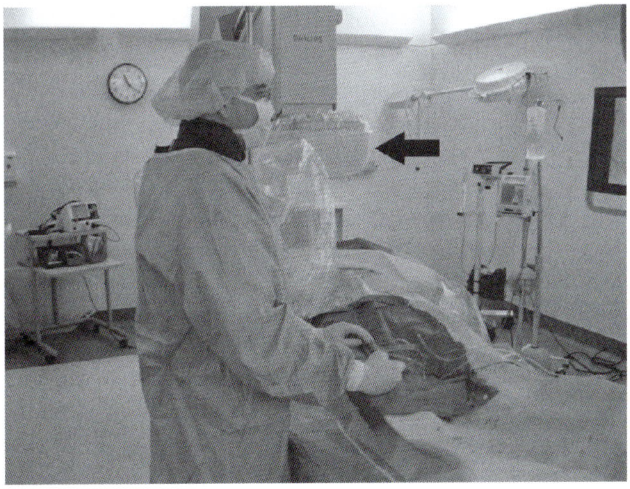

Figure Q3-17

(A) The operator has placed an air gap between the patient and the image detector to reduce his dose of scatter radiation
(B) The operator has placed an air gap between the patient and the image detector to improve image quality
(C) The operator should lower the detector to the patient's chest in order to reduce the skin entrance dose
(D) The operator should lower the table as much as possible to minimize the skin entrance dose

3.18 Which of the following statements about radiation safety terminology is TRUE?

(A) ALARA is the adjusted lifetime average of radiation accumulated
(B) The unit of measure for the quantity of radiation absorbed is the roentgen (R)
(C) The unit of measure for radiation exposure is the sievert (Sv)
(D) The unit of measure for the quantity of radiation absorbed is the gray (Gy)

3.19 A 23-year-old woman has developed pulmonary edema during her second trimester of pregnancy. Echocardiography demonstrates critical rheumatic mitral stenosis, and the patient is referred for balloon valvotomy. Which of the following statements is TRUE regarding radiation exposure during pregnancy?

(A) Pregnancy is an absolute contraindication to cardiac fluoroscopy
(B) The procedure can be performed safely as long as proper shielding is applied to the abdomen and pelvis
(C) The radiation hazard to the fetus is very small, and shielding is not necessary
(D) The most likely adverse effect is intrauterine growth retardation because rapidly growing tissues are extremely sensitive to small doses of ionizing radiation

3.20 Which of the following statements about the device shown in Figure Q3-20 is TRUE?

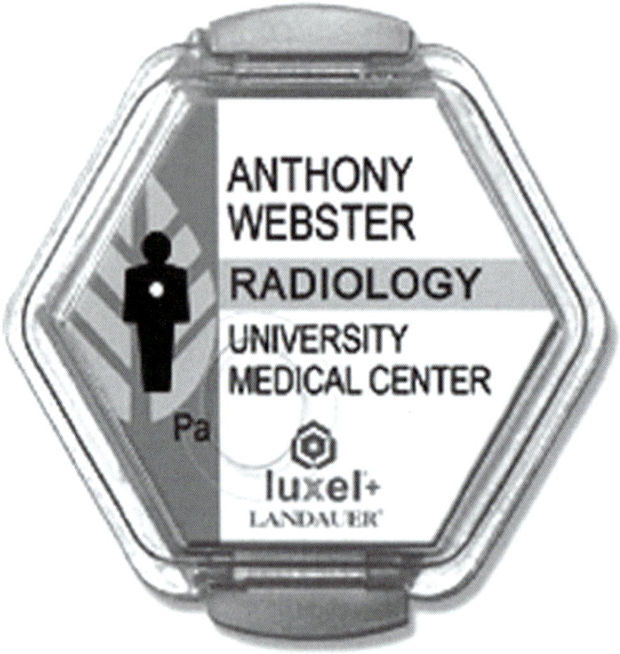

Figure Q3-20

(A) If a single film badge is worn, it should be placed under the apron at waist level
(B) If a single film badge is worn, it should be placed on the outside of the apron at waist level
(C) If a single film badge is worn, it should be placed on the outside of the thyroid collar on the side closest to the source of scatter radiation
(D) Acceptable readings indicate that the operator is using safe radiologic practices
(E) This device protects the operator against cumulative doses of radiation that are above the threshold for stochastic effects

3.21 Figure Q3-21 depicts coronary arteriograms obtained from two different patients utilizing the same radiographic equipment. In Panel A, the arteries are well opacified with excellent contrast between contrast-filled vessels and background structures. In Panel B, the arteries are not as dark, and they do not stand out as well against the background. Which of the following statements best explains the difference?

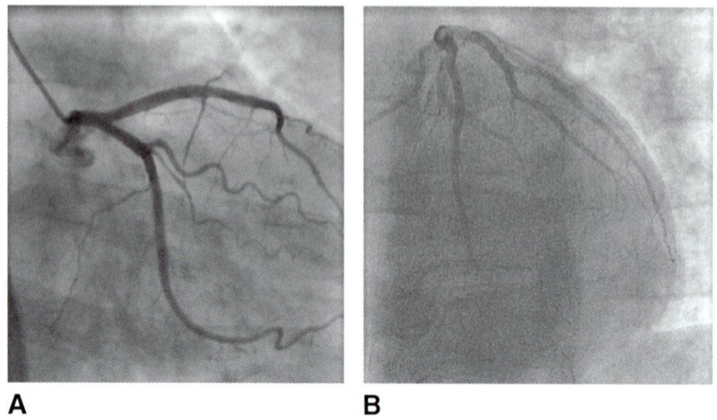

Figure Q3-21

(A) The operator injected less contrast agent in Panel B, so fewer iodine atoms are available to absorb x-rays
(B) A higher mA setting was used in Panel B
(C) A shorter pulse width was used in Panel A
(D) A higher kVp setting was used in Panel B

3.22 X-rays have variable tissue-penetrating power depending on certain factors. This process, named attenuation or beam modulation, is the basis for a generation of contrasted images of diagnostic quality. Among the following factors, identify those directly influencing x-rays attenuation.

(A) Tissue molar mass, tissue thickness, x-ray photon energy, and tissue density
(B) X-rays photon energy, atomic number of the atoms composing the tissue, tissue density, and tissue thickness
(C) Atomic number of the atoms composing the tissue, tissue density, tissue thickness, and electrical current applied to the tube (mA)
(D) Tissue density, x-ray photon speed, tissue thickness, and atomic number of the atoms composing the tissue

3.23 Which of the following patients would you be most concerned for potentially developing a malignancy from radiation exposure?

(A) A 78-year-old female undergoing CT of the head and neck and then undergoing carotid angiography with ad hoc angioplasty and bilateral stent placement
(B) A 17-year-old male undergoing CT of the chest and abdomen/pelvis following a motor vehicle accident
(C) A 52-year-old male with recurrent sinus infections requiring repeat head CT
(D) A 49-year-old female undergoing a barium enema for a suspected colonic mass

3.24* Figure Q3-24 is a schematic diagram of a simple x-ray tube along with a plot of the energy it produces. Which of the following statements is TRUE?

(A) Arrow *A* marks the kVp of the x-ray tube
(B) The x-rays were made with a peak filament current of 70 mA
(C) Arrow *B* indicates the power rating of the tube
(D) Up to 70,000 V was applied to this tube

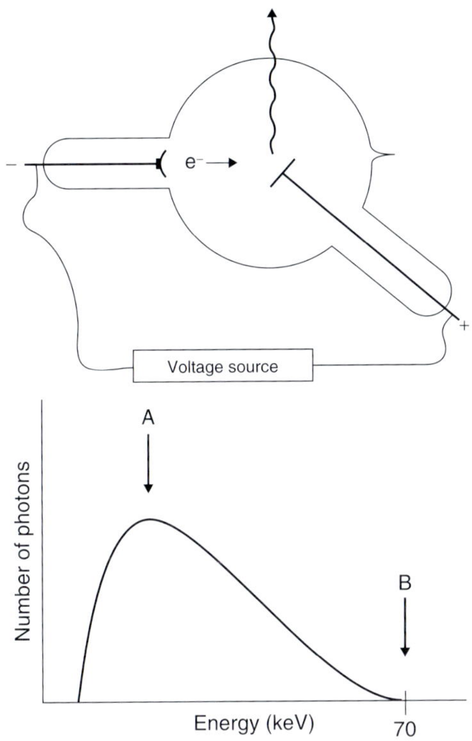

Figure Q3-24

3.25 Concerning the optimization process of radiation use during image acquisition, which of the following is FALSE?

(A) Reducing the frame rate from 15 to 10 fps is not associated with a clinically significant reduction in image quality during fluoroscopy loops
(B) Reducing the dose per pulse during cine-acquisition loops probably has the greatest impact on patient exposure
(C) Reducing the frame rate from 15 to 7.5 fps during fluoroscopy is associated with a 50% reduction in both operator and patient exposure
(D) Switching fluoroscopy on and off every time the operator looks at his hands is an effective way of reducing his exposure

3.26 The patient in Figure Q3-26 complained to his family physician about an uncomfortable "rash" on his right lower back that appeared 3 weeks after he was hospitalized for chest pain. Which of the following statements is TRUE?

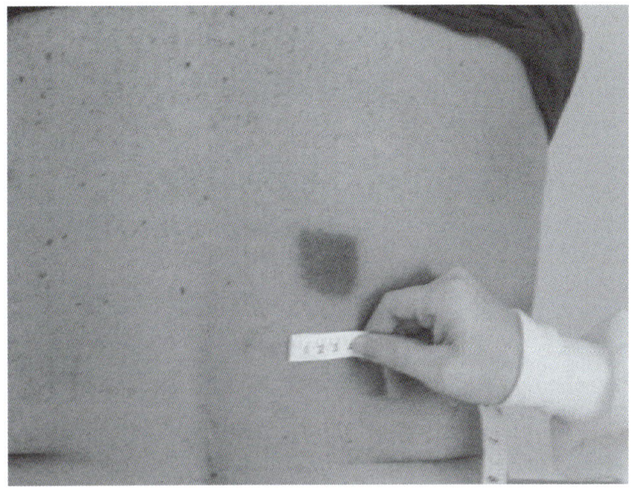

Figure Q3-26

(A) The photograph illustrates a deterministic effect of radiation
(B) This type of injury is very unpredictable
(C) The delayed appearance makes radiation skin injury unlikely
(D) The photograph illustrates a stochastic effect of radiation

3.27 A 56-year-old man has been referred to you for a second attempt at catheter-based repair of a chronic, total circumflex artery occlusion. He had not seen a physician until 1 week ago when he presented with heart failure and angina. During the past week, he underwent diagnostic coronary arteriography, an unsuccessful PCI, and successful implantation of a biventricular defibrillator. The transfer records note hyperglycemia and obesity (weight: 329 lb). You realize that two of the three procedures performed during the past week probably involved prolonged fluoroscopy, so radiation skin injury is a very real possibility. Before beginning another procedure, which of the following should you do?

(A) Examine the back of the chest for signs of hair loss (epilation)
(B) Examine the back of the chest for signs of telangiectasia
(C) Examine the back of the chest for signs of dermal atrophy or necrosis
(D) Examine the back of the chest for signs of moist desquamation
(E) None of the above

3.28 Various worldwide institutions have implanted diagnostic reference levels (DRLs) to provide guidance to health care professionals using radiation for diagnostic purposes. Concerning DRLs, which of the following is TRUE?

(A) DRLs are used to restrict radiation usage on a daily basis for individual patients and can be applied as dose thresholds that should not be overpassed
(B) DRLs are a useful marker to identify patients at risk of developing radiation-induced side effects
(C) Their use is mandatory by law in Europe and in the United States
(D) DRLs are calculated using the arithmetic mean of the distribution of doses in a specific location (e.g., hospital)

3.29 While obtaining consent with your patient concerning a percutaneous coronary procedure for STEMI that will most likely require angioplasty, he asks you: "Doctor, I've read on the Internet that the procedure can cause cancer. Is that true?" Which of the following does not correctly describe PCI-associated cancer risk?

(A) For a standard coronary angiography (5 to 10 mSv), the risk may be described as low but should nonetheless be discussed with the patient
(B) For an uncomplicated angioplasty procedure (10 to 20 mSv), the additional attributable cancer risk is between 1:1,000 and 1:100
(C) If a patient undergoes two PCIs separated from 10 or more years, the cancer risk they carry is not cumulative
(D) The risk of dying from a motor vehicle accident is 20 times higher than from a radiation-induced cancer attributable to a coronary angiography (10 mSv)

3.30 Individual radiation exposure is attributable to various sources, both environmental and man-made. In the past decades, medical radiation exposure has grown significantly, reaching an individual dose of 3 mSv per annum in the United States. A significant part of this increase is directly attributable to cardiovascular diagnostic modalities. Concerning the evolution of medical exposure attributable to interventional cardiology, which of the following sentences is FALSE?

(A) About 40% of medical radiation exposure is attributable to cardiovascular imaging
(B) About 10% of medical radiation exposure is attributable to interventional cardiology, and this percentage is declining
(C) Most of medical radiation exposure is attributable to CT scans
(D) Nuclear medicine now constitutes more than two-thirds of individual medical exposure in the United States

ANSWERS AND EXPLANATIONS

3.1 Answer D. The MATRIX trial is the latest large-scale randomized controlled trial comparing radial and femoral access in 8,404 acute coronary syndrome (ACS) patients (Valgimigli M, et al. *Lancet* 2015;385(9986):2465–2476). Authors reported a mortality reduction from 2.2% to 1.6% ($p = 0.045$) with radial access. They also performed a meta-analysis of all major trials comparing radial and femoral access updated with MATRIX data and found a risk ratio of 0.72 (95% CI 0.60 to 0.88; $p = 0.0011$) for all-cause mortality favoring radial access. The authors subsequently published the RAD-MATRIX substudy, which specifically focused on radiation exposure, and found a 1-minute absolute increase in fluoroscopy time with radial access and a 6 Gy·cm^2 increase in radiation dose (Sciahbasi A, et al. *J Am Coll Cardiol* 2017;69(20):2530–2537). These results are in the same magnitude as those published in a recent meta-analysis of all trials comparing radial and femoral access since inception of radial access until 2014 (1-minute of supplemental fluoroscopy with radial access and 1.72 Gy·cm^2 dose increase) (Plourde G, et al. *Lancet* 2015;386(10009):2192–2203).

3.2 Answer A. In digital subtraction angiography, a non-contrast-filled (mask) image is subtracted from a contrast-filled (live) image. Constant densities, such as bone, are neutralized, leaving only the contrast column. The pattern created by random noise is different on the mask and live images, so subtraction accentuates the noise inherent in low-dose images. To suppress noise, each frame of a subtraction study requires a substantially larger dose of radiation than is needed for a cardiac cine frame. A typical subtraction study can deliver more than ten times the dose per frame to the patient. Scatter exposure to the operator and room staff is increased commensurately. Subtraction studies are usually acquired at low frame rates of 1 to 6 per second, but this only partially mitigates the higher dose per frame. Subtraction cannot create image detail that was not present in the original image.

3.3 Answer A. In recent years, the scope and complexity of interventional procedures has expanded greatly. Although it is true that refinements to imaging systems have reduced x-ray exposure rates, the greater duration of therapeutic procedures has actually *increased* the potential for radiation exposure to patients and operators. Even procedures that only utilize fluoroscopy are capable of delivering skin doses sufficient to cause severe burns.

The recognition that diagnostic x-ray systems can cause skin injury to patients is a relatively recent phenomenon. The first US Food and Drug Administration (FDA) advisory was published in 1994, and the first reports of radiation skin necrosis due to fluoroscopy did not appear in the medical literature until 1996 (Shope TB. *Radiographics* 1996;16(5):1195–1199). Even modern properly calibrated systems are capable of causing radiation skin injury. The risk is greatest with prolonged or repeated procedures, heavy patients, and when body parts are positioned close to the x-ray tube.

The FDA limits the maximum exposure rate for diagnostic fluoroscopy, but this does not guarantee patient safety. Body parts that are positioned close to the x-ray tube (such as the arm in a lateral projection) can receive much more than the calibrated 88 mGy per minute limit (10 R per minute). Prolonged exposures can further increase the risk of injury.

3.4 Answer A. Scatter radiation is the main source of exposure to the operator, to laboratory staff, and to patient body parts outside the x-ray beam. Most scatter to the operator originates from the beam entry point, where incoming x-rays strike the table and body surface. In Panel B, the source of scatter is farther from the operator, so exposure is reduced as predicted by the inverse square law. In addition, the patient's body is positioned as a shield between the source of scatter and the operator. By choosing Panel B, this operator can estimate a tenfold reduction in personal exposure.

The primary beam is collimated to the size of the image receptor. Therefore, the operator in these illustrations would not be exposed to the primary beam.

Finally, his personal exposure could be reduced by stepping back when using fluoroscopy whenever possible.

3.5 Answer D. X-rays and visible light are both forms of electromagnetic radiation, and the energy they carry is characterized as discrete packets or quanta named photons. The background granularity of the image on the left is known as "quantum mottle" or "image noise." It is due to random variation in the distribution of x-ray photons striking the image detector, and it is most apparent when very few photons are available to generate an image (i.e., when the x-ray dose decreases).

Quantum mottle degrades the detectability of vessel edges and low-contrast structures. Increasing the tube filament current (mA) or the pulse width would generate more x-ray photons and thereby minimize quantum mottle.

Small amounts of x-rays are used during fluoroscopy, whereas larger amounts of x-rays are used to produce archive-quality images ("cine mode"), such as the one on the right.

Quantum mottle does not indicate a lack of focus or any other problem with the equipment. In fact, the ability to appreciate quantum mottle should reassure the operator that the fluoroscopic dose settings are appropriately low.

The image on the left was obtained with "low-dose" fluoroscopy, whereas that on the right was obtained in the "cine" acquisition mode. The difference in x-ray dose to the patient and operator was approximately 10- to 15-fold.

3.6 Answer D. An increase in filament current (mA) increases the number of photons produced without altering the distribution of photon energies, as depicted in Panel A. An increase in kVp shifts the energy spectrum toward the right, increasing the proportion of high-energy photons (Panel B).

High-energy photons have more penetrating power and therefore are less likely to be absorbed by surrounding tissues and to contribute to patient dose. On the other hand, low-energy photons have less penetrating power and are readily absorbed by the skin at the beam entry point, deposing all their energy into tissues without contributing to image production.

Copper and aluminum filters are routinely utilized to absorb the low-energy x-rays (a process named "hardening the beam") that would otherwise contribute to the skin dose but not to image production (Panel C). Beam filtration does not affect the filament current (mA) or the energy of the x-ray beam.

3.7 Answer C. Tube filament current (mA) is directly proportional to the number of x-ray photons being produced. Doubling the mA will double the patient's skin entry dose, and it will also double the amount of scatter radiation for operators and room staff.

3.8 Answer B. Medical radiation exposure is a progressively worrisome issue. Diagnostic and therapeutic modalities requiring radiation use are becoming increasingly available and patients are being exposed at a younger age. Since 2006, medical radiation exposure has surpassed individual annual background exposure in the United States, which is estimated at 2.4 mSv per annum. A typical coronary angiography has an effective dose (ED) of 7 mSv and a PCI of 15 mSv. In comparison, a chest radiograph has an ED of approximately 0.02 mSv.

3.9 Answer A. Collimators are lead shutters that restrict the size and shape of the x-ray beam as it leaves the tube. The amount of radiation exiting the tube is directly proportional to the area of the beam.

The uncollimated beam used to create the image on the left exposes tissues outside the area of interest to useless radiation. This creates scatter radiation that unnecessarily exposes the operator, patient, and room staff. Moreover, scatter radiation reaching the detector reduces contrast and quality of the image.

The exposed area of the collimated image on the right is less than half of the uncollimated image. This means that exposure for everyone in the room is less than half of what it would have been without collimation.

Although collimation reduces the exposed skin area, it does not reduce the absorbed dose by skin cells within the irradiated area. In some cases, tight collimation can actually increase the skin dose. This happens if the collimator blades fall within the sampling area for automatic brightness compensation.

3.10 Answer E. The black line represents the energy *emission* spectrum of an x-ray tube. The dotted line represents the x-ray *absorption* spectrum of iodine. A sudden jump in absorption occurs when the incident photon energy is just above the binding energy of the K-shell electron of the iodine atom. The process is known as *photoelectric absorption* and constitutes the second source of tissue attenuation in the diagnostic range after the Compton effect.

Iodine is a good agent for contrast angiography because it is relatively safe and has a K-shell binding energy of 33.2 keV, which is close to the peak output spectrum of medical x-ray machines. In comparison, barium has an interesting K-edge binding energy of 37.4 keV, but it is more toxic than iodine.

X-rays are produced when electrons emitted from the cathode are accelerated toward a rotative anode generally made of tungsten. When high-speed electrons approach a dense, positively charged tungsten nucleus, most are deflected and slowed, and their kinetic energy is released in the form of heat (99%) and x-ray photons (1%). This process is called *bremsstrahlung*, a German word meaning "breaking radiation." Almost all the x-rays produced by a medical x-ray system are issued from the *bremsstrahlung* process.

A few of the high-speed electrons interacting with the target cause the ejection of orbital electrons from shells close to the tungsten nucleus. When an electron from a higher shell drops down to fill the void, the difference in the binding energy between the two shells is released in the form of an x-ray photon. These "characteristic x-rays" always have the same wavelength, which is a chemical property of the target metal and the specific shells involved. The production of *bremsstrahlung* and characteristic x-rays is illustrated in Figure A3-10A and B.

Many of the x-rays produced by a fluoroscopy unit have energies that are either too low to penetrate the patient or too high to be absorbed by iodine. Copper filters screen out the low-energy photons that would contribute to skin dose but have no imaging value. An ideal x-ray beam for angiography would contain photons in the range between 30 and 70 keV.

Compton scattering is the most significant source of tissue attenuation in the diagnostic energy range. It occurs when the incoming x-ray photons' energy is much greater than the binding energy of

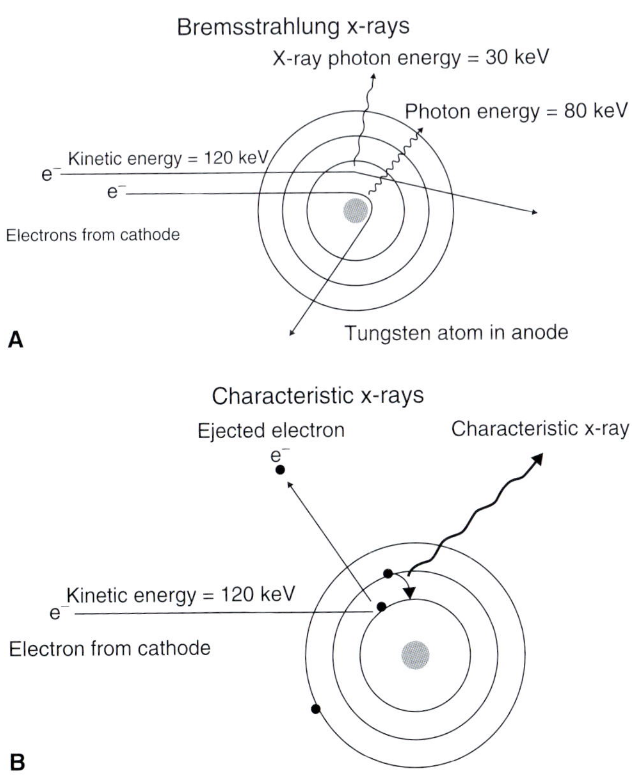

Figure A3-10

electrons composing body tissues. The incoming photon transfers enough energy to completely eject an electron from its atom and then continues as a lower energy x-ray in a different direction (momentum and energy conservation principles). Most of the scatter radiation in a catheterization laboratory comes from Compton interactions.

3.11 Answer C. A movable leaded acrylic shield should be part of every catheterization laboratory. Because most scatter radiation originates from the area where the x-ray beam first strikes the patient's chest wall, the shield should be positioned between the beam entry port and the operator's face and as close to the patient and the operator as possible. It is important to remember that scatter radiation comes from the patient, not from the image detector. A well-positioned acrylic shield will reduce exposure to the operator's eyes, chest, and thyroid by 90%.

An assistant who stands in the "shadow" of the primary operator can reduce his exposition by >90%. In addition to increasing the distance from the primary beam, such a position requires that scatter rays first penetrate the operator's body, plus two layers of lead, before reaching the assistant.

3.12 Answer B. Radiation exposure-associated risks can be divided in two categories: stochastic and deterministic (tissue reactions). While a single 5 mGy acute exposure comprises a greater deterministic risk than five repeated 1 mGy exposures, the stochastic risk associated to a single or cumulative 5 mGy exposure is approximately the same.

Recent evidence states that operator cataract risk is increased after a single 0.5 mSv exposure, but there is no evidence below this threshold.

The NCI divides radiation-induced skin damage into four levels. Level 2 dermatitis may result in dermal atrophy and telangiectasia lasting over 40 weeks.

Radiation-induced cancer is a rare, albeit dreadful consequence of radiation exposure. The British Royal College of Radiology suggests an exposure threshold of 1 mSv (equivalent to an additional cancer risk of 1:10,000) to discuss cancer risks with patients. These recommendations are seldom used in practice, but clinicians should at least discuss radiation exposure risks while planning a long or complex intervention.

3.13 Answer C. In about two-thirds of cases, x-ray-induced DNA damage results from free radical formation (indirect damage) rather than direct structure alteration. DNA is more prone to damage when it is unpacked, which happens more frequently in cells with high metabolic activity or replication rate. Hence, since breast tissue is mostly glandular, it is particularly radiosensitive.

A higher rate of chromosomal aberrations in circulating lymphocytes has been observed in interventional cardiologists who were compared to unexposed, matched health care workers. This leads some authors to suggest it might become a useful biomarker of radiation hazard in health care professionals and patients. However, it is not yet accepted as a valid prognostic tool for long-term radiation-induced carcinogenesis.

3.14 Answer A. Energy transfer from x-rays to tissue is commonly estimated with two metrics: air KERMA and DAP. These are derived from direct measures made in an ionization chamber placed within the beam inside the x-ray tube.

Air KERMA is calculated for a reference point at the skin surface when considering the heart as the isocenter. During a procedure, the cumulative air KERMA is displayed on the monitor and is a fairly good estimate of skin dose, which is otherwise difficult to measure directly. The air KERMA will overestimate the skin dose when multiple projections are used because of the dose spreading over several entry ports. On the other hand, it will underestimate the skin dose (and the subsequent risk of injury) whenever the body is placed close to the x-ray tube because it does not take scatter into account.

DAP, also named kerma-area product, is the product of the air KERMA and the beam cross-sectional area. The cumulative DAP is a good estimate of the total amount of radiation absorbed by the patient. It is also a good indicator of total room exposure.

Collimation reduces the beam area, the DAP, the total patient dose, and the room exposure.

3.15 Answer A. A standard diagnostic coronary angiography exposes a patient to about 7 mSv, equivalent to 2 to 4 years of natural background exposure. A PCI exposes patients to about 15 mSv per procedure, which is equivalent to 6 years of natural background exposure.

A single-isotope SPECT exposes a patient to 10 mSv on average, which is equivalent to 10 years of natural background exposure. The dual-isotope SPECT is performed less nowadays due to its high radiation burden; a single study exposes a patient to 24 mSv, which is equivalent to 10 years of natural background exposure.

The PET myocardial perfusion imaging and the calcium score CT are associated with a 2 to 3 mSv exposure on average, roughly equivalent to 1 year of natural background exposure.

3.16 Answer C. Normal aortic arch anatomy includes the right carotid artery originating from the innominate artery (bifurcation of the innominate artery into the subclavian and carotid arteries) with the left carotid artery and left subclavian artery originating separately and directly from the aorta. The most frequent variant is a common origin of the innominate artery and left carotid artery. This is erroneously referred to as a "bovine arch." Technically, cattle have a single brachiocephalic trunk from which all arch vessels originate.

3.17 Answer C. The table height and detector position are key technical determinants of x-ray exposure under the operator's control.

Raising the detector, as shown in the photograph, forces the generator control computer to increase the x-ray output to compensate for lost image brightness. This markedly increases the patient's skin dose and the scatter dose in the room. The computer is also forced to increase the kVp, which in turn diminishes image contrast. Hence, the detector should always be placed as close to the patient as possible to optimize radiation exposure.

Lowering the table will place the patient's skin in the most intense part of the x-ray beam, thereby increasing skin dose rates. Some medical x-ray tubes have permanent spacers to keep the patient's body away from the intense beam.

3.18 Answer D. Concerning the interaction between radiation and organic matter, three distinct dimensions must be taken into account: intensity of exposure, absorption, and biologic effects.

The Roentgen is an old unit of equivalent and effective dose, now replaced by the Sievert (1 Sv = 1 J/kg). The Sievert is a weighted measure of the biologic effect on the whole body of one or many absorbed doses. It can be used to estimate the long-term risk of cancer.

The Gray, also equivalent to 1 J/kg, is a measure of the absorbed dose, which refers to the quantity of energy transferred to a tissue.

ALARA stands for As Low as Reasonably Achievable. It serves as a guiding principle for anyone who uses x-rays in a medical setting.

3.19 Answer C. Pregnancy is not an absolute contraindication to necessary cardiac catheterization procedures.

External shielding is considered useless since the fetus is not exposed to the primary beam, but rather to the scattered radiation originating from the mother's chest. Most of these scattered doses are absorbed by the abdominal viscera, and the very small doses reaching the pelvis are not expected to cause any cell damage that could lead to intrauterine growth retardation. However, even the smallest dose of ionizing radiation could increase the future risk of malignancy in an unpredictable manner (stochastic risk).

Since fetuses and newborns are known to be at least onefold more susceptible to radiation-induced malignancy than adults, the risk is not to be neglected.

When planning to expose a pregnant woman to radiation, an operator should discuss the very small cancer risk with the patient and utilize the smallest amount of radiation needed to conduct the procedure safely (ALARA principle). The operator should limit the beam to the chest and use fluoroscopy instead of cine mode acquisition whenever possible.

3.20 Answer C. This film badge is a type of dosimeter that records the accumulated dose of scatter radiation over a period of time. Ideally, two badges should be worn, one over the thyroid collar and one under the apron at the waist level. If a single badge is used, it should be placed on the outside of the thyroid collar on the side closest to the source of scatter radiation. Acceptable readings do not indicate safe practice. An operator who performs a limited number of procedures can expose his patient, his room staff, and himself to unnecessary radiation while recording low readings. According to the linear-no-threshold model, there is no safe dose for the prevention of stochastic effects.

A dosimeter will not protect anyone. The best protection is a good understanding of radiation safety practices.

3.21 Answer D. The difference in image quality stems from the greater thickness and density of tissue that must be penetrated in Panel B. The image in Panel A was obtained from an average-sized patient in a shallow right anterior oblique (RAO) projection with the lung as the background. The image in Panel B was obtained from a large patient in a cranial projection with the spine as the background.

When steep projections are used in large patients, the generator control system automatically increases the kVp, often to >90 kVp, in an attempt to maintain image brightness. This produces more energetic photons that are able to penetrate tissues better. Unfortunately, many of these photons are too energetic to be absorbed by iodine and hence contribute to decreased image contrast.

It might seem that the iodine concentration is too low in Panel B, but in fact the same contrast medium was used and both arteries were well injected. The problem is not the intra-arterial iodine concentration, but rather the transparency of iodine in the presence of high-energy photons (K-edge absorption peak of 33.2 keV). This "washed out" image is characteristic of a high kVp.

3.22 Answer B. The attenuation phenomenon, or beam modulation, is the basis for a generation of contrasted images of diagnostic quality. Attenuation is proportional to four factors: x-ray photon beam energy, atomic number of the atoms composing the tissue, tissue density (g/cc), and tissue thickness.

3.23 Answer B. All radiation exposure potentially adds to the lifetime risk of developing a malignancy. This risk is cumulative according to effective doses of exposure and time of the exposure. As such, younger patients are of particular concern when receiving radiation-exposing diagnostic studies. In this series of patients, it is known that a head CT scan has the lowest typical effective dose (2 to 3 mSv), whereas CT scans of the abdomen/pelvis produce an effective dose several times higher (8 to 10 mSv). While patient A may have a slightly higher total effective dose than patient B, given that patient B is markedly younger, he is the patient with the greatest lifetime risk.

3.24 Answer D. This type of simple x-ray tube was used in the late 1890s by Roentgen and other pioneers to produce amazingly high-quality radiographs. A high voltage accelerates electrons from the cathode until they collide with the metal anode. The maximum voltage applied to the tube determines the maximum energy of the x-ray photons spectrum produced. In this example, a 70,000 V peak (70 kVp) produces x-rays with energies up to 70 keV.

Modern cardiovascular tubes use the same principle, with a few refinements to increase the output of x-rays. The cathode consists of a white-hot filament that boils off the large quantities of electrons needed to produce x-rays. The anode consists of a rotating tungsten disk that absorbs and dissipates heat much better than a stationary target, which would quickly melt if used for the complex procedures of contemporary interventional cardiology.

X-ray production is very inefficient. Approximately 1% of the electrical energy delivered to the tube is converted into x-rays; the remaining 99% is converted to heat that must be dissipated. For years, heat dissipation was a major technical challenge for physical engineers. The problem has largely been solved by liquid cooling systems that work a lot like automobile radiators.

3.25 Answer C. Recent data arising from both observational studies and randomized trials suggest that reducing the number of frames per second during fluoroscopy and cine-acquisition is not associated with image quality reduction. However, it is an effective way of reducing both patient and operator radiation exposure.

In addition to reducing frame rate, decreasing the dose per pulse (especially during cine-angiography acquisition) is probably the best way to reduce patient radiation exposure.

Switching fluoroscopy on and off each time the operator looks at his hands is another excellent way of reducing radiation exposure. Indeed, exposing the patient during that time is useless (and even harmful) since x-rays reaching the patient do not contribute to the generation of a diagnostic image, albeit they contribute to the patient dose.

3.26 Answer A. Stochastic effects are attributable to DNA injury that increases the probability of chromosomal aberrations, mutations, and cancer at some point in the future. Theoretically, even a single x-ray photon can induce DNA injury in a single cell that leads to fatal lymphoma 20 years later. A greater exposure and one of a longer duration will increase the probability of a stochastic effect, but there is no "safe dose" since the consequences are unpredictable. Moreover, the severity of stochastic effects is not influenced by exposure: a cancer caused by a single x-ray photon is just as bad as one caused by the cumulative effect of multiple exposures to millions of photons.

Deterministic effects are attributable to cell death that occurs shortly (hours to months) after a threshold dose of radiation is exceeded. Skin injury is the most common deterministic effect of x-ray exposure. Because skin cells divide continuously, they are susceptible to injury from large doses of radiation that can occur at the beam entrance port. The injury becomes apparent weeks to months after the exposure when cells lost by normal desquamation are no longer replaced. Because of the delay, patients and physicians may not link the injury with a past radiation exposure.

The photograph illustrates radiation skin injury from fluoroscopy used during a PCI. The size and location indicate that the operator worked in the left anterior oblique (LAO) projection and utilized square collimators. This type of injury can progress for months, sometimes leading to deep, nonhealing ulcers that require grafting. It is important to recall that deterministic effects are predictable and, therefore, preventable.

3.27 Answer E. Because of his obesity, this patient will receive substantially increased skin entry doses during cardiac fluoroscopy. The recent exposures will lower the threshold for skin injury with the next procedure. Diabetes may further increase the susceptibility to skin injury. In addition to discussing the risks and benefits, and considering the alternatives to another fluoroscopic procedure, this operator should examine the patient carefully for signs of radiation skin injury.

All the answers list deterministic effects of radiation. However, hair loss does not appear until 3 weeks after the exposure, and the latent period is even longer for desquamation (4 weeks), dermal atrophy or necrosis (3 months), and telangiectasia formation (1 year). Erythema can develop within hours to days.

3.28 Answer B. The International Commission on Radiological Protection (ICRP) introduced DRLs in 1990. They have been implanted to control radiation exposure on a population level and as an investigation threshold for the appropriateness of potentially harmful exposures. DRLs are usually set to the 75th percentile of the dose distribution for a specified center (hospital) or population. They should not be used for occupational or public exposures, nor as individual dose limits or constraints.

Many international institutions, including the American College of Radiology, suggest DRL use, but it is only mandatory by law in Europe.

3.29 Answer C. The radiation-induced cancer risk refers to the stochastic effects of ionizing radiation, which are cumulative regardless of the timing of exposure. The British Royal College of Radiology has proposed specific terms that should be used with patients to quantify the radiation-induced risks. For both coronary angiography and angioplasty, the risk could be quantified as low but should nonetheless be discussed with the patient since the average exposure is over 1 mSv (the threshold suggested to discuss such risks with patients).

3.30 Answer D. About 40% of medical radiation exposure is attributable to cardiovascular imaging, and 10% of total exposure is directly attributable to interventional cardiology.

In contemporary practice, most of medical radiation exposure is attributable to CT scans.

Recently updated data are lacking to estimate the actual contribution of nuclear medicine, but it represents between a quarter and a third of medical radiation exposure in the United States.

4 Inflammation and Arterial Injury

Jay Giri and Harold L. Dauerman

QUESTIONS

4.1 A 54-year-old man presents to your office 2 weeks after sirolimus-eluting stent (SES) placement with diffuse hives and pruritus. There is no wheezing, and his blood pressure is stable. The patient is on chronic aspirin therapy and was started on an angiotensin-converting enzyme (ACE) inhibitor, statin, and clopidogrel during his recent hospitalization. The patient shows you a journal article given to him by a physician who is a family friend. He asks if the problem reported in the article (Fig. Q4-1) is the cause of his "rash." You review the article and advise him to:

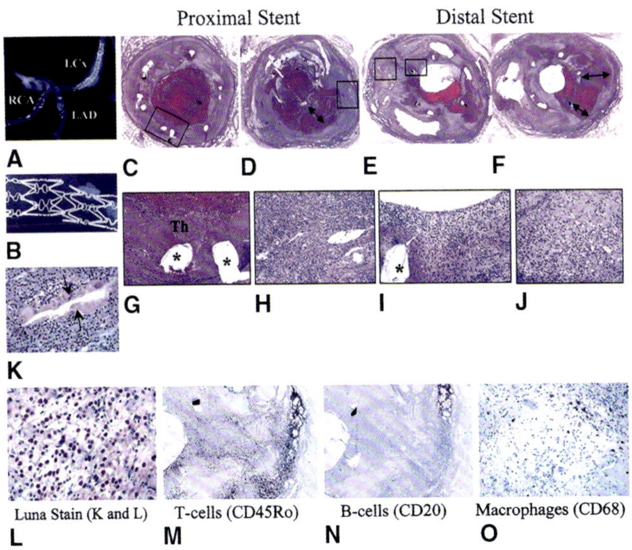

Figure Q4-1 (With permission from Virmani R, et al. *Circulation* 2004;109(6):701–705.)

(A) Discontinue clopidogrel
(B) Discontinue aspirin
(C) Start antihistamines and steroids
(D) Stop the statin and ACE inhibitor, consider changing from clopidogrel to prasugrel, and start antihistamines and possibly oral steroids

4.2 A 43-year-old woman presents for elective cardiac catheterization and asks that you use ticagrelor as opposed to clopidogrel if stenting is required. Data that support the patient's request include which of the following?

(A) Ticagrelor suppresses postpercutaneous coronary intervention (PCI) inflammation to a greater degree than clopidogrel
(B) Ticagrelor decreases cardiovascular events compared to clopidogrel in a population of patients with acute coronary syndrome (ACS)
(C) Ticagrelor is a more potent inhibitor of the glycoprotein (GP) IIb/IIIa receptor than clopidogrel
(D) Ticagrelor decreases ischemic cardiovascular events compared to clopidogrel in patients with stable coronary syndromes undergoing PCI

4.3 A 65-year-old woman comes to your office after seeing a television report about stents, and she is concerned that her drug-eluting stent is a "ticking time bomb in my chest." She wants proof that drug-eluting stents (DES) are at the same risk as bare metal stents (BMS) for late stent thrombosis. She has done some research and shows you a figure

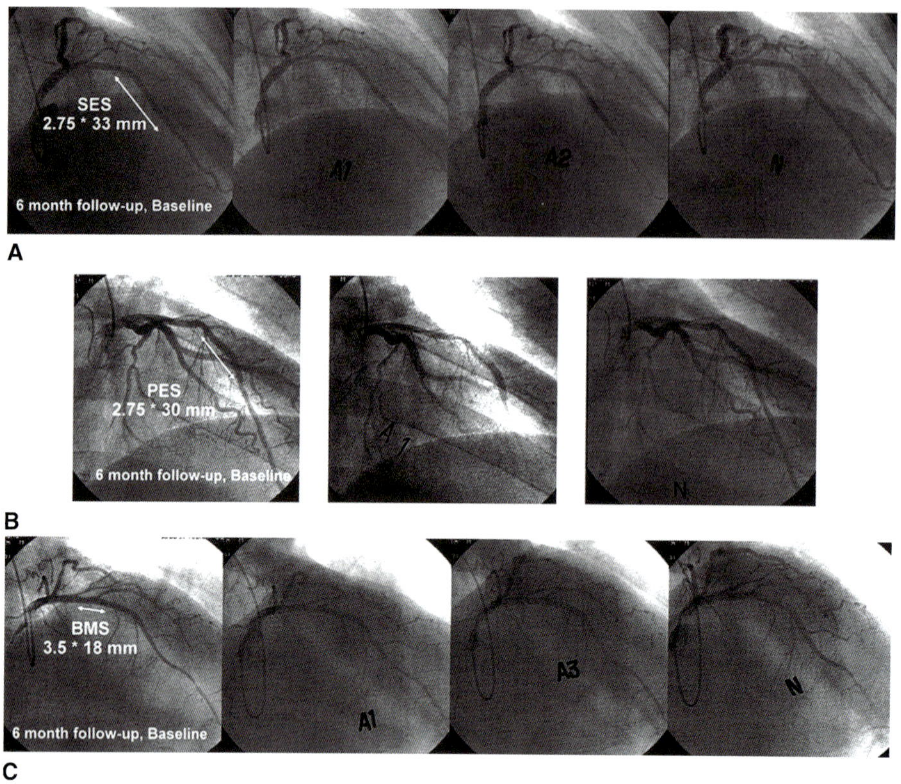

Figure Q4-3 (With permission from Pendyala LK, et al. *JACC Cardiovasc Interv* 2009;2(12): 1169–1177.)

(Fig. Q4-3) that depicts the impact of intracoronary acetylcholine and nitroglycerin administered 6 months after BMS and DES (implantation). Your interpretation of this experiment is:

Note: A, acetylcholine; N, nitroglycerin; PES, paclitaxel-eluting stent; SES, sirolimus-eluting stent.

(A) BMS and DES have a similar acute vasodilatory response to acetylcholine consistent with a similar chronic risk of inflammation and stent thrombosis

(B) First-generation DES (sirolimus and paclitaxel) demonstrate an enhanced risk of chronic endothelial dysfunction compared to BMS, which is consistent with the patient's concerns about chronically enhanced inflammation and thrombotic risk with DES

(C) First-generation DES (sirolimus and paclitaxel) have similar risk of chronic endothelial dysfunction, and thus there is no increased risk of inflammation and thrombosis with DES

(D) First-generation DES (sirolimus and paclitaxel) cause more chronic endothelial dysfunction, but this dysfunction is only at the proximal edges of the stent and should not cause any increased inflammation or thrombotic risk in the distal vasculature

4.4 The same 65-year-old woman as in the previous question is now more concerned than ever about her lifetime risk of stent thrombosis. She has looked up her stent type and found it to be a second-generation (zotarolimus-eluting) stent. You show her Figure Q4-4 and explain the experiment as follows:

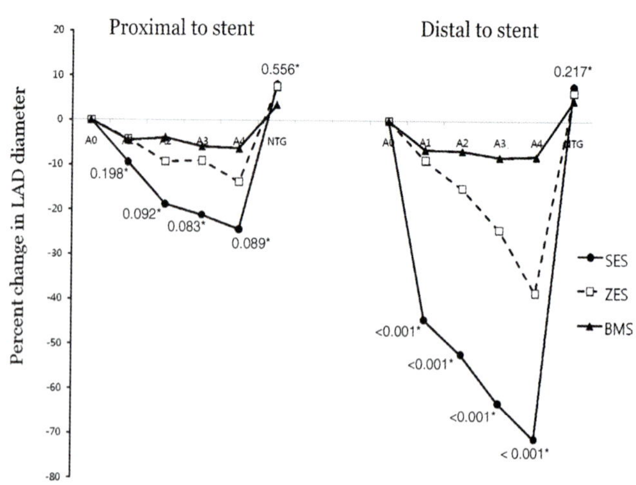

Figure Q4-4 (With permission from Kim JW, et al. *J Am Coll Cardiol* 2009;53(18):1653–1659.)

(A) Risks of acute, late, and very late stent thrombosis are the same with sirolimus- vs. zotarolimus-eluting stents (ZES)
(B) ZES causes more chronic endothelial dysfunction than SES
(C) BMS cause the most chronic endothelial dysfunction and thus have the highest likelihood of chronic inflammation and thrombosis
(D) While ZES cause more chronic inflammation than BMS, the chronic endothelial dysfunction and thus inflammatory response are better than SES, and this may translate into a lower risk of late thrombosis

4.5 Assuming identical and guideline-directed antiplatelet therapies, which of the following are TRUE regarding stent thrombosis rates with BMS and late-generation cobalt chromium (CoCr) everolimus-eluting stents (EES)?

(A) BMS have lower rates of subacute stent thrombosis (<30 days) and similar rates of late stent thrombosis compared to CoCr EES
(B) BMS have similar rates of subacute and late stent thrombosis as CoCr EES
(C) BMS have similar rates of subacute stent thrombosis (<30 days) but lower rates of late stent thrombosis compared to CoCr EES
(D) BMS have higher rates of subacute stent thrombosis (<30 days) and higher rates of late stent thrombosis compared to CoCr EES

4.6 Which of the following is TRUE regarding polymers on DES?

(A) Newer generation durable polymers, unlike older generation durable polymers, are not associated with inflammation
(B) Polymers on DES modulate the elution characteristics of the drug
(C) Stents with biodegradable polymers have superior 1-year clinical outcomes in comparison with durable polymer CoCr or platinum chromium DES
(D) After complete drug release, durable polymers serve as an additional mechanism to prevent neoatherosclerosis and late in-stent restenosis

4.7 After coronary stenting, which of the following cell types would NOT be part of the initial injury response?

(A) Platelets
(B) Lymphocytes and macrophages
(C) Alpha-actin–positive smooth muscle cells
(D) Neutrophils

4.8 How does arterial injury caused by balloon angioplasty differ from injury due to DES placement?

(A) Negative remodeling may be a major factor in DES-related healing
(B) DES abolishes the early phases of platelet activation and inflammatory cytokines increase
(C) Polymer coating of the stent limits migration of smooth muscle cells
(D) Both neointimal hyperplasia and negative remodeling play major roles in the long-term healing response to balloon angioplasty

4.9 All of the following may contribute to arterial injury and inflammation, EXCEPT:

(A) Stent coating with selected polymers/drugs
(B) Increased stent strut thickness and specific geometric factors
(C) Stent deployment with struts in contact with damaged media or lipid core
(D) Stent deployment with struts in contact with fibrous plaque

4.10 Consider the photomicrographs in Figure Q4-10. Panel A is a histopathologic section from a rabbit artery stented with polymer and a high dose of paclitaxel. Panel B is from an artery stented with polymer alone. How did the high dose of paclitaxel influence the healing response?

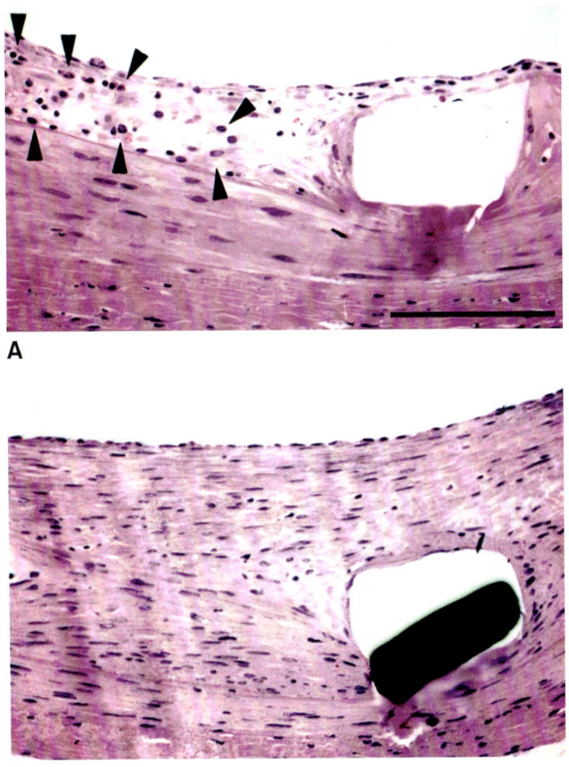

Figure Q4-10 (With permission from Farb A, et al. *Circulation* 2001;104(4):473–479.)

(A) Decreased intimal hyperplasia in the paclitaxel polymer-coated stent
(B) Increased inflammatory reaction in the polymer-only stent
(C) Decreased intimal hyperplasia in the polymer-only stent
(D) Persistent fibrin deposition in the polymer-only stent

4.11 Figure Q4-11 shows a histopathologic analysis 1 day after implantation of a coronary artery stent. What does the asterisk (*) indicate?

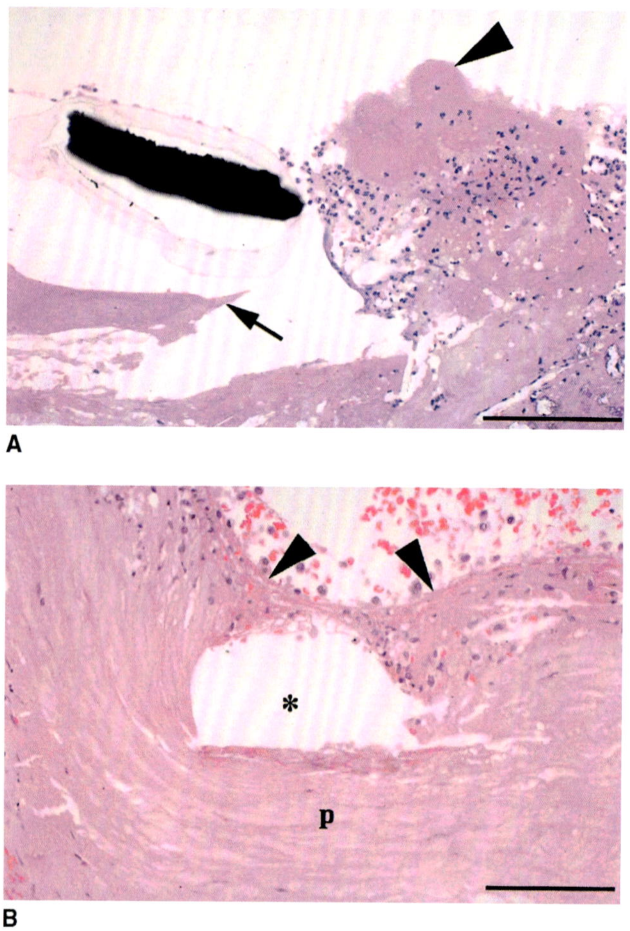

Figure Q4-11 (With permission from Farb A, et al. *Circulation* 1999;99(1):44–52.)

(A) Platelet-rich thrombus
(B) Lipid-rich vulnerable plaque
(C) Site of stent strut
(D) Fibrous plaque

4.12 Late stent thrombosis after first-generation DES placement has been associated with which of the following?

(A) Warfarin anticoagulation in addition to dual antiplatelet therapy (DAPT)
(B) A localized, hypersensitivity (eosinophilic, giant cell) reaction to the polymer
(C) Implantation of DES in the setting of ST-segment elevation myocardial infarction (STEMI)
(D) Geographic miss during DES implantation

4.13 A patient develops acute chest pain and the electrocardiogram (ECG) changes within 1 minute of stent implantation. What type of arterial injury is shown just distal to the stent (Fig. Q4-13)?

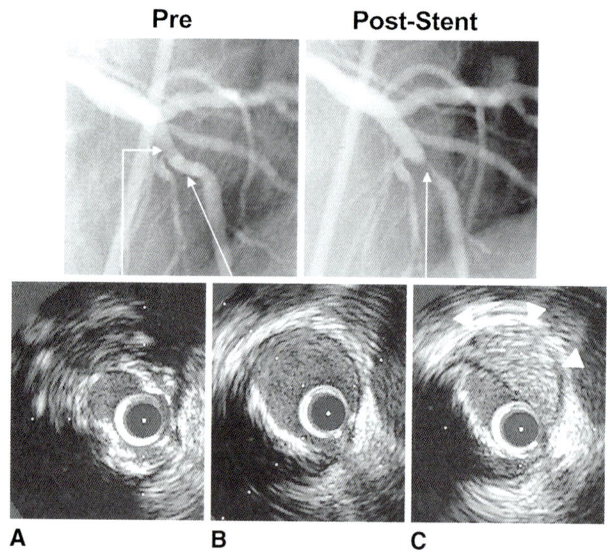

Figure Q4-13 (With permission from Maehara A, et al. *Circulation* 2002;105(17):2037–2042.)

(A) Acute intramural hematoma
(B) Intraprocedural stent thrombosis
(C) Spontaneous rupture of distal lipid-rich plaque
(D) Acute platelet-rich thrombus due to stent-mediated hypersensitivity

4.14 Arterial injury due to stent placement induces a systemic inflammatory response. Figure Q4-14 shows the systemic rise of which inflammatory marker after stenting?

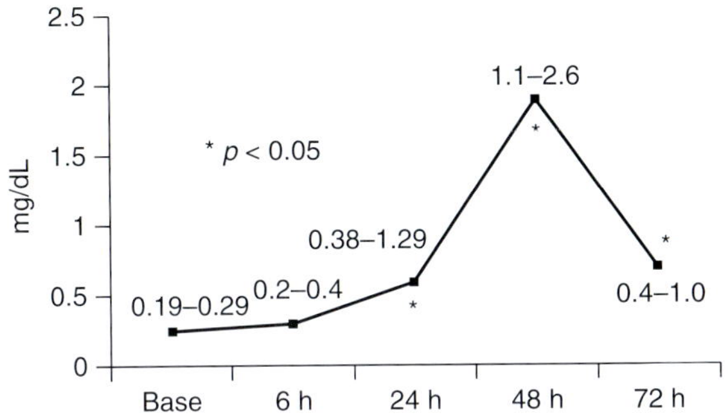

Figure Q4-14 (With permission from Gaspardone A, et al. *Am J Cardiol* 1998;82(4):515–518.)

(A) Serum amyloid A
(B) C-reactive protein (CRP)
(C) Soluble CD40 ligand
(D) Interleukin (IL)-6

4.15 Which of the following improvements in stent design has NOT been associated with decreased stent thrombosis rates?

(A) Thinner strut sizes
(B) Bioresorbable drug-eluting scaffolds
(C) More potent antiproliferative agents such as everolimus
(D) Novel metal alloys

4.16 Optical coherence tomography (OCT) is performed on a patient 12 months after DES implantation. Figure Q4-16 shows what phenomenon and what potential mechanisms are a reasonable explanation of this occurrence?

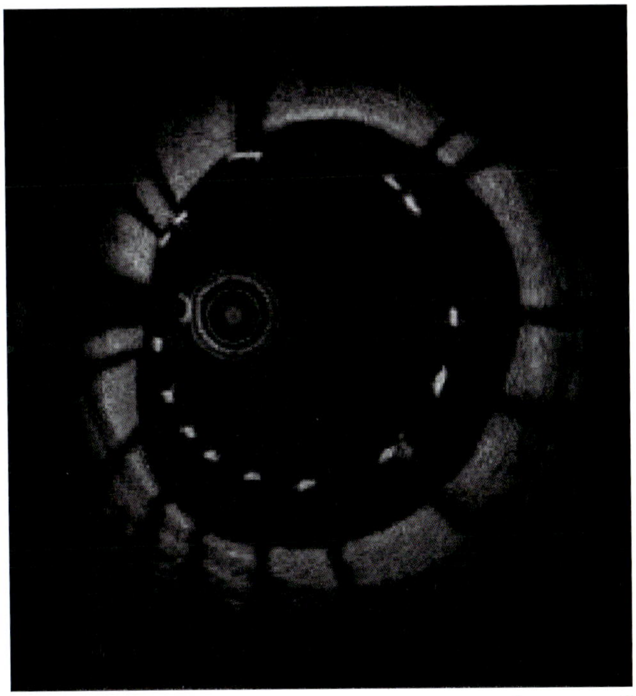

Figure Q4-16 (With permission from Garg S, et al. *J Am Coll Cardiol* 2010;56(10):S1–S42.)

(A) Persistent intramural hematoma caused by extensive coronary dissection
(B) A predominantly eosinophilic inflammatory response that is associated with increased risk of incomplete stent apposition
(C) Spontaneous dissection postprocedure that is associated with overexpansion or a stent diameter in great excess to the reference vessel diameter
(D) Pseudoaneurysm associated with inappropriate extent of anticoagulation during the procedure

4.17 Activated macrophages recruited after arterial injury secrete which of the following systemic mediators of inflammation?

(A) CRP
(B) Soluble CD40 ligand
(C) IL-1 and IL-6
(D) P selectin

4.18 A 56-year-old woman with anterior ischemia on stress testing is found to have a long segment of left anterior descending (LAD) artery disease. The lesion length is 23 mm. You have the option of using one 28 mm DES or two 15 mm DES. Figure Q4-18 is from a porcine model and shows the consequences of your choice and is best interpreted as follows:

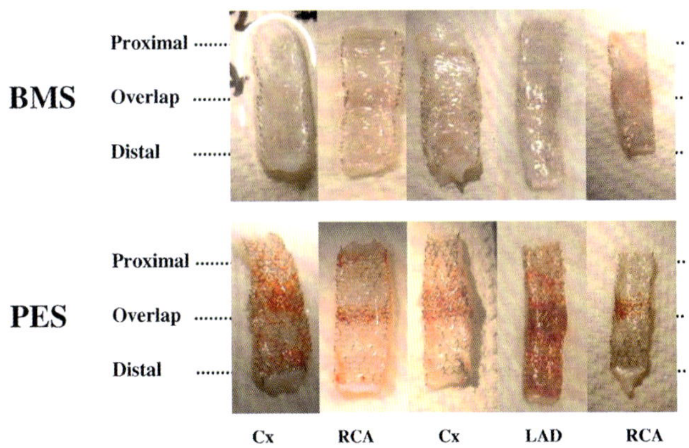

Figure Q4-18 (With permission from Chen JP, et al. *JACC Cardiovasc Interv* 2009;2(7):583–593.)

(A) A single long DES has an enhanced inflammatory response compared to two shorter DESs
(B) Overlap of DES may cause a heightened inflammatory response at the overlap sites with increased rates of in-stent restenosis
(C) Drug-elution patterns are similar at overlap sites as compared to nonoverlap sites
(D) You should use a BMS to avoid increased risk of stent thrombosis due to overlapping DES

4.19 Arterial injury leads to a cascade of platelet activation followed by local and systemic inflammation. Figure Q4-19 demonstrates vasoconstriction occurring after exercise in a patient who received an SES more than 6 months prior to the stress test. Which of the following is INCORRECT?

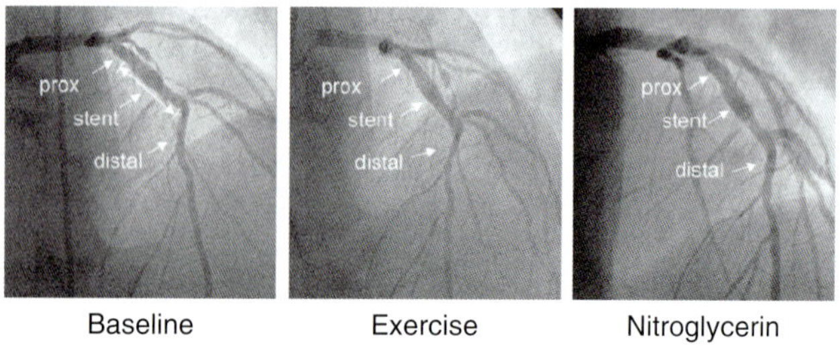

Figure Q4-19 (With permission from Togni M, et al. *J Am Coll Cardiol* 2005;46(2):231–236.)

(A) The patient might also have abnormal flow-independent dilation of the brachial artery
(B) The patient might also have abnormal flow-mediated dilation of the brachial artery
(C) DES lead to delay in endothelial regeneration after injury
(D) Chronic endothelial dysfunction suggests durable polymers lead to chronic inflammation

4.20 Figure Q4-20 demonstrates a similar extent of DES- and BMS-induced systemic inflammation after PCI. If inflammation after arterial injury is important in developing restenosis, which of the following partially contributes to the 50% reduction in restenosis with DES vs. BMS?

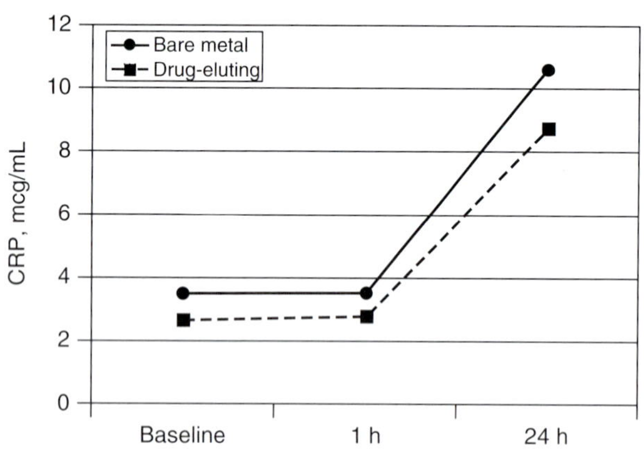

Figure Q4-20 (With permission from Gogo PB, et al. *J Thromb Thrombolysis* 2005;19(2):87–92.)

(A) DES decrease initial and chronic platelet activation compared to BMS
(B) DES decrease the early systemic inflammatory response to stenting compared to BMS
(C) DES decrease systemic inflammation occurring between 24 hours and 9 months after stenting
(D) DES decreases the local, but not systemic, impact of stenting on inflammation

4.21 An enhanced systemic inflammatory response may occur after PCI for cardiogenic shock. This inflammatory response may lead to:

(A) Upregulation of nitric oxide synthase leading to vasodilation and hypotension
(B) Severe vasoconstriction resulting in a decreased cardiac output
(C) A downregulation of nitric oxide synthase leading to pulmonary edema
(D) Upregulation of natriuretic peptides leading to hypotension via excessive diuresis

4.22 All of the following drugs have been shown to have a potential favorable impact on the acute inflammatory response after PCI, EXCEPT:

(A) Atorvastatin
(B) Clopidogrel
(C) Abciximab
(D) Beta-blockers

4.23 Which of the following is NOT a hypothesized mechanism for stent thrombosis with drug-eluting bioresorbable vascular scaffolds?

(A) Increased strut sizes
(B) Inadequate lesion preparation
(C) Everolimus coating
(D) Intraluminal masses

4.24 Which of the following do you expect at 5 years after implantation of a bioabsorbable vascular scaffold in a patient who had no coronary events in the intervening years after initial placement?

(A) Return of normal endothelin-independent vasomotion in the previously stented segment as compared to adjacent undiseased and unstented areas
(B) No discernible scaffold struts seen on intravascular imaging
(C) Similar endothelin-independent coronary vasomotion in the previously stented segment at 3 and 5 years after BVS placement
(D) Thin-capped neointima over the area of prior BVS placement when evaluated with OCT

4.25 Eptifibatide and tirofiban have been shown to have which effects after PCI?

(A) Decrease intimal hyperplasia via a direct effect on macrophage accumulation
(B) Decrease intimal hyperplasia via inhibition of smooth muscle cell hyperplasia
(C) Decrease the rise of CRP and IL-6 in the first 24 hours after PCI compared to heparin alone
(D) Decrease platelet aggregation and the incidence of periprocedural myonecrosis

ANSWERS AND EXPLANATIONS

4.1 Answer D. The figure incidentally shows a case of intense eosinophilic reaction to a DES associated with late stent thrombosis. The patient is correct that DES can elicit a chronic inflammatory response even after the drug has fully eluted. This reaction is generally localized and hypothesized to be associated with an increased risk of very late stent thrombosis. In this patient's case, a systemic allergic response is much more likely to be drug mediated and careful alteration of medications is warranted. A chronic systemic reaction to the permanent components of the stent (nickel and polymer) is extremely rare but is a potential explanation for the symptoms if medication changes do not relieve the hypersensitivity reaction (Virmani R, et al. *Circulation* 2004;109(6):701-705).

4.2 Answer B. Ticagrelor is a more potent platelet $P2Y_{12}$ receptor antagonist than clopidogrel. In the PLATO trial, cardiovascular events were decreased with ticagrelor as compared to clopidogrel among a population of patients with ACS. Neither ticagrelor nor prasugrel have been demonstrated to reduce cardiovascular events in patients undergoing PCI with stable coronary artery disease (CAD). While more potent inhibition of $P2Y_{12}$ receptor-mediated platelet activation could plausibly impact platelet-monocyte interactions and post-PCI inflammation, a positive impact on arterial injury mediated inflammation has not yet been demonstrated (Wallentin L, et al. *N Engl J Med* 2009;361(11):1045-1057).

4.3 Answer B. The figure demonstrates significantly more proximal and distal vasoconstriction with PES and SES vs. BMS among patients tested with ascending doses (A1, A2) of intracoronary acetylcholine 6 months after stent implantation. Non-endothelium-dependent vasodilation (N = nitrates) is similar among all three groups. It should be appreciated that any drug should have fully eluted 6 months after DES implantation, so this chronic endothelial dysfunction likely represents a chronic inflammatory response to permanent polymer. This pathophysiologic finding has not been clearly linked to an increased risk of clinical late stent thrombosis (Pendyala LK, et al. *JACC Cardiovasc Interv* 2009;2(12):1169-1177).

4.4 Answer D. Vasoreactivity is abnormal for both SES (sirolimus) and ZES (zotarolimus) 6 months after stent implantation compared to BMS. But the relative vasoconstriction is much more intense proximally and distally with the first-generation SES. This suggests more intense endothelial dysfunction due to chronic inflammation with the SES vs. ZES stent. Similar results have been noted with regard to second-generation EES. Of note, the BASKET-PROVE trial compared SES vs. second-generation EES and did not show a difference in death, infarction, or stent thrombosis despite a possible difference in inflammatory responses based on the generation of the DES.

4.5 Answer D. A seminal meta-analysis of randomized controlled trials (RCTs) demonstrated dramatically reduced rates of definite stent thrombosis at all time points with CoCr EES compared to BMS. No other tested DES had lower definite stent thrombosis than BMS at 2-year follow-up. Importantly, platinum chromium EES was not evaluated in this study, though subsequent trials and observational data suggest similar positive results with this platform (Palmerini T, et al. *Lancet* 2012;379(9824):1393-1402).

4.6 Answer B. Polymers serve to modulate the elution characteristics of the drug on DES. They do not have an independent positive effect on neoatherosclerosis or in-stent restenosis rates. Newer generation durable polymers cause less inflammation than first-generation polymers, but the inflammatory response is not completely eliminated. Stents using biodegradable polymers have demonstrated similar results in randomized trials to durable CoCr or platinum chromium DES (Kereiakes DJ, et al. *Circ Cardiovasc Interv* 2015;8(4):e002372).

4.7 Answer C. Coronary stenting is a model for arterial injury, and the healing response proceeds in phases. Phase I is de-endothelialization followed by deposition of platelets and fibrin. Via platelet activation and cytokine increases, acute inflammatory cells are then recruited in the first few days after stenting. Phase II involves release of growth factors from platelets and leukocytes driving proliferation and migration of smooth muscle cells and chronic inflammatory cells. Phase III (weeks to months after injury) is characterized by migration of alpha-actin-positive smooth muscle cells into the neointima, extracellular matrix deposition, and re-endothelialization of the stent (Grewe PH, et al. *J Am Coll Cardiol* 2000;35(1):157–163; Welt FG, et al. *Arterioscler Thromb Vasc Biol* 2002;22(11):1769–1776).

4.8 Answer D. All forms of arterial injury lead to platelet activation, inflammation, and smooth muscle cell-mediated chronic healing. Paclitaxel and sirolimus decrease the amount of neointimal hyperplasia compared to BMS, but the underlying polymer has no favorable effect on the healing process. All stents in general abolish two adverse components of the healing response: an acute decrease in vessel diameter (recoil) and a chronic decrease in the external elastic membrane dimension (negative remodeling). Incomplete stent apposition may rarely occur as part of the healing process after stenting. This is related to positive remodeling during the healing process and does not contribute to restenosis after BMS or DES (Kimura T, et al. *Circulation* 1997;96(2):475–483; Mintz GS, et al. *Circulation* 2003;107(21):2660–2663).

4.9 Answer D. The inflammatory response to stent-mediated arterial injury determines adverse healing responses. Among the factors that may increase inflammation and restenosis are (a) certain polymers/drugs, (b) stent strut thickness and geometric factors, and (c) medial injury or lipid core penetration by stent struts. Deployment of stents in fibrous plaque without causing medial damage reduces the inflammatory response to stenting (Virmani R, et al. *Circulation* 2002;106(21):2649–2651; Pache J, et al. *J Am Coll Cardiol* 2003;41(8):1283–1288).

4.10 Answer A. Paclitaxel successfully reduced the thickness of intimal hyperplasia in the top picture as compared to polymer alone. This is a major benefit of various other drugs (sirolimus, everolimus, and zotarolimus) eluted from stents as well. At this high dose of paclitaxel, though, the inflammatory response is augmented (*arrowheads*) as compared to polymer alone. Adverse events related possibly to chronic inflammation and delayed healing due to high-dose paclitaxel were seen with the QuaDS QP-2 stent. Similar adverse clinical events were not seen using the different polymer/paclitaxel dosing regimen in the TAXUS-IV trial (Farb A, et al. *Circulation* 2001;104(4):473–479; Stone GW, et al. *N Engl J Med* 2004;350(3):221–231).

4.11 Answer C. Both panels show acute response to arterial injury. In the top panel (A), platelet-rich thrombus (*arrowhead*) is seen. Numerous acute inflammatory cells are also present within the thrombus; focal fibrous cap disruption is also demonstrated (*arrow*). In Panel B, an asterisk shows the site of the stent strut with associated fibrin-rich thrombus (*arrowheads*). Fibrous plaque (*p*) is present below the strut.

4.12 Answer B. The major cause of DES thrombosis is early cessation of DAPT. But case reports demonstrate rare hypersensitivity reactions after implantation of SES that may be associated with stent thrombosis. While other causes of hypersensitivity reactions may occur (i.e., clopidogrel or aspirin allergies), an eosinophilic reaction can occur at the site of the stent strut and be associated with fatal stent thrombosis. This could be due to either the drug or polymer, but early drug elution suggests that an allergic reaction to the permanent polymer may be implicated in some cases of late stent thrombosis (Iakovou I, et al. *JAMA* 2005;293(17):2126–2130).

4.13 Answer A. Arterial injury can manifest itself angiographically immediately after stent deployment. Causes of acute vessel closure in the stent era include intraprocedural stent thrombosis, extensive dissection, or intramural hematoma formation (Chieffo A, et al. *Circulation* 2004;109(22):2732–2736). Intramural hematoma complicates approximately 7% of PCI procedures, and the angiogram may show stenosis, dissection, or even a normal appearance. In intravascular ultrasound (IVUS), intramural hematomas are crescent shaped, homogenous, hyperechoic areas with an entry site from dissection into the media.

4.14 Answer B. The most extensively studied systemic marker of inflammation is CRP; the magnitude of pre-and post-PCI levels of CRP has been associated with adverse events after stenting. The systemic rise in CRP after injury is fairly slow, with no rise appreciated until at least 24 hours after PCI. The slow systemic rise of CRP after stenting is most consistent with production of CRP primarily in the liver and a downstream role of this cytokine in the response to injury.

4.15 Answer B. Newer generation metallic DES have demonstrated progressively decreasing rates of both early and late stent thrombosis in observational studies and randomized trials compared to their early-generation counterparts. Proposed mechanisms for this include thinner struts, everolimus coatings, and the utilization of CoCr or platinum chromium. Bioresorbable drug-eluting scaffolds are associated with significantly higher rates of subacute stent thrombosis than current-generation metallic DES (Cassese S, et al. *Lancet* 2016;387(10018):537–544).

4.16 Answer B. Late acquired incomplete stent apposition is more common after DES than BMS (and not related to underdeployment of stents at time of implantation). While the exact mechanism is unknown, the clinical consequences of incomplete apposition may be an increased risk of stent thrombosis. Potential mechanisms of increased risk of incomplete apposition after DES include inflammation, delayed healing, underlying soft plaque, and a chronic eosinophilic response to DES implantation.

4.17 Answer C. CRP is an acute-phase reactant produced by the liver. IL-6 is the main hepatic stimulus for CRP production and is produced by macrophages. CRP in turn stimulates further production of inflammatory cytokines such as IL-1, IL-6, and tumor necrosis factor (TNF)-alpha by macrophages. P selectin is stored in the alpha granules of platelets. CD40 ligand, a transmembrane protein, was originally identified on CD4+ T cells and recently found on activated platelets. Both membrane-bound and soluble forms of this ligand may interact with CD40, which is expressed on vascular cells, resulting in a variety of inflammatory responses (Aukrust P, et al. *Circulation* 1999;100(6):614–620; Moliterno DJ, et al. *Am Heart J* 2003;145:563–566).

4.18 Answer B. While lesion length and multiple DES may be predictors of DES stent thrombosis, the clinical results of overlapping DES are not entirely clear. Overlapping DES, though, is clearly associated with variable drug elution and an enhanced chronic inflammatory response at the overlap sites as shown in this porcine PES histology. Since BMS do not elute drugs, there is no increased inflammatory response at BMS overlap sites, but intimal hyperplasia is abundant. Use of a single longer DES obviates both the altered drug elution and increased inflammation associated with overlapping multiple DES.

4.19 Answer A. Flow-mediated dilation of the brachial artery reflects systemic endothelial dysfunction while flow-independent dilation reflects smooth muscle function. Patients have abnormal endothelial function early after PCI, but it is somewhat surprising that abnormal endothelial function can be seen >6 months after DES placement. As sirolimus is no longer present on the stent at that time, the etiology of this longer term endothelial dysfunction is most likely related to durable polymer (Togni M, et al. *J Am Coll Cardiol* 2005;46(6):231–236; Blum A, et al. *Am J Cardiol* 2004;94(11):1420–1423; Hofma SH, et al. *Eur Heart J* 2006;27(2):166–170).

4.20 Answer D. While prior literature has suggested that the post-PCI rise of cytokines is predictive of restenosis, this has not been confirmed in the DES era. In fact, it appears that systemic cytokine rise after PCI is marked and similar for both DES and BMS. No difference in platelet activation has been shown for various stent types. Given the markedly lower restenosis rates for DES, it is likely local drug delivery works via local suppression of inflammation and smooth muscle cell migration despite a similar systemic inflammatory response (Gogo PB Jr, et al. *J Thromb Thrombolysis* 2005;19(2):87–92; Dibra A, et al. *Am Heart J* 2005;150(2):344–350).

4.21 Answer A. Cardiogenic shock has traditionally been thought of as massive myonecrosis leading to reduced cardiac output and compensatory vasoconstriction. In the SHOCK trial, though, systemic vascular resistance was not markedly elevated in most cardiogenic shock patients. Newer evidence suggests that shock induces a systemic inflammatory response leading to nitric oxide synthase overproduction. This leads to inappropriate vasodilation and may play an important role in the refractory hypotension associated with cardiogenic shock (Hochman JS. *Circulation* 2003;107(24):2998–3002; Cotter G, et al. *Eur Heart J* 2003;24(14):1287–1295).

4.22 Answer D. Atorvastatin, clopidogrel, and abciximab may blunt the inflammatory response after PCI as one mechanism of their beneficial impact on PCI. Abciximab blunted the rise of CRP and IL-6 after PCI in a subset of patients in the EPIC trial. Clopidogrel may attenuate the increased risk associated with PCI among patients with high CRP levels. Similarly, statin therapy prior to PCI seems to have the most benefit among patients with the highest level of pre-PCI inflammation. While none of these systemic medications clearly impacts long-term healing (stent restenosis), local applications of statin drugs may be promising given their potential effects on inflammation and smooth muscle cell migration (Chew DP, et al. *Am J Cardiol* 2001;88(6):672–674; Chan AW, et al. *Circulation* 2003;107(13):1750–1756; Nannizzi-Alaimo L, et al. *Circulation* 2003;107:1123–1128; Gaspardone A, et al. *Am J Cardiol* 2002;90(7):786–789).

4.23 Answer C. Several mechanisms have been proposed for the increased stent thrombosis rates seen with bioresorbable scaffolds. These include thicker strut sizes, poorer radial strength that necessitates more aggressive prestent lesion preparation, and visualized intraluminal masses on follow-up intravascular imaging that might represent early thrombi or late malapposed struts. Everolimus coatings have not been independently implicated given their association with lower stent thrombosis rates when used on traditional metallic alloy stents.

4.24 Answer B. In follow-up studies from the ABSORB trials, no residual struts were seen at 5 years in patients who received bioabsorbable vascular scaffolds. While dilation of the stented segment to intracoronary nitroglycerin (endothelin-independent coronary vasomotion) improved between years 3 and 5, this did not return completely to normal when compared to adjacent undiseased coronary segments which still dilated more at both time points. Intravascular imaging has revealed thick capped neointima over the areas of prior bioabsorbable vascular scaffolds (Dudek D, et al. *JACC Cardiovasc Interv* 2017;10(8):786–795; Serruys PW, et al. *J Am Coll Cardiol* 2016;67(7):766–776).

4.25 Answer D. GP IIb/IIIa inhibitors decrease platelet aggregation and periprocedural myonecrosis. While the EPIC trial suggests that abciximab decreased the rise of CRP and IL-6 after PCI as compared to heparin alone, there are little data to suggest that eptifibatide or tirofiban significantly suppress the inflammatory response to PCI. It is possible that the inferiority of tirofiban compared to abciximab in the TARGET trial may relate to both inadequate tirofiban dosing and lack of tirofiban anti-inflammatory effects. None of the GP IIb/IIIa inhibitors have been clearly shown to prevent intimal hyperplasia and in-stent restenosis (Topol EJ, et al. *N Engl J Med* 2001;344(25):1888–1894; Schneider DJ, et al. *Am J Cardiol* 2003;91(3):334–336).

5 Antiplatelet, Antithrombotic, and Thrombolytic Agents

David J. Moliterno and Tracy E. Macaulay

QUESTIONS

5.1 You are called regarding a 63-year-old male who underwent successful percutaneous coronary intervention (PCI) and placement of a femoral arteriotomy closure suture approximately 20 minutes ago. He had a coughing paroxysm and now has an enlarging hematoma. Local pressure has been applied to the hematoma and you ask that intravenous (IV) protamine be administered. Which of the following statements BEST describes protamine?

(A) Regular use of neutral protamine Hagedorn (NPH) insulin is not a contraindication to taking protamine
(B) It is a potent anticoagulant as well as a reversing agent for heparin
(C) Doses >50 mg should be avoided
(D) Patients allergic to fish are not at risk for anaphylactoid reactions to protamine

5.2 Which of the following BEST describes why prasugrel provides more potent and consistent platelet aggregation inhibition than clopidogrel?

(A) It is absorbed over a broader gastric pH range and is therefore less affected by proton-pump inhibitors
(B) Clopidogrel is affected by multiple foods, such as grapefruit juice, whereas prasugrel is not
(C) The active metabolite is formed by a single oxidative step
(D) Morphine and similar drugs more negatively impact clopidogrel absorption

5.3 Which anticoagulant is represented in Figure Q5-3?

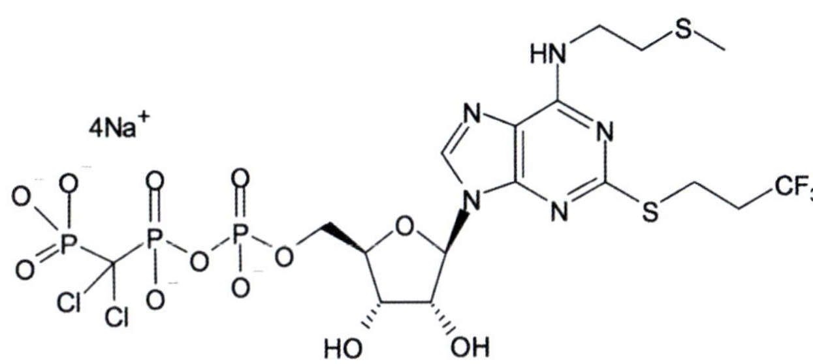

Figure Q5-3 (Courtesy of Chiesi, USA, Inc.)

(A) Bivalirudin
(B) Cangrelor
(C) Fondaparinux
(D) Eptifibatide
(E) Recombinant tissue plasminogen activator (rtPA)

5.4 Which of the following is NOT an absolute contraindication for thrombolytic therapy for the treatment of ST-segment elevation myocardial infarction (STEMI)?

(A) Ischemic stroke >1 year prior
(B) Suspected aortic dissection
(C) Intracranial arteriovenous malformation
(D) Recent, severe head trauma

5.5 A 63-year-old Caucasian male was found to have a positive stress test during preoperative evaluation. He subsequently underwent successful implantation of a paclitaxel-eluting stent (PES) into the left anterior descending (LAD) coronary artery. Approximately 4 weeks later, the patient's orthopedic surgeon contacts you. He wishes to proceed with a planned knee-replacement surgery. Your recommendations are:

(A) Proceed with the planned surgery, but discontinue clopidogrel at least 5 days in advance
(B) Postpone surgery for 1 month
(C) Postpone surgery for 11 months
(D) Discontinue clopidogrel, and after 2 days, admit the patient to the hospital for fondaparinux injections

5.6 Which of the following characteristics accurately describes bivalirudin?

(A) 20 amino acids; 25-minute half-life; hepatic clearance
(B) 20 amino acids; 25-minute half-life; <25% removal with dialysis
(C) 65 amino acids; 75-minute half-life; immunogenic
(D) 65 amino acids; 75-minute half-life; leech derivative

5.7 Several large-scale randomized trials (CHAMPION-PCI, CHAMPION-PLATFORM, and CHAMPION-PHOENIX) tested cangrelor vs. placebo or clopidogrel among patients undergoing PCI. A patient-level pooled analysis (N = 24,910) of these trials assessed major adverse cardiovascular events (MACE) (i.e., death, myocardial infarction [MI], ischemia-driven revascularization, and stent thrombosis) and bleeding (GUSTO severe) at 48 hours. As compared with placebo or clopidogrel, the use of cangrelor resulted in:

(A) Approximately 20% reduction in severe bleeding and no difference in MACE
(B) Approximately 20% reduction in severe bleeding but an increase in MACE
(C) Approximately 20% reduction in MACE and no difference in severe bleeding
(D) Approximately 20% reduction in MACE but an increase in severe bleeding

5.8 Which of the following factors associated with coagulation is NOT released from activated platelets?

(A) Fibrinogen (factor I)
(B) Adenosine diphosphate (ADP)
(C) Plasminogen activator inhibitor-1 (PAI-1)
(D) Tissue plasminogen activator (tPA)
(E) Soluble CD40 ligand (sCD40L)

5.9 You receive a call from a dentist who has a patient taking ticagrelor and wonders how this drug is administered, as well as its antiplatelet effect and mechanism. Which of the following BEST describes the administration and activity of ticagrelor?

(A) Oral, irreversible, direct-acting $P2Y_{12}$ receptor antagonist
(B) Oral, reversible, direct-acting $P2Y_{12}$ receptor antagonist
(C) Oral, irreversible, indirect-acting $P2Y_{12}$ receptor antagonist
(D) Oral, reversible, indirect-acting $P2Y_{12}$ receptor antagonist

5.10 One of your colleagues refers his father to you for outpatient catheterization and ad hoc PCI. He is a thin 82-year-old man with hypertension and hypercholesterolemia. He has never used tobacco products. When talking with you, he relates that he is fearful about the risk of major bleeding described to him by a friend. You explain that you will use his radial artery for access, and major bleeding, as defined by the thrombolysis in myocardial infarction (TIMI) study criteria, reportedly occurs in what percentage of radial artery cases in large observational registries?

(A) <1%
(B) Between 1% and 2%
(C) Between 2% and 3%
(D) >3%

5.11 In the scenario above, the patient tells you that his friend had a bleeding event and was hospitalized with a heart attack when he had his complication; the doctors "went into his groin area" for the procedure. In the MATRIX trial, where 8,404 acute coronary syndrome (ACS) patients were randomized to radial vs. femoral access, the investigators used the Bleeding Academic Research Consortium (BARC) classification as an endpoint. In what percentage of patients in the femoral-access group did BARC major bleeding occur?

(A) <1%
(B) Between 1% and 2%
(C) Between 2% and 3%
(D) >3%

5.12 Historically, which of the following practices in interventional cardiology has MOST reduced the occurrence of bleeding associated with PCI?

(A) Using weight-based heparin dosing
(B) Decreasing arterial sheath size
(C) Removing sheaths on the same day of the procedure
(D) Avoiding the use of heparin after the procedure
(E) All of the above

5.13 Which factor is LEAST important in assessing whether patients being treated with enoxaparin have adequate anticoagulation during percutaneous coronary revascularization?

(A) The milligram dose of enoxaparin being given
(B) Timing of the last enoxaparin dose
(C) The number of subcutaneous doses of enoxaparin received
(D) The current activated clotting time (ACT)

5.14 Which of the following drugs is NOT known to be associated with antibody formation?

(A) Unfractionated heparin (UFH)
(B) Low molecular weight heparin (LMWH)
(C) Cangrelor
(D) Lepirudin
(E) Abciximab

5.15 Which of the following statements accurately describes heparin-induced thrombocytopenia (HIT)?

(A) The diagnosis of HIT is a clinical one and should be suspected when the platelet count is below 150,000 per mm^3 or has decreased 50% from baseline
(B) The likelihood of HIT substantially increases for patients receiving heparin for ≥24 hours
(C) Antibodies related to HIT remain present for about 1 to 2 years
(D) All of the above

5.16 In the Platelet Inhibition and Patient Outcomes (PLATO) trial comparing ticagrelor to clopidogrel in patients with an ACS, how did ticagrelor affect the rates of mortality and noncoronary artery bypass grafting (CABG) major bleeding?

(A) Decreased mortality, decreased non-CABG bleeding
(B) Decreased mortality, increased non-CABG bleeding
(C) Unchanged mortality, increased non-CABG bleeding
(D) Unchanged mortality, decreased non-CABG bleeding

5.17 Which of the following is NOT an action of thrombin?

(A) Converts fibrinogen to fibrin
(B) Activates factors V and XII
(C) Causes normal endothelium to vasoconstrict
(D) Stimulates platelet aggregation

5.18 A 68-year-old African American gentleman presents for an ACS-PCI. He has stage III chronic kidney disease (CKD). Which of the following drugs should have its dose adjusted if it is being used in a patient with moderate renal impairment?

(A) Argatroban
(B) Tirofiban
(C) Abciximab
(D) Cangrelor

5.19 Pharmacotherapies known to reduce the occurrence of death or MI among patients with non-STEMI (NSTEMI) include all of the following, EXCEPT:

(A) Aspirin
(B) Clopidogrel
(C) LMWH
(D) Fibrinolytic agents

5.20 Which anticoagulant is represented in Figure Q5-20?

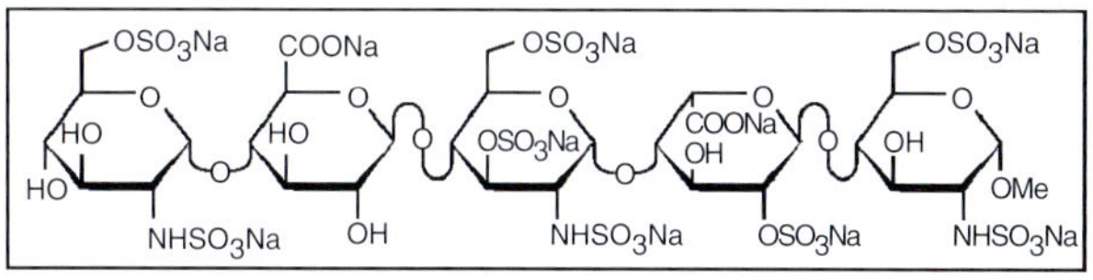

Figure Q5-20

(A) UFH
(B) Enoxaparin
(C) Fondaparinux
(D) Bivalirudin
(E) Eptifibatide

5.21 A 68-year-old woman weighing 72 kg undergoes a PCI for a severe mid-LAD stenosis with an irregular surface. For procedural anticoagulation, bivalirudin is used. Soon after stent deployment, haziness is noted within the stent. The patient develops chest pain, and the TIMI flow becomes frankly decreased in the stented vessel. Bailout abciximab is added, and repeat balloon angioplasty with optical coherence tomography (OCT) inspection of the stented area is performed. The patient's chest pain resolves and the antegrade coronary blood flow is noted to be normal. The OCT shows appropriate stent expansion and no residual abnormalities. Unfortunately, following the procedure, the patient is found to be hypotensive and tachycardiac, and a retroperitoneal hemorrhage is diagnosed. Which of the following measures would be the next step in her treatment to reverse the effects of abciximab?

(A) Transfuse random donor platelets
(B) Administer IV protamine
(C) Request fresh frozen plasma from the blood bank
(D) IV bolus of cryoprecipitate

5.22 A 72-year-old retired lawyer presents with a NSTEMI, and at angiography, a severe right coronary artery (RCA) stenosis with a large thrombus is found. You plan to use a glycoprotein (GP) IIb/IIIa inhibitor, though the patient comments he has heard a lot of negative information about those drugs. Which of the following statements is FALSE concerning GP IIb/IIIa inhibitors?

(A) Bleeding is infrequent although it usually occurs in hollow organs (gastrointestinal, genitourinary, and vascular)
(B) TIMI major bleeding is increased by approximately 1% when using a GP IIb/IIIa inhibitor, and this is predominately due to an increase in intracranial hemorrhage
(C) Severe thrombocytopenia occurs in approximately 1% of patients
(D) Thrombocytopenia is more frequent with abciximab, especially with early repeat administration

5.23 A 48-year-old male was transferred to your facility after being medically treated for an ACS. He was found to have complex left main coronary artery disease (CAD) and is awaiting CABG. He had been receiving clopidogrel, and the surgical team discontinued the clopidogrel in plans for his upcoming surgery. He has also been receiving UFH over the past several days. This morning you notice that his platelet count has dropped from a baseline of 246,000/mL to 142,000/mL, and you suspect he may have developed HIT. Which of the following drugs should NOT be used in the treatment of HIT?

(A) Fondaparinux
(B) Bivalirudin
(C) Dicoumarol
(D) Enoxaparin

5.24 Which of the following characteristics accurately describes cangrelor?

(A) Small molecule (ATP analogue), rapidly activated in serum
(B) Small molecule (cyclic adenosine monophosphate [cAMP] analogue), rapidly activated in serum
(C) Small molecule (ATP analogue), rapidly degraded in serum
(D) Small molecule (cAMP analogue), rapidly degraded in serum

5.25 The TRITON-TIMI 38 (Trial to Assess Improvement in Therapeutic Outcomes by Optimizing Platelet Inhibition With Prasugrel-Thrombolysis In Myocardial Infarction 38) trial compared prasugrel with clopidogrel among patients with an ACS and intending to undergo PCI. At >1-year follow-up, how did the occurrence of ischemic events (cardiovascular death, MI, and stroke) and major non-CABG bleeding events with prasugrel treatment compare with clopidogrel?

(A) Increased, no change
(B) Increased, decreased
(C) Decreased, no change
(D) Decreased, increased

5.26 Among patients with an ACS who are undergoing PCI, which of the following are appropriate strategies to minimize bleeding risk?

(A) Discontinue novel oral anticoagulants for 24 hours (skipping 1 day of therapy) among those undergoing elective or nonemergent procedures
(B) Preferred use of the radial artery for access
(C) Minimize the duration of polypharmacy anticoagulation to 1 to 3 months among those with concomitant atrial fibrillation and receiving a drug-eluting stent (DES)
(D) Allow the prothrombin time international normalized ratio (INR) to fall below 2.0 for elective cases
(E) All of the above

5.27 The PIONEER AF-PCI trial randomized approximately 2,100 patients with atrial fibrillation and undergoing PCI to rivaroxaban or warfarin with both groups receiving dual antiplatelet therapy (DAPT) for prespecified variable durations. At 1-year follow-up, what were the main findings?

(A) Stent thrombosis rates were similar and approximately 2.0% among the treatment groups
(B) Irrespective of DAPT or rivaroxaban dose, warfarin was associated with higher rates of clinically significant bleeding
(C) The frequency of major ischemic events, including death, MI, and stroke tended to be higher with warfarin
(D) Together, ticagrelor and prasugrel were more commonly used than clopidogrel as part of DAPT

5.28 Which of the following bleeding reversal strategies is likely ineffective?

(A) Use of idarucizumab among patients treated with dabigatran
(B) A bolus plus infusion of andexanet-alpha for a patient on rivaroxaban
(C) Platelet transfusion for a patient receiving eptifibatide
(D) IV protamine for a patient taking enoxaparin

5.29 Several large registries and a few small, randomized clinical trials have compared triple therapy (oral anticoagulant plus DAPT) vs. double therapy (oral anticoagulant plus single antiplatelet) for patients requiring anticoagulation (often for atrial fibrillation) and antiplatelet therapy following DES implantation. In these studies, what is the relative increase of serious bleeding with triple therapy vs. double therapy over a tested treatment course?

(A) 0% to 10%
(B) 11% to 20%
(C) 21% to 30%
(D) 31% to 40%
(E) >40%

5.30 The DAPT trial randomized 9,961 patients who had received a DES 12 months prior and who were free from major adverse events during the interval to an additional 18 months of DAPT or to placebo. As compared with those receiving DAPT for 12 months, those who received DAPT for 30 months had:

(A) Less stent thrombosis, but more BARC ≥2 bleeding
(B) Less stent thrombosis, and less BARC ≥2 bleeding
(C) More stent thrombosis, and more BARC ≥2 bleeding
(D) More stent thrombosis, but less BARC ≥2 bleeding

5.31 You are asked to see a 72-year-old African American woman who is referred for preoperative assessment. She is planning to have a breast mass removed. Her past medical history is remarkable for successful placement of a stent in her RCA approximately 3 years ago. Eight years ago, she had aortic valve replacement using a St. Jude mechanical prosthesis. As part of her evaluation, a treadmill nuclear stress test was performed. This revealed a large anterolateral reversible defect at a moderate workload with preserved left ventricular (LV) systolic function. Her INR is 2.7. Which of the following plans should be implemented for her to undergo coronary angiography?

(A) Discontinue warfarin 2 to 3 days before outpatient catheterization and measure the INR on the day of planned catheterization
(B) Continue warfarin and use a 6-Fr diagnostic coronary artery catheter via the radial artery
(C) Administer fresh frozen plasma on the day of planned catheterization
(D) Admit the patient to hospital, discontinue warfarin, and begin enoxaparin

ANSWERS AND EXPLANATIONS

5.1 Answer C. Protamine is currently synthesized by way of biotechnology but was originally produced from fish products. Patients with a strong fish allergy or those who take NPH insulin should avoid protamine due to the increased risk of a histamine-mediated reaction. Theoretically, protamine in higher doses can act as an anticoagulant; for usual doses, this effect would be weak. Doses >50 mg should be avoided.

5.2 Answer C. Prasugrel and clopidogrel both require hepatic cytochromes for oxidation to generate their active drug metabolite. Whereas prasugrel requires only a single oxidative step involving CYP2C19, clopidogrel requires two oxidative steps. Both drugs can be affected by morphine by delaying gastric emptying.

5.3 Answer B. The diagram shows a modified adenosine triphosphate (ATP) analogue, cangrelor.

5.4 Answer A. The absolute contraindications for thrombolytic therapy are centered on life-threatening bleeding such as intracranial hemorrhage. Any history of previous *hemorrhagic* stroke is an absolute contraindication. *Ischemic stroke* history is not a contraindication for thrombolysis in STEMI unless the stroke occurred in the last 3 months. This is not to be confused with the use of thrombolytics for acute ischemic strokes (within 3 hours of stroke occurrence).

5.5 Answer C. The need for surgery in the early weeks to months following DES placement is a vexing problem. No large-scale prospective data are available. It is well recognized that premature discontinuation of adequate antiplatelet therapy markedly increases the risk for stent thrombosis. In one large-scale registry, it was found that premature antiplatelet therapy discontinuation was associated with a hazard ratio of 90 (95% CI, 30 to 270) for stent thrombosis (Iakovou I, et al. *JAMA* 2005;293(17):2126–2130). Current expert consensus suggests 12 months of DAPT after first-generation DES, though some data suggest a decreasing benefit beyond 6 months. Newer-generation DES have the best safety profile evidence for short course (i.e., 6 months) of DAPT. In current practice, this patient would have likely received a zotarolimus-eluting or everolimus-eluting stent (EES) with a thinner strut design and a better safety profile with a short course of DAPT.

5.6 Answer B. Bivalirudin is a short amino acid sequence with the shortest half-life among the IV direct thrombin inhibitors. It is poorly dialyzable. Answer C is a description for lepirudin. Answers A and D do not accurately characterize any of the direct thrombin inhibitors.

5.7 Answer C. In individual studies of cangrelor vs. clopidogrel, each given 30 minutes before ACS-PCI, the primary endpoint of ischemic events at 48 hours was not different between study groups. In a patient-level analysis of the above three trials and considering different endpoints, cangrelor was found to reduce the odds of MACE by 19% with no difference in GUSTO severe bleeding. Cangrelor was associated with more GUSTO minor bleeding (Steg PG, et al. *Lancet* 2013;382(9909): 1981–1992).

5.8 Answer D. Many factors associated with coagulation, inflammation, or cell repair and growth are released from platelets. Most factors either accelerate coagulation (i.e., ADP and fibrinogen) or promote inflammation (i.e., sCD40L). Platelets do not contain tPA but rather release PAI-1 (the natural inhibitor of tPA) when activated.

5.9 Answer B. Ticagrelor is the first orally available $P2Y_{12}$ receptor antagonist that reversibly affects the receptor. Other currently available oral antiplatelet agents (e.g., aspirin, clopidogrel, and prasugrel) are irreversible, and it takes several days for an adequate number of new platelets to be generated for effective platelet function in the absence of these drugs. Cangrelor is the first IV reversible agent affecting the $P2Y_{12}$ receptor. Other IV agents, such as tirofiban and eptifibatide, are also quickly reversible though differ from cangrelor in that they block the platelet glycoprotein (GP) IIb/IIIa receptors.

5.10 Answer A. Major bleeding for a presumably non-ACS catheterization and possible PCI should be <1%, particularly for radial access. Large-scale reports have shown radial access in elective angiography and PCI to be as low as 0.1% (Jolly SS, et al. *Am Heart J* 2009;157(1):132–140).

5.11 Answer C. Major bleeding in most studies has been shown to be higher with the femoral approach than the radial approach, particularly among ACS patients. Various definitions have been used. The most stringent or lowest frequency occurring definition of major or severe bleeding is from the original TIMI trial, which assessed the use of thrombolytic agents in patients with acute MI, whereas more contemporary or PCI-trial-specific definitions of bleeding have focused on more clinically relevant and more frequently occurring bleeding outcomes—such as the definition utilized in ACUITY or similar definitions developed by an academic interventional consortium, such as the BARC major bleeding criteria. In the MATRIX trial, femoral and radial access were associated with a frequency of BARC major bleeding of 2.3% and 1.6%, respectively ($p = 0.013$) (Valgimigli M, et al. *Lancet* 2015;385(9986):2465–2476). These definitions are arguably more relevant.

5.12 Answer E. The rate of major bleeding in randomized clinical trials and in practice has substantially decreased over the last decade from 2% to 4% to <1%. Many changes in practice have resulted in this decrease in bleeding despite the use of multiple antiplatelets and anticoagulants (i.e., aspirin, clopidogrel, GP IIb/IIIa inhibitors, and potent antithrombins). While large-scale trials and registries have compared bivalirudin vs. heparin and radial vs. femoral access, little data exist for the other stepwise changes that have occurred to reduce bleeding, though they followed a natural evolution in techniques and equipment.

5.13 Answer D. Several factors are important when deciding if a patient remains adequately anticoagulated with enoxaparin. These include the dose of enoxaparin given and the number of hours since the dose. Likewise, patients who have received only one subcutaneous dose of enoxaparin will be therapeutic for a shorter interval than patients who have reached steady state following several subcutaneous doses. It is also important whether the patient has received IV or subcutaneous enoxaparin. The ACT is an unreliable measure of the extent of anticoagulation provided by enoxaparin. Since the primary excretion for LMWH is renal, the creatinine clearance can have an important influence on the extent and duration of the anticoagulant effect.

5.14 Answer C. Both UFH and fractionated or LMWH, by interacting with platelet factor 4, can lead to antibody formation. Abciximab, having a protein-antibody structure, can act as an antigen and cause antibody formation. Hirudin and lepirudin are polypeptides and may lead to relevant antibody formation, whereas cangrelor is a modified ATP analogue and has not been found to cause antibody formation.

5.15 Answer A. The suspicion and diagnosis of HIT should be made solely on clinical grounds. Laboratory-based assays for HIT can be diagnostic but should be confirmatory. While UFH is much more likely than LMWH to cause HIT, all heparins can cause and exacerbate HIT. Fondaparinux has not been associated with HIT. The mechanism of HIT is antibody generation in response to a heparin–platelet factor complex. This antibody formation usually takes several days of exposure (>96 hours) of heparin to occur, and the antibody remains present for 3 to 6 months.

5.16 Answer B. PLATO randomized 18,624 patients with an ACS to 12 months of ticagrelor or clopidogrel. Ticagrelor significantly reduced the primary end point of death from vascular causes, MI, or stroke. Impressively, death from vascular causes was significantly reduced (HR 0.79; 95% CI, 0.69 to 0.91). While overall bleeding was not increased, the rate of non–CABG-related major bleeding was increased from 3.8% to 4.5% (HR 1.19; 95% CI, 1.02 to 1.38) (Wallentin L, et al. *N Engl J Med* 2009;361(11):1045–1057).

5.17 Answer C. Among the primary activities of thrombin is facilitating the conversion of fibrinogen to fibrin and activating other coagulation pathway factors, including V, VIII, and XII, as it autoamplifies its production. Normal endothelium, in response to thrombin, releases tPA and vasodilates. Abnormal endothelium vasoconstricts (through endothelin) in response to thrombin. Another important activity of thrombin is that it is one of the most potent stimulators of platelet aggregation.

5.18 Answer B. Argatroban is hepatically metabolized. Abciximab is largely cleared by the reticuloendothelial system and not by the kidney. Therefore, the dose does not need to be adjusted for renal insufficiency. This is in contrast to the small-molecule GP IIb/IIIa inhibitors, such as tirofiban and eptifibatide, especially when given as a prolonged infusion. Cangrelor, while renally excreted, is deactivated rapidly in the serum prior to excretion, and therefore, its dose does not need to be adjusted for renal insufficiency.

5.19 Answer D. Placebo-controlled trials have shown many antiplatelet and antithrombin therapies to reduce death or MI among patients with NSTEMI. Several early studies, including TIMI-IIIB, showed patients with NSTEMI-ACS receiving fibrinolytic therapy to have a worse outcome—primarily a higher rate of MI (Antman EM, et al. *Circulation* 1999;100(15):1593–1601).

5.20 Answer C. The diagram shows a five-sugar unit entity, namely, a pentasaccharide (fondaparinux).

5.21 Answer A. Abciximab, being a monoclonal antibody, avidly binds to platelet receptors. Protamine would be a useful treatment to reverse the effects of heparin; however, it will have no effect on abciximab. Administering cryoprecipitate or plasma products will be of little to no value because of the mechanism of abciximab binding. Rather, transfusion of platelets will provide additional GP IIb/IIIa receptors to facilitate appropriate coagulation. In addition, abciximab can migrate among platelets, and the transfused platelets will aid in decreasing the number of abciximab molecules on the originally affected platelets, thereby allowing their earlier recovery. Bivalirudin has a very short half-life and its effect should be gone rapidly.

5.22 Answer B. Although TIMI major bleeding is increased by approximately 1%, this is not due to an increase in intracranial hemorrhage. Intracranial hemorrhage occurs in 0.1% of patients undergoing PCI, and this is not particularly increased with the use of GP IIb/IIIa inhibitors.

5.23 Answer D. Each of the agents is established in the care HIT except for enoxaparin. While dicoumarol (warfarin) would not be appropriate for this patient about to undergo bypass surgery, it could be appropriate following surgery. Patients undergoing bypass surgery in the setting of HIT are at increased risk for acute graft closure and other thrombotic events. All LMWHs (e.g., enoxaparin) are heparin derivatives and can cause or worsen heparin-induced platelet aggregation and therefore must be avoided.

5.24 Answer C. Cangrelor is a modified ATP derivative, which irreversibly inhibits the ADP receptor of platelets. It does not require modification for effect (i.e., it is an active compound). It is rapidly degraded in the circulation and primarily excreted by the kidneys. It has a half-life of several minutes and platelet function should return fully to normal in less than an hour.

5.25 Answer D. In the TRITON trial, at an average follow-up of 15 months, the composite ischemic end point *decreased* from 12.1% to 9.9% ($p < 0.001$) with prasugrel vs. clopidogrel. In contrast, the major bleeding rate *increased* from 1.8% to 2.4% ($p = 0.03$) with prasugrel as compared to clopidogrel (Wiviot SD, et al. *N Engl J Med* 2007;357(20):2001–2015).

5.26 Answer E. Each of the above approaches has been deemed reasonable based on clinical trial evidence or expert consensus.

5.27 Answer B. The incidence of stent thrombosis was similar among the treatment groups, though it was well under 1%. The occurrence of major ischemic events was similar among the treatment groups, though the study was not powered or designed for primary assessment of ischemic events. Simply counting ischemic events, more occurred with rivaroxaban, but again, this is not an appropriate conclusion. Clopidogrel was used in >90% of cases, and this is appropriate since experience with combinations of new oral anticoagulant drugs and newer thienopyridines is limited and likely to be associated with a particularly heightened risk of bleeding.

5.28 Answer C. While not approved worldwide, idarucizumab and andexanet have been shown in multicenter investigations to effectively reverse the effects of anti-IIa and anti-Xa oral agents, respectively. Adexanet should also reverse the anti-Xa component of enoxaparin; so too, protamine reverses the anti-IIa component of enoxaparin (as it does with UFH). Therefore, both adexanet and protamine will partially reverse the effects of LMWHs. In contrast, eptifibatide is given in a several hundred-fold excess of platelet receptors due to its pharmacokinetics and pharmacodynamics such that platelet transfusions are not helpful. Fortunately, the drug is quickly cleared by the kidneys.

5.29 Answer E. The DANISH Health System tracks all prescriptions and hospitalizations and has shown bleeding-related hospitalizations to be increased with a hazard ratio of 1.41 among those receiving triple therapy (Lamberts M, et al. *Circulation* 2012;126(10):1185–1193). The ISAR TRIPLE trial randomized patients requiring oral anticoagulation to 6 weeks vs. 6 months of clopidogrel on a background of aspirin and oral anticoagulation and showed that BARC ≥ 2 bleeding increased from 7.6% to 12.2% (approximately 60% increase) with the extended duration of clopidogrel (Fiedler KA, et al. *J Am Coll Cardiol* 2015;65(16):1619–1629). The WOEST trial maintained a background of oral anticoagulation with clopidogrel and randomized patients to receive aspirin (triple therapy) or not (double therapy). At 1-year follow-up, bleeding occurred more than twice as often in the triple therapy group (44.4% vs. 19.4%) (Dewilde WJM, et al. *Lancet* 2013;381(9872):1107–1115).

5.30 Answer A. Because of evolutions in treatment practice and in stent designs, the US Food and Drug Administration (FDA) requested manufacturers and clinical trialists conduct the DAPT study. Like many other studies, antithrombotic benefit was seen with the prolongation of DAPT, particularly among patients at increased risk, yet at the cost of increased bleeding events. With prolonged antiplatelet therapy, major adverse cardiac and cerebrovascular events (MACCE) were reduced from 9% to 4.3% ($p < 0.001$), though GUSTO moderate or severe bleeding was increased from 1.6% to 2.5% ($p = 0.001$). Interestingly, in both treatment groups, the occurrence of stent thrombosis and MI was increased in the first 3 months after stopping clopidogrel (Mauri L, et al. *N Engl J Med* 2014;371(23):2155–2166).

5.31 Answer A. The patient's stent placement was done many years before so there is no concern for stent thrombosis. Perioperative UFH therapy is recommended for patients in whom the risk of postprocedure bleeding with oral anticoagulation is high and the risk of thromboembolism without anticoagulation is also high (i.e., mechanical valve in the mitral position, a Bjork-Shiley valve, recent [i.e., <1 year] thrombosis or embolus, or three or more of the following risk factors: atrial fibrillation, previous embolus at any time, hypercoagulable condition, mechanical prosthesis, and LV ejection fraction <30%). For patients between these two extremes, physicians must assess the risk and benefit of reduced anticoagulation vs. perioperative heparin therapy. Since the patient's INR is 2.7, it is reasonable to simply discontinue the warfarin and measure the INR on the second or third morning. If the patient's INR remains elevated (>1.5 or for some >2.0), using a particularly small arterial sheath (5-Fr) in the radial artery should be considered. An arteriotomy closure device could also be considered.

6 Pharmacogenomics and Drug–Drug Interactions

Timir K. Paul

QUESTIONS

6.1 Which of the following mechanisms leads to the inhibition of platelet function following treatment with $P2Y_{12}$ receptor inhibitors such as clopidogrel?

(A) Reduction of cyclic adenosine monophosphate (cAMP) levels
(B) Increased phosphorylation status of vasodilator-stimulated phosphoprotein (VASP-P)
(C) Inhibition of phospholipase C (PLC)
(D) Inhibition of adenylyl cyclase
(E) Inhibition of protein kinase C (PKC)

6.2 Proton pump inhibitors (PPIs) such as omeprazole have been shown to reduce the pharmacokinetic (PK) and pharmacodynamic (PD) effects of clopidogrel by modulating the effects of which of the following?

(A) Glycoprotein (GP) IIb/IIIa receptor expression
(B) Cytochrome P450 (CYP) 2C19 enzymatic activity
(C) CYP 3A4 enzymatic activity
(D) Intestinal P-glycoprotein transport activity

6.3 A 56-year-old male with a history of smoking, hypertension, and dyslipidemia who has not followed up with any doctor in last 5 years presents to the emergency department (ED) with severe midsternal chest pain. He is diaphoretic with a blood pressure (BP) of 110/64 mm Hg and heart rate (HR) of 98 beats per minute (bpm). Electrocardiogram (EKG) shows inferior ST-segment elevation myocardial infarction (STEMI). He was given 2 mg of morphine twice on the way to ED due to severe chest pain; it reduced his chest pain a little. He was given 4,000 intravenous (IV) units of heparin in the ED and 325 mg of aspirin. Emergent heart catheterization showed proximal right coronary artery (RCA) total thrombotic occlusion, which was stented with a bare metal stent (BMS). He was loaded with 180 mg of ticagrelor at the end of the procedure. Which of the following is a possible drug–drug interaction between ticagrelor and morphine?

(A) Although morphine delays absorption, it does not reduce active metabolite of ticagrelor
(B) Morphine lowers the active metabolite of ticagrelor but has no effect on antiplatelet activity
(C) Although morphine delays the onset of action of ticagrelor, it does not reduce antiplatelet effect
(D) Platelet reactivity is high when ticagrelor is coadministered with morphine
(E) There is a difference in residual platelet reactivity between ticagrelor and prasugrel when coadministered with morphine

6.4 The U.S. Food and Drug Administration (FDA) has issued a genetic-related boxed warning for clopidogrel. This boxed warning derives from studies showing that clopidogrel at recommended doses forms less of its metabolite and has a smaller effect on platelet function in patients who are CYP2C19 "poor metabolizers." In addition, "poor metabolizers" with acute coronary syndrome (ACS) or undergoing percutaneous coronary intervention (PCI) treated with clopidogrel at recommended doses exhibit higher cardiovascular event rates than patients with normal CYP2C19 function. Which of the following represents a CYP2C19 genotype identifying a clopidogrel "poor metabolizer"?

(A) wt/wt (wt: wild type)
(B) wt/*2
(C) wt/*17
(D) *2/*17
(E) *2/*2

6.5 Which of the following guideline recommendations has been given for platelet function testing and genotyping for a CYP2C19 in clopidogrel-treated patients?

(A) Both are Class I but level of evidence B
(B) Platelet function testing is Class IIa, but genotyping is Class IIb
(C) Both are Class IIb
(D) Both are Class IIa
(E) Platelet function testing is Class IIb, but genotyping is Class IIa

6.6 A 70-year-old Caucasian female with a history of hypertension, transient ischemic attack (TIA), dyslipidemia, and diabetes was admitted with chest pain and a stress test showing anterolateral ischemia with a left ventricular ejection fraction (LVEF) of 50% to 55%. She did not have any previous history of gastrointestinal (GI) bleeding. Her home medications included lisinopril 40 mg, rosuvastatin 20 mg, and insulin. Her diabetes was well controlled. BP on admission was 148/80 mm Hg and HR was 90 bpm. She had a coronary angiogram showing a proximal left anterior descending (LAD) 75% stenosis, a proximal obtuse marginal (OM) 60% stenosis, and a mid-RCA 50% stenosis. She was given 325 mg of aspirin before the angiogram. She received a drug-eluting stent (DES) and an immediate post-PCI ticagrelor loading dose of 180 mg was given; 90 mg bid was prescribed. She was started on metoprolol, 25 mg two times a day, and aspirin, 325 mg daily. Which of the following statements is true regarding the dose of aspirin in this patient?

(A) There is evidence of decreased platelet inhibiting activity with ≥300 mg of aspirin as compared to ≤100 mg when concurrently used with ticagrelor in the North American population
(B) There is no recommended dose of aspirin when concomitantly used with ticagrelor
(C) Despite interaction between ticagrelor and aspirin, 162 to 324 mg of daily aspirin is still effective in this patient
(D) This patient should receive prasugrel
(E) Despite dose-dependent interaction between aspirin and ticagrelor, a neutral effect on antiplatelet benefit of ticagrelor is observed across geographic region

6.7 Platelet function testing comparing prasugrel with clopidogrel has shown which of the following?

(A) Prasugrel 60 mg loading dose is associated with more potent platelet inhibition compared with a 300-mg clopidogrel loading dose, but not a 600-mg clopidogrel loading dose
(B) Prasugrel 60 mg loading dose and 10 mg maintenance dose is associated with more potent platelet inhibition compared with clopidogrel, irrespective of the clopidogrel loading (300 to 600 mg) or maintenance (75 to 150 mg) dose used
(C) Prasugrel 60 mg loading dose is associated with more potent platelet inhibition compared with a clopidogrel 600 mg loading dose but has slower effects
(D) Prasugrel 60 mg loading dose is associated with more potent platelet inhibition compared with a clopidogrel 600 mg loading dose but has similar effects when transitioning to maintenance therapy

6.8 A 66-year-old male with a history of HIV, dyslipidemia, and diabetes presents with palpitations and chest pain that radiates to arm. His HR is 110 bpm, and EKG shows sinus rhythm. His peak troponin is 0.92 ng/dL. Home medications include ritonavir, insulin, and pravastatin 20 mg daily. Catheterization showed moderate diffuse coronary artery disease with a 75% mid-posterior descending artery (PDA) stenosis. He remained chest pain-free and medical management was recommended. He was started on low-dose metoprolol, aspirin 81 mg daily, ticagrelor 180 mg loading dose, and 90 mg bid was recommended for 1 year. Which of the following statements is true regarding ticagrelor and ritonavir drug–drug interaction?

(A) Ritonavir is a strong inducer of CYP3A4
(B) Ritonavir is a potent inhibitor of CYP2C9
(C) Ritonavir increases the bleeding risk when coadministered with ticagrelor
(D) Ritonavir increases risk of thrombosis
(E) There is no potential drug–drug interaction

6.9 A patient comes to your clinic and informs you that he participated in a research study in which he was found to be "aspirin resistant." The patient had a DES implanted in his mid-RCA 8 months ago and is currently asymptomatic on treatment with aspirin (81 mg/day), clopidogrel (75 mg/day), and atorvastatin (40 mg/day). What do you believe should be the most appropriate therapeutic approach in this patient?

(A) Given the history of aspirin resistance, the patient should have the dose of aspirin increased to overcome resistance
(B) Given the history of aspirin resistance, the patient should maintain clopidogrel and stop aspirin at 1 year post-PCI
(C) Given the history of aspirin resistance, the patient may also be clopidogrel resistant and should be tested for this
(D) Although the patient has shown aspirin resistance, no changes in his medical management should be made at the current time; ensure that the patient is compliant to his medication

6.10 A 77-year-old female with hypertension, dyslipidemia, and diabetes presented to the ED with intermittent new-onset chest pain for the last few hours. Her initial BP was 160/72 mm Hg and HR was 110 bpm. EKG showed T inversions in the lateral leads. Initial troponin was 0.61 ng/mL. She received 4 mg of IV morphine in the ED, and her chest pain subsided. She was given a full dose of enoxaparin and 325 mg of aspirin in the ED. She was loaded with 600 mg of clopidogrel. Optimal medical management was initiated with serial troponin and a coronary angiogram was planned for the next day. Which of the following statements is true regarding the effects of morphine on platelets when coadministered with clopidogrel?

(A) Residual platelet aggregation is higher but has no effect on maximal platelet inhibition
(B) Morphine causes delayed maximal inhibition of platelets
(C) Morphine delays absorption of clopidogrel but has no effect on residual platelet aggregation
(D) Morphine lowers plasma concentration of active metabolite of clopidogrel but has no effect on maximal platelet inhibition
(E) Morphine delays absorption but does not reduce plasma concentration of active metabolite of clopidogrel

6.11 Which of the following has been shown to be the most important determinant of inadequate clopidogrel-induced antiplatelet effects?

(A) Genetic polymorphisms of the P2Y12 receptor
(B) Interaction with atorvastatin
(C) Upregulation of nonpurinergic signaling pathways
(D) Noncompliance and underdosing
(E) Accelerated platelet turnover

6.12 A 76-year-old female with dyslipidemia, smoking, atrial fibrillation, and a history of gastric ulcer was admitted with chest pain. EKG showed no acute ischemic changes. Lipid profile showed an LDL of 112 mg/dL and HDL of 42 mg/dL. She was taking 40 mg of atorvastatin and 5 mg of Coumadin daily. Initial BP was 142/82 mm Hg. Troponin was 2.2 ng/dL and hemoglobin was 11.6 g/dL, which is chronic and stable. She denied any recent bleeding events. In the ER, she received aspirin 324 mg. International normalized ratio (INR) was 2.5. Coumadin was held until INR became <2.0. Catheterization showed a 99% long OM lesion, a 40% LAD stenosis, and an RCA free of disease. She received a 2.75- × 32-mm DES. Post-PCI, she was started on clopidogrel 75 mg daily and aspirin 81 mg daily and resumed Coumadin. Due to remote GI bleeding history, the primary admitting team started omeprazole. The patient read about the possible adverse effects of clopidogrel when used with omeprazole and other PPIs. She is seeking your opinion as a cardiologist on possible drug–drug interactions. Based on the current evidence, what would you tell this patient who is concurrently taking a PPI and clopidogrel?

(A) Studies showed omeprazole decreased the antiplatelet effect of clopidogrel
(B) Clopidogrel should be changed to prasugrel because of potential interaction
(C) There are significant clinical cardiovascular adverse effects observed when omeprazole and clopidogrel are coadministered
(D) Existing data showed class effect of PPI on clopidogrel
(E) Although studies revealed pharmacodynamics interaction between omeprazole and clopidogrel, there is no study on clinical outcomes to assess this interaction

6.13 True statements about aspirin include all of the following, EXCEPT:

(A) The antiplatelet effects of aspirin can be diminished with concomitant nonsteroidal anti-inflammatory drug (NSAID) use
(B) Aspirin exerts its antiplatelet effects through inhibition of the platelet thrombin receptor (PAR) for the lifespan of the platelet
(C) Aspirin is a relatively weak inhibitor of platelet aggregation in vitro
(D) When chewed or solubilized, the full antiplatelet effects of aspirin can be achieved in approximately 15 minutes
(E) Aspirin exerts its antiplatelet effects through irreversible blockade of the COX-1 enzyme

6.14 A 48-year-old male with history of kidney transplant, hypertension, and dyslipidemia presents with typical chest pain. His vitals are otherwise stable. He is currently on ketoconazole for prophylaxis, lisinopril 40 mg daily, and rosuvastatin 10 mg daily as an outpatient. Coronary angiogram showed mild diffuse coronary artery disease in the LAD and left circumflex (LCx) with an 80% proximal RCA stenosis. He underwent PCI with a DES to the RCA. He was started on 81 mg of aspirin and 75 mg of daily clopidogrel dose after giving a loading dose of both in the catheterization lab. What is the potential drug–drug interaction you may be concerned about with this patient?

(A) Ketoconazole decreases the antiplatelet effect of clopidogrel
(B) Ketoconazole increases bleeding risk when coadministered with clopidogrel
(C) Ketoconazole is a strong inducer of CYP3A4
(D) Ketoconazole is a potent CYP2C9 inhibitor
(E) There is no significant interaction between ketoconazole and clopidogrel

6.15 Which of the following platelet function tests assessing antiplatelet drug response has been mostly associated with adverse outcomes and considered the gold standard assay?

(A) VerifyNow assay
(B) PFA-100
(C) P-selectin assessed by whole blood cytometry
(D) Light transmittance aggregometry
(E) GP IIb/IIIa activation assessed by whole blood cytometry

6.16 A 60-year-old male presented to the ER with severe typical chest pain and diaphoresis. EKG showed ST depressions in the anterolateral leads. Initial troponin in the ER was 1.4 ng/dL. He has a history of hypertension, but BP is controlled with carvedilol 6.25 bid. Echocardiogram showed a 55% ejection fraction (EF) and catheterization revealed severe proximal LAD stenosis for which he received a DES. He was loaded with 600 mg of clopidogrel at the end of the procedure. He was started on atorvastatin 40 mg daily, aspirin 81 mg, and clopidogrel 75 mg daily. Due to a proximal LAD stent, a genotyping of clopidogrel was ordered and the lab reported a CYP2C19 genotype *2/*2. The primary team called a cardiologist for further management given this genotype result. Which of the following is your response to this result?

(A) He is at high bleeding risk and should be on a PPI
(B) The patient is a poor metabolizer of clopidogrel and at higher risk of future cardiovascular events
(C) He is a good responder to clopidogrel
(D) He is a poor responder and at higher risk of future cardiovascular events
(E) He is an ultrametabolizer, but bleeding risk is unknown

6.17 Polymorphisms of which of the following genotypes can modulate intestinal absorption of several cardiovascular drugs?

(A) ABCB1 (also known as multidrug resistance-associated protein [MDR]-1)
(B) Cytochrome P450 enzymes
(C) *PlA* polymorphisms
(D) Vitamin K epoxide reductase (*VKOR*)

6.18 Antithrombotic agents with linear pharmacokinetics (PK) have a more predictable pharmacodynamic (PD) response. Which of the following antithrombotic agents has the BEST PK/PD response profile?

(A) Unfractionated heparin
(B) Low molecular weight heparin
(C) Bivalirudin
(D) Warfarin

6.19 Which of the following statements is correct with regard to heparin dosing and activated clotting time (ACT) monitoring in patients undergoing PCI who do not receive GP IIb/IIIa inhibitors?

(A) Unfractionated heparin (UFH) should be given during coronary angioplasty to achieve an ACT of 250 to 300 seconds with the HemoTec device and 300 to 350 seconds with the Hemochron device
(B) A weight-adjusted bolus heparin (70 to 100 IU/kg) can be used to avoid excess anticoagulation
(C) If the target values for ACT are not achieved after a bolus of heparin, additional heparin boluses (2,000 to 5,000 IU) can be given
(D) All of the above

6.20 A 72-year-old male with past medical history of hypertension, diabetes, gout, and chronic arthritis presents with a non-STEMI. He is on amlodipine, metformin, and insulin and taking daily ibuprofen for his severe arthritis. His BP is 124/68 mm Hg and HR is 88 bpm. He is given 324 mg of aspirin in the ED, and a full-dose enoxaparin subcutaneous (SQ) bid is started. Coronary angiogram shows 40% proximal RCA, 30% mid-LCx, and 80% mid-LAD lesions. He undergoes PCI to the mid-LAD without any complications. Bivalirudin is used during PCI. He is started on aspirin 81 mg daily, Lipitor 40 mg, metoprolol 12.5 mg bid, and clopidogrel 75 mg daily. He is educated on the increased risk of bleeding with concomitant use of ibuprofen, aspirin, and clopidogrel. He reports that without ibuprofen, he will have limited functional ability. What advice do you give to this patient?

(A) As he needs ibuprofen, he should continue without any cardiovascular risk except some increased risk of bleeding
(B) He should take aspirin 6 hours after taking ibuprofen
(C) He should take aspirin 30 minutes before taking ibuprofen
(D) He should take aspirin and ibuprofen at night at the same time
(E) There is no drug–drug interaction between aspirin and ibuprofen

ANSWERS AND EXPLANATIONS

6.1 Answer B. The active metabolite of clopidogrel inhibits the ADP $P2Y_{12}$ receptor. The downstream effects of this are an increase in cAMP levels and VASP-P. This overall inhibits platelet activation and thus aggregation processes. Activation of ADP $P2Y_{12}$ receptor signaling inhibits adenylyl cyclase, which reduces cAMP levels and thus the status of VASP-P. PLC and PKC are part of the $P2Y_1$ receptor signaling pathway (Fig. A6-1) (Angiolillo DJ, et al. *J Am Coll Cardiol* 2007;49(14):1505–1516).

6.2 Answer B. Several factors have been associated with reduced PK and PD response profiles to clopidogrel. Among these, a drug interaction between PPIs, in particular omeprazole and clopidogrel, has been demonstrated. This drug–drug interaction is due to the common metabolic pathway of these agents, which involves the cytochrome P450 (CYP) 2C19 enzyme (Angiolillo DJ, et al. *Clin Pharmacol Ther* 2011;89(1):65–74). This drug interaction is also reflected in a boxed warning issued by the FDA. The CYP2C19 isoenzyme is of particular importance since it is involved in both oxidation steps required for clopidogrel prodrug to generate its active metabolite. Therefore, intrinsic (e.g., genetic polymorphisms) or extrinsic (e.g., drugs) factors modulating the activity of this enzyme may affect active metabolite levels and thus the platelet inhibitory effects of clopidogrel. Other drugs may interfere with different targets involved in clopidogrel metabolism (Fig. A6-2) (Bates ER, et al. *J Am Coll Cardiol* 2011;57(11):1251–1263).

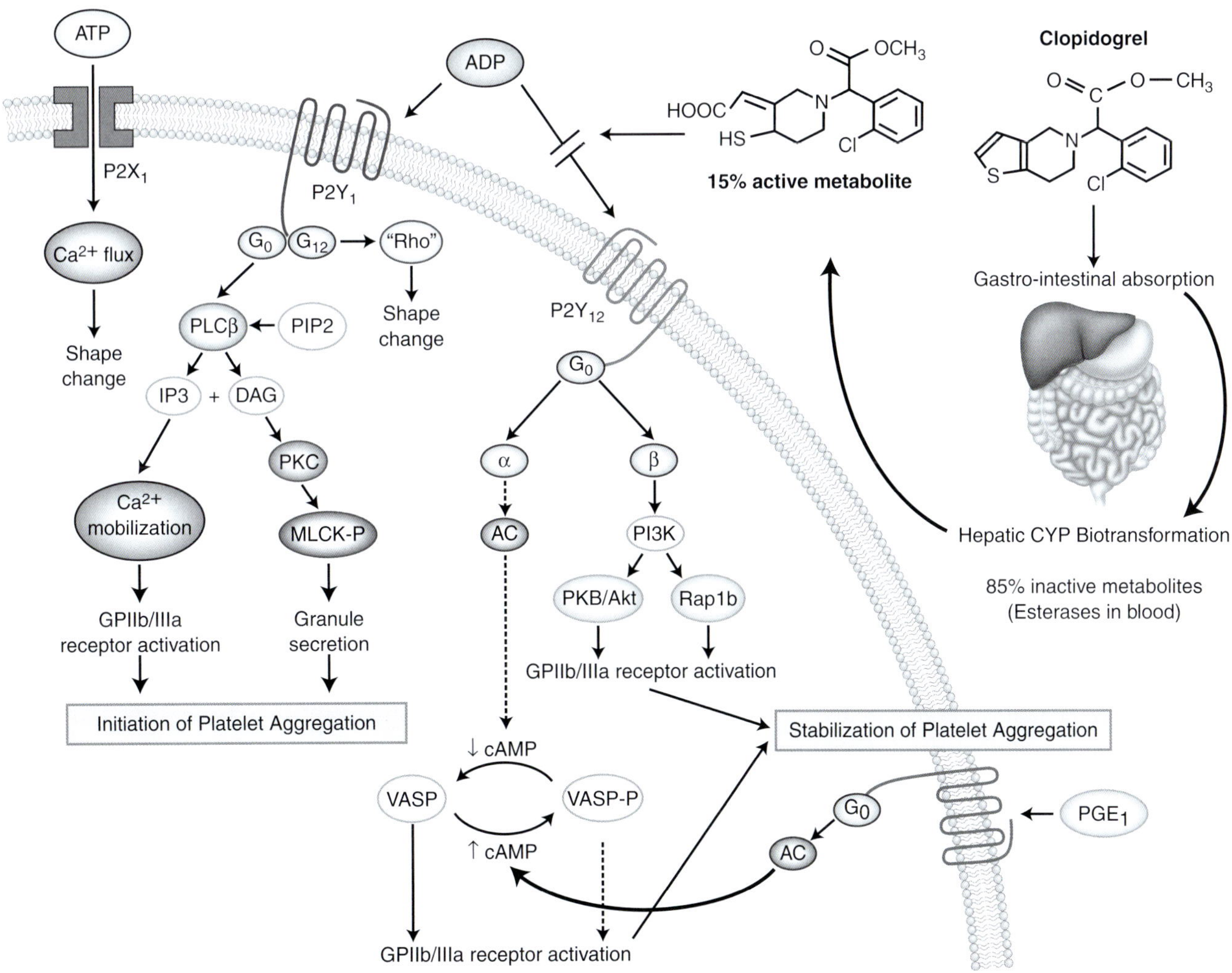

Figure A6-1 (Reproduced from Angiolillo DJ, et al. *J Am Coll Cardiol* 2007;49(14):1505–1516, with permission.)

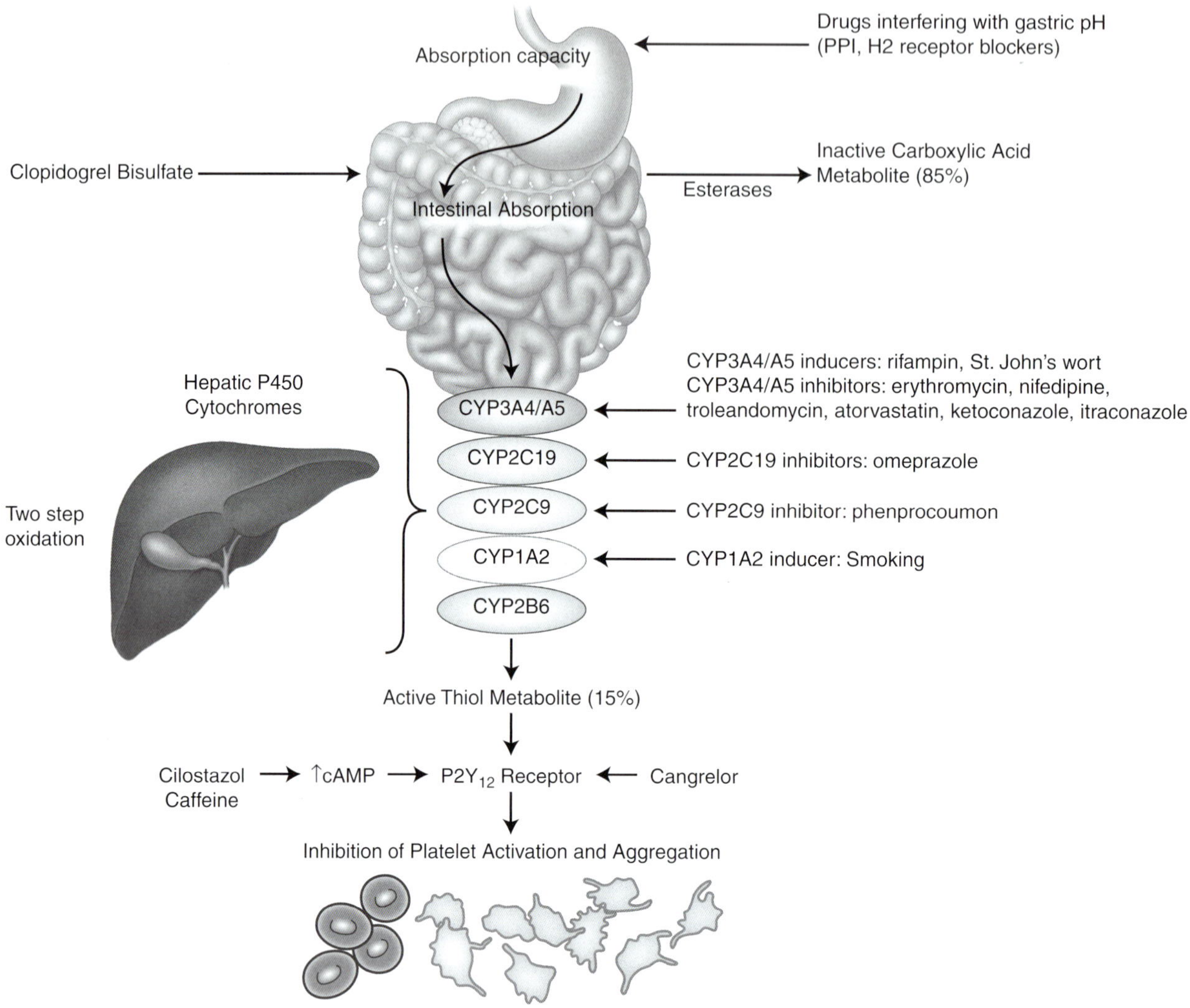

Figure A6-2 (Adapted from Bates ER, et al. *J Am Coll Cardiol* 2011;57(11):1251–1263, with permission.)

6.3 Answer D. Morphine reduces the antiplatelet effects of ticagrelor and prasugrel and delays the onset of action with high-residual platelet reactivity in ACS, especially in STEMI when platelet reactivity is already high. This may not be applicable in stable ischemic patients and if patients are already taking $P2Y_{12}$ receptor antagonists. Several recently published studies showed these interactions between morphine and ticagrelor or prasugrel in ACS patients, although there is no updated specific recommendation in this regard in American College of Cardiology (ACC)/American Heart Association (AHA) guidelines.

A single-center randomized trial including patients with non-STEMI and STEMI showed morphine lowers the total exposure to ticagrelor and its active metabolite by 37% and delays the maximal plasma concentration of ticagrelor 4 hours vs. 2 hours, as compared to placebo with higher platelet reactivity (Kubica J, et al. *Eur Heart J* 2016;37(3): 245–252). Morphine administration was associated with delayed onset of action of ticagrelor in patients who underwent primary PCI for STEMI (Silvain J, et al. *Thromb Haemost* 2016;116(2):369–378). The similar high-residual platelet reactivity was noted in patients receiving either ticagrelor or prasugrel when coadministered with morphine. A multicenter patent-level integrated analysis from 5 observational studies of 300 STEMI and post-PCI patients who received either prasugrel or ticagrelor loading dose showed high-residual platelet reactivity ($P2Y_{12}$ reactivity units ≥ 208) at 2 hours in 53% and 29% patients with and without morphine, respectively, and no difference noted between prasugrel and ticagrelor. The independent predictor of high-residual platelet reactivity at 2 hours was use of morphine (Parodi G, et al. *Circ Cardiovasc Interv* 2014;8(1). pii:e001593; Parodi G, et al. *J Am Coll Cardiol* 2013;61(15): 1601–1606).

6.4 Answer E. The genes that encode the CYP enzymes are polymorphic, with certain alleles demonstrated to confer reduced enzymatic function, thereby interfering with production of the drug metabolites. These reduced-function alleles, particularly in CYP2C19, have been shown to affect the PK and PD responses to clopidogrel. Moreover, in the setting of treatment with clopidogrel, patients carrying reduced-function CYP2C19 alleles compared with noncarriers have substantially higher rates of major adverse cardiovascular events, including stent thrombosis (Mega JL, et al. *N Engl J Med* 2009;360(4):354–362). The boxed warning issued by the FDA is for poor metabolizers only. Poor metabolizer status is defined by the presence of 2 reduced-function alleles. The most common reduced-function allele is *2, and the most common poor metabolizer status is *2/*2, which has a prevalence of approximately 3% among Caucasians, 5% in African Americans, and up to 15% in Asians. Other reduced-function alleles are shown in the table below. An increased function allele has also been identified (*17). The wild-type (wt) allele is indicated as *1. The table below indicates the classification of CYP2C19 metabolic status.

1. Ultrarapid: *1/*17, *17/*17
2. Extensive: *1/*1
3. Intermediate: *1/*2-*8, *17/*2-*8
4. Poor: *2-*8/*2-*8

6.5 Answer C. The recent 2011 American College of Cardiology Foundation (ACCF)/AHA focused update (Wright RS, et al. *J Am Coll Cardiol* 2011;57(19):1920–1959) provides new recommendations for platelet function and genetic testing. Both new recommendations are Class IIb but differ in level of evidence. Guidelines state the following: (a) platelet function testing to determine platelet inhibitory response in patients with unstable angina/non-STEMI (or after ACS and PCI) on thienopyridine therapy may be considered if results of testing may alter management (*level of evidence B*); and (b) genotyping for a CYP2C19 loss of function variant in patients with unstable angina/non-STEMI (or after ACS and with PCI) on clopidogrel therapy might be considered if results of testing may alter management (*level of evidence C*). Routine use of platelet function and genetic testing to screen patients who underwent PCI and are treated with clopidogrel is not recommended (Class III, *level of evidence C*) (Levine GN, et al. *J Am Coll Cardiol* 2011;58(24):e44–e122).

6.6 Answer A. When concomitantly using ticagrelor, the higher dose of aspirin may decrease the antiplatelet effect and potential benefits of ticagrelor in certain populations. There exists a significant interaction between treatment and region, and a post hoc analysis in the PLATO (Platelet Inhibition and Patient Outcomes) trial showed no benefit of ticagrelor as compared to clopidogrel in North American patients as compared to the rest of the world, and decreased efficacy of ticagrelor with a higher dose of aspirin (≥300 mg daily) as compared to ≤100 mg aspirin daily (Mahaffey KW, et al. *Circulation* 2011;124(5):544–554). The FDA has added a boxed warning to the ticagrelor label and recommended that the daily maintenance dose of aspirin should be 75 to 100 mg when used with ticagrelor (http://www.accessdata.fda.gov/drugsatfda_docs/label/2011/022433s000lbl.pdf). Prasugrel is relatively contraindicated in patients with a history of TIA or stroke.

6.7 Answer B. Pharmacodynamic studies in which various platelet function tests have been used have shown a 60-mg loading dose of prasugrel to be more potent than clopidogrel loading, even when clopidogrel is used at high doses (≥600 mg). More potent antiplatelet effects are achieved more rapidly and are sustained in the maintenance phase using a 10-mg maintenance dose of prasugrel compared with clopidogrel, irrespective of maintenance clopidogrel dosing (75 to 150 mg) (Wiviott SD, et al. *Circulation* 2007;116(25):2923–2932).

6.8 Answer C. Ticagrelor is metabolized through the liver, primarily via the CYP3A4 system. In clinical practice, the commonly encountered strong CYP3A4 inhibitors are azole antifungals (ketoconazole, voriconazole, itraconazole, fluconazole), protease inhibitors (ritonavir, saquinavir, nelfinavir, indinavir, atazanavir), clarithromycin, telithromycin, and nefazodone. CYP3A4 inhibitors decrease elimination of ticagrelor and might significantly increase risk of bleeding; use of these drugs are contraindicated with ticagrelor. Strong CYP3A4 inducers such as rifampin, dexamethasone, phenytoin, carbamazepine, and phenobarbital increase metabolism of ticagrelor via CYP3A4 and might result in increased risk of thrombotic events, including in-stent thrombosis. Coadministration of strong *CYP3A4* inhibitors or strong *CYP3A4* inducers is not recommended (Brilinta. [package insert] Wilmington, Delaware: AstraZeneca, LP, 2011. Available at http://www.accessdata.fda.gov/drugsatfda_docs/label/2011/022433s000lbl.pdf).

6.9 Answer D. Although some small studies have shown that increasing the dose of aspirin may overcome aspirin resistance, most studies have not. In fact, increasing the dose of aspirin does not further inhibit the COX-1 enzyme. Recent studies have shown that the most important cause of aspirin resistance is noncompliance to medication. Therefore, compliance to antiplatelet therapy should be evaluated in patients shown to be resistant in a platelet function test. Importantly, there are no studies showing that increasing the dose of aspirin in these patients or switching treatment is clinically beneficial. Increasing the dose of aspirin is known to increase the risk of bleeding, in particular in patients concomitantly treated with clopidogrel. Although some functional studies have shown that patients with aspirin resistance may also be clopidogrel resistant, there is no indication to test for this in routine clinical practice. At the current time, the patient should maintain without modifications his dual antiplatelet dose regimen. The patient should maintain aspirin indefinitely and clopidogrel up to 1 year (Angiolillo DJ. *Am J Cardiol* 2009;103(3 Suppl):27A–34A).

6.10 Answer B. A randomized placebo-controlled crossover trial of 24 healthy subjects received 600-mg loading dose of clopidogrel, and 5 mg of IV morphine showed delayed absorption, reduced active metabolite, and delayed maximal inhibition of platelet aggregation on average by 2 hours with higher residual platelet aggregation (Hobel EL, et al. *J Am Coll Cardiol* 2014;63(7):630–635). Although there is insufficient evidence on clinical outcomes of concomitant use of morphine and clopidogrel, it has been shown that the use of morphine is associated with higher mortality and major adverse cardiovascular events in patients with non-STEMI (Meine TJ, et al. *Am Heart J* 2005;149(6):1043–1049). Despite these pharmacodynamics and pharmacokinetic interactions between morphine and clopidogrel, there is no specific clinical recommendation that can be given until more randomized trials are available.

6.11 Answer D. Numerous factors account for inadequate clopidogrel-induced antiplatelet effects. These include genetic, cellular, and clinical factors. However, noncompliance and underdosing seem to play the most important role. Dose-finding studies supporting currently recommended dosages of clopidogrel were designed to achieve a degree of platelet inhibition similar to 250 mg bid of ticlopidine. Importantly, these studies did not take into consideration the prothrombotic milieu of high-risk subjects, such as those with ACS or undergoing PCI. Numerous platelet function studies have shown that when increasing the loading and maintenance dose of clopidogrel, enhanced antiplatelet effects are achieved (Angiolillo DJ. *Am J Cardiol* 2009;103(3 Suppl):27A–34A).

6.12 Answer A. Although there are controversial results on the use of PPIs concurrently with clopidogrel, based on the current evidence, patients on dual antiplatelet or triple therapy who have GI bleeding history or are at risk of GI bleeding can continue or start taking PPIs, including omeprazole. A placebo-controlled trial showed omeprazole significantly reduced the antiplatelet effect of clopidogrel (Gilard M, et al. *J Am Coll Cardiol* 2008;51(3):256–260). Prasugrel is relatively contraindicated and has a black box warning in patients more than 75 years of age or with a prior history of TIA or stroke. Although PD interaction exists, there are no meaningful clinical adverse effects observed, as evidenced by the TRITON study on clinical impact of PPI use on the efficacy or safety of prasugrel or clopidogrel (O'Donoghue ML, et al. *Lancet* 2009;374(9694):989–997).

Another randomized study (COGENT trial) that included patients who need dual antiplatelet assessed the effectiveness of clopidogrel in combination with omeprazole vs. placebo showing no significant cardiovascular interaction between clopidogrel and omeprazole and no difference in ischemic outcomes, but combined use decreased GI bleeding and events (Bhatt DL, et al. *N Engl J Med* 2010;363(20):1909–1917). Although omeprazole consistently showed that it decreased the antiplatelet effect of clopidogrel, studies revealed that the interaction between PPIs and clopidogrel is not a class effect (Sibbing D, et al. *Thromb Haemost* 2009;101(4):714–719; Angiolillo DJ, et al. *Clin Pharmacol Ther* 2011;89(1):65–74). A prospective randomized study showed that patients receiving pantoprazole and clopodogrel had a significantly better platelet inhibition compared to omeprazole and clopidogrel and there were more clopidogrel nonresponders in the omeprazole group than in the pantoprazole group (44% vs. 23%) (Cuisset T, et al. *J Am Coll Cardiol* 2009;54(13):1149–1153).

Although, the FDA has recommended avoiding the use of clopidogrel and omeprazole or esomeprazole simultaneously (https://www.accessdata.fda.gov/drugsatfda_docs/label/2011/022456s004lbl.pdf), the ACCF/American College of Gastroenterology/AHA's consensus document on the evidence of clopidogrel and PPI interaction gives a recommendation that PPIs might still be used in high-risk patients receiving dual antiplatelet therapy (DAPT) (Abraham NS, et al. *J Am Coll Cardiol* 2010;56(24):2051-2066). The current ACCF/AHA PCI guideline gives a Class I recommendation for PPI use in patients with a history of prior GI bleeding who require DAPT and Class IIa recommendation in patients who are at increased risk of GI bleeding (e.g., advanced age, concomitant use of warfarin, steroids, NSAIDs, and *Helicobacter pylori* infection) who require DAPT (Levine GN, et al. *Circulation* 2011;124(23):e574-e651). Clopidogrel is the P2Y12 inhibitor of choice in patients receiving triple therapy (Levine GN, et al. *Circulation* 2016;134(10):e123-e155).

6.13 Answer B. Concomitant use of NSAIDs, such as ibuprofen, indomethacin, and naproxen, can prevent aspirin from acetylating the platelet COX-1 enzyme. COX-1 inhibition (and not PAR inhibition) is the mechanism through which aspirin exerts its effects and blocks platelet's ability to synthesize thromboxane A2. While it is a weak inhibitor of platelet aggregation in vitro, it does decrease the incidence of peri-PCI thrombotic events by up to 75%. Chewing 162 to 325 mg of aspirin allows for the achievement of its full effects within approximately 15 minutes (Patrono C, et al. *N Engl J Med* 2005;353(22):2373-2383).

6.14 Answer A. Azole antifungal drugs (e.g., ketoconazole, itraconazole, fluconazole, and voriconazole) are used to treat fungal infections and long-term fungal prophylaxis in organ transplants, including heart transplant patients. CYP3A4 inhibitors decrease and CYP3A4 inducers increase the antiplatelet activity of clopidogrel. Ketoconazole is a potent inhibitor of both CYP3A4 and CYP3A5. The azole antifungals inhibit the isoenzyme CYP3A4 variably (Dvorak Z. *Toxicol Lett* 2011;202(2):129-132) with ketoconazole possibly the strongest inhibitor and fluconazole a moderate inhibitor (Lazar JD, et al. *Semin Oncol* 1990;17(3 Suppl 6):14-18). Azole antifungals may interfere with the efficacy of clopidogrel as both act via CYP3A4 and clopidogrel partially converts through the CYP3A4 system to its active metabolite. In one study, patients who were taking clopidogrel with concomitant use of ketoconazole showed decreased formation of the active metabolite of clopidogrel with significantly reduced platelet inhibition, but that effect was not observed in prasugrel-treated patients (Farid NA, et al. *Clin Pharmacol Ther* 2007;81(5):735-741). Another CYP3A4 inhibitor, itraconazole, significantly reduced the inhibitory effect of clopidogrel on platelet aggregation (Suh JW, et al. *CMAJ* 2006;174(12):1715-1722). However, there is a lack of evidence on the clinical outcomes of clopidogrel-treated patients with azole antifungals, and there is no currently available therapeutic recommendation in this regard.

6.15 Answer D. The vast majority of data available in the scientific literature associating antiplatelet drug resistance with clinical outcomes have utilized light transmission aggregometry (LTA), which, despite its numerous pitfalls, is still considered the gold standard assay for platelet function. Although point-of-care assays (VerifyNow and PFA-100) and platelet membrane receptors (assessed by flow cytometry) have also been utilized in determining adverse clinical outcomes, the degree of evidence is less robust compared to LTA (Angiolillo DJ. *Am J Cardiol* 2009;103(3 Suppl):27A-34A).

6.16 Answer B. Clopidogrel is a prodrug and needs two-step metabolism to convert its active metabolite. CYP2C19 isoenzyme plays a central role in clopidogrel metabolism and carriers of loss of function alleles have lower clopidogrel active metabolite (Mega JL, et al. *N Engl J Med* 2009;360(4):354-362). CYP2C19*1/*2 and *2/*2 carriers of loss of function alleles are poor metabolizers, and clopidogrel may not be fully effective in inhibiting platelets in these patients due to diminished active metabolite of clopidogrel. The genotyping test of CYP2C19 indicates that this patient is a poor metabolizer and thus at higher risk of cardiovascular events (Mega JL, et al. *JAMA* 2010;304:1821-1830), but it does not measure the response to clopidogrel. The clopidogrel responsiveness is measured by platelet function test. CYP2C19*17/*17 vs. CYP2C19*1/*1 carriers are ultrametabolizers and regular metabolizers, respectively. The incidence of major bleeding is higher with clopidogrel in ultrametabolizers vs. regular metabolizers (Siller-Matula JM, et al. *J Thromb Haemost* 2012;10(4):529-542; Sibbing D, et al. *Circulation* 2010;121(4):512-518).

6.17 Answer A. A key protein involved in thienopyridine absorption is the efflux pump P-glycoprotein, which is encoded by *ABCB1* (also known as *MDR1*, located on chromosome 7). P-glycoprotein is an ATP-dependent efflux pump that transports various molecules across extracellular and intracellular membranes. It is expressed, among other places, on intestinal epithelial cells where increased expression or function can affect bioavailability of drugs that are substrates. Studies have shown that following clopidogrel administration, individuals with genetic variants in *ABCB1* (specifically those who are TT homozygotes for the 3435C→T variant) have reduced concentrations of the active drug metabolite and increased rates of adverse clinical outcomes (Mega JL, et al. *Lancet* 2010;376(9749):1312–1319). Polymorphisms of cytochrome P450 enzymes have been implied in modulating clopidogrel response through its hepatic metabolism. Controversial data exist on the modulating role of *Pl^A* polymorphisms on antiplatelet agents, which encode for the platelet GP IIb/IIIa receptor. *VKOR* polymorphisms are involved in modulating warfarin effects (Fig. A6-17) (Marin F, et al. *J Am Coll Cardiol* 2009;54(12):1041–1057).

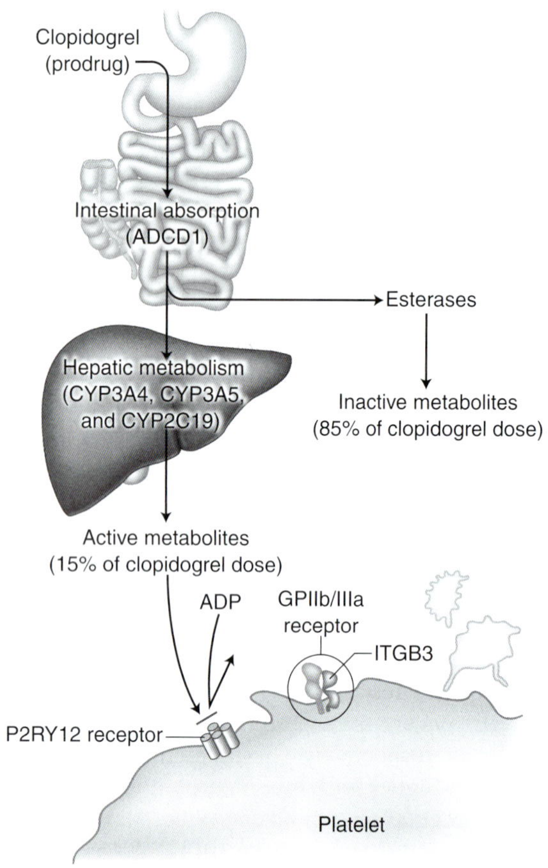

Figure A6-17 (Adapted from Simon T, et al. *N Engl J Med* 2009;360(4):363–375.)

6.18 Answer C. UFH, low molecular weight heparin, bivalirudin, and warfarin are all anticoagulant agents. PK studies have shown that bivalirudin has a linear dose-plasma concentration relationship (Topol EJ, et al. *Circulation* 1993;87(5):1622–1629). This translates into more predictable anticoagulant effects as assessed in PD studies. The effects of UFH, low molecular weight heparin, and warfarin are influenced by multiple factors, which ultimately lead to broad variability in intersubject anticoagulant effects.

6.19 Answer D. In patients undergoing PCI who do not receive GP IIb/IIIa inhibitors, guidelines (Smith SC Jr, et al. *Circulation* 2006;113(7):e166–e286) recommend that (a) UFH should be given during coronary angioplasty to achieve an ACT of 250 to 300 seconds with the HemoTec device and 300 to 350 seconds with the Hemochron device; (b) a weight-adjusted bolus heparin (70 to 100 IU/kg) can be used to avoid excess anticoagulation; and (c) if the

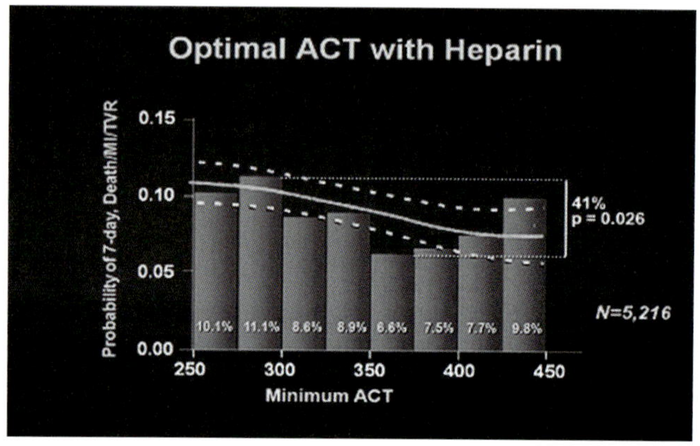

A

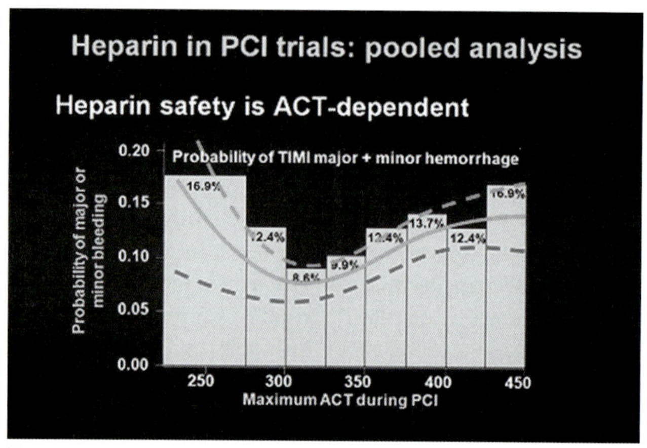

B

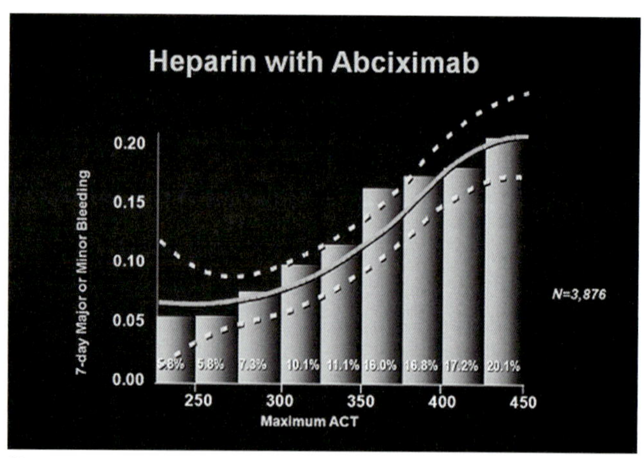

C

Figure A6-19 (A–C: Adapted from Chew DP, et al. *Circulation* 2001;103(7):961–966.)

target values for ACT are not achieved after a bolus of heparin, additional heparin boluses (2,000 to 5,000 IU) can be given (Chew DP, et al. *Circulation* 2001;103(7):961–966). No large randomized study has established the optimal dose of heparin or target ACT, especially in the contemporary device and drug era. Many interventionalists begin with a 50-IU/kg bolus of heparin (Fig. A6-19A and B).

In patients undergoing PCI receiving GP IIb/IIIa inhibitors, guidelines recommend that the UFH bolus should be 50 to 70 IU/kg in order to achieve a target ACT of 200 seconds, irrespective of the device that is being used to measure ACT. Higher doses of UFH (70 to 100 IU/kg) have been associated with increased risk of bleeding and should be reserved for patients undergoing PCI without the use of GP IIb/IIIa inhibitors. A fixed (non-weight-based) bolus of 5,000 IU, without ACT monitoring, is subject to broad variability in ACT levels. Oftentimes, an ACT of >200 seconds can be achieved with a low dose (50 IU/kg) of heparin (Fig. A6-19C).

6.20 **Answer C.** Ideally, in patients with coronary artery disease or history of myocardial infarction (MI), ibuprofen or other NSAIDs—except aspirin—should be avoided when possible. If they have to take ibuprofen, then immediate release or non-enteric-coated aspirin should be taken 30 minutes before or 8 hours after taking ibuprofen for full antiplatelet benefit of aspirin (http://www.fda.gov/Drugs/DrugSafety/PostmarketDrugSafetyInformationforPatientsandProviders). NSAIDs can cause or potentiate ACS and adverse cardiovascular outcomes in patients with coronary artery disease. One study revealed that patients taking ibuprofen had a significantly higher risk of all-cause mortality compared with patients not taking ibuprofen (MacDonald TM, et al. *Lancet* 2003;361(9357):573–574). Studies showed that there is a PD interaction between ibuprofen and low doses of aspirin.

Aspirin and NSAIDs both inhibit the cyclooxygenase-1 (COX-1) enzyme. Competitive inhibition of COX-1 by other NSAIDs might reduce the antiplatelet effectiveness of aspirin, especially non-COX-2 selective drugs, and may have adverse cardiovascular events if aspirin is primarily used for cardioprotection. Studies showed that the antiplatelet effect of aspirin was significantly reduced when ibuprofen was given 2 hours before aspirin (Catella-Lawson F, et al. *N Engl J Med* 2001;345(25):1809–1817; Renda G, et al. *Clin Pharmacol Ther* 2006;80(3):264–274).

Although there is insufficient evidence on other NSAIDs, in general, other nonselective NSAIDs (e.g., indomethacin and naproxen) also interfere with the antiplatelet effects of aspirin, similarly as with ibuprofen, but more COX-2 selective agents (e.g., celecoxib, diclofenac, and meloxicam) are less likely to interfere with the effectiveness of aspirin (Meek IL, et al. *Eur J Clin Pharmacol* 2013;69(3):365–371; Schuijt MP, et al. *Br J Pharmacol* 2009;157(6):931–934; Gladding PA, et al. *Am J Cardiol* 2008;101(7):1060–1063). The AHA suggests that this interaction between aspirin and other COX-1 inhibitors might be clinically significant (Antman EM, et al. *Circulation* 2007;115(12):1634–1642).

7 Antiarrhythmics, Sedatives, and Lipid-lowering Agents

Steven P. Dunn and David J. Moliterno

QUESTIONS

7.1 A 68-year-old Caucasian male with a history of hypertension, diabetes, and hyperlipidemia presents 6 hours after the onset of substernal chest pressure. An electrocardiogram (ECG) shows ST elevation in leads V4 to V6. He is seen in the emergency department and then taken to the catheterization suite for coronary angiography and possible percutaneous coronary intervention (PCI). After injecting the left coronary artery, the nurse notifies you of a rapid heart rate (Fig. Q7-1). The aortic pressure is noted to be 65/30 mm Hg, and the patient does not respond to questions. What is the best treatment?

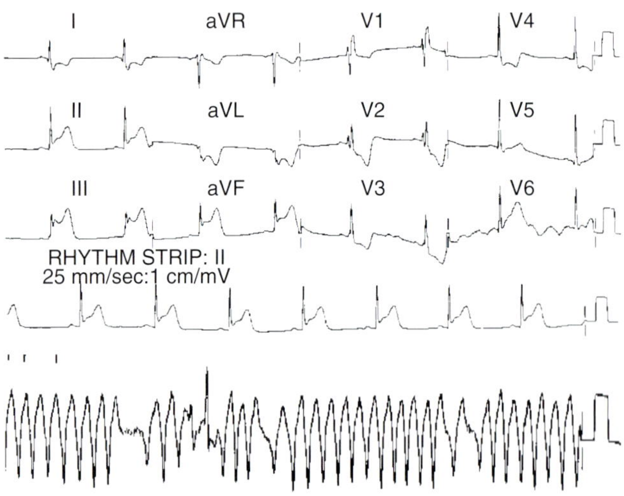

Figure Q7-1

(A) Immediate lidocaine 100 mg intravenous (IV) bolus
(B) Electrical cardioversion
(C) Rapid atrial pacing
(D) Give metoprolol 5 mg IV push
(E) Load with IV amiodarone 300 mg

7.2 Which of the following is the most appropriate description of amiodarone dosing for stable ventricular tachycardia (VT) (assume long-term continuation)?

(A) A 300-mg IV bolus, followed by a 200-mg daily maintenance dose
(B) A 150-mg IV bolus, followed by a 1-mg/min IV infusion for 6 hours, followed by a 0.5-mg/min IV infusion for 18 hours, followed by an oral loading dose for 5 to 7 days followed by a 400-mg oral maintenance dose
(C) A 1-mg/min IV infusion for 6 hours, followed by a 0.5-mg/min IV infusion for 18 hours
(D) A 400-mg oral maintenance dose

7.3 Which of the following methods of administration for amiodarone is most likely to cause hypotension?

(A) Amiodarone oral loading dose
(B) Amiodarone continuous IV infusion
(C) Amiodarone maintenance dose
(D) Amiodarone IV bolus

7.4 Accumulating evidence has demonstrated that the development of new atherosclerotic lesions, as opposed to the treatment of restenosis or previously intervened upon lesions, is a leading cause for recurrent coronary artery disease (CAD) and symptoms. As such, it is crucial following PCI to aggressively treat lipid abnormalities. Assuming you are treating a patient naïve to medical therapy who is undergoing initial PCI, which of the following lipid-lowering therapies would you prescribe to achieve the greatest risk reduction of both stable and unstable coronary artery lesions, irrespective of abnormalities on the patient's lipid panel?

(A) Atorvastatin
(B) Fenofibrate
(C) Niacin
(D) Omega-3 fatty acids
(E) Evolocumab

7.5 An 87-year-old woman undergoes left heart catheterization and diagnostic angiography following suspected unstable angina. The night prior to the procedure, she was anxious and had difficulty sleeping. She received 5 mg of zolpidem for sleep and 2 mg of lorazepam for anxiety. The morning of the catheterization, she received 25 mg of diphenhydramine orally. Near the time her femoral arterial sheath was placed, she complained of back pain and received two tablets of oxycodone/acetaminophen 5 mg/325 mg since there was a PRN order. Prior to obtaining arterial access, conscious sedation procedures are initiated with 50 mcg of IV fentanyl. Over the next several minutes, her oxygen saturation decreases to <80% and she is difficult to arouse. Her vital signs are stable except her respiratory rate is decreased. The next appropriate step would be to administer:

(A) Midazolam
(B) Atropine
(C) Flumazenil
(D) Naloxone
(E) Epinephrine

7.6 Atropine is used in the cardiac catheterization laboratory, particularly among patients who are experiencing vasovagal bradycardia and/or hypotension. Which of the following statements is true for the use of atropine in the cardiac catheterization laboratory?

(A) It should be used in caution among patients with a history of diabetes
(B) It may cause anticholinergic side effects
(C) It should be used among patients who have a substantial decrease in heart rate
(D) It should be used in small doses (<0.4 mg), especially among patients with diabetes
(E) It should be given in large doses (>2 mg) among patients with a large body mass index (BMI) (>30)
(F) All of the above

7.7 On your morning rounds, you plan to discharge an 85-year-old man who had been admitted several days prior with non-ST-segment elevation myocardial infarction (NSTEMI). He underwent successful angioplasty and bare-metal stent (BMS) placement to the proximal left anterior descending (LAD) artery. You notice his fasting cholesterol profile reveals the total cholesterol to be 332 mg/dL, triglycerides (TG) 600 mg/dL, and high-density lipoprotein (HDL) 48 mg/dL. The low-density lipoprotein (LDL) is unable to be calculated. Which of the following lipid-lowering therapies would be appropriate for this patient?

(A) Simvastatin
(B) Niacin
(C) Gemfibrozil
(D) Simvastatin plus ezetimibe
(E) Simvastatin plus fenofibrate

7.8 Assuming you are ready to discharge the patient in Question 7.7 home, the medical resident on your team presents the following as his medication regimen upon discharge: aspirin 81 mg daily, ticagrelor 90 mg bid, simvastatin 80 mg nightly, metoprolol 25 mg twice daily, gemfibrozil 600 mg twice daily, and lisinopril 5 mg daily. Which of the following combinations represents a clinically important drug–drug interaction that requires therapeutic modification?

(A) Ticagrelor–Simvastatin
(B) Simvastatin–Gemfibrozil
(C) Aspirin–Ticagrelor
(D) Aspirin–Lisinopril
(E) None of the above

7.9 A 65-year-old male with known atherosclerotic cardiovascular disease (ASCVD)—he had two coronary stents 5 years prior and myocardial infarction (MI)—presents for follow-up. He has been doing very well with no anginal symptoms but is interested in maximizing his nonpharmacologic and pharmacologic regimen to prevent any future events. To this end, he has quit smoking and is contemplating other lifestyle changes. His fasting lipid panel reveals the following: total cholesterol (TC) 170 mg/dL, HDL 30 mg/dL, TG 100 mg/dL, LDL 65 mg/dL. His medication regimen is as follows: acetylsalicylic acid (ASA) 81 mg daily, ticagrelor 60 mg twice daily, rosuvastatin 40 mg daily, metoprolol XL 50 mg daily, and lisinopril 10 mg daily. Which of the following is true regarding the use of HDL-increasing therapies for this patient?

(A) Niacin should be added to this patient's regimen to raise HDL and reduce risk of recurrent MI
(B) Niacin has not been demonstrated to be of benefit in reducing cardiovascular events when added to statin therapy

(C) Niacin should be avoided as it results in a clinically significant drug interaction with aspirin
(D) Niacin should be avoided in favor of the addition of ezetimibe, which increases HDL to a greater extent

7.10 A 75-year-old man with a past medical history of stroke, CAD, ischemic cardiomyopathy, hypertension, and chronic kidney disease (CKD) with a creatinine clearance of 42 mL/min undergoes angioplasty and direct stent placement, which are successful. However, he develops atrial fibrillation overnight, and further discussion with the patient reveals a history of palpitations over the past several months. Which antiarrhythmic medication(s) would be reasonable treatment options for this patient at this time?

(A) Sotalol
(B) Flecainide
(C) Mexiletine
(D) Dofetilide

7.11 A 62-year-old woman with renal insufficiency, atrial fibrillation, and a CHA_2DS_2-Vasc score of 4 is being discharged after a hospitalization where she received a drug-eluting stent (DES). Your resident informs you of the final medication regimen at discharge, which includes aspirin 325 mg daily, clopidogrel 75 mg daily, warfarin 5 mg daily, simvastatin 40 mg nightly, amiodarone 200 mg daily, digoxin 125 mcg daily, and metoprolol 25 mg twice daily. Which of the following is a clinically significant drug–drug interaction, requiring either increased monitoring or therapeutic intervention?

(A) Amiodarone–Digoxin
(B) Amiodarone–Simvastatin
(C) Amiodarone–Warfarin
(D) All of the above

7.12 Which of the following should NOT be routinely monitored during chronic amiodarone therapy?

(A) Chest x-ray or pulmonary function tests
(B) Thyroid function tests
(C) Magnetic resonance imaging (MRI) of the brain
(D) Eye exams
(E) Liver function tests

7.13 Which of the following lipid-lowering therapies does not result in a drug–drug interaction when given with warfarin?

(A) Ezetimibe
(B) Evolocumab
(C) Lovastatin
(D) Simvastatin

7.14 A 56-year-old man with a positive nuclear stress test and exertional angina is referred for coronary angiography and possible stent placement. The patient is prepped, and local anesthesia is administered around the access site. At this time, which of the following medications is appropriate for inducing conscious sedation?

(A) Lidocaine 100 mg IV
(B) Midazolam 2 mg IV
(C) Diphenhydramine 50 mg IV
(D) Succinylcholine 100 mg IV
(E) None of the above

7.15 Assuming the patient in Question 7.14 has an allergy to benzocaine, which of the following actions with local anesthesia initiation is appropriate?

(A) Abandon the procedure since cross-allergenicity is possible with all anesthetics
(B) Administer larger doses than usual of fentanyl in order to "make up" for the lack of a local anesthetic
(C) Proceed with administration of lidocaine, but choose a preservative-free solution without vasoconstrictor components
(D) None of the above

7.16 Which of the following patient parameters most closely describes characteristics of the level of sedation recommended for cardiac catheterization procedures?

(A) Purposeful response to commands
(B) Maintenance of pulmonary ventilation and oxygenation
(C) Maintenance of cardiovascular function
(D) All of the above
(E) None of the above

7.17 Which of the following local anesthetics is associated with the most adverse effects on the cardiovascular system?

(A) Lidocaine
(B) Ropivacaine
(C) Bupivacaine
(D) Benzocaine

7.18 An 82-year-old African American male with a history of CAD, hypertension, diabetes, and CKD presents with an inferolateral STEMI and receives primary PCI to the right coronary artery (RCA). Following the procedure, he remains bradycardic with a heart rate around 40 beats per minute (bpm) and hypertensive with a systolic blood pressure of 140 to 150 mm Hg. His serum creatinine at baseline is 2.3 mg/dL but is found to be now 3.0 mg/dL after obtaining labs post-PCI. The decision is made to try to increase his heart rate in an attempt to improve renal perfusion. He declines consent for a temporary pacing wire due to lack of desire for further invasive procedures, so he must be paced using pharmacologic measures. Which of the following would be the least appropriate method for pharmacologic pacing at this time?

(A) Isoproterenol
(B) Dopamine
(C) Dobutamine
(D) None of the above

7.19 The patient's serum creatinine in the above question eventually returns to baseline and pharmacologic pacing is withdrawn several days following his acute MI. He does not appear to require a permanent pacemaker (and would refuse if one was offered), but his heart rate remains in the 50 bpm. Prior to discharge, the patient develops atrial fibrillation with a slow ventricular response on telemetry for which he feels light-headed and dizzy, despite normal hemodynamics. This rhythm resolves spontaneously. Which of the following medications would be the optimal choice to maintain the patient in sinus rhythm, assuming such a strategy is used?

(A) Amiodarone
(B) Diltiazem
(C) Dofetilide
(D) Metoprolol

7.20 Which of the following is true regarding the chronic use of dofetilide?

(A) Dofetilide is preferred due to its minimal potential for drug interactions relative to amiodarone
(B) Dofetilide can only be prescribed by certain physicians and dispensed by certain pharmacies who have completed extra training
(C) The patient must be hospitalized for the first 3 days of therapy to monitor for QT prolongation and torsades
(D) None of the above

ANSWERS AND EXPLANATIONS

7.1 Answer B. Figure Q7-1 shows a tracing of VT that is associated with hypotension and reduced mental status (the patient does not respond to your question). In this scenario, the best treatment is direct current cardioversion to immediately restore sinus rhythm. Although amiodarone and lidocaine are Advanced Cardiovascular Life Support (ACLS) drugs of choice for hemodynamically stable VT, the goal in this patient is to rapidly convert the ventricular tachycardia to a more stable rhythm (Link MS, et al. 2015 American Heart Association Guidelines Update for Cardiopulmonary Resuscitation and Emergency Cardiovascular Care Part 7: Adult advanced cardiovascular life support. *Circulation* 2015;132: S444–S464). Metoprolol would be less desirable in a hypotensive patient.

7.2 Answer B. Amiodarone is a complex drug to administer, requiring a bolus followed by a prolonged loading period. Answers A and D are incorrect due to the lack of an appropriate total loading dose (usually 8 to 10 g weeks for VT). Answer C is also incorrect due to the lack of an initial IV dose to attempt to terminate the rhythm and also due to cessation of therapy beyond the 24-hour infusion period. Therefore, B is the most appropriate answer, assuming amiodarone is continued beyond the short-term period. The use of a 150-mg loading dose is appropriate assuming stable VT, whereas a higher loading dose (300 mg) may be preferred in a pulseless scenario.

7.3 Answer D. IV amiodarone contains a polysorbate compound that is known to cause hypotension upon rapid infusion. While all methods of amiodarone administration are associated with some impact on hemodynamic parameters due to beta and calcium channel antagonism, the IV bolus is most consistently the cause of hemodynamically significant hypotension. Additionally, aqueous amiodarone solutions are also now available, which may be associated with less hypotension during the bolus phase of administration.

7.4 Answer A. HMG-CoA reductase inhibitors ("statins") have been extensively shown to reduce the secondary development of both unstable and stable CAD. Intensive statin therapy has also shown regression in coronary artery plaque. While other therapies on this list may alter lipid parameters, none have demonstrated reduction in events similar to statin drugs and are indicated in virtually all patients with known CAD. PCSK9 inhibitors or other LDL reducing agents such as ezetimibe have demonstrated cardiovascular risk reduction as adjunctive therapy but not in place of a statin.

7.5 Answer D. Pharmacologic reversal is indicated due to her decreased respiratory rate and oxygen saturation and altered mental status. Midazolam would be inappropriate in this scenario as benzodiazepines can further reduce respiratory efforts, an effect that can also be synergistic in combination with opiate analgesics. Atropine additionally has no indication in this scenario due to the stable hemodynamics. Flumazenil would potentially be indicated if the patient had received IV benzodiazepines for sedation, but from this scenario, only fentanyl had been given. The lorazepam from the previous evening is probably not significantly present in the body at this time. Epinephrine is also not indicated due to the stable hemodynamic profile. Naloxone would be the most appropriate choice to block the respiratory depression observed immediately after the administration of IV opiate therapy (Table A7-5).

Table A7-5 Reversal agents for conscious sedation procedures

	Dose	Peak Effect	Duration of Effect
Flumazenil (benzodiazepine antagonist)	0.2 mg initial; maximum (total) 1 mg	6–10 min	1–4 h
Naloxone (opioid antagonist)	0.4 mg initial; maximum (total) 2 mg	5–10 min	45 min–3 h

7.6 Answer B. Atropine is a valuable drug in the cardiac catheterization laboratory and can quickly reverse the bradycardia and hypotension sometimes associated with infarction, ischemia, and inappropriate vagal tone. Diabetes is not a concern when administering atropine. Additionally, the relative degree of decrease in heart rate is not a significant factor when deciding whether or not to administer atropine; rather bradycardia with hemodynamic compromise should be the indication. Doses <0.4 mg should not be administered due to potential for a paradoxical bradycardic reaction. Finally, a patient's body weight does not influence the initial dose of atropine given. Atropine does, however, antagonize muscarinic receptors and exerts its therapeutic effect via anticholinergic mechanisms. Therefore, other anticholinergic effects may be present with the use of atropine, but these should dissipate within a few hours and not be considered a significant barrier to its use.

7.7 Answer E. This patient has severe dyslipidemia that will require combination therapy to achieve optimal levels. Niacin seems reasonable, as it will potentially affect LDL, HDL, and TG but will not be enough by itself, and its primary target, HDL, is already at goal. Statins are certainly indicated for risk reduction and due to the patient's age, a moderate-intensity statin such as simvastatin would be reasonable. Gemfibrozil will not significantly change LDL levels or reduce recurrent events to the extent that statin therapy will. As the patient's TGs are significantly elevated (>500), such that there is acute risk for pancreatitis, combination therapy with a statin plus a potent TG-reducing agent is reasonable. Therefore, E is the best answer.

7.8 Answer B. The combination of statin and fibrates may be utilized, but multiple reports exist describing the increased risk of muscle toxicities, including rhabdomyolysis, associated with the combination. Therefore, the choice of fibrate and the dose of statin make a clinically significant difference. Gemfibrozil inhibits certain proteins that uptake statins into the liver and therefore will increase levels of virtually all statin medications. Simvastatin may be utilized in combination, but it is recommended to be dosed no higher than 10 mg daily. Additionally, fenofibrate affects statin bioavailability to a lesser degree and may be more safely utilized with statin therapy. Statin therapy does not appear to interact with ticagrelor therapy, despite many statins being cometabolized through CYP3A4, making A incorrect. Aspirin and ticagrelor do increase the risk of bleeding but are therapeutically indicated in this patient due to the recent stent, which makes C incorrect. Aspirin has also been shown to interfere with the vasodilating effects of angiotensin-converting enzyme inhibitors (ACEI), but not enough data exist to suggest modification of therapy in this patient, making D incorrect. Therefore, B is the correct answer.

7.9 Answer B. Per the American College of Cardiology (ACC)/American Heart Association (AHA) guidelines (Stone NJ, et al. *Circulation* 2014;129(25 suppl 2):S1–S45), the primary basis for prevention of ASCVD in this high-risk patient is the use of statin therapy. The use of niacin as adjunctive therapy to statins has not demonstrated clinical benefit (HPS2-THRIVE Collaborative Group, et al. *N Engl J Med* 2014;371(3):203–212; AIM-HIGH Investigators, et al. *N Engl J Med* 2011;365(24):2255–2267) and is therefore not recommended. While niacin does raise HDL levels effectively, it does not reduce cardiovascular events, making Answer A incorrect. The use of niacin and aspirin together does not result in a drug interaction and may be of clinical benefit to reduce the flushing reaction associated with niacin, making Answer C incorrect. Finally, ezetimibe does not increase HDL levels, making answer D incorrect.

7.10 Answer D. The decision to use an antiarrhythmic in a patient with extensive cardiovascular disease and altered organ function is complex. Sotalol could initially be considered, but is not recommended for use in patients with heart failure. Mexiletine is not effective for atrial arrhythmias. Flecainide is also not recommended for patients with structural heart disease due to risk of proarrhythmia. As such, it is very reasonable to treat this patient with either amiodarone, which is entirely metabolized by the liver, or dofetilide, which is primarily eliminated by the kidney but can be adjusted for renal dysfunction to a certain extent. Both agents can be used successfully not only in acute atrial fibrillation but also as prophylactic agents to prevent recurrent atrial fibrillation. Additionally, both amiodarone and dofetilide are the only recommended antiarrhythmic drugs to be used chronically in patients with a history of heart failure.

7.11 Answer D. All of the above are significant drug–drug interactions, which require either increased monitoring or therapeutic intervention. Amiodarone inhibits P-glycoprotein, which partially metabolizes digoxin prior to absorption. Therefore, amiodarone initiation in a patient receiving digoxin will necessitate a dose reduction of digoxin. Amiodarone inhibits CYP3A4, a major metabolic pathway for simvastatin and warfarin. The maximum dose of simvastatin recommended with warfarin is 20 mg/day. Additionally, initiation of warfarin in a patient receiving amiodarone will require close monitoring, and it is recommended that an empiric 50% reduction in the dose of warfarin be performed.

7.12 Answer C. While amiodarone may result in a number of neurologic toxicities, they do not result in anatomic changes such that an MRI would be a useful monitoring tool; therefore, it is not generally recommended as a screening tool. Amiodarone does result in the potential for lung, thyroid, liver, and ocular toxicities, making periodic screening an essentially component of long-term follow-up.

7.13 Answer B. Many lipid-lowering therapies inhibit metabolism of warfarin (such as many statins) or, in the case of cholestyramine, absorption of warfarin, both of which can affect the resultant anticoagulant effect of warfarin. Evolocumab is a monoclonal antibody of PCSK9 but does not undergo metabolic elimination and would therefore not be subject to interaction potential with warfarin (Page MM, Watts GF. *Expert Opin Drug Metab Toxicol* 2015;11(9):1505–1515).

7.14 Answer B. Short-acting, IV benzodiazepines are the method of choice to induce conscious/moderate sedation in patients undergoing catheterization. The table below (Table A7-14) illustrates potential benzodiazepine options in the catheterization lab. IV lidocaine would have no effect on the level of sedation. Diphenhydramine is often administered to patients undergoing catheterization as a premedication to induce a baseline level of sedation, but this ideally should be done at least 30 minutes prior to the procedure. Succinylcholine is a neuromuscular blocker that would be inappropriate to give for sedation and would additionally result in a loss of respiratory function.

7.15 Answer C. True local anesthetic allergies are uncommon. However, amine-containing anesthetics (benzocaine, prilocaine, or tetracaine) do contain a potentially immunogenic substitution. Amide-containing anesthetics (such as lidocaine) should not be cross-reactive in patients with "amine" allergies. In addition, preservative-free solutions of lidocaine can also be utilized. Patients also may have allergic reaction to sulfite compounds in vasoconstrictors, which can also be avoided in a patient with a local anesthetic allergy. While similar anesthesia may be obtained with IV opiates, this should be considered a less preferential pathway due to the potential for oversedation and respiratory dysfunction. Therefore, C is the best answer.

7.16 Answer D. Conscious (or moderate) sedation is the recommended level of sedation for cardiac catheterization procedures. This level of sedation is a drug-induced depression of consciousness that still allows for the patient to respond to commands and for maintenance of pulmonary and cardiovascular function. The patient's ability to respond to commands is particularly critical in the catheterization laboratory since patient symptoms can often be the first indicator of procedural success or complications.

7.17 Answer C. Bupivacaine is widely regarded as the local anesthetic with the most potential for cardiotoxicity. Cardiotoxicity with local anesthetics typically results from the same nerve blocking mechanism extending to the myocardial conduction system, resulting in potential bradyarrhythmias. Additionally, anesthetics may promote ventricular arrhythmias via unidirectional block and reentry pathways. Lidocaine is typically considered the local anesthetic of choice due to its rapid onset, offset, and minimal potential for cardiotoxic effects.

7.18 Answer B. In general, all of the above medications are options for pharmacologic pacing due to the fact that all of these options stimulate β-1 receptors, which should result in an increase in both inotropic and chronotropic effects. However, dopamine is inappropriate in this situation given

Table A7-14 Benzodiazepines in conscious sedation

		Dose	Peak Effect	Duration of Effect	Metabolic Pathway	Active Metabolite	Protein Binding (%)
Midazolam	**Oral:** NA	**IV:** 0.5–2 mg: Max 5–10 mg	3–5 min	30–80 min	Oxidation	Yes	95
Diazepam	**Oral:** 5 mg	**IV:** 2–5 mg; Max 10 mg	**Oral:** 30 min **IV:** 8–10 min	2–4 h	Oxidation	Yes	80
Lorazepam	**Oral:** 4 mg	**IV:** 2 mg; Max 4 mg	**Oral:** 60–90 min **IV:** 15–20 min	6–8 h	Conjugation	No	85

that the patient is already hypertensive at baseline. Dopamine stimulates dopaminergic, β-1, and α-1 receptors in a dose-dependent manner and is the most likely drug to further increase the patient's blood pressure. Isoproterenol and dobutamine would be better choices due to the lack of alpha-stimulating activity. Both isoproterenol and dobutamine stimulate β-1 and β-2 receptors, which may actually result in hypotension.

7.19 Answer C. A rhythm-control strategy may be reasonable in this patient, since he is symptomatic in atrial fibrillation despite a slow ventricular rate. Diltiazem and metoprolol would be primarily rate-control strategies, although they may have some benefit in maintaining the patient in sinus rhythm, particularly metoprolol. However, both would be contraindicated in this patient with bradycardia due to effects on atrioventricular (AV) and sinoatrial (SA) node conduction. Amiodarone would be an effective antiarrhythmic but also has effects on beta and calcium channels (and therefore heart rate), which would not be desirable. Since the patient's serum creatinine has returned to baseline, dofetilide would be an ideal choice as a pure potassium channel antagonist since it does not affect chronotropy in any significant way.

7.20 Answer C. As part of the dofetilide prescribing label, the patient must be hospitalized for the first 3 days of therapy due to the potential for QT prolongation and potentially fatal ventricular arrhythmias. Both dofetilide and amiodarone have numerous contraindicated drug interactions, making answer A incorrect. The traditional U.S. Food and Drug Administration Risk Evaluation and Mitigation Strategies (REMS) program recently has also been updated and no longer mandates that only certified physicians and pharmacies can prescribe and dispense dofetilide, making answer B incorrect.

8 Inotropes, Vasopressors, and Vasodilators

Tracy E. Macaulay and David J. Moliterno

QUESTIONS

8.1 A 57-year-old male presents to the emergency room complaining of chest pain, and his electrocardiogram (ECG) is consistent with ST-segment elevation myocardial infarction (STEMI). Upon arrival to the cardiac catheterization laboratory, the patient's systolic blood pressure (SBP) is 85 mm Hg, and his heart rate (HR) is 115 beats per minute (bpm). An emergent right heart catheter is inserted while the patient is being prepared for the intervention. The cardiac index (CI) is 1.7 L/min/m^2, and the pulmonary capillary wedge pressure (PCWP) is 19 mm Hg. An intra-aortic balloon pump (IABP) is placed; however, BP and CI remain low. Which of the following medications have been shown to decrease the risk of death in cardiogenic shock? *Note: Table contains the answer choices.*

(A) Dopamine
(B) Epinephrine
(C) Norepinephrine
(D) Milrinone
(E) Vasopressin

8.2 Which of the following scenarios would be most appropriate for initiation of milrinone, 0.375 mcg/kg/min, in a patient undergoing a right heart catheterization? Hemodynamic parameters include mean pulmonary arterial pressure (MPAP), mean arterial pressure (MAP), CI, systemic vascular resistance (SVR), pulmonary capillary wedge pressure (PCWP), and HR. *Note: Table contains the answer choices.*

8.3 A 72-year-old female patient with known heart failure with reduced left ventricular ejection fraction (LVEF) (20% to 30%) is undergoing elective percutaneous coronary intervention (PCI) for progressive anginal symptoms. During the procedure, she begins to experience hypotension (MAP 55 mm Hg) and shortness of breath. A quick examination reveals pulmonary edema, and her mixed venous oxygen saturation (SVO_2) is 65%. Which of the following is the most appropriate pharmacotherapy?

(A) Nesiritide 0.01 mcg/kg/min
(B) Dopamine 10 mcg/kg/min
(C) Nitroprusside 15 mcg/min
(D) Milrinone 0.5 mcg/kg/min

8.4 No reflow can be a significant problem for patients with high thrombus burden or who are undergoing vein graft PCI. Which one of the following agents has NOT offered therapeutic benefit when infused into the coronary artery?

Table Q8-2

	MPAP (mm Hg)	MAP (mm Hg)	CI (L/min/m^2)	SVR (dynes × s/cm^5)	PCWP (mm Hg)	HR (bpm)
(A)	22	55	4.0	800	8	110
(B)	22	70	3.5	1,000	8	90
(C)	38	70	2.0	1,600	36	110
(D)	38	55	2.0	1,000	36	105

(A) Adenosine
(B) Hydralazine
(C) Nicardipine
(D) Papaverine
(E) Verapamil

8.5 You are using a radial approach to perform PCI on a proximal left anterior descending (LAD) lesion in a 61-year-old woman. Following performance of balloon angioplasty, slow flow remains, and the entire vessel appears constricted. Which of the following agents would NOT be appropriate to administer?

(A) Acetylcholine
(B) Diltiazem
(C) Nitroglycerin
(D) Sodium nitroprusside
(E) Verapamil

8.6 A 38-year-old with scleroderma presents to the cardiology clinic with marked limitations in physical activity secondary to progressive shortness of breath. Thus far, workup has revealed a normal ECG and echocardiographic changes consistent with pulmonary arterial hypertension. For further diagnosis, you decide to perform a right heart catheterization and a vasodilatory study. Which vasodilatory regimen would be appropriate?

(A) Nifedipine 10 mg sublingual (SL) every 10 minutes
(B) Nitroglycerin 50 to 100 mcg/min as a continuous infusion
(C) Inhaled nitric oxide (NO) at 80 parts per million (ppm) with 90% oxygen for 10 minutes
(D) Treprostinil 2 ng/kg/min subcutaneous (SQ) titrated every 5 minutes to a maximum of 10 ng/kg/min
(E) Verapamil 20 mg intravenous (IV) bolus, followed by 10 mg/h continuous infusion

8.7 Which of the following statements best describes the activity of norepinephrine?

(A) Norepinephrine, similar to epinephrine, primarily exerts its effect on the β_1 receptors resulting in potent cardiostimulatory effects
(B) Norepinephrine and phenylephrine are preferred over epinephrine in vasodilatory shock as they produce more vasoconstrictive than cardiostimulatory effects
(C) Norepinephrine exhibits vasodilatory effects at low doses, inotropic effects at moderate doses, and vasoconstrictive effects at high doses
(D) Norepinephrine is favored over vasopressin among patients with low pH and cardiopulmonary arrest

8.8 Which one of the following statements is most correct about contrast media-induced anaphylactoid reactions and their treatment?

(A) Urticaria should be immediately treated with SQ epinephrine
(B) IV steroid injection is effective at ameliorating the acute hemodynamic effects of contrast-mediated anaphylactoid reactions
(C) Angioedema should be treated with 0.3 mL of 1:1,000 epinephrine given IV push
(D) Significant anaphylactoid reactions to contrast media occur in 2% to 3% of all patients undergoing selective coronary angiography, and IV diphenhydramine is the initial treatment of choice
(E) Vasodilatory shock should be treated with a 10-mcg IV bolus of epinephrine followed by continuous infusion of 1 to 4 mcg/min as needed

8.9 While PCI was being performed on a 74-year-old male, he developed diffuse vasoconstriction in the target vessel. This was successfully ameliorated with intracoronary nitroprusside (400 mcg). Subsequently, the patient developed hypotension (MAP 52 mm Hg) and tachycardia (HR 106 bpm). In addition to IV fluids, which of the following is the BEST agent to reverse hypotension in this patient?

(A) Dobutamine
(B) Dopamine
(C) Epinephrine
(D) Isoproterenol
(E) Phenylephrine

8.10 A 62-year-old male with a history of hypertension, hyperlipidemia, and pulmonary arterial hypertension secondary to HIV presents with the onset of severe chest pain. His ECG reveals new ST-segment depression. His initial BP is 132/88 mm Hg and HR is 93 bpm. Caution should be exercised with administration of which of the following?

(A) Aspirin 325 mg chewed or crushed and then swallowed
(B) Enoxaparin 1 mg/kg SQ every 12 hours
(C) Metoprolol 12.5 mg orally every 12 hours
(D) Nitroglycerin continuous infusion starting at 10 to 20 mcg/min
(E) Unfractionated heparin (UFH) 60 units/kg bolus followed by 12 units/kg/h

8.11 A 37-year-old male is brought to the emergency department after a witnessed cardiac arrest. He had return of spontaneous rhythm following advanced cardiac life support including cardiopulmonary resuscitation and defibrillation. At the time of arrival, his BP is 75/40 mm Hg, and his HR is 55 bpm. In the emergency department, he is started on dopamine at 15 mcg/kg/min and placed on a mild therapeutic hypothermia protocol. The ECG is consistent with inferior STEMI with second-degree atrioventricular (AV) block. In the cardiac catheterization laboratory, an IABP is placed with 2:1 augmentation; the patient remains hypotensive with a SBP < 90 mm Hg. Which of the following will be most helpful?

(A) Switch dopamine to epinephrine
(B) Administer IV fluid boluses
(C) Change IABP 1:1 augmentation to provide better SBP support
(D) Add milrinone to increase his HR, cardiac output, and BP
(E) Add IV nitroglycerin to prevent recurrent ischemia

8.12 Nitric oxide (NO) has many physiologic effects on vascular endothelium and the underlying smooth muscle. Which of the following is NOT correct about NO?

(A) NO inhibits neutrophil adhesion by decreasing production of neutrophils
(B) NO inhibits platelet aggregation
(C) NO inhibits adhesion molecule production by vascular endothelial cells
(D) NO decreases cyclic guanosine monophosphate (cGMP) in vascular smooth muscle cells

8.13 While performing PCI for unstable angina on a 55-year-old male with a past medical history of hypertension and type II diabetes mellitus, the patient develops chest pain. His BP steadily climbs to 195/107 mm Hg with an HR of 120 bpm. The patient then develops flash pulmonary edema. Which of the following treatments would be best for this acute situation?

(A) Diltiazem 5 mg/h continuous infusion
(B) Fenoldopam 0.1 to 1 mcg/kg/min continuous infusion
(C) Labetalol 10 to 20 mg IV push every 5 to 10 minutes as needed
(D) Nitroglycerin 5 mcg/min continuous infusion
(E) Phentolamine 1 mg/h continuous infusion

8.14 Which of the following statements best describes the use of sodium nitroprusside?

(A) It is particularly useful in patients with low-output, left-sided heart failure because of balanced arteriole and venous vasodilation
(B) Sodium nitroprusside has a long elimination half-life, which precludes its use in acute settings
(C) Cyanide toxicity is only seen at very high doses with prolonged infusion
(D) It is the treatment of choice for patients with cardiorenal syndrome

8.15 A 38-year-old alcoholic female patient complains of recurrent episodes of chest pain. An exercise stress test reveals negative U waves, which were not present at rest. You suspect she has coronary artery spasm (CAS) and recommend angiography with provocative testing. Methylergonovine is the "gold standard" vasoactive agent for the diagnosis of this condition. Which of the following is TRUE regarding methylergonovine?

(A) Methylergonovine is a vasopressin agonist that directly activates the coronary vascular smooth muscle in patients prone to coronary artery spasm
(B) Methylergonovine causes coronary vasoconstriction by upregulated thromboxane production in abnormal vascular endothelium but not in segments with normal endothelium
(C) Methylergonovine stimulates abnormal vascular endothelium to produce endothelin, causing vasoconstriction
(D) Methylergonovine is a serotonin receptor agonist that causes vasodilation if normal endothelium is present but vasoconstriction in the presence of unhealthy endothelium

8.16 A 49-year-old male undergoing PCI for inferior STEMI begins to experience hypotension and bradycardia during the procedure. He is adequately volume resuscitated and you decide to add dopamine. Which of the following is the appropriate dose?

(A) 50 mcg/kg bolus followed by 5 mcg/kg/min continuous infusion
(B) 7.5 mcg/kg/min continuous infusion
(C) 15 mcg/kg/min continuous infusion
(D) 75 mcg/kg bolus followed by 20 mcg/kg/min continuous infusion
(E) 30 mcg/kg/min continuous infusion

8.17 Which of the following is TRUE of low-dose dopamine?

(A) It results in an increase in mucosal perfusion and a higher pH
(B) Extravasation does not result in tissue sloughing; therefore, administration can safely occur through peripheral IV
(C) It has been proven to decrease incidence of acute renal failure
(D) Low doses stimulate the dopamine receptor and may resolve oliguria
(E) Low doses can be used to prevent contrast-induced nephropathy

8.18 A patient undergoing emergent left heart catheterization for STEMI develops hypotension and an epinephrine infusion is started. During the case, it is noticed that the peripheral IV where epinephrine was being administered has infiltrated. Which of the following may be useful in treating the extravasation?

(A) Hyaluronidase
(B) Hydralazine
(C) Sodium thiosulfate
(D) Normal saline
(E) Phentolamine

8.19 A 62-year-old male with known ischemic cardiomyopathy (LVEF 20% to 25%) undergoes a right heart catheterization for progressive heart failure symptoms and recurrent hospitalizations with symptoms of volume overload. During the procedure, she becomes extremely short of breath, and urine output decreases despite increasing doses of diuretics. Her right heart catheterization shows a CI of 1.8 L/min/m^2 and a PCWP of 32 mm Hg. Her HR is 95 bpm and MAP is 65 mm Hg. Her repeat basic metabolic panel shows increasing serum creatinine (SCr) from 2.5 to 3.0 mg/dL earlier in the day. Which of the following should be initiated?

(A) Dobutamine
(B) Dopamine
(C) Esmolol
(D) Milrinone
(E) Norepinephrine

8.20 A 63-year-old female patient is undergoing primary PCI for an anterior STEMI. She has received aspirin, ticagrelor, UFH infusion, and nitroglycerin at 20 mcg/min. Her BP is 162/89 mm Hg and HR is 75 bpm. She continues to have ischemia. Which of the following changes is most appropriate?

(A) Decrease nitroglycerin to 10 mcg/min
(B) Increase nitroglycerin to 30 mcg/min
(C) Switch nitroglycerin to sodium nitroprusside
(D) Add metoprolol 5 mg IV every 5 minutes for three doses
(E) Add morphine 2 to 4 mg IV bolus

ANSWERS AND EXPLANATIONS

8.1 Answer C. Based on hemodynamic data given, the patient is in cardiogenic shock (SBP < 90 mm Hg, CI < 2.2 L/min/m^2, PCWP > 12 mm Hg). According to the subgroup analysis from the SOAP II trial, patients with cardiogenic shock (n = 280) who were randomized to receive norepinephrine had decreased rates of death compared to those who were randomized to receive dopamine (p = 0.03). This may have been related to a decrease in arrhythmic events in patients treated with norepinephrine compared to dopamine (De Backer D, et al. *N Engl J Med* 2010;362(9):779–789). The other agents (i.e., epinephrine, milrinone, and vasopressin) have not been shown to improve survival in STEMI patients with cardiogenic shock.

8.2 Answer C. Milrinone is a phosphodiesterase inhibitor that induces positive inotropic effects via inhibition of the breakdown of cyclic adenosine monophosphate (cAMP), which causes an intracellular shift of calcium ion to produce an increase in myocardial contractility. It also has a dose-dependent vasodilatory effect by inducing relaxation of the peripheral vasculature. This effect is not present with other inotropic agents (dobutamine, isoproterenol, or dopamine), making it the ideal choice in patients with low CI and elevated systemic vascular resistance, as well as elevated pulmonary artery pressures. Patient D has a low MAP and milrinone may worsen this.

8.3 Answer B. All are potential options for patients with LV systolic dysfunction in certain clinical circumstances. Nitroprusside and nesiritide are vasodilators and therefore should be avoided in patients that are exhibiting signs of shock. Milrinone may increase this patient's SVO_2; however, given its peripheral vasodilatory properties, it may further lower the patient's MAP. In this case, dopamine, given at a dose that results in both inotropy and vasoconstriction, is the most appropriate choice.

8.4 Answer B. No reflow occurs in 1% to 4% of all percutaneous interventions. It happens when oxygen reperfusion to ischemic tissue results in formation of reactive oxygen species and a sequel of events, including oxygen radical-mediated cell injury, cell edema, and platelet plugs. Embolization of thrombotic material related to an ACS or atherosclerotic material during vein graft interventions can initiate such events. Microvascular vasospasm and endothelial dysfunction also contribute to no reflow; therefore, certain vasodilators administered intracoronary may offer therapeutic relief. Useful medical therapies include adenosine, diltiazem, nicardipine, papaverine, verapamil, and sodium nitroprusside. There is limited evidence that "combination therapy" with adenosine and nitroprusside is better than adenosine alone. Infusion of vasodilators into the distal vascular bed—instead of through the guide catheter—using a pulse spray method (perfusion catheter) may also improve angiographic outcome. However, angiographic improvement does not clearly alter subsequent morbidity and mortality (Hillegass WB, et al. *J Am Coll Cardiol* 2001;37(5):1335–1343; Fischell TA, et al. *Catheter Cardiovasc Diagn* 1998;45(4):360–365; Michaels AD, et al. *J Invasive Cardiol* 2002;14(6):299–302; Huang RI, et al. *Catheter Cardiovasc Interv* 2006;68(5):671–676).

8.5 Answer A. This patient's response is suggestive of diffuse vasospasm. The treatment of choice for vasospasm is administration of a vasodilator, such as diltiazem, verapamil, sodium nitroprusside, or nitroglycerin (Fig. A8-5). These agents are all preferred over acetylcholine, as they are endothelium-independent vasodilators, whereas acetylcholine is an endothelium-dependent vasodilator. In patients such as this with CAD, endothelial dysfunction is common, and agents such as acetylcholine are ineffective or may cause further vasoconstriction (Ludmer PL, et al. *N Engl J Med* 1986;315(17):1046–1051).

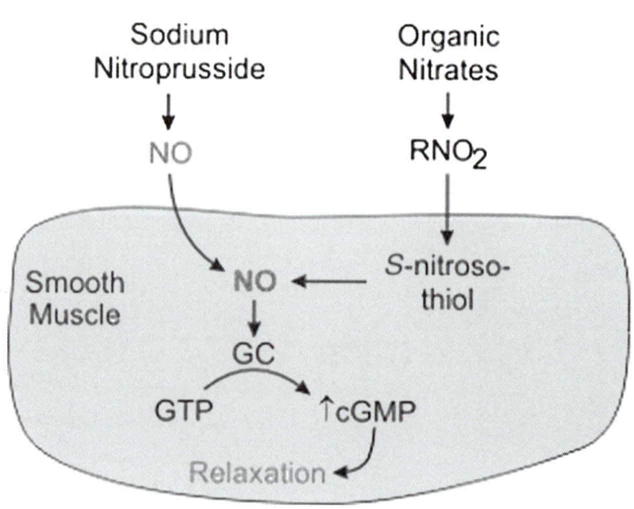

Figure A8-5

8.6 Answer C. Multiple agents have been used for acute vasodilatory challenges in patients undergoing evaluation of pulmonary arterial hypertension. An ideal agent has short biologic half-life, is safe (and relatively free of systemic side effects), and easily administered. Immediate-release nifedipine has a half-life of 2 to 5 hours and administration of this formulation has been associated with stroke and death. Both verapamil and diltiazem also have a longer half-life making titration to maximal effect challenging and often resulting in systemic hypotension. Prostacyclin has been used, particularly epoprostenol intravenously, and some studies have evaluated other prostacyclin analogs given intravenously as well as inhaled iloprost. Administration of treprostinil subcutaneously would offer challenges and unnecessary patient discomfort. Additionally, IV adenosine has been used. The best answer is inhaled NO, as among these options it has a rapid onset (<10 s) and produces little rebound hypertension. Inhaled options also offer the advantage of avoiding systemic effects (Ghofrani HA, et al. *Circulation* 2008;118(11):1195–1201).

8.7 Answer B. Norepinephrine is an important vasoactive medication with mixed effects on the α_1 and β_1 receptors across all doses. Due to the potent effects on the α_1 receptors, administration increases SVR, PAWP, MAP, and HR, but has a somewhat neutral effect on cardiac output. The usual starting dose is 2 mcg/min and ranges up to 30 mcg/min. Norepinephrine, often in combination with vasopressin, appears to be the drug of choice in septic shock. In cardiogenic shock, recent studies have suggested that norepinephrine may decrease mortality compared to dopamine (De Backer D, et al. *N Engl J Med* 2010;362(9):779–789). Norepinephrine and phenylephrine are preferred over epinephrine in vasodilatory shock as they produce more vasoconstrictive than cardiostimulatory effects due to predominantly their α_1 effect.

8.8 Answer E. Anaphylactoid reactions secondary to contrast media rarely occur (<0.5%) in patients undergoing coronary angiography. Early treatment should include IV steroids; however, it will take several hours for steroids to have an effect; therefore, they should not be used alone in severe reactions. If hypotension (vasodilatory shock) is evident, epinephrine should be administered in bolus doses of 10 mcg every minute until MAP is >60 mm Hg. A 10-mcg dose can be easily made by diluting 0.1 mL of 1:1,000 (1 mg/mL) epinephrine in 9.9 mL of 0.9% normal saline, resulting in a final concentration of 10 mcg/mL. If continued epinephrine support is needed, then 1 to 4 mcg/min continuous infusion may be given. For minor or moderate reactions, epinephrine can be administered subcutaneously with 0.3 mL of 1:1,000 solution (0.3 mg) every 15 minutes up to a total dose of 1 mg. Minor reactions such as isolated urticaria can be treated with IV diphenhydramine, 25 to 50 mg. Of note, anaphylactic reactions occur much more frequently (17% to 35%) in patients with previous sensitivity. Identification of patients with prior reaction and pretreatment with steroid and antihistamines are important for preventing this potentially serious reaction.

8.9 Answer E. Phenylephrine is a pure alpha agonist with no to minimal beta-adrenergic effects. Therefore, it can be administered without increasing heart rate. Isoproterenol is incorrect as it is a chronotropic agent (i.e., increases heart rate) with minimal vasoconstrictor activity. While dopamine and epinephrine will help increase SVR, they have mixed beta activity (at all doses with epinephrine and at doses required for vasoconstriction with dopamine); therefore, they may further increase HR. Finally, dobutamine does not result in vasoconstriction and is best utilized in patients with low CI or evidence of hypoperfusion without profound hypotension.

8.10 Answer D. Before administration of nitroglycerin, this patient should be questioned about medical management of his pulmonary arterial hypertension. A common treatment in patients with pulmonary arterial hypertension is phosphodiesterase inhibitors, which have the potential to interact with nitrates. Nitrates stimulate cGMP production, while phosphodiesterase inhibitors inhibit cGMP degradation. When combined, these two drug classes greatly potentiate cGMP levels, which can lead to hypotension and impaired coronary perfusion. All other therapies listed here would be appropriate for management of his ACS.

8.11 Answer B. This patient is having an inferior wall MI possibly with right ventricular involvement. Switching from high-dose dopamine to epinephrine is unlikely to be beneficial. Increasing the rate of IABP will not affect SBP, but will increase the diastolic pressure. Milrinone could increase myocardial ischemia and worsen hypotension. The initial treatment for hypotension associated with inferior wall and right ventricular infarction is generous IV volume administration. Administration of nitroglycerin is relatively contraindicated in patients with hypotension, particularly with right ventricular compromise.

8.12 Answer D. NO diffuses rapidly from endothelial cells into the surrounding vascular smooth muscle cells and increases the production of cGMP, which initiates a cascade of events leading to vascular smooth muscle relaxation. NO is a potent inhibitor of platelet aggregation in conjunction with endothelial-derived prostacyclin. NO also inhibits adhesion of neutrophils by at least two mechanisms: reducing the expression of adhesion molecules in normal vascular endothelium and via a direct effect on neutrophils, preventing adhesion.

8.13 Answer C. Labetalol is a beta-blocker with α_2 vasodilatory properties. Along with esmolol, labetalol is considered the preferred treatment of hypertensive crisis in patients with cardiac ischemia. Nitroglycerin is an excellent adjunct therapy, especially in patients with evidence of pulmonary edema, although it is not the preferred first-line therapy as its utility is often limited by side effects. Phentolamine is useful in patients with catecholamine-induced hypertension, such as those with pheochromocytoma. Unlike dihydropyridine calcium channel blockers, diltiazem is more useful in patients needing control of HR as opposed to BP. Fenoldopam is a selective dopamine-1 receptor agonist approved for the management of severe hypertension. It may be useful as an adjunct in this setting (for hypertension uncontrolled by labetalol and nitroglycerin) or as a first line in patients with acute renal injury in hypertensive emergency.

8.14 Answer A. Sodium nitroprusside has an immediate onset and a very short half-life that make it easily titratable. Sodium nitroprusside contains 44% cyanide by weight, which is released nonenzymatically from nitroprusside. Both cyanide and its renally eliminated metabolite, thiocyanate, can cause toxicity, including respiratory failure, coma, delirium, psychosis, and hypothyroidism. However, given the potential cyanide toxicity, it should be used at the lowest effective dose for the shortest duration possible, ideally <72 hours. It has demonstrated utility in the management of heart failure with reduced ejection fraction (EF) for rapid afterload reduction in patients with low-output and volume overload (Mullens W, et al. *J Am Coll Cardiol* 2008;52(3):200–207).

8.15 Answer D. Methylergonovine is a serotonin receptor agonist and has effects on both the vascular endothelium and the vascular smooth muscle. When the vascular endothelium is healthy, methylergonovine produces vasodilation through an endothelium-dependent (NO-mediated) mechanism that dominates the direct vasoconstrictor effects on the vascular smooth muscle. However, if the endothelium is abnormal, the direct smooth muscle vasoconstrictor action is unopposed, thereby causing "spasm" in the coronary artery segment. Methylergonovine has no effect on vasopressin receptors, thromboxane, or endothelin. Acetylcholine may also be used to diagnose CAS. Nitroglycerin should be readily available at the time of provocative testing to relieve CAS.

8.16 Answer C. Dopamine's beta1-adrenergic, alpha-adrenergic, and dopaminergic effects are based on the dosing rate (Table A8-16). At low doses (<5 mcg/kg/min), dopamine primarily affects the dopamine receptor. This may increase urine output and renal blood flow. Between 5 and 10 mcg/kg/min (moderate doses), heart rate is increased, along with cardiac contractility and cardiac output. Doses > 10 mcg/kg/min also stimulate the alpha-1 receptor, providing increase in BP. In this patient, 15 mcg/kg/min would likely increase HR and BP. Given the short half-life, no bolus is needed with initiation or titration.

Table A8-16 Dopamine pharmacologic and clinical effects

Dopamine Dose	α	β_1	β_2	DA	VC	VD	INT
1–5 mcg/kg/min	–	+	–	++++	–	+	++
5–10 mcg/kg/min	–	++++	++	++++	–	+	++++
>10–20 mcg/kg/min	+++	++++	+	–	+++	–	+++

DA, dopamine receptor; INT, inotropic; VC, vasoconstriction; VD, vasodilation.

8.17 Answer D. At low-doses, <5 mcg/kg/min, dopamine primarily exerts its effects on the dopamine receptors (D1 and D2). D1 increases intracellular cAMP and directly mediates vasodilation; the presynaptic D2 receptor inhibits the release of norepinephrine release, resulting indirectly in vasodilation. While it was once believed that low-dose (or renal dose) dopamine would be renal protective and/or decrease the incidence of renal failure, it has been demonstrated that it may just help resolve oliguria without improving other renal outcomes. Data do not support its prophylactic use in the prevention of kidney injury during catheterization procedures, as it is no more effective than adequate hydration. Related to extravasation, the alpha-1 vasoconstriction properties of the medication and the local drug concentration—and not the rate of infusion—affect tissue ischemia and sloughing when infiltration occurs. Therefore, whenever possible, medications with vasoconstricting properties should be administered through a central line (Kellum JA, et al. *Crit Care Med* 2001;29(8):1526-1531; Gare M, et al. *J Am Coll Cardiol* 1999;34(6):1682-1688).

8.18 Answer E. In general, once extravasation is observed, the infusion should be discontinued, followed by slow aspiration of as much of the drug as possible. Although other medications may respond to cold or warm compresses, catecholamines (i.e., dopamine, epinephrine, phenylephrine and norepinephrine) should be treated immediately with phentolamine. This alpha-adrenergic blocker can be used to the block the hypertensive effects of pheochromocytoma and, in turn, is useful in the diagnosis of this condition. As in this case, it is also useful for counteracting the effects of alpha-adrenergic stimulants. Phentolamine is prepared by diluting 5 mg in 10 mL of normal saline and injecting subcutaneously into the affected area. Hyaluronidase and sodium thiosulfate are antidotes for other drug extravasations.

8.19 Answer A. Given this patient's low cardiac output, an agent with positive inotropic support is indicated. This patient would likely respond best to dobutamine, an inotropic agent (beta agonist), which would not have significant impact on afterload. Although dopamine is also a strong beta agonist, it can also increase SVR; however, this patient is not currently in shock (adequate MAP). Milrinone is a phosphodiesterase inhibitor that does increase inotropy; however, it also causes significant vasodilation, which may lower this patient's MAP. It also has a long half-life (2 to 4 hours), which is further increased in renal failure (20 hours). Although certain beta-blockers have been demonstrated to prolong survival in chronic heart failure, esmolol produces bradycardia and hypotension, decreases cardiac output, and is contraindicated in this clinical scenario. Likewise, norepinephrine would likely increase SVR (which tends to be elevated in heart failure with reduced EF), and it is not as potent an inotrope as dobutamine.

8.20 Answer B. At low doses (<30 mcg/min), nitroglycerin is primarily a venodilator. At doses of 30 mcg/min and above, it begins to exhibit balanced venous and arterial dilation as well. Therefore, with an increased dose, it is likely that the patient's BP will begin to decrease, and she will have an improvement in ischemic symptoms. Studies comparing nitroprusside and nitroglycerin show an increase in coronary collateral flow with nitroglycerin and a decrease in flow with nitroprusside. In the modern era, early IV metoprolol has not been shown to reduce infarct size in patients experiencing STEMI. Morphine should be reserved for pain unrelieved by nitroglycerin. This patient does not exhibit nitroglycerin adverse drug reactions; therefore, uptitration of nitroglycerin should be prioritized over administration of morphine. Morphine also may interfere with antiplatelet onset and effectiveness.

9 Guide Catheter Selection for Coronary Interventions

Timothy A. Mixon and Elizabeth M. Holper

INTRODUCTION

Intelligent guide catheter selection and use are areas of interventional cardiology that frequently rely on the *art* of medicine more than the *science* of medicine. Although there are reports describing specific types of guide catheters and their use, there are almost no randomized trials. In fact, more than most other elements of the catheterization laboratory experience, guide catheter selection is influenced less by evidence-based medicine and more by the habits and biases of the operator's mentors or by specific institutional availability of equipment. Furthermore, it is likely that most operators have learned or improved their guide catheter selection by *trial and error*.

The guide catheter has several functions during coronary intervention, including:

1. Arterial pressure monitoring throughout the procedure
2. Delivery of radiographic contrast to visualize the vessel, stenoses, and device positioning during the intervention
3. Providing adequate axial support, or "backup," to allow delivery of interventional devices to the diseased area
4. Serving as a conduit for passage of the coronary guidewire and all interventional equipment

The development of diagnostic and guide catheters has occurred in three progressive phases:

Phase I: Limited catheter choices with the need for operators to shape catheters using "shaping" instruments and applying heat to "fix" the shape

Phase II: Development and adoption of preformed catheters, but types and sizes were limited to many of the basic shapes (Judkins left and right, Amplatz left and right, etc.)

Phase III: Proliferation of new and unique shapes, such as the Q-curve and Voda/XB/EBU shape, in addition to multiple specialized shapes (Fig. 9) designed to improve coaxial fit, enhance support, and allow radial artery intervention, as well as improve catheter characteristics such as softer, less traumatic tips, and larger usable lumens.

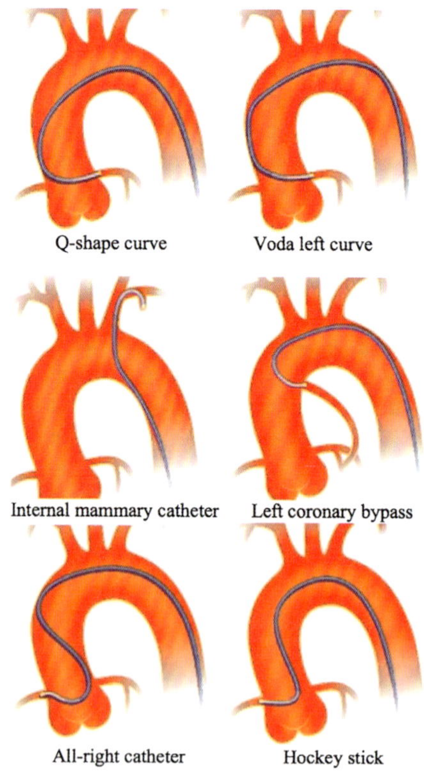

Figure 9 Illustration of the proliferation of catheter shapes. Various vendors have slight variations. For example, the Q curve is similar to the XB-LAD (Cordis) and the JCL (Medtronic) catheters. The Voda left is similar to the XB (Cordis) and EBU (Medtronic) catheters. (Image courtesy of Boston Scientific, Natick, MA.)

STRUCTURE AND CHARACTERISTICS OF A GUIDE CATHETER

Catheters are engineered to maximize multiple properties, although there may be competing interests, for example, maximum stiffness vs. atraumatic design. The ideal guide catheter will maximize lumen size to allow easy passage of interventional equipment with sufficient space to allow accurate pressure monitoring and injection of contrast. In contrast to diagnostic catheters, this is accomplished by designing guide catheters with thinner walls, although adequate *torque control* must be maintained. The ideal guide should balance good *flexibility* while maintaining *kink resistance* and *shore hardness* (i.e., the relative resistance to indentation by a specific force). Additionally, *biocompatibility*, adequate *lubricity*, and *resistance to thrombogenicity* are desirable characteristics.

Guide catheters have a three-layer design. The outer layer is typically a synthetic polymer such as polyurethane, polyether-ester, or other proprietary compounds. The inner layer is smooth and lubricious (e.g., may be lined with polytetrafluoroethylene [PTFE] or other similar compounds), while the middle layer is a wire or nylon braid. Advanced engineering has allowed this middle braid to become stronger yet flatter, which has yielded larger lumen guides that still maintain adequate torque control and support.

Sizing of guide catheters

The size of a guide catheter is referenced to its outer diameter (OD) expressed as French (Fr) size. One Fr is 0.33 mm; thus, a 6 Fr guiding catheter has an OD of 2 mm, a 7 Fr is 2.33 mm, etc.

In contrast, the size of a sheath is referenced to its inner diameter (ID). Therefore, a 7 Fr sheath has an ID of 2.33 mm and thus can accommodate a 7 Fr guide, while the sheath's outer diameter is of necessity larger. This distinction is especially important for peripheral vascular intervention where cases may be performed through sheaths alone, without a guide catheter. As a general rule, a device will require a guiding catheter two French sizes larger than the corresponding sheath size used. For example, if a carotid stent can be passed through a 6 Fr sheath but a guiding catheter is required to complete the procedure, an 8 Fr guide catheter should be selected.

QUESTIONS

9.1 You are performing coronary angiography from the femoral approach on a 56-year-old commercial airline pilot who has atypical chest pain, but a small inferior perfusion defect. After attempting to cannulate the left main with a Judkins left (JL) 4 catheter, the following coronary angiogram is obtained (Fig. Q9-1). The most likely diagnosis and a maneuver to obtain additional images of the left coronary tree is:

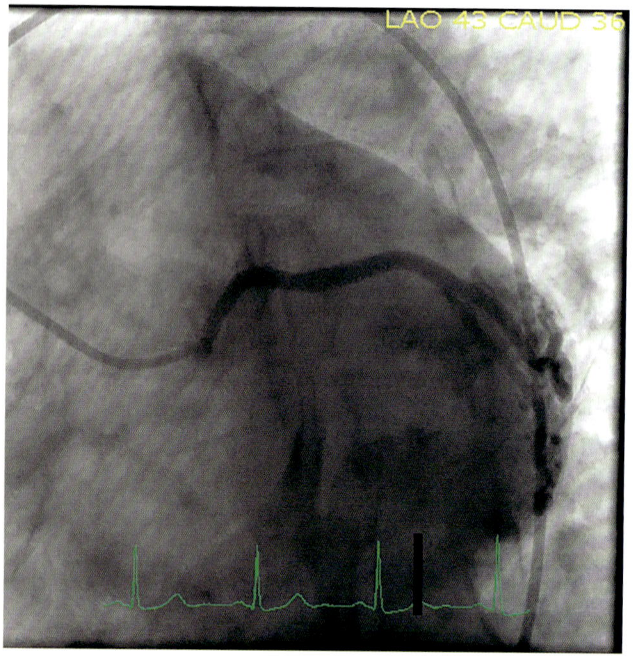

Figure Q9-1

(A) Anomalous origin of a coronary artery from the right sinus of Valsalva; change to a multipurpose catheter and look for the anomalous artery in the right cusp
(B) Separate coronary ostia; change to a JL 3.5
(C) Separate coronary ostia; change to a JL 4.5
(D) Anomalous origin of a coronary artery from the pulmonary artery; perform a pulmonary angiogram
(E) Stop the procedure and perform a computed tomography (CT) coronary angiogram

9.2 Treatment of a distal left anterior descending (LAD) stenosis through a long, tortuous left internal mammary (IM) artery bypass graft is most likely to be successful using the following guide catheter:

(A) Standard IM-A curve guide catheter
(B) Newer, IM-C curve guide catheter
(C) Judkins right (JR) 4 guide catheter
(D) 90 cm IM guide catheter
(E) A left radial approach with a standard IM guide catheter

9.3 Angiography is performed in a patient with a remote history of coronary artery bypass surgery, which included a vein graft to the right coronary artery (RCA). After imaging the RCA with a JR 4 catheter, you seek the vein graft with the same catheter and obtain the image shown in Figure Q9-3. The angiogram obtained is felt to be inadequate. The best alternative catheter choice for more selective images would be:

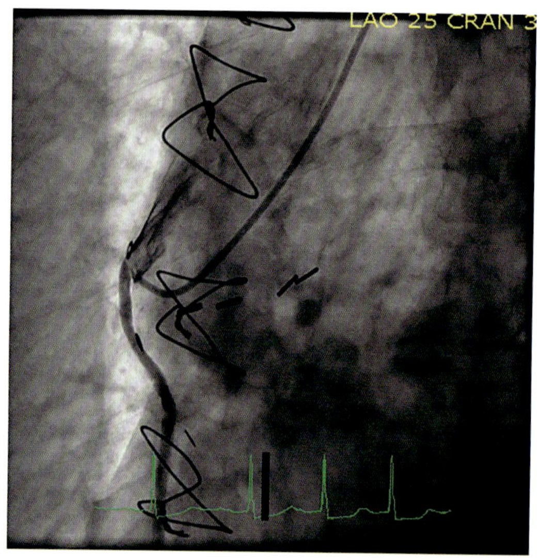

Figure Q9-3

(A) Amplatz left (AL) 1
(B) Multipurpose (MP) 1
(C) No-torque right (NTR)
(D) Hockey stick (HS)
(E) IM-A curve

9.4 You are asked to perform percutaneous coronary intervention (PCI) on a diffuse stenosis in the left circumflex (LCx) and obtuse marginal artery of a woman with an occluded bypass graft to the first obtuse marginal (OM1) branch. You note that the vessel is somewhat tortuous and moderately calcified (Fig. Q9-4), so you anticipate the need for good guide catheter support. Diagnostic angiography was performed from the right radial artery. Which of the following is the most reasonable plan for guide catheter support during PCI?

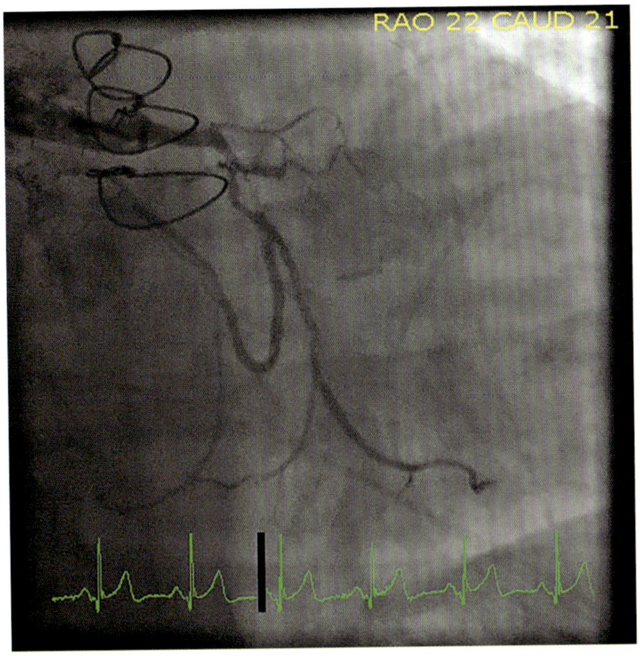

Figure Q9-4

(A) Continue from the radial approach using a 6 Fr system with plans to enhance support using a 6 Fr GuideLiner or Guidezilla if necessary
(B) This is unlikely to be successful from the radial approach due to the lesion length and tortuosity; convert to a femoral approach
(C) This can be done from the radial approach using a 6 Fr JL 4
(D) Upsize to a 8 Fr system for enhanced support and proceed from the radial site
(E) Continue from the radial approach, but use a guide catheter with side holes and deep seat the catheter into the mid-LCx

9.5 Which of the following is a concern that should be considered when selecting larger French size guide catheters over smaller diameter guide catheters?

(A) Increased potential for trauma at the ostium of the artery selected for intervention
(B) Larger arteriotomy site with increased risk of bleeding and delay to ambulation
(C) Increased contrast volume use
(D) Increased potential for embolization of atherosclerotic debris from the aortic wall
(E) All of the above

9.6 You are performing coronary angiography in a 52-year-old man with typical angina and a reversible lateral wall defect demonstrated on a stress myocardial perfusion study. There were no coronary stenoses seen in the LAD, which arose normally from the left main, but the circumflex was not visualized. The RCA has minimal atherosclerotic narrowing; an anomalous origin of the LCx is seen near the RCA ostium (Fig. Q9-6) with a high-grade obstruction identified in the mid-LCx. Since the lesion found matches the area of abnormal perfusion, you proceed with PCI. Which of the following would be a POOR choice for a guide catheter in this case?

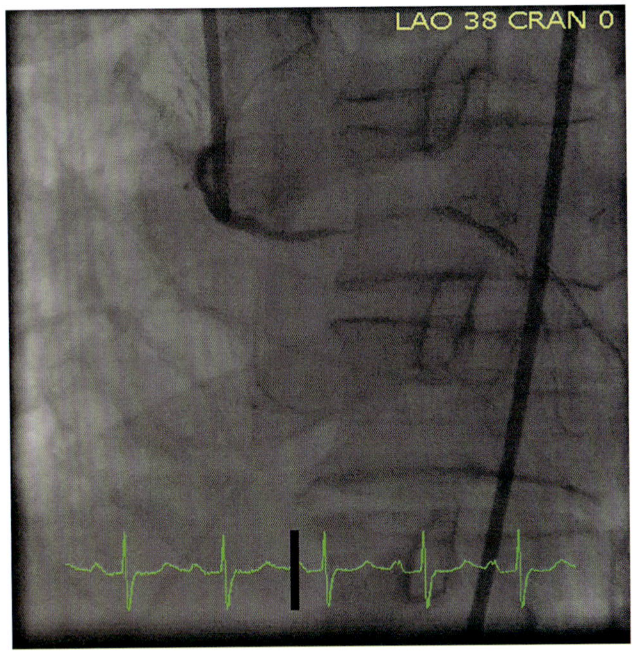

Figure Q9-6

(A) JR 4
(B) MP 1
(C) Amplatz right (AR) 1
(D) Voda left (VL) 4
(E) HS

9.7 You are asked to perform PCI on a heavily calcified mid-LAD stenosis in a 76-year-old woman with exertional angina and an abnormal stress test. She is 5 ft 4 in. tall and weighs 112 lb. Her diagnostic catheterization was done via radial artery access. What is the largest Rotablator burr recommended by the manufacturer that can be used with a 6 Fr guide catheter?

(A) 1.25-mm burr
(B) 1.5-mm burr
(C) 1.75-mm burr
(D) 2-mm burr
(E) 2.15-mm burr

9.8 A 55-year-old woman with diabetes and prior stenting of her RCA 6 years ago presents with exertional angina. Angiography reveals occlusion of her mid-RCA stent (type 4 in-stent restenosis) as seen in Figure Q9-8. In planning PCI, an appropriate guide catheter choice might include:

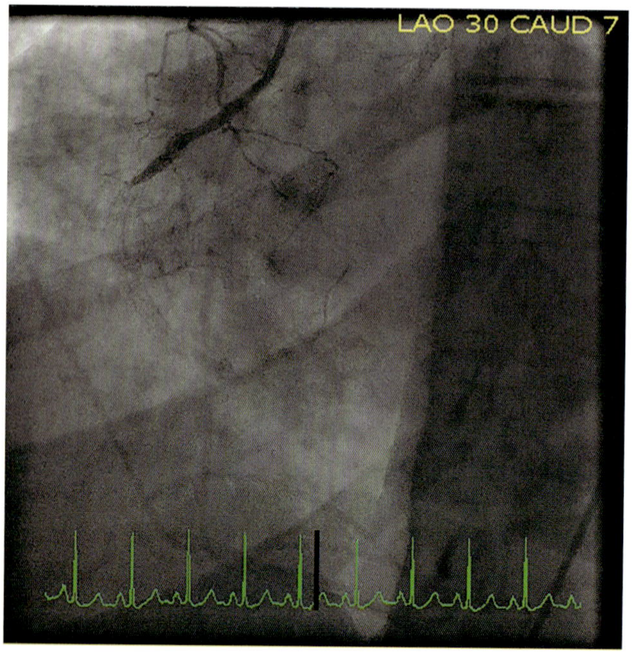

Figure Q9-8

(A) IM
(B) AL 1
(C) JR 4
(D) allRight (ART) 1
(E) AR 1

9.9 You are performing coronary angiography before possible PCI in a 60-year-old man who presented late after an inferior myocardial infarction (MI). He now has angina during his daily activities. He is 5-ft-10 in. tall, has a normal build, and no history of hypertension. You are planning access from the right radial artery since his Allen's test is normal. Acceptable catheter choices include all of the following, EXCEPT:

(A) JL 3.5
(B) Jacky catheter
(C) Kimny catheter
(D) JR 3.5
(E) Ikari left catheter

9.10 You are asked to treat a bifurcation stenosis that consists of two approximately equal-sized branches with disease primarily located at the ostium of each branch (Medina classification 0,1,1). You elect a strategy of simultaneous kissing stents. Which of the following is the smallest French guide catheter that would provide an adequate lumen size for your planned approach?

(A) 6 Fr guide catheter
(B) New generation large lumen 7 Fr guide catheter
(C) 8 Fr guide catheter
(D) 5 Fr guide catheter
(E) 8 Fr large lumen guide catheter

9.11 A 45-year-old construction worker presents with progressive angina for the past year. He has been reluctant to seek medical attention because of fear he will lose his job, but he can no longer perform his regular work duties because of angina. After obtaining an abnormal stress test, coronary angiography is performed showing an occluded mid-LAD. One of your colleagues has unsuccessfully attempted to open the chronic total occlusion (CTO) via an antegrade approach, so the patient is referred to you to consider a retrograde approach through one of the septal collateral channels (Fig. Q9-11A and B). When considering guide catheter choice, you should consider all of the following, EXCEPT:

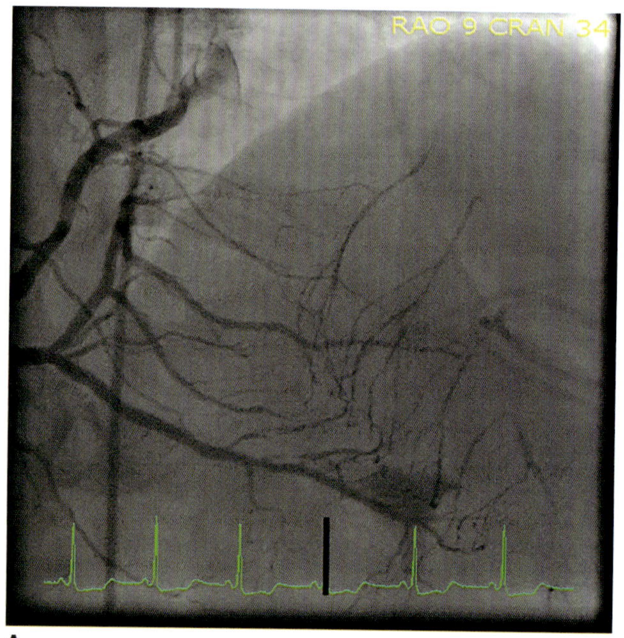

A

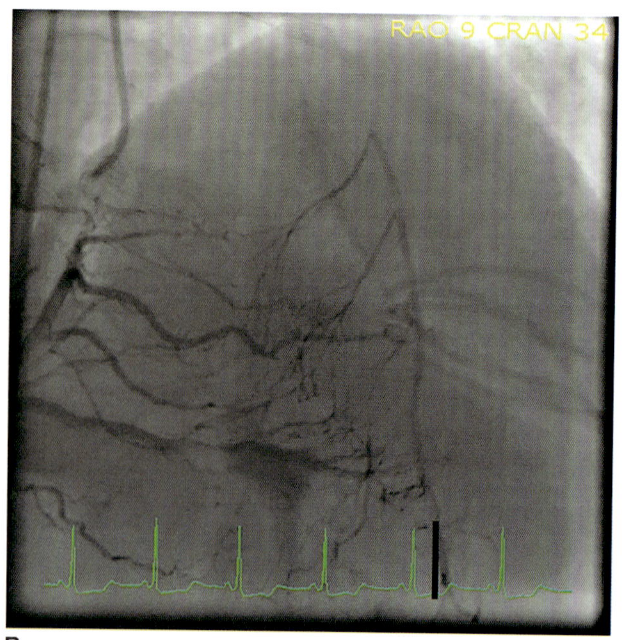

B

Figure Q9-11

(A) Shortening the retrograde guide catheter in anticipation of a longer distance for CTO wires and microcatheters due to the retrograde approach
(B) Use an 8 Fr guide catheter for enhanced support
(C) Use a 6 Fr JR 4 to minimize vessel trauma
(D) Use a 90-cm length guide catheter in the retrograde guide
(E) Use two 8 Fr guide catheters to allow visualization of the occluded vessel from an antegrade and retrograde view

9.12 An 84-year-old man with a prior CoreValve placed for severe symptomatic aortic stenosis presents with escalating angina despite maximal medical therapy. Prior to his transcatheter aortic valve replacement (TAVR), he had undergone PCI of his proximal LCx. Diagnostic catheterization was challenging to successfully engage the left main (Fig. Q9-12A–C), but ultimately demonstrated significant in-stent restenosis of the proximal LCx stent. Which of the following is FALSE regarding guide catheter choice for this case?

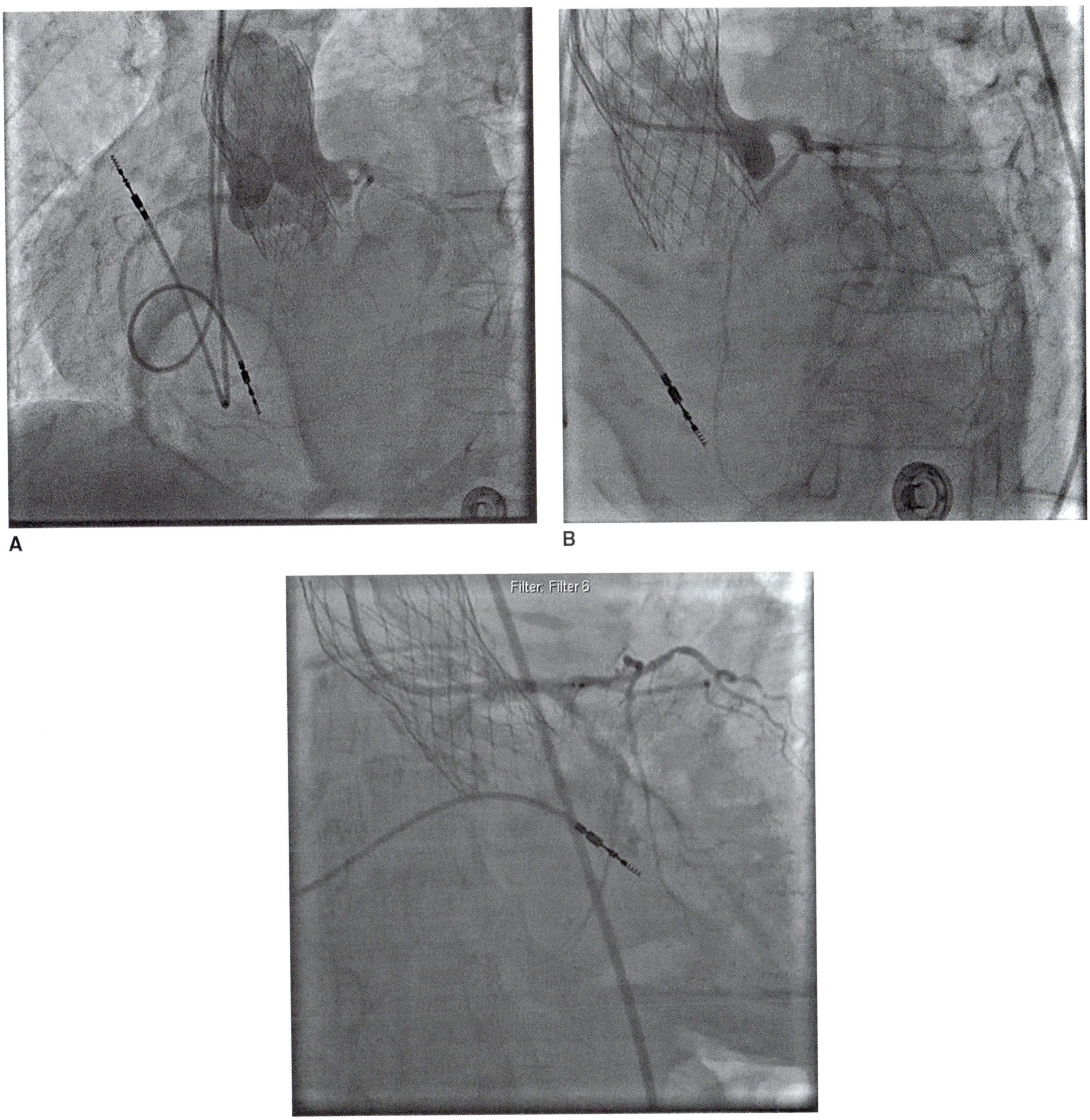

Figure Q9-12 (Courtesy of Timothy Mixon and Elizabeth Holper.)

(A) Engagement of the left main coronary artery may be more challenging with a CoreValve compared to an Edwards Sapien valve placed below the coronary ostia
(B) The open-cell configuration of the CoreValve is designed to cover the ostia of the coronary arteries
(C) It may require several guide attempts to successfully engage the left main coronary artery through the struts of the valve
(D) Femoral access or left radial access may facilitate easier engagement of the left main
(E) Care must be taken not to damage the Nitinol frame or valve leaflets of the TAVR bioprosthesis

9.13 You initially have difficulty cannulating the left main artery in a woman who is 5 ft 0 in. and weighs 245 lb. Your assessment of the JL 4 catheter shows the tip to consistently lie in the left cusp just inferior to the origin of the left main origin (Fig. Q9-13). Which of the following maneuvers is most likely to engage the left main?

(A) Change to a JL 5
(B) Have the patient take a deep breath and attempt to engage the left main again

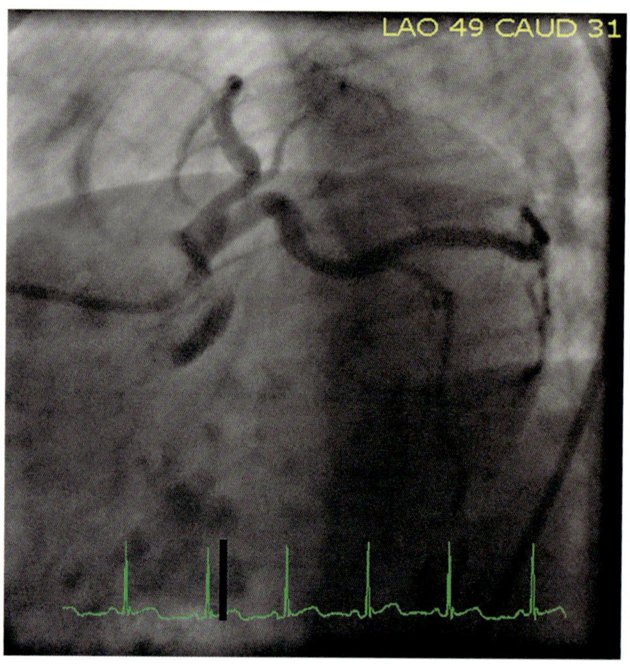

Figure Q9-13

(C) Change to a MP 1
(D) Change to an AL 2
(E) Change to a VL 4

9.14 A 56-year-old man with a history of prior bypass surgery presents with increasing exertional angina. During a stress test, he develops 2 mm of horizontal ST-segment depression in the anterior leads at a heart rate of 104 beats per minute (bpm). Diagnostic angiography shows a severe stenosis in the body of the vein graft to the LAD. Which of the following guide catheters is least likely to cannulate the vein graft and provide adequate support for PCI?

(A) NTR
(B) JR 4
(C) HS
(D) Left coronary bypass (LCB) or left graft seeker
(E) AL 1

9.15 A 64-year-old man with a recent transient ischemic attack (TIA) is found to have a 90% stenosis of his proximal right internal carotid artery. He has a prior history of surgery and radiation for a squamous cell carcinoma of the neck and is deemed to be high risk for carotid endarterectomy. He is referred to you for carotid stenting. His initial aortogram is shown (Fig. Q9-15). Which of the following is the best guide catheter to cannulate the innominate artery?

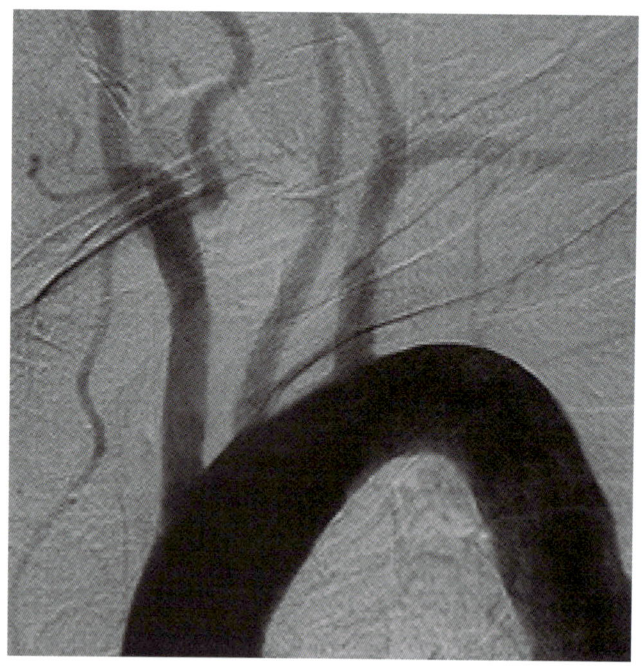

Figure Q9-15

(A) JR 4
(B) IM
(C) Simmons 1
(D) Vertebral catheter
(E) JB 1

9.16 You are asked to treat a heavily calcified mid-RCA stenosis. Considerations for proper guide catheter selection before rotational atherectomy includes all of the following, EXCEPT:

(A) Adequate French size to accommodate the anticipated required burr
(B) Presence of side holes
(C) Coaxial positioning at the vessel ostium
(D) Deep seating potential to allow maximum support
(E) Adequate catheter tip stiffness to maintain position in the coronary ostium

9.17 You are asked to intervene on a small Asian woman (59 in. tall) who has a simple, short, mid-LAD stenosis and suffers from predictable angina, despite adequate medical therapy. Your partner performed angiography with a 5 Fr diagnostic catheter via the right radial approach, but noted—based on ultrasound-guided access—that her radial artery was quite small. Which is the least desirable option?

(A) Perform PCI using a 5 Fr guiding system
(B) Perform PCI with a 6.5 Fr Sheathless Eaucath system
(C) Switch to a femoral approach using a 6 Fr guiding catheter
(D) Use a 6 Fr guide catheter through a 6 Fr Glidesheath Slender sheath
(E) Switch to a left radial approach

9.18 After diagnostic angiography with a 5 Fr system, you are asked to treat a focal stenosis in the mid-LAD. Upon placement of a 7 Fr JL 4 guide catheter, you notice significant dampening of the pressure waveform (Fig. Q9-18). Which of the following is the best course of action?

(A) Manipulate the catheter in the left main in an attempt to improve the waveform
(B) Change to a catheter with side holes
(C) Perform intravascular ultrasound (IVUS) to better understand the geometry and presence of any disease in the left main
(D) Downsize to a 6 Fr guide catheter
(E) Proceed with the PCI, but disengage the guide once the wire is across the stenosis

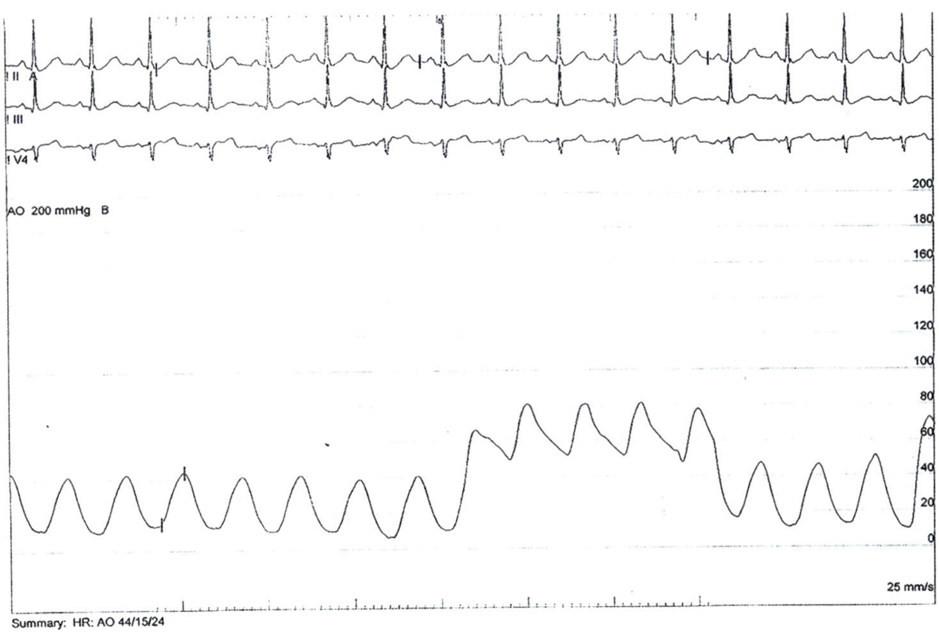

Figure Q9-18

9.19 You are asked to intervene on a mid-LAD and diagonal branch in a 78-year-old Asian woman (Fig. Q9-19A). Your partner has performed angiography from a femoral approach, having to use a JL 4.5 to cannulate the left main. You choose a 6 Fr Extra Backup (EBU) 4.0 as a guide. As you are placing the first stent, the invasive pressure reading declines significantly. The following image is obtained (Fig. Q9-19B). What is the likely cause of the decreased pressure reading?

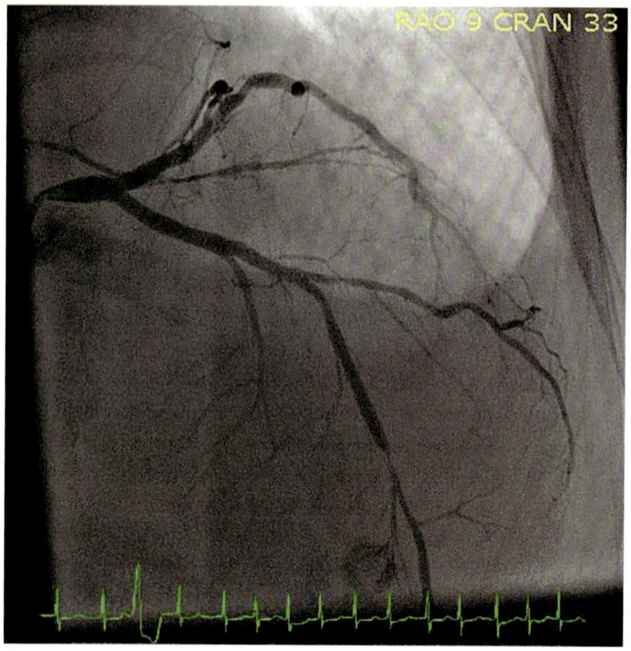

A

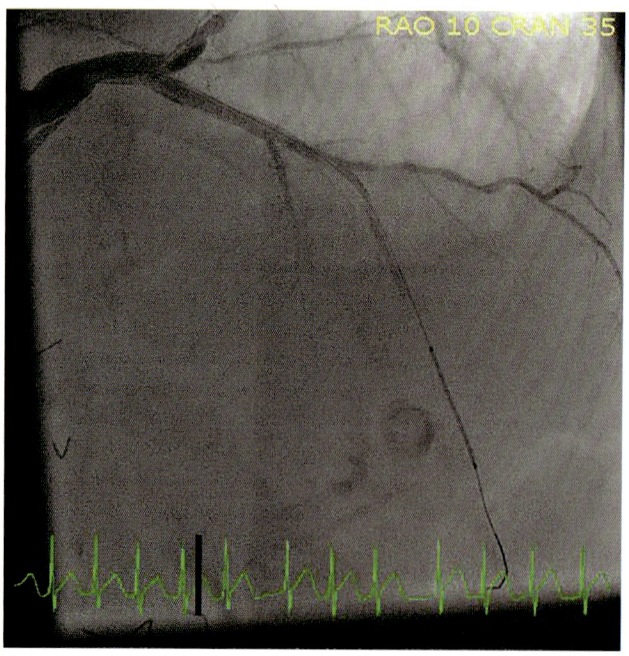

B

Figure Q9-19 (Courtesy of Timothy Mixon and Elizabeth Holper.)

(A) Air within the guide catheter causing "dampening"
(B) Lack of coaxial guide catheter positioning
(C) It is likely an artifact related to a stent catheter being within the guide
(D) Left main catheter-induced dissection
(E) Suspect retroperitoneal hemorrhage

9.20 You are asked to perform PCI to correct a severe stenosis in a large third marginal branch of a tortuous LCx. Which of the following catheters is least likely to provide adequate backup support?

(A) XB 3.5
(B) EBU 4
(C) AL 2
(D) VL 3.5
(E) JL 4

9.21 A 60-year-old woman presents with atypical angina. A dobutamine echocardiogram showed mild hypokinesis of the inferior wall. Coronary angiography showed no disease in the left coronary, but an anomalous RCA originating superior to the usual location and midway between the left coronary and the usual position of the RCA ostium. The operator performing the diagnostic study had considerable difficulty engaging the anomalous RCA, but the angiograms showed a severe stenosis in the mid-to-distal RCA. Which of the following types of guide catheters is least likely to successfully cannulate the RCA?

(A) JR family
(B) Voda (XB, EBU)
(C) JL family
(D) AL family
(E) Q-curve catheter

9.22 After diagnostic angiography, PCI is requested of a mid-RCA stenosis. The diagnostic operator had difficulty accessing the aorta from the femoral artery and subsequently "kinked" a 6 Fr JR 4 catheter while attempting to rotate it into the RCA ostium. Angiography of the iliac vessels (Fig. Q9-22) reveals extremely tortuous, although widely patent, vessels. Which of the following options is least likely to result in a smooth and successful procedure?

(A) Convert to a radial artery approach
(B) Using a stiff Amplatz wire, exchange the short diagnostic sheath for a 7 Fr 45 cm sheath
(C) Upsize to a short, 8 Fr sheath and use an 8 Fr guide catheter
(D) Use a long 8 Fr sheath and a 7 Fr JR 4 guide catheter
(E) Use a 6 Fr JR 4 guide catheter

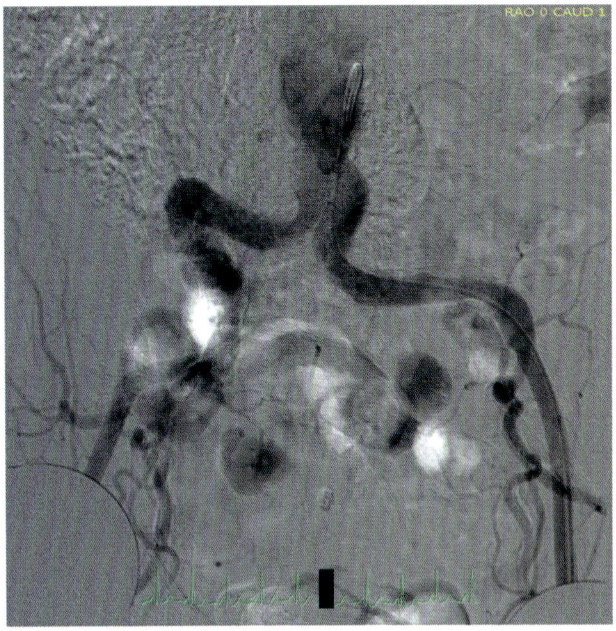

Figure Q9-22

9.23 Upon placement of a 6 Fr guide catheter into the ostium of the coronary artery with a significant stenosis, the waveform seen in Figure Q9-23 is observed. The catheter is immediately removed from the ostium but the waveform remains the same. What is the most likely explanation for this waveform?

(A) Kinking of the guide catheter
(B) Excessively deep intubation into the coronary artery
(C) Unappreciated significant stenosis at the ostium
(D) Obstruction of the guide lumen or pressure tubing with air or thrombus
(E) This is a normal waveform

9.24 You are asked to assist a colleague who has been unable to pass an embolic protection device into a tortuous, proximal vein graft to a circumflex marginal artery (Fig. Q9-24). A 6 Fr JR 4 guide catheter was being used but the guide catheter repeatedly disengaged from the graft ostium when the protection device was advanced. In addition to upsizing to an 8 Fr guide catheter, which of the following strategies would you recommend?

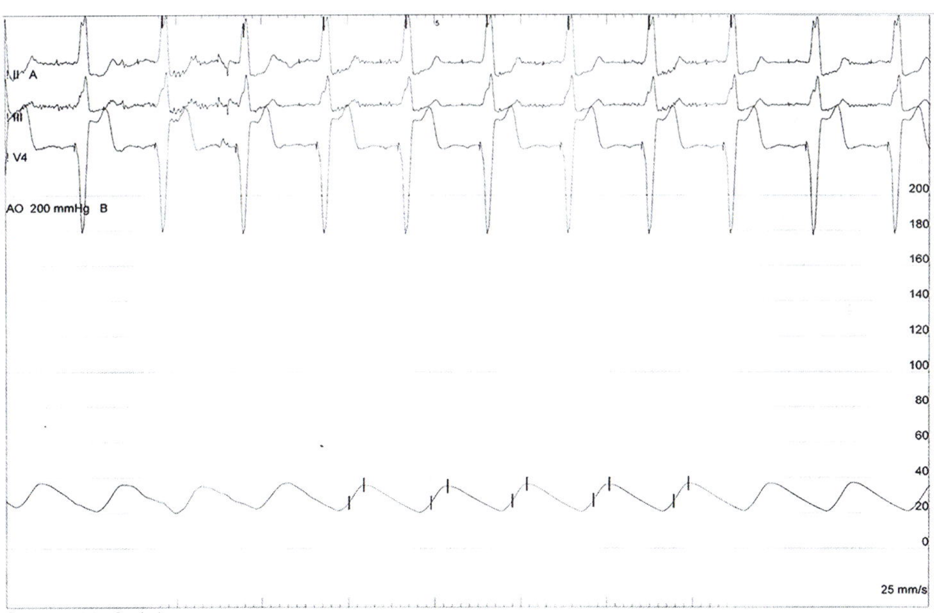

Figure Q9-23

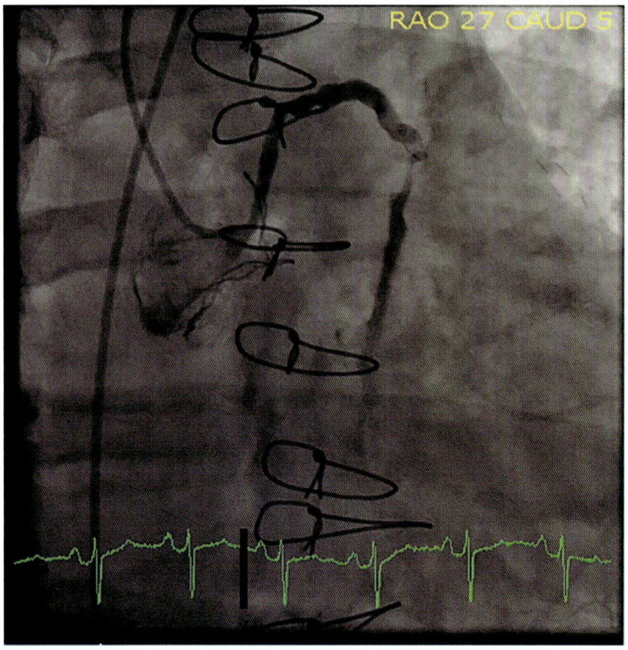

Figure Q9-24

(A) Change to an AL 1 guide
(B) A JR 4 guide in 8 Fr size will be adequate
(C) IM guide
(D) JL 5
(E) Any of the above is likely to be successful in an 8 Fr size

9.25 To achieve optimal support and coaxial alignment in treating a RCA with a "shepherd's crook" (upward takeoff) configuration, which of the following guide catheters would be best?

(A) AR 1
(B) JR 4
(C) AL 1
(D) HS
(E) NTR (Modified Williams)

9.26 A 62-year-old man with diabetes and a history of smoking presents with an inferior ST-segment elevation myocardial infarction (STEMI). You recommend a right radial artery approach. Based on the electrocardiogram (ECG), it is uncertain whether the etiology of the infarction is a RCA or LCx occlusion. Based on your uncertainty of the infarct artery and wanting to image the left coronary system first to assure that he does not have left main disease given his risk factors, you wish to use a catheter that will allow you to image both coronary arteries quickly and then also perform PCI, if necessary, through it. Which of the following catheters would be the best choice?

(A) JL 3.5
(B) Ikari left 3.5 (IL 3.5)
(C) AL 2
(D) JR 4
(E) EBU 4

ANSWERS AND EXPLANATIONS

9.1 Answer B. Separate ostia of the left coronary artery or a very short left main artery is one of the most common coronary anomalies (occurring in approximately 1% of patients) and must be recognized by the operator. In this circumstance, it is often better to selectively cannulate and obtain separate angiograms of the LCx and LAD than to obtain inadequate angiograms of both vessels by a suboptimal catheter position. In this patient, a JL 4 catheter selectively entered the LCx. The most likely maneuver to selectively cannulate the LAD is to change to the next smaller Judkins curve size, in this case, a JL 3.5 (Fig. A9-1A–C). Other maneuvers that may work are to withdraw the JL 4 slightly and apply clockwise rotation, which will direct the tip anteriorly, allowing cannulation of the LAD. Additionally, a smaller backup guide, such as an XB 3.0 or EBU 3.5, may allow engagement of each separate ostia selectively. A longer Judkins catheter (JL 4.5) would place the tip inferior to the LCx ostium. CT coronary angiography can be very helpful to define the course of anomalous coronary arteries in difficult cases, but there is no reason to abort the case at this point without trying other maneuvers. This patient was found to have no significant coronary stenoses.

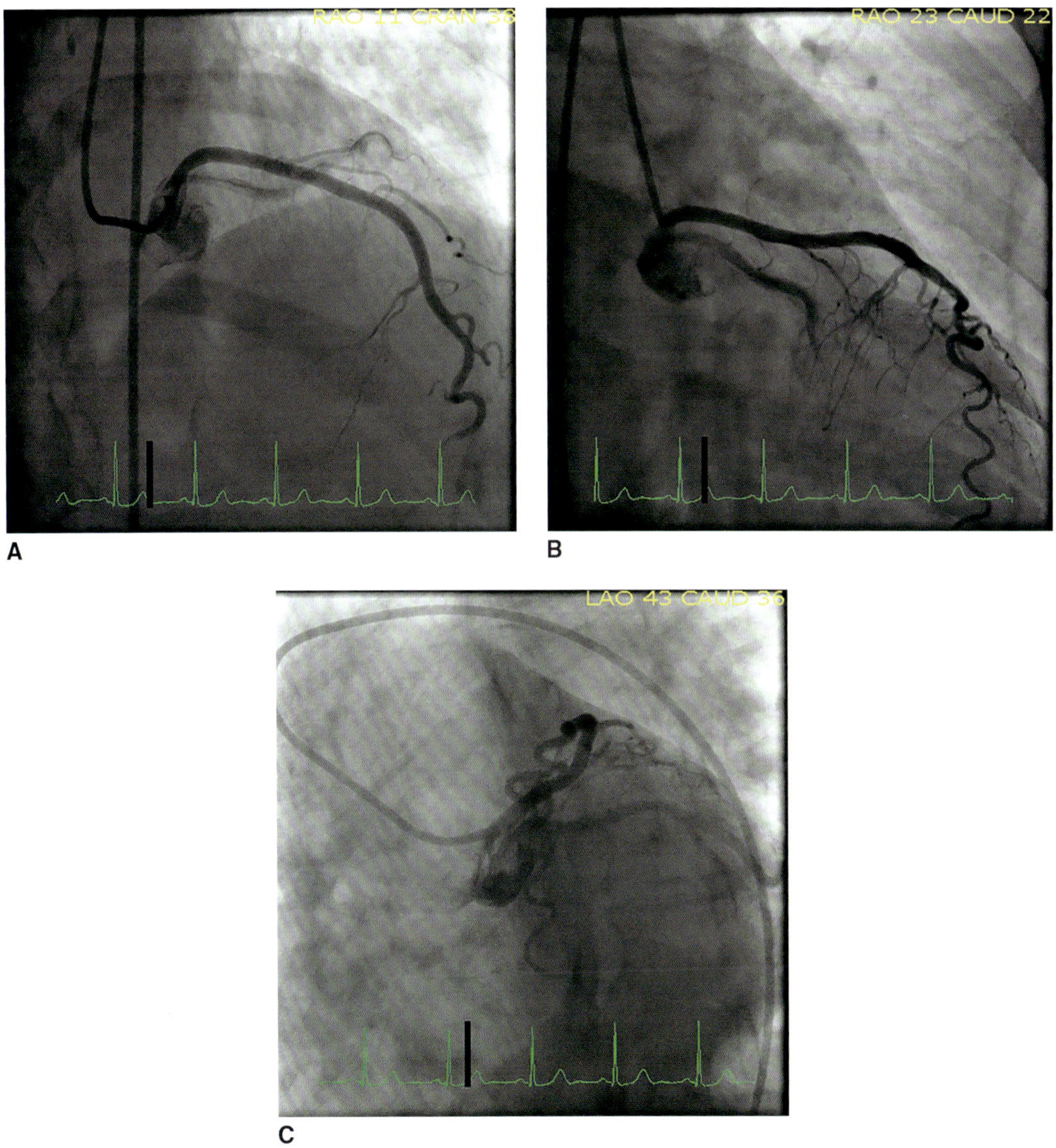

Figure A9-1

9.2 Answer D. When treating a stenosis that is very distal in the coronary artery or if it is necessary to approach the stenosis through a bypass conduit, a common technical limitation is the shaft length of the balloon or stent catheter (typically 135 cm). If a 90-cm guide is used, 10 additional centimeters of working length is preserved and may allow successful completion of the procedure. Alternatively, some balloons and stents may be obtained on longer shafts (e.g., 143 to 150 cm). Although not the only route to success, a left radial approach has gained popularity and could be utilized, but there would still be the need for a shorter guide catheter.

9.3 Answer B. Frequently, a JR 4 catheter can be used to cannulate many vein grafts, including those to the left or right coronary system. However, vein grafts to the RCA usually have an inferiorly directed origin with an acute angle from the aorta, such that the distal curve of the JR 4 may not allow selective cannulation. In this case, a catheter with a downward directed and longer tip is needed; an MP catheter is usually ideal (Fig. A9-3). In this example, it was placed at the ostium, which was adequate for diagnostic angiograms. With rotation, the tip can often be engaged deeper in the graft for more support during PCI. The NTR and IM-A have tips of inadequate length and shape to reach the ostium. In a normal aorta, the HS and AL 1 generally have the tip pointed in a cephalad direction, which would not be ideal for this graft origin.

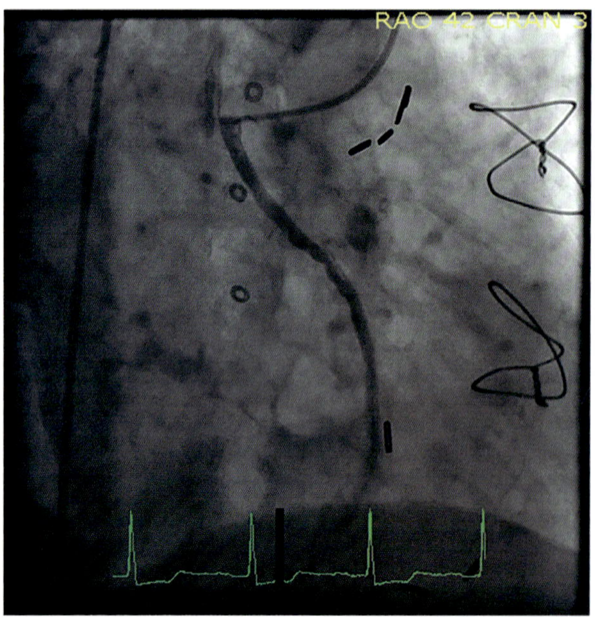

Figure A9-3

9.4 Answer A. Radial interventions are commonly performed in Europe and gradually gaining popularity in the US market. With more experience, operators are able to approach increasingly complex interventions with good success rates, thus immediate conversion to a femoral approach is rarely required. Nonetheless, adequate guide catheter support is required, and a 6 Fr JL 4 is unlikely to provide the necessary support in this case. Radial arteries are smaller than femoral arteries and rarely allow 8 Fr sheaths without increasing local complication rate (e.g., dissection, ischemia, thrombosis, or even vessel rupture). While deep seating the guide catheter can enhance support, it is utilized less frequently now and associated with an increased risk of vessel complication. A "guide within a guide," or telescoping technique, will greatly increase the support that a 6 Fr guide provides. Currently, this can be achieved using the GuideLiner system (Vascular Solutions, Minneapolis, MN), or the Guidezilla device (Boston Scientific, Maple Grove, MN). With either system, the additional support catheter goes inside of the guide catheter and can be placed within the proximal or even mid vessel (see Fig. A9-4 and note the GuideLiner placed into the proximal LCx). This not only enhances the performance of the parent guide catheter but also allows enhanced delivery of devices through the proximal and midvessel with less resistance. There are downsides and risks associated with such guide extenders, including (a) the reduction in the internal lumen of the guide catheter, which may limit the number or size of interventional equipment (e.g., bifurcation stenting, imaging or atherectomy equipment); (b) the risk of dissection of the proximal coronary artery from physically placing the guide extender through it; and (c) the risk of a hydraulic dissection due to contrast injection through the extender (Mamas MA, et al. *Catheter Cardiovasc Interv* 2010;76(1):102–111; Waterbury TM, et al. *Catheter Cardiovasc Interv* 2016;88(7):1057–1065).

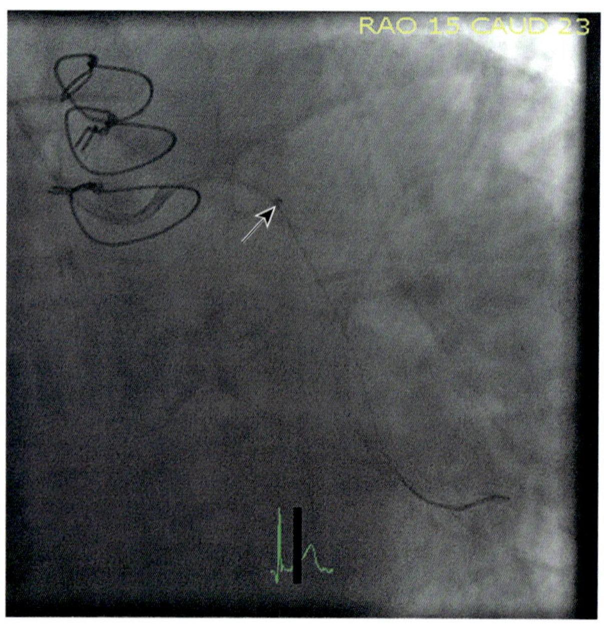

Figure A9-4

9.5 Answer E. Larger lumen catheters require larger introducer sheaths and thus have an increased potential for complications at the puncture site as well as the origin of the target vessel. Larger lumen catheters require a larger volume of contrast to fill the catheter and are associated with higher contrast loads. Care should be taken to limit contrast loads in patients with underlying renal dysfunction when larger diameter catheters are needed. Larger lumen catheters, especially 8 Fr, have been associated with more trauma to the aorta and the potential for producing atherosclerotic debris. This is especially true for certain shapes of catheters, including the JL, VL, and MP (Grossman PM, et al. *JACC Cardiovasc Interv* 2009;2(7):636-644; Eggebrecht H, et al. *Catheter Cardiovasc Interv* 2000;49(4):389-394; Keeley EC, et al. *J Am Coll Cardiol* 1998;32(7):1861-1865).

9.6 Answer D. Figure Q9-6 shows an anomalous circumflex arising from a separate ostium near the origin of the RCA. An anomalous circumflex is one of the most common coronary anomalies encountered among patients referred for angiography (prevalence 0.18% to 0.67%), and the anomalous vessel may be affected by atherosclerosis. Therefore, it is important to understand guide catheter options that can be used to cannulate this anomalous artery. The anomalous LCx can arise from a separate ostium near the ostium of the RCA, from an ostium shared with the RCA, or from the proximal RCA. Its course is posterior to the aorta toward the posterior atrioventricular (AV) groove. An MP curve or JR catheter often will engage the ostium of the anomalous circumflex although backup support may not be ideal. An AR (1 or 2 curve) or HS curve are reasonable backup options. Although designed for LCx interventions in an anatomically normal LCx, a VL 4 is unlikely to engage this artery adequately. Figure A9-6 shows this artery after successful stent placement through a multipurpose guide catheter (Morgan KP, et al. *Cardiovasc Revasc Med* 2012;13(6):335-340; West NE, et al. *Catheter Cardiovasc Interv* 2006;68(6):882-890).

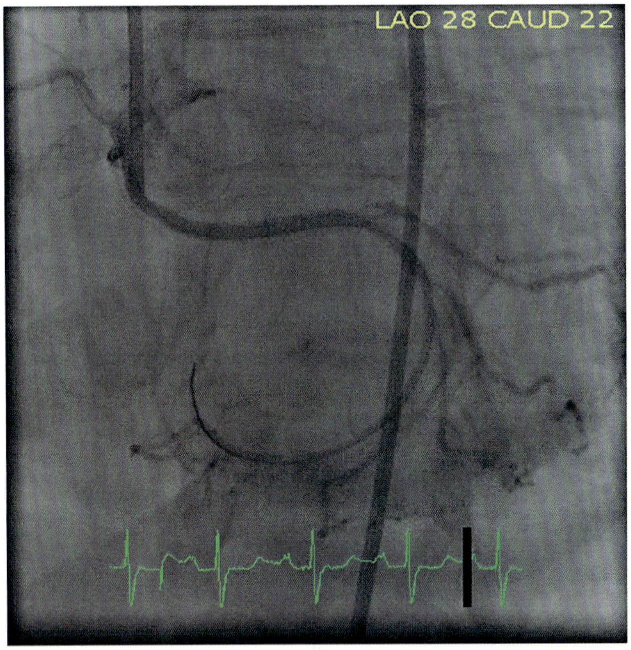

Figure A9-6

9.7 Answer B. An essential component in planning a rotational atherectomy case is knowledge of the maximum burr size, which can be used in the chosen guide catheter. Table A9-7 is from the manufacturer, which recommends a minimum guide size 0.004-in. larger than the burr.

There is some variation in the internal diameters of guide catheters from various manufacturers so it is appropriate to anticipate the burr sizes you will need and make certain you are using a guide catheter of sufficient size. However, neither a 6 Fr system nor a radial approach is a contraindication to rotational atherectomy.

Guide Catheter Selection & Sizing

Guide sizes are based on larger lumen catheters.

Burr (mm)	Diameter (Inches)	Minimum Recommended Guide Catheter Internal Diameter (Inches)	Recommended Guide Catheter (French)*
1.25	0.049	0.060†	6.0
1.50	0.059	0.063	6.0
1.75	0.069	0.073	7.0
2.00	0.079	0.083	8.0
2.15	0.085	0.089	8.0
2.25	0.089	0.093	9.0
2.38	0.094	0.098	9.0
2.50	0.098	0.102	10.0

* Inside guide catheter diameter and french size may differ among manufacturers. Ensure guide is compatible with the largest burr intended to be used.
† Sheath size is the determinant of the minimum ID on the 1.25 mm burr.
‡ Add 0.004" to burr diameter to calculate minimum ID needed

Recommended Guide Catheter Curves
Right: FR4, Multipurpose **Left:** Q-Curve™, CLS™, Left Back-Up
(Guide catheters with side holes can help to improve flow.)

Recommended Burr Speed
Small Burrs (1.25 mm–2.0 mm): 160,000–180,000 RPM
Large Burrs (≥ 2.15 mm): 140,000–160,000 RPM

Source: http://www.bostonscientific.com/content/dam/bostonscientific/Interventional%20Cardiology/portfolio-group/Plaque-Modification/Rotablator-System-Reference-Guide_IC-193906-AA.pdf. Accessed: April 18, 2017.

9.8 Answer E. The diagnostic angiogram shows an inferiorly directed origin of the RCA. Of the provided guide catheter choices, the IM, AL 1, and ART 1 are best suited for a RCA with a horizontal or superiorly directed origin. While the JR 4 would likely fit, the need for enhanced backup support in treating the occlusion should be anticipated and would not be provided by a JR catheter. The best selection would be the AR 1 (Fig. A9-8A and B), which should fit coaxially and provide adequate support. Other options would include the HS or MP catheters.

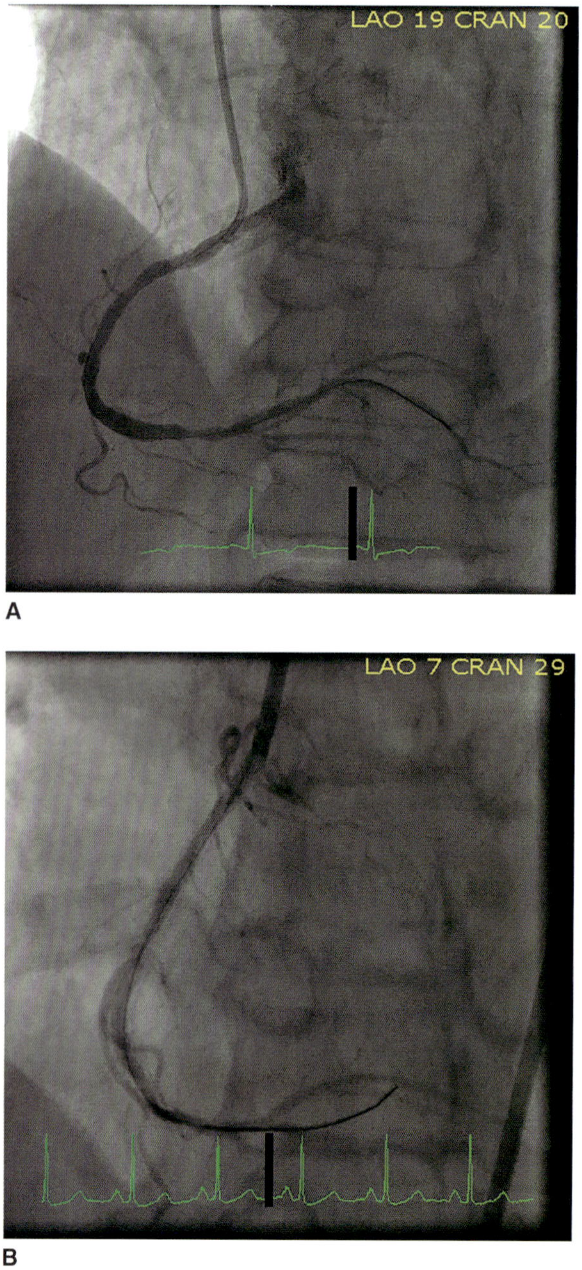

Figure A9-8

9.9 Answer D. When choosing Judkins catheters for a right radial approach, traditional teaching is that the JL catheters should be downsized by 0.5 cm (e.g., JL 3.5 in place of the usual JL 4.0), while the JR should be upsized (JR 4.5 or JR 5 in place of the usual JR 4.0). Therefore, a JR 3.5 is not likely to be a good and successful choice in this case. Alternatively, dedicated radial catheters have been developed, which may allow cannulation of both the left and right coronary with the same catheter, such as the Jacky, Kimny, or Barbeau catheters (Fig. A9-9A and B shows cannulation of the left and right coronary artery with the same Jacky catheter [Terumo Medical Somerset, NJ]) (Bertrand OF, et al. *JACC Cardiovasc Interv* 2010;3(10):1022–1031).

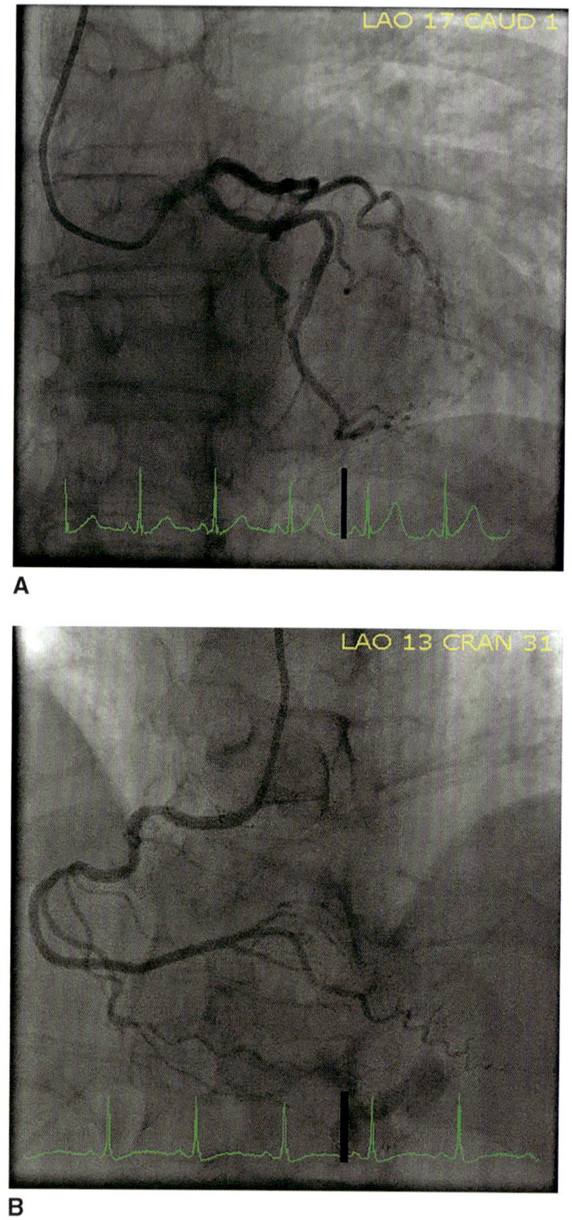

Figure A9-9

9.10 Answer A. With the increasing popularity of radial artery interventions, operators have adapted ways to complete many types of complex interventions via 6 Fr guide catheters. Frequently, radial arteries cannot safely accommodate sheaths larger than 6 Fr. To complete this procedure with a 6 Fr guide catheter, monorail or "rapid exchange" equipment would be required. Two monorail balloons or stents systems can simultaneously pass through most current generation 6 Fr guides. In addition to bifurcation stenting, other complex interventions can usually be performed through 6 Fr systems (e.g., rotational atherectomy up to a 1.50-mm burr, thrombectomy with appropriate-sized catheters, IVUS, etc.). However, opacification of the target vessel may be suboptimal when larger devices are used through a 6 Fr system.

9.11 Answer C. Guide catheter selection in CTO cases is critical to achieving success in these challenging interventions. While minimizing vessel trauma is always important, the need for adequate visualization and support in complex cases does require more aggressive guide catheter size and shape as outlined above; thus, a JR 4 guide is not an optimal choice for CTO PCI. Factors to consider to optimize success include larger French size and supportive shapes to optimize wire and device crossing. The vast majority of such cases require dual injections via an anterograde and retrograde guiding catheter to image the antegrade occlusion as well as the target vessel filling via retrograde collaterals. If a primary retrograde approach is chosen for the PCI, it is necessary to have a shorter retrograde guiding catheter to allow the microcatheters and CTO wires to reach the anterograde guide catheter or guide extender. A retrograde guide that is 90 cm in length or one that is manually shortened will achieve this goal.

If a manufactured 90 cm guide is not available, or a length <90 cm is required, it may be necessary to create one by shortening a 100 cm catheter. This can be done by removing the desired excess length (typically 10 to 20 cm) near the back end of the catheter. It is best to remove and patch the guide catheter in a location that will not enter the body in the event that the catheter disarticulates. The most common method excises the desired length approximately 5 cm from the hub (Fig. A9-11A and B). A piece of sheath 1 Fr size smaller is used to reconnect the guide (Fig. A9-11C and D). Alternatively, the terminal 10 to 15 cm of the catheter, including the hub, can be removed and attached to a sheath 1 Fr smaller using the diaphragm that is part of the sheath (Thompson CA, et al. *JACC Cardiovasc Interv* 2009;2(9):834-842; Moses JW, et al. *Catheter Cardiovasc Interv* 2010; 75(Suppl 1):S21-S27).

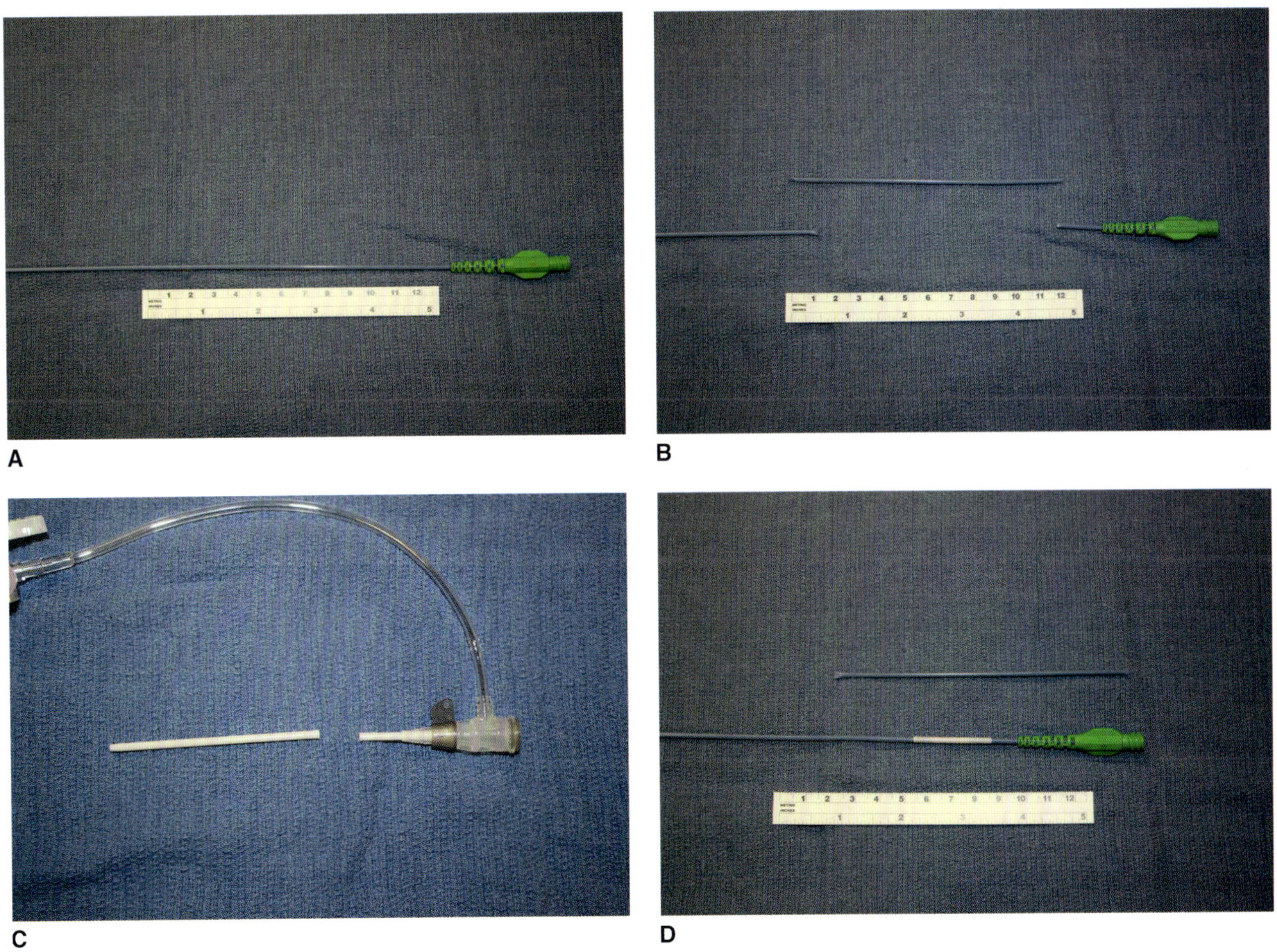

Figure A9-11

9.12 Answer B. The two commercially available transcatheter aortic valve bioprostheses in the United States include the balloon-expandable Edwards Sapien 3 valve and the Medtronic CoreValve Evolut. The Sapien 3 valve is designed to be positioned below the coronary ostia, while the CoreValve device extends well above the coronary ostia. The design of the CoreValve is to allow protection of the coronary ostia with its open-cell configuration—not covering of the ostia as in Answer B. However, placing a guide through the valve struts may be more challenging in this situation. Strategies, including using a short-tip guide to initially engage or a longer tip catheter to completely cross the valve struts, both have been advocated. The primary goal of guide placement for intervention is to minimize guide catheter manipulation to avoid damaging the Nitinol frame or valve leaflets. In our case (Fig. Q9-12B and C), an EBU 3.5 guide was used to successfully perform PCI. An alternative image of a PCI after Sapien XT TAVR is also demonstrated (Fig. A9-12) (Chakravarty T, et al. *J Am Coll Cardiol* 2016;67(8):951-960; Blumenstein J, et al. *Clin Res Cardiol* 2015;104(8):632-639; Greenberg G, et al. *J Invasive Cardiol* 2013;25(7):361-363).

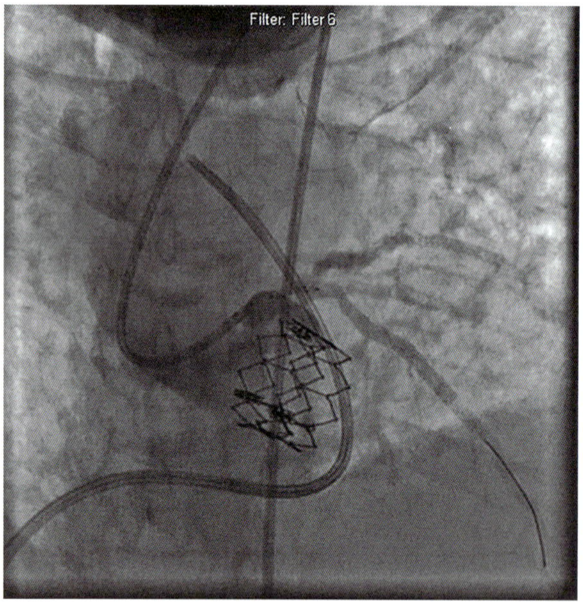

Figure A9-12 (Courtesy of Timothy Mixon and Elizabeth Holper.)

9.13 Answer B. When the tip of a Judkins catheter lies just inferior to the left main ostium, one must recognize that the curve size of the Judkins catheter is too large. This is commonly encountered in patients who are of short stature (regardless of weight). Sometimes, gentle clockwise rotation of the catheter will allow engagement of the left main, especially if the left main ostium is slightly out of the normal plane. A JL 5, AL 2, and Voda 4 are "longer" than the JL 4 and thus are not expected to fit. An MP catheter might work, but the easiest thing to try first is another attempt to engage the LM with the patient taking a deep breath. As the diaphragm moves downward, the heart and aorta also move and the ostium of the LM is "pulled" downward. If the tip of the JL catheter is slightly below the LM, this simple maneuver often allows engagement of the LM. This occurs frequently when angiography is performed from the right radial approach.

9.14 Answer A. Saphenous vein bypasses to the left coronary (LAD or LCx) most frequently arise from the

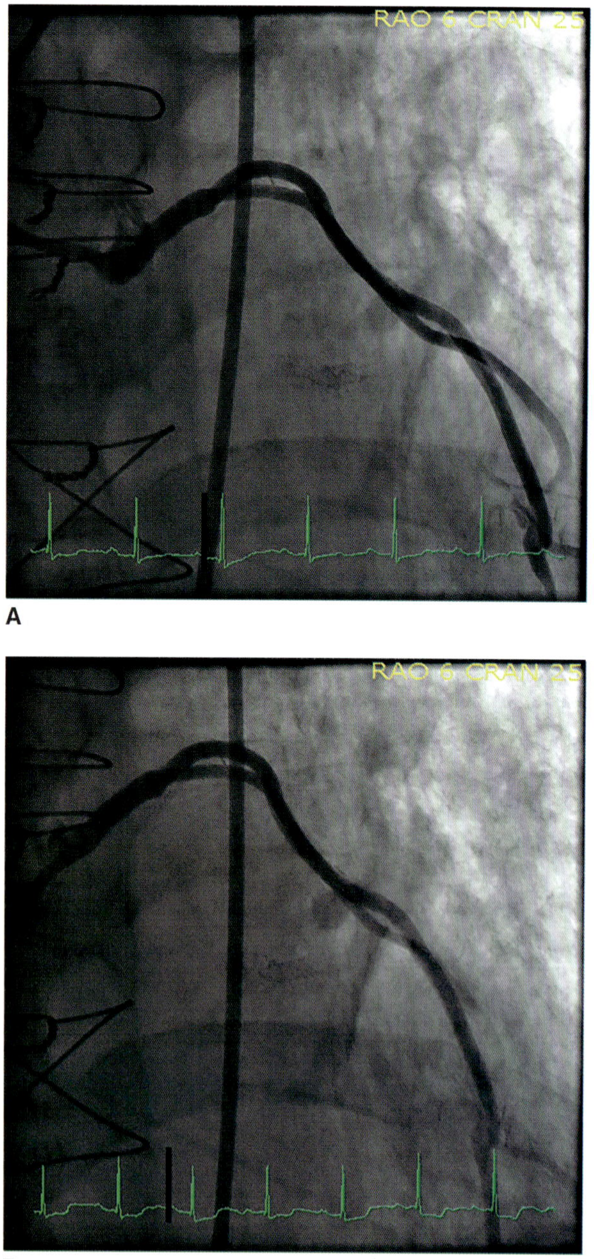

Figure A9-14

left anterior surface of the aorta, superior to the native vessels, and usually superior to a bypass graft to the RCA. The JR 4 and LCB catheters will often engage left-sided bypass grafts but do not necessarily provide robust backup support. An HS and AL catheter can be expected to provide additional support and backup compared to those. The NTR catheter (Williams catheter) was designed for the RCA and generally would be directed to the opposite wall of the aorta; it likely would not reach the saphenous vein graft (SVG) and certainly would not provide backup support. Figure A9-14A and B is from a different patient and show a typical superior directed origin of a saphenous vein Y-graft anastomosed to branches of the left coronary artery, with cannulation by an AL1.

9.15 Answer C. The image represents a type III aortic arch (with the innominate and left common carotid arising from the ascending aorta). In this type of arch configuration, a simple (or so-called passive) curve catheter such as a JR 4, IM, or vertebral catheter will not reach into the ostium of the innominate to allow wire access. An "intermediate" catheter, such as a JB 1, is popular for type I and type II arches, but is unlikely to allow access to the innominate artery of a type III arch. The best choice would be a Simmons catheter, which comes in various tip lengths (i.e., Simmons 1, Simmons 2, etc.). Such a "reverse angle," or so-called "active," catheter requires reformation and then manipulation in the aorta to engage the innominate artery. Originally, reformation was accomplished by placing the catheter tip in the left subclavian artery and then prolapsing the catheter forward to recreate the shape. Alternate techniques were subsequently developed including clockwise rotation in the arch, advancement to the sinus of Valsalva, and counterclockwise rotation or reforming the tip by deflecting the J-wire off of the aortic valve and then tracking the catheter over this wire to the proximal ascending aorta (Berg R, Lim M. Diagnostic angiographic catheters: Coronary and vascular. In: Mukherjee D, Bates ER, Roffi M, Moliterno DJ, eds. *Cardiovascular catheterization and intervention*. New York: Informa, 2010:202-204; Simmons CR, et al. *Am J Roentgenol Radium Ther Nucl Med* 1973;119(3):605-612; Smith DC, et al. *Radiology* 1985;155(1):247-248).

9.16 Answer D. When performing rotational atherectomy, the operator must be aware of certain equipment requirements. The guide catheter must be large enough (French size) to accommodate the needed atherectomy burr (see explanation to Question Q9.7). To help facilitate washout of the debris created by the burr, it is important that good flow is maintained down the vessel, so many routinely use a guiding catheter with side holes. Coaxial positioning at the ostium is always important but especially for easy advancement of the burr; the guide catheter tip should be stiff enough to remain engaged in the ostium throughout the procedure. However, with rotational atherectomy, deep seating is not necessary or particularly desirable. The operator should slowly advance the burr allowing it to engage and debulk the stenosis rather than force the burr into the stenosis using a great amount of forward pressure.

9.17 Answer E. Radial arteries can be quite small in some patients and may not allow standard 6 Fr sheaths. Many PCI operators report success using 5 Fr guiding systems, although more complex PCI and optimal radiopacity may be limited. Switching to a left radial approach is unlikely to yield a significantly larger artery. Sheathless systems were initially "homemade" but are now available in the United States, Europe, and Japan. These include the SheathLess Eaucath system (Asahi Medical), which allows one to realize the luminal size of a 6.5 F guide catheter with an outer diameter equivalent to a 5F sheath. Switching to a femoral approach is reasonable, although not likely necessary and may increase the bleeding rate. Finally, industry has innovated new approaches, such as the Terumo Glidesheath Slender sheath, which has the outer diameter of a 5 Fr sheath, but allows for passage of a 6 Fr guiding catheter. Although it did not establish noninferiority to a 5 Fr sheath in regard to radial artery occlusion rates, it is unknown how it may compare to standard 6 Fr sheath for ischemic complication rates (Tada N, et al. *J Invasive Cardiol* 2015;27(5):237-241; Cheaito R, et al. *Catheter Cardiovasc Interv* 2015;86(1):51-58; Aminian A, Saito S, Takahashi A, et al. Comparison of a new slender 6 Fr sheath with a standard 5 Fr sheath for transradial coronary angiography and intervention: RAP and BEAT (Radial Artery Patency and Bleeding, Efficacy, Adverse evenT), a randomised multicentre trial. *EuroIntervention* 2017;13(5):e549-e556.).

9.18 Answer C. When angiography is performed with a 4 or 5 Fr diagnostic catheter, it is possible for important left main disease to be missed. Left main disease may be suspected when a larger French size guide catheter is placed and pressure dampening or "ventricularization" occurs (see the first three beats of Fig. A9-23B for an example of ventricularization).

While this can occur in the absence of obstructive disease, such as when the catheter is not coaxial, or when the left main has an angulated takeoff, this should be investigated to assure the patient does not have significant left main disease. IVUS is an excellent way to understand the mechanism of pressure dampening. If significant obstructive disease is identified, the treatment plan for the patient may need to be modified. Changing to a side hole guide catheter or to a smaller guide system may minimize the ischemia experienced by the patient, but could deprive the patient of the correct diagnosis. Simply proceeding with the PCI is not the best course if there is uncertainty about important left main disease. (Baim DS. Coronary angiography. In: Baim DS, ed. Grossman & Baim's *cardiac catheterization, angiography, and intervention*, 8th ed. Philadelphia: Lippincott Williams & Wilkins, 2013:295–334)

9.19 Answer D. Diagnostic or guide catheters can induce ostial coronary artery dissections either in the setting of severe pre-existing disease or with mild, insignificant disease—especially if the guide is not in a coaxial position. It is also important to check the pressure waveform prior to each injection, as a dampened pressure (either based on the presence of atherosclerotic disease or noncoaxial catheter placement) would increase the risk of a hydraulic dissection with contrast injection. Air within the system, noncoaxial catheter placement, and other "artifacts" could be a cause, but should not be entertained until other life-threatening possibilities, such as left main dissection or other forms of shock, are excluded. Retroperitoneal hemorrhage is more likely to appear after sheath removal. Recognizing a left main dissection, maintaining wire position, and being prepared to immediately stent the dissection (or refer to emergent surgery) are essential to assuring optimal patient outcome. Figure Q9-19B shows dissection of the left main extending into the proximal LAD and into the proximal LCx.

9.20 Answer E. The Amplatz catheter shape, the XB family of curves (Cordis), the EBU family of curves (Medtronic), or the Voda curves (Boston Scientific) should all provide substantial backup for delivery of stents and/or larger devices. The JL 4 shape provides minimal backup, and frequently, operators rely on catheter manipulation or support wires to complete even straightforward interventions when a JL guide is used.

9.21 Answer A. The anomalous RCA originating above the usual location and between the left and right cusps is often very challenging to cannulate. Standard left catheters (i.e., JL 3.5, JL 4, JL 5, AL 1, and AL 2) can sometimes be utilized. Both a Voda curve and Q-curve catheter can also be used successfully to cannulate such an anomalous RCA and can provide reasonable backup support (Fig. A9-21A). However, JR catheters are too short and are not likely to work in this situation. It is important to understand the route of the anomalous RCA as some variants course directly between the aorta and pulmonary artery and have been associated with sudden cardiac death. While its course may be determined with some certainty in the catheterization laboratory, CT or magnetic resonance (MR) angiography is very helpful in determining the course of an anomalous artery. In this instance, a JL 3.5 seems to selectively cannulate the ostium the best, though it is still suboptimal. After passing the guidewire, a guide extender was used, as seen in Figure A9-21B (intraprocedurally) and Figure A9-21C (completion angiogram with guide extender deeply intubated into the RCA) (Sarkar K, et al. *J Interv Cardiol* 2009;22(3):234–239; Qayyum U, et al. *Catheter Cardiovasc Interv* 2003;60(3):382–388).

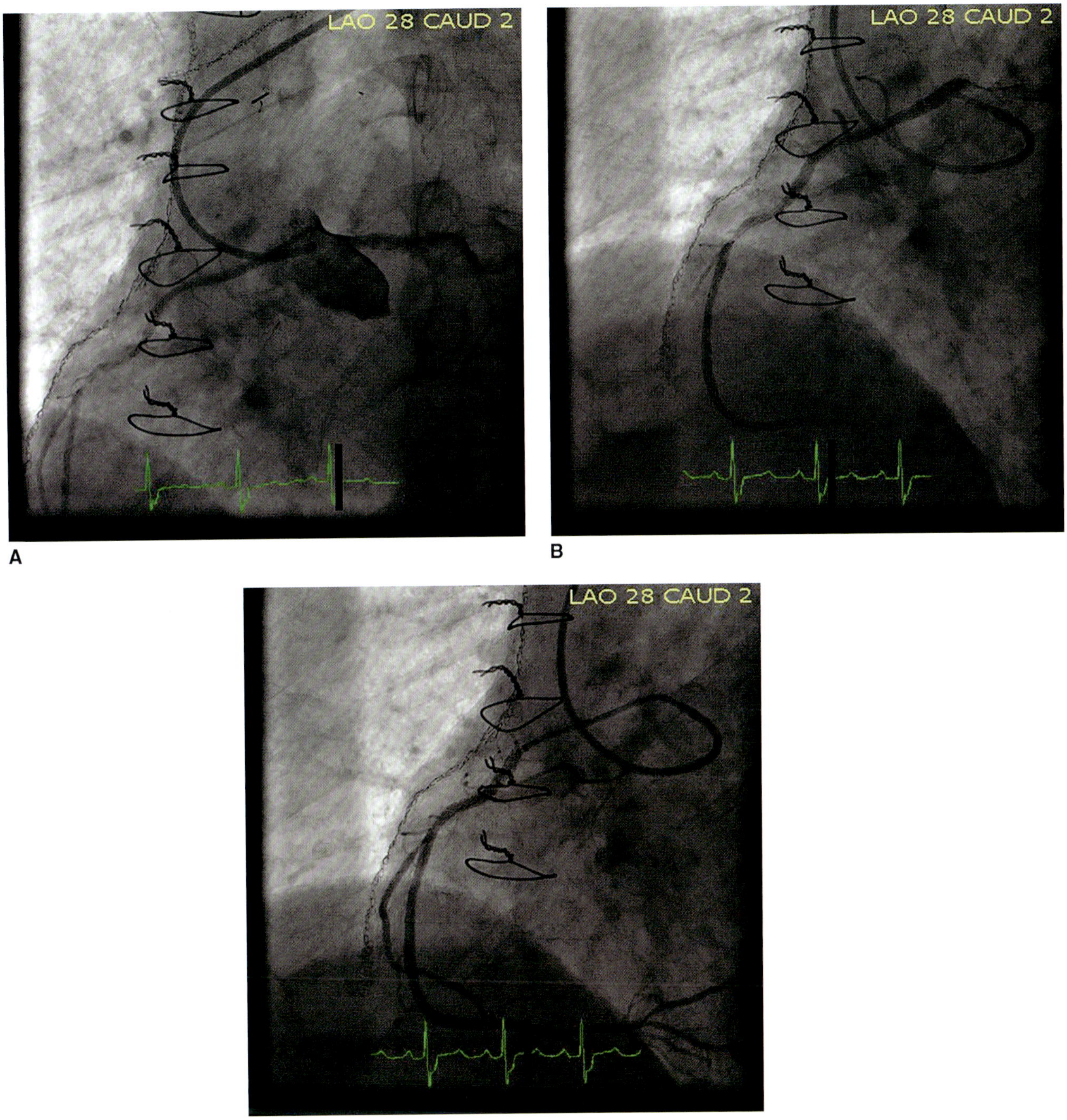

Figure A9-21

9.22 Answer E. In the presence of a tortuous iliac artery, diagnostic or guide catheters can become kinked when attempting to rotate them into the RCA ostium. This is recognized by dampening or even complete loss of the pressure waveform. If this occurs, the operator should rotate the catheter in the opposite direction (usually counterclockwise) in an attempt to "unkink" the catheter. Once kinking of the catheter has occurred, it is best to remove this catheter using a stiff wire. Kinking of a catheter can occur with tortuous vessels in the absence of obstructive disease. A good solution is to place a stiff 0.035-in. wire (Amplatz, SupraCor, or other) through the diagnostic catheter into the aorta and then change the short sheath for a longer sheath (25 cm may suffice or 40 to 45 cm to reach all the way into the abdominal aorta)—often a larger sheath size (6 to 8 Fr) is better for support. This will partially straighten the iliac vessel and "absorb" the contact of the iliac vessels, allowing better movement of the guide catheter. Alternatively, conversion to radial artery catheterization would likely be successful. Using a short 8 Fr sheath and system might be successful with a larger guide being somewhat less likely to become kinked and compressed. A 6 Fr JR 4 guide will run into the same issues as the diagnostic catheter.

9.23 Answer D. The waveform recorded from the guide catheter should be monitored frequently by the physician, as well as the cardiovascular technician monitoring the patient. Particular attention is necessary during all maneuvers that could change the guide position, especially (a) when first seating the guide catheter, (b) before each injection, and (c) when passing interventional equipment in or out of the guide catheter. In this case, the pressure waveform displays a significant loss of systolic pressure, although it does not have the typical

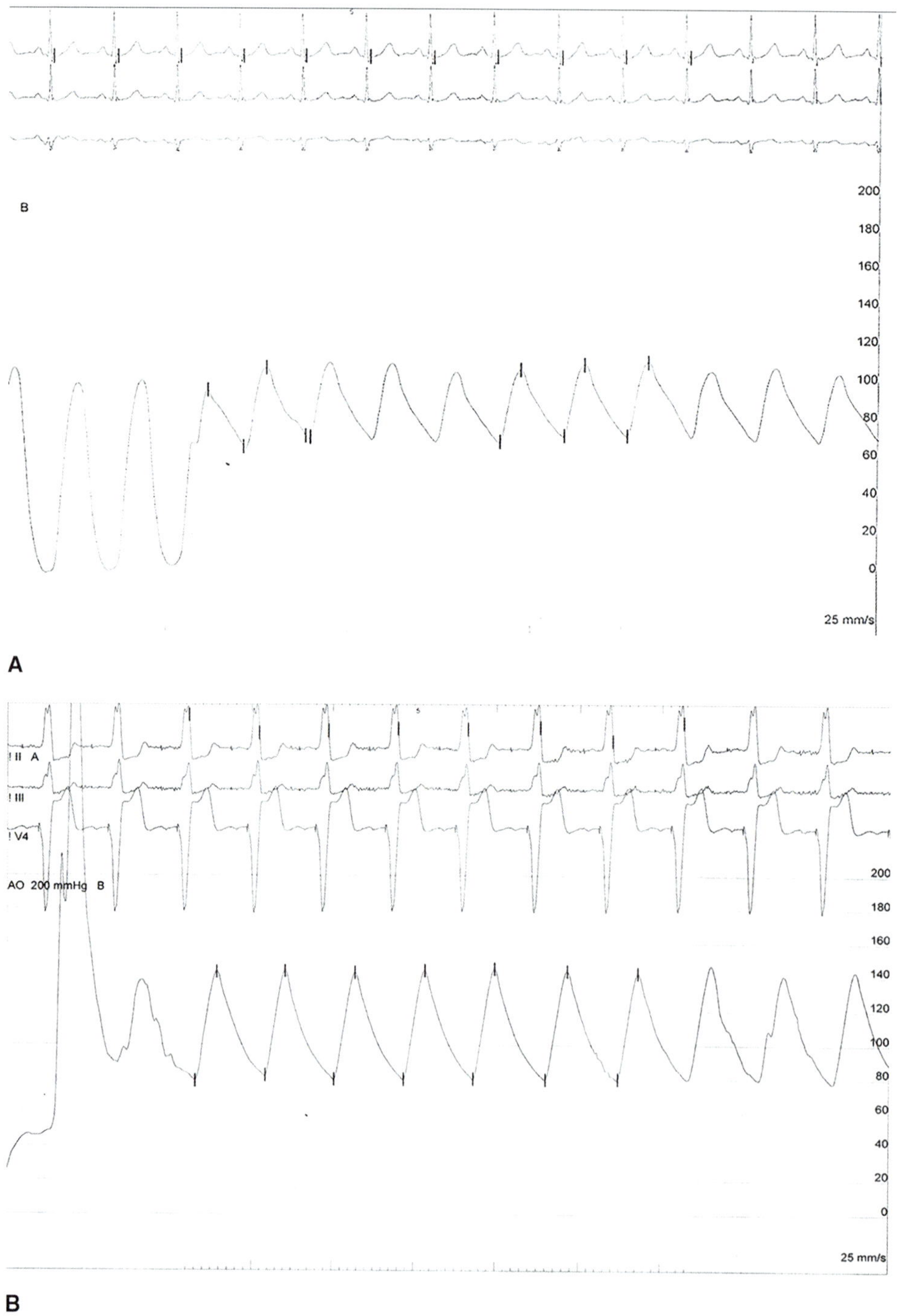

Figure A9-23

shape of "ventricularization." (See first three beats in Figure A9-23B.)

While this could represent pressure dampening from placing the catheter in a very small or diseased artery, in this case, the pressure did not improve after ensuring the catheter was free within the aorta, and it did not correlate with noninvasive pressures. Therefore, this is most likely due to obstruction within the fluid filled pressure line such as can occur when thrombus or air becomes entrapped. An injection should not occur until the catheter is thoroughly aspirated and then flushed with care taken not to allow air back into the system. Figure A9-23A shows restoration of a normal waveform and pressure after aspirating and flushing the pressure line. A kinked guide catheter will typically have a very low-pressure reading with a very narrow "pulse pressure" (see Fig. A9-23B). Deep intubation and an unappreciated ostial stenosis are associated with systolic dampening or "ventricularization," although these possibilities should be considered in all such cases. (Baim DS. Coronary angiography. In: Baim DS, ed. *Grossman's cardiac catheterization, angiography, and intervention*, 8th ed. Philadelphia: Lippincott Williams & Wilkins, 2013:295–334)

9.24 Answer A. For enhanced support with a left-sided SVG, an AL guide (AL 1, AL 1.5, or AL 2, depending on the size of the aorta) should allow for adequate support (Fig. A9-24). Alternatively, an LCB or HS catheter may provide additional support. A JR catheter and IM catheter, while having the correct tip shape, are not long enough to rest against the contralateral aortic wall and seat securely in the ostium. The JL catheters are not suitable for SVG cannulation. (Baim DS. Coronary angiography. In: Baim DS, ed. *Grossman's cardiac catheterization, angiography, and intervention*, 8th ed. Philadelphia: Lippincott Williams & Wilkins, 2013:295–334)

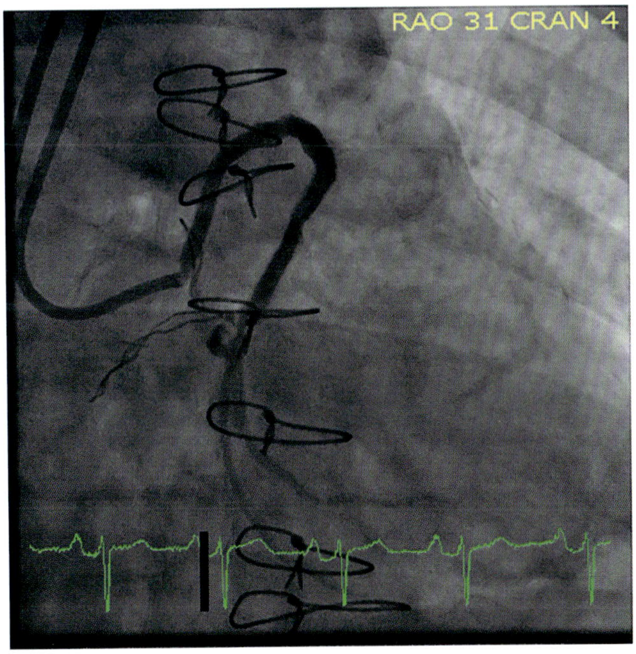

Figure A9-24

9.25 Answer C. An RCA with an upward takeoff can frequently present difficulties in device passage around the proximal bends; thus, optimal coaxial alignment and backup support is desirable. Of the catheters listed, the AL 1 is the best choice (Fig. A9-25). The AR 1 and HS are best suited for a horizontal or downward takeoff. The JR 4 and NTR may seat coaxially, but would not provide much support.

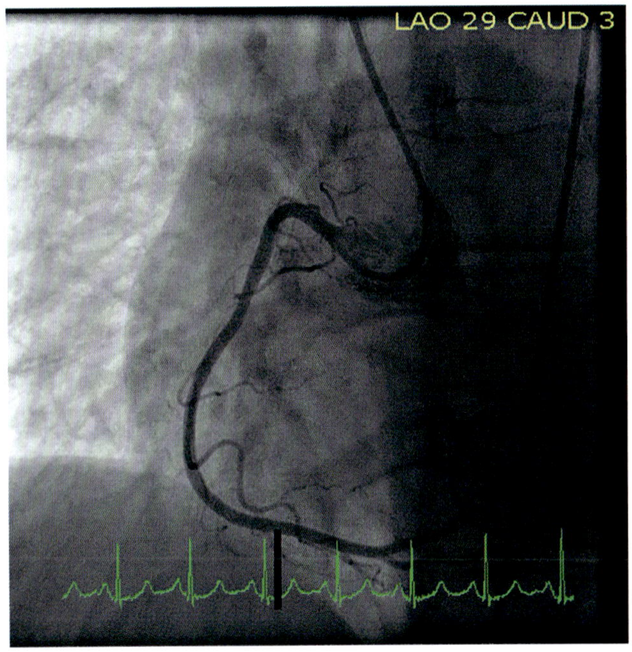

Figure A9-25

9.26 Answer B. The Ikari left guide is well suited to cannulate and image both the left and right coronary arteries. This can facilitate rapid angiography prior to PCI in the setting of STEMI. The AL 2 would likely be too long to cannulate the RCA well, although it is possible. The JR 4 would not cannulate the left main, while the JL 3.5 would not easily cannulate the RCA. The EBU 4 guide is routinely used for left coronary intervention (Youssef AA, et al. *EuroIntervention* 2008;3(4):475–481; Chow J, et al. *J Interv Cardiol* 2012;25(3):235–244).

10 Intravascular Contrast Agents

John J. Lazarus and Brahmajee K. Nallamothu

QUESTIONS

10.1 A 68-year-old man with a history of four-vessel coronary artery bypass surgery to the right posterior descending artery, the obtuse marginal branch of the left circumflex (LCX) artery, the left anterior descending (LAD) artery, and the diagonal branch of the LAD artery presents with progressive stable angina and inferior ischemia on stress testing. His diagnostic angiogram and cardiac rhythm are shown in Figure Q10-1. What is the best next step?

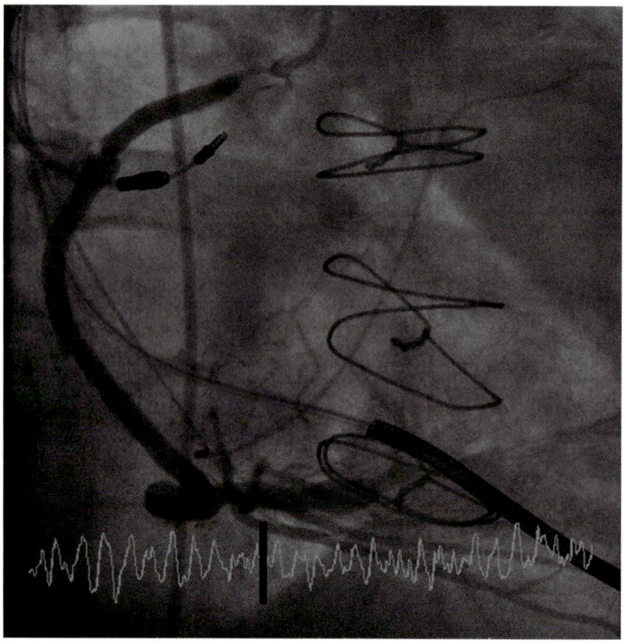

Figure Q10-1

(A) Switch to iso-osmolar contrast in order to minimize contrast cardiotoxicity
(B) Disengage the diagnostic catheter and instruct the patient to cough
(C) Switch to power injection in order to optimize bypass graft visualization
(D) Insert a transvenous pacemaker

10.2 A 75-year-old woman with lifestyle-limiting angina, diabetes mellitus, and chronic renal insufficiency with a serum creatinine (SCr) of 2.3 mg/dL is scheduled for elective cardiac catheterization with possible percutaneous coronary intervention (PCI). Which is a preferred contrast agent in this setting?

(A) Ioxaglate (Hexabrix)
(B) Iodixanol (Visipaque)
(C) Diatrizoate (Hypaque, Renografin, Angiovist)
(D) Carbon dioxide

10.3 A 66-year-old male with stable angina, anterior ischemia on nuclear stress echocardiogram, and asthma presents for diagnostic cardiac catheterization. For which of these scenarios should he receive corticosteroids prior to coronary angiography with low-osmolar contrast?

(A) He has a history of anaphylaxis to penicillin
(B) He has a shell food allergy (angioedema)
(C) He has diabetes and a SCr of 2.7 mg/dL
(D) He had hives and wheezing when undergoing a computed tomography (CT) scan with high-osmolar contrast 20 years ago

10.4 A 74-year-old male with a history of diabetes and stage III chronic kidney disease (CKD) presents to the catheterization lab with exertional angina. Nuclear stress test reveals inferior ischemia and an ejection fraction of 55%. His creatinine is 1.8 mg/dL on the day of catheterization, which is at his baseline. What strategy will best help reduce the risk of contrast-induced nephropathy in this patient?

(A) Use of high-osmolar contrast during catheterization
(B) Renal-dose dopamine prior to the procedure
(C) Checking left ventricular end-diastolic pressure (LVEDP) followed by hemodynamic-guided fluid administration
(D) Performing right coronary angiography alone and staging left coronary angiography 72 hours later

10.5 An 87-year-old male with a history of hypertension (HTN), previous coronary artery bypass grafting (CABG), and a baseline creatinine of 0.94 undergoes successful transcatheter aortic valve replacement (TAVR). Thoracic aortic aortography after deployment of the valve confirmed mild paravalvular regurgitation. His urine output decreased to 50 mL over 12 hours and his creatinine increased to 2.5 mg/dL on postoperative day 1. Which of these findings is not consistent with atheroembolic acute kidney injury?

(A) Cutaneous findings, such as purpura and livedo reticularis, after the procedure
(B) Abdominal pain 12 hours after the procedure with elevated lactate and CT findings concerning for mesenteric ischemia
(C) Peripheral hypereosinophilia and eosinophiluria
(D) Recovery of SCr to baseline within 14 days

10.6 Typical doses of contrast agents for left ventriculography and thoracic aortography during routine cineangiography include:

(A) 30 to 40 mL injected at a rate of 10 mL/s and 80 to 100 mL injected at a rate of 40 mL/s, respectively
(B) 30 to 40 mL injected at a rate of 10 mL/s and 40 to 60 mL injected at a rate of 20 mL/s, respectively
(C) 20 to 30 mL injected at a rate of 5 mL/s and 20 to 40 mL injected at a rate of 20 mL/s, respectively
(D) 60 to 80 mL injected at a rate of 20 mL/s and 40 to 60 mL injected at a rate of 20 mL/s, respectively

10.7 A 52-year-old man with a history of hypertension, diabetes, and unstable angina develops pruritis, urticaria, wheezing, a heart rate of 95 beats per minute (bpm), and hypotension with a systolic blood pressure of 70 mm Hg after his first injection of contrast for diagnostic cardiac catheterization despite 500-mL intravenous (IV) bolus of normal saline. What is the best next step?

(A) Hydrocortisone 200 mg IV
(B) Diphenhydramine 50 mg IV
(C) 0.01 mg of 1:10,000 epinephrine IV
(D) Albuterol nebulizer

10.8 A 49-year-old man with exertional dyspnea, mitral valve prolapse with a flail leaflet, and severe mitral regurgitation confirmed by transesophageal echocardiography (TEE) is referred for preoperative coronary angiography. Coronary angiogram through the femoral artery is normal. He then develops pruritus, urticaria, and respiratory distress with wheezing, angioedema, and severe stridor. His blood pressure is 120/70 mm Hg and heart rate is 115 bpm. His oxygen saturation is 95% on a 3-L nasal cannula. What is the best next step?

(A) Albuterol nebulizer
(B) Intra-aortic balloon pump and furosemide IV
(C) Continuous positive airway pressure
(D) Prepare for emergent endotracheal intubation

10.9 A 67-year-old female with a history of hypertension, diabetes, and stage III CKD with baseline creatinine of 1.9 comes to see you for an evaluation. Surface echocardiogram reveals bicuspid aortic valve without aortic stenosis or regurgitation and a 5.6-cm dilated ascending aortic root. She is referred for coronary angiography prior to valve sparring root replacement (David procedure). She is 60 kg and her LVEDP prior to contrast exposure is 16 mm Hg. What is the optimal hydration strategy to minimize contrast-induced nephropathy (CIN) in this patient?

(A) 180 mL/h of normal saline 1 hour preprocedure and 180 mL/h of normal saline during the procedure and for 4 hours afterward
(B) Prehydration with 90 mL/h of 5% dextrose in ½ normal saline for 1 hour
(C) Use of furosemide drip to maintain steady urine output during the procedure
(D) Hydration with 100 mL/h of normal saline for 4 hours after the procedure

10.10 When compared to high-osmolar contrast agents, which of the following statements regarding low-osmolar contrast agents is the most CORRECT?

(A) Low-osmolar agents increase the risk of thrombotic complications
(B) Low-osmolar agents reduce the risk of bradyarrhythmias
(C) Low-osmolar agents increase the risk of post-procedure renal failure
(D) Low-osmolar agents increase the risk of anaphylactoid reactions

10.11 A 45-year-old female presents to the catheterization lab with non–ST-elevation myocardial infarction (NSTEMI). Surface echocardiogram shows an ejection fraction of 25% and findings concerning for Takotsubo cardiomyopathy. Her coronary injection of the right coronary artery (RCA) is shown in Figure Q10-11, and her blood pressure is 70/45 mm Hg. Which of the following will NOT reduce the risk of contrast-related cardiotoxicity (i.e., myocardial ischemia and arrhythmia) in this patient?

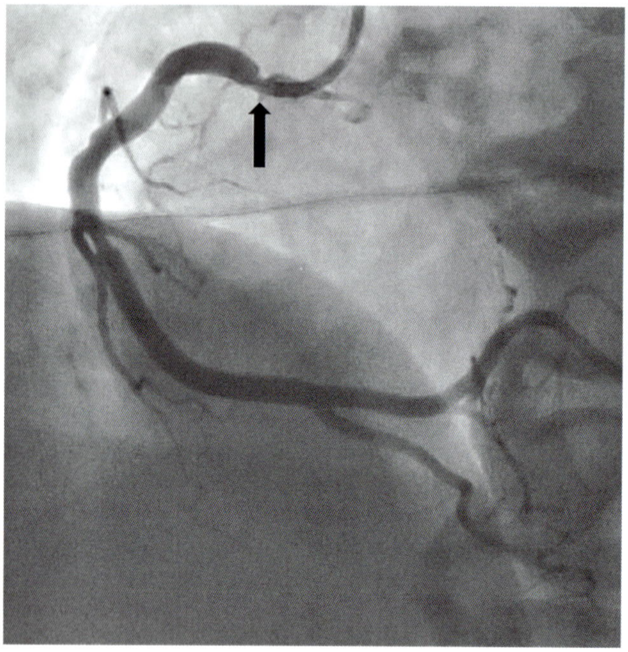

Figure Q10-11 (Courtesy of John Lazarus.)

(A) Limiting number of injections and volume of contrast per injection
(B) Giving intracoronary nitroglycerin to relieve coronary vasospasm prior to further angiography
(C) Disengaging the coronary catheter after injection of contrast to allow anterograde perfusion
(D) Switching to high-osmolar iodinated contrast for coronary angiography

10.12 What is the incidence of life-threatening reactions to contrast agents?

(A) 1:100
(B) 1:1,000
(C) 1:100,000
(D) 1:1,000,000

10.13 Which of the following patients has the highest risk of developing CIN following cardiac catheterization and/or PCI?

(A) A 72-year-old woman with diabetes mellitus and a SCr of 2.0 mg/dL who presents with STEMI and hypotension
(B) A 48-year-old man without diabetes mellitus and a SCr of 2.6 mg/dL undergoing elective PCI
(C) An 80-year-old man with diabetes mellitus and a SCr of 1.0 mg/dL who is also taking metformin
(D) A 45-year-old woman with a history of a solitary kidney and a SCr of 0.9 mg/dL who is undergoing a right- and left-heart catheterization for a suspected atrial septal defect (ASD)

10.14 A 56-year-old man with a history of five-vessel CABG, insulin-dependent diabetes, and stage III CKD (baseline creatinine of 1.9 mg/dL) presents with NSTEMI and hypotension. Echocardiography reveals a left ventricular ejection fraction (LVEF) of 25%. He undergoes coronary angiography and percutaneous intervention to the left internal mammary artery (LIMA) graft. Two days after the procedure, his creatinine increased to 2.8 mg/dL despite LVEDP-guided volume resuscitation. Which of the following statements is FALSE about CIN?

(A) Recovery of SCr usually occurs within 2 weeks
(B) CIN is associated with increased in-hospital mortality and renal failure
(C) CIN is associated with increased risk of post-procedural bleeding
(D) Fractional excretion of sodium reliably distinguishes CIN from prerenal azotemia

10.15 A 63-year-old woman with a history of diabetes mellitus and a 55-pack-year smoking history is referred to your clinic for a management of her atrial fibrillation. On questioning, she describes lifestyle-limiting claudication. Her baseline creatinine is 2.5 mg/dL. Which of the following techniques would NOT be advised in planning and performing peripheral angiography?

(A) Noncontrast-enhanced magnetic resonance angiography (MRA) to assess peripheral arterial anatomy and location of stenosis
(B) Use of trace subtract fluoroscopy (i.e., road mapping)
(C) Use of a nontraditional contrast agent, such as CO_2
(D) Noncontrasted lower extremity CT scan to assess peripheral arterial anatomy and location of stenosis

10.16 Which is CORRECT regarding the mechanism of action of an anaphylactoid reaction to contrast media?

(A) It is due to immunoglobulin E (IgE)-mediated degranulation of mast cells
(B) It is due to chemokine release from memory T cells, which causes degranulation of mast cells
(C) It involves iodine binding of vitronectin receptors and basophil degranulation
(D) It involves degranulation of basophils and tissue mast cells by direct complement activation

10.17 Which is correct regarding the contrast agent iodixanol (Visipaque)?

(A) It has consistently been shown to be superior to the low-osmolar, nonionic contrast agent, iopamidol (Isovue), in reducing the incidence of CIN
(B) It may cause less discomfort than ionic contrast agents in patients undergoing peripheral angiography
(C) It is a low-osmolar, nonionic contrast agent
(D) It is associated with a higher risk of catheter thrombosis compared to high-osmolar contrast agents

10.18 All of the following are clear indications for using low-osmolar contrast agents for coronary angiography, EXCEPT:

(A) Severe coronary artery disease (e.g., left main disease)
(B) Severe emphysema
(C) Severe aortic stenosis
(D) Moderate to severe left ventricular dysfunction

10.19 A 55-year-old man with diabetes, nonischemic cardiomyopathy with an ejection fraction of 20%, and CKD with a baseline creatinine of 1.7 mg/dL is seen in the office in preparation for coronary angiography after a positive stress test. He is an internist and inquires about strategies to reduce incidence of CIN. Which one of the following statements is TRUE?

(A) *N*-acetylcysteine reduces risk of procedural myocardial ischemia and arrhythmia
(B) Routine use of oral *N*-acetylcysteine following the procedure reduces the risk of contrast-induced nephropathy
(C) Preprocedure and postprocedure hydration with IV normal saline will reduce the risk of CIN
(D) Staging PCI for 3 to 4 hours after diagnostic coronary angiography

10.20 In which of the following scenarios should you consider switching from low-osmolar to iso-osmolar contrast medium?

(A) To minimize cardiotoxicity in a patient with severe left ventricular dysfunction
(B) To minimize the risk of an anaphylactoid reaction in a patient with multiple drug allergies
(C) To minimize patient discomfort associated with a peripheral angiogram
(D) To optimize visualization of the coronary arteries in a morbidly obese patient

10.21 The mechanism of CIN is thought to be related to which of the following?

(A) Inhibition of preglomerular prostaglandin synthesis
(B) Deposition of T lymphocytes and monocytes in the renal interstitium
(C) Direct cellular toxicity and hypoxia due to renal vasoconstriction and hyperviscosity
(D) Immunoglobulin deposition and complement activation within renal glomeruli

10.22 A 58-year-old man with poorly controlled hypertension presents with acute onset of severe "tearing" chest pain that radiates to his midback. Electrocardiogram (ECG) shows sinus tachycardia, left ventricular hypertrophy, and no evidence of myocardial ischemia or injury. SCr is 3.9. Which test would you order next to establish a diagnosis?

(A) CT aortogram with IV contrast
(B) TEE
(C) Magnetic resonance imaging (MRI) of the aorta with and without gadolinium
(D) Coronary angiography

10.23 A 37-year-old man with hypertensive nephropathy and a baseline SCr of 3.5 mg/dL is found to have a 70% ostial RCA stenosis on diagnostic angiography in the context of exertional chest pain. Which of these statements is FALSE with regard to his planned PCI and CIN?

(A) Staging the intervention for at least 72 hours later and use of biplane angiography will reduce risk of CIN
(B) Use of a JR 4 guide catheter with side holes for this percutaneous intervention could increase volume of contrast used
(C) CIN defined as an absolute increase of SCr > 0.3 mg/dL and a relative increase of SCr > 50% is highly predictive of inpatient mortality
(D) Calculating the estimated glomerular filtration rate (eGFR) via the Cockcroft-Gault equation is the most accurate in predicting adverse outcomes associated with PCI

10.24 A 63-year-old woman suffered bronchospasm during diagnostic coronary angiography with a high-osmolar contrast agent 2 years ago. She presents for repeat coronary angiography secondary to angina and a positive stress test. What is the likelihood of another reaction when exposed to a nonionic low-osmolar contrast agent?

(A) <1%
(B) <10%
(C) <25%
(D) <50%

ANSWERS AND EXPLANATIONS

10.1 Answer B. This patient has a severe ostial stenosis of the vein graft to the right posterior descending artery and ventricular fibrillation with contrast injection. The best initial steps are to stop the injection, disengage the catheter, and instruct the patient to cough (if he is still conscious) to clear contrast from the myocardium. The other options do not immediately address the arrhythmia.

10.2 Answer B. High-osmolar agents (diatrizoate) cause more contrast-induced nephropathy than low-osmolar or iso-osmolar agents (Barrett BJ, et al. *Radiology* 1993;188(1):171–178) and are less commonly used in current practice. The nonionic iso-osmolar iodixanol is one of the preferred agents in this setting. It has been proven to be less nephrotoxic than the ionic low-osmolar ioxaglate, but data in comparison to other ionic low-osmolar agents are less clear (Jo SH, et al. *J Am Coll Cardiol* 2006;48(5):924–930). There is no role for carbon dioxide above the diaphragm given the risk of cerebral embolization.

10.3 Answer D. Although risk of repeat reaction with low-osmolar contrast is lower, any patient with a prior hypersensitivity reaction to contrast should receive a "prep" that includes corticosteroids. Patients with multiple drug allergies may be at increased risk of a contrast reaction, but routine pretreating of patients with a penicillin allergy is not indicated. It had been proposed in the 1970s that shellfish allergy confers a higher risk of contrast allergy because shellfish contains iodine, although this theory has been debunked. In fact, the allergen within shellfish is tropomyosin, a protein not present in contrast media. Diabetes and renal dysfunction do not increase the risk of a hypersensitivity reaction to contrast.

10.4 Answer C. Contrast-induced nephropathy occurred less frequently (6.7% vs. 16.3%; relative risk 0.41; CI 0.22 to 0.79; $p = 0.005$) in patients with LVEDP-guided hydration compared to the control group who received standard hydration of 1.5 mL/kg/h in the POSEIDON randomized controlled trial (Brar SS, et al. *Lancet* 2014;383(9931):1814–1823). High-osmolar contrast has been associated with increased risk of CIN. Renal-dose dopamine has not shown consistently to reduce nephrotoxicity. Staging right and left coronary angiography would expose the patient to increased risk of complication from repeat catheterizations and delay reperfusion strategy for inferior ischemia and chest pain.

10.5 Answer D. Transcatheter aortic valves are anchored within calcified native aortic valve during TAVR, and atheroembolism can be a complication. In this case, a rapid rise in creatinine with concomitant mesenteric ischemia is suggestive of an atheroembolic cause of renal failure. Cutaneous findings and peripheral eosinophilia or eosinophiluria should also raise suspicions for atheroembolic renal failure, although they are not consistently present. Skin findings occur in 50% of patients and eosinophiluria or peripheral eosinophilia can be seen in 10% to 15% of individuals. Eosinophiluria or peripheral eosinophilia can be transient and missed on diagnostic testing. Recovery of SCr to baseline at 2 weeks is a strong clinical finding that favors CIN. A continuously raised SCr 3 to 8 weeks following the procedure raises suspicion of atheroembolic failure.

10.6 Answer B. Adequate visualization of the left ventricle and thoracic aorta requires rapid delivery of large amounts of contrast agents through power injectors. Typical rates for these procedures are listed in (B), but these may be modified on the basis of the heart size or cardiac output, the catheter being used (e.g., lower flow rates with end-hole catheters), or the use of digital subtraction imaging in the case of aortic imaging.

10.7 Answer C. This patient is having a severe anaphylactoid reaction to contrast and should receive IV epinephrine immediately. Corticosteroids are reasonable to help prevent a delayed hypersensitivity reaction but take hours to work. Diphenhydramine and albuterol may also be given, but these are a lower priority than systemic epinephrine.

10.8 Answer D. This patient's stridor and angioedema in the setting of a hypersensitivity reaction indicates severe laryngeal edema and impending airway collapse. Delay in endotracheal intubation could result in complete airway collapse and need for emergent cricothyroidotomy. The other options will not treat laryngeal edema.

10.9 Answer A. The answer above is based on the POSEIDON randomized controlled trial. CIN occurred less frequently (6.7% vs. 16.3%; relative risk 0.41; CI 0.22 to 0.79; $p = 0.005$) in patients with LVEDP-guided hydration (5 mL/kg/h for LVEDP < 13 mm Hg, 3 mL/kg/h for LVEDP 13 to 18 mm Hg, and 1.5 mL/kg/h for LVEDP > 18 mm Hg) compared to the control group who had standard hydration of 1.5 mL/kg/h during the catheterization and for 4 hours afterward. All patients in the POSEIDON trial received 3 ml/kg of fluid for at least 1 hour prior to the cardiac catheterization prior to randomization into LVEDP guided hydration or the control group. Use of furosemide will reduce preload (thus having the opposite effect of normal saline).

10.10 Answer B. Low-osmolar nonionic contrast agents are better tolerated by patients and produce fewer episodes of bradycardia, transient hypotension, renal dysfunction, and both mild and serious anaphylactoid reactions. There are no clear differences in the incidence of thrombotic complications between these agents.

10.11 Answer D. This patient has catheter-induced spasm of the RCA, which could result in stasis of contrast within the coronary, and raises the risk of cardiotoxicity (i.e., myocardial ischemia and arrhythmia). Strategies to mitigate this coronary artery spasm would be catheter manipulation to allow coaxial/proximal engagement of the RCA, intracoronary nitroglycerin if systemic pressures allow to relieve spasm, minimizing contrast volume injection, and disengaging the catheter after contrast injection to allow anterograde blood flow. The use of high-osmolar iodinated contrast increases the risk of cardiotoxicity when compared with low or iso-osmolar contrast and would be not indicated in this case.

10.12 Answer C. Fatal reactions to contrast agents are rare and are most often quoted as being between 1:75,000 and 1:170,000 procedures (Katayama H, et al. *Radiology* 1990;175(3):621–628).

10.13 Answer A. Risk factors for contrast-associated nephropathy include pre-existing chronic renal insufficiency, diabetes mellitus, advanced age, hemodynamic instability, intra-aortic balloon pump placement, congestive heart failure, anemia, volume depletion, and the volume of contrast used. The 72-year-old woman has several of these risk factors (Mehran R, et al. *J Am Coll Cardiol* 2004;44(7):1393–1399). In addition, it is likely that a SCr of 2.0 mg/dL represents a more substantial decline in glomerular filtration rate in an elderly woman than a higher SCr in a younger (and presumably larger) man. Metformin does not increase the risk of contrast-related nephropathy, but its continued use in that setting is contraindicated due to the risk of metabolic acidosis from impaired renal clearance.

10.14 Answer D. The fractional excretion of sodium may be low or high, depending of prerenal hypo perfusion vs. actual tubular injury, and is not a reliable way to distinguish CIN from prerenal azotemia. In CIN, creatinine typically peaks at 48 to 72 hours and renal function typically recovers within 2 weeks, whereas acute kidney injury (AKI) from atheroembolic disease often continues to be raised for 3 to 8 weeks after insult. Increased in-hospital mortality, renal failure, and bleeding can occur in patients with CIN after PCI (Thomas T, et al. *J Am Coll Cardiol Intv* 2014;7(1):1–9).

10.15 Answer D. Although noncontrasted lower extremity CT scan could estimate arterial calcium, it would not provide adequate information on lower extremity arterial anatomy or extent of stenosis. All the other choices take advantage of the relatively static nature of many peripheral vascular structures. In road mapping and digital subtraction angiography (DSA), this static nature allows of the generation of baseline images in which radiopaque structures (i.e., bone) are subtracted out.

Nontraditional agents such as CO_2 can be used in this setting but vascular imaging may be suboptimal. The risk of nephrogenic systemic fibrosis, which can occur with exposure to gadolinium in patients with GFR < 30 mL/min/1.73 m^2 (Grobner T. *Nephrol Dial Transplant* 2006;21(4):1104–1108) is ameliorated with non-contrast-enhanced MRA, which has been shown to be a useful imaging modality in diagnosis of peripheral vascular disease (Mihai G, et al. *Cardiol Clin* 2011;29(3):341–350).

10.16 Answer D. Contrast media can cause direct complement activation with the degranulation of basophils and mast cells. This is considered an "anaphylactoid" reaction (Wittbrodt ET, et al. *Ann Pharmacother* 1994;28(2):236–241).

10.17 Answer B. Iodixanol is an iso-osmolar, nonionic agent. It causes less discomfort during peripheral angiography than ionic higher-osmolar agents. The largest randomized controlled trial comparing iodixanol to iopamidol found no difference in the incidence of CIN (Solomon RJ, et al. *Circulation* 2007;115:3189–3196). There is no increase in catheter thrombosis when compared to high-osmolar agents (Bertrand ME, et al. *Circulation* 2000;101:131–136).

10.18 Answer B. Severe emphysema is not an indication for low-osmolar contrast agents. All other conditions listed in the preceding text make patients more susceptible to the hemodynamic effects associated with high-osmolar contrast agents.

10.19 Answer C. Preprocedure and postprocedure hydration is a universally accepted prophylaxis against CIN. Oral *N*-acetylcysteine does not reduce risk of cardiac toxicity. Oral *N*-acetylcysteine has been shown to be beneficial in some small studies if begun 1 day before injection of intravascular contrast (Birck R, et al. *Lancet* 2003;362(9384):598–603), but not in a more recent large randomized controlled trial (i.e., the ACT trial in Berwanger O, et al. *Circulation* 2011;124(11):1250–1259). Minimizing contrast volume with the use of staged (>24 hours) interventions and biplane angiography is another effective strategy to reduce the risk of CIN.

10.20 Answer C. Of the choices listed, the most clearly established reason to use iso-osmolar contrast media instead of low-osmolar contrast is to minimize discomfort during a peripheral procedure. Iso-osmolar contrast may actually result in *less* optimal visualization than low-osmolar contrast, particularly in a morbidly obese person.

10.21 Answer C. Renal hypoperfusion due to renal vasoconstriction and hyperviscosity in the small renal arterials as well as direct renal toxicity are proposed mechanisms of CIN. The other choices describe the mechanism of renal injury due to nonsteroidal anti-inflammatory drugs (A), interstitial nephritis (B), and glomerulonephritis (D).

10.22 Answer B. The history is consistent with an acute aortic dissection. TEE will establish the diagnosis without risk of CIN or gadolinium-induced nephrogenic systemic fibrosis.

10.23 Answer D. The Cockcroft-Gault equation is no longer recommended for calculating eGFR as it was developed before the standardization of creatinine assays and is less accurate. Studies have shown major clinical implications for predicting adverse outcomes after PCI and for drug-dosing recommendations when using the Modification of Diet in Renal Disease (MDRD) and CKD-Epidemiology Collaboration (EPI) formulas to calculate GFR (Parsh J, et al. *J Am Coll Cardiol* 2015;65(25):2714–2723). All other choices are true with regard to PCI planning and CIN. Staging the intervention will allow time for contrast from the diagnostic procedure to clear this patient's system and reduce the risk of CIN. The use of a guide catheter with side holes may minimize pressure dampening during PCI of ostial lesions but typically results in more contrast use because a significant amount of contrast is injected into the aorta. In a recent publication by Parsh et al., CIN defined by an absolute increase of SCr > 0.3 mg/dL and a relative increase of SCr > 50% was optimal compared to other standard definitions and was highly predictive of and specific for inpatient mortality after PCI (Parsh J, et al. *Am Heart J* 2016;175:160–167).

10.24 Answer A. Even without pretreatment using steroids and histamine blockers, the incidence of severe cross-reactions between ionic and nonionic contrast agents is extremely low (Ritchie JL, et al. *J Am Coll Cardiol* 1993;21(1):269–273).

11 Elective Coronary Intervention

Rajesh V. Swaminathan

QUESTIONS

CASE NO. 1 (FOR QUESTIONS Q11.1 THROUGH Q11.9)

A 66-year-old man with progressive exertional angina is transferred to your institution for cardiac catheterization. His past medical history includes a myocardial infarction (MI) with subsequent catheterization and three-vessel coronary artery bypass grafting (CABG) 9 years ago. He is currently taking aspirin and clopidogrel, losartan and diltiazem for hypertension, and simvastatin for hyperlipidemia. He admits to occasionally missing doses of his medications, and he continues to smoke cigarettes. He has normal left ventricular (LV) systolic function by a recent echocardiogram, and his creatinine is chronically elevated in the range of 1.7 to 2.2 mg/dL. Although he gives no history of neurologic problems, a recent carotid Doppler study demonstrated bilateral high-grade internal carotid stenoses (80% to 99%). A recent sestamibi was interpreted as "multiple reversible defects over anterior and lateral walls suggestive of multivessel coronary artery disease (CAD)." He experienced one episode of angina at rest on the day prior to transfer and activated emergency medical services, which took him to his local hospital that does not have catheterization facilities. His chest pain resolved with intravenous (IV) nitroglycerin, and he was ruled out for acute MI with serial cardiac markers.

Diagnostic angiography was performed with a total of 80 mL of x-ray contrast after vigorous prehydration with normal saline and bicarbonate. The following findings were obtained:

- The left internal mammary artery (LIMA) to left anterior descending (LAD) artery was widely patent with good anastomosis and good flow. There was approximately 70% eccentric stenosis of the native LAD shortly after insertion of the LIMA (Fig. Q11-1A).
- A saphenous vein graft (SVG) to the posterior descending artery (PDA) was patent with good distal anastomosis and good flow. The native vessel was <2.0 mm with additional discrete high-grade stenosis downstream from the graft insertion (Fig. Q11-1B).
- An SVG to the obtuse marginal (OM) was shaggy and irregular with angiographic suggestion of thrombus; there were high-grade lesions both in the body of the SVG and at the distal anastomosis; the native vessel was also of small caliber (Fig. Q11-1C).

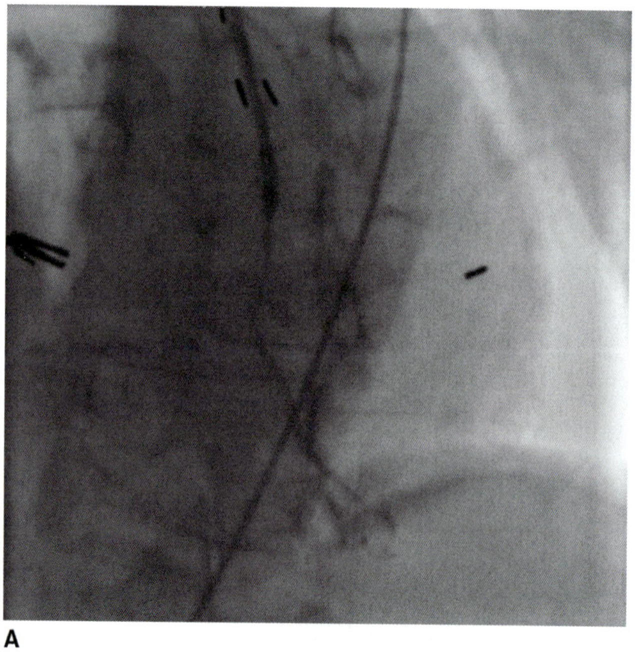

A

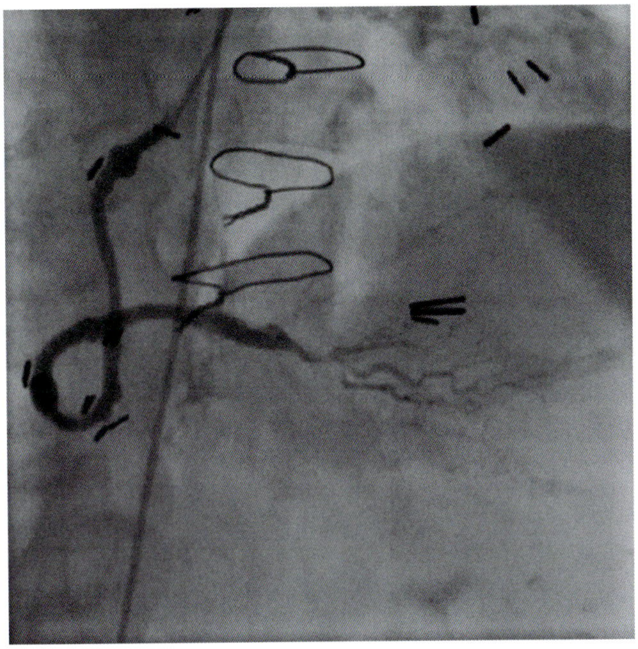

B

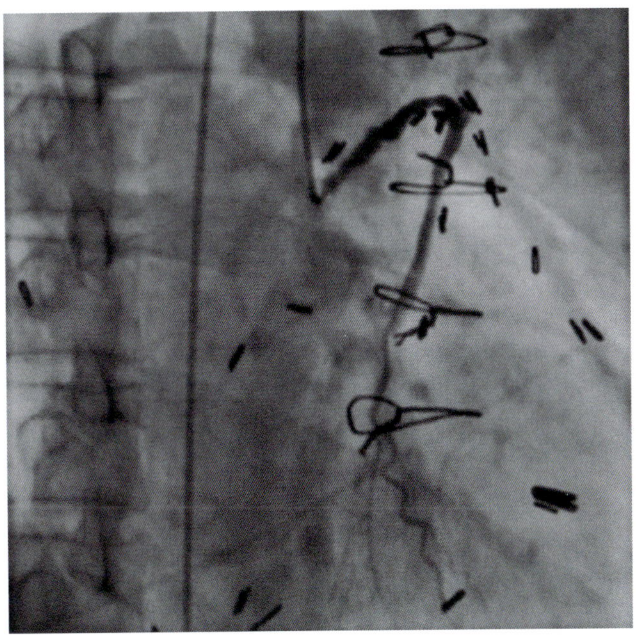

C

Figure Q11-1

11.1 What clinical and anatomic features weigh against a reoperation (repeat CABG) in this patient?

(A) Patent internal mammary graft to the LAD artery
(B) Three patent grafts
(C) Bilateral severe carotid vascular disease
(D) Chronic renal insufficiency
(E) Risk of second CABG is approximately three times higher than first CABG
(F) All of the above

11.2 What clinical and anatomic features weigh against percutaneous coronary intervention (PCI) for this patient?

(A) Noncompliance causes concern for the use of dual antiplatelet therapy (DAPT) if the patient were to receive a drug-eluting stent (DES)
(B) Noncompliance with statins and antihypertensive agents increases likelihood of adverse outcomes after PCI
(C) Chronic renal insufficiency increases risk of bleeding and restenosis
(D) Multivessel disease increases likely dye load and attendant contrast-associated nephropathy
(E) SVG disease is associated with decreased likelihood of procedural success and increased likelihood of distal embolization with attendant morbidity and/or mortality
(F) All of the above

11.3 How soon is the creatinine elevation seen in contrast-associated nephropathy?

(A) <24 hours
(B) 24 to 48 hours
(C) 48 to 72 hours
(D) 72 to 96 hours
(E) 96 to 120 hours

11.4 Risk factors for contrast-associated nephropathy after PCI include all of the following, EXCEPT

(A) Total dye dose from procedure
(B) Multiple dye procedures within 1 week
(C) Diabetes
(D) Elevated creatinine before catheterization
(E) Number of coronary arteries with >70% stenosis

11.5 Which of the following are established means (supported by a Class IIa or higher recommendation in published guidelines) of reducing the likelihood of contrast-associated nephropathy?

(A) Hydration with normal saline
(B) Use of iso-osmolar contrast agents
(C) Fenoldopam
(D) *N*-acetylcysteine
(E) Dopamine infusion in a "renal perfusion" dose (<5 mcg/kg/min)
(F) A and B
(G) A and D

11.6 With regard to PCI of the native LAD lesion in this patient, which of the following concepts is usually CORRECT?

(A) PCI through the native LAD (were it possible) would be less likely to injure the internal mammary artery
(B) PCI of the distal LIMA-LAD anastomosis is one of the few anatomic settings where stents have not been shown to reduce restenosis
(C) Straightening of the LIMA with a PCI wire can produce pseudolesions
(D) With a regular-length LIMA guide and a long internal mammary vessel, it is possible to "run out of catheter length" when trying to treat native LAD lesions
(E) All are correct

11.7 With regard to PCI of the SVG-OM artery in this patient, which of the following concepts is CORRECT?

(A) The use of glycoprotein (GP) IIb/IIIa inhibitors has not been shown to reduce the incidence of major adverse cardiac events (MACE) after PCI of an SVG
(B) Randomized controlled trial (RCT) data do not support the use of "distal protection" in old (>3 years) SVG lesions when technically feasible
(C) The use of rotational atherectomy for treating SVG lesions is associated with a reduction in MACE over the use of stents
(D) Thrombectomy devices have been shown to be superior to balloon angioplasty in SVG lesions
(E) Stents have been shown to be superior to balloon angioplasty in SVG lesions
(F) A and E
(G) A, B, and E

11.8 With regard to PCI of the SVG-PDA in this patient, which of the following is likely to be CORRECT?

(A) The PDA is too small for even the smallest drug-eluting stent (DES)
(B) This is not likely the source of anterior or lateral ischemia
(C) There is no "landing zone" for distal protection
(D) All are correct

11.9 What is the most evidence-based approach for this patient?

(A) Smoking cessation clinic
(B) Repeat CABG
(C) PCI of the SVG-PDA and SVG-OM with distal protection to address the anterior ischemia
(D) Optimize doses of β-blocker, angiotensin-converting enzyme (ACE) inhibitors, and statins and follow clinically for anginal symptoms
(E) A and D

CASE NO. 2 (FOR QUESTIONS Q11.10 THROUGH Q11.16)

A 59-year-old man with hypertension, current tobacco use, strong family history of CAD, diabetes mellitus type 2, and Class II angina was evaluated in the clinic for his chest pain. His blood pressure (BP) was 110/85, heart rate (HR) was 60, and oxygen saturation was 99%. His physical exam was unremarkable. A 12-lead electrocardiogram (ECG) showed normal sinus rhythm with an incomplete right bundle-branch block (RBBB). A transthoracic echocardiogram (TTW) revealed an ejection fraction (EF) of 50% with mild inferior wall hypokinesis. He was taking aspirin, atorvastatin, metoprolol succinate, and lisinopril, and isosorbide mononitrate was added to his regimen. An exercise nuclear stress test was scheduled; however, prior to completion, the patient called 2 weeks later with continued symptoms. He was then referred for direct cardiac catheterization.

A right radial approach was taken for the diagnostic catheterization, which revealed tandem lesions in the right coronary artery (RCA) (a proximal, focal 50% lesion followed by a diffuse, mid 60% lesion). The RCA was dominant with a reference vessel diameter of 3 mm in the proximal and mid segments. Only mild disease was found in the left main, left circumflex (LCx), and LAD artery.

Fractional flow reserve (FFR) with a pressure wire across the tandem lesions in the RCA was performed using systemic adenosine infusion and was found to be significant at 0.77.

11.10 What is the optimal FFR strategy to determine which lesion to treat first in tandem intermediate stenoses?

(A) If the combined FFR is significant, treat the lesion that is angiographically the most significant, and then repeat FFR to determine if the second lesion requires intervention
(B) Treat the distal lesion first and then repeat the FFR to determine if the proximal lesion requires intervention
(C) Perform a "pullback" during the adenosine infusion across the sequential lesions and treat whichever lesion has the greatest pressure gradient first. Then, repeat the FFR to determine if the remaining lesion requires intervention
(D) Treat the proximal lesion first and then repeat FFR to determine if the distal lesion requires intervention

11.11 In tandem lesions, as the distal lesion becomes more severe, what is the influence on the FFR measurement of the more proximal lesion?

(A) The FFR of the proximal lesion increases (becomes less severe)
(B) The FFR of the proximal lesion decreases (becomes more severe)
(C) There is no influence of the distal lesion on the FFR of the proximal lesion
(D) The influence on the proximal lesion is unknown

11.12 The operator treated the distal lesion first with a single new generation DES. Repeat FFR with a pressure wire in the distal RCA is now 0.92. What is known about the relationship between immediate post-PCI FFR and clinical outcomes?

(A) Post-PCI FFR values are not associated with differences in long-term outcomes
(B) Post-PCI FFR values ≥0.95 are paradoxically associated to high rates of death, MI, and target vessel revascularization (TVR) at 6 months
(C) Post-PCI FFR values ≥0.90 are associated with reduced rates of repeat interventions and MACE
(D) Post-PCI FFR can distinguish between stent malapposition, underexpansion, and stent edge dissection

11.13 All of the following are true regarding FFR assessments of lesions EXCEPT

(A) Intermediate lesions in more proximal segments of an epicardial vessel will have greater physiologic significance than the same degree of stenosis in a more distal segment of the vessel due to the amount of myocardium supplied
(B) An anatomically obstructive lesion by intravascular ultrasound (IVUS) can be FFR negative if supplying infarcted myocardium
(C) FFR cannot be used to assess an ostial left main lesion
(D) FFR can be an important tool in the treatment of bifurcation lesions to determine whether a pinched side branch requires further intervention

11.14 According to the 2017 multisociety "Appropriate Use Criteria," the above patient underwent an "appropriate" PCI because

(A) Ischemic symptoms were present
(B) He was taking two antianginal medications
(C) His FFR was ≤0.80
(D) All of the above

11.15 According to the 2017 multisociety "Appropriate Use Criteria (AUC)," if the above patient was treated in a similar fashion, but was only taking one antianginal medication at the time of PCI, the AUC classification would

(A) Be appropriate
(B) May be appropriate
(C) Rarely be appropriate
(D) Be inappropriate

11.16 All of the following are potential advantages of a transradial approach for coronary interventions compared with a transfemoral approach, EXCEPT

(A) Reduction in major bleeding
(B) Reduction in major vascular complications
(C) Lower risk of all-cause mortality
(D) Lower rates of stroke

CASE NO. 3 (FOR QUESTIONS Q11.17 THROUGH Q11.23)

An 84-year-old male is referred to you for angiography. He has a history of severe peripheral arterial disease with a known infrarenal abdominal aortic aneurysm (AAA) and complete occlusions of both iliac arteries. In addition, he has a history of diabetes mellitus, hypertension, and oxygen-requiring chronic obstructive pulmonary disease (COPD) with an FEV1 < 1 L. He is not very active but walks up and down his street, which is approximately the distance of one city block. Over the past 3 months, he has noticed exertional chest tightness that has increased in frequency and intensity. A dobutamine multigated acquisition (MUGA) scan demonstrated a significant decrease in his LV function with stress. You perform angiography via the right radial artery approach, which demonstrates a nondominant RCA, a focal 90% stenosis of the distal left main with nonsignificant disease in the LAD and LCx arteries (Fig. Q11-17).

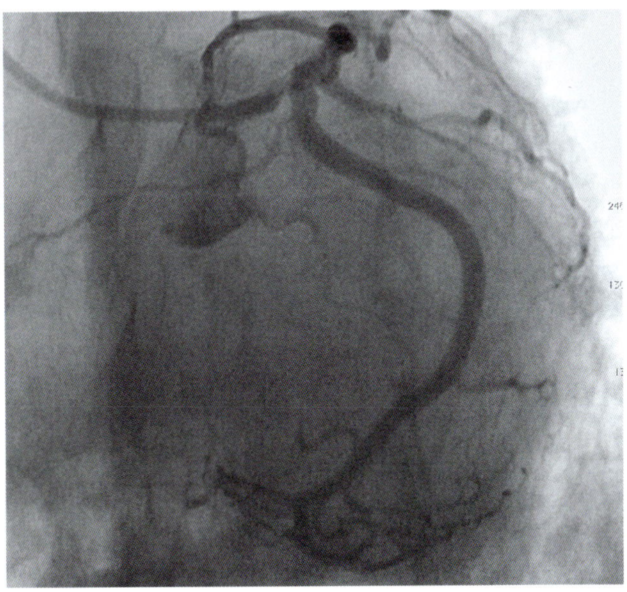

Figure Q11-17

11.17 Under which of the following scenarios is revascularization appropriate in the presence of left main stenosis?

(A) No symptoms
(B) Canadian Cardiovascular Society (CCS) Class I or II angina, low-risk findings on noninvasive imaging
(C) CCS Class III angina
(D) CCS Class III angina, high-risk findings on noninvasive imaging
(E) All of the above

11.18 In the SYNTAX trial, which strategy (CABG or PCI) was associated with a significantly lower rate of MACE (i.e., death, MI, stroke, or repeat revascularization) at 5-year follow-up for all patients with left main stenosis?

(A) CABG
(B) PCI
(C) PCI was associated with a higher rate of repeat revascularization but a lower rate of stroke, resulting in no significant difference between the two strategies
(D) Hybrid revascularization with a LIMA to the LAD and a DES to the LCx and RCA lesions

11.19 In the SYNTAX trial, at 5-year follow-up, PCI was associated with a significantly higher rate of MACE in which subset of patients with left main stenosis?

(A) Ostial left main stenosis, SYNTAX score of 12
(B) Midshaft left main stenosis, SYNTAX score 25
(C) Distal bifurcation left main, SYNTAX score 30
(D) Ostial left main stenosis, SYNTAX score 35

11.20 The patient in the described scenario was calculated to have a SYNTAX score of 13 and a Society of Thoracic Surgeons (STS) score of 5.2%. The 2012 guidelines from the American College of Cardiology (ACC), American Heart Association (AHA), and the Society for Cardiovascular Angiography and Interventions (SCAI), and the 2014 Focused Update for the diagnosis and management of patients with stable ischemic heart disease, gives which recommendation to PCI for this left main stenosis?

(A) Class I
(B) Class IIa
(C) Class IIb
(D) Class III

11.21 The ACC/AHA/SCAI 2012 guidelines and the 2014 Focused Update for the diagnosis and management of patients with stable ischemic heart disease gives which recommendation regarding left main revascularization?

(A) A heart team approach is reasonable in patients with unprotected left main or complex CAD (Class IIa)
(B) A heart team approach is recommended in patients with unprotected left main or complex CAD (Class I)
(C) Calculation of the STS and SYNTAX scores is reasonable in patients with unprotected left main and complex CAD (Class IIa)
(D) Calculation of the STS and SYNTAX scores is recommended in patients with unprotected left main and complex CAD (Class I)
(E) A and C
(F) A and D
(G) B and C
(H) B and D

11.22 Which angiographic view is most likely to help assess the left main, LAD, and circumflex anatomic relationships?

(A) Left anterior oblique (LAO) caudal
(B) Left lateral
(C) LAO cranial
(D) 60 degrees LAO
(E) All of the above

11.23 You decide to proceed with PCI of this patient's left main stenosis based on the fact that his chronic lung disease makes him a poor surgical candidate. The procedure is successful both angiographically and clinically. At what point should you schedule the patient for repeat angiography?

(A) In 2 to 6 months, regardless of the patient's symptoms
(B) Routine repeat angiography is no longer recommended by the guidelines
(C) Every 6 months
(D) Annually

CASE NO. 4 (FOR QUESTIONS Q11.24 THROUGH Q11.28)

A 54-year-old man presents to your catheterization laboratory for diagnostic angiography to evaluate progressive exertional chest pain. He has a history of type 2 diabetes mellitus, hypertension, peripheral arterial disease, and CAD. He underwent CABG 7 years ago with a LIMA to the LAD and SVGs to the left PDA, the ramus, the third OM artery, and the second diagonal artery. Three years after his CABG, he developed recurrent angina and underwent angiography that demonstrated a patent LIMA but complete occlusion of all of his vein grafts. He underwent PCI with a BMS to the proximal, mid, and distal LCx artery. He did well without recurrent symptoms until 3 weeks prior to presentation when he developed exertional angina. He progressed to the point where he was seen by his primary care physician who referred him to you. Based on his prior history of CABG and PCI, you decide to proceed with diagnostic angiography. This reveals a left dominant system, patent LIMA, occluded vein grafts, an occluded mid-LAD, a diffuse 50% in-stent restenosis of the proximal LCx, and a 90% in-stent restenosis of the mid-LCx (Fig. Q11-24).

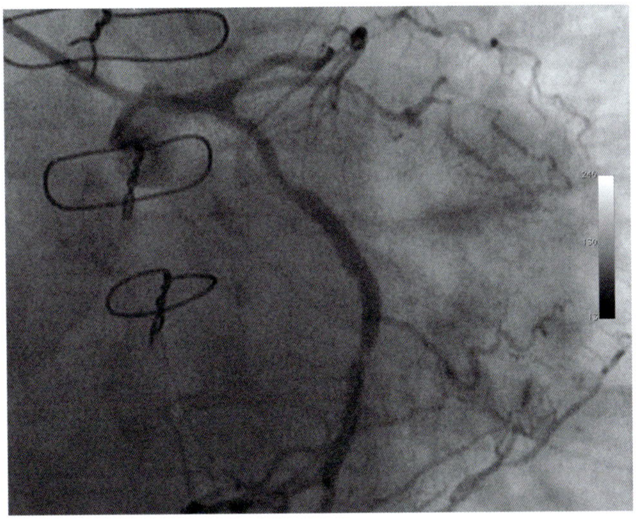

Figure Q11-24

11.24 What would be the BEST approach to revascularizing this patient?

(A) Repeat CABG
(B) PCI of the chronically occluded LAD
(C) PCI of the mid-LCx artery and then FFR assessment of the 50% proximal LCx lesion
(D) B and C

11.25 In the FAME trial of FFR-guided PCI vs. conventional angiography-guided PCI, the rate of 12-month death, nonfatal MI, or repeat revascularization showed which pattern between the two arms?

(A) Higher rate of the composite end point among patients assigned to FFR-guided PCI
(B) Significantly lower in the FFR-guided PCI arm
(C) No difference between the two arms
(D) Nonsignificantly higher death rate but lower rate of repeat revascularization in the FFR-guided PCI arm, resulting in an overall slightly higher event rate in the FFR-guided PCI arm

11.26 In which of the following instances can PCI of the proximal LCx artery stenosis be safely deferred?

(A) Coronary flow reserve (CFR) = 3.0
(B) Relative coronary flow reserve (rCFR) = 1.9
(C) FFR = 0.86
(D) All of the above
(E) Prophylactic PCI should be performed to avoid future ischemic events independent of invasive physiologic data

11.27 If the patient has a history of prior MI in the area supplied by the LCx, which of the following findings are indications for PCI?

(A) CFR = 3.0, rCFR = 2.0, FFR = 0.86
(B) CFR = 1.5, rCFR = 0.6, FFR = 0.82
(C) CFR = 2.5, rCFR = 0.7, FFR = 0.91
(D) CFR = 2.3, rCFR = 2.0, FFR = 0.70

11.28 Which of the following are adenosine-free techniques that have been studied for correlation to adenosine FFR of an intermediate coronary lesion?

(A) Resting Pd/Pa (distal coronary pressure to aortic pressure)
(B) Instantaneous flow reserve (iFR)
(C) Contrast fractional flow reserve (cFFR)
(D) All of the above
(E) A and B only

CASE NO. 5 (FOR QUESTIONS Q11.29 THROUGH Q11.35)

A 77-year-old female is scheduled for elective coronary angiography for invasive risk stratification after a non–ST-segment elevation myocardial infarction (NSTEMI). She presented yesterday with chest pain at rest. On initial exam, she had a body mass index (BMI) of 34 (body weight of 90 kg), and her oxygen saturation was 98% on room air. Her vital signs showed an HR of 90 beats per minute in a regular rhythm, a BP of 180/90 mm Hg, and a respiratory rate of 18 breaths per minute. Her initial ECG demonstrated 1 mm of downsloping ST-segment depression in leads I and II and aVF, and her bedside qualitative troponin value was elevated. Her initial laboratory values showed a hemoglobin value of 10 g/dL, creatinine of 1.8 mg/dL, platelet count of 430,000, creatine kinase-MB (CKMB) of 36 ng/mL (upper limit of normal 9 ng/mL), and a troponin I of 4.0 ng/mL (upper limit of normal 0.10 ng/mL). Her medical history is significant for hypertension, hyperlipidemia, ongoing cigarette smoking, and chronic kidney disease (CKD) with a baseline creatinine of 1.7 to 2.0 mg/dL. Her current medications include aspirin 81 mg daily, furosemide 40 mg daily, simvastatin 40 mg daily, and a multivitamin. She is adherent with her medical regimen. A transthoracic echocardiogram reveals an EF of 50% with anterior wall hypokinesis.

11.29 What clinical features of the case should prompt consideration of invasive risk stratification?

(A) Low thrombolysis in myocardial infarction (TIMI) risk score
(B) Hypertension on admission
(C) Anemia, which could be the cause of her MI
(D) Elevated cardiac markers
(E) None of the above

11.30 The patient is treated initially with two sublingual nitroglycerin tablets, which relieve her chest pain, unfractionated heparin (UFH), and 300 mg of clopidogrel orally. What clinical features of this patient are associated with high bleeding risk?

(A) Age
(B) Female sex
(C) Renal insufficiency
(D) Body weight
(E) All of the above
(F) A, B, and C

11.31 You decide to proceed with cardiac catheterization using a 6-Fr system. This reveals nonsignificant disease in the RCA and the LCx arteries. The LAD has a complex 70% to 80% lesion that extends from the proximal to the mid segment, across a large second diagonal, which also has a 90% lesion in its ostium (Fig. Q11-31). Based on the available evidence, what is the best treatment for this patient?

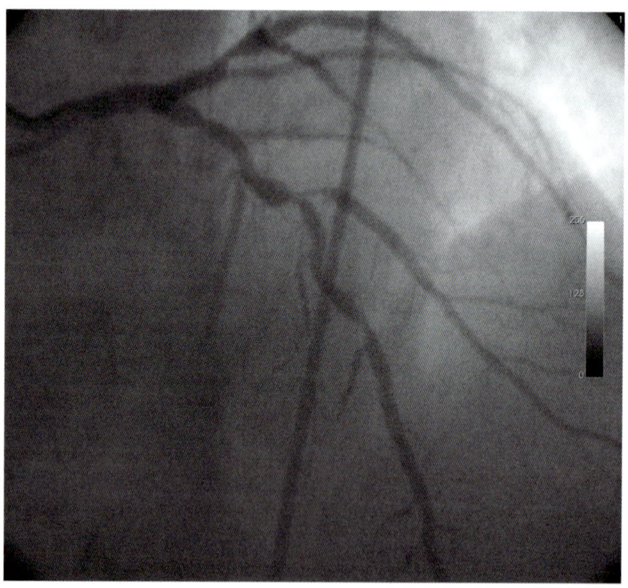

Figure Q11-31

(A) Control of risk factors
(B) Maximal medical therapy, secondary prevention, and revascularization of the LAD system
(C) Smoking cessation and antianginal therapy
(D) FFR of the second diagonal branch

11.32 If you decide to proceed with PCI of the LAD system, what does the totality of the clinical evidence suggest about bifurcation stenting?

(A) The best approach for true bifurcation disease is culotte stenting with DES
(B) Using a DES in the main branch and a BMS in the side branch is associated with reduced mortality compared to CABG
(C) Most of the evidence supports a strategy of stenting the main branch with provisional stenting of the side branch for dissections, reduced TIMI flow, or symptoms
(D) Simultaneous kissing stents with DES has been proven to be superior to CABG with respect to long-term death, MI, or repeat revascularization

11.33 You decide to proceed with PCI of the LAD diagonal bifurcation and place a 28-mm DES followed by an 18-mm DES in the LAD. After deployment of the LAD stent, flow in the second diagonal is reduced to TIMI 2, and the patient begins to complain of chest pain. You quickly place a 0.014-in. angioplasty wire into the diagonal branch and proceed with kissing balloon inflation of the LAD and diagonal, which reestablishes TIMI 3 flow in the diagonal. You notice that there is a visible dissection in the proximal portion of the diagonal with contrast staining. You then place a 15-mm DES in the diagonal using a "T" stent technique. After placement of the diagonal stent, the dissection is no longer visible and the result is excellent angiographically. You decide to stop the procedure and remove the guidewires and take your final pictures. Which of the following features of this case are independently associated with increased risk of DES thrombosis?

(A) Radial approach
(B) Bifurcation stenting
(C) Renal failure
(D) Diabetes
(E) Age >70 years
(F) B, C, and D

11.34 Which of the following strategies can be used to facilitate stent delivery through tortuous or calcified coronary arteries?

(A) Upsizing the guide catheter size
(B) Using a stiffer guidewire
(C) Aggressive guide manipulation ("deep throating the guide")
(D) Using a guide extension catheter
(E) Using a buddy wire
(F) Using a buddy balloon
(G) All of the above

11.35 Stable ischemic heart disease patients undergoing workup and management for renal transplant often proceed to coronary angiography. In which clinical setting is revascularization with *PCI* considered appropriate in a nondiabetic patient?

(A) Asymptomatic patient, not on antianginal therapy, with two-vessel CAD and no proximal LAD involvement, with intermediate- or high-risk noninvasive findings
(B) Asymptomatic patient, not on antianginal therapy, with two-vessel CAD, including proximal LAD involvement, with low-risk noninvasive findings
(C) Symptomatic patient, on maximal antianginal therapy, with two-vessel CAD and no proximal LAD involvement, with low-risk noninvasive findings
(D) Asymptomatic patient, not on antianginal therapy, with left main and/or three-vessel CAD, with intermediate- or high-risk noninvasive findings (SYNTAX > 22)

ANSWERS AND EXPLANATIONS

11.1 Answer F. Both a patent LIMA and three patent grafts (to each major vascular territory: anterior, lateral, and inferior) reduce the potential benefit of a reoperation (Edwards FH, et al. *Ann Thorac Surg* 1994;57(1):27–32). The CABG Guideline lists the effect of reoperation in terms of operative mortality as threefold. Renal disease and cerebrovascular disease are risk factors for CABG mortality (Jones RH, et al. *J Am Coll Cardiol* 1996;28(6): 1478–1487), and cerebrovascular disease is an additional risk for cerebral morbidity with CABG (Roach GW, et al. *N Engl J Med* 1996;335(25):1857–1863).

11.2 Answer F. A number of trials have demonstrated the superiority of DAPT over aspirin alone or Coumadin as adjuncts to stenting (Serruys PW, et al. *N Engl J Med* 1991;324(1):13–17; Cutlip DE, et al. *Circulation* 2001;103(15):1967–1971; Leon MB, et al. *N Engl J Med* 1998;339(23):1665–1671; Schömig A, et al. *N Engl J Med* 1996;334(17): 1084–1089). Failure to continue taking antiplatelet therapy is potentially a greater problem with DES, which inhibits endothelialization. In addition to the wealth of data showing hard endpoint clinical benefits in patients with CAD with lipid-lowering and hypertension control, specific evaluation of post-PCI patients, as in the LIPS trial of statins, demonstrates the importance of ongoing medical management (Serruys PW, et al. *JAMA* 2002;287(24):3215–3222). Chronic renal insufficiency is a PCI risk factor for multiple reasons, including both increased bleeding diathesis and increased restenosis (Mehran R, et al. *J Am Coll Cardiol* 2004;44(7):1393–1399). SVG intervention is associated with increased risk of distal embolization, which is part of the rationale for "distal protection," and not necessarily ameliorated by GP inhibitors (Stone GW, et al. *Circulation* 2003;108(5):548–553).

11.3 Answer C. Contrast-induced nephropathy (CIN) is defined as the impairment of renal function and measured as either a 25% increase in serum creatinine (SCr) from baseline or a 0.5 mg/dL (44 μmol/L) absolute increase in SCr value typically within 48 to 72 hours after IV contrast administration (Kidney Disease Improving Global Outcomes (KDIGO) Acute Kidney Injury Work Group. KDIGO Clinical Practice Guideline for acute kidney injury. *Kidney Int Suppl* 2012;2(Suppl 1):1–138). The creatinine usually starts to decline within 3 to 7 days (Rich MW, et al. *Arch Intern Med* 1990;150(6):1237).

11.4 Answer E. The risk for contrast-associated nephropathy is dependent on the timing and volume of contrast administered and preexisting kidney disease or diabetes (Maeder M, et al. *J Am Coll Cardiol* 2004;44(9):1763–1771; Parfrey PS, et al. *N Engl J Med* 1989;320(3):143–149). CAD burden is not a predictor of contrast-associated nephropathy (Taliercio CP, et al. *Ann Intern Med* 1986;104(4):501–504).

11.5 Answer F. Both hydration with normal saline and the use of iso-osmolar contrast agents or low osmolar contrast agents are recommended by the ACC guidelines and SCAI (King SB III, et al. *J Am Coll Cardiol* 2008;51(2):172–209; Schweiger MJ, et al. *Catheter Cardiovasc Interv* 2007;69(1):135–140). Clinical trials of *N*-acetylcysteine have come to conflicting conclusions. Neither fenoldopam nor "renal-dose" dopamine has been found to be beneficial (Sudarsky D, et al. *Int J Nephrol Renovasc Dis* 2011;4:85–99).

11.6 Answer E. All choices are potential issues when performing PCI of the LAD in the patient with a preexisting LIMA graft (Gruberg L, et al. *J Am Coll Cardiol* 2000;35(4):944–948).

11.7 Answer F. A meta-analysis of randomized trials of GP inhibitors in the setting of PCI found no advantage to the addition of GP inhibitors to UFH (Roffi M, et al. *Circulation* 2002;106:3063–3067). In addition, a post hoc analysis from the REPLACE-2 trial showed that bivalirudin is just as efficacious as the combination of heparin and GP inhibitors at reducing the composite end point of death, MI, or TVR, with a significant reduction in bleeding complications (Kao J, et al. *Catheter Cardiovasc Interv* 2006;68(3):352–356). The use of rotational atherectomy or thrombectomy is not recommended for SVG PCI, while the use of distal protection devices when technically feasible has been proven to be associated with significant reductions in MACE. In addition, stents are more effective than balloon angioplasty in SVG (Maluenda, et al. *Interv Cardiol Clin* 2013;2(2):307–313).

11.8 Answer D. The PDA is <2.25 mm in diameter and the smallest diameter DES available commercially is 2.25 mm. Because the PDA supplies the inferior wall, the presence of stenoses in it would not explain the stress test findings. There is no significant lesion in the vein graft to the PDA; therefore, distal protection is not necessary (Bhatt DL, et al. *Am J Med* 2000;108:176–177).

11.9 Answer E. There are no RCT data to support survival benefit or MI reduction from either repeat CABG or PCI in a patient who has already had one or more CABG. PCI of both the SVGs to the circumflex and RCA territories are unlikely to relieve the ischemia documented in the anterior distribution; accordingly, any PCI strategy should likely include the LAD artery stenosis. There are survival benefit data from RCTs of statins, beta-blockers, ACEI, and smoking cessation (*Lancet* 2002;360(9326):7–22; *N Engl J Med* 1998;339(19):1349–1357).

11.10 Answer C. Assessing FFR values for individual lesions when in tandem can lead to inaccurate values due to the interdependence of flow physiology that each lesion has on the other. For example, a distal stenosis can falsely raise the FFR value of a more proximal lesion (less significant) if measured in isolation (pressure wire parked just beyond the proximal lesion, but not including the distal lesion). The optimal treatment strategy is to measure the combined FFR of both lesions and perform a pullback across each lesion during hyperemia to evaluate the relative pressure drop. Treatment is directed toward the lesion with the highest-pressure gradient, followed by repeat measurement, and final treatment if the vessel FFR remains significant.

11.11 Answer A. As described above, there is interdependence of flow physiology between sequential lesions. If measuring only the FFR of a proximal lesion, the value will increase (become less severe) as a distal lesion becomes more severe (Pijls NHJ, et al. *Circulation* 2000;102:2371).

11.12 Answer C. The immediate post-PCI FFR, although not routinely performed, has been shown to correlate with long-term outcomes. Specifically, values ≥0.90 are associated with reduced rates of repeat interventions and MACE (Pijls NH, et al. *Circulation* 2002;105(25):2950–2954; Rimac G, et al. *Am Heart J* 2017;183:1–9). There is no paradoxical impact at high FFR values. Post-PCI FFR cannot distinguish characteristics of malapposition, underexpansion, or stent edge dissection, which would all require intravascular imaging such as IVUS or optical coherence tomography (OCT).

11.13 Answer C. FFR can be used to assess the physiologic significance of an ostial left main lesion; however, careful technique must be employed. The pressure wire should be equalized in the aorta, the guide catheter should not be fully engaged against the lesion, careful monitoring for dampening during the study should be performed, and a drift check at the end of the procedure should also be routine.

11.14 Answer D. The 2017 Appropriate Use Criteria takes into consideration patient symptoms, optimal antianginal medical therapy, and results of noninvasive imaging studies or intraprocedure physiologic assessment (i.e., FFR) to classify appropriateness of procedures. This patient underwent an appropriate PCI because he was symptomatic on two antianginal medications and had a positive FFR (Patel MR, et al. *J Am Coll Cardiol* 2017;69(17):2212–2241).

11.15 Answer B. If only taking one antianginal medication, then the patient is not optimized on medical therapy. The procedure is now deemed "may be appropriate." There are instances when patients cannot tolerate a second antianginal medication for medical reasons (i.e., side effects or hypotension). It is important to document these reasons in the patient's medical records. The wording "inappropriate" is no longer part of the classification for Appropriate Use Criteria (Patel MR, et al. *J Am Coll Cardiol* 2017;69(17):2212–2241).

11.16 Answer D. Numerous studies, including randomized trials and meta-analyses, comparing the transradial approach with transfemoral across a spectrum of clinical presentations, from elective cases to STEMI, demonstrate that the radial approach is associated with reduced bleeding, vascular complications, and rates of mortality. There is no significant difference in the rates of stroke (Ferrante G, et al. *JACC Cardiovasc Interv* 2016;9(14):1419–1434).

11.17 Answer E. According to the published Appropriateness Criteria for Revascularization (Patel MR, et al. *J Am Coll Cardiol* 2009;53(6):530–553), the presence of left main stenosis should prompt consideration of revascularization regardless of symptoms. Importantly, this does not mean PCI; instead, it means either CABG or rarely PCI depending on other issues, such as patient comorbidities, anatomical features, etc.

11.18 Answer C. The SYNTAX trial randomized 1,800 patients with three-vessel or left main CAD to either CABG or PCI (Serruys PW, et al. *N Engl J Med*

2009;360(10):961–972). The primary end point was 12-month all-cause death, MI, stroke, or repeat revascularization. PCI failed to meet the noninferiority criteria in comparison with CABG for the entire cohort. PCI was associated with a reduction in stroke but an increase in repeat revascularization. In the left main subset, a similar pattern was seen resulting in no significant difference between the two strategies. This finding should be interpreted with caution given that it is a subgroup analysis. Hybrid revascularization was not addressed in the SYNTAX trial. Five-year results of the left main subset showed similar trends (Mohr FW, et al. *Lancet* 2013;381(9867):629–638).

11.19 Answer D. When stratified by SYNTAX score tertiles, high SYNTAX scores (≥33) were associated with significantly higher MACE for PCI (first-generation DES) vs. CABG (46.5% vs. 29.7%, $p = 0.003$). There was no significant difference in revascularization strategies for low/intermediate SYNTAX scores (0 to 32) (Mohr FW, et al. *Lancet* 2013;381(9867):629–638).

11.20 Answer B. Based on the evolution of contemporary left main trials with newer-generation DES, guidelines have upgraded the recommendation for left main PCI in certain patients over time. Stable ischemic heart disease patients with favorable left main anatomic lesions for PCI, low SNYTAX scores, and who are high risk for surgical intervention now have a Class IIa level of recommendation (Fihn SD, et al. *J Am Coll Cardiol* 2012;60(24):e44–e164; Fihn SD, et al. *J Am Coll Cardiol* 2014;64(18):1929–1949).

11.21 Answer G. Updated guidelines on left main revascularization in stable ischemic heart disease provide a strong recommendation for a heart team approach to patients with unprotected left main or complex CAD (Class I) and indicate that it is reasonable (Class IIa), in the context of determining which approach is best for revascularization, to calculate the STS and SYNTAX score (Fihn SD, et al. *J Am Coll Cardiol* 2012;60(24):e44–e164; Fihn SD, et al. *J Am Coll Cardiol* 2014;64(18):1929–1949).

11.22 Answer A. Of the choices provided, the LAO caudal view provides the best separation of the LAD and LCx arteries in most cases.

11.23 Answer B. The 2005 PCI guidelines recommended routine angiographic follow-up 2 to 6 months after unprotected left main stenting. However, routine angiography is no longer recommended (removed in 2009) after left main PCI based on the inability of angiography to predict acute, sudden stent thrombosis, and the risks associated with repeat angiography in a patient who has undergone placement of a left main stent (Kushner FG, et al. *J Am Coll Cardiol* 2009;54(23):2205–2241). Moreover, the results of the SYNTAX trial suggest good intermediate-term results for PCI in left main patients.

11.24 Answer C. The 2009 Focused Update to the PCI guidelines give a Class IIa (Level of Evidence A) to use intracoronary physiologic measurements (i.e., FFR) as an alternative to noninvasive functional testing to guide PCI. In this patient, the proximal LCx artery stenosis is of intermediate severity (defined in the guidelines as 30% to 70%) and should be evaluated further with FFR. This should be done after stenting of the 90% (severe) distal lesion. Repeat CABG is not indicated in this patient with a patent LIMA. Recanalizing the chronically occluded LAD is also not indicated because the LIMA is patent.

11.25 Answer B. The FAME trial randomized 1,005 patients with multivessel CAD to PCI guided by conventional angiographic assessment or PCI guided by FFR (*N Engl J Med* 2009;360(3):213–224). Patients assigned to the angiography-guided PCI had all lesions stented, while patients assigned to the FFR-guided PCI strategy had only those lesions with an FFR value ≤0.80 stented. The FFR-guided strategy was associated with a significantly lower rate of death, nonfatal MI, or repeat revascularization at 12 months (13.2% vs. 18.3%, $p = 0.02$).

11.26 Answer D. CFR is measured distal to a lesion and is the ratio of the flow distal to a lesion before and after vasodilation ($Q_{dil}/Q_{initial}$). The rCFR compares the CFR in a normal vessel to one that has the lesion of interest. Values below 2.0 for the CFR and below 0.8 for the rCFR indicate a hemodynamically significant lesion. An FFR value ≤0.80 indicates a hemodynamically significant lesion.

11.27 Answer D. The key to this question is the history of prior MI in the territory supplied by the artery in question. Only the FFR is reliable in the presence of a prior MI; therefore, the FFR value of 0.70 indicates a hemodynamically significant lesion regardless of the CFR and rCFR values.

11.28 Answer D. As there are potential risks associated with adenosine administration for induction of hyperemia during FFR measurement, several novel adenosine-free methods have emerged and been tested against traditional adenosine FFR. These modalities are generally safer and may provide a more rapid assessment of physiologically significant lesions (Johnson NP, et al. *JACC Cardiovasc Interv* 2016;9(8):757–767).

11.29 Answer D. This patient has a TIMI risk score of 5, giving her a 26% incidence of death, MI, or urgent revascularization within 14 days. This indicates a high-risk situation and the presence of elevated cardiac markers should prompt invasive risk stratification.

11.30 Answer F. Several analyses have examined risk factors for bleeding complications in patients with acute coronary syndrome (ACS) undergoing PCI. These have demonstrated that age, female sex, and renal insufficiency are major risk factors for hemorrhagic complications. Low body weight is also a risk, but the patient described in the case is overweight (Rao SV, et al. *Eur Heart J* 2007;28(10):1193–1204; Mehran R, et al. *J Am Coll Cardiol* 2010;55(23):2556–2566).

11.31 Answer B. Revascularization of the presumed culprit artery is indicated in high-risk patients with ACS. This patient has a high TIMI risk score, and the results of her echocardiogram correlate with significant stenosis on the coronary angiogram. Choices A and C are not the best answer because they do not include revascularization. FFR is indicated for lesions of intermediate severity (30% to 70%).

11.32 Answer C. Most of the retrospective studies and prospective randomized trials support a strategy of provisional stenting of side branches for true bifurcation lesions (Al Suwaidi J, et al. *J Am Coll Cardiol* 2000;35(4):929–936; Iakovou I, et al. *J Am Coll Cardiol* 2005;46(8):1446–1455).

11.33 Answer F. A prospective cohort study of 2,229 patients who underwent DES demonstrated that independent predictors of cumulative stent thrombosis include premature cessation of antiplatelet therapy, renal failure, bifurcation stenting, diabetes, and LV dysfunction (Iakovou I, et al. *JAMA* 2005;293(17):2126–2130). Age was a univariate predictor but was not independently associated with stent thrombosis after multivariable adjustment.

11.34 Answer G. All are techniques that can facilitate stent delivery through tortuous or calcified coronary arteries. In general, deep throating the guide catheter should be avoided to avoid trauma to proximal vessel.

11.35 Answer C. The updated 2017 Appropriate Use Criteria addressed situations of revascularization in the setting of renal transplant. Note that revascularization can include either CABG or PCI. Choices A and B are classified as "May Be Appropriate." D "May Be Appropriate" for PCI and "Appropriate" for CABG. Only C is "Appropriate" for PCI (Patel MR, et al. *J Am Coll Cardiol* 2017;69(17): 2212–2241).

12 Percutaneous Coronary Intervention for Acute Coronary Syndromes

Madhan Shanmugasundaram

QUESTIONS

12.1 A 70-year-old man came to the emergency room (ER) for evaluation after his family "talked" him into seeking medical attention. He claims that he had severe pressure-type nonexertional chest pain that woke him up from his sleep 3 days ago; it persisted for hours, but he has not had any symptoms since. His daughter who is a nurse wanted him to come for an evaluation because he has been fatigued since. His presentation electrocardiogram (ECG) showed age indeterminate inferior ST-segment elevation myocardial infarction (STEMI). Admission lab work was unremarkable, except for a troponin T of 10 ng/mL. Coronary angiogram shows 100% occluded mid-right coronary artery (RCA) and mild nonobstructive disease in the left system. What is the recommended treatment for this gentleman?

(A) Drug-eluting stent (DES) to the mid-RCA
(B) Bare metal stent (BMS) to the mid-RCA
(C) Thrombectomy followed by balloon angioplasty only as he is asymptomatic
(D) Medical therapy with aspirin, beta-blockers, statins, and angiotensin-converting enzyme (ACE) inhibitors
(E) Coronary artery bypass graft (CABG) surgery with a vein graft to RCA

12.2 A 75-year-old woman was admitted with a non-STEMI to a non-percutaneous coronary intervention (PCI)-capable hospital where she was started on standard medical therapy that included aspirin, clopidogrel, metoprolol, and atorvastatin. She was maintained on enoxaparin 1 mg/kg subcutaneously twice a day. Her lab work showed an elevated troponin T of 3 ng/mL. The cardiologist who evaluated her the following day transferred her to another hospital for coronary angiogram, which showed critical stenosis of the left circumflex (LCx) artery. She had been on enoxaparin for 24 hours, and the last dose was 10 hours ago. What would be the ideal antithrombotic strategy for this patient's PCI?

(A) Enoxaparin 0.3 mg/kg intravenous (IV) once
(B) Unfractionated heparin (UFH) with a goal activated clotting time (ACT) of 300 seconds
(C) Additional dose of enoxaparin 1 mg/kg administered subcutaneously
(D) No additional anticoagulant needed as the last dose was only 10 hours ago
(E) Bivalirudin 0.75 mg/kg IV bolus followed by 1.75 mg/kg/h infusion

12.3 Fondaparinux is not recommended as a sole anticoagulant to support PCI because:

(A) It is significantly more expensive than UFH and confers no additional therapeutic advantage
(B) Unlike UFH, its therapeutic efficacy cannot be monitored during PCI
(C) There is a significant increase in catheter-related thrombosis with fondaparinux
(D) There is an increase in stent thrombosis with fondaparinux
(E) All of the above

12.4 A 70-year-old man with no prior cardiac history, but with multiple atherosclerotic risk factors and end-stage renal disease (ESRD), was admitted on a Saturday to the coronary care unit with 6 hours of worsening chest pain and an ECG showing non-specific ST-T wave changes. His admission lab work showed a troponin T of 2 ng/mL. His medical therapy includes aspirin, a loading dose of clopidogrel, UFH, and atorvastatin. He has persistent chest pain on nitroglycerin infusion. What would be the next step in his care?

(A) Proceed with coronary angiography with intent to revascularize
(B) Increase nitroglycerin infusion with a plan for angiography on Monday
(C) Start glycoprotein (GP) IIb/IIIa inhibitor eptifibatide
(D) Obtain bedside echocardiogram to look for regional wall motion abnormalities
(E) Switch UFH to enoxaparin for better antithrombotic effects

12.5 A 55-year-old diabetic man presents to a non-PCI-capable hospital with chest pain and an ECG showing anterior STEMI. The ER physician decided to thrombolyze him as the closest PCI facility is 2 hours away. He also received UFH, aspirin, a clopidogrel loading dose, metoprolol, and atorvastatin. Post thrombolytic ECG showed near complete resolution of ST elevation in the anterior leads. He arrives at your facility, which has PCI capability, 2 hours later. The ER doctor at your facility who received the patient calls you to see what he should do.

(A) Tell him to activate the catheterization immediately as the patient had anterior STEMI and, hence, by definition, is high risk
(B) Patient should be admitted to the coronary care unit so your team can evaluate him to make a decision
(C) Ask him to start the patient on a GP IIb/IIIa inhibitor of his choice
(D) Cardiology consultation is not necessary as his treatment is complete
(E) Nuclear stress test should be obtained immediately and patient can be referred for angiography if there is ischemia in the anterior wall

12.6 An 80-year-old man presents with 3 hours of angina to the ER where ECG shows inferior STEMI and a Mobitz type I atrioventricular (AV) block. After appropriate medical therapy is initiated, the STEMI team was paged. Coronary angiography showed 100% thrombotic occlusion of the mid-RCA that was treated successfully with a DES. There is also another 80% mildly calcific stenosis of the mid left anterior descending artery (LAD). This is your partner's case, and he calls you for a second opinion with the patient on the table. He wants to see if you recommend proceeding with PCI of the LAD. Your response should be:

(A) Patient is not in cardiogenic shock, so there is no indication for PCI of the LAD
(B) Nuclear stress test the following day to assess for ischemia
(C) PCI of non-infarct-related artery during STEMI is contraindicated
(D) PCI of the LAD may be considered either at the time of primary PCI or as a planned, staged procedure as it has been shown to decrease major adverse cardiac events (MACE)
(E) PCI of the LAD is recommended only if the patient has postinfarct angina

12.7 In current day practice, the accepted indication for a GP IIb/IIIa inhibitor includes

(A) Patients with low-risk acute coronary syndrome (ACS) that are being managed conservatively
(B) Patients with intermediate- to high-risk ACS who were adequately loaded with a $P2Y_{12}$ inhibitor in preparation for early invasive approach
(C) Patients with ACS who are considered for early invasive approach who were not adequately preloaded with a $P2Y_{12}$ inhibitor
(D) Routine use in combination with UFH in patients with ACS to decrease risk of myocardial infarction (MI) or death
(E) Patients with high-risk ACS in a prehospital setting to decrease adverse cardiovascular events

12.8 A 65-year-old woman with diabetes and hypertension presented to the hospital with 3 hours of chest pain and light-headedness. On presentation, ECG showed 4-mm ST elevation in the inferior and lateral leads with anterior precordial ST-segment depression. Vitals show a blood pressure (BP) of 86/54 mm Hg that did not respond to intravenous fluid (IVF) boluses, and hence, Dopamine was started. Her jugular venous pressure (JVP) was elevated with S3 noted on cardiac exam. The nearest PCI-capable hospital is 3 hours away. She has no contraindications to thrombolytic therapy. What is the best course of management?

(A) Transfer her to the nearest PCI facility
(B) Thrombolyze her and then transfer her in 48 to 72 hours after stabilization
(C) Thrombolyze her and transfer her immediately
(D) Request a do not resuscitate (DNR) and do not intubate (DNI) and treat her medically as she has a poor prognosis
(E) Add a GP IIb/IIIa inhibitor to the treatment regimen

12.9 A 70-year-old diabetic man presents with 4 hours of crushing chest pain and ECG showing anterior STEMI. He is hemodynamically stable and received 324 mg of aspirin, 180 mg loading dose of ticagrelor, and 5,000 units of UFH and was referred for emergent angiography. The anteroposterior (AP) cranial projection shows 100% thrombotic occlusion of the mid-LAD at the site of takeoff of a large-sized diagonal branch. There is also high-grade stenosis of the mid-RCA. This is your young partner's first STEMI after fellowship, and he wants your recommendation for the next step:

(A) As the artery is completely occluded and he is hemodynamically stable, advise him to treat the patient medically
(B) Refer him for emergent CABG, as he is a diabetic with multivessel coronary artery disease (CAD)
(C) Start a GP IIb/IIIa inhibitor to decrease the thrombus burden and defer PCI for 24 hours
(D) Aspiration thrombectomy is indicated to reduce infarct size and improve outcomes
(E) Proceed with angioplasty and stent placement to mid LAD.

12.10 A 55-year-old woman sustains an out-of-hospital ventricular fibrillation (VF) cardiac arrest and was resuscitated successfully with bystander CPR and defibrillation. She is brought into the ER after being intubated in the field and is sedated on arrival. Not much history is available, but a postresuscitation ECG is shown Figure Q12-10.

As the on-call interventional cardiologist, you decide to take the patient for emergent coronary angiography with intent to revascularize. The ER physician attempted to place a nasogastric (NG) tube repeatedly without much success. She received aspirin rectally. You decide to move her to the catheterization lab. Angiography confirms your suspicion of 100% thrombotic occlusion of the proximal LAD. The LCx and RCA appear free of high-grade stenosis. It was decided to use bivalirudin as the anticoagulant for PCI. What would be the ideal antiplatelet strategy for her?

(A) Proceed with PCI and administer clopidogrel later in the coronary care unit after they place an NG tube
(B) Stop the procedure and try to place an NG tube to give clopidogrel
(C) IV cangrelor loading followed by an infusion for 4 hours, to be transitioned to ticagrelor
(D) Proceed with GP IIb/IIIa inhibitors that will be continued until she is awake
(E) None of the above

12.11 A 79-year-old man with CAD and prior CABG 15 years ago with the left internal mammary artery (LIMA) to LAD and a vein graft to the obtuse marginal (OM) 1 and distal RCA was admitted to the hospital with worsening angina. His lab work was remarkable for elevated creatinine of 1.8 mg/dL, which was close to his baseline renal function and troponin T that peaked at 5 ng/mL. Echocardiogram showed mild left ventricular (LV) systolic dysfunction with an estimated ejection fraction of 45% and a hypokinetic inferior wall. He was previously noted to have preserved systolic function by an echocardiogram that was completed over a year ago. After initial medical stabilization with aspirin, clopidogrel, metoprolol, lisinopril, atorvastatin, and

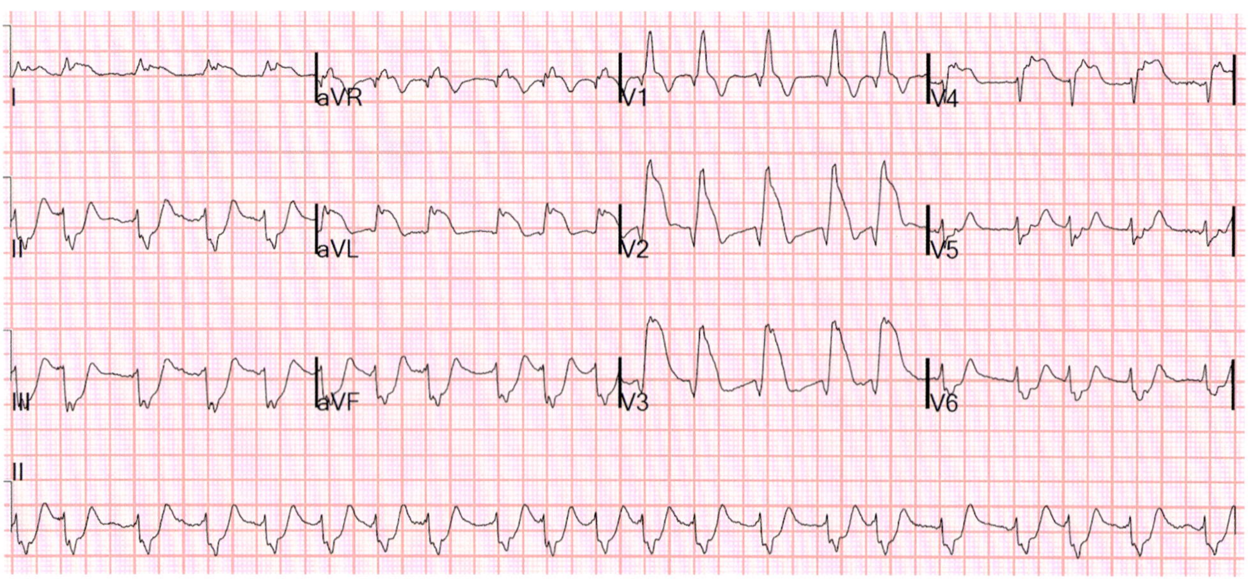

Figure Q12-10 (Courtesy of Madhan Shanmugasundaram.)

IV UFH, he was referred for coronary angiography. This showed a chronic total occlusion (CTO) of the mid-LAD and proximal circumflex, and a high-grade moderately calcific long stenosis of the mid-RCA. The LIMA to LAD and vein graft to OM-1 was patent without significant stenosis; however, the vein graft to distal RCA was noted to be 100% occluded in the proximal body. What would be the next step in his care?

(A) Treat him medically as there are no targets for percutaneous revascularization
(B) Attempt PCI of the occluded vein graft to distal RCA
(C) PCI of the mid-RCA with DES
(D) PCI of the LCx occlusion with BMS given his age
(E) There is no clear culprit lesion identified in this angiography, and there is nothing you can do to reduce his future cardiac events

12.12 A 65-year-old man with CAD and prior CABG with two grafts (LIMA to the LAD and a saphenous vein graft [SVG] to the posterior descending artery [PDA]) was admitted to the hospital with unstable angina. After initial medical stabilization, he was referred for angiography due to persistent angina. Angiogram showed a CTO of the mid-LAD and a proximal RCA with no high-grade stenosis in the circumflex system. The LIMA to LAD was patent, but there was a 90% focal stenosis of the body of the SVG to PDA. It is decided to proceed with PCI of this SVG. Which of the following is indicated to reduce periprocedural MI and improve outcomes in this PCI?

(A) Distal embolic protection with a filter
(B) GP IIb/IIIa inhibitors infusion
(C) Adenosine and nicardipine administered intragraft before PCI to prepare the microvasculature
(D) Attempt to direct stent the lesion in the SVG to avoid distal embolization
(E) Since this is an old SVG, attempt to open the RCA CTO

12.13 An 83-year-old woman with hypertension, diabetes, atrial fibrillation, and prior stroke was admitted with NSTEMI and troponin of 6 ng/mL. She was maintained on warfarin for stroke prophylaxis that she stopped recently for an elective surgery. Her international normalized ratio (INR) at presentation was 1.1. Angiography shows a thrombotic 95% lesion in the mid-LAD with a thrombolysis in myocardial infarction (TIMI) grade 2 flow (culprit lesion) that was treated with a DES. This was performed on UFH, acetylsalicylic acid (ASA), and clopidogrel loading dose. What would be the ideal antiplatelet and anticoagulant combination for her after the PCI with lowest bleeding risk?

(A) Aspirin, clopidogrel, and warfarin
(B) Aspirin, ticagrelor, and warfarin
(C) Clopidogrel and rivaroxaban
(D) Aspirin and clopidogrel only
(E) Aspirin and warfarin

12.14 A 60-year-old diabetic man presents to the hospital with unrelenting chest pain and a troponin of 4 ng/mL. He has a history of extensive smoking and peripheral artery disease (PAD) with a left superficial femoral artery (SFA) stent that was placed 2 years ago. His admission ECG shows ischemic changes. Your noninterventional colleague is on call and wants your opinion on the best $P2Y_{12}$ inhibitor for this patient. He is currently chest pain–free and is scheduled to undergo coronary angiography the following day with you. His current medical regimen includes aspirin, enoxaparin, metoprolol, lisinopril, and rosuvastatin. Which antiplatelet agent would you recommend?

(A) Clopidogrel 600 mg loading dose as he is a low vascular–risk patient
(B) Prasugrel 60 mg loading dose as he is a diabetic with PAD and prasugrel has better bioavailability as it does not need two-step activation like clopidogrel
(C) Ticagrelor 180 mg loading dose
(D) Recommend waiting until angiogram is completed to decide on antiplatelet agent as he can have multivessel disease requiring CABG
(E) There is no evidence for early and routine $P2Y_{12}$ inhibitor use in NSTEMI

12.15 A 75-year-old woman with a recent history of DES PCI (everolimus-eluting stent 3.0 × 23 mm) to the RCA in the setting of NSTEMI 10 days ago presents to the ER with inferior STEMI and 2 hours of chest pain. Her previous medical regimen included aspirin, clopidogrel, metoprolol, and atorvastatin. She has had a stroke 2 years ago with no significant residual neurologic sequelae. She claims that she was very compliant with her medications; she, in fact, recalled all her drugs with correct dosing. Emergent coronary angiography confirms your suspicion of subacute stent thrombosis. She undergoes successful angioplasty followed by optical coherence tomography (OCT) examination of the RCA that shows adequately expanded and well-apposed previous stent with some residual thrombus. No distal edge dissections noted. Since she was on a maintenance dose of clopidogrel, the ER physician did not reload her with a $P2Y_{12}$ agent. You decide to place another DES (zotarolimus-eluting stent 3.0 × 18 mm). What should her antiplatelet regimen be?

(A) Assume that she is not telling the truth and continue clopidogrel
(B) Assume that she is a clopidogrel nonresponder and switch her to prasugrel
(C) The stent thrombosis was unique to the everolimus-eluting stent. Now that she has a different DES, it is safe to continue clopidogrel
(D) Assume that she is a clopidogrel nonresponder and switch her to ticagrelor
(E) Perform platelet function testing to see if there is a high on treatment platelet reactivity and then switch her to another agent if it is confirmed
(F) Perform genetic testing to confirm that she is a clopidogrel nonresponder before switching her to another agent

12.16 An 87-year-old woman is transferred to your facility for catheterization and possible PCI after presenting with chest pain with ST-segment depressions and an elevated troponin level. Her creatinine level is 1.9 mg/dL, and she weighs 58 kg. The patient is started on aspirin, 600 mg clopidogrel, enoxaparin, and eptifibatide. All of the following are independently associated with an increased risk of major bleeding, EXCEPT

(A) Renal dysfunction
(B) Female gender
(C) Previous CABG
(D) Advanced age

12.17 A 70-year-old diabetic man with chronic kidney disease (CKD) (baseline creatinine 2.4 mg/dL) was admitted to the hospital with NSTEMI and ongoing chest pain. You are called in as the interventional cardiologist in the group to evaluate him. His troponin T was 8 ng/mL and is trending up. After initial medical stabilization, you decide to proceed with angiography with intent to revascularize. His creatinine on the day of the procedure was 2.5 mg/dL and estimated glomerular filtration rate (eGFR) is 25. As you are discussing the risks of the procedure, including contrast-induced nephropathy (CIN), he sustains a VT cardiac arrest and is successfully resuscitated. What is the best strategy to avoid CIN in this patient?

(A) Use the CIN risk calculator and give the patient a percentage risk of CIN so that he will refuse the procedure
(B) Delay the angiography and attempt to hydrate him before the procedure
(C) Minimize the amount of contrast use for the procedure
(D) There is nothing that you can do; his risk of CIN is 100%
(E) Administer 600 mg of *N*-acetylcysteine and a sodium bicarbonate infusion

12.18 A patient returns to your clinic for follow-up after you performed a PCI for single-vessel CAD in the setting of an NSTEMI. He has done very well and has had no evidence of recurrent angina or congestive heart failure (CHF). He is known to have normal LV systolic function following the intervention. He asks about the benefit of future stress testing and wonders if he should periodically have such a noninvasive evaluation performed. What should you tell him?

(A) Stress ECG is a simple and sensitive way to predict and identify the presence of restenosis following PCI
(B) All patients with documented CAD who undergo PCI should have yearly stress testing performed to evaluate functional capacity and to look for objective evidence of ischemia
(C) Stress testing in asymptomatic patients is indicated only for patients with high-risk features when trying to find objective evidence of ischemia
(D) Only the presence of recurrent symptoms justifies stress testing in patients who have undergone PCI
(E) After PCI, the only way to assess for ischemia is fractional flow reserve (FFR)

12.19 A diagnosis of ACS was made in a very active 70-year-old woman who still manages her own restaurant. Her cardiovascular risk profile is significant for hypertension, well controlled on amlodipine 5 mg daily, and hyperlipidemia on atorvastatin 20 mg daily. During the last 14 months, she has required intermittent antibiotic treatment for recurrent episodes of urinary tract infection. Initial evaluation had revealed a residual urinary volume of 147 mL, mild prolapsed bladder, and urethral strictures. She was admitted 2 days ago with severe urinary tract infection and a temperature of 39°C. Her BP was 137/85 mm Hg and heart rate was 100 beats per minute (bpm). Her weight was 52 kg. Laboratory data showed a creatinine of 1.5 mg/dL, a white blood cell (WBC) count of 12,700, and hemoglobin 12 g/dL. She developed intermittent chest pressure during her first night in the hospital. There were no ST-segment changes on the ECG. Troponins were followed and found to be abnormal. Following an early invasive pathway, the patient is planned to undergo angiographic evaluation. In the event a PCI is needed and if the bleeding risk of anticoagulation is to be minimized, which would be the most appropriate anticoagulation strategy?

(A) UFH at 60 U/kg with concomitant GP IIb/IIIa inhibitor
(B) IV enoxaparin and as a single bolus of 0.75 mg/kg
(C) Bivalirudin 0.75 mg/kg IV bolus followed by 1 mg/kg/h infusion for the duration of PCI
(D) Fondaparinux 2.5 mg

12.20 A 65-year-old man with no prior cardiac history was brought to the ER with chest pain, dizziness, and fatigue. He appears somnolent and the history was mostly obtained from his family. They claim that he has been having these symptoms for 48 hours but was refusing to seek medical attention. His vital signs are significant for tachycardia (heart rate 120 bpm) and hypotension (80/50 mm Hg) with cold extremities. He was given IVF that did not significantly improve his BP. He was started on IV norepinephrine that increased his BP to 90/60 mm Hg. He required escalating doses of norepinephrine to maintain his BP and his labs showed a troponin T of 20 ng/mL. You are called in for an emergent coronary angiography. Apart for early revascularization, what else would you consider at this point that will significantly help this patient?

(A) GP IIb/IIIa inhibitors
(B) Intubate and sedate the patient so he does not decompensate during PCI
(C) Proceed with emergent angiography and PCI as indicated
(D) Start dobutamine, in addition to norepinephrine, to improve his hemodynamics before the angiogram
(E) After diagnostic angiogram, consider placing a hemodynamic support device before PCI

12.21 A 70-year-old man comes to your office for a follow-up visit after PCI to the mid-LAD for NSTEMI. His past history includes diabetes, hypertension, and hyperlipidemia. His medical regimen includes aspirin, ticagrelor, lisinopril, metoprolol, and atorvastatin. Echocardiogram post PCI showed preserved LV systolic function with mild septal hypokinesis. He seemed to have recovered very well and is eager to discuss his treatment goals with you. He wants to know what other therapy you can prescribe that will make him live longer after his ACS.

(A) Reassure him that his survival was not altered by the acute MI and is comparable to the rest of the population as it was successfully treated with PCI.
(B) Routine annual stress test to look for ischemia and revascularize as soon as it turns positive
(C) Refer him to a supervised cardiac rehabilitation program
(D) Rivaroxaban 2.5 mg twice a day has been shown to improve survival in post MI patients
(E) There is nothing you can do to improve his survival since his LV ejection fraction is normal

Questions 12.22 through 12.27 are Optical coherence tomography (OCT) images. Match the image with the most appropriate answer.

12.22 See Figure Q12-22.

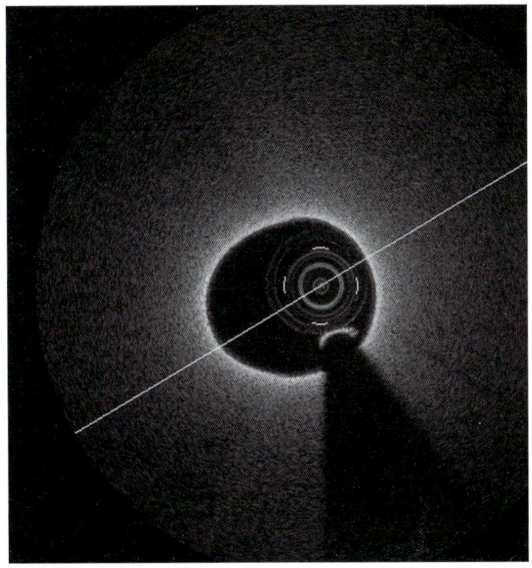

Figure Q12-22

(A) Normal vessel anatomy
(B) Unstable angina
(C) Guiding catheter
(D) Stable angina
(E) Side branch
(F) ACS if rupture occurs

12.23 See Figure Q12-23.

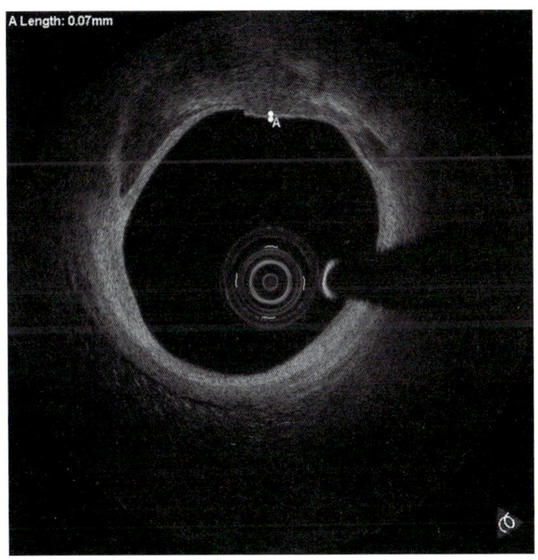

Figure Q12-23

(A) Normal vessel anatomy
(B) Unstable angina
(C) Guiding catheter
(D) Stable angina
(E) Side branch
(F) ACS if rupture occurs

12.24 See Figure Q12-24.

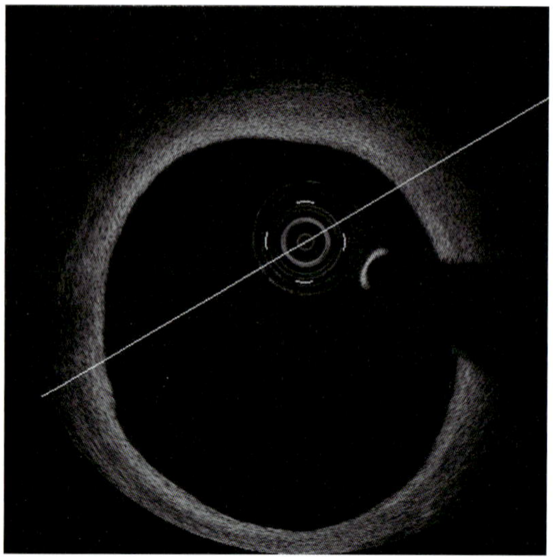

Figure Q12-24

(A) Normal vessel anatomy
(B) Unstable angina
(C) Guiding catheter
(D) Stable angina
(E) Side branch
(F) ACS if rupture occurs

12.25 See Figure Q12-25.

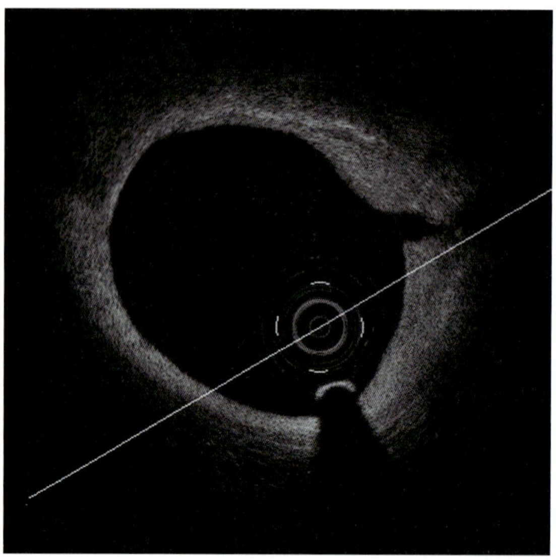

Figure Q12-25

(A) Normal vessel anatomy
(B) Unstable angina
(C) Guiding catheter
(D) Stable angina
(E) Side branch
(F) ACS if rupture occurs

12.26 See Figure Q12-26.

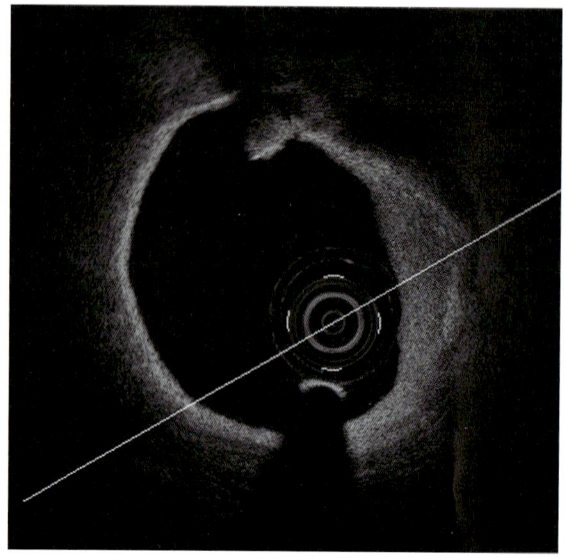

Figure Q12-26

(A) Normal vessel anatomy
(B) Unstable angina
(C) Guiding catheter
(D) Stable angina
(E) Side branch
(F) ACS if rupture occurs

12.27 See Figure Q12-27.

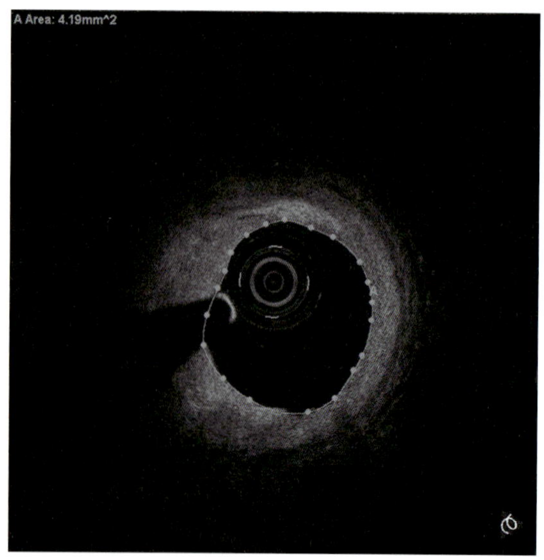

Figure Q12-27

(A) Normal vessel anatomy
(B) Unstable angina
(C) Guiding catheter
(D) Stable angina
(E) Side branch
(F) ACS if rupture occurs

ANSWERS AND EXPLANATIONS

12.1 Answer D. Medical therapy with aspirin, beta-blockers, statins, and ACE inhibitors. PCI of a completely occluded infarct-related artery after 24 hours of onset of STEMI should not be performed in asymptomatic patients with no ECG or clinical evidence of ongoing ischemia. This was studied in the Occluded Arteries Trial (OAT) that randomized over 2,000 patients who had total occlusion of the infarct-related artery 3 to 28 days after MI and who met a high-risk criterion (an ejection fraction of <50% or proximal occlusion) to either PCI with medical therapy or medical therapy alone. This trial concluded that there was no benefit with PCI in regard to death, reinfarction, or reduction in heart failure at 4-year follow-up in patients who presented late with STEMI (Hochman JS, et al. *N Engl J Med* 2006;355(23):2395–2407).

12.2 Answer A. Enoxaparin 0.3 mg/kg IV once. Patients who have received multiple doses of subcutaneously administered enoxaparin who undergo PCI within 8 hours of the last subcutaneous dose generally have adequate degree of anticoagulation to undergo PCI, but the degree of anticoagulation may diminish in the 8- to 12-hour period after the last subcutaneous dose. In such patients, as well as in patients who have received only one subcutaneous dose of enoxaparin, the addition of enoxaparin (0.3 mg/kg IV) at the time of PCI provides an additional degree of anticoagulation and has become standard practice. An additional dose of 0.3 mg/kg IV enoxaparin should be administered at the time of PCI to patients who have received fewer than two therapeutic subcutaneous doses (e.g., 1 mg/kg) or received the last subcutaneous enoxaparin dose 8- to 12-hours before PCI per guidelines from the American College of Cardiology Foundation (ACCF) (Levine GN, et al. *J Am Coll Cardiol* 2011;58(24):e44–e122). Patients who undergo PCI 12 hours after the last subcutaneous dose are usually treated with full-dose anticoagulation using full-dose UFH, enoxaparin, or bivalirudin (Cohen M, et al. *Catheter Cardiovasc Interv* 2010;75(6):928–935).

12.3 Answer C. There is a significant increase in catheter-related thrombosis with fondaparinux. Fondaparinux is an indirect inhibitor of factor X_a with no effect on thrombin. Multiple randomized trials that examined the use of fondaparinux in ACS patients showed a significant increase in catheter thrombosis during PCI (Yusuf S, et al. *N Engl J Med* 2006;354(14):1464–1476; Yusuf S, et al. *JAMA* 2006;295(13):1519–1530). Hence, the latest American College of Cardiology (ACC), American Heart Association (AHA), and Society of Cardiovascular Angiography and Interventions (SCAI) PCI guidelines give fondaparinux use during PCI a Class III (harm) recommendation (Levine GN, et al. *J Am Coll Cardiol* 2011;58(24):e44–e122). However, fondaparinux is still recommended for patients with ACS who are treated conservatively. If these patients are referred for PCI, then it is recommended to use standard-dose UFH (85 or 60 U/kg with GP IIb/IIIa inhibitors) (Group FO-T, et al. *JAMA* 2010;304(12):1339–1349).

12.4 Answer A. Proceed with coronary angiography with intent to revascularize. Early angiography is indicated in patients who have refractory angina or hemodynamic or electrical instability without serious comorbidities or contraindications to such procedures. Early invasive strategy is also indicated for patients with unstable angina/NSTEMI who were initially stabilized with medical therapy but are determined to be at a high risk of adverse cardiac events (Levine GN, et al. *J Am Coll Cardiol* 2011;58(24):e44–e122). The term "early" generally means within 24 hours. There is no added benefit in performing angiography within the first few hours of presentation in unstable angina and NSTEMI ACS. Switching from UFH to enoxaparin would result in stacking of anticoagulants and, hence, increased bleeding. Eptifibatide is typically contraindicated in patients with end-stage renal disease. High-risk features that support an "early invasive" strategy include:

- Recurrent angina/ischemia at rest or with low-level activities, despite intensive anti-ischemic therapy
- Elevated TnT or TnI
- New or presumably new ST-segment depression
- Recurrent angina/ischemia with symptoms, an S_3 gallop, pulmonary edema, worsening rales, or new or worsening mitral regurgitation
- High-risk findings on noninvasive stress testing
- Depressed systolic function (e.g., ejection function < 0.40 on noninvasive study)

- Hemodynamic instability
- Sustained ventricular tachycardia
- PCI within 6 months
- Prior CABG

12.5 Answer B. Patient should be admitted to the coronary care unit so your team can evaluate him to make a decision. Patient just received full-dose thrombolytic 2 hours ago; angiography should be considered within 3- to 24-hours after the thrombolysis. Immediate angiography (in the first 3 hours) has been shown to increase the bleeding risk significantly (White HD. *Circulation* 2008;118(3):219–222). Patients presenting to hospitals without PCI capability should be transferred to a PCI-capable hospital where the door-to-balloon time would be <120 minutes. If this cannot be achieved, then the recommendation is to thrombolyze and then transfer the patient. In stable patients who were thrombolyzed with good response, it is recommended to proceed with angiography within 24 hours to reduce reinfarction and recurrent ischemia (Cantor WJ, et al. *N Engl J Med* 2009;360(26):2705–2718). The clinical diagnosis of failed fibrinolysis is difficult but is best made when there is <50% ST-segment resolution 90 minutes after initiation of therapy in the lead showing the greatest degree of ST-segment elevation at presentation.

12.6 Answer D. PCI of the LAD may be considered either at the time of primary PCI or as a planned, staged procedure as it has been shown to decrease MACE. The PCI guidelines that were last updated in 2011 gave a Class III (harm) recommendation for PCI of a non-infarct-related artery due to concerns over additional contrast use, radiation exposure, and performing PCI in a prothrombotic state that might result in higher complication rate. However, there were two recent trials that confirmed the safety and efficacy of PCI of a non-infarct-related artery. The PRAMI trial showed that compared to PCI of an infarct-related artery only, complete revascularization resulted in a significant reduction in death from cardiac causes, MI, or refractory angina (Wald DS, et al. *N Engl J Med* 2013;369(12):1115–1123). The CvLPRIT trial demonstrated that complete revascularization resulted in a significant reduction in all-cause death, MI, heart failure, or ischemia-driven revascularization at 12 months compared to PCI of a infarct-related artery only. Although both these studies did not show a reduction in death or MI separately, the difference was driven by revascularization. This resulted in a change in the 2015 STEMI guidelines that assigned a Class IIb recommendation for non-infarct-related PCI—although the timing of PCI was less clear, but generally within the same admission (Levine GN, et al. *J Am Coll Cardiol* 2016;67(10):1235–1250).

12.7 Answer C. Patients with ACS who are considered for early invasive approach that are not adequately preloaded with a $P2Y_{12}$ inhibitor. GP IIb/IIIa inhibitors are strong IV antiplatelet agents that were mostly studied in the era of balloon angioplasty and before the routine use of clopidogrel. In ACS, it was shown to reduce MI; however, it caused more bleeding than standard approach, which was UFH alone. The advantage of GP inhibitors is the rapid achievement of potent antiplatelet activity that was not established by oral $P2Y_{12}$ inhibitors. In the era of routine $P2Y_{12}$ inhibitor use, the role of GPI is limited. Certainly, the guidelines do not support routine use of GP inhibitors in ACS. In patients who are treated conservatively or with low-risk ACS, the bleeding risk outweighs the benefit. In today's practice, GP inhibitors are reserved for patients who are considered for early invasive approach that were not adequately preloaded with a $P2Y_{12}$ inhibitor. In patients with intermediate- to high-risk ACS undergoing PCI, if they are noted to have a large thrombus burden, then it is reasonable to add GP inhibitors despite $P2Y_{12}$ use. Small molecule agents, such as eptifibatide and tirofiban, are favored over abciximab (Levine GN, et al. *J Am Coll Cardiol* 2011;58(24):e44–e122).

12.8 Answer C. Thrombolyze her and transfer her immediately. The patient is in cardiogenic shock, which is ideally treated with PCI, but in this case, that is not the best option given the PCI facility is 3 hours away. This patient has inferior STEMI with cardiogenic shock; hence, the best option is to thrombolyze and transfer ("drip and ship") immediately to a PCI-capable facility as she might need invasive treatment and/or hemodynamic support (Levine GN, et al. *J Am Coll Cardiol* 2011;58(24):e44–e122).

12.9 Answer E. Proceed with angioplasty and stent placement to mid LAD. Large thrombus burden may cause distal embolization with microvascular obstruction and edema that has been shown to result in poor cardiovascular outcomes. This paved the way for a variety of thrombectomy devices that have become quite popular. The TAPAS trial was the original trial that showed significant improvement in myocardial blush grade with aspiration thrombectomy plus PCI compared to conventional PCI alone (Svilaas T, et al. *N Engl J Med* 2008;358(6):557–567). At 1-year follow-up, this trial showed a significant reduction in the primary end point of cardiac death or nonfatal MI with aspiration thrombectomy plus PCI compared to PCI alone (5.6% vs. 9.9%, HR 1.81; 95% CI 1.16 to 2.84; $p = 0.009$) (Vlaar PJ, et al. *Lancet* 2008;371(9628): 1915–1920). It should be noted that this was a single center study that resulted in an increase in aspiration thrombectomy use. Two large multicenter randomized trials that were published following TAPAS (TASTE and TOTAL) showed no benefit with routine thrombus aspiration. TASTE showed no reduction in all-cause mortality or recurrent MI at 30- to 1-year follow-up (Lagerqvist B, et al. *N Engl J Med* 2014;371(12):1111–1120). The TOTAL trial showed no reduction in the primary composite outcomes of cardiovascular death, recurrent MI, cardiogenic shock, or New York Heart Association (NYHA) Class IV heart failure at 180 days with aspiration thrombectomy. On the contrary, there was a significant increase of stroke in patients who underwent thrombectomy (Jolly SS, et al. *N Engl J Med* 2015;372(15):1389–1398). Although GP IIb/IIIa inhibitors can be used to reduce thrombus burden, PCI cannot be deferred for later as he has ongoing chest pain. Along the same line, since he has ongoing clinical and ECG evidence of ischemia, he should undergo emergent PCI and not be treated medically or referred for emergent CABG.

12.10 **Answer C.** IV cangrelor loading followed by an infusion for 4 hours, to be transitioned to ticagrelor. This would be the most ideal strategy among the options presented. It has been shown that patients undergoing PCI, especially with ACS, should be given a loading dose of $P2Y_{12}$ inhibitors. Even though the pharmacokinetics of these $P2Y_{12}$ inhibitors have been well established in non-ACS patients, it has been shown that in patients with ACS, it takes longer duration even for the novel $P2Y_{12}$ inhibitors (prasugrel or ticagrelor). This has resulted in a search for an ideal antiplatelet agent that will achieve rapid and predictable levels of platelet inhibition in ACS patients. Cangrelor is a reversible $P2Y_{12}$ platelet receptor inhibitor that blocks adenosine diphosphate-mediated platelet activation and aggregation. The antiplatelet effects of cangrelor are almost immediate with extensive platelet inhibition occurring within 2 minutes of drug administration. Cangrelor and ticagrelor, unlike the thienopyridines prasugrel and clopidogrel, do not require metabolic conversion to become active and can therefore directly inhibit the $P2Y_{12}$ receptor. The CHAMPION group of trials studied cangrelor use against clopidogrel in different clinical scenarios. CHAMPION PCI (Harrington RA, et al. *N Engl J Med* 2009;361(24):2318–2329) and PLATFORM (Bhatt DL, et al. *N Engl J Med* 2009;361(24):2330–2341) were negative trials in that there was no significant reduction in death, MI, or ischemia-driven revascularization at 48 hours in patients receiving cangrelor compared to clopidogrel. However, the CHAMPION PHOENIX trial that included patients with stable CAD and ACS undergoing PCI showed a significant reduction in death, MI, urgent revascularization, or stent thrombosis at 48 hours in patients receiving cangrelor compared to clopidogrel, mostly driven by a reduction in stent thrombosis (Bhatt DL, et al. *N Engl J Med* 2013;368(14):1303–1313). Cangrelor is ideally suited for patients who couldn't be adequately loaded with $P2Y_{12}$ inhibitors before PCI and in whom GP inhibitors are not used. Clopidogrel given hours after the procedure in this patient is less ideal as it puts her at a risk of stent thrombosis and the PCI cannot be postponed to place an NG tube. Since bivalirudin was used, it is less desirable to use GP IIb/IIIa inhibitors as it negates the bleeding risk reduction provided by bivalirudin. Cangrelor was recently approved for use and it remains to be seen how this fits in our clinical practice.

12.11 **Answer C.** PCI of the mid-RCA with DES. The echocardiogram shows newly reduced LV function with regional wall motion abnormalities in the RCA territory. It is most likely that the vein graft to the RCA occlusion is the culprit lesion for his NSTEMI. However, reopening occluded vein grafts is not recommended as it is associated with low success rates, high risk for complications, and poor long-term patency rates (de Feyter PJ, et al. *Am J Cardiol* 1989;64(1):88–90; Al-Lamee R, et al. *Am J Cardiol* 2010;106(12):1721–1727). This has resulted in a Class III recommendation for PCI of completely occluded vein grafts in the PCI guidelines (Levine GN, et al. *J Am Coll Cardiol* 2011;58(24):e44–e122). In these situations, native-vessel PCI has favorable short- and long-term outcomes when performed.

12.12 **Answer A.** Distal embolic protection with a filter. Vein graft interventions are high risk due to embolic risks that result in slow flow or no-reflow, increasing MACE (Hoffmann R, et al. *Coron Artery Dis* 2007;18(7):559–564). One randomized trial showed a significant reduction in the composite primary end point of death, MI, emergent CABG, or target-vessel revascularization at 30 days in the distal embolic protection arm compared to no distal protection arm. This was primarily driven by reduction in MI. Other randomized trials showed similar results (Mauri L, et al. *J Am Coll Cardiol* 2007;50(15):1442-1449; Stone GW, et al. *Circulation* 2003;108(5):548-553). GP IIb/IIIa inhibitors have shown to be of no benefit in SVG interventions (Roffi M, et al. *Circulation* 2002;106(24):3063-3067). Several drugs, such as nicardipine, nitroprusside, and adenosine, have shown to be useful in treating no-reflow once it occurs. However, none of these drugs given pre-PCI have been shown to prevent no-reflow (Fischell TA, et al. *J Invasive Cardiol* 2007;19(2):58-62). This distinction is important as some operators believe they can skip distal embolic protection device use if they empirically pretreat before the PCI, but this has never been shown to be beneficial.

12.13 **Answer A.** Aspirin, clopidogrel, and warfarin. Atrial fibrillation patients undergoing PCI present a unique challenge post procedure as they often need an anticoagulant for stroke prophylaxis in addition to dual antiplatelet therapy (DAPT)—often referred to as "triple" therapy. It is no surprise that those patients on triple therapy have high bleeding risk. Triple therapy increases bleeding risk to a range of 10% to 14% from 4% to 6% with DAPT (Hansen ML, et al. *Arch Intern Med* 2010;170(16):1433-1441). In the recent years, there have been some trials addressing this issue. The WOEST (What is the Optimal Antiplatelet and Anticoagulant Therapy in Patients With Oral Anticoagulation and Coronary Stenting) trial was a randomized, open-label trial of 563 patients (approximately 25% of whom had ACS) receiving oral anticoagulant therapy and undergoing coronary stenting. Patients randomized to single antiplatelet treatment with clopidogrel had significantly fewer bleeding complications and no increase in thrombotic events compared with those randomized to DAPT with aspirin and clopidogrel (Dewilde WJ, et al. *Lancet* 2013;381(9872): 1107-1115). Of note, the WOEST trial was small (only 279 patients received oral anticoagulation plus clopidogrel and, of these, only approximately 180 received a DES) and was not powered to detect risk of stent thrombosis. PIONEER AF-PCI (Open-Label, Randomized, Controlled, Multicenter Study Exploring Two Treatment Strategies of Rivaroxaban and a Dose-Adjusted Oral Vitamin K Antagonist Treatment Strategy in Subjects with Atrial Fibrillation who Undergo Percutaneous Coronary Intervention) was a recently published study that randomized AF patients undergoing PCI into one of the three groups: low-dose rivaroxaban plus clopidogrel, very low-dose rivaroxaban plus DAPT, or warfarin plus DAPT. This trial showed that there was significantly reduced bleeding in patients randomized to the rivaroxaban plus clopidogrel arm with similar rates of death from cardiovascular causes, MI, or stroke compared to the two other arms in the study. Of note, the very low dose of rivaroxaban (2.5 mg twice daily), as used in the PIONEER AF-PCI trial, is not approved for use in this setting in the United States. Furthermore, the PIONEER AF-PCI trial was underpowered to exclude an increased risk for stroke (Gibson CM, et al. *N Engl J Med* 2016;375(25):2423-2434). The ACC/AHA guidelines (January CT, et al. *J Am Coll Cardiol* 2014;64(21):e1-e76) recommend initial triple oral antithrombotic therapy (aspirin plus clopidogrel plus warfarin) as opposed to any other antithrombotic strategy. Newer data may modify this recommendation in the future.

12.14 **Answer C.** Ticagrelor 180 mg loading dose. It is a Class I recommendation to give a loading dose of $P2Y_{12}$ inhibitor to patients with NSTEMI in whom early invasive strategy is considered. There is a choice of three drugs that are available, including thienopyridines (clopidogrel and prasugrel) and pyrimidine derivative (ticagrelor). Thienopyridines are prodrugs requiring conversion to active molecules (two-step process for clopidogrel and one-step activation for prasugrel), thus explaining the variability in time to peak effect and their bioavailability. Ticagrelor, on the other hand, does not require activation and achieved its maximal antiplatelet effect much sooner than the other agents. The PLATO (The Study of Platelet Inhibition and Patient Outcomes) study demonstrated a significant reduction in the composite end point of death from vascular causes, MI, or stroke at 12 months in patients with ACS who received ticagrelor compared to clopidogrel (Wallentin L, et al. *N Engl J Med* 2009;361(11):1045-1057). Prasugrel loading dose can be given only after the coronary anatomy is defined. This patient with diabetes and prior peripheral artery disease is a high vascular-risk patient, and hence, ticagrelor is the best choice compared to clopidogrel.

12.15 **Answer D.** Assume that she is a clopidogrel nonresponder and switch her to ticagrelor. She clearly had subacute stent thrombosis while on clopidogrel, which would indicate she is a clopidogrel failure or nonresponder. This warrants switching her to one of the other $P2Y_{12}$ inhibitors. Prasugrel is contraindicated in her because of her age (over 70 years) and prior stroke (increased intracranial bleeding risk). Thus, ticagrelor is the ideal choice $P2Y_{12}$ inhibitor. Platelet function testing or genetic testing is currently not indicated routinely. There was a considerable interest in platelet function testing with a variety of commercially available tests that measured treatment platelet reactivity (adenosine diphosphate [ADP]-mediated platelet aggregation on drugs) in order to tailor antiplatelet therapy to patients. However, even though it was shown that patients high on treatment platelet reactivity had increased adverse cardiac events, higher-dose clopidogrel use did not show any added benefit. In GRAVITAS (Gauging Responsiveness With A VerifyNow Assay-Impact On Thrombosis And Safety), treatment with high-dose clopidogrel for 6 months in patients with high platelet reactivity on standard-dose clopidogrel was not beneficial (Price MJ, et al. *JAMA* 2011;305(11):1097–1105). At the present time, the evidence base is insufficient to recommend routine platelet function testing (Levine GN, et al. *J Am Coll Cardiol* 2011;58(24):e44–e122).

12.16 Answer D. Previous CABG. The best data evaluating the risk of in-hospital bleeding in an ACS population come from an analysis of over 24,000 patients in the Global Registry of Acute Coronary Events (Moscucci M, et al. *Eur Heart J* 2003;24(20):1815–1823). The analysis showed an incidence of major bleeding in 4.7% of the NSTEMI population and identified four independent predictors of an increased risk of major bleeding: advanced age, female gender, a history of bleeding, and renal insufficiency. As has been found in subsequent studies, major bleeding was associated with a significant increase in mortality.

12.17 Answer C. Minimize the amount of contrast used for the procedure.

CIN is one of the leading causes of acute kidney injury (AKI) in hospitalized patients. Major predictors of CIN include advanced age, pre-existing CKD, diabetes, volume of contrast, and CHF. Mehran et al. developed a simple calculator that can be used to estimate the risk of CIN, including CIN needing hemodialysis (Mehran R, et al. *J Am Coll Cardiol* 2004;44(7):1393–1399). The two strategies shown to be beneficial in reducing CIN are infusion of normal saline (1 to 1.5 mL/kg/h for 3 to 12 hours before and 6 to 24 hours after the procedure) and minimizing contrast use. Several other therapies, including sodium bicarbonate infusion, saline with mannitol, saline with furosemide, and *N*-acetylcysteine, have been tried but none of them show a consistent benefit in CIN risk reduction. The correlation between the volume of contrast media and the risk of contrast-induced AKI has been documented in several studies (Marenzi G, et al. *Ann Intern Med* 2009;150(3):170–177; McCullough PA, et al. *Am J Med* 1997;103(5):368–375). Thus, minimization of contrast media volume is important to prevent contrast-induced AKI in patients undergoing angiography. The volume of contrast already administered during diagnostic catheterization is an important factor when considering possible "ad hoc" PCI such as in this patient.

12.18 Answer C. Stress testing in asymptomatic patients is indicated only for patients with high-risk features when trying to find objective evidence of ischemia.

Routine periodic stress testing of patients who have undergone PCI with no high-risk features and who are asymptomatic received a Class III recommendation from the ACC/AHA (Levine GN, et al. *J Am Coll Cardiol* 2011;58(24):e44–e122). High-risk patients generally include those with decreased LV function, multivessel CAD, proximal LAD disease, previous sudden death, diabetes mellitus, hazardous occupations, and suboptimal percutaneous transluminal coronary angioplasty PCI results. In the presence of such high-risk features, exercise testing within 12 months of PCI to detect restenosis is a Class IIb recommendation, indicating additional studies are needed to confirm efficacy and safety of this approach. The only Class I recommendation for stress testing after revascularization is for recurrent symptoms that suggest ischemia. Another potential use for postrevascularization stress testing is to assist with activity counseling and to guide exercise training as part of a comprehensive cardiac rehabilitation program.

12.19 Answer C. Bivalirudin 0.75 mg/kg IV bolus followed by 1 mg/kg/h infusion for the duration of the PCI. Bivalirudin would be the most appropriate anticoagulant agent. The calculated creatinine clearance is 28.65 mL/min. The loading dose of bivalirudin remains the same (0.75 mg/kg), but the maintenance dose is dependent on eGFR or creatinine clearance. For creatinine clearance >30 mL/min, no dose adjustment is necessary (1.75 mg/kg/h). For creatinine clearance <30 mL/min, 1 mg/kg/h dose is used; and for dialysis-dependent patients, a 0.25-mg/kg/h dose is recommended. Further analyses of the ACUITY (Acute Catheterization and Urgent Intervention Triage strategY) trial compared various antithrombotic strategies in patients with NSTE-ACS in two important subgroups of patients, namely, those managed without revascularization (Goto K, et al.

Circulation 2010;121(7):853–862) and patients with CKD (Mehran R, et al. *JACC Cardiovasc Interv* 2009;2(8):748–757). Large and consistent reductions in bleeding complications with bivalirudin monotherapy compared to heparin with GP IIb/IIIa inhibitors were reported at 1 year with no difference in ischemic end points. In the ISAR-REACT (Intracoronary Stenting and Antithrombotic Regimen: Rapid Early Action for Coronary Treatment) 3 trial, bivalirudin was compared with UFH in 4,570 patients with stable or UA and normal levels of troponin T and CKMB who underwent PCI. Patients randomized to bivalirudin experienced less bleeding and had similar rates of ischemic complications through 1 year compared with those who received UFH (Schulz S, et al. *Eur Heart J* 2010;31(5):582–587). Of note, in this trial, all patients were pretreated with clopidogrel 600 mg more than 2 hours before PCI, and no GP IIb/IIIa inhibitors were used in combination with bivalirudin. When compared to UFH or low molecular weight heparin (LMW) plus a GP IIb/IIIa inhibitor in patients with ACS undergoing PCI, bivalirudin is as effective and associated with a lower bleeding risk. Whether bivalirudin reduces bleeding compared with heparin monotherapy is not well established (Valgimigli M, et al. *N Engl J Med* 2015;373(11):997).

12.20 Answer E. After diagnostic angiogram, consider placing a hemodynamic support device before PCI. This patient has cardiogenic shock on presentation, and the most important treatment strategy is emergent angiography and revascularization as indicated. However, this patient is on escalating doses of IV norepinephrine, indicating he may not be stable enough for the PCI. Use of hemodynamic support devices in patients with cardiogenic shock is indicated when patients are refractory to pharmacologic measures. There are a variety of devices that are currently available, but in a cardiogenic shock situation, the ideal device is the one that is readily available in the catheterization lab and easy to implant and maintain with less complications. The intra-aortic balloon pump is one such device that has been around for a long time and used in these situations. It is a very useful device to improve diastolic coronary blood flow and thus treat ischemia, but does not provide a meaningful cardiac output in patients with pump failure. The Impella is a percutaneous LV assist device that is placed via a 13-Fr or 14-Fr sheath in a retrograde fashion across the aortic valve into the LV. This device provides a forward flow of up to 2.5 L (Impella 2.5) or 3.5 L (Impella CP). It has been used in patients with cardiogenic shock with good success. It should be noted that none of the hemodynamic support devices have shown to improve outcomes in cardiogenic shock in randomized clinical trials. Observational data have shown improvement in hemodynamics with support devices. Also, if one is considering a hemodynamic device, it is recommended that it be placed before the PCI, thus achieving maximal support for the most challenging part of the procedure. The only strategy that has been consistently shown to improve outcomes in cardiogenic shock is early revascularization.

12.21 Answer C. Refer him to a supervised cardiac rehabilitation program.

Supervised cardiac rehabilitation programs are associated with a significant reduction in all-cause mortality and cardiovascular mortality as shown in multiple studies (Goel K, et al. *Circulation* 2011; 123(21):2344–2352; Taylor RS, et al. *Am J Med* 2004; 116(10):682–692). This therapy should particularly be considered in intermediate- to high-risk patients such as the one in this case. Cardiac rehabilitation is also associated with improvements in exercise tolerance, cardiac symptoms, lipid levels, cigarette smoking cessation rates (in conjunction with a smoking cessation program), stress levels, improved medical regimen compliance, and improved psychosocial well-being. This is precisely the reason why it was given a Class I recommendation in the PCI and NSTEMI guidelines (Levine GN, et al. *J Am Coll Cardiol* 2011;58(24):e44–e122; Amsterdam EA, et al. *J Am Coll Cardiol* 2014; 64(24):e139–e228).

12.22 Answer C. Guiding catheter. There are no vessel wall structures seen.

12.23 Answer F. Evidence of a thin fibrotic cap large atheromatous burden. Most likely would provoke an ACS in the event of rupture.

12.24 Answer A. Normal vessel anatomy with very mild atherosclerotic changes.

12.25 Answer E. Side branch.

12.26 Answer B. Unstable angina. Shows plaque rupture/dissection.

12.27 Answer D. Significant atheromatous burden with a decrease in mean lumen area. Most likely would be associated with stable angina.

13 Primary, Rescue, and Facilitated Angioplasty

Amit N. Vora and Michael H. Sketch, Jr.

QUESTIONS

13.1 The currently accepted ideal maximum first medical contact (FMC) to initial device deployment time for patients with ST-segment elevation myocardial infarction (STEMI) presenting to a PCI-capable hospital is:

(A) 30 minutes
(B) 60 minutes
(C) 90 minutes
(D) 120 minutes
(E) 360 minutes

13.2 A 76-year-old man presents with an acute anterior wall myocardial infarction (MI). Emergency coronary angiography reveals a completely occluded left anterior descending (LAD) artery with Thrombolysis In Myocardial Infarction (TIMI) 0 flow (Fig. Q13-2A) and a 70% to 80% stenosis of the right coronary artery (RCA) with TIMI 3 flow (Fig. Q13-2B). Left ventriculogram shows anterolateral hypokinesis. His heart rate (HR) is 88 and blood pressure (BP) is 127/78 with an oxygen saturation of 98% on room air. Optimal management of this patient will include:

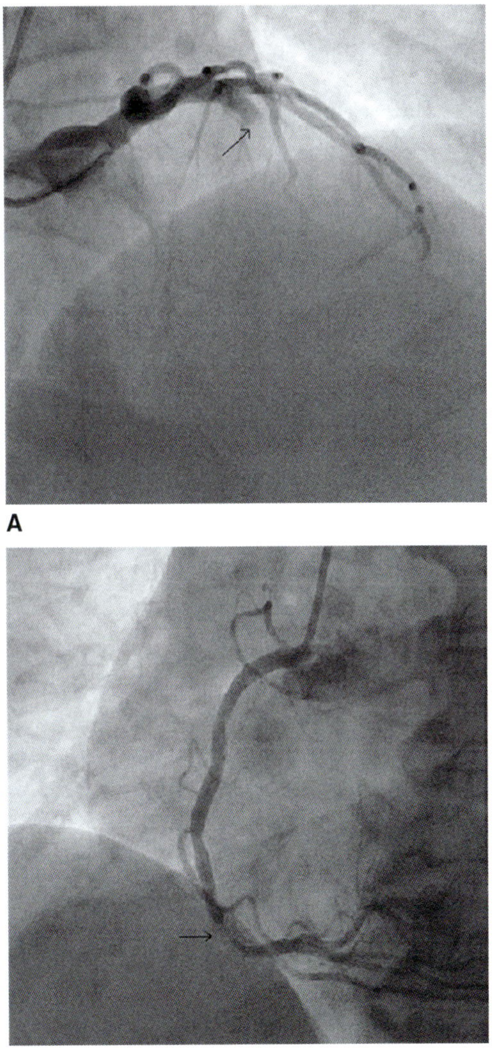

A

B

Figure Q13-2

(A) Bypass surgery because he has two-vessel disease involving the LAD artery
(B) Percutaneous coronary intervention (PCI) of the LAD artery only and consideration of PCI of the RCA at a later date (staged PCI)
(C) PCI of the LAD and referral for bypass of the RCA
(D) PCI of the LAD and measurement of fractional flow reserve (FFR) of the RCA to assess hemodynamic significance followed by PCI if indicated

13.3 A 57-year old man with hypertension and hypercholesterolemia is at the airport when he suddenly collapses. No breathing or pulse is noted, and bystander CPR is immediately initiated. An automated external defibrillator (AED) is applied and defibrillates the patient for ventricular fibrillation, and a pulse is regained, though the patient is still unconscious. Immediate postprocedure electrocardiogram (EKG) reveals 2 mm anterior ST-segment elevation. Which of the following is the next appropriate step in the management of this patient?

(A) The patient should be transferred to a PCI-capable facility for emergent primary PCI with a goal of FMC to device time of 120 minutes
(B) The patient should undergo therapeutic hypothermia and primary PCI as soon as possible
(C) The patient should undergo therapeutic hypothermia and undergo cardiac catheterization once target temperature is achieved
(D) Therapeutic hypothermia should be deferred, and the patient should undergo primary PCI

13.4 A 68-year-old woman presents to your office for evaluation of chest discomfort she had the previous evening. The discomfort lasted for approximately 30 to 40 minutes and subsequently resolved. Currently, she is pain free with a HR of 74 and a BP of 118/71. Her lungs are clear to auscultation and you do not hear any significant murmurs on cardiac exam. EKG reveals an evolving STEMI. On further questioning, she states discomfort started at approximately 7 PM the evening before and lasted until 7:45 PM or so. It is now 10 AM the next morning. Appropriate management would include:

(A) Admission to the hospital and treatment with aspirin, heparin, clopidogrel, statin, and β-blocker
(B) Admission to the cardiac catheterization laboratory for emergency angiography with a goal of primary PCI
(C) Administration of full-dose fibrinolysis, admission to hospital, and treatment with aspirin, heparin, clopidogrel, statins, and β-blockers
(D) Administration of full-dose fibrinolytics and then admission to the catheterization laboratory for emergency angiography

13.5 An 82-year-old woman presents with 2 hours of acute, substernal chest discomfort. She has a prior history of hypertension, hyperlipidemia, and a transient ischemic attack (TIA) 3 years ago. She weighs 65 kg. Her initial EKG reveals 2 mm of inferior ST elevation. Which of the following is an appropriate strategy for the administration of a $P2Y_{12}$ inhibitor prior to primary PCI?

(A) Load 90 mg ticagrelor and continue at a dose of 60 mg twice daily
(B) Load 60 mg prasugrel and continue at a dose of 10 mg daily
(C) Load 180 mg ticagrelor and continue at a dose of 90 mg twice daily
(D) Defer loading $P2Y_{12}$ inhibitor until after the PCI is complete

13.6 In patients with STEMI, compared with fibrinolysis, primary PCI lowers the (relative) odds of death at 1 year by:

(A) 5%
(B) 10%
(C) 15%
(D) 20%
(E) 25%

13.7 The role of embolic protection devices in primary PCI is BEST characterized as being:

(A) Strongly recommended for all patients undergoing primary PCI (Class I recommendation)
(B) Strongly recommended for primary PCI only in patients with large thrombus burden (Class I recommendation)
(C) Currently not recommended for primary PCI
(D) Recommended for patients with no reflow after PCI

13.8 A 67-year-old man undergoes bypass surgery for severe three-vessel coronary artery disease (CAD). Approximately 12 hours after the surgery, he becomes short of breath and has 3 mm ST elevation in the inferolateral leads. The BEST management strategy at this time is:

(A) Conservative management without coronary angiography
(B) Coronary angiography intending to manage the patient with a catheter-based treatment strategy (i.e., immediate PCI)
(C) Coronary angiography intending to manage the patient with a surgical-based treatment strategy (i.e., emergency redo coronary artery bypass graft [CABG] surgery)
(D) Coronary angiography followed by conservative treatment

13.9 A 56-year-old man with a history of hypertension, type II diabetes, and obesity presents with 1 hour of crushing substernal chest discomfort and is found to have anterior ST elevations on ECG. The patient is taken emergently to the cardiac catheterization laboratory for primary PCI. He has received aspirin 325 mg and ticagrelor 180 mg. His creatinine is 1.1 mg/dL. A glycoprotein (GP) IIb/IIIa inhibitor is not used during the PCI. Which of the following is an appropriate anticoagulation strategy during primary PCI?

(A) Unfractionated heparin (UFH) at a dose of 50 units/kg
(B) UFH at a dose of 130 units/kg
(C) Bivalirudin 0.75 mg/kg bolus and 1.75 mg/kg/h infusion
(D) Fondaparinux 2.5 mg intravenous (IV)

13.10 A 47-year-old man with hypertension and type II diabetes presents to a regional community hospital with acute chest pain and is found to have 3 mm inferior ST-segment elevation. The nearest primary PCI facility is 45 minutes away. What is the recommended maximum time interval that the patient should spend at the primary facility before transferring to the PCI-capable facility (the door-in-door-out time)?

(A) 10 minutes
(B) 30 minutes
(C) 45 minutes
(D) 60 minutes

13.11 A 44-year-old man presents with chest heaviness and 0.5 mm ST-segment elevation in ECG leads I and aVL Coronary angiogram is performed (Fig. Q13-11). The most likely etiology of his chest pain is:

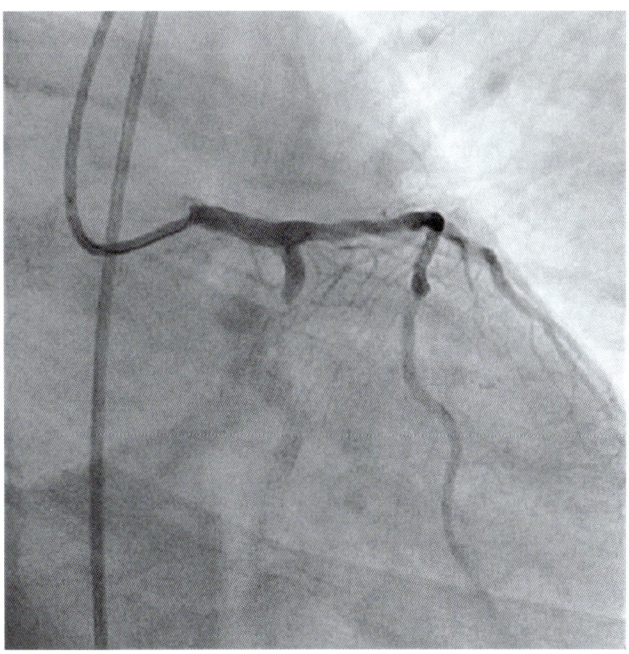

Figure Q13-11

(A) Pericarditis
(B) Occluded coronary artery
(C) Anomalous coronary artery
(D) Kawasaki's disease
(E) Congenital coronary artery fistula

13.12 A 63-year-old woman presents with an acute STEMI. Emergency coronary angiography reveals a completely occluded RCA with large thrombus burden (Fig. Q13-12). Optimal management of this lesion includes:

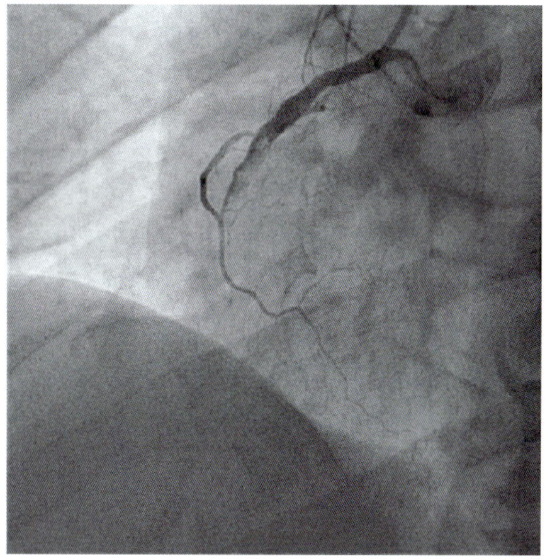

Figure Q13-12

(A) Rheolytic thrombectomy
(B) Emboli protection device
(C) Balloon angioplasty followed by stenting
(D) Medical therapy

13.13 A 57-year-old man presents with an acute anterior wall MI. The patient is administered aspirin, clopidogrel, and eptifibatide and undergoes emergency coronary angiography (Fig. Q13-13). The BEST management strategy in this individual is:

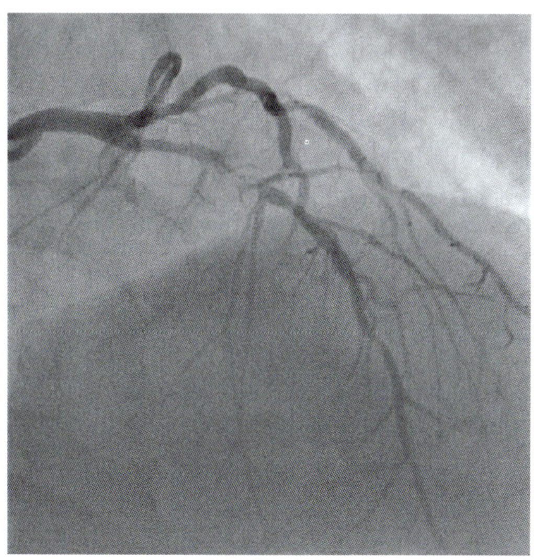

Figure Q13-13

(A) Balloon angioplasty
(B) Fibrinolytic therapy followed by PCI in 3 to 4 days
(C) Bare-metal stent (BMS) implantation
(D) Drug-eluting stent (DES) implantation

13.14 A 34-year-old female lawyer presents with chest discomfort after a particularly challenging tennis match. ECG reveals a 1 mm ST-segment elevation in leads II, III, and aVF. An emergency coronary angiogram is performed (Fig. Q13-14). The most likely etiology of her chest pain is:

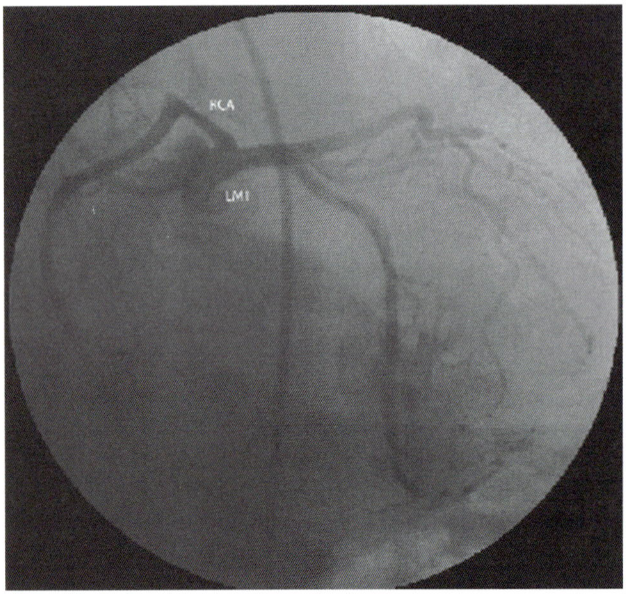

Figure Q13-14

(A) Anomalous coronary artery
(B) Musculoskeletal chest pain
(C) Coronary artery dissection
(D) Coronary embolus

13.15 You are asked to consult on an 83-year-old woman for possible PCI. Eight days ago, she was admitted to the hospital with chest pain and ST elevation in leads V2 to V4. She was diagnosed with an acute anterior MI. However, she was not given thrombolytic therapy because of her history of stroke 4 months before admission, and she refused cardiac catheterization. She was treated with aspirin, heparin, clopidogrel, simvastatin, metoprolol, and lisinopril. She responded well to the treatment, and her chest pain eventually resolves. Her ECG now has Q waves in the anterior leads. She has been free of chest pain since hospital day 1 and hemodynamically stable without any arrhythmias. Her echocardiogram on hospital day 4 was unremarkable except for anterior wall hypokinesis and left ventricular ejection fraction (LVEF) of 35%. Her physician son has come in from out of town and wants her to undergo cardiac catheterization and possible PCI. What will be the effect of delayed PCI of a persistently occluded infarct-related artery in this setting?

(A) Delayed PCI will result in long-term improvement in the LVEF, greater freedom from adverse in-hospital clinical events, and a reduced incidence of long-term MI and death from CAD
(B) Delayed PCI will result in long-term improvement in the LVEF and greater freedom from adverse in-hospital clinical events but will not decrease the incidence of subsequent MI or death from CAD
(C) There are no convincing data to support the routine use of late PCI days after MI in patients who did not receive reperfusion therapy
(D) There are no convincing data to support the routine use of late PCI days after MI in patients who did not receive reperfusion therapy, but it does reduce recurrent angina

13.16 A 61-year-old woman is brought to the emergency room by paramedics with chest pain for 2 hours. She is found to have ST elevation anteriorly. Her initial BP is 95/60 with a HR of 100. The closest hospital with an interventional catheterization laboratory is 2 hours away. Which of the following options is the most appropriate initial strategy?

(A) Reteplase plus abciximab and transfer for PCI only if ongoing chest pain
(B) Abciximab alone with subsequent transfer for PCI
(C) Reteplase with transfer for PCI as soon as possible
(D) Half-dose reteplase plus abciximab and transfer for PCI

13.17 Each community should develop a STEMI system of care that follows standards at least as stringent as those developed by the American Heart Association (AHA)'s national initiative (Mission: Lifeline) to include which of the following?

(A) Multidisciplinary team meetings
(B) A process for prehospital identification and activation
(C) Destination protocols for STEMI receiving centers
(D) Transfer protocols for patients arriving at STEMI referral centers
(E) All of the above

13.18 A 57-year-old woman presented with an anterior STEMI to a rural facility where primary PCI is not available. She receives tenecteplase and is transferred to a primary PCI facility. In addition to 325 mg aspirin, what is the appropriate concomitant $P2Y_{12}$ therapy for this patient?

(A) Clopidogrel 300 mg and 75 mg thereafter
(B) Clopidogrel 600 mg and 75 mg thereafter
(C) Prasugrel 60 mg and 10 mg thereafter
(D) Ticagrelor 180 mg and 90 mg twice daily thereafter

13.19 A 71-year-old man is admitted to the hospital after promptly receiving a fibrinolytic agent, heparin, aspirin, and clopidogrel for an inferior wall MI. Primary angioplasty was not performed because the catheterization laboratory was not readily available at 2 AM when he presented. The patient's chest pain gradually resolved over several hours, and you see him later that morning when making rounds. He remains free of chest pain though he complains of dyspnea. His BP is 110/68 with a pulse rate of 92 and a respiratory rate of 20. On physical examination, a third heart sound is faintly heard, and crackles are noted over the lower third of the posterior lung fields. Although he is free of chest pain, you decide to urgently send him for coronary angiography. In the catheterization laboratory, the RCA is found to be completely occluded with faint left-to-right collateral. No other severe CAD is noted, and the LVEF is 40% to 45%. Which of the following would be the appropriate treatment?

(A) The MI is completed; therefore, place a Swan-Ganz catheter and return the patient to the intensive care unit for diuretic therapy and initiation of angiotensin-converting enzyme (ACE) inhibitors
(B) Perform PCI and give an appropriate anticoagulant plus antiplatelet agent
(C) Begin IV GP IIb/IIIa inhibition and have the patient return tomorrow for follow-up angiography and possible PCI
(D) Consult cardiothoracic surgery for consideration of bypass grafting to the RCA

13.20 In the HORIZONS-AMI trial, which compared bivalirudin with heparin plus a GP IIb/IIIa inhibitor, which of the following was TRUE?

(A) No differences in the rate of acute (≤24 hours) or subacute (24 hours to 30 days) stent thrombosis in either group
(B) Higher acute and subacute stent thrombosis with bivalirudin compared with heparin
(C) Lower acute and subacute stent thrombosis with bivalirudin compared with heparin
(D) Higher acute stent thrombosis but similar overall stent thrombosis through 30 days with bivalirudin

13.21 In patients presenting with STEMI undergoing primary PCI, which of the following is correct with respect to radial access?

(A) Lower bleeding but higher mortality
(B) Higher bleeding but lower mortality
(C) Higher bleeding and higher mortality
(D) Lower bleeding and lower mortality

13.22 A 57-year-old man with a history of hypertension and hyperlipidemia presents to a rural, community hospital with 2 hours of acute chest pain. EKG reveals 4 mm inferior ST elevations but the closest primary PCI center is 2 hours away. The patient is administered tenecteplase with resolution of his ST-segment changes. The patient weighs 80 kg and his creatinine clearance is 95 mL/min. Which of the following is an appropriate adjunctive anticoagulation strategy for this patient?

(A) IV UFH bolus of 20 units/kg followed by an infusion of 10 units/kg/h
(B) Enoxaparin 30 mg IV bolus then 80 mg twice daily subcutaneously
(C) Fondaparinux 5 mg IV daily
(D) Enoxaparin 100 mg twice daily

13.23 A 69-year-old man with diabetes presents with 2 mm inferior ST-segment elevation. The closest primary PCI facility is 150 minutes away, so fibrinolytic therapy is considered. Which of the following is NOT an absolute contraindication to fibrinolysis for this patient?

(A) Suspected aortic dissection
(B) Ischemic stroke 6 months ago
(C) Known cerebral arteriovenous malformation (AVM)
(D) Prior subarachnoid hemorrhage

13.24 A 62-year-old homeless man presents with 2 days of substernal discomfort that has now resolved. His ECG demonstrates inferior Q-waves but no persistent ST-segment elevation. His HR is 80 beats per minute (bpm) and his BP is 132/64. His troponin is elevated to 4.62 (upper reference limit 0.045). Transthoracic echocardiogram (TTE) demonstrates inferior akinesis. He is taken to the cardiac catheterization lab and is found to have an occluded proximal RCA. Which of the following is the appropriate treatment strategy?

(A) Perform PCI of the occluded RCA
(B) Continue medical management with dual antiplatelet therapy (DAPT), beta-blocker, ACE inhibitor, and statin
(C) Recheck troponin and perform PCI if increasing
(D) Continue medical management and plan for relook cardiac catheterization in 2 weeks

13.25 A 46-year-old woman with no prior medical history presents with acute chest pain that awoke her from sleep. EKG demonstrates anterior ST-segment elevation. In the emergency room, her HR is 120 bpm and her BP is 80/50. Emergent coronary angiography demonstrates spontaneous coronary artery dissection (SCAD) in the mid-LAD. Which of the following is the most appropriate management strategy?

(A) Conservative therapy with medical management
(B) Referral for emergency CABG
(C) PCI of the LAD lesion
(D) Extracorporeal membranous oxygenation (ECMO) therapy with no revascularization

13.26 A 65-year-old man presents with 2 hours of crushing substernal chest pressure to the emergency room. ECG reveals complete AV block and ST elevation in leads I, II, III, aVF, aVL, and V5 to V6. On physical examination, he is cool, diaphoretic, and hypotensive with a systolic BP of 80 mm Hg. Appropriate pharmacotherapy is administered and you place a transvenous pacemaker and perform emergency coronary angiography. This reveals a RCA that is occluded in its midportion, normal left main and LAD arteries, and an occluded midleft circumflex (LCx) artery. Which of the following is the best therapeutic option?

(A) Intra-aortic balloon pump (IABP) placement and referral for bypass surgery
(B) Primary PCI of the LCx artery with staged PCI of the RCA in 30 days
(C) Primary PCI of the RCA, followed by attempted PCI of the LCx artery if chest pain and hemodynamic instability continue after RCA PCI
(D) Primary PCI of the RCA only, with IABP support for continued chest pain and hemodynamic instability after RCA PCI

13.27 A 64-year-old man presents with acute chest pain that started 2 hours prior. EKG reveals anterior ST-segment elevation. He was given aspirin, heparin, and clopidogrel. His past medical history is significant for an ischemic stroke 2 months ago. His HR is 115 bpm and his BP is 70/30. He is started on dopamine infusion with minimal improvement in his BP. Which of the following is the most appropriate next step in the management of this patient?

(A) Primary PCI of the LAD with no hemodynamic support
(B) Emergency bypass surgery
(C) Emergent placement of an IABP followed by primary PCI of the LAD
(D) Fibrinolytic therapy with tenecteplase and admission to the cardiac intensive care unit

13.28 A 54-year-old type I diabetic (HbA1c 7%) without other known medical problems presents with an acute anterior STEMI. He is a Medicaid-receiving patient. Following emergency coronary angiography and subsequent thrombus aspiration of the LAD artery, you are about to select a stent. Assessment of the proximal LAD lesion by quantitative coronary angiography suggests a reference vessel diameter of 2.4 mm and lesion length of at least 15 mm. Which of the following devices is most appropriate?

(A) 2.5 × 15 mm BMS
(B) 2.5 × 18 mm BMS
(C) 2.5 × 18 mm DES
(D) 2.25 × 18 mm DES

13.29 An emergency room physician calls you about a 72-year-old female with diabetes mellitus, hypertension, and a history of embolic stroke 2 years ago, who has presented to the emergency room with several hours of crushing substernal chest discomfort. Physical examination reveals a thin woman (weight: 58 kg) with ongoing chest pain, tachycardia (rate 110), and BP 100/70 mm Hg. ECG demonstrates ST elevation in the anterior precordial leads. The emergency room physician has already given aspirin 325 mg, morphine 2 mg IV, and a heparin bolus, and has started a nitroglycerin drip. He is now asking for advice on which thienopyridine regimen you would like the patient to receive before you perform cardiac catheterization. You recommend:

(A) Prasugrel 60 mg loading dose, followed by 10 mg daily
(B) Clopidogrel 75 mg daily
(C) Prasugrel 10 mg daily
(D) Clopidogrel 600 mg loading dose, followed by 75 mg daily

13.30 All of the following are absolute contraindications to thrombolytic therapy for STEMI, EXCEPT:

(A) History of intracranial hemorrhage
(B) Intrascapular pain associated with hypotension and >60 mm Hg BP differential between the left and the right arm
(C) Bronchial carcinoma with intracranial metastatic disease
(D) Traumatic and prolonged cardiopulmonary resuscitation lasting >30 minutes
(E) Significant facial trauma 2 weeks ago

13.31 A 47-year-old male presents with chest pain to his local community emergency room. A 12-lead ECG shows 4 mm ST elevation in the inferior leads. He is tachycardic, and his systolic BP is 90 mm Hg. The nearest PCI facilities are 3 hours away. What is the next most appropriate step in the management of this patient?

(A) Full-dose thrombolysis followed by transfer to the nearest PCI facility only if ongoing chest pain or <50% resolution of the ST segments at 60 to 90 minutes
(B) Full-dose thrombolysis followed by immediate transfer to the nearest PCI facility
(C) Half-dose thrombolysis plus abciximab followed by PCI
(D) Full-dose abciximab followed by PCI

13.32 You are asked to see a 68-year-old female who describes an episode of chest pressure, which radiated to her jaw, diaphoresis, and shortness of breath that occurred 29 hours ago at home. She did not seek medical attention at the time but now presents to the emergency room at the insistence of her husband. She is currently pain free with an ECG that demonstrates normal sinus rhythm with 2 mm ST elevation in leads II, III, and aVF and pathologic Q waves. Her BP is 110/70 mm Hg and her O_2 saturations are 98% on room air. You recommend diagnostic angiography, which demonstrates a RCA that is occluded in its midsegment with some left-to-right collaterals. She is also found to have an 80% lesion in her mid-LAD. What is the most appropriate next step in the management of this patient?

(A) Aspiration thrombectomy of the RCA followed by PCI
(B) Balloon angioplasty followed by stenting of the LAD
(C) Medical management
(D) Aspiration thrombectomy of the RCA followed by PCI of RCA and LAD

13.33 In the TRANSFER-AMI trial, 1,059 high-risk STEMI patients presented to a non-PCI hospital and were treated with tenecteplase thrombolysis within 12 hours of chest pain. The patients were randomized to either urgent transfer for cardiac catheterization (PCI within 6 hours after fibrinolysis) or to standard care (transfer for rescue and/or urgent PCI or for routine catheterization after 24 hours). Patients were eligible for inclusion in the study either if they had ST-segment elevation of ≥2 mm in two anterior leads or if they had ST-segment elevation of ≥1 mm in two inferior leads and at least one of the predefined high-risk characteristics. High-risk features in this trial included all of the following, EXCEPT:

(A) Systolic BP < 100 mm Hg
(B) Prior CABG
(C) Killip class II or III
(D) Heart rate > 100 bpm
(E) ≥2-mm anterior ST depression or ≥1-mm ST elevation in V_4R

13.34 In patients with STEMI with known chronic kidney disease (not on hemodialysis) undergoing coronary angiography for primary PCI, which of the following contrast media is recommended?

(A) Ioxaglate
(B) Iohexol
(C) Iodixanol
(D) A nonionic hyperosmolar agent
(E) An ionic hyperosmolar agent

ANSWERS AND EXPLANATIONS

13.1 Answer C. The 2013 American College of Cardiology (ACC) and AHA guidelines recommend that PCI for acute STEMI should be performed as quickly as possible, with a goal of FMC-to-balloon—or door-to-balloon—time within 90 minutes (O'Gara PT, et al. *J Am Coll Cardiol* 2013;61(4):e78–e140). An additional 30 minutes is allowed if the patient initially presents to a non-PCI-capable facility and requires transfer for primary PCI. Symptom onset to reperfusion remains an important predictor of patient outcome even with PCI.

13.2 Answer B. The 2013 ACC/AHA guidelines clearly state that elective PCI should not be performed in a non-infarct-related artery at the time of primary PCI of the infarct-related artery in patients without hemodynamic compromise; this is considered a contraindication (O'Gara PT, et al. *J Am Coll Cardiol* 2013;61(4):e78–e140). In the 2013 recommendations, complete revascularization at the time of the index PCI was considered a Class III recommendation. However, two recent trials have demonstrated the potential value of PCI in severe stenoses of nonculprit vessels (CvLPRIT and PRAMI) in the STEMI setting, but the timing for complete revascularization is currently unclear. As such, the current recommendation is to consider PCI of the nonculprit vessels, but this carries a Class IIb recommendation. Although bypass surgery is an alternative in elective patients with severe multivessel disease, particularly diabetes, waiting for bypass is not an option in this patient with an occluded LAD artery and a large amount of myocardium at jeopardy.

13.3 Answer B. The 2013 ACC/AHA guidelines offer a Class I recommendation for the initiation of therapeutic hypothermia in patients with out of hospital cardiac arrest due to ventricular tachycardia (VT) or fibrillation (VF) and emergent primary PCI. Although PCI should not be delayed in order to initiate therapeutic hypothermia, there is no reason to delay hypothermia initiation until after the PCI. Choice A is incorrect because the goal for FMC-device is ≤90 minutes, not 120 minutes.

13.4 Answer A. 2013 guidelines state that primary PCI should not be performed in asymptomatic patients who are hemodynamically and electrically stable more than 12 hours after the onset of STEMI (American College of Emergency Physicians, et al. *J Am Coll Cardiol* 2013;61(4):e78–e140). She should be admitted for management of MI and be referred for semielective cardiac catheterization. However, she does not meet criteria for either emergency cardiac catheterization or fibrinolytic therapy for management of an acute STEMI.

13.5 Answer C. In patients with acute STEMI, $P2Y_{12}$ inhibitor should ideally be given as early as possible to ensure some degree of platelet inhibition during the primary PCI. The correct dose for ticagrelor is 180 mg as a loading dose followed by 90 mg twice daily. The benefit for ticagrelor in these patients was demonstrated in the PLATO Trial. This patient is not a candidate for prasugrel given her prior history of TIA. Prasugrel was not shown to be beneficial in patients that weighed <60 kg or were ≥75 years of age in the TRITON-TIMI 38 trial and is generally not recommended in these patients.

13.6 Answer E. Primary PCI with stenting has been compared with fibrinolytic therapy in 12 randomized clinical trials. These investigations demonstrate that PCI-treated patients experience lower mortality rates (5.9% vs. 7.7%, OR 0.75, 95% CI 0.60 to 0.94, p = 0.013), fewer reinfarctions (1.6% vs. 5.1%, OR 0.31, 95% CI 0.21 to 0.44, p = 0.0001), and fewer hemorrhagic strokes than those treated by fibrinolysis (Fig. A13-6) (Keeley EC, et al. *Lancet* 2003;361(9351):13–20). Compared with percutaneous transluminal coronary angioplasty alone, intracoronary stents achieve a better immediate angiographic result with a larger arterial lumen, less reclosure of the infarct-related artery, and fewer subsequent ischemic events.

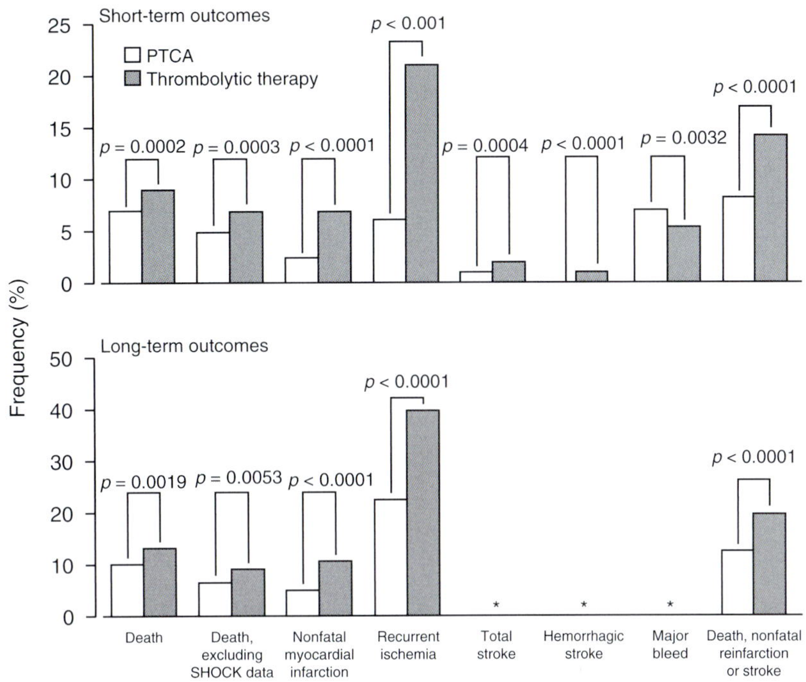

Figure A13-6 Short-term and long-term clinical outcomes in individuals treated with primary percutaneous coronary interventions vs. fibrinolytic therapy. (With permission from Keely EC, et al. *Lancet* 2003;361(9351):13–20.)

13.7 Answer C. Embolic protection devices have not shown benefit in the setting of primary PCI for STEMI, as noted in the Enhanced Myocardial Efficacy and Recovery by Aspiration of Liberated Debris (EMERALD) trial (GuardWire) (Stone GW, et al. *JAMA* 2005;293(9):1063–1072). Subsequent trials, such as the PCI Treatment of Myocardial Infarction for Salvage of Endangered Myocardium (PROMISE) study, have also failed to show benefit with these devices (Gick M, et al. *Circulation* 2005;112:1462–1469). Embolic protection devices are not currently recommended for native-vessel primary PCI.

13.8 Answer B. The best approach to managing acute graft failure after CABG has been unclear for some time. However, a 2006 study compared primary PCI, emergency reoperation, and conservative therapy in a cohort of patients who developed an acute MI shortly after bypass surgery. The study reported that re-revascularization with emergency PCI may limit the extent of myocardial cellular damage compared with the surgical-based treatment strategy in patients with acute perioperative myocardial ischemia because of early graft failure following CABG. When technically feasible, percutaneous revascularization of the native coronary vessel affected by the acutely occluded graft vessel should be considered.

13.9 Answer C. UFH should be used at a dose of 70 to 100 units/kg to achieve a therapeutic activated clotting time (ACT). Choices A and C are likely to lead to underdose and overdose, respectively. The efficacy and safety of bivalirudin was demonstrated in the HORIZONS-AMI trial. Fondaparinux should not be used as the sole anticoagulant during primary PCI due to the risk of catheter thrombosis as demonstrated in the OASIS 6 Trial (Yusuf S, et al. *JAMA* 2006;295(13):1519–1530).

13.10 Answer B. When a patient with STEMI presents to a non–PCI-capable facility, an assessment should be made whether he or she can be transferred to a primary PCI facility within a maximum FMC to device time of ≤120 minutes. If the patient is to be transferred, the goal for the maximum time in the first facility (the door-in-door-out time) should be ≤30 minutes. If the FMC-device time is estimated to be ≥120 minutes and the patient does not have contraindication to fibrinolytic therapy, fibrinolysis should be performed within 30 minutes (door-to-needle time ≤ 30 minutes).

13.11 Answer B. The coronary angiogram reveals acute occlusion of the LCx artery consistent with his symptoms and a (relatively) electrocardiographically silent lateral MI. ECG changes are often subtle in patients with LCx artery disease. Although pericarditis should be considered in the differential diagnosis of chest pain in a relatively young individual, the presence of an occluded coronary artery rules out this diagnosis. The angiogram does not reveal any coronary anomalies or arteriovenous fistula (AVF). Patients with Kawasaki's disease are younger and typically have coronary artery aneurysms rather than occlusions.

13.12 Answer C. There is no consistent evidence that rheolytic (AngioJet) thrombectomy or the emboli protection devices are useful in native coronary arteries with thrombus. A study conducted using AngioJet in acute STEMI failed to demonstrate a reduction in infarct size or other improvement in clinical outcome measures (the AngioJet Rheolytic Thrombectomy in Patients Undergoing Primary Angioplasty for STEMI [AiMI] trial). Regarding embolic protection devices, neither the EMERALD nor PROMISE trials demonstrated a benefit in thrombus-containing native coronary arteries. Of note, several trials of thrombus aspiration have been positive, and this should be strongly considered whenever technically feasible and meta-analysis has supported aspiration thrombectomy (De Luca G, et al. *Eur Heart J* 2008;29(24):3002–3010). Regardless, an attempt at revascularization is indicated in all patients with STEMI and medical therapy alone would not be appropriate in this situation.

13.13 Answer D. Available data suggest that compared with conventional BMS, DES implantations are not associated with increased risk when used for primary PCI in patients with STEMI. Postprocedure vessel patency, biomarker release, and the incidence of short-term adverse events were similar in patients receiving sirolimus-eluting stent (SES) or BMS. Thirty-day event rates of death, reinfarction, or revascularization were 7.5% vs. 10.4%, respectively ($p = 0.4$) (Lemos PA, et al. *J Am Coll Cardiol* 2004;43(4):704–708). Hofma et al. reported the safety and efficacy of currently available DES in patients with acute MI and demonstrated that there were no significant differences in major adverse cardiac outcomes-free survival at 1 year between SES and paclitaxel-eluting stents for the treatment of AMI with very low rates of reintervention for restenosis with both (Hofma SH, et al. *Heart* 2005;91:1176–1180). In this patient with a relatively proximal LAD artery stenosis, absent a contraindication, a DES rather than BMS or balloon angioplasty is the best option to reduce the likelihood of neointimal hyperplasia and in-stent restenosis. There is no reason to administer fibrinolytic therapy after performing coronary angiography in this patient.

13.14 Answer A. The angiogram reveals an anomalous RCA. Subsequent computed tomography (CT) angiogram revealed a course between the aorta and pulmonary artery. She developed ST-segment elevation on vigorous exercise with a treadmill. Table A13-14 lists the common congenital coronary anomalies and their clinical manifestations.

Table A13-14 Common coronary artery anomalies and their potential clinical manifestations

Coronary Artery Anomaly	Incidence (%)	Potential Clinical Manifestations
Separate origin of the LAD and LCx	0.31	—
Ectopic origin of the LCx from the RCA	0.25	—
Ectopic origin of the LCx from the right sinus	0.13	—
Myocardial bridge	0.11	UA, AMI, MA, SD
Ectopic origin of the LCA from the right sinus	0.098	UA, AMI, MA, SD
Single coronary artery	0.098	SA, UA, SD
Atresic coronary artery	0.039	SI
Dual LAD type IV	0.039	—
Ectopic origin of the RCA from the left sinus	0.039	UA, AMI, MA, SD
Coronary artery fistula	0.039	HF, UA, AMI, SYC
Ectopic origin of the RCA from the PA	0.020	SD
Ectopic origin of the LCA from the PA	0.020	HF, SA, UA
Total	1.21	

Abbreviations: AMI, acute myocardial infarction; HF, heart failure; LAD, left anterior descending coronary artery; LCA, left coronary artery; LCx, left circumflex coronary artery; MA, malignant arrhythmias; PA, pulmonary artery; RCA, right coronary artery; SA, stable angina; SD, sudden death; SI, silent ischemia; SYC, syncope; UA, unstable angina.

13.15 Answer C. There are no data to support the routine use of late (days to weeks) PCI days after MI in patients who did not receive reperfusion therapy. This patient had her event 8 days ago and is now stable without recurrent ischemic symptoms, hemodynamic compromise, or arrhythmia. Specifically, the Occluded Artery Trial documented no difference, with a trend toward harm, in stable patients post-STEMI who were randomized to reperfusion of an occluded artery 3 to 30 days following the STEMI. Cardiac catheterization is thus not indicated in this patient (Hochman JS, et al. *N Engl J Med* 2006;355(23):2395–2407).

13.16 Answer C. Based on results from the FINESSE trial (Ellis SG, et al. *N Engl J Med* 2008;358(21):2205–2217), in anticipation of urgent PCI for patients with STEMI, the use of a facilitated pharmacologic strategy for reperfusion with either abciximab alone or abciximab plus reduced-dose reteplase did not improve clinical outcomes. Primary PCI with abciximab administered in the catheterization laboratory provided a better benefit-to-risk ratio than the two facilitated strategies among patients with STEMI who underwent PCI within 4 hours after the FMC. The TRANSFER-AMI Study (Cantor WJ, et al. *N Engl J Med* 2009;360(26):2705–2718) evaluated a strategy of fibrinolysis with immediate transfer vs. standard therapy and found that the primary endpoint of composite of death, reinfarction, recurrent ischemia, new or worsening congestive heart failure, or cardiogenic shock within 30 days occurred in 11.0% of immediate transfer patients vs. 17.2% of standard therapy patients (HR 0.64, 95% CI 0.47 to 0.87, $p = 0.004$). Based partly on this trial, the 2013 ACC/AHA Guidelines recommend early transfer to a PCI facility after administration of fibrinolytic therapy.

13.17 Answer E. The 2013 STEMI/PCI Guidelines (Kushner FG, et al. *J Am Coll Cardiol* 2009;54(23):2205–2241) underline the importance of regional systems of STEMI care to include encouraging the participation of key stakeholders in collaborative efforts to evaluate care, measuring outcomes and adherence to evidence-based processes (Class I recommendation). The AHA has also promoted its "MissionLifeline" initiative, which was developed to encourage closer cooperation and trust among prehospital emergency services and cardiac care professionals.

13.18 Answer A. According to the 2013 ACC/AHA STEMI guidelines, in conjunction with fibrinolytic therapy, clopidogrel 300 mg should be administered initially as the $P2Y_{12}$ agent of choice if the patient is ≤75 years of age; only 75 mg should be given if the patient is >75 years of age. The coadministration of the other $P2Y_{12}$ agents (prasugrel and ticagrelor) with fibrinolytic therapy has not been studied prospectively.

13.19 Answer B. According to the 2013 ACC/AHA STEMI guidelines, it is reasonable for high-risk patients who receive fibrinolytic therapy as primary reperfusion therapy to undergo early PCI with an appropriate antithrombotic regimen. The most recent trials to support this recommendation include the CARESS-in-AMI trial (Di Mario C, et al. *Lancet* 2008;371(9612):559–568) and the TRANSFER-AMI trial (Cantor WJ, et al. *N Engl J Med* 2009;360(26):2705–2718), both of which defined patients with Killip Class II as high risk.

13.20 Answer D. The HORIZONS-AMI trial compared bivalirudin vs. heparin plus a GP IIb/IIIa inhibitor in patients presenting with STEMI and found a reduction in net adverse clinical events with bivalirudin due primarily to a lower rate of major bleeding. The rate of protocol defined stent thrombosis was similar in the bivalirudin and heparin/GP inhibitor arms (2.5% vs. 1.9%, $p = 0.30$); however, the risk of acute stent thrombosis within 24 hours was significantly higher with bivalirudin compared with heparin/GP inhibitors (1.3% vs. 0.3%, $p < 0.001$). This finding was further confirmed in the EUROMAX trial, which evaluated prehospital administration of bivalirudin in patients with STEMI (Steg PG, et al. *N Engl J Med* 2013;369(23):2207–2217).

13.21 Answer D. Radial access in patients undergoing primary PCI for STEMI was studied in the RIFLE-STEACS (Radial Versus Femoral Randomized Investigation in ST-Elevation Acute Coronary Syndrome) Trial (Romagnoli E, et al. *J Am Coll Cardiol* 2012;60(24):2481–2489), which randomized 1,001 patients presenting with STEMI to transradial ($n = 500$) or transfemoral (501) access. The primary outcome of composite death/MI/stroke/target vessel revascularization (TVR)/non-CABG bleeding occurred in 13.6% of radial access patients vs. 21.0% of femoral access patients ($p = 0.003$) with decreased mortality (5.2% vs. 9.2%, $p = 0.02$) and bleeding (7.8% vs. 12.2%, $p = 0.026$) in the radial access arm. A subsequent meta-analysis (Karrowni W, et al. *JACC Cardiovasc Intv* 2013;6(8):814–823) demonstrated a lower risk of mortality and bleeding with radial vs. femoral access, though with slightly longer procedure time.

13.22 Answer B. In conjunction with fibrinolytic therapy, appropriate anticoagulant therapies can include UFH, enoxaparin, or fondaparinux. UFH is dosed at a weight-based bolus of 60 U/kg (max 4,000 U) followed by an infusion of 12 U/kg/h (max 1,000 U). For patients <75 years of age, enoxaparin is dosed with an IV bolus of 30 mg followed by 1 mg/kg subcutaneously every 12 hours; for patients ≥75 years, there is no bolus and the dose is 0.75 mg/kg. Additionally, if the creatinine clearance is <30 mL/min, the dose is 1 mg/kg subcutaneously every 24 hours. Fondaparinux is dosed 2.5 mg IV initially, then 2.5 mg subcutaneously the following day. Fondaparinux is contraindicated if CrCl < 30 mL/min.

13.23 Answer B. According to the 2013 ACC/AHA STEMI guidelines, choices A, C, and D are absolute contraindications to the administration of fibrinolytic therapy in patients with STEMI. Choice B is correct because ischemic stroke within 3 months is an absolute contraindication to lytic therapy; an ischemic stroke >3 months prior is a relative contraindication.

13.24 Answer B. This patient is >24 hours from his initial event. The 2013 ACC/AHA guidelines offer a Class III (no benefit) recommendation for delayed PCI in an asymptomatic patient with no electrical or hemodynamic instability who has no evidence of severe ischemia. This is based on the Occluded Artery Trial (OAT), which demonstrated no difference in the composite end point of death/repeat MI/Class IV heart failure in patients managed medically vs. with PCI. Additionally, reinfarction rates were higher in the PCI group.

13.25 Answer C. This patient has cardiogenic shock as a result of poor flow in the LAD territory. If the patient is stable and does not have any high-risk features (i.e., left main dissection, ongoing chest pain/ischemia, ventricular tachycardia or fibrillation, or cardiogenic shock), conservative therapy is indicated. If the patient has a high-risk feature, PCI is reasonable if it is a feasible option. In this case, the patient has an isolated lesion in the mid-LAD territory. She has cardiogenic shock, so PCI of the LAD is indicated. The patient may require mechanical circulatory support, but revascularization is also necessary (Saw J, et al. *J Am Coll Cardiol* 2016;68(3):297–312).

13.26 Answer C. In general, PCI should not be performed in a noninfarct artery at the time of primary PCI (Class III, Level of Evidence C). However, in patients with more than one potential infarct-related artery and evidence of hemodynamic compromise or cardiogenic shock, multivessel PCI may be considered.

13.27 Answer C. The patient requires reperfusion to the LAD territory, but at this point, he is currently in cardiogenic shock. The 2013 ACC/AHA guidelines offer a Class IIa recommendation for the use of IABP counterpulsation in patients with cardiogenic shock after STEMI that does not improve with pharmacologic therapy. Given this patient's history of recent ischemic stroke, fibrinolytic therapy is contraindicated in this situation.

13.28 Answer C. There does not appear to be a significant difference between BMS and DES in mortality rates of MI or stent thrombosis, with DES having the advantage of a reduction in TVR rates as compared to BMS. It is reasonable to use a DES as an alternative to BMS for primary PCI in STEMI (Class IIa, Level of Evidence B) especially if clinical and anatomic considerations such as small vessel diameter, longer lesion length, or diabetes mellitus are present. The most significant practical challenge is usually trying to determine, in an emergency setting, if the patient is a candidate for DAPT. If there is evidence of financial limitations, patient noncompliance, increased bleeding risk, and upcoming surgical procedures, DES should be avoided. In this case, however, the patient is insured and, at least by HbA1c, the patient appears to be compliant and without any obvious bleeding concerns. A DES would be preferred given the lesion location and length, vessel diameter, and history of diabetes.

13.29 Answer D. A loading dose of thienopyridine is recommended for STEMI patients in whom PCI is planned (Class I, Level of Evidence C). Clopidogrel at a loading dose of 300 to 600 mg or prasugrel 60 mg should be given as soon as possible before or at the time of primary PCI. However, prasugrel is relatively contraindicated in patients ≥75 years of age and with a body weight <60 kg or those with a history of TIA or stroke. Patients weighing <60 kg have an increased exposure to the active metabolite of prasugrel and an increased risk of bleeding. Data from the TRITON-TIMI 38 trial (Wiviott SD, et al. *N Engl J Med* 2007;357(20):2001–2015) that randomized high-risk ACS/STEMI patients to prasugrel 60 mg load, 10 mg maintenance vs. clopidogrel 300 mg load, and 75 mg maintenance dose showed superior efficacy in major predefined subgroups. However, a post hoc analysis suggested that patients with prior cerebrovascular accident/TIA had net harm from prasugrel and patients with a body weight <60 kg and ≥75 years of age had no net benefit from prasugrel.

13.30 **Answer D.** Traumatic or prolonged (>10 minutes) cardiopulmonary resuscitation is a relative contraindication. All other responses are absolute contraindications to thrombolytic therapy.

13.31 **Answer B.** High-risk STEMI patients (≥2 mm of ST-segment elevation in two anterior leads or ST elevation of at least 1 mm in inferior leads with at least one of the following: systolic BP < 100 mm Hg, heart rate ≥ 100 bpm, Killip Class II to III, ≥2 mm of ST-segment depression in the anterior leads, or ≥1 mm of ST elevation in right-sided lead V4 indicative of right ventricular involvement) presenting to non–PCI-capable facilities who are not close enough to be transferred for primary PCI within 90 minutes should receive thrombolytic therapy as the primary reperfusion strategy and then be moved immediately to a PCI-capable facility for diagnostic catheterization and consideration of PCI without waiting to determine whether reperfusion has occurred. This strategy is based on evidence from both the CARESS-in-AMI trial (Di Mario C, et al. *Lancet* 2008;371(9612):559–568) and the TRANSFER-AMI trial (Cantor WJ, et al. *N Engl J Med* 2009;360(26):2705–2718). Data from both trials support early diagnostic angiography and possible revascularization (Class IIa, Level of Evidence B).

13.32 **Answer C.** PCI of a totally occluded infarct artery >24 hours after STEMI is not recommended in asymptomatic patients with one- or two-vessel disease if they are hemodynamically and electrically stable and do not have evidence of severe, ongoing ischemia (Class III, Level of Evidence B). Further, in the absence of hemodynamic compromise or cardiogenic shock, PCI should not be performed in a noninfarct artery in the acute setting (Class III, Level of Evidence C) (Canadian Cardiovascular Society, et al. *J Am Coll Cardiol* 2008;51(2):210–247).

13.33 **Answer B.** Key exclusion criteria for the TRANSFER-AMI trial included cardiogenic shock before randomization, PCI within the previous month, previous coronary artery bypass surgery, and the availability of primary PCI with an anticipated door-to-balloon time of <60 minutes. All other options were inclusion criteria for the trial. Among high-risk STEMI patients who were treated with fibrinolysis, transfer for PCI within 6 hours after fibrinolysis was associated with significantly fewer ischemic complications than standard treatment (Cantor WJ, et al. *N Engl J Med* 2009;360(26):2705–2718).

13.34 **Answer C.** In patients with chronic kidney disease undergoing angiography who are not undergoing chronic dialysis, either an iso-osmolar contrast medium, that is, iodixanol (Class I, Level of Evidence A) or a low-molecular-weight contrast medium, other than ioxaglate or iohexol, is indicated (Class I, Level of Evidence B). This is based on a number of trials, including the moderate-sized randomized clinical trial RECOVER (Jo SH, et al. *J Am Coll Cardiol* 2006;48(5):924–930) that compared the isosmolar agent iodixanol and ioxaglate and favored the former, as well as the CARE trial (Solomon RJ, et al. *Circulation* 2007;115(25):3189–3196), which compared iodixanol and the low-osmolar agent iopamidol and found no difference. However, several larger randomized trials have been published more recently that reported no difference in contrast-induced nephropathy when iodixanol was compared with various other low-osmolar contrast media other than iohexol (Kuhn MJ, et al. *AJR Am J Roentgenol* 2008;191(1):151–157; Rudnick MR, et al. *Am Heart J* 2008;156(4):776–782; Thomsen HS, et al. *Invest Radiol* 2008;43(3):170–178). A pooled comparison of iodixanol with all nonionic low-osmolar contrast media indicated equivalent safety (Reed M, et al. *J Am Coll Cardiol Intv* 2009;2(7):645–654).

14 Periprocedural Myocardial Infarction, Emboli Protection, and Mechanical Thrombectomy

Terence Hill and Mehdi H. Shishehbor

QUESTIONS

14.1 Cardiac catheterization performed on a 69-year-old female who presented with unstable angina revealed a long diffuse lesion extending from the mid to distal atrioventricular (AV) left circumflex (LCx) coronary artery (Fig. Q14-1A). The first angiogram after balloon angioplasty and stenting is shown (Fig. Q14-1B). Which of the following mechanisms explains the findings seen on this angiogram?

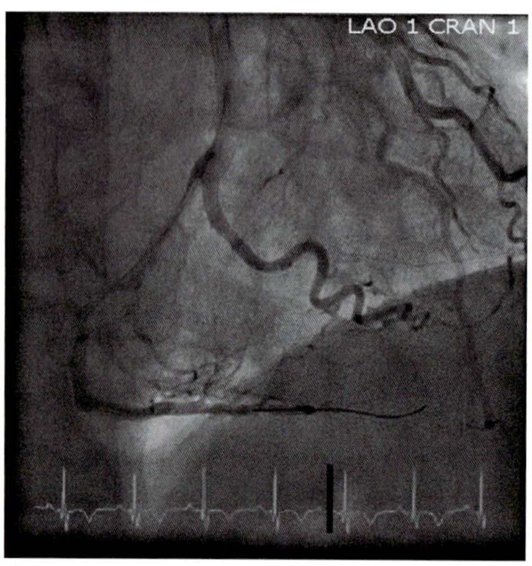

A

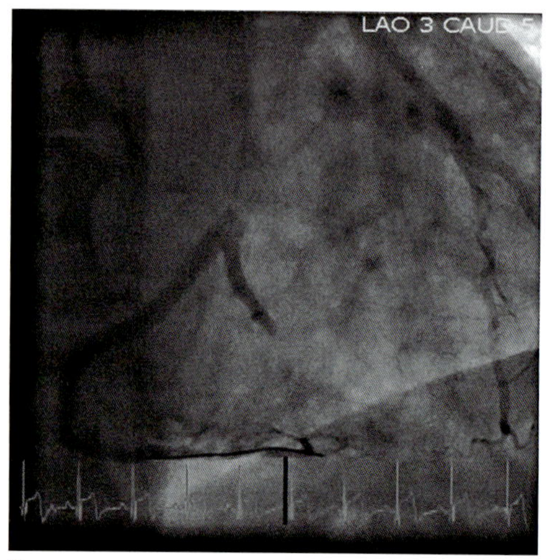

B

Figure Q14-1

(A) Side-branch closure with embolization
(B) Occlusive dissection
(C) Microvascular obstruction due to embolization
(D) Epicardial obstruction due to thrombus formation

14.2 You are performing percutaneous coronary intervention (PCI) on a patient who had coronary artery bypass surgery 5 years ago and has a severe lesion at the distal anastomosis of the saphenous vein graft (SVG) to the first obtuse marginal (OM) branch. What would be the best procedural approach?

(A) Balloon dilate, place a FilterWire, stent, and then postdilate
(B) Direct stent
(C) Balloon dilate, stent, and postdilate

14.3 Which of the following devices would be a good choice for embolic protection in a patient with an aorto-ostial SVG lesion?

(A) Boston Scientific FilterWire
(B) ev3 Spyder
(C) Medtronic GuardWire
(D) Either A or B

14.4 The use of a distal embolic protection device (EPD) during PCI of saphenous vein aortocoronary bypass grafts has been shown to reduce which of the following?

(A) Death
(B) Myocardial infarction (MI)
(C) Emergency bypass
(D) All of the above
(E) None of the above

14.5 Which of the following treatments has been shown to significantly reduce the risk of periprocedural MI?

(A) Rotational atherectomy, if performed for <2 minutes
(B) Pretreatment with intragraft verapamil before SVG intervention
(C) Thrombectomy using the AngioJet device before stent implantation in SVG intervention
(D) Pretreatment with atorvastatin before elective coronary intervention
(E) Intracoronary urokinase when given 15 minutes before PCI

14.6 In which of the following SVG lesions would an EPD be expected to provide the LEAST benefit?

(A) A long complex midshaft lesion
(B) A focal midshaft lesion in a 7-year-old vein graft
(C) In-stent restenosis of a previously placed SVG stent 2 years ago
(D) A short lesion at the distal anastomosis of an 18-month-old vein graft
(E) C and D

14.7 Use of an EPD during PCI has a guideline-recommended Class I indication for which of the following interventions?

(A) Direct stenting of the left main trunk
(B) PCI of a native coronary artery in the setting of ST-segment elevation myocardial infarction (STEMI)
(C) PCI of a native coronary artery in the setting of non-STEMI
(D) PCI of a native coronary artery in the setting of unstable angina
(E) PCI of an SVG to LCx artery

14.8 The likelihood of an adverse event occurring at 30 days when using EPD during PCI of an SVG is around:

(A) >60%
(B) 46% to 60%
(C) 31% to 45%
(D) 16% to 30%
(E) 0% to 15%

14.9 Which of the following procedure characteristics is NOT associated with a higher risk of periprocedural MI?

(A) Bifurcation treatment
(B) Multivessel procedure
(C) Lesion length
(D) Lesion angulation

14.10 Which of the following is the least effective pharmacologic therapy for "no reflow" after percutaneous intervention?

(A) Intracoronary (IC) nitroglycerin
(B) IC adenosine
(C) IC nitroprusside
(D) IC nicardipine

14.11 Which of the following patient characteristics may increase the risk of periprocedural myonecrosis?

(A) Increased arterial inflammation
(B) Aspirin resistance
(C) Clopidogrel resistance
(D) Genetic predisposition
(E) All of the above

14.12 In clinical practice, creatine kinase-MB (CK-MB) elevations (less than five times the upper normal limits) occur after what percentage of technically successful PCIs?

(A) 0% to 15%
(B) 15% to 30%
(C) 31% to 45%
(D) 46% to 60%
(E) >60%

14.13 There is a dose–response relationship between periprocedural CK elevation and mortality.

(A) True
(B) False

14.14 All of the following outcomes listed below are associated with periprocedural myonecrosis, EXCEPT:

(A) Immediate in-hospital mortality
(B) Short-term (<30 days) mortality
(C) Long-term (>1-year) mortality
(D) Stroke
(E) All of the above

14.15 Which of the following factors is associated with a decreased risk of periprocedural MI?

(A) Statin therapy
(B) Clopidogrel therapy
(C) Aspirin therapy
(D) Prasugrel therapy
(E) All of the above

14.16 You are planning an elective intervention on an 82-year-old male with a 90% mid-right heavily calcified mid-right coronary artery (RCA) lesion. In order to assess the likelihood of distal embolization, you perform an intravascular ultrasound (IVUS) assessment. All of the following findings by IVUS have been shown to be associated with higher periprocedural CK elevations, EXCEPT:

(A) Plaque burden
(B) Lesion site calcification
(C) Cross-sectional narrowing at the lesion site by IVUS
(D) Lumen dimension at the lesion site
(E) Positive remodeling

14.17 According to the 2015 American College of Cardiology (ACC) and American Heart Association (AHA) guidelines for primary percutaneous coronary intervention for patients with STEMI, what is the recommendation regarding aspiration thrombectomy?

(A) Class III (no benefit) for all patients
(B) Class IIa (reasonable) for all patients
(C) Class III (no benefit) for routine use and Class IIb (not unreasonable) in selected situations
(D) Class I (recommended) if extensive thrombus is seen on angiography and Class IIb (not unreasonable) for routine use

14.18 All of the following factors have been shown to be independent predictors of distal embolization during SVG interventions, EXCEPT:

(A) Undersizing of stents
(B) Presence of thrombus
(C) Diffusely diseased vein grafts
(D) Balloon angioplasty followed by stenting

14.19 A 78-year-old female underwent PCI of a totally occluded RCA (Fig. Q14-19A). After percutaneous intervention is performed on the occlusion, the patient is discovered to have another abnormality in the RCA (Fig. Q14-19B). What is the abnormality shown at the arrow in Figure Q14-19B?

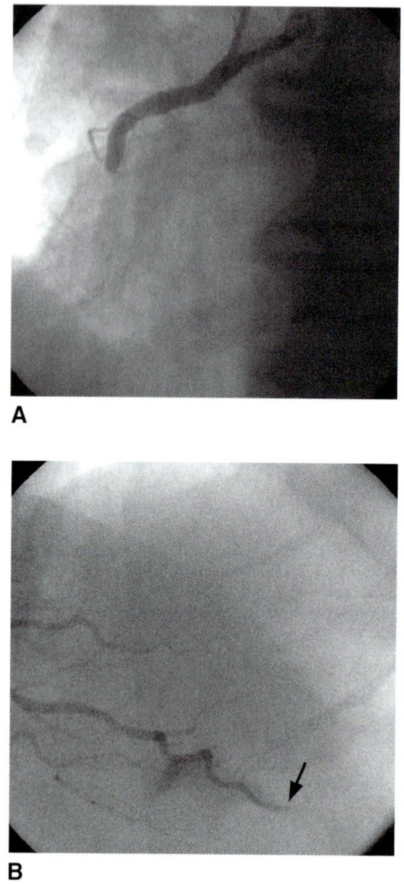

Figure Q14-19

(A) Vasospasm
(B) Dissection
(C) Perforation
(D) Distal embolization and cutoff
(E) Stenosis

14.20 In randomized clinical trials, mechanical thrombectomy for STEMI has been shown to reduce the risk of which of the following?

(A) Death
(B) Reinfarction
(C) Congestive heart failure
(D) Hospital length of stay
(E) Low myocardial blush score

14.21 The risk of which of the following may potentially be increased with the use of aspiration thrombectomy in STEMI?

(A) Stroke
(B) Myocardial infarct size
(C) No reflow
(D) Death
(E) Arrhythmia

14.22 In the TAPAS Trial, atherothrombotic material was retrieved in what percentage of cases?

(A) 10% to 20%
(B) 30% to 40%
(C) 50% to 60%
(D) 60% to 70%
(E) 70% to 80%

14.23 Arrange the following aspiration thrombectomy catheters in order of increasing tip diameter:

a. Medtronic Export
b. Terumo Priority One
c. Vascular Solutions Pronto LP

(A) a, b, c
(B) a, c, b
(C) b, a, c
(D) b, c, a
(E) c, a, b
(F) c, b, a

14.24 Which of the following represents optimal technique when performing aspiration thrombectomy?

(A) Start aspiration distal to the obstruction and stop at the guiding catheter
(B) Start aspiration proximal to the obstruction and continue until the device is removed from the body
(C) Start aspiration proximal to the obstruction and stop at the guiding catheter
(D) Start aspiration proximal to the obstruction and stop distal to the obstruction

14.25 All of the following trials evaluated the utility of thrombus aspiration in the setting of primary PCI, EXCEPT:

(A) EMERALD
(B) REMEDIA
(C) AIMI
(D) TAPAS
(E) BOOST

ANSWERS AND EXPLANATIONS

14.1 Answer A. This angiogram shows abrupt closure with embolization of the OM branch after stenting the AV LCx artery. The other answers are known causes of periprocedural MI. The major mechanism for periprocedural MI is embolization of microscopic debris with subsequent platelet activation and inflammation leading to impairment in microvascular flow.

14.2 Answer B. Distal embolic protection devices require a distal landing zone in the SVG to provide for safe placement. In the case of a distal anastomotic lesion, there is no safe landing zone for a filter wire. In this case, the best practice to reduce the degree of embolization is to perform direct stenting without pre- or postdilation. The Proxis proximal protection system, which involves a proximal balloon to stop flow, followed by aspiration prior to balloon removal, was formerly an option in these lesions but is no longer commercially available in the United States.

14.3 Answer D. A filter device would be preferred in an aorto-ostial lesion to a balloon occlusion device (such as the Medtronic GuardWire). With the latter device, embolic debris can be embolized to the systemic circulation.

14.4 Answer B. The randomized trial of a DEP device during PCI of saphenous vein aortocoronary bypass grafts (Baim DS, et al. *Circulation* 2002;105(11):1285–1290) showed a significant reduction in the composite end point of death, MI, emergency bypass, or target lesion revascularization (TLR) at 30 days among those who received distal protection (9.6%) compared to the control group (16.5%) (p = 0.004). However, this was mainly driven by lower rates of MI and the "no-reflow" phenomenon (3% distal embolic protection vs. 9% control, p = 0.02).

14.5 Answer D. In the Atorvastatin for Reduction of Myocardial Damage During Angioplasty (ARMYDA) trial (Pasceri V, et al. *Circulation* 2004;110(6): 674–678), atorvastatin (40 mg/day) administered 7 days before elective coronary intervention had a significant reduction in all markers for myocardial injury—including CK-MB, troponin I, and myoglobin—measured 8 and 24 hours after the procedure when compared with patients who did not receive atorvastatin. Postprocedural MI measured by CK-MB occurred in 5% of patients who received atorvastatin vs. 18% in patients in the placebo group (p = 0.025). Intragraft verapamil before PCI in SVG was examined in a small study and verapamil was shown to decrease the rate of "no reflow" and improve flow rate in the vessel; however, there was no difference in postprocedural cardiac enzyme release (Kereiakes DJ, et al. *J Invasive Cardiol* 2002;14(6):303–304). In a study of 797 patients with diseased SVG or thrombus-containing native coronary arteries, routine thrombectomy before stent implantation did not decrease the incidence of periprocedural MI when compared with stent implantation without thrombectomy (Stone GW, et al. *J Am Coll Cardiol* 2003;42(11):2007–2013). Many studies have shown increased rates of distal embolization and periprocedural MI with directional and rotational atherectomy.

14.6 Answer E. Recently placed (<2-year-old) vein grafts have had less time to degenerate and theoretically should have less embolic potential. A short, simple lesion also could be addressed in a procedurally simple manner, further lessening the risk for embolization. In-stent restenosis is largely due to fibrosis, which would also be expected to produce less embolic material. Older vein grafts with increased lesion complexity would be expected to have a higher potential for distal embolism.

14.7 Answer E. In the SAFER trial (Baim DS, et al. *Circulation* 2002;105(11):1285–1290), 801 patients undergoing percutaneous intervention to stenotic SVGs were randomly assigned to stent placement over the shaft of the PercuSurge GuardWire balloon occlusion and aspiration system vs. stent placement over a conventional angioplasty guidewire. Use of the distal protection device resulted in a 42% relative risk reduction in the primary end point, which was a composite of death, MI, emergency bypass, or TLR by 30 days. Analysis of the individual components of the primary end point revealed a statistically significant reduction in MI and "no reflow." Therefore, the use of EPD for SVG intervention has a Class I indication in the current guidelines. EPD is not indicated for any of the other interventions listed.

14.8 Answer E. The MACE rate with use of the current EPDs (including distal filters, proximal devices, and distal balloon occlusion/aspiration systems) is 7% to 12% depending upon the device. The SAFER trial, which evaluated a distal balloon occlusion and aspiration system (PercuSurge GuardWire), had a 9.6% MACE rate at 30 days. In the FilterWire EX Randomized Evaluation (FIRE) trial (Stone GW, et al. *J Am Coll Cardiol* 2002;40(10):1882-1888), which assessed the utility of a distal filter device (FilterWire EX), there was a 30-day MACE rate of 11.3%. The Protection Devices in PCI Treatment of Myocardial Infarction for Salvage of Endangered Myocardium (PROMISE) trial (unpublished, presented at the Transcatheter Cardiovascular Therapeutics 2005 meeting) examined the efficacy of a proximal balloon and occlusion system (Proxis) and had 9.2% of MACE at 30 days. The Protection During Saphenous Vein Graft Intervention to Prevent Distal Embolization (PRIDE) trial (Carrozza JP, et al. *J Am Coll Cardiol* 2005;46(9):1677-1683), which examined the use of a balloon-protection flush and extraction system (TriActiv System), found 11.2% of MACE at 30 days.

14.9 Answer D. In a retrospective study of 3,371 patients (Zhao D, et al. *Catheter Cardiovasc Interv* 2017; 89(S1):534-540), bifurcation lesions, multivessel procedures, and overall lesion treated length were shown to be independent predictors of periprocedural MI.

14.10 Answer A. Nitroglycerin must metabolize to active nitric oxide by the vascular wall to provide vasodilation. The microvascular arterioles are not able to effectively metabolize the nitroglycerin, and therefore, it is less effective than the other options. Sodium nitroprusside also acts via a nitric oxide mechanism but is direct acting and therefore has a larger effect on the microvasculature.

14.11 Answer E. Genetic predisposition, aspirin and clopidogrel resistance, and increased arterial inflammation are factors believed to increase the risk of periprocedural myonecrosis (Decker RS, et al. *Circulation* 2005;111(7):906-912).

14.12 Answer A. In clinical practice, asymptomatic CK-MB elevations (less than five times the upper normal limits) occur after 3% to 11% of technically successful PCIs (Thygesen K, et al. *Circulation* 2007;116(22):2634-2653).

14.13 Answer A. The EPIC trial (Topol EJ, et al. *JAMA* 1997;278(6):479-484) was one of the first trials to demonstrate the association between periprocedural MI and increased mortality in the intermediate period after percutaneous intervention. The study demonstrated a direct relationship between the degree of CK elevation postprocedure and 3-year mortality. Patients with CK elevations ten-, five- and three-fold the normal CK level had an estimated mortality rate at 3 years of 16.5%, 14.8%, and 13.1%, respectively. As compared with those with normal CK levels, patients with CK levels greater than once the upper limit of normal also had an increased mortality rate at 3 years (10.2% vs. 7.3%).

14.14 Answer D. The association between periprocedural MI and PCI has been established by numerous studies and meta-analysis (Bhatt DL, et al. *Circulation* 2005;112(6):906-915; discussion 923). However, periprocedural MI has not been linked to increased stroke risk.

14.15 Answer E. Antiplatelet and antithrombotic therapies including aspirin, clopidogrel, prasugrel, and glycoprotein (GP) IIb/IIIa inhibitors have been shown to attenuate the impact of embolization during PCI, leading to reductions in periprocedural MI. Similarly, as noted previously, statins have also been shown to significantly reduce the risk of periprocedural MI when given before PCI.

14.16 Answer D. IVUS assessment of 2,256 patients undergoing PCI of native coronaries identified plaque burden at the lesion, lesion site calcification, positive remodeling, cross-sectional narrowing at the lesion, and reference sites to be associated with periprocedural CK-MB elevations. In the multivariable analysis, age, sex, diabetes mellitus, and lumen dimension at the lesion site before and after intervention were not predictive of CK-MB elevation (Mehran R, et al. *Circulation* 2000;101(6):604-610).

14.17 Answer A. In 2015, the ACC/AHA recommendation for aspiration thrombectomy for STEMI was changed from the 2013 recommendation. Previously, aspiration thrombectomy was recommended as Class IIa (reasonable) for all patients undergoing primary PCI based on the TAPAS study (Svilaas T, et al. *N Engl J Med* 2008;358(6): 557-567). Subsequent larger randomized controlled trials and meta-analyses concluded there was no benefit and a possible trend towards increased stroke.

14.18 Answer A. Observational studies and case reports have shown lower distal embolization with less aggressive stent sizing in SVGs. However, the long-term safety and efficacy of this approach is not well established. The CAVEAT-II was a prospective, multicenter trial comparing percutaneous transluminal coronary angioplasty vs. directional coronary angiography in patients with SVG lesions. The use of directional coronary angiography and the presence of thrombus in this clinical trial were both independent predictors of distal embolization (Leftkovits J, et al. *Circulation* 1995;92(4):734–740). Other angiographic predictors of distal embolization after balloon angioplasty of SVGs included diffusely diseased vein grafts and large plaque volume (Liu MW, et al. *Am J Cardiol* 1993;72(7):514–517). Graft age is also a predictor of distal embolization.

14.19 Answer D. The angiogram shows distal embolization and cutoff in the distal PDA after intervention was performed to the complete occlusion in the midsegment of the RCA.

14.20 Answer E. The TAPAS (Thrombus Aspiration during Primary Percutaneous Coronary Intervention) trial examined the utility of manual aspiration using a 6-Fr Export Aspiration Catheter (Medtronic) (*cited above*). The primary end point was the postprocedural frequency of a myocardial blush grade of 0 or 1. In this study, the Export Aspiration Catheter was shown to be superior to conventional treatment for primary end point. While there was a trend toward lower clinical events with manual aspiration, this did not reach statistical significance. Subsequent larger trials did not show any difference in "hard" clinical outcomes with aspiration thrombectomy.

14.21 Answer A. Following the 1,071 patient TAPAS trial (referenced above), the TASTE trial (Jolly SS, et al. *N Engl J Med* 2015:372(15):1389–1398) enrolled 10,732 patients with STEMI undergoing primary PCI to aspiration thrombectomy vs. no aspiration thrombectomy. No change in the primary outcome (i.e., death, recurrent MI, cardiogenic shock, or New York Heart Association [NYHA] Class IV heart failure at 180 days) was observed, and an increased risk of stroke (0.7% vs. 0.3%, HR 2.1) was observed. A subsequent meta-analysis of 20,960 patients (Elgendy IY, et al. *Circ Cardiovasc Interv* 2015:8(7):e002258) confirmed no difference in death or MI and a nonstatistically significant increase in the risk of stroke.

14.22 Answer E. In the TAPAS trial (Svilaas T, et al. *N Engl J Med* 2008;358(6):557–567), 73% of those who underwent manual aspiration had atherothrombotic material extracted.

14.23 Answer F. The Pronto LP is the smallest with a tip diameter of 1.34 mm, followed by the Priority One with a tip diameter of 1.68 mm. The Export is the largest with a tip diameter of 1.73 mm. All catheters are 6-Fr guide compatible.

14.24 Answer B. Continuous aspiration from prior to the lesion until the catheter is out of the body is important to minimize the risk of peripheral embolization.

14.25 Answer E. The EMERALD trial (Stone GW, et al. *JAMA* 2005;293(9):1063–1072) randomized 501 patients presenting with ST-segment MI to receive PCI with a balloon occlusion and aspiration distal microcirculatory system vs. angioplasty without any distal protection. There was no difference among the treatment groups with respect to either of the coprimary end points, which were ST-segment resolution measured 30 minutes after PCI by continuous Holter monitoring, and infarct size measured by single-photon emission computed tomography (SPECT) imaging between days 5 and 14. There was also no improvement in microvascular flow or success of reperfusion. The Randomized Evaluation of the Effect of Mechanical Reduction of Distal Embolization by Thrombus-Aspiration in Primary and Rescue Angioplasty (REMEDIA) trial was a single-center, prospective, randomized study that was designed to determine the safety and efficacy of the *Diver CE* catheter for thrombus aspiration in ST-segment elevation acute MI patients vs. standard PCI. The primary end point was myocardial blush score >2 and ST-segment resolution >70%. REMEDIA showed that thrombus aspiration prior to PCI resulted in an improvement in myocardial blush score and ST resolution compared to PCI alone. The AIMI (AngioJet Rheolytic Thrombectomy in Patients Undergoing Primary Angioplasty for Acute Myocardial Infarction) trial evaluated 480 patients and failed to show a significant difference in ST resolution. Furthermore, those who underwent thrombectomy had a larger infarct size and 1-month MACE rate. The TAPAS trial has been described above. The BOOST (intracoronary autologous bone-marrow cell transfer after MI) randomized controlled clinical trial did not test thrombus aspiration.

15 Chronic Total Occlusions

David E. Kandzari and Dimitri Karmpaliotis

QUESTIONS

15.1 Compared with percutaneous revascularization of nonocclusive coronary lesions, which statement best characterizes outcomes among patients with chronic total occlusions (CTOs) when using bare metal stents (BMS)?

(A) CTOs have higher rates of restenosis and reocclusion
(B) Restenosis is higher with total occlusions, but reocclusion rates are similar
(C) Reocclusion is more frequent among total coronary occlusions, but restenosis rates are similar
(D) Rates of both restenosis and reocclusion are similar

15.2 Which variable best predicts improvement in left ventricular (LV) function following successful recanalization of a CTO?

(A) History of prior myocardial infarction (MI)
(B) Baseline LV dysfunction
(C) Angiographic presence of collateral flow
(D) Duration of occlusion

15.3 Compared with conventional BMS, treatment with a drug-eluting stent (DES) following recanalization of CTOs is associated with all of the following, EXCEPT:

(A) Reductions in restenosis
(B) Decrease in repeat target lesion revascularization (TLR)
(C) Improved survival
(D) Decreased rates of reocclusion

15.4 Compared with procedural failure to recanalize CTOs, successful percutaneous revascularization of CTOs is associated with all of the following, EXCEPT:

(A) Improved long-term survival
(B) Increased need for repeat revascularization procedures
(C) Reduced angina
(D) Improved LV function

15.5 The most common reason for failure of percutaneous revascularization of a CTO is:

(A) Guidewire entry into a subintimal dissection plane
(B) Inability to cross the occluded segment
(C) Inability to deliver an angioplasty balloon
(D) Coronary artery perforation

15.6 Which of the following statements regarding coronary perforation in revascularization of CTOs is TRUE?

(A) In-hospital mortality is similar among patients who do and do not experience cardiac tamponade
(B) Cardiac tamponade often develops hours following the interventional procedure
(C) Guidewire perforation most commonly occurs distal to the occluded segment
(D) Absence of angiographic evidence of contrast extravasation excludes the diagnosis of cardiac tamponade

15.7 A 73-year-old Caucasian male is referred to you for percutaneous coronary intervention (PCI) of a chronically occluded right coronary artery (RCA) (Fig. Q15-7A). The procedure is successful (Fig. Q15-7B), and the interventional cardiology fellow asks you which of the following statements regarding collateral flow in CTOs is NOT true?

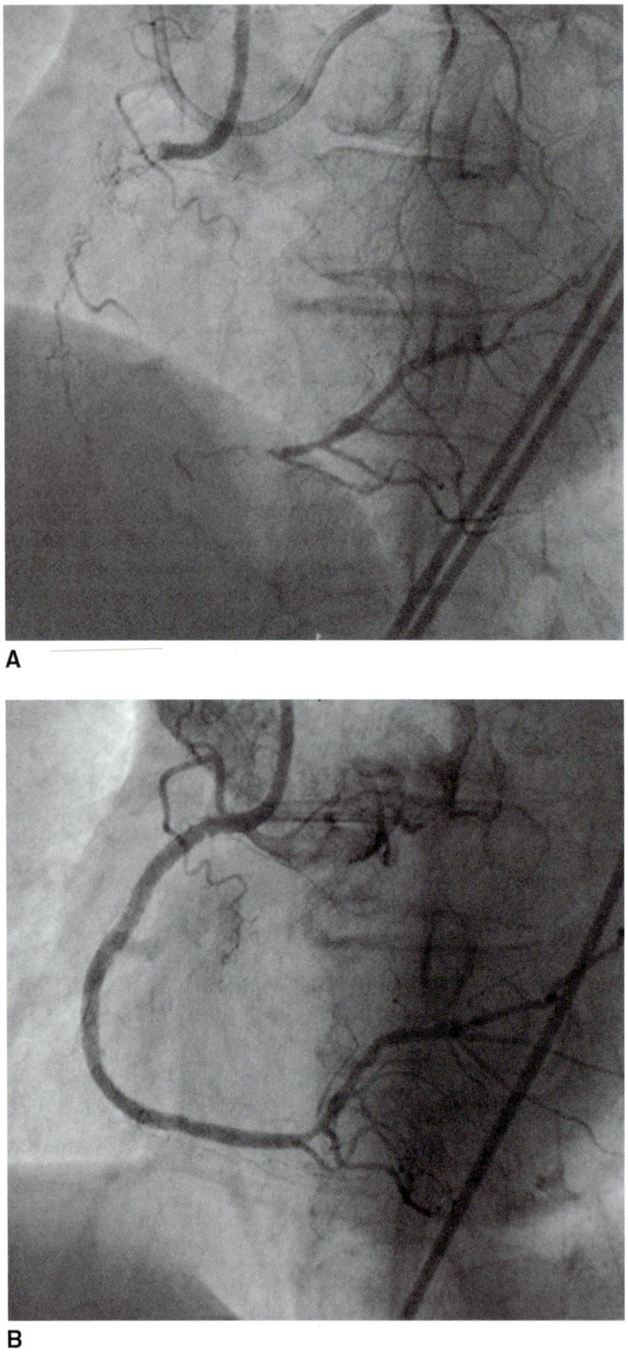

Figure Q15-7 A: Chronic total occlusion of the right coronary artery. B: Right coronary artery following PCI.

(A) Collateral function is worse in patients with impaired regional wall motion
(B) The presence and extent of collateral flow predicts improvement in ventricular function following revascularization
(C) Collateral function regresses after recanalization of CTOs
(D) Growth factor expression is related to collateral function and the duration of occlusion

15.8 Which of the following technologies/strategies has demonstrated significantly higher procedural success over coronary guidewires in a randomized trial?

(A) Excimer laser guidewire
(B) Fibrinolytic infusion
(C) Optical coherence tomography (OCT) guidewire
(D) None of the above

15.9 Advances in coronary guidewires for CTOs include all of the following, EXCEPT:

(A) Tapered tip
(B) Hydrophilic coating
(C) Increased tip stiffness
(D) Absence of coiled tip

15.10 Which characteristic is NOT a predictor of procedural failure in chronic total coronary occlusion revascularization?

(A) Presence of side branch at the site of occlusion
(B) Tapered stump of occlusion
(C) Bridging collaterals
(D) Duration of total occlusion

15.11 Compared with more traditional guidewire techniques, a "hybrid" method that incorporates antegrade, retrograde, and dissection/re-entry methods is associated with which of the following?

(A) Decreasing use of retrograde technique
(B) Increased radiation exposure and contrast utilization
(C) Higher procedural success
(D) All of the above

15.12 CTOs:

(A) Are present in approximately one-half of patients with other severe coronary artery disease
(B) Are identified in approximately one-third of all diagnostic coronary angiograms following abnormal stress testing

(C) Account for <10% of all percutaneous revascularization procedures
(D) All of the above

15.13 Chronic total coronary occlusions are most prevalent in which vessel?

(A) The left anterior descending (LAD) artery
(B) The left circumflex (LCx) artery
(C) The RCA
(D) The left main artery

15.14 The pathophysiology of CTOs includes which of the following?

(A) Adventitial neovascularization
(B) Expression of collagen types I and III
(C) Organized thrombus
(D) All of the above

15.15 Angiographic collateral flow is a predictor of:

(A) Improvement in LV function
(B) Restenosis
(C) Reocclusion
(D) None of the above

15.16 Compared with femoral artery access, CTO guidewire recanalization (technical success) performed with radial artery access is:

(A) Similar between vascular access strategies
(B) Significantly lower than femoral access
(C) Significantly higher than femoral access
(D) Limited to antegrade only techniques

15.17 Which statement best characterizes the histology of chronic total coronary occlusions?

(A) Approximately one-half of CTOs are <99% stenotic despite their angiographic appearance
(B) The severity of lumen stenosis is related to lesion age
(C) Collagen-rich fibrous tissue is most dense in the mid segment of the total occlusion
(D) Inflammation is most prevalent in the adventitia

15.18 In patients with ST-segment elevation myocardial infarction (STEMI) who do not receive reperfusion therapy, a total occlusion is identified in approximately what percent of patients at 1 month?

(A) 10%
(B) 25%
(C) 50%
(D) 75%

15.19 In patients with CTOs who undergo attempted revascularization, which factor is most predictive of increased long-term mortality risk?

(A) Chronic kidney disease (CKD)
(B) Diabetes mellitus
(C) Multivessel coronary disease
(D) Procedural failure

15.20 For treatment of long CTO lesions requiring extensive stenting ("full metal jacket"), predictors of target lesion failure over late follow-up include which of the following:

(A) Number of stents placed
(B) Japan CTO score
(C) Persistent luminal narrowing distal to the stents
(D) A and C

15.21 Among patients presenting with acute STEMI, the presence of a CTO in a noninfarct-related artery (non-IRA) is:

(A) A stronger predictor of 5-year mortality than the presence of multivessel disease (MVD)
(B) Less predictive of 5-year mortality after STEMI than the presence of MVD and diabetes mellitus
(C) Not independently associated with increased 5-year mortality after adjustment for other angiographic and clinical variables
(D) A predictor of late-term (>1 year) mortality, but not at earlier time points

15.22 Among patients with MVD and a CTO, successful CTO PCI ("complete" revascularization) compared to no CTO revascularization is associated with:

(A) Neutral effect on long-term survival but lower incidence of MI at 2 years
(B) Improved 2-year survival in patients with MVD
(C) Worse 2-year survival in patients with MVD
(D) Improved 2-year survival only in patients with CTO involvement of the RCA

15.23 Grade III coronary perforation is:

(A) Most commonly caused by a guidewire
(B) Associated with a high rate of in-hospital adverse cardiovascular events, but not late-term events following hospital discharge
(C) Associated with high in-hospital and late-term adverse cardiovascular events
(D) Most commonly treated with emergency coronary bypass surgery

ANSWERS AND EXPLANATIONS

15.1 Answer A. CTO revascularization with a BMS is associated with considerably higher rates of restenosis and reocclusion compared with stenting of nonocclusive lesions. In the Total Occlusion Study of Canada (TOSCA)-1 (Buller CE, et al. *Circulation* 1999;100(3):236–242), the rates of restenosis and reocclusion at 6-month angiographic follow-up were 55% and 11%, respectively, among patients assigned to treatment with BMS. In the Stenting in Chronic Coronary Occlusion trial (Sirnes PA, et al. *J Am Coll Cardiol* 1996;28(6):1444–1451), the reocclusion rate was 16% in the stent cohort.

15.2 Answer B. Compared with patients with normal or regional impairment of LV function and CTOs, patients with global LV dysfunction derive the greatest relative improvement in the percent ejection fraction (EF) and decrease in wall motion severity index following successful revascularization. In a recent study of patients with angiographic follow-up, baseline LV dysfunction was an independent predictor of improvement in LV function (Werner GS, et al. *Am Heart J* 2005;149(1):129–137). Variables including angiographic collateral flow, duration of occlusion, or history of MI were not predictive of improvement. Recent studies with cardiac magnetic resonance angiography have also identified dysfunctional but viable myocardium as the most significant predictor of improvement in the LVEF and wall motion severity index (Baks T, et al. *J Am Coll Cardiol* 2006;47(4):721–725). Finally, TOSCA examined the influence of successful revascularization on LVEF and regional wall motion (Dzavik V, et al. *Am Heart J* 2001;142(2):301–308). Although an occlusion duration of ≤6 weeks was independently predictive of a significant increase in the percent EF, the greatest improvement was among patients with a baseline EF < 60%.

15.3 Answer C. Several recent studies have examined the safety and efficacy of DES in CTO revascularization. In most instances, nonrandomized observational studies have compared angiographic and clinical outcomes with historical controls of patients with CTOs treated with BMS. A consistent finding among these trials is a significant reduction in angiographic binary restenosis, reocclusion, and the need for repeat target-vessel revascularization (TVR). In the only randomized trial to date comparing sirolimus-eluting stents (SES) and BMS, treatment with SES was associated with an 81% relative reduction in in-stent restenosis at 6-month angiographic follow-up (36% vs. 7%, $p < 0.0001$) (Suttorp MJ, et al. *Circulation* 2006;114(9):921–928). There were no differences in survival between patients treated with BMS or DES.

15.4 Answer B. Several observational studies examining the influence of attempted percutaneous revascularization of CTOs have demonstrated that compared with failed attempts, successful revascularization is associated with improved long-term survival, reduced angina, and improvements in LVEF and regional wall motion (Olivari Z, et al. *J Am Coll Cardiol* 2003;41(10):1672–1678; Suero JA, et al. *J Am Coll Cardiol* 2001;38(2):409–414). Successful total occlusion revascularization is not associated with an increased need for repeat revascularization but instead with a significant improvement in event-free survival from bypass surgery.

15.5 Answer B. The most common mode of failure is inability to successfully pass a guidewire across the occluded segment into the distal true lumen of the vessel. Among 397 patients undergoing attempted total occlusion revascularization (Kinoshita I, et al. *J Am Coll Cardiol* 1995;26(2):409–415), the most common reasons for procedural failure were inability to cross the lesion with a guidewire (63% of cases), long intimal dissection with creation of a false lumen (24%), dye extravasation (11%), failure to cross with a balloon or dilate (2%), and thrombus formation (1.2%).

15.6 Answer B. In a series of patients who developed cardiac tamponade from complications related to PCI, cardiac tamponade was diagnosed on an average of 4.4 hours following completion of the procedure (Fejka M, et al. *Am J Cardiol* 2002;90(11):1183–1186). The occurrence of cardiac tamponade is associated with a high likelihood of in-hospital death and MI. Guidewire perforation typically occurs at the site of the occluded segment; however, perforation may occur in the distal segment of the vessel, underscoring the need to exchange stiff, tapered, or hydrophilic guidewires for soft, less traumatic guidewires after successful crossing. Absence of contrast extravasation does not exclude the possibility of cardiac tamponade. Therefore, if perforation is suspected although not angiographically evident, important measures include serial echocardiography and hemodynamic monitoring.

15.7 Answer B. Recovery of impaired LV function after revascularization of a CTO is not directly related to the extent of collateral function (Werner GS, et al. *Am Heart J* 2005;149(1):129–137). Growth factor expression, in particular, fibroblast growth factor, has been related to both the duration of occlusion and collateral function (Werner GS, et al. *Circulation* 2004;110(14):1940–1945). Collateral function is better in patients with a total coronary occlusion and normal regional wall motion than in patients with impaired regional function (Werner GS, et al. *Circulation* 2001;104:2784–2790). Collateral function also regresses during long-term follow-up after successful recanalization and may not be readily recruitable in the event of acute occlusion (Werner GS, et al. *Circulation* 2003;108(23):2877–2882).

15.8 Answer D. Of the techniques listed, only the laser wire has been compared with conventional coronary guidewires in a randomized trial. In the Total Occlusion Trial with Angioplasty by using a Laser Wire trial (Serruys PW, et al. *Eur Heart J* 2000;21(21):1797–1805), 303 patients with CTOs were randomized to treatment with either the laser wire or conventional wire technique. Successful lesion crossing was achieved in 53% of the laser wire cohort vs. 47% in the conventional wire group ($p = 0.33$).

15.9 Answer D. Guidewires with a tapering tip diameter of 0.009 to 0.011 in. may facilitate wire engagement in microchannels of CTOs. Similarly, guidewires with incremental tip stiffness may penetrate the occluded segment more easily and provide greater shape retention. Hydrophilic wires typically advance with minimal resistance, are easily maneuverable in tortuous vessels, and are therefore used by some operators in CTOs. However, hydrophilic wires must also be used with caution because they are more likely to penetrate beneath the plaque and cause dissection and more frequently select small vessel branches, increasing the likelihood of perforation (Stone GW, et al. *Catheter Cardiovasc Interv* 2005;66(2):217–236).

15.10 Answer B. Compared with a blunted appearance of the occlusion or side branch presence at the site of occlusion, angiographic appearance of a tapered occlusion has been associated with an increased likelihood of procedural success (Noguchi T, et al. *Catheter Cardiovasc Interv* 2000;49(3):258–264; Olivari Z, et al. *J Am Coll Cardiol* 2003;41(10):1672–1678; Stone GW, et al. *Catheter Cardiovasc Interv* 2005;66(2):217–236; Tan KH, et al. *Br Heart J* 1993;70(2):126–131). Increasing duration of the occlusion and the presence of bridging collaterals are also associated with increased procedural failure.

15.11 Answer C. The hybrid algorithm employs guidewire antegrade, retrograde, and dissection/re-entry techniques based on the assessment of four variables: lesion length, proximal CTO cap ambiguity, suitability of the distal vessel for re-entry, and presence/absence of collaterals for retrograde crossing (King SB III. *J Am Coll Cardiol Interv* 2012;5(4):367–379). Compared with traditional guidewire techniques, the hybrid approach has been associated with decreased contrast and radiation use, increased application of retrograde methods, and higher procedural success (Michael TT, et al. *Catheter Cardiovasc Interv* 2015;85(3): 393–399; Michael TT, et al. *Am J Cardiol* 2013; 112(4):488–492).

15.12 Answer D. Overall, a CTO is identified in approximately one-third of all diagnostic coronary angiograms, yet attempted percutaneous revascularization of a total occlusion accounts for <10% of all PCIs (Kahn JK. *Am Heart J* 1993;126 (3 Pt 1):561–564; Srinivas VS, et al. *Circulation* 2002;106(13):1627–1633). However, in a summary of 8,004 patients presenting for diagnostic cardiac catheterization over a 10-year period, a CTO was identified in 52% of patients with significant disease (≥70% stenosis) in another major epicardial vessel (Christofferson RD, et al. *Am J Cardiol* 2005;95(9):1088–1091).

15.13 Answer C. According to the National Heart, Lung, and Blood Dynamic Registry (Srinivas VS, et al. *Circulation* 2002;106(13):1627–1633), CTOs are most prevalent in the RCA and least common in the LCx artery. The frequency of total occlusions also increases with advancing age. Total occlusion of the RCA was identified in 18.2%, 21.3%, and 22.8% of patients <65 years, 65 to 79 years, and ≥80 years of age, respectively (Cohen HA, et al. *Am Heart J* 2003;146(3):513–519).

15.14 Answer D. CTOs most commonly develop from thrombotic occlusion followed by thrombus organization and collagen deposition (in particular, types I and III) (Katsuragawa M, et al. *J Am Coll Cardiol* 1993;21(3):604–611). Neovascularization is also prominent and begins within the adventitia. As total occlusions age, angiogenesis becomes more extensive, and the number and size of capillaries in the intima and adventitia become similar.

15.15 Answer D. The presence and extent of angiographic collateral flow have been associated with the presence of viable and functional myocardium, but it does not predict the improvement in regional wall motion, the occurrence of restenosis, or reocclusion following successful revascularization (Werner GS, et al. *Am Heart J* 2005;149(1):129–137).

15.16 Answer A. Radial artery access (including bilateral radial artery approaches) for CTO PCI permits both antegrade and retrograde strategies and overall has been associated with similar technical success compared with femoral access methods (Rinfret S, et al. *Catheter Cardiovasc Interv* 2011;78(3):366–374; Alaswad K, et al. *Catheter Cardiovasc Interv* 2015;85(7):1123–1129; Tanaka Y, et al. *J Am Coll Cardiol Interv* 2017;10(3):235–243). However, in selected, more complex cases, radial approaches may have a higher failure rate; in one recent study, catheter size <7 Fr, calcification, and lesions longer than 20 mm predicted higher transradial CTO PCI failure.

15.17 Answer A. By histology, approximately one-half of CTOs are <99% stenotic despite the angiographic appearance of thrombolysis in MI-0 flow. Inflammation is most prevalent in the intima of CTOs, regardless of the lesion age (Katsuragawa M, et al. *J Am Coll Cardiol* 1993;21(3):604–611). No relationship exists between the severity of stenosis and either plaque composition or lesion age. The concentration of collagen-rich fibrous tissue is particularly dense at the proximal and distal ends of the lesion with a mid segment characterized by soft lipid core and organized thrombus.

15.18 Answer C. In patients with STEMI not treated with reperfusion therapy, an occluded infarct-related artery has been identified in 87% of patients within 4 hours, 65% within 12 to 24 hours, 53% at 15 days, and 45% at 1 month (Bertrand ME, et al. *Am Heart J* 1979;97(1):61–69; Betriu A, et al. *Circulation* 1982;65(6):1099–1105; DeWood MA, et al. *N Engl J Med* 1980;303(16):897–902).

15.19 Answer D. Several observational studies have demonstrated increased long-term mortality among patients with failed attempts at total occlusion revascularization compared with successful revascularization (Hoye A, et al. *Eur Heart J* 2005;26(24):2630–2636; Olivari Z, et al. *J Am Coll Cardiol* 2003;41(10):1672–1678; Suero JA, et al. *J Am Coll Cardiol* 2001;38(2):409–414). In a multivariable model in 1,118 patients with CTOs in the British Columbia Cardiac Registry, only the factors of end-stage renal disease and LV dysfunction were more predictive of late mortality than procedural failure. Table A15-19 shows consistently higher mortality among patients undergoing failed vs. successful percutaneous revascularization of CTOs.

Table A15-19

Trial	Success (N)	Failure (N)	Follow-Up Duration (years)	Mortality (%)		
				Success	Failure	*p* Value
British Columbia Cardiac Registry[a]	1,118	340	6	10.0	19.0	<0.001
Suero et al.[b]	1,491	514	10	26.0	35.0	0.001
TOAST-GISE[c]	286	83	1	1.1	3.6	0.13
Aziz et al.[d]	377	166	2.4	2.5	7.3	0.049
Hoye et al.[e]	568	306	5	6.5	12.0	0.02

[a]*Am Heart J* 1979;97:61–69.
[b]*Circulation* 1982;65:1099–1105.
[c]*Circulation* 1999;100:236–242.
[d]*Am J Cardiol* 2005;95:1088–1091.
[e]*Am Heart J* 2003;146:513–519.

15.20 Answer D. In a recent survey of 406 patients undergoing CTO revascularization with extensive stenting (mean stent length 76.8 ± 14.6 mm), target lesion failure over a median follow-up period of 5.1 years was 16.0% (Lee PH, et al. *JACC Cardiovasc Interv* 2017;10(14):1405–1412). Repeat TLR was favorably low (8.6%) despite lesion complexity. In multivariable analysis, both number of stents implanted and persistent luminal narrowing were identified as predictors of target lesion failure. Whether persistent luminal narrowing reflects negative vessel remodeling or instead extensive distal vessel atherosclerotic disease is uncertain.

15.21 Answer A. The presence of a CTO in a non-IRA is a strong and independent predictor of 5-year mortality. Particularly in the high-risk subgroup of STEMI patients with diabetes mellitus, MVD has prognostic significance only if a concomitant CTO is present (Claessen BE, et al. *Heart* 2010;96(24):1968–1972). During the first 30 days following STEMI, the presence of a CTO (hazard ratio [HR] 3.6; 95% confidence interval [CI] 2.6 to 4.7) was the strongest predictor of mortality only after the presence of cardiogenic shock (HR 7.4; 95% CI 5.8 to 9.6) (Claessen BE, et al. *JACC Cardiovasc Interv* 2009;2(11):1128–1134).

15.22 Answer B. In a retrospective analysis of 486 patients with MVD, Valenti et al. reported a survival advantage for patients undergoing "complete" revascularization that involved successful treatment of the CTO (Valenti R, et al. *Eur Heart J* 2008;29(19):1336–1342). In an analysis of 2,608 patients undergoing attempted CTO revascularization, Safley and colleagues reported that successful CTO recanalization of the LAD artery—but not the LCx or RCA—was associated with improved survival (Safley DM, et al. *JACC Cardiovasc Interv* 2008;1(3):295–302).

15.23 Answer C. Among 24,465 patients undergoing PCI, Al-Lamee et al. described outcomes among 56 patients who had grade III coronary perforation (Al-Lamme R, et al. *JACC Cardiovasc Interv* 2011;4(1):87–95). The device causing perforation was the intracoronary balloon in 50% of the cases, the intracoronary guidewire in 17.9% of the cases, rotablation in 3.6% of the cases, and directional atherectomy in 3.6%. Following perforation, immediate treatment and success rates, respectively, were prolonged balloon inflation 58.9% and 54.5%; covered stent implantation 46.4% and 84.6%; coronary artery bypass graft surgery and surgical repair 16.0% and 44.4%; and coil embolization 1.8% and 100%. In-hospital mortality was 14.8%. The combined procedural and in-hospital MI rate was 42.9%, and the MACE rate was 55.4%. At late-term clinical follow-up (median: 38.1 months), 4.3% of patients experienced MI, 4.3% required coronary bypass surgery, and 15.2% died. The TLR rate was 13%, TVR in 19.6%, and MACE in 41.3%.

16 Ostial and Bifurcation Lesions

Antonio Colombo and Azeem Latib

QUESTIONS

16.1 The operator performing percutaneous coronary intervention (PCI) on this right coronary artery (RCA) (Fig. Q16-1) utilized a 6-Fr Judkins right guiding catheter with side holes. Which of the following would be very suggestive of an aorto-ostial lesion?

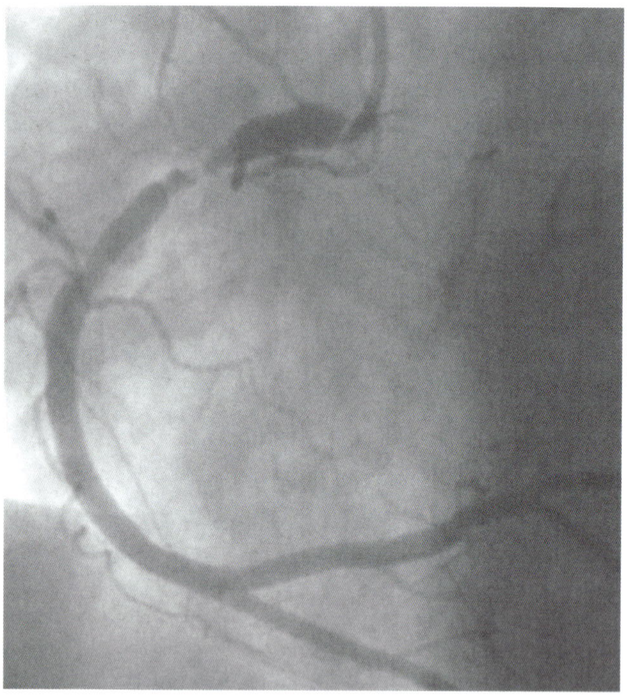

Figure Q16-1

(A) Pressure damping
(B) Absence of backflush of dye into the aorta
(C) Fractional flow reserve (FFR) measurement after intracoronary adenosine
(D) Angiographically visible stenosis

16.2 When performing ostial left main stenting, which of the following are associated with deformation of the stent?

(A) Advancing the guide catheter when one of the guidewires is jailed
(B) Pulling out a jailed guidewire
(C) Pulling back a partially deflated balloon
(D) All of the above

16.3 Among the devices listed, which one has been proposed as the most suitable device to treat calcified non–aorto-ostial lesions?

(A) Cutting balloon
(B) Excimer laser
(C) Rotational atherectomy
(D) Compliant balloon

16.4 A 57-year-old man presenting with chest pain, elevated troponin, and inferior T-wave inversion on electrocardiogram (ECG) underwent coronary angiography. The left coronary artery (LCA) was without significant stenosis, and the RCA is shown in Figure Q16-4. The main difference between stent treatment of this aorto-ostial lesion and a non–aorto-ostial stenosis is:

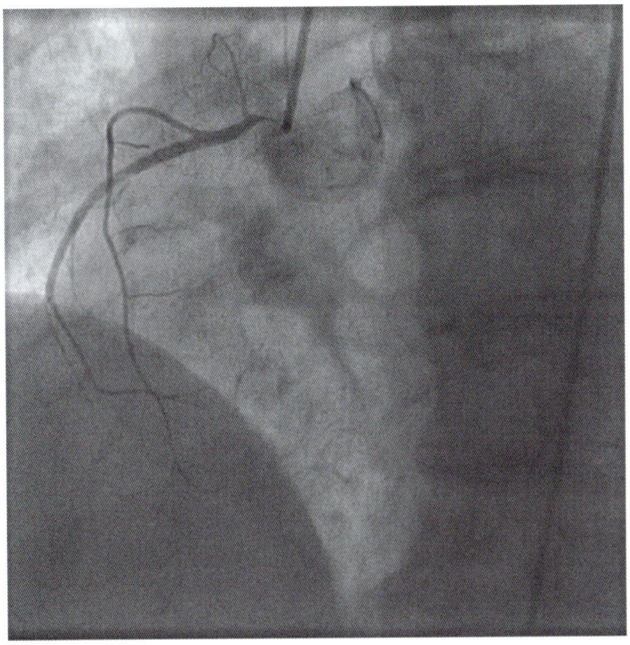

Figure Q16-4 (Courtesy of Andrew MacIsaac.)

(A) There is no specific difference
(B) When treating a lesion at the aorto-ostial location, the stent should protrude a few millimeters into the aorta
(C) The need to have the stent protrude proximally a few millimeters applies also to non-aorto-ostial lesions
(D) Non-aorto-ostial lesions should be treated routinely with a cutting balloon

16.5 The lesion in the above question was treated with an implantation of a 3.0- × 12-mm drug-eluting stent (DES) inflated to 14 atmospheres (atm), utilizing an Amplatz left 1 guide catheter. Which of the following is the best description for the angiographic and intravascular ultrasound (IVUS) result at the ostium shown in Figure Q16-5?

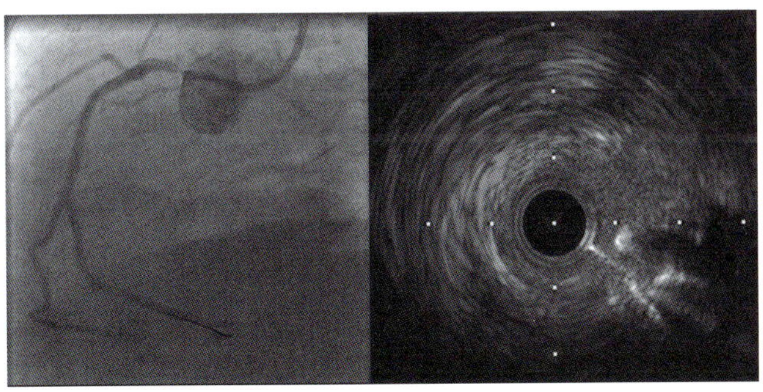

Figure Q16-5 (Courtesy of Andrew MacIsaac.)

(A) The stent is underexpanded at the ostium
(B) Satisfactory stent deployment
(C) Stent strut malapposition
(D) Another stent is required

16.6 The ______________ classification of bifurcation lesions is shown in Figure Q16-6:

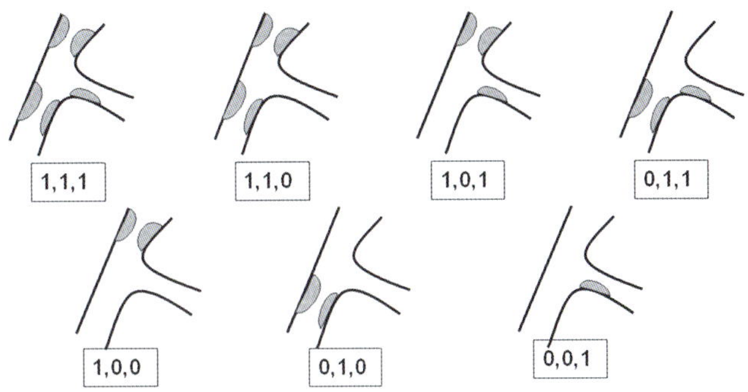

Figure Q16-6

(A) Lefevre
(B) Medina
(C) Duke
(D) Sanborn

16.7 A 68-year-old patient with new-onset chest pain during moderate effort undergoes stress echocardiography that demonstrates inducible ischemia of the anterior wall. Coronary angiography demonstrates the following bifurcation lesion (Fig. Q16-7). Based on the Nordic Bifurcation Study, which of the following would be TRUE about the interventional strategy in this patient?

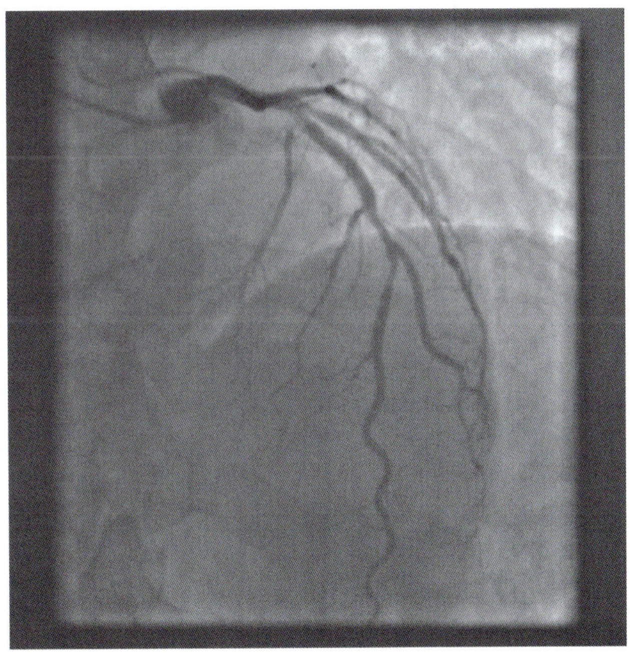

Figure Q16-7

(A) Stenting both branches of the bifurcation is associated with reduced target lesion revascularization (TLR) rates during follow-up
(B) A provisional side-branch stenting approach is associated with lower side-branch restenosis at angiographic follow-up
(C) Elective stenting of both branches of the bifurcation is associated with higher rates of stent thrombosis
(D) A provisional side-branch approach is associated with lower contrast volumes and fluoroscopy time but similar event rates at follow-up, as compared to an elective two-stent approach

16.8 The bifurcation in the previous question was treated with a provisional approach, and the main branch was stented with a 3.0- × 24-mm zotarolimus-eluting stent (ZES). Coronary angiography reveals a residual stenosis at the side-branch ostium (Fig. Q16-8). The operator decided to perform fractional flow reserve (FFR) to evaluate this stenosis. Which of the following statements is TRUE about the measurement of FFR on side branches with >50% angiographic residual narrowing after stent implantation on the main branch?

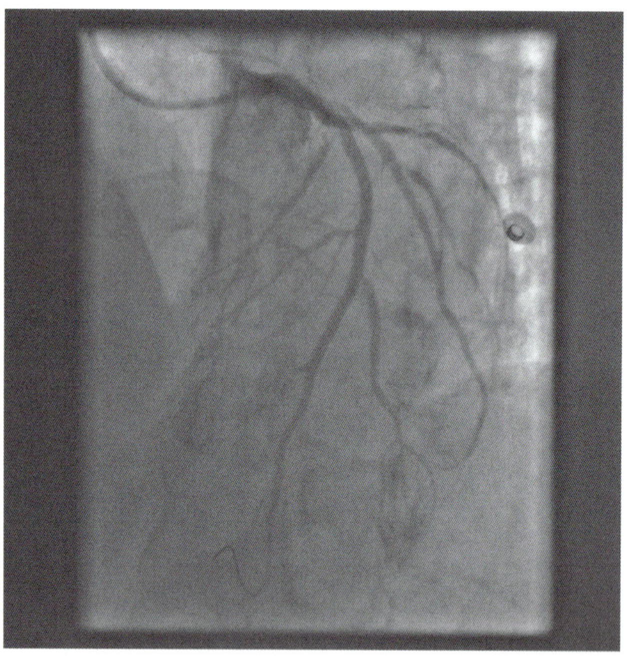

Figure Q16-8

(A) All the lesions have a reduced value of FFR (<0.75), indicating the functional significance of the narrowing in all cases
(B) Angiographic evaluation is sufficient and the residual stenosis in the side branch should be treated further
(C) Most lesions have normal values of FFR (>0.75), indicating the absence of functional significance of the narrowing in the majority of cases
(D) The measurement of FFR in this setting should be avoided due to the high rate of complications when recrossing through stent struts with the pressure guidewire

16.9 FFR evaluation of the jailed side branch in the previous question after adenosine-induced maximal hyperemia is shown (Fig. Q16-9). Based on this finding, what would be the most appropriate strategy for the side branch?

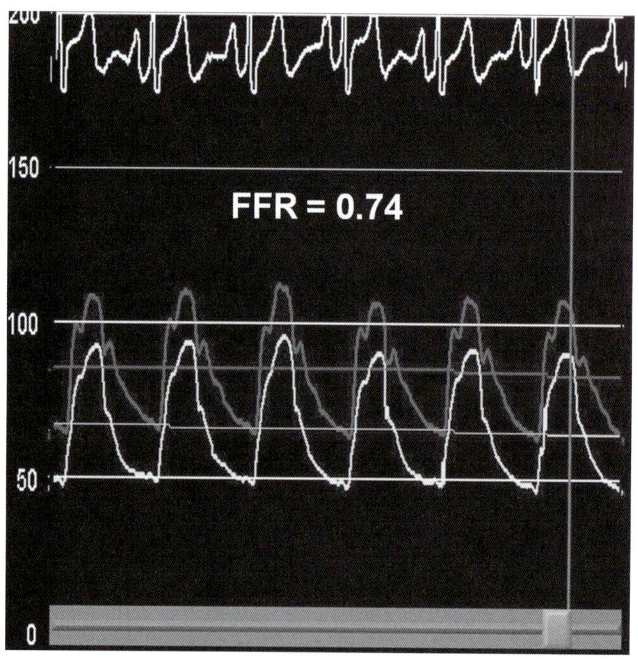

Figure Q16-9

(A) Stent implantation
(B) Kissing balloon inflation
(C) Medical therapy
(D) None of the above

16.10 A 60-year-old man with hypertension and dyslipidemia undergoes coronary angiography for effort-induced angina and a positive exercise stress test. On angiography, the RCA shows no significant stenosis, and the LCA is shown (Fig. Q16-10). Based on the findings of the CACTUS study, which of the following is CORRECT about the percutaneous strategy in this patient?

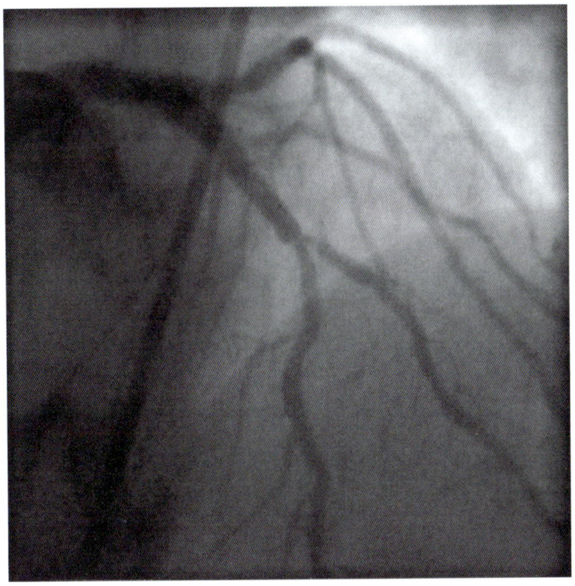

Figure Q16-10

(A) Provisional side-branch stenting is associated with a lower rate of myocardial infarction (MI) and death during follow-up
(B) Additional stenting on the side branch in the provisional group occurred in 50% of lesions
(C) Final kissing inflation was performed in less than half of bifurcations treated in this study
(D) Implantation of two stents in this bifurcation was not associated with a higher incidence of adverse events at 6 months

16.11 When performing the crush technique with everolimus-eluting stents (EES), which of these is important?

(A) It can only be performed with an 8-Fr guide catheter
(B) Perform two-step final kissing balloon inflation
(C) Restenosis and thrombosis rates are influenced by the performance of final kissing balloon inflation
(D) The most frequent site for restenosis is the body of the side branch

16.12 In regard to the crush technique, which of the following statements is FALSE?

(A) In the Nordic Bifurcation Study, the crush technique was associated with similar rates of death, MI, or revascularization as compared to the culotte technique
(B) The crush technique should be avoided in bifurcations with an angle >50 degrees
(C) In the DKCRUSH-II study, the double kissing crush technique was associated with lower rates of restenosis and TLR as compared to the provisional technique
(D) The double kissing crush technique requires at least a 7-Fr guide and has no advantage over the standard step crush technique

16.13 A 55-year-old man with a long-standing smoking history presenting with angina at rest but normal troponin undergoes coronary angiography. For the lesion shown (Fig. Q16-13), which is the best treatment strategy?

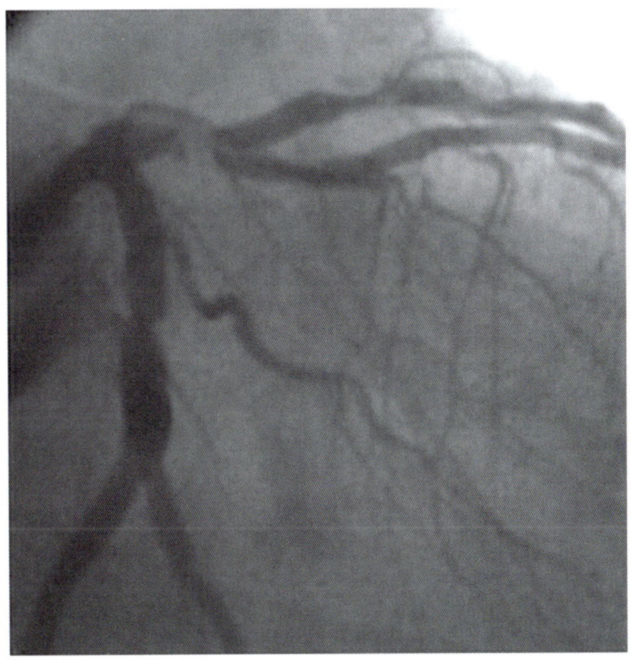

Figure Q16-13

(A) Culotte stenting
(B) Crush stenting
(C) Provisional side-branch stenting
(D) Any of the above

16.14 Which of the following is TRUE about Culotte stenting?

(A) It does not provide complete coverage of the carina and side-branch ostium
(B) In the Nordic Stent Technique Study, culotte stenting was associated with lower in-stent restenosis rates as compared to crush stenting
(C) Culotte stenting is associated with lower major adverse cardiac event (MACE) rates as compared to crush stenting
(D) It can be performed in all types of bifurcation anatomy

16.15 A 55-year-old man undergoes coronary angiography and PCI via the right radial artery using a 6-Fr guide catheter that demonstrates the following Medina 1,1,1 bifurcation lesion with marked angulation of the side branch (Fig. Q16-15). A floppy workhorse guidewire is placed in the main branch, and after great difficulty, the side branch was eventually wired. What would your bifurcation strategy be for this lesion?

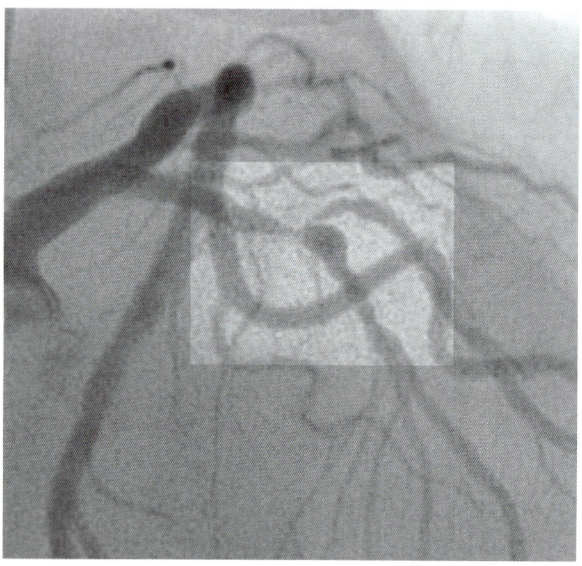

Figure Q16-15

(A) Provisional stenting
(B) V-stenting
(C) Culotte stenting
(D) Classical crush stenting

16.16 The angiographic images show preintervention and postintervention images of a Medina 1,1,0 bifurcation treated with DES implantation on the main branch (Fig. Q16-16). What would your approach be toward the side branch?

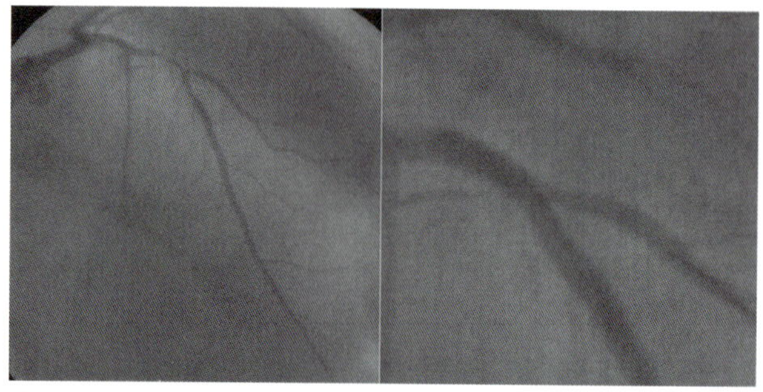

Figure Q16-16

(A) No further treatment of the side branch
(B) Routine final kissing inflation
(C) Side-branch–only dilatation
(D) Elective double stent implantation

16.17 A 65-year-old man presents with exertional angina and anteroapical ischemia on stress echocardiography. Coronary angiography demonstrates a critical stenosis of the mid–left anterior descending (LAD) artery involving the bifurcation with a large second diagonal (Fig. Q16-17). What would your interventional approach be to this lesion?

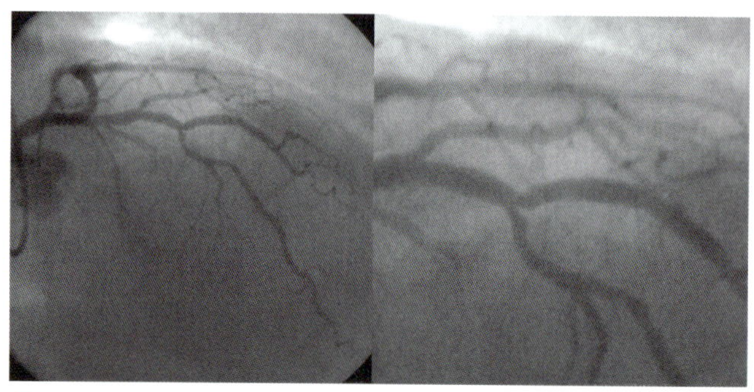

Figure Q16-17

(A) Elective double stenting of the LAD diagonal bifurcation
(B) Placing a guidewire only in the LAD, followed by stenting across the ostium of the diagonal
(C) Wire both branches, followed by stenting of the LAD across the bifurcation
(D) Placing a guidewire only in the LAD, followed by stenting of the LAD distal to the ostium of the diagonal

16.18 A 60-year-old man with a critical stenosis of the LAD-diagonal bifurcation undergoes treatment of the bifurcation with the provisional technique. After stent implantation on the LAD, he develops chest pain with ST elevation in leads I and AVL. Angiography demonstrates a subtotal occlusion of the diagonal branch (Fig. Q16-18A) and the

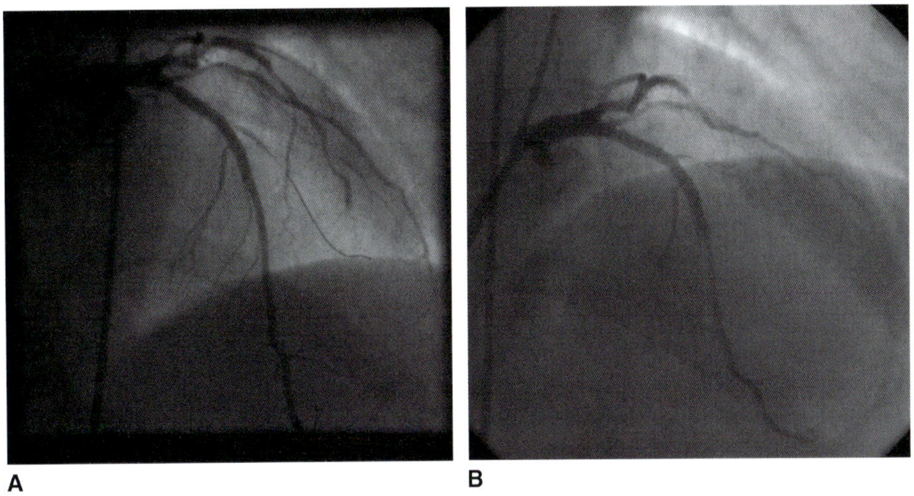

Figure Q16-18 (Courtesy of Antonio Colombo and Azeem Latib.)

operator attempts to recover the side branch with a Pilot 50 wire. The patient develops hypotension and repeat coronary angiography (Fig. Q16-18B) demonstrates:

(A) Complete occlusion of the side branch
(B) Acute stent thrombosis of the LAD
(C) Distal perforation of the diagonal branch
(D) Catheter dissection of the left main

16.19 When performing an optimal provisional technique on the bifurcation in Figure Q16-19, which of the following considerations are important?

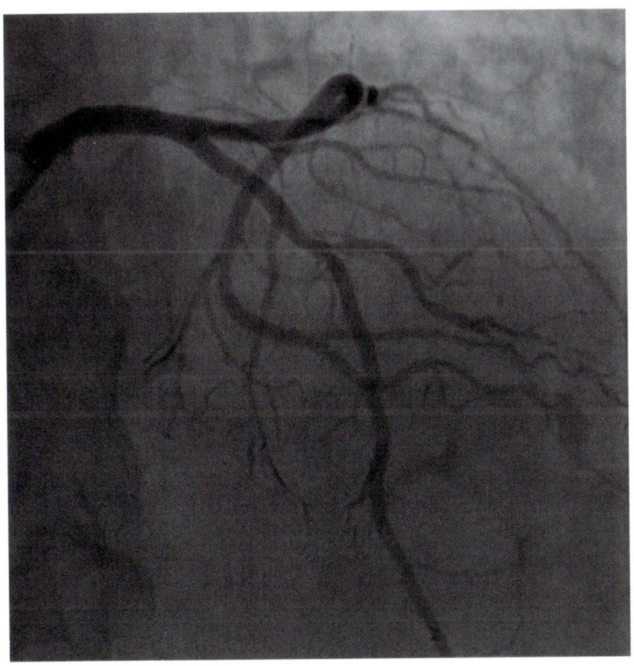

Figure Q16-19

(A) The stent size should be based on the diameter of the distal main branch
(B) The proximal optimization technique should be used to correct stent underexpansion in the proximal main branch
(C) The approximate diameter of the proximal main branch is equal to two-thirds of the sum of the diameters of the side branch and distal main branch
(D) All of the above

16.20 Figure Q16-20 (Koo BK, et al. *Circ Cardiovasc Interv* 2010;3(2):113–119) demonstrates an angiogram (left), a cross-sectional IVUS image at the level of the carina (middle), and a longitudinal IVUS image (right) before (upper panels) and after (lower panels) main-branch stent implantation. What is the explanation for the angiographic and IVUS findings of aggravation of the side-branch ostial stenosis after main-branch stent implantation?

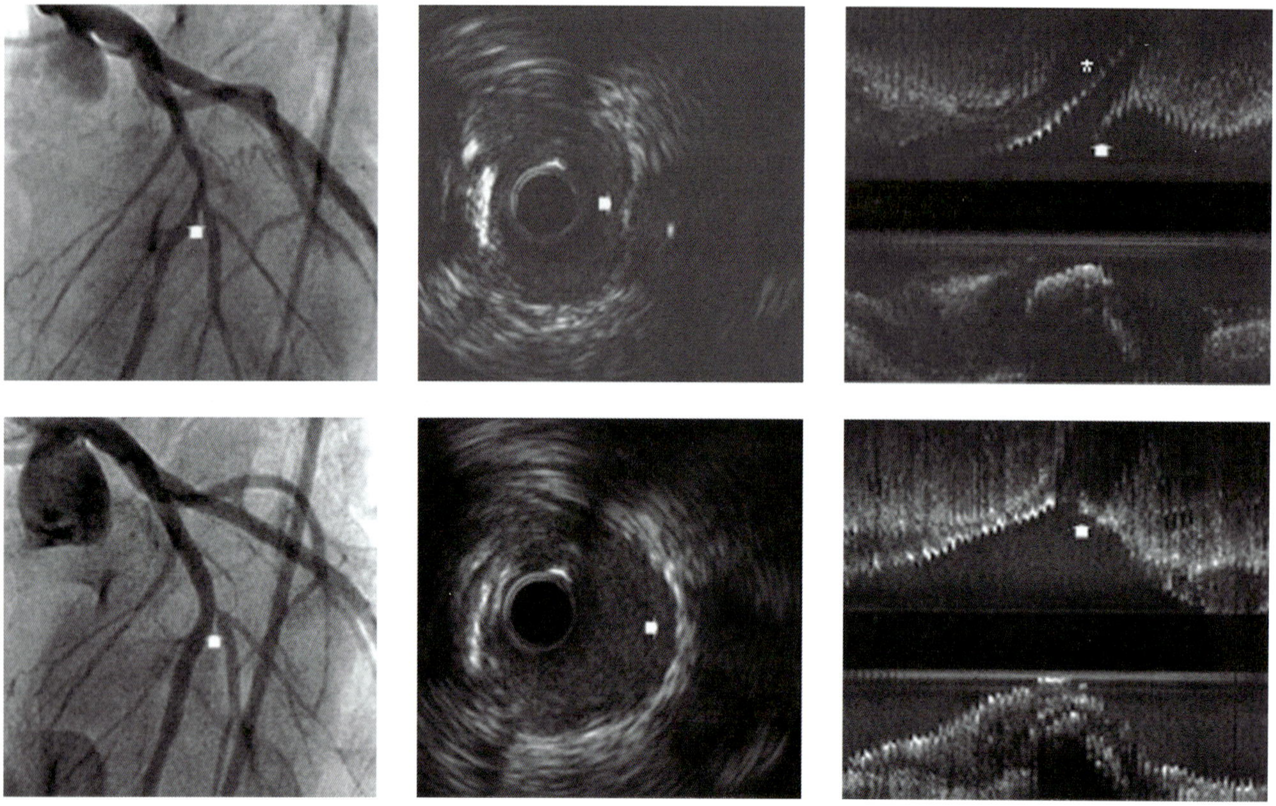

Figure Q16-20 (Courtesy of Bon-Kwon Koo.)

(A) Plaque shift
(B) Thrombus
(C) Dissection
(D) Carina shift

16.21 In regard to the proximal optimization technique (POT), which of the following statements is FALSE?

(A) The POT technique should be routinely performed when performing the provisional technique to restore the geometry of the bifurcation and correct proximal MB underexpansion
(B) The POT technique has been shown to reduce restenosis and TLR
(C) The POT technique facilitates wire recrossing and balloon crossing into the side branch
(D) The balloon used for the POT should not cover the ostium of the side branch

16.22 Figure Q16-22A demonstrates a LAD diagonal bifurcation treated with the provisional approach of main-branch DES implantation followed by kissing balloon inflation. Figure Q16-22B shows the angiographic result after kissing inflation, which resulted in a dissection of the diagonal ostium. In regard to the approach to crossover to stenting the diagonal branch after a provisional approach, which of the following is CORRECT?

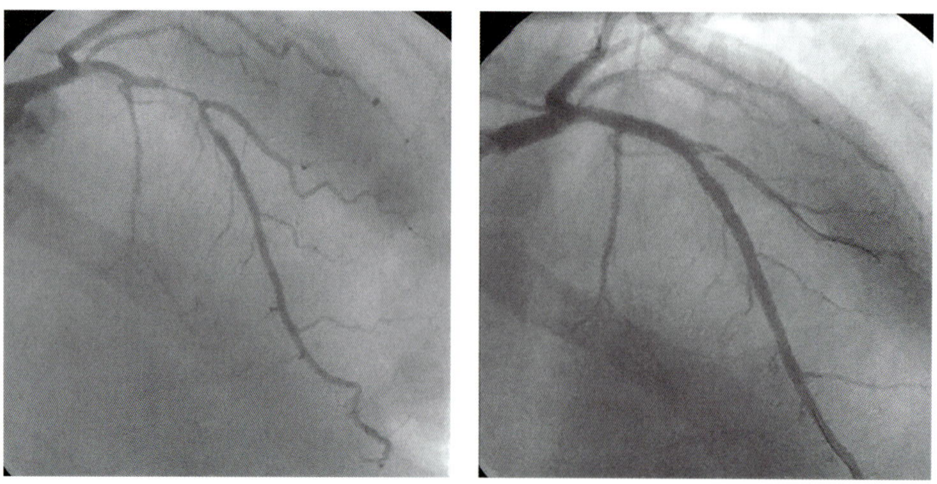

A B

Figure Q16-22 (Courtesy of Antonio Colombo and Azeem Latib.)

(A) The technique chosen is based only on the operator's preference and is not influenced by the bifurcation anatomy or angle
(B) The reverse crush technique is the simplest to perform because it guarantees complete coverage of the ostium
(C) The T-stenting And small Protrusion (TAP) technique is the easiest to perform as it does not require wire recrossing of stent struts
(D) Final kissing inflation is not mandatory after implanting the side-branch stent as it was already performed after the provisional approach

16.23 The TAP technique (Fig. Q16-23) is a useful technique for stenting the side branch after main-branch stenting. Which of the following statements regarding the TAP is FALSE?

(A) When TAP is performed on bifurcations with a shallow angle ≤30 degrees, significant protrusion of the stent into the main branch may occur to ensure ostial side-branch coverage
(B) Final kissing inflation is mandatory to remodel the main branch correcting protrusion of the side-branch struts into the main branch
(C) In the Bifurcations Bad Krozingen (BBK) II randomized bifurcation trial, TAP stenting was associated with a higher incidence of angiographic restenosis compared to culotte stenting
(D) When performing kissing inflation after stent implantation, the side-branch balloon should always be deflated first

16.24 If stent implantation is considered a clinically appropriate procedure in a patient with a lesion involving an unprotected left main coronary artery (Fig. Q16-24), the best approach is:

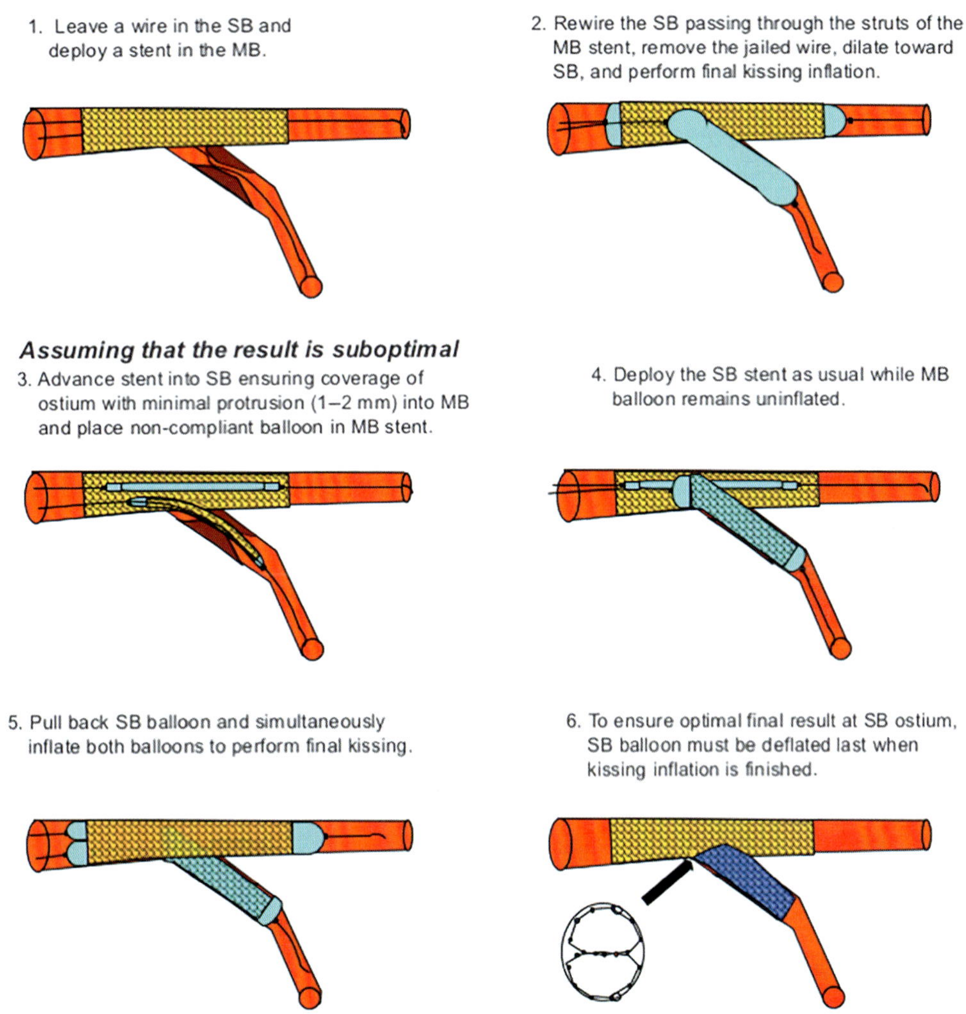

Figure Q16-23 (Courtesy of Antonio Colombo and Azeem Latib.)

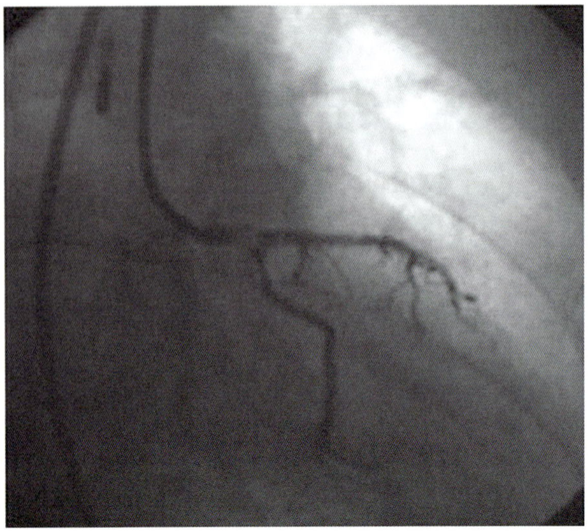

Figure Q16-24

(A) Perform directional atherectomy and then implant two bare-metal stents (BMS)
(B) Implant a DES toward the LAD artery leaving implantation of a second stent toward the circumflex as a possible option
(C) Proceed with implantation of two BMS, one in the LAD artery and the other in the circumflex
(D) Perform balloon angioplasty only in this lesion given its unique complexity

16.25 A 72-year-old man with a history of previous coronary artery bypass graft (CABG) and occluded bypass grafts (two vein grafts and a left internal mammary artery) presented with an acute coronary syndrome (ACS). Baseline coronary angiography (Fig. Q16-25A) demonstrated a severe stenosis in the distal left main coronary artery (LMCA) bifurcation involving both the LAD and the left circumflex (LCx), a subtotally occluded and diffusely diseased LAD, and severe stenosis of the first diagonal branch (D1). An intra-aortic balloon pump (IABP) was electively inserted and the patient underwent PCI with a paclitaxel-eluting stent (PES) implantation on the mid-LAD and first diagonal and crush stenting of the LMCA bifurcation with two 3.5- × 32-mm stents. Two-step kissing inflation was performed with two 3.5- × 15-mm noncompliant balloons. The angiographic and IVUS images (Fig. Q16-25B) taken after final kissing inflation demonstrate:

(A) Dissection
(B) Thrombus
(C) Stent underexpansion
(D) Stent malapposition
(E) Good final result

16.26 What is the role of IVUS-guided DES implantation in coronary bifurcation lesion treatment?

(A) IVUS-guided PCI has no role in bifurcation PCI
(B) IVUS-guided PCI is associated with higher periprocedural complication rates
(C) IVUS-guided PCI has been shown to reduce revascularization rates and stent thrombosis after DES in randomized trials
(D) IVUS-guided PCI may improve long-term outcomes in coronary bifurcations, especially if involving the LMCA

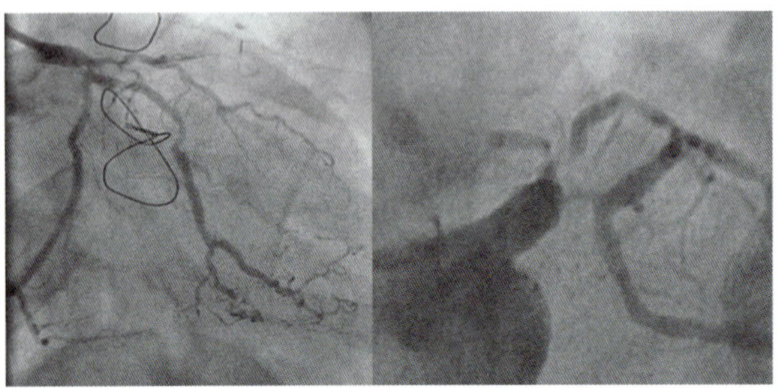

A

Figure Q16-25

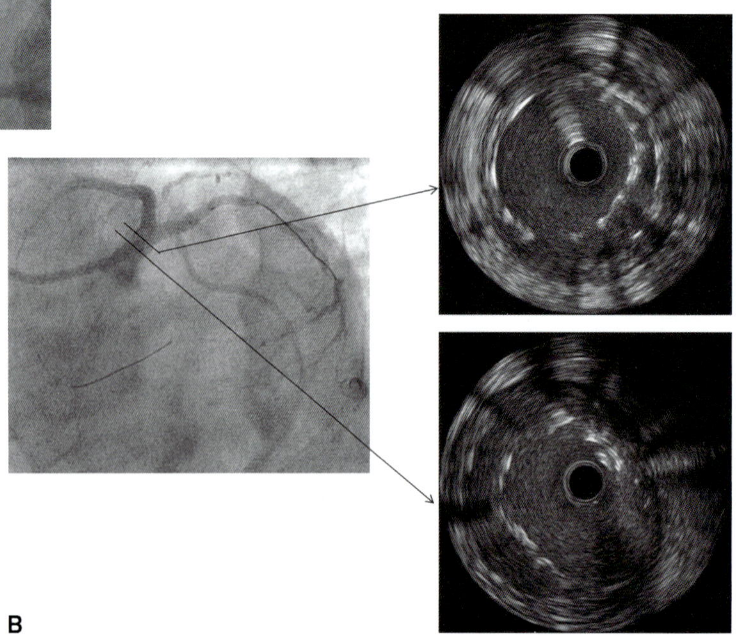

B

ANSWERS AND EXPLANATIONS

16.1 Answer B. On the baseline image, there is clearly a proximal lesion, but the ostial lesion is not clearly evident. However, the absence of a good backflush into the aorta during contrast injection is suggestive of an ostial lesion. Pressure damping is also valuable but may be misleading when utilizing a guiding catheter with side holes. The presence of a pressure gradient after adenosine may be useful but is difficult to interpret in the presence of the proximal lesion and when utilizing a guiding catheter with side holes. Figure A16-1 shows the final angiogram after implantation of a 4- × 24-mm DES to treat the ostial and proximal lesion. The presence of backflow at the final angiogram is an important sign supporting a good final result and satisfactory treatment of the aorto-ostial lesion.

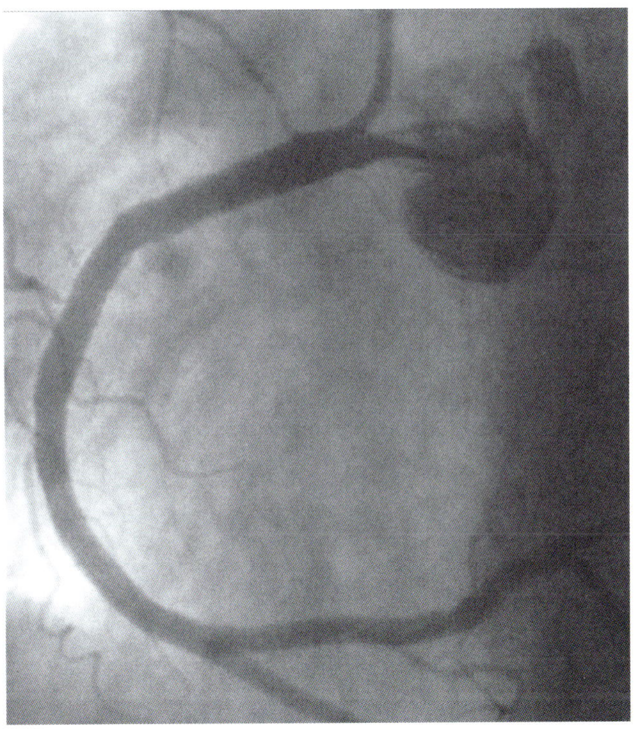

Figure A16-1

16.2 Answer D. If not properly performed, aorto-ostial stenting can result in significant complications, including stent deformation, accidental crushing of the stent when recrossing a left main bifurcation stent into a branch, missing the ostium, and retrograde dissection of the left main that involves the aorta. Second- and third-generation DES have provided improved acute and long-term results, but the thinner struts of these stents have made them more prone to stent deformation. When performing ostial left main stenting, the operator needs to be careful with guide manipulation and be aware that the following maneuvers can result in stent deformation: (1) advancing the guide catheter after stent implantation with one of the guidewires jailed, as this will bias the guide away from the center of the stent, (2) pulling out jailed guidewires or partially deflated balloons, and (3) advancing the guide catheter without fully expanding the stent by postdilating the proximal part with a larger noncompliant balloon.

16.3 Answer C. The cutting balloon as a stand-alone device is very unlikely to cross the lesion. A number of single-center studies (Colombo A, et al. *J Invasive Cardiol* 1999;11(4):231–232; Kurbaan AS, et al. *Heart* 1997;77(4):350–352; Muramatsu T, et al. *J Invasive Cardiol* 1999;11(4):201–206) have reported the feasible combination of stenting when preceded by cutting balloon dilatation. In bifurcation lesions, in which there is a large fibrotic plaque at the ostium of the side branch, use of the cutting balloon as a predilatation strategy before stenting does seem reasonable. The Restenosis reduction by Cutting balloon Evaluation (REDUCE) III trial evaluated the role of cutting balloon predilatation before stenting vs. standard balloon predilatation in a variety of lesions. This trial reported a lower restenosis rate when lesions were predilated with the cutting balloon. The excimer laser is not effective in severely calcified lesions. Even if more specifically applied for calcific lesions, rotational atherectomy (rotablator) is the most appropriate answer.

16.4 Answer B. Aorto-ostial lesions are more frequently difficult to dilate and are more prone to recoil than non–aorto-ostial lesions. This is due to more fibrous and elastic tissue in the aortic wall than within the coronary arteries. High-speed rotational atherectomy and cutting balloons have been advocated for difficult to dilate ostial lesions, especially when they are calcified. Precise stent placement is critical to ensure satisfactory procedural outcomes. Determining the exact location of the vessel ostium can prove difficult, especially after predilatation of the lesion. Appropriate guide catheter positioning is critical. Deep engagement of the vessel ostium may lead to distal stent deployment, that is, geographical miss. Alternatively, disengaging the guide catheter from the vessel ostium can result in poor vessel opacification, poor guide catheter support, and geographic miss. The most appropriate way to treat lesions located at the aorto-ostial location is to place a stent, which will slightly protrude into the aorta. This approach will guarantee adequate coverage of the ostium. Protrusion of more than a few millimeters increases the risk of stent embolization as well difficulty in reengaging the vessel ostium for future angiography. Geographic miss of the ostium may predispose to stent recoil and restenosis.

16.5 Answer D. The angiogram demonstrates a hazy appearance of the right coronary ostium post-stent deployment. The IVUS demonstrates that there are no stent struts at the vessel ostium that has significant concentric plaque, thus confirming geographic miss of the ostial lesion. Another stent is required to cover the aorto-ostial lesion and protrude a few millimeters into the aorta. In this case, the position of the ostium was clarified by the IVUS, ensuring that the second stent was accurately positioned. Figure A16-5 demonstrates the final angiographic result and IVUS, confirming that stent struts are protruding into the aorta.

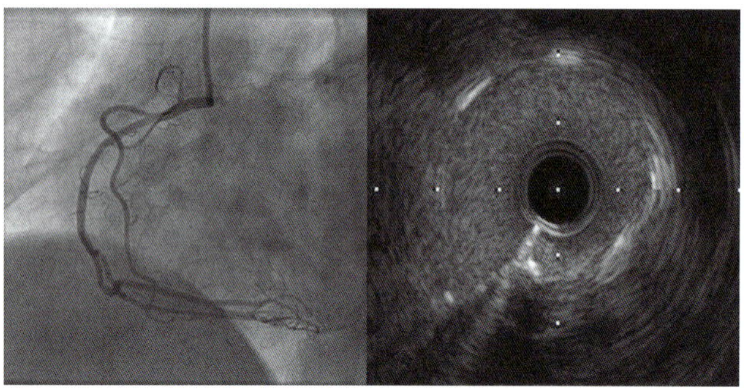

Figure A16-5

16.6 Answer B. The classification shown is the Medina classification (Medina A, et al. *Rev Esp Cardiol* 2006;59(2):183). Currently, there are at least seven classifications that have been proposed for bifurcation lesions (Latib A, et al. *JACC Cardiovasc Interv* 2008;1(3):218–226). The Medina is the only classification that indicates the position of lesions and does not require memorization. It is comprised of three numbers separated by two commas. The first number represents the proximal main branch, the second number is for the distal main branch, and the third number is for the side branch. The number may be either "1" or "0," indicating the presence or absence of a >50% lesion.

16.7 Answer D. The Nordic Bifurcation Study randomized 413 patients to DES implantation in both branches (n = 206) with crush, culotte, Y, or other techniques vs. provisional stenting (n = 207). At 8-month angiographic follow-up, there was no significant difference in restenosis of the bifurcation (22.5% vs. 16%, p = 0.15) or side branch (19.2% vs. 11.5%, p = 0.062) in the one- vs. two-stent group, respectively. At 6 months, the rates of MACE (3.4% vs. 2.9%) and stent thrombosis (0% vs. 0.5%) were similar between the double stenting and provisional groups, respectively. A two-stent strategy was associated with higher contrast usage (283 mL of contrast vs. 233 mL with one stent, $p < 0.0001$) and longer fluoroscopy times (21 minutes vs. 15 minutes with one stent, $p < 0.0001$).

16.8 Answer C. Angiographic evaluation overestimates the severity of jailed side branches during the provisional strategy, and thus, FFR evaluation is recommended in important side branches with significant residual stenosis. Indeed, many lesions at the ostium of a side branch do not demonstrate signs of ischemia. Among 97 bifurcation lesions evaluated with FFR on both branches, none of the 21 lesions with <75% stenosis had FFR < 0.75; and among the 73 lesions with >75% stenosis, only 20 were functionally significant (Koo BK, et al. *J Am Coll Cardiol* 2005;46(4):633–637). The unreliability of angiography in estimating the severity of side-branch stenosis was highlighted by the same group in a recent study in which FFR assessment of the side branch after intervention revealed that a hemodynamically significant side-branch stenosis was present only in 54.5% of lesions classified as severe by angiography and that 29.4% of angiographically nonsignificant side-branch lesions were associated with an abnormal FFR. Furthermore, in both of these studies, FFR measurement in jailed side-branch lesions was shown to be safe and feasible.

16.9 Answer B. In a study by Koo et al. (Koo BK, et al. *Eur Heart J* 2008;29(6):726–732), kissing balloon angioplasty performed in 26 of 28 side-branch lesions with an FFR < 0.75 was successful in improving FFR to ≥0.75, even though the final mean residual stenosis was 69 ± 10%. During follow-up, there were no changes in side-branch FFR, and the rate of functional restenosis (FFR < 0.75) at 6-month follow-up was only 8%.

In this patient, kissing balloon angioplasty was performed and resulted in an excellent angiographic and hemodynamic result (Fig. A16-9).

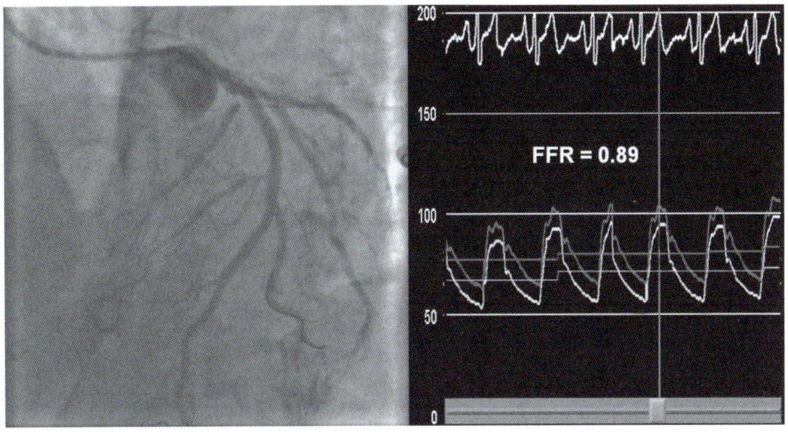

Figure A16-9

16.10 **Answer D.** The CACTUS (Coronary bifurcations: Application of the Crushing Technique Using Sirolimus-eluting stents) trial randomized 350 patients with true bifurcation lesions to either elective crush stenting or provisional side-branch stenting. The rate of angiographic restenosis at 6 months was similar between the crush (4.6% and 13.2% in the main branch and side branch, respectively) and provisional stenting groups (6.7% and 14.7% in the main branch and side branch, respectively; p = NS). Furthermore, the rates of MACE, including (15.8% vs. 15%, p = NS) MI (10.7% vs. 8.6%, p = NS), death (0% vs. 0.5%), and TLR (7.3% vs. 6.3%, p = NS), were similar between the crush and the provisional groups. This study, in conjunction with other randomized trials, confirmed that provisional side-branch stenting is effective in most true nonreplaced left main bifurcations. The need to implant a second stent on the side branch occurred in 31% of cases, and we believe that in a real-world setting, additional side-branch stenting is required in 10-20% of cases. Final kissing inflation was mandatory in CACTUS and successfully performed in over 90% of cases in both groups. A subanalysis suggested that kissing inflation was associated with a lower incidence of angiographic restenosis at the main and side branch of the bifurcation.

16.11 **Answer B.** The classical crush technique in which stents are positioned on the side branch and main branch simultaneously requires at least a 7-Fr guide catheter, although we prefer using an 8-Fr guide catheter. However, when there is need to perform the minicrush technique and a 6-Fr guiding catheter is the only available approach (e.g., radial approach), the "step crush" or "the modified balloon crush" techniques can be used. The final result is similar to that obtained with the standard crush technique, with the only difference being that each stent is advanced and deployed separately, with the side-branch stent crushed by a balloon placed on the main branch prior to side-branch stent deployment. When performing the crush technique, it is important to perform final kissing inflation following recrossing into the side branch. This maneuver lowers the risk of restenosis at the ostium of the side branch but does not seem to affect the risk of thrombosis (Ge L, et al. *J Am Coll Cardiol* 2005;46(4):613-620). When performing the crush technique, it is very important to perform the so-called two-step kissing inflation, which consists of high-pressure balloon inflation in the side branch before performing the true final kissing inflation at medium pressures. Ormiston et al. (Ormiston JA, et al. *JACC Cardiovasc Interv* 2008;1(4):351-357) recently demonstrated through imaging of bench deployments that (1) recrossing the crushed stent for kissing postdilatation, the most difficult part of the procedure, is technically easier with minicrush than with classical crush; (2) traditional one-step kissing postdilatation leaves considerable residual metallic stenosis that may not be visible on angiography and may predispose to thrombosis because of eddy currents, stasis, altered shear stress, and foreign body presence; and (3) side-branch ostial coverage and residual stenosis by metal struts is significantly reduced by two-step kissing inflation (Fig. A16-11). Finally, irrespective of the bifurcation technique utilized, the most frequent site of bifurcation restenosis remains the ostium of the side branch.

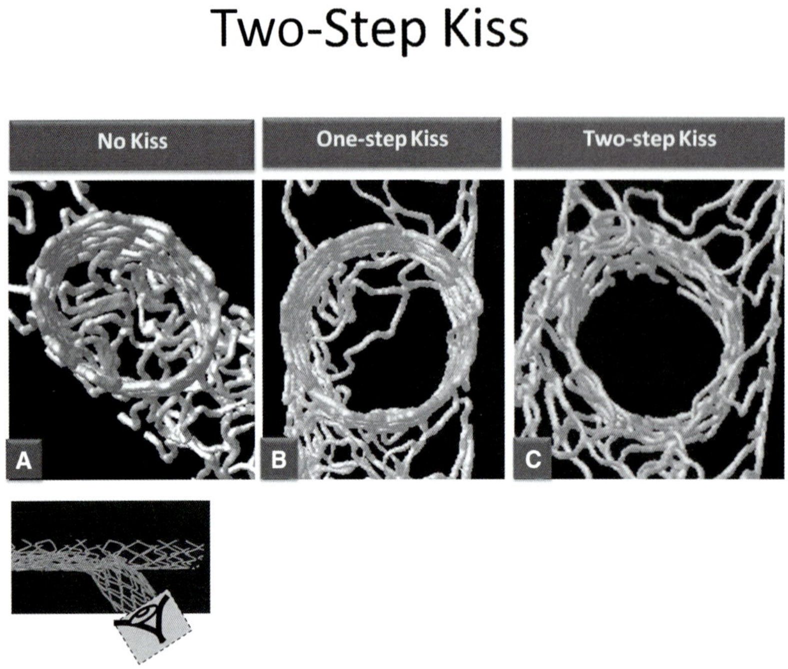

Figure A16-11 (Courtesy of John Ormiston.)

16.12 **Answer D.** The double kissing (DK) crush technique is a modification of the step crush, with each stent advanced and deployed separately and where kissing balloon inflation is performed twice: first after the side-branch stent is crushed by the main-branch balloon and then the routine final kissing balloon inflation (FKBI) at the end of the procedure. Thus, it can be performed with a 6-Fr guide. DK crush may result in less stent distortion and improved stent apposition and facilitate FKBI. This technique may be superior to the classic crush technique in optimizing acute procedural results and possibly also improves clinical outcomes by facilitating FKBI in all patients (Chen SL, et al. *Eur J Clin Invest* 2008;38(6):361–371). We recommend that the DK crush should be the default two-stent technique when this approach is selected as intention to treat. This technique was evaluated in the DKCRUSH-II study (Chen SL, et al. *J Am Coll Cardiol* 2011;57(8):914–920) that was the first and only randomized trial to suggest that double stenting may be superior to provisional stenting and associated with a lower rate of restenosis and repeat revascularization. In this study, 370 true bifurcations were randomly assigned to treatment with either provisional stenting or the DK crush technique. The DK crush was associated with a reduction in restenosis, especially in the side branch (4.9% vs. 22.2%, $p < 0.001$) and TLR (4.3% vs. 13%, $p = 0.005$), but not in MACE (10.3% vs. 17.3%, $p = 0.07$). How do we reconcile the contradictory findings of the DKCRUSH-II study with those of the other six bifurcation studies that showed no advantage of double stenting over provisional stenting? In our opinion, this study reconfirms the importance of bifurcation technique and optimization of the final result (in this case, a refinement of the standard crush technique), which is extremely important with double stenting techniques and appears to be directly related to long-term outcomes. Nevertheless, we see no rationale to make a procedure more complex when similar immediate and medium term follow-up results can be obtained with a more simple approach. Finally, Dzavik et al. have demonstrated that a bifurcation angle ≥50 degrees between the two branches may be an independent predictor of MACE after crush stenting (Dzavik V, et al. *Am Heart J* 2006;152(4):762–769).

16.13 **Answer D.** There is no recognized standard approach in the treatment of bifurcation lesions except for the preference of provisional side-branch stenting with a final kissing balloon when possible (Latib A, et al. *JACC Cardiovasc Interv* 2008;1(3):218–226). In this specific example, there is significant stenosis involving both branches with a reasonable reference vessel diameter (3.0 mm or more). In such a lesion, the usage of two DES as intention to treat appears a reasonable approach.

16.14 **Answer B.** The culotte technique provides near-perfect coverage of the carina and side-branch ostium at the expense of an excess of metal covering the proximal end. It will give the best immediate angiographic result, and theoretically, it may guarantee a more homogeneous distribution of the struts and drug at the site of the bifurcation. The only anatomic limitation to the culotte technique is when there is a large mismatch between the proximal main-branch and the side-branch diameters due to the risk of incomplete side-branch stent apposition to the proximal main branch. The Nordic Stent Technique Study was the first randomized trial comparing two different double stent techniques that result in complete coverage of the side-branch ostium (Erglis A, et al. *Circ Cardiovasc Interv* 2009;2(1):27–34). In this study, 424 patients were randomized to either crush or culotte stenting utilizing sirolimus-eluting stents (SES) (77% of which were true bifurcation lesions). At 6-month clinical follow-up, there were no significant differences between the two groups in terms of death, MI, or revascularization (crush 4.3% vs. culotte 3.7%, $p = 0.87$). Procedure and fluoroscopy times and contrast volumes were also similar in the two groups. Angiographically, there was a trend toward less in-segment restenosis (6.6% vs. 12.1%; $p = 0.10$) and significantly reduced in-stent restenosis following culotte stenting (4.5% vs. 10.5%; $p = 0.046$).

16.15 Answer C. There are no certain data supporting a specific technique over another in this type of bifurcation. The unfavorable takeoff angle of the side branch may impede recrossing into the side branch with a wire, balloon, or stent after main-branch stenting, and thus, the majority of operators would favor a two-stent approach with stenting of the side branch first rather than a provisional stenting. As this procedure is being performed via the radial artery with a 6-Fr guide catheter, two-stent techniques, such as V-stenting and classical crush stenting, that require the placement of a stent in the side and main branch simultaneously are not possible. The culotte stenting technique can be performed via a 6-Fr guide catheter and would be the preferable approach. However, if the operator wants to perform one of the other bifurcation techniques described above, the guiding catheter could be upsized to 7 Fr, which would allow implantation of the newer second-generation DES.

16.16 Answer A. In this nontrue bifurcation (i.e., no disease in the side branch), the result in the side branch after main branch is good without any evidence of side-branch compromise. The decision to perform no further treatment on the side branch is supported by the Nordic-Baltic Bifurcation Study III (Niemelä M, et al. *Circulation* 2011;123(1):79–86), which randomized 477 patients with bifurcation lesions undergoing main vessel stenting to final kissing inflation ($n = 238$) or no final kissing inflation ($n = 239$). The 6-month MACE rates were 2.1% and 2.5% ($p = 1.0$) in the final kissing and no final kissing groups, respectively. At 8 months, the rate of angiographic restenosis in the entire bifurcation lesion was 11.0% vs. 17.3% ($p = 0.11$), 3.1% vs. 2.5% in the main vessel ($p = 0.68$), and 7.9% vs. 15.4% in the side branch ($p = 0.039$), in the final kissing vs. no final kissing groups, respectively. The lower restenosis rate in the side branch was due to the efficacy of FKBI in reducing angiographic restenosis in true bifurcation lesions, where the side-branch restenosis rate was 7.6% vs. 20.0% ($p = 0.024$) in the final kissing and no final kissing groups, respectively. This study supports the simple approach of only main vessel stenting without routine FKBI in nontrue bifurcation lesions. However, in true bifurcation lesions that are treated with the provisional approach, routine FKBI should be performed, as it is associated with improved angiographic outcomes in the side branch.

16.17 Answer C. The most appropriate strategy in this patient would be to place a guidewire in both branches of the bifurcation and stent across the ostium of the diagonal. Stenting distal to the ostium would risk a suboptimal result in the LAD as well as in the diagonal branch. In this particular case, the operator only placed a guidewire in the main branch and not the side branch. Figure A16-17 shows the result after main vessel stenting with occlusion of the side branch (*arrow*). This case highlights the importance of protecting side branches with guidewires to prevent their closure as it has been shown that side-branch compromise is not inconsequential. Occlusion of side branches >1 mm can be associated with 14% incidence of MI (Arora RR, et al. *Cathet Cardiovasc Diagn* 1989;18(4):210–212) and compromise of large side branches (≥2 mm). During a provisional approach, it can be associated with a large periprocedural MI (Chaudhry EC, et al. *J Thromb Thrombolysis* 2007;24(1):7–13). This approach of wiring both branches during bifurcation stenting is important in protecting the side branch from closure due to plaque shift, carina shift, and/or stent struts during main vessel stenting. The jailed side-branch wire also facilitates rewiring of the side branch (if side-branch post-dilatation/stenting or FKBI is needed or if the side branch occludes) by widening the angle between the main branch and the side branch, by acting as a marker for the side-branch ostium, and by changing the angle of side-branch takeoff. Finally, in the case of side-branch occlusion, the side-branch wire can be used to reopen the side branch by pushing a small balloon between the stent and the wall of the vessel. The jailed wire technique is also supported by data from the COBIS II Registry (COronary BIfurcation Stenting) (Hahn JY, et al. *J Am Coll Cardiol* 2013;62(18):1654–1659) demonstrating that the jailed wire in the side branch is associated with flow recovery of side branches that occlude after main-branch stenting (74.8% vs. 57.8%, $p = 0.02$).

There is no need to remove the jailed wire during high-pressure stent dilatation in the main vessel. It is preferable to avoid jailing hydrophilic guidewires as there is a risk of removing the polymer coating. Accurate handling of the guiding catheter to prevent migration into the ostium of the coronary vessel will allow removal of the jailed wire.

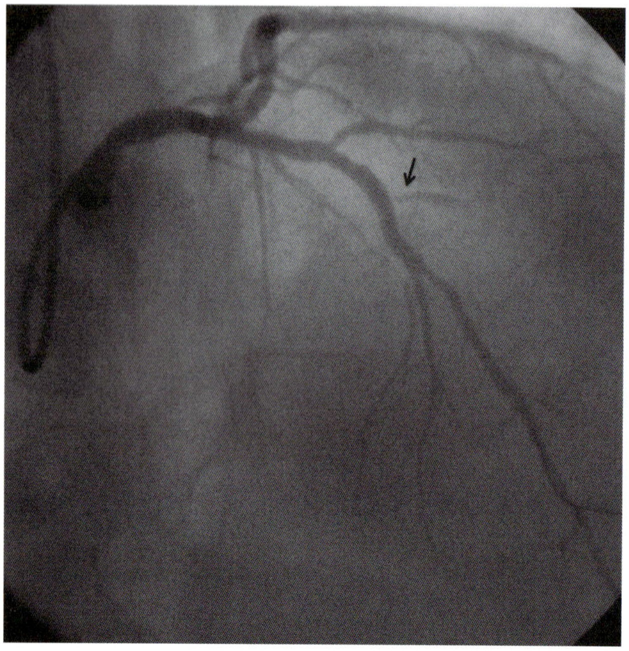

Figure A16-17

16.18 Answer C. The differential diagnosis of acute hypotension during bifurcation PCI includes both complications related to the bifurcation but also related to the procedure itself. Thus, all of the responses listed are conceivable complications. In this specific case, the angiography reveals a distal wire perforation caused by a hydrophilic guidewire resulting in cardiac tamponade that requires urgent pericardiocentesis. In Figure A16-18, note the visible contrast in the pericardium on the diaphragmatic border of the heart and pigtail catheter in the pericardial space. When attempting to recover an occluded side branch after main-branch stenting, if a workhorse wire fails, wire escalation in the following manner is recommended: polymer jacket or double coil, such as a Fielder FC or Sion blue, followed by a stiff controllable wire, such as an Intermediate or Miracle 3g. In some cases, where rewiring of a small occluded side branch is not possible, a conservative approach may be advisable. Special care and attention needs to be taken with hydrophilic guidewires because of the risk of distal wire perforation, especially if the wire enters the subintimal space.

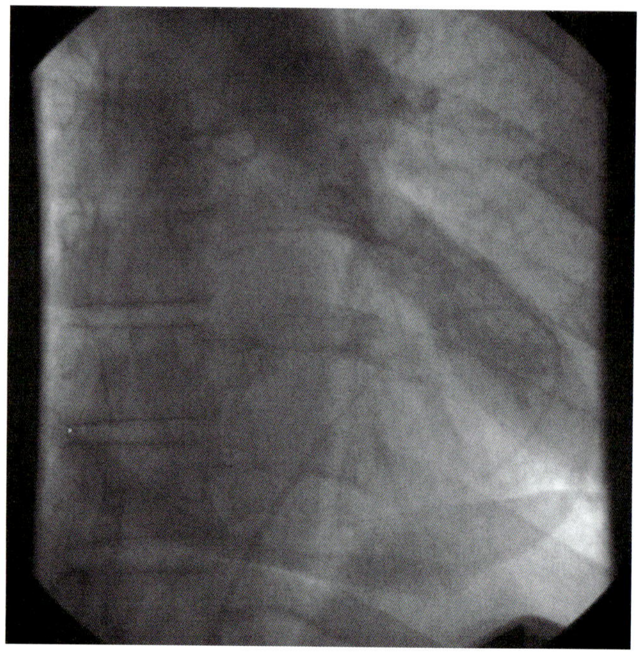

Figure A16-18 (Courtesy of Antonio Colombo and Azeem Latib.)

16.19 Answer D. The coronary tree is an object of pseudofractal geometry and branches off into asymmetrical bifurcations and increasingly smaller bifurcations with a clear mathematical relationship between the diameters of the main branch and side branch (Sawaya FJ, et al. *JACC Cardiovasc Interv* 2016;9(18):1861–1878). This complex mathematical relationship can be simplified and expressed by Finet's formula as follows: proximal main diameter = 0.678 × (distal main diameter + side-branch diameter). Respecting the relationship between these diameters restores the normal physiologic anatomy and prevents side branch compromise when implanting a main-branch stent and is helpful in selecting the correct kissing balloon size to prevent overstretching of the proximal main branch. Selecting the main-branch stent diameter according to the proximal main diameter results in carina shift and compromise of the side-branch ostium (Fig. A16-19A). In order to prevent carina shift, the stent diameter should be selected according to the diameter of the distal main branch, but this results in underexpansion of the stent proximal to the carina (Fig.A16-19B) that should be corrected with the proximal optimization technique.

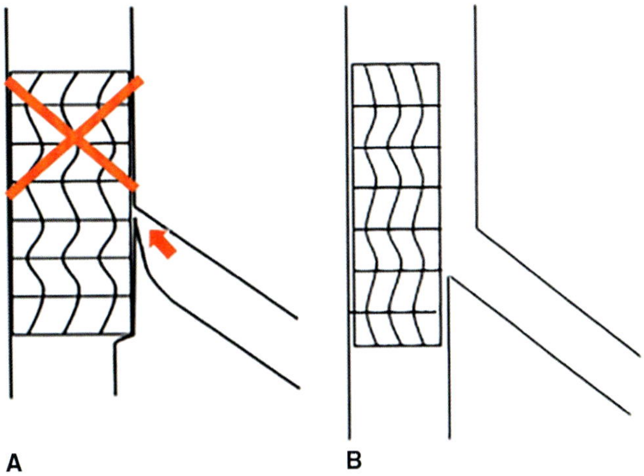

Figure A16-19 (A,B: Courtesy of Olivier Darremont and Goran Stankovic.)

16.20 Answer D. The images demonstrate that there is an alteration in the location and geometry of the carina. The carina is shifted to the side-branch side, and this shift results in an eccentric luminal narrowing of the side-branch ostium. There has been considerable debate as to whether the appearance of a new stenosis or aggravation of an existing stenosis at the side-branch ostium after main-branch stenting is due to plaque shift or carina shift. A recent study (Koo BK, et al. *Circ Cardiovasc Interv* 2010;3(2):113–119) of IVUS evaluation after main-branch stent implantation showed (1) a significant increase in the vessel and lumen volume index in both the proximal and the distal segments of the main branch, (2) a significant decrease in the plaque volume index in the proximal segment of the main branch, and (3) no change in the plaque volume index in the distal segment of the main branch after stenting. These results suggest that the lumen increase in the distal main branch is primarily due to enlargement of the vessel and not plaque shift, supporting the concept that part of the luminal narrowing of a side branch after stenting the main branch is explained by carina shift. However, in the proximal main-branch, plaque area changed significantly after stent implantation, particularly in the region closest to the ostium of the side branch. Although plaque shift to the side-branch ostium was not observed directly, these data provide indirect evidence of plaque shift from the proximal segment of the main branch into the side-branch ostium after main vessel stent implantation. Thus, both plaque shift from the main branch and carina shift contribute to the creation/aggravation of a side-branch ostial lesion after main vessel stent implantation. Carina shift resulting in side-branch occlusion may be prevented by selecting the main-branch stent diameter according to the distal main-branch diameter.

16.21 Answer B. When performing the POT, the main-branch stent diameter is usually selected according to the distal main diameter in order to prevent carina shift. However, this results in the proximal stent being malapposed, which should be corrected with the proximal optimization technique (i.e., a short larger diameter balloon sized to the proximal main branch and positioned with the distal marker of the balloon in front of the carina) (Fig.A16-21). The POT also changes the orientation of the side-branch ostium and projection of struts in the side-branch ostium, thus facilitating wire recrossing into the most distal strut, balloon crossing, and, if necessary, a stent in the side branch. POT is especially useful in bifurcation lesions with a large side branch because a marked difference in the diameter of the proximal and distal main branch is observed. The main-branch stent should be implanted sufficiently proximal to the side branch to accommodate a short, large diameter balloon sized to the proximal main at least 6 or 8 mm in length. The distal marker of this balloon must be positioned in front of the carina. Optimization of the proximal stent segment allows strut protrusion into the side branch with larger strut opening, as well as no or limited carinal shifting for easier guidewire exchange.

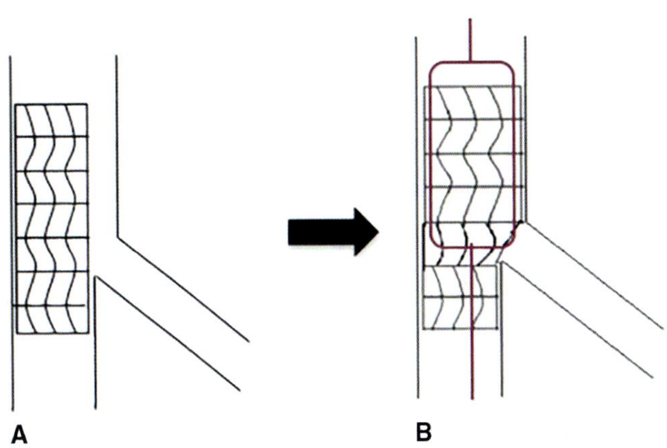

Figure A16-21 (Courtesy of Olivier Darremont and Goran Stankovic.)

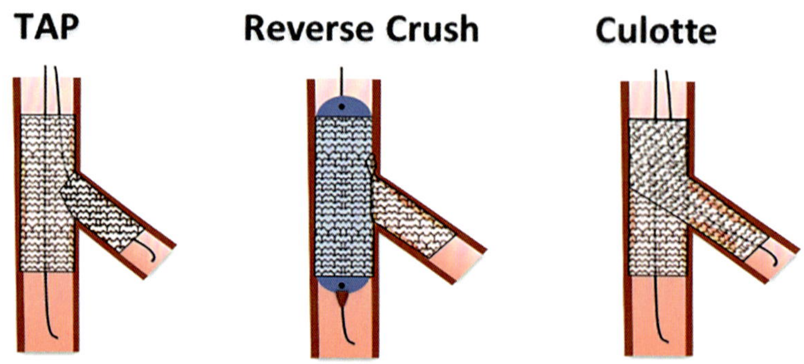

	TAP	Reverse Crush	Culotte
Advantages	Easy to perform No recrossing	Complete coverage of ostium Any anatomy	Complete coverage of ostium
Disadvantages	Struts protruding into main branch	Recrossing into SB 3 layers of struts	More labourious Rewiring both branches Double stent layer

Figure A16-22 (Courtesy of Antonio Colombo and Azeem Latib.)

16.22 Answer C. Crossover to stenting the side branch should be considered when the angiographic result remains unsatisfactory after main-branch stenting and balloon dilatation of the side branch (i.e., >75% residual stenosis, dissection, thrombolysis in myocardial infarction [TIMI] flow grade <3, or FFR < 0.75 in a side branch ≥2.5 mm). Crossover to side-branch stenting can be performed with the TAP, reverse crush, or reverse (provisional) culotte techniques. The main advantages and disadvantages of each technique are shown in Figure A16-22. Clearly, the TAP technique is the easiest to perform as the wire in the side branch can be immediately used for advancing and deploying the side-branch stent, whereas in the crush and culotte technique, recrossing stent struts with the wire and balloon is unavoidable. FKBI is always mandatory after all two-stent techniques.

16.23 Answer D. The TAP technique is the simplest and easiest to perform technique for side-branch stent implantation after a provisional approach. In wider-angle bifurcations, the TAP results in minimal strut protrusion into the main branch. However, shallow angles result in more protrusion and this technique may be inappropriate. Registry data (Naganuma T, et al. *JACC Cardiovasc Interv* 2013;6(6):554–561) have shown excellent clinical outcomes with low TLR rates of 5.1%. However, the only randomized controlled trial to evaluate this technique, randomized 300 bifurcations requiring a side-branch stent to culotte stenting and demonstrated that binary restenosis rates were 6.5% with culotte and 17% with TAP ($p = 0.006$). FKBI is mandatory after implanting the side-branch stent to prevent the protruding side-branch stents from obstructing the main branch. However, it is very important to remember that the side-branch balloon should never be deflated first because this will allow the main-branch balloon to deform or crush the side-branch stent (Fig. A16-23).

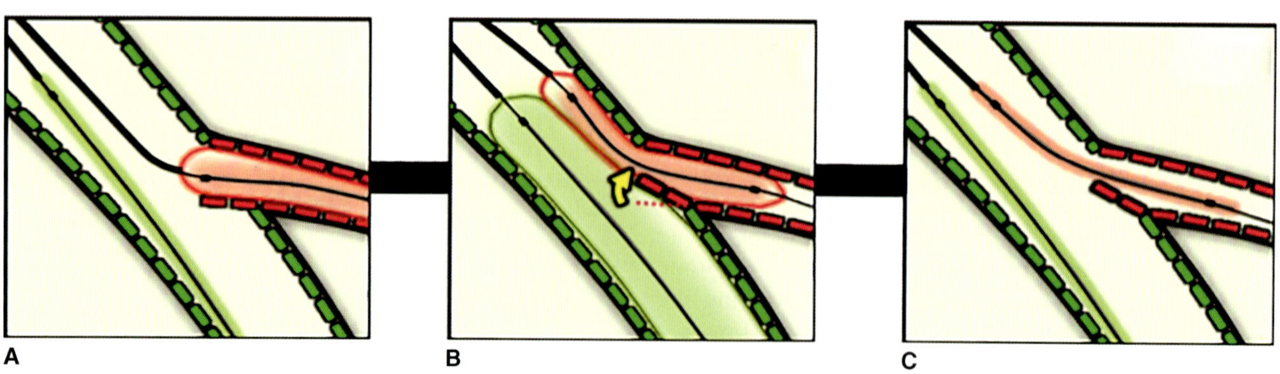

Figure A16-23 (Courtesy of Antonio Colombo and Azeem Latib.)

16.24 **Answer B.** The lesion presented is a complex stenosis involving a left main coronary artery. Presently, these lesions can be treated with stenting only in selected conditions, such as the presence of a contraindication to the standard approach for left main stenosis, which is CABG. If the patient needs to be treated with a percutaneous technique, the most favored approach is for a DES (Chieffo A, et al. *Circulation* 2005;111(6):791–795; Park SJ, et al. *J Am Coll Cardiol* 2005;45(3):351–356). While some operators may perform directional atherectomy, this approach is not considered standard in most coronary lesions; in addition, the stenosis presented here is likely to be calcific, a feature that makes directional atherectomy likely to fail.

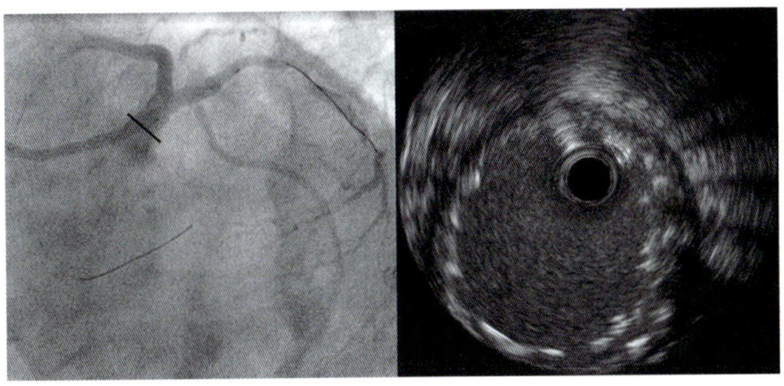

Figure A16-25

16.25 **Answer D.** Although the angiographic result appeared good, the IVUS images demonstrated marked malapposition of the stent in the distal LMCA. We thus performed further postdilatation with noncompliant balloons: 4.0 × 15 mm at 18 atm toward the LAD, 3.5 × 12 mm at 18 atm toward the LCx, and 4.5 × 20 mm at 18 atm on the LMCA. Repeat angiography and IVUS confirmed good stent apposition (Fig. A16-25). This case highlights the value of IVUS in complex lesions such as bifurcations, in particular the LMCA bifurcation.

16.26 **Answer D.** Although the repeat revascularization rates at coronary bifurcations have significantly decreased after the introduction of DES, there still remain many challenges in optimizing outcomes in this complex lesion subset, which may be related to factors such as the variability in bifurcation anatomy, the large number of possible anatomical permutations, the dynamic changes in anatomy during treatment, and the flow dynamics and shear stresses related to a bifurcation.

Although the majority of IVUS studies have been underpowered or otherwise limited by selection bias or suboptimal technique, the collective results from numerous randomized and registry BMS studies (with rare exception) have demonstrated that IVUS guidance compared with angiographic guidance alone likely results in improved freedom from target vessel revascularization and MACE. Indeed, IVUS-guided PCI may be more beneficial if limited to complex lesions. Park et al. (Park SJ, et al. *Circ Cardiovasc Interv* 2009;2(3):167–177) have reported the findings from a post hoc analysis from the MAIN-COMPARE (revascularization for unprotected left MAIN coronary artery stenosis: COMparison of Percutaneous coronary Angioplasty vs. surgical REvascularization) multicenter registry in which the nonrandomized outcomes of IVUS guidance and angiography guidance for LMCA stenting were evaluated in 975 patients. Among 145 propensity-matched pairs of patients receiving DES, the 3-year incidence of mortality was 61% lower with IVUS guidance as compared with angiographic guidance. After multivariable adjustment, this difference just missed statistical significance ($p = 0.055$). However, the risk of MI and TLR was not lowered by the use of IVUS guidance. Furthermore, Kim et al. (Kim JS, et al. *Am Heart J* 2011;161(1):180–187) showed that in patients treated with DES for bifurcation lesions, IVUS-guided PCI was associated with a lower incidence of death and MI at 3-year follow-up compared to angiography-guided PCI. Although the exact mechanisms of eventual clinical benefits using IVUS at bifurcation lesions is not clearly explained, this imaging modality may help to better define bifurcation morphology, geometry, and plaque distribution for selecting an optimal stenting strategy. Furthermore, IVUS may help to obtain an optimal final result after stent implantation by ensuring optimal stent expansion, adequate lesion coverage, and full stent apposition. The meticulous approach to these procedural aspects may help to reduce future adverse clinical events (i.e., stent thrombosis, MI, and death). Although these data are promising, they have been derived exclusively from retrospective observational studies and no amount of statistical adjustment can correct for major imbalances in unmeasured confounders. Only one randomized trial has been performed in the DES era in complex lesions (AVIO, angiographic versus IVUS optimization) and that was underpowered to show reductions in clinical outcome.

17 Long Lesions and Diffuse Disease

Subhash Banerjee

QUESTIONS

17.1 Which of the following statements associated with diffuse epicardial coronary artery disease (CAD) is TRUE?

(A) Unlike severe focal stenoses, diffuse coronary atherosclerosis does not increase the severity of inducible myocardial ischemia
(B) Presence of diffuse epicardial CAD is not associated with a high risk for serious adverse events
(C) Coronary flow reserve integrates the hemodynamic effects of diffuse epicardial CAD, epicardial focal coronary stenosis, diffuse atherosclerosis, and microvascular dysfunction on myocardial perfusion
(D) Fractional flow reserve (FFR) allows an operator to distinguish between upstream focal and diffuse CAD
(E) All of the above

17.2 Data on outcomes of coronary artery bypass graft (CABG) surgery in patients with diffuse epicardial CAD are scarce. However, based on current evidence, which of the following best describes clinical outcomes following CABG in patients with diffuse CAD?

(A) Patients with diffuse CAD do not demonstrate an improvement in angina symptom severity or maximum oxygen uptake
(B) Significantly lower occlusion rate is noted for internal mammary artery grafts compared with saphenous vein grafts (SVGs)
(C) Annual graft occlusion rate in patients with diffuse CAD is significantly higher in non-left anterior descending (LAD) territories compared with LAD territories
(D) Complete revascularization is often accomplished in this patient subgroup
(E) None of the above

17.3 More recent outcomes of percutaneous coronary intervention (PCI) studies have provided important insights into the interventional treatment of diffuse epicardial CAD and can be best described by which of the following?

(A) PCI in patients with small vessel diffuse CAD demonstrate comparable short-term clinical outcomes with drug-eluting balloons (DEB) and drug-eluting stents (DES)
(B) Studies exploring DEB use with DES (hybrid approach) have not been promising for the treatment of diffuse CAD
(C) Use of DEB in small-caliber diffuse coronary lesions is associated with an unacceptably high bail out stent rate
(D) In patients with diffuse CAD, stenting and DEB use leads to similar residual stenosis and acute luminal gains
(E) None of the above

17.4 Which of the following statements best summarize the findings of the LONG DES III trial?

(A) For patients with long native diffuse CAD, everolimus-eluting stent (EES) implantation was associated with significantly better clinical outcomes compared to the sirolimus-eluting stent (SES)
(B) SES implantation was associated with greater angiographic in-segment late loss and higher rates of in-segment restenosis compared to EES

(C) In-segment binary restenosis rate was higher in the EES group than in the SES group
(D) ST rates at 1 month and 12 months were significantly higher in the SES group
(E) The study was powered for both angiographic and clinical end points

17.5 Full metal jacket (FMJ) stent implants are often used to treat diffuse flow-limiting coronary lesions and such procedures are associated with which of the following?

(A) FMJ procedures are generally associated with high success rates and very low in-hospital complications
(B) Long-term cardiac death or myocardial infarction (MI)-free survival rates approach 85% at 8 years
(C) Left ventricular (LV) dysfunction and a stent length >80 mm are significantly related to cardiac death/MI
(D) ST rates associated with FMJ are approximately 0.5% per year
(E) All of the above

17.6 In response to a question from your clinical cardiology colleague regarding FMJ stenting of the coronary vessel shown in Figure Q17-6, which of the following is most consistent with the current evidence base?

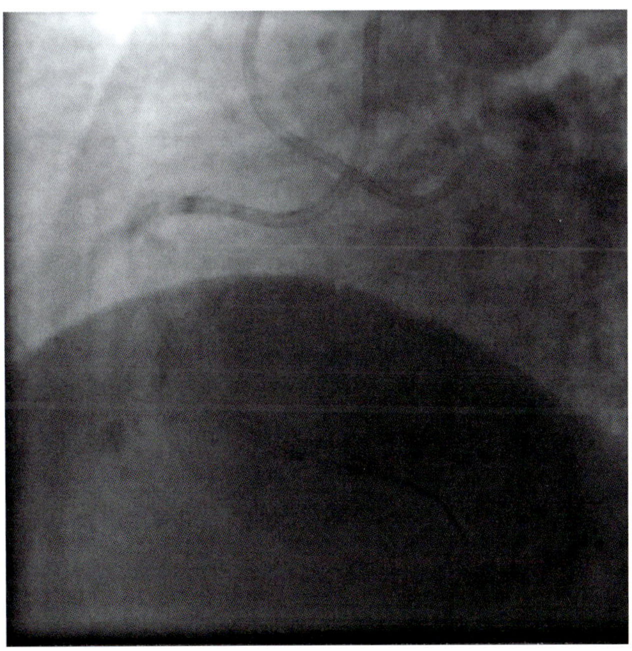

Figure Q17-6 (Courtesy of Subhash Banerjee.)

(A) FMJ is arbitrarily defined as placement of coronary stents in one or more coronary arteries with a cumulative stent length of ≥60 mm
(B) FMJ stenting is exclusively performed with bioresorbable scaffolds for not precluding future coronary bypass options
(C) Definite or probable acute stent thrombosis rates are high and exceed 5% and therefore require more prolonged and more intensive dual antiplatelet therapy (DAPT)
(D) Long-term target lesion revascularization (TLR) rates approach 30% at 6 years and diabetes mellitus, smoking, and left ventricular ejection fraction (LVEF) are independent predictors of major adverse cardiac events (MACE)
(E) Most FMJ stenting is performed in the LAD coronary artery distribution in patients at high risk for coronary bypass surgery

17.7 Treatment of long diffuse coronary lesions with bioresorbable vascular scaffolds (BVS) often requires placement of overlapping BVS. Of the following options related to optimal overlapping BVS deployment, select the best option.

(A) BVS strut thickness of 100 μm is thicker than that of newer-generation DES; therefore, strut overlap should be minimized
(B) BVS stents have distal markers that are located at the very edges (proximal and distal) of the BVS and serve as important landmarks during overlapping deployments
(C) Distal marker of the proximal scaffold should be just next to the proximal marker of the distal scaffold, resulting in <1 mm of overlap in most cases
(D) Distal marker of the proximal scaffold should be overlapped with the proximal marker of the distal scaffold for optimal positioning
(E) BVS edge platinum markers are completely superimposed over the balloon markers and hence are detectable only postimplantation and following removal of the deployment balloon

17.8 Which of the following maneuvers is NOT appropriate for performing transradial orbital atherectomy of long, heavily calcified and tortuous coronary lesions?

(A) A 7-Fr guiding catheter is a must for orbital atherectomy procedures
(B) Use of a sheathless guide system since the outer diameter of a 5-Fr sheath (2.28 mm)

parallels that of a 7-Fr guide (2.31 mm). The sheathless approach may reduce the incidence of associated spasm and allow use of larger-caliber guiding catheters

(C) In the absence of a sheathless guide catheter, a 7-Fr sheath may be used by inserting only 1 cm of sheath into the radial artery to allow for atraumatic entry of the 7-Fr guide into the radial artery

(D) A guiding catheter extension may improve selective coronary engagement during orbital atherectomy procedures

(E) Each run (spin time) should be limited to 30 seconds. Longer lesions require additional runs, not longer runs. The rest time between each run should be equal to or longer than the run time

(F) Advancement of the knob at a maximum of 1 cm/s and not ending the run in the middle of a lesion. Never force the crown through the lesion

17.9 What is the American College of Cardiology (ACC)/American Heart Association (AHA) criteria for the definition of a "long" lesion in the coronary circulation?

(A) <5 mm of length
(B) >5 mm of length
(C) >20 mm of length
(D) >10 mm of length

17.10 Which of the following statements is TRUE regarding the influence of lesion length on the AHA/ACC classification of lesion type?

(A) A lesion >2 cm in length represents an AHA/ACC type B1 lesion
(B) A lesion <10 mm in length represents an AHA/ACC type A lesion
(C) A lesion >2 cm in length represents an AHA/ACC type B2 lesion
(D) A lesion 10 to 20 mm in length represents an AHA/ACC type C lesion

17.11 A 62-year-old diabetic male undergoes coronary stenting of his right coronary artery (RCA) chronic total occlusion (CTO) with multiple overlapping DES shown in Figure Q17-11. The *arrowheads* indicate the stented coronary segment. Which of the following factors have been shown to independently predict long-term target lesion failure (TLF) at 5 years?

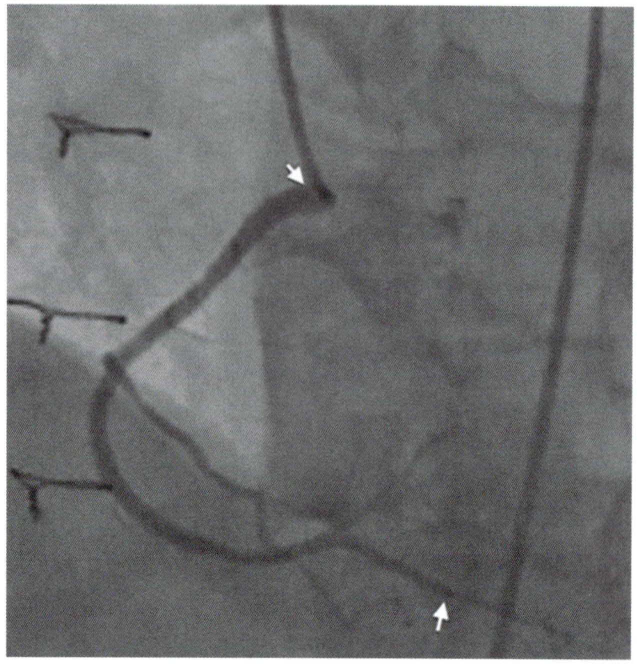

Figure Q17-11 (Courtesy of Subhash Banerjee.)

(A) Diabetes mellitus
(B) Coronary J-CTO score
(C) LVEF
(D) Average stent diameter
(E) Persistent distal vessel narrowing

17.12 A 58-year-old male who underwent heart transplantation 5 years ago due to an ischemic cardiomyopathy has a recent coronary angiogram characterized by diffuse and severe concentric narrowing of the coronary arteries. Regarding the diagnosis, prognostic significance, and treatment of this condition, all of the following statements are true EXCEPT:

(A) Intravascular ultrasound (IVUS) offers earlier detection and better characterization when compared with routine angiography
(B) The presence of angiographic coronary disease posttransplantation is highly predictive of subsequent coronary disease-related events
(C) Flow-limiting lesions requiring intervention generally occur >5 years posttransplantation
(D) Primary procedural success for the interventional treatment of transplant vasculopathy lesions is less than for the treatment of native atherosclerosis
(E) Transplant vasculopathy is the second leading cause of death in cardiac transplant patients beyond 1 year from the time of transplantation

17.13 While considering PCI of the long, diffusely diseased LAD coronary artery depicted in Figure Q17-13, which of the following procedural factors have NOT been shown to be an independent risk factor for in-stent restenosis?

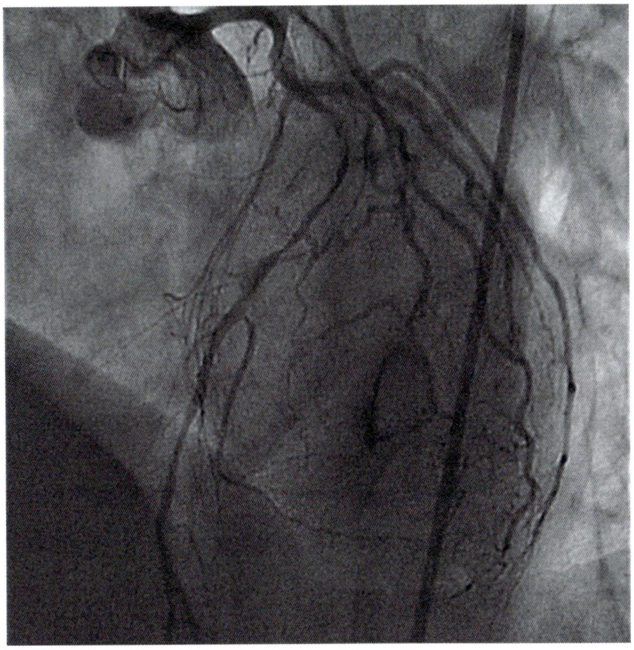

Figure Q17-13

(A) Lesion length
(B) Vessel diameter and postprocedural minimal luminal diameter
(C) Chronic occlusion
(D) Number of stent overlaps
(E) Stent length

17.14 Which one of the following criteria is traditionally used to define coronary FMJ stenting?

(A) ≥60-mm stent length in a single coronary artery without gaps
(B) ≥38-mm stent length in a single coronary artery without gaps
(C) ≥60 mm of total stent length in one or more coronary arteries
(D) ≥60-mm stent length in a single coronary artery with <5-mm gap between stents
(E) ≥38-mm stent length in a single coronary artery implanted within preexisting stents to treat in-stent restenosis

17.15 Regarding the relationships between the incidence of stent thrombosis and both stent length and lesion length, which of the following statements is TRUE?

(A) With the use of bare-metal stents (BMS), increased stent length is not predictive of an increased risk of stent thrombosis
(B) With the use of BMS, increased lesion length is predictive of an increased risk of stent thrombosis
(C) With the use of DES, increased lesion length is predictive of an increased risk of stent thrombosis
(D) With the use of DES, increased stent length is predictive of an increased risk of stent thrombosis

17.16 During performance of coronary stenting of long and diffusely diseased stable lesions, which of the following medical interventions has been associated with improved clinical outcomes?

(A) Maintenance of activated clotting time (ACT) >280 seconds
(B) Use of bivalirudin
(C) Periprocedural infusion of tirofiban
(D) Preloading with $P2Y_{12}$ agents in addition to aspirin therapy
(E) None of the above

17.17 Treatment of long and diffuse coronary lesions, especially in the LAD coronary artery, with BVS may offer some putative advantages, including preservation of future CABG surgery options. Which of the following most accurately describe outcomes following overlapping BVS implantation to treat long coronary artery lesions?

(A) Use of BVS compared with DES in long lesions has been reported by multiple randomized controlled trials
(B) Overlapping BVS implantation is not approved by the device instruction for use and is therefore off-label
(C) Hybrid implantation of BVS and DES to treat long lesions with bifurcations has demonstrated durable long-term outcomes
(D) Stent thrombosis rate of BVS is exclusively related to the length of the implanted scaffold
(E) BVS > 60 mm in lengths have been associated with high TLF rates

17.18 A 61-year-old diabetic male presents with stable angina refractory to standard medical therapy. Myocardial perfusion imaging shows a large defect in the anterior wall of moderate severity. Angiography reveals a long LAD lesion with diffuse disease. Prior to stenting, your interventional colleague prompts you to use IVUS. Which of these arguments is CORRECT?

(A) IVUS evaluation is a very useful tool for selecting the most appropriate-sized stent
(B) IVUS allows the operator to discern negative vessel remodeling from plaque burden in diffuse disease
(C) IVUS decreases the risk of undersizing a stent
(D) IVUS decreases the risk of oversizing a stent and thus reduces the risk of vessel rupture
(E) In the context of diffuse disease, it is common to see segments with negative and positive remodeling
(F) All of the above

ANSWERS AND EXPLANATIONS

17.1 Answer C. Diffuse coronary atherosclerosis is highly prevalent among patients with CAD. It increases the severity of inducible myocardial ischemia and risk for serious adverse events. In contrast to FFR, which is unable to distinguish between upstream focal and diffuse CAD, coronary flow reserve (CFR)—calculated as the ratio of hyperemic to rest absolute myocardial blood flow—integrates the hemodynamic effects of focal epicardial coronary stenosis, diffuse atherosclerosis, and microvascular dysfunction on myocardial perfusion (Gould KL, et al. *J Am Coll Cardiol* 2013;62(18):1639-1653).

17.2 Answer B. In patients with diffuse CAD, incomplete CABG revascularization is common and still results in a significant clinical improvement with an acceptable (19%) graft occlusion rates at 1 year. There is significant improvement in angina severity, maximum oxygen uptake, and reduction in the use of long-acting nitrates. Graft occlusion rate is not significantly different between LAD and non-LAD territories, and a lower occlusion rate is noted for the internal mammary artery grafts compared with SVGs in the LAD distribution. Overall, the use of venous graft is a predictor of graft occlusion at 1 year (Dourado LO, et al. *Thorac Cardiovasc Surg* 2017. doi: 10.1055/s-0037-1601306).

17.3 Answer A. Initial experience with DEB, either alone in smaller-diameter vessels or in combination with DES for very long disease, has emerged as an acceptable approach for the treatment of diffuse CAD. DEB is associated with MACE, TVR, and TLR rates similar to those seen with a DES-alone approach at long-term follow-up (Costopoulos C, et al. *JACC Cardiovasc Interv* 2013;6(11):1153-1159).

17.4 Answer C. For patients with long, diffuse native CAD, EES implantation was associated with greater angiographic in-segment late loss and higher rates of in-segment restenosis compared with SES implantation, albeit with similar clinical outcomes and no difference in ST rates (Park DW, et al. *JACC Cardiovasc Interv* 2011;4(10):1096-1103).

17.5 Answer E. Long-term outcomes after FMJ procedures are favorable. LV dysfunction and a stent length >80 mm are significant predictors of MACE. ST rate after FMJ is low, and procedural success is above 97%. These findings may help identify patients suitable for FMJ for diffuse epicardial CAD. FMJ, especially in the LAD distribution, can limit feasibility of future CABG. Event-free survival rate for cardiac death, MI, or TLR is approximately 72% at 8 years (Lee CW, et al. *Catheter Cardiovasc Interv* 2014;84(3):361-365).

17.6 Answer D. FMJ is arbitrarily defined as placement of overlapping coronary stents in at least one coronary artery with total stent length of ≥60 mm. Some studies have, in addition, classified FMJ into complete and incomplete based on the presence of nonstented vessel within the long stented coronary segment. Most FMJs are in the RCA distribution. Although the use of bioresorbable scaffolds provides an inherent advantage related to preservation of future coronary bypass option, most contemporary procedures are performed with new generation DES. Longer-term clinical outcomes and stent thrombosis rates are favorable. During the median follow-up of 6.2 years, the rates of cardiac death, MI, and TLR were 5.8%, 6.2%, and 27.3%, respectively. The rate of definite and probable stent thrombosis was 3.6% (Whan Lee C, et al. *Catheter Cardiovasc Interv* 2014;84(7):1051-1052).

17.7 Answer C. The struts are 156 μm thick (twice the size of present-generation DES). It is nearly invisible and its presence can be detected by the two platinum markers at each end of the device, placed at approximately 0.7 mm from the edge of the scaffold. The BVS deployment balloon extends beyond these platinum markers. The distal marker of the proximal scaffold should be just next to the proximal marker of the distal scaffold, resulting in <1 mm of overlap for optimal deployment of overlapping BVS in long diffusely diseased coronary vessels (Seth A, et al. *EuroIntervention* 2015;11(2):131-135).

17.8 Answer A. Orbital atherectomy can be used through a 6- or 7-Fr guide catheter. In addition to the above maneuvers, ultrasound measurement of the radial artery with sublingual nitroglycerin can be helpful to determine the sheath and guide size that can be used without increasing the incidence of spasm or asymptomatic radial artery occlusion. A 6-Fr system can be used when the radial artery size is <2.2 mm and a 7-Fr system when the diameter is >2.2 mm (Ruisi M, et al. *J Invasive Cardiol* 2015;27(11):E252–E255).

17.9 Answer C. According to the ACC/AHA and the Society for Coronary Angiography and Interventions (SCAI) lesion classifications system, lesions <10 mm in length are discrete, lesions of 10 to 20 mm in length are referred to as tubular, and lesions >20 mm in length are considered long (Krone RJ, et al. *Am J Cardiol* 2003;92(4):389–394).

17.10 Answer B. Type A lesions are discrete and <10 mm in length. In terms of lesion length, both type B1 and B2 lesions are 10 to 20 mm in length. Type B2 lesions have two or more type B characteristics (i.e., eccentric, moderate tortuosity of proximal segment, moderately angulated segment [45 to 90 degrees], irregular contour, moderate to heavy calcification, ostial in location, bifurcation lesions requiring double guidewires, some thrombus present, and total occlusion <3 months old). Type C lesions are considered diffuse and have a length of >2 cm (Krone RJ, et al. *Am J Cardiol* 2003;92(4):389–394).

17.11 Answer E. A recent study by Lee et al. reported that TLF of 16% and TLR or occlusion rates of 8.6% over a median of 5 years are well within the accepted range for complex PCI with contemporary DES (Lee PH, et al. *JACC Cardiovasc Interv* 2017;10(14):1405–1412). The same can be said about periprocedural MI (MI; 2.5%), overall stent thrombosis (ST; 1.2%), cardiovascular death (5.7%), and nonfatal spontaneous MI (2.2%) rates reported in this study. These findings may provide reassurance and alleviate concerns regarding FMJ stenting, which include potential loss of side branches, especially with dissection re-entry, implantation of additional stent layers to treat TLF, loss of coronary bypass surgery options, and associated high TLF and ST rates. Finally, two independent predictors of TLF were identified: number of target vessel DES (per 1 increment; multivariable hazard rate or HR, 1.72; 95% confidence interval or CI, 1.16 to 2.54) and persistent distal luminal narrowing (≥50% narrowing compared with distal stent edge and ≥20 mm in length; HR, 2.73; 95% CI, 1.66 to 4.47) (Banerjee S, et al. *JACC Cardiovasc Interv* 2017;10(14):1413–1414).

17.12 Answer D. Traditional noninvasive modalities are insensitive in the detection of transplant vasculopathy. Although conventional coronary angiography is the most commonly employed method for the detection of transplant vasculopathy, it is less sensitive than IVUS, which is the gold standard for the detection of this pathology. Significant flow-limiting lesions due to transplant vasculopathy are unusual in the first 5 years posttransplantation but show an exponential rise after this time point. Interventional strategies, including angioplasty and stenting, have been reported for the treatment of these lesions, with similar primary procedural success compared with the treatment of native coronary atherosclerosis. There is a high rate of repeat procedures in this group due to a combination of late restenosis at the treatment site and progression of transplant vasculopathy. Beyond 1 year from the time of cardiac transplantation, transplant vasculopathy is the second leading cause of death, with malignancy being the most common cause. In patients with end-stage transplant vasculopathy, the only treatment option currently is repeat transplantation. Attenuated-signal plaque (ASP) progression appears to reflect chronic inflammation related to acute cellular rejection and is an independent predictor of long-term mortality after heart transplantation (Tuzcu EM, et al. *J Am Coll Cardiol* 2005;45(9):1538–1542; Okada K, et al. *J Am Coll Cardiol* 2016;68(4):382–392).

17.13 Answer D. While lesion length, vessel diameter, chronic occlusion, stent length, and postprocedural minimal lumen diameter are known to be risk factors of in-stent restenosis, Hong et al. reported that the most important factor for in-stent restenosis in long stenoses was stent lumen cross-sectional area by IVUS regardless of the stent length in a relatively large vessel. Other studies demonstrated that distal vessel diameter <2.5 mm was a powerful predictor of restenosis after long coronary stenting. Kastrati et al. reported that overlapping stents was an independent risk factor of in-stent restenosis; it has been found to provide an outcome comparable to a single long stent by several investigators with newer-generation DES (Kastrati A, et al. *Am J Cardiol* 1999;83(12):1617–1622; Ortega-Paz L, et al. *EuroIntervention* 2017;13(5):e557–e563; Lee SH, et al. *Catheter Cardiovasc Interv* 2004;62(3):298–302).

17.14 Answer A. In published literature, FMJ is defined as a ≥60-mm stent length without gaps (Lee CW, et al. *Catheter Cardiovasc Interv* 2014;84(3):361–365).

17.15 Answer D. Increased stent length, both with BMS and DES, predicts an increased risk of stent thrombosis. In an analysis of six BMS trials, Cutlip et al. demonstrated a 30% increase in the risk of stent thrombosis per 10 mm of BMS (Cutlip DE, et al. *Circulation* 2001;103(15):1967–1971). In a large prospective observational series of patients receiving DES, Iakovou et al. demonstrated a similar magnitude of risk of increased stent thrombosis per 10 mm of DES length (Iakovou I, et al. *JAMA* 2005;293(17):2126–2130). Lesion length does not appear to predict an increased risk of stent thrombosis (Moreno R, et al. *J Am Coll Cardiol* 2005;45(6):954–959).

17.16 Answer C. Of all the above listed medical interventions, infusion of tirofiban during PCI has been shown to reduce the occurrence of periprocedural MI and MACE at 1 year in stable CAD patients undergoing elective PCI for long lesions with overlapping stent implantation in the prospective, randomized, multicenter PETITION study (Zhang Q, et al. *Catheter Cardiovasc Interv* 2015;85(Suppl 1):762–769).

17.17 Answer E. The comparative efficacy of BVS and DES in long lesions is a question for ongoing randomized clinical studies: ABSORB-LONG (Everolimus-Eluting Bioresorbable Scaffolds Versus Everolimus-Eluting Metallic Stents for Diffuse Long Coronary Artery Disease [NCT02831205]) and Compare Absorb (ABSORB Bioresorbable Scaffold vs. Xience Metallic Stent for Prevention of Restenosis in Patients at High Risk of Restenosis [NCT02486068]).

Treatment of very long coronary lesions (scaffold length ≥ 60 mm) with BVS was associated with a high 12-month TLF rate of 14.3% in the GHOST-EU registry (Schnorbus B, et al. *EuroIntervention* 2017; pii: EIJ-D-16-00568). The TLF rates reported in the UNDERDOGS study were a mean scaffold length on average of 30 mm shorter than GHOST-EU. The rate of TLF in patients with scaffold lengths between 30 and 60 mm enrolled in the GHOST-EU registry was more reassuring (4.5%) and comparable to that observed in the UNDERDOGS study (Biscaglia S, et al. *Int J Cardiol* 2016;208:40–45).

The 12-month incidence of definite scaffold thrombosis was 2.6% in acute coronary syndrome (ACS) patients. In a multivariate analysis, ACS was a predictor of stent thrombosis (hazard rate or HR, 2.51; 95% confidence interval or CI, 1.13 to 5.60; $p = 0.025$).

A hybrid FMJ approach involving stenting of the LAD with overlapping metal DES and bioresorbable scaffolds has been described. Although this approach offers some putative advantages in terms of preserving future left internal mammary artery anastomosis options for surgical bypass, its technical feasibility, safety, and durability are yet to be rigorously tested in well-designed clinical studies.

17.18 Answer F. In the context of diffuse disease, IVUS evaluation is a useful tool for selecting an appropriate stent. Visual estimation of a long lesion in diffuse disease does not allow for an accurate evaluation of negative remodeling vs. plaque burden. This visual estimation may result in the undersizing of the stent. Long diffuse disease can have areas of negative and positive remodeling (Takagi K, et al. *Int J Cardiol* 2013;168(4):3791–3796).

18 Restenosis and Percutaneous Options

Craig R. Narins

QUESTIONS

18.1 A 61-year-old woman with diabetes mellitus and hypertension presents with unstable angina. Coronary angiography demonstrates single-vessel coronary artery disease (CAD) as displayed in Figure Q18-1. A 2.5 × 12 mm everolimus-eluting stent (EES) was placed at the ostium of the right coronary artery (RCA). Which of the following factors is NOT a predictor of higher restenosis following drug-eluting stent (DES) placement in this patient?

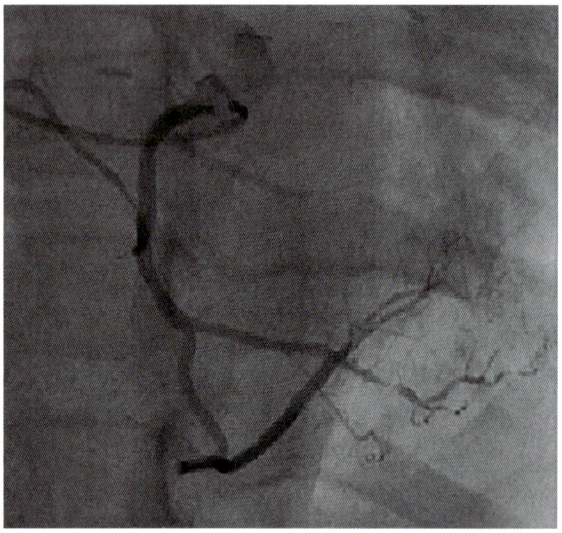

Figure Q18-1

(A) Ostial lesion location
(B) Diabetes mellitus
(C) Smaller reference vessel diameter
(D) Use of a bioabsorbable polymer-coated EES instead of a durable polymer coated EES

18.2 Which of the following is TRUE regarding differences between in-stent restenosis following DES vs. bare metal stent (BMS) implantation?

(A) BMS in-stent restenosis tends to present later than DES in-stent restenosis
(B) In-stent restenosis within a BMS tends to demonstrate a lower volume of intimal hyperplasia than within a DES
(C) Longer stent length is a predictor of in-stent restenosis following BMS but not DES implantation
(D) Incomplete stent strut apposition is more common with DES compared to BMS in-stent restenosis

18.3 Which of the following statements regarding the pathogenesis of coronary atherosclerosis vs. coronary restenosis is TRUE?

(A) Vessel wall inflammation, which is a major component in the formation of coronary atherosclerosis, plays little role in the development of restenosis
(B) Lipid-rich pools are commonly found in both atherosclerotic and restenotic lesions
(C) Genetic susceptibility plays a role in the occurrence of both atherosclerosis and restenosis
(D) Plaque rupture and acute thrombosis serve as predominant mechanisms for clinical events caused by both atherosclerotic and restenotic lesions

18.4 Which of the following is TRUE regarding the use of animal models for the study of restenosis?

(A) Smooth muscle cell proliferation and migration from media to intima are features of all animal models of restenosis
(B) Animals subjected to hyperlipidemic diets typically demonstrate histologic features of atherosclerosis identical to those seen in human atherosclerosis, including ulceration, intraplaque hemorrhage, and thrombosis
(C) The use of large mammals—particularly canine and porcine models—permits accurate study of complex human phenotypes that predispose to restenosis, such as diabetes
(D) Development of hemodynamically significant lesions following balloon-induced vascular injury is a feature common to all animal models of restenosis

18.5 Which of the following is TRUE regarding the use of paclitaxel-eluting balloon (PEB) angioplasty for the treatment of in-stent restenosis within a DES?

(A) PEB angioplasty is less effective at preventing recurrent in-stent restenosis than the placement of a paclitaxel-eluting stent
(B) PEB angioplasty is associated with lower target vessel revascularization (TVR) rates when used for diffuse rather than focal patterns of in-stent restenosis
(C) Compared to DES placement, PEB angioplasty is associated with higher rates of stent thrombosis when used for the treatment of in-stent restenosis
(D) PEB angioplasty is associated with less angiographic late loss compared to noncoated balloon angioplasty

18.6 A 57-year-old man is referred for coronary angiography following a non–ST-elevation myocardial infarction (STEMI). The angiogram demonstrates a severe stenosis of the mid-RCA and a 3.5 × 18 mm zotarolimus-eluting stent is placed. Online quantitative coronary angiography (QCA) performed before and after stenting reveals the measurements listed below (Table Q18-6). Six months later, the patient experienced two episodes of chest discomfort, and an exercise nuclear stress test suggested mild ischemia of the inferior wall. Angiography with QCA demonstrated a patent stent with measurements as described. What is the in-stent late loss in this individual?

Table Q18-6 Quantitative coronary angiography (QCA) measurements

	Present	Poststent	6-Month Follow-up
Vessel reference diameter (mm)	3.52	3.52	3.68
Minimum luminal diameter (mm)	1.08	3.40	2.98

(A) 0.32 mm
(B) 1.90 mm
(C) 0.54 mm
(D) 0.16 mm
(E) 0.42 mm

18.7 What is the late loss index for the patient described in Question 18.6 (Table Q18-6)?

(A) 0.18
(B) 3.49
(C) 1.90
(D) 0.66
(E) 0.39

18.8 Compared to balloon angioplasty, BMS implantation is associated with a lower likelihood of restenosis as a result of which one of the following biologic mechanisms?

(A) Reduced degree of neointimal formation
(B) Reduced vascular smooth muscle cell proliferation
(C) Increased collagen deposition
(D) Reduced degree of negative remodeling
(E) All of the above

18.9 A 44-year-old man who underwent orthotopic heart transplantation 6 years ago for treatment of dilated cardiomyopathy presents with increasing dyspnea, exertion, and fatigue. He denies chest discomfort and has been compliant with his immunosuppressant medications. Coronary angiography demonstrates a severe focal stenosis in the proximal left circumflex (LCx) artery (Fig. Q18-9) that is treated with stent placement. Which of the following statements regarding restenosis following percutaneous coronary intervention (PCI) among patients with transplant arteriopathy is correct?

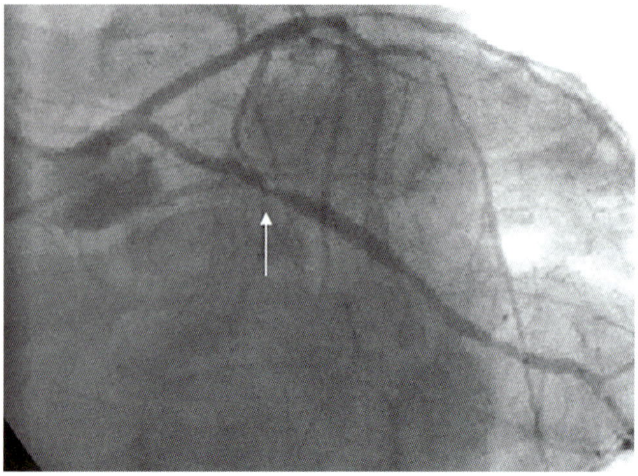

Figure Q18-9

(A) Restenosis rates following balloon angioplasty are equivalent to those following stent placement
(B) Successful PCI is associated with increased longevity of the transplanted heart
(C) The likelihood of restenosis following PCI is reduced with higher doses of antiproliferative immunosuppressant drugs
(D) Restenosis rates following PCI are similar in the setting of transplant arteriopathy and native atherosclerotic disease

18.10 Which one of the following best describes the biologic mechanism of action of paclitaxel for the prevention of restenosis?

(A) Blocks cell cycle progression at the G1- to S-phase transition in vascular smooth muscle cells
(B) Stabilizes microtubule assembly
(C) Enhances microtubule breakdown
(D) Functions as a macrolide antibiotic

18.11 When comparing first- and second-generation DES, which of the following statements is TRUE?

(A) EES are associated with lower rates of angiographic and clinical restenosis compared to sirolimus-eluting stents (SES)
(B) The incidence of stent fractures has decreased significantly with second-generation DES compared to first-generation DES and BMS
(C) Zotarolimus eluting stents (ZES) coated with a polymer that allows a longer duration of drug elution are associated with lower target vessel revascularization rates than ZES preparations with a polymer that results in a shorter duration of release
(D) Cessation of $P2Y_{12}$ inhibitor therapy at 6 months following ZES implantation is associated with greater late loss than cessation at 12 months

18.12 Figure Q18-12 is a frequency distribution curve from a hypothetical trial comparing two stents, "Stent A" and "Stent B." Based on the figure, which one of the following statements is TRUE?

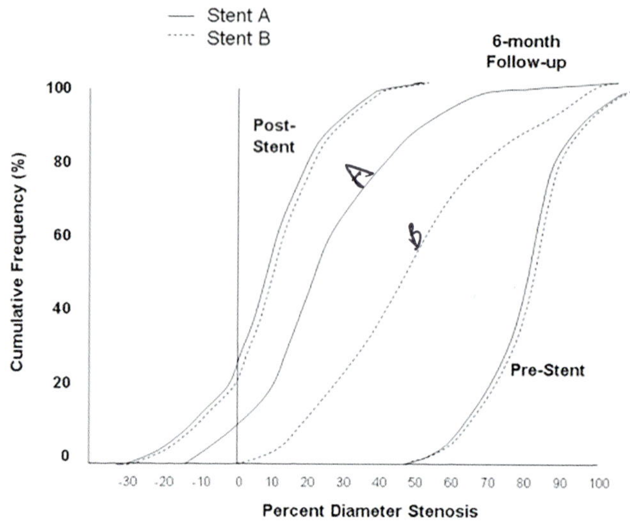

Figure Q18-12

(A) Late loss is greater for Stent B than for Stent A
(B) The incidence of angiographic restenosis, defined as a stenosis severity of ≥50% at 6-month follow-up, is approximately 25% for Stent B
(C) The differences in 6-month restenosis rates between the two stents can be attributed to better acute gain with Stent A
(D) The median stent length was greater for patients treated with Stent A than Stent B

18.13 Which of the following statements regarding the formation of neoatherosclerosis within a stent is NOT true?

(A) Neoatherosclerosis tends to occur earlier following BMS than DES implantation
(B) Optical coherence tomography (OCT) is often able to differentiate neoatherosclerosis from fibrointimal hyperplasia within a stent
(C) Neoatherosclerosis is characterized by lipid-laden macrophages within neointimal tissue
(D) Late stent failure caused by neoatherosclerosis is more likely to present as an acute coronary syndrome (ACS) than stent failure related to fibrointimal hyperplasia

18.14 Which of the following statements regarding the time course of restenosis within BMS is TRUE?

(A) The degree of intimal hyperplasia within a stent usually reaches its peak within the first 3 months following stent implantation
(B) Between 6 months and 3 years following stent implantation, there is often lessening in the degree of luminal narrowing within the stent
(C) Early stent recoil is a phenomenon that often contributes to the development of in-stent restenosis
(D) Patients presenting with in-stent restenosis <3 months following initial stent placement have a more favorable response to repeat PCI than patients presenting with restenosis at a later time

18.15 A 76-year-old man with diabetes mellitus, hypertension, and renal insufficiency (glomerular filtration rate [GFR] = 46 mL/min) presented with an acute anterior wall STEMI and underwent successful primary PCI with placement of a 3.0 × 18 mm ZES in his proximal left anterior descending (LAD) artery. Angiography at the time of the myocardial infarction (MI) also demonstrated a 70% proximal stenosis of a large obtuse marginal (OM)-1 branch and proximal occlusion of a dominant RCA, which received brisk collateral flow from the LCx artery. A postdischarge thallium single-photon emission-computed tomography (SPECT) scan showed mild inferior ischemia, a small anterior fixed perfusion defect, no transient ischemic dilation, and a left ventricular ejection fraction (LVEF) of 50%. He was treated medically and completed phase-2 cardiac rehabilitation without angina. Four months following his MI, he experienced two episodes of chest discomfort at rest of similar quality and location as the pain associated with his MI. He was hospitalized and his troponin I level was elevated at 1.1 ng/mL. A coronary angiogram demonstrated diffuse severe in-stent restenosis of the LAD (Fig. Q18-15). There was no change in the severity of the LCx or RCA disease, and the LVEF had decreased to 40% with hypokinesis of the anterolateral and apical segments. Which of the following is the preferred treatment strategy at this time?

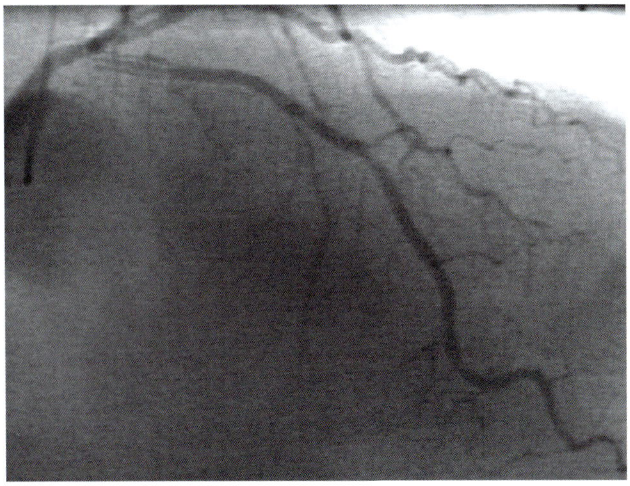

Figure Q18-15

(A) Treatment of the in-stent lesion in the LAD with a DES and continued medical management of the LCx and RCA disease
(B) Treatment of the LAD, LCx, and RCA lesions with DES
(C) Augmented medical therapy with provisional DES placement in the LAD if his anginal symptoms are refractory to medications
(D) Referral for coronary artery bypass grafting surgery (CABG)

18.16 Which of the following patterns of BMS in-stent restenosis is associated with the highest likelihood of recurrent restenosis following repeat percutaneous intervention? The white lines in Figure Q18-16 indicate the edges of the stents.

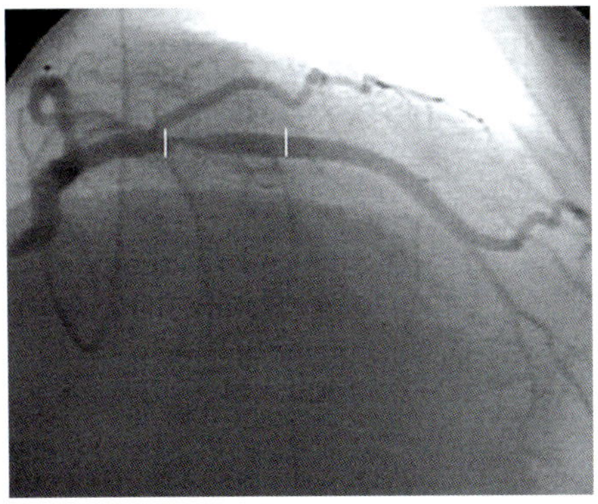

A

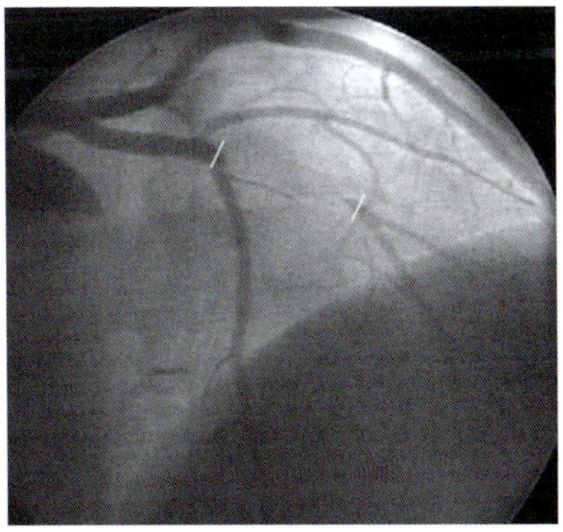

B

Figure Q18-16

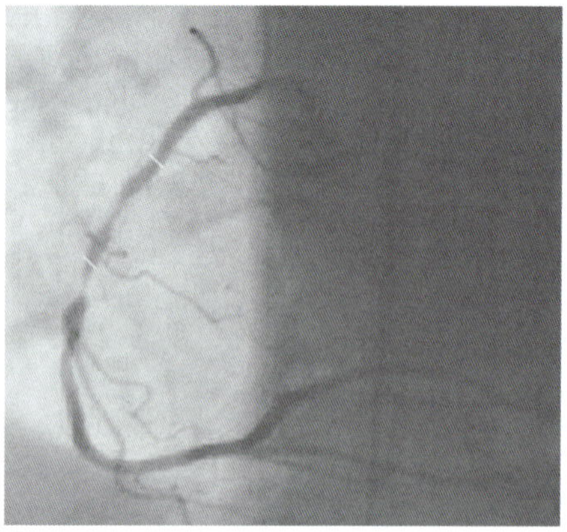

C

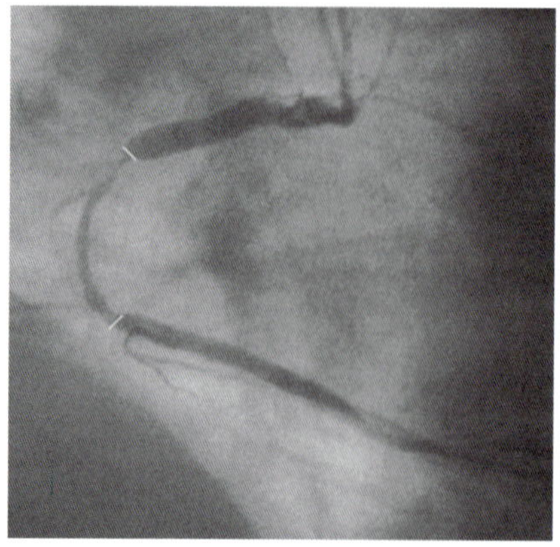

D

(A) Panel A
(B) Panel B
(C) Panel C
(D) Panel D

18.17 Which of the following statements regarding the biologic characteristics of BMS vs. DES restenosis is TRUE?

(A) On pathologic examination, BMS restenosis is more likely to be associated with organized thrombus and fibrinous material than DES restenosis
(B) Elevated pre-PCI serum inflammatory marker levels such as C-reactive protein are predictive of restenosis following DES, but not BMS, placement
(C) Eosinophil infiltrates, indicative of allergic hypersensitivity, are often observed within restenotic tissue surrounding struts of DES but not BMS
(D) Late development of neointimal hyperplasia ≥1 year following stent placement has been observed in multiple studies of DES placement

18.18 Compared to guidance by angiography alone, is intravascular ultrasound (IVUS) guidance following stent implantation associated with reductions in TVR rates following BMS placement, DES placement, both, or neither?

	Lower TVR post-BMS	Lower TVR post-DES
(A)	Yes	Yes
(B)	Yes	No
(C)	No	Yes
(D)	No	No

18.19 Which one of the following modifications to stent design had been associated with increased rates of in-stent restenosis?

(A) Use of a slotted tubular rather than a coil design
(B) Use of a cobalt chromium platform instead of stainless steel
(C) Heparin coating
(D) Gold coating
(E) Thinner stent struts

18.20 Which of the following statements is TRUE regarding restenosis following balloon valvotomy used for the treatment of valvular heart disease?

(A) Balloon aortic valvuloplasty is associated with very high (>80%) rates of restenosis at 1 year in both adults with calcific aortic stenosis and children with noncalcific congenital aortic stenosis
(B) Balloon valvotomy for discrete aortic subvalvular or supervalvular membranes is associated with lower rates of restenosis than for valvular aortic stenosis and is indicated in younger individuals without concomitant valvular aortic stenosis
(C) Pulmonary balloon valvotomy is associated with restenosis rates in the 20% to 40% range at 10-year follow-up
(D) A lower echo score is predictive of both lower procedural complication rates and a lower risk of restenosis following mitral balloon valvotomy

18.21 Which of the following clinical and angiographic risk factors is NOT associated with resistant in-stent restenosis, defined as multiply recurrent in-stent restenosis of the same coronary lesion after multiple interventions?

(A) Lesion calcification
(B) Diffuse (rather than focal) pattern of restenosis
(C) Bifurcation lesion
(D) Chronic kidney disease

18.22 Which of the saphenous vein graft (SVG) lesions depicted below is associated with the lowest likelihood of restenosis following BMS placement (Fig. Q18-22)?

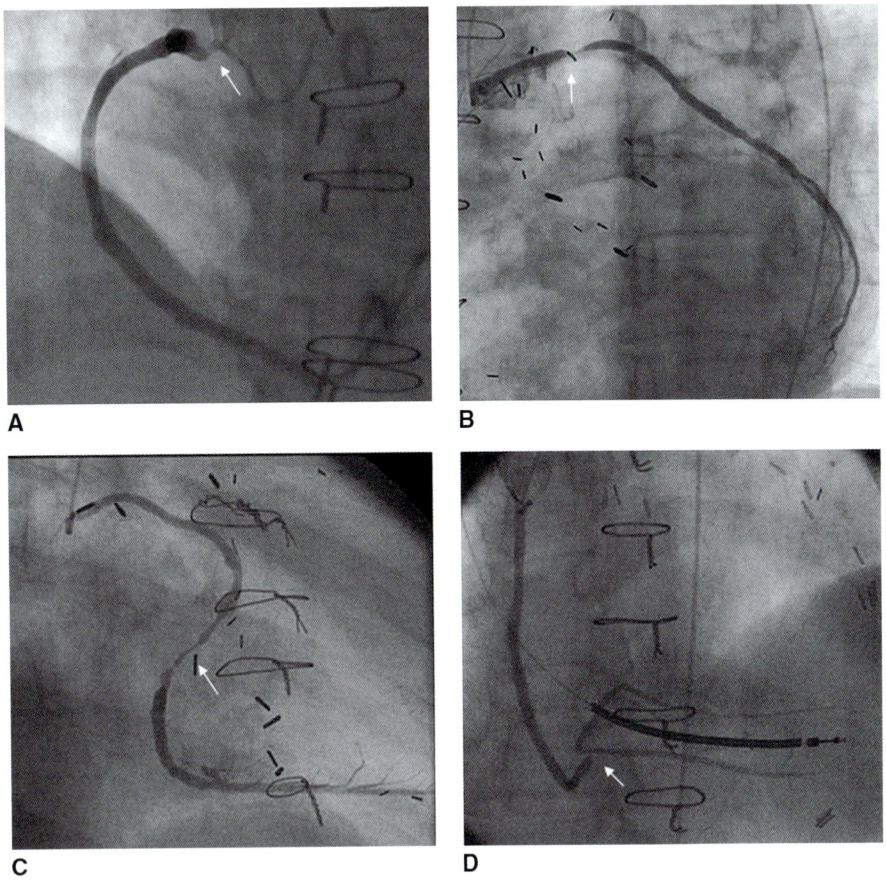

Figure Q18-22

(A) Panel A
(B) Panel B
(C) Panel C
(D) Panel D

18.23 Which statement is true regarding the use of DES placement vs. vascular brachytherapy for the treatment of restenosis within a BMS?

(A) Unlike DES, intracoronary brachytherapy is ineffective for treatment of diffuse (>30 mm in length) in-stent restenosis
(B) Brachytherapy is associated with similar efficacy as DES placement for the treatment of in-stent restenosis
(C) "Geographic mismatch" is a potential mode of failure for both DES and vascular brachytherapy
(D) There is a 4% to 5% incidence of late aneurysm formation following coronary brachytherapy for in-stent restenosis, which is substantially greater than that observed following DES

18.24 Which of the following statements is true regarding restenosis following carotid artery stenting?

(A) Randomized trials of carotid stenting vs. carotid endarterectomy have not shown higher rates of repeat TVR among patients treated with carotid stenting
(B) Among individuals with asymptomatic carotid artery in-stent restenosis of >70% in severity, clinical trials have demonstrated reduced stroke rates with repeat stenting compared to medical therapy
(C) Minimizing residual stenosis during carotid stenting by aggressive postdilation (balloon to artery ratio 1.1:1) is the preferred approach to reduce the likelihood of subsequent restenosis
(D) Restenosis following carotid bifurcation stenting is more likely when self-expanding stents are used instead of balloon-expandable stents

18.25 A 68-year-old woman with diabetes, ongoing tobacco use, and prior CABG underwent placement of a BMS in a SVG to the distal RCA following a non-STEMI. Nine months later, she presents with unstable angina, and angiography is performed demonstrating in-stent restenosis. Her previous and current angiographic images are as shown below (Fig. Q18-25). Which of the following clinical features is NOT a predictor of restenosis in this patient?

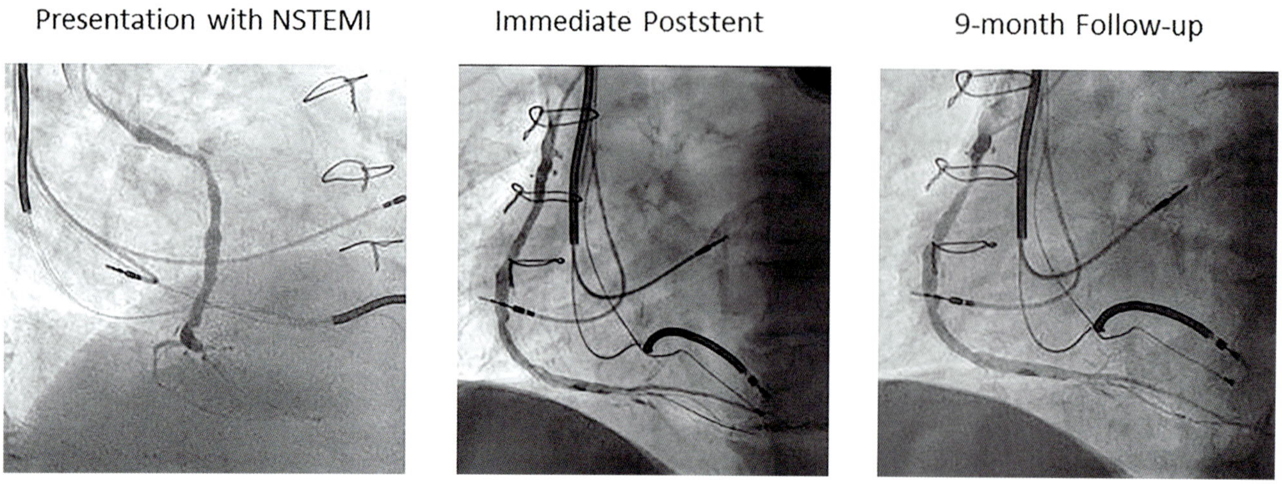

Figure Q18-25 (Courtesy of Craig Narins.)

(A) SVG location
(B) Female gender
(C) ACS
(D) Ongoing cigarette smoking

18.26 Which statement is NOT true regarding the mechanism of action of sirolimus and its analogues everolimus and zotarolimus?

(A) Sirolimus and its analogues bind to the mTOR protein, which functions as a kinase that regulates cellular growth
(B) Sirolimus exhibits antifungal, antibiotic, and anti-inflammatory properties
(C) The "limus" drugs result in arrest of the cell cycle at the G1 phase
(D) Sirolimus and its analogues inhibit vascular smooth muscle cell proliferation rather than cellular migration

18.27 A 71-year-old man underwent implantation of a ZES in his mid-to-distal LAD for treatment of unstable angina. He returns 9 months later with a non-STEMI, and angiography is performed as demonstrated in Figure Q18-27. Which of the following statements regarding late stent fracture following DES implantation is TRUE?

(A) The incidence of late stent fracture is <1%
(B) The probability of stent fracture is significantly greater for stents placed in the LAD artery than for stents placed in the LCx or RCA
(C) The presence of a stent fracture is associated with increased rates of both in-stent restenosis and target lesion revascularization (TLR)
(D) Shorter stent length is a risk factor for stent fracture

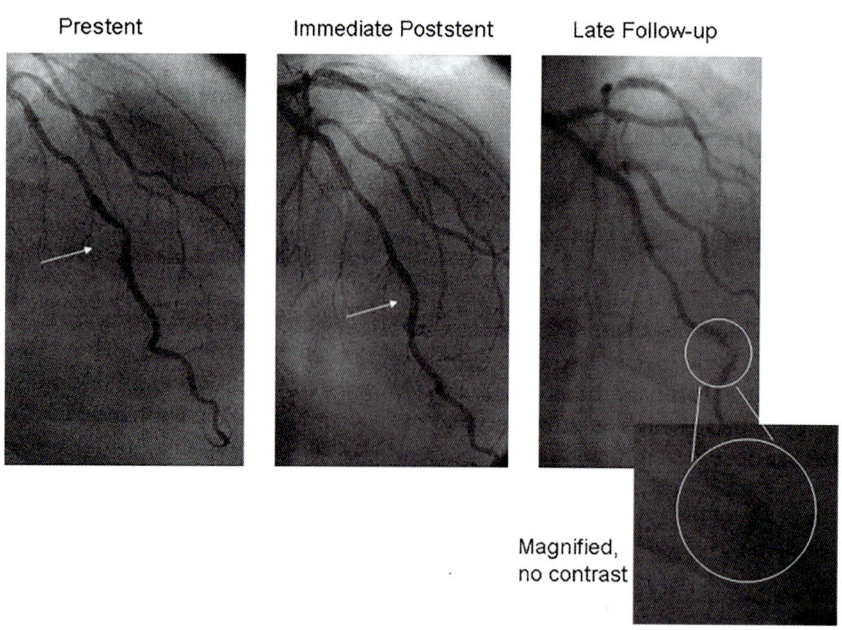

Figure Q18-27

18.28 A 63-year-old man with hypertension, dyslipidemia, and ongoing tobacco use underwent stenting of his left common iliac and superficial femoral arteries 9 months earlier. He presents to your office with ischemic rest pain of the left foot. The left femoral pulse is easily palpable, but the left dorsalis pedis and posterior tibial pulses are absent. The left ankle-brachial index is 0.40, and Doppler analysis of the left superficial femoral artery stent demonstrates an end systolic velocity of 588 cm/s and an end diastolic velocity of 117 cm/s. A subsequently obtained angiographic image of the left superficial femoral artery is shown (Fig. Q18-28), and PCB angioplasty is performed. Regarding the use of PCB angioplasty for treatment of femoral-popliteal level arterial disease, which of the following statements is TRUE?

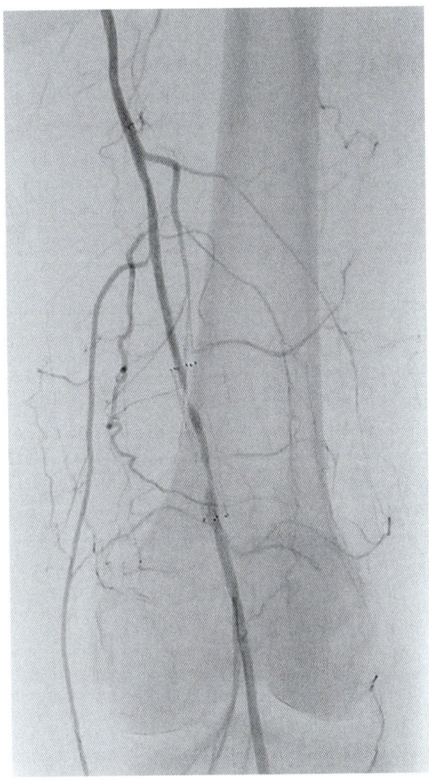

Figure Q18-28 (Courtesy of Craig Narins.)

(A) Compared to standard balloon angioplasty for treatment of de novo disease, PCB angioplasty is associated with lower rates of angiographic restenosis (late loss and binary restenosis) but similar rates of clinical restenosis (TLR)

(B) Higher-dose paclitaxel delivery is associated with lower rates of clinical restenosis than lower-dose delivery

(C) PCB angioplasty is more effective than standard balloon angioplasty for preventing restenosis for shorter (≤60 mm), but not longer, de novo lesion lengths

(D) PCB angioplasty is associated with lower rates of TLR when used for de novo lesions, but not when used for treatment of in-stent restenosis

18.29 A 69-year-old woman developed recurrent low threshold angina 4 months following BMS placement in her mid-LAD coronary artery. Coronary angiography demonstrated diffuse in-stent restenosis, and IVUS interrogation of the stent was performed. Which of the following statements regarding the IVUS image in Figure Q18-29 is TRUE?

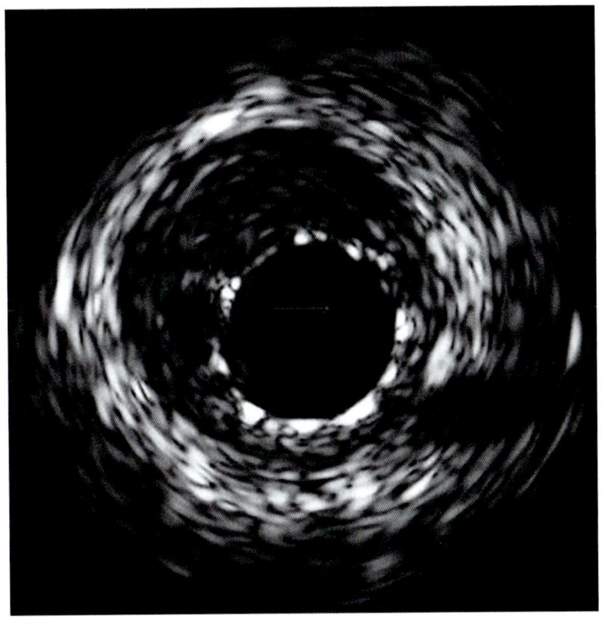

Figure Q18-29

(A) Incomplete apposition of several stent struts is apparent

(B) Heavy vessel wall calcification is present

(C) The stent is well apposed but under-expanded relative to the size of the vessel

(D) Negative vascular remodeling is the likely cause of restenosis in this patient

18.30 A 23-year-old man presents for evaluation of refractory hypertension. On examination, an ejection click is present and there is a systolic murmur heard under the left scapula. A femoral artery pulse delay is detected and the ankle-brachial index is 0.80 bilaterally. A transthoracic echocardiogram

(TTE) demonstrates a bicuspid aortic valve without significant stenosis or regurgitation and confirms a coarctation of the aorta distal to the origin of the left subclavian artery with a peak velocity of 3.1 m/s across the stenosis. After a "heart team" evaluation is undertaken, the patient undergoes successful stent placement with elimination of the pressure gradient across the coarctation; however, 1 year later, he returns with recurrent hypertension and a velocity of 2.5 m/s across the stent on echo. Which of the following statements is TRUE regarding recoarctation (restenosis) following percutaneous or surgical treatment of aortic coarctation?

(A) Recoarctation is more common in children than adults following successful angioplasty
(B) Indications for repeat revascularization for recoarctation include a resting gradient across the coaction of ≥20 mm Hg if symptomatic and ≥30 mm Hg if asymptomatic
(C) Surgical correction is the procedure of choice if recoarctation develops following catheter-based therapy
(D) Covered stent placement for coarctation is associated with lower rates of restenosis and localized pseudoaneurysm formation compared to noncovered stent placement

ANSWERS AND EXPLANATIONS

18.1 Answer D. Most of the clinical and anatomical predictors of restenosis following BMS placement also serve as risk factors for restenosis after DES implantation. Such variables include diabetes mellitus, ostial or SVG lesion location, prior restenosis, smaller reference vessel diameter, smaller postintervention minimum luminal diameter, longer lesions, and greater total stent length (Dangas GD, et al. *J Am Coll Cardiol* 2010;56(23):1897-1907). Comparison of a bioabsorbable polymer-coated everolimus-eluting coronary stent and a durable polymer-coated everolimus stent was undertaken in the randomized EVOLVE II trial and demonstrated no significant differences in TVR or stent thrombosis rates between the stents (Kereiakes DJ, et al. *Circ Cardiovasc Interv* 2015;8(4):e002372).

18.2 Answer A. In a study of 298 in-stent restenosis lesions that underwent IVUS analysis, restenosis within BMS presented significantly later after stent implantation and was associated with greater volumes of neointimal hyperplasia but shorter lesion lengths compared to restenosis within DES. No differences were noted in the completeness of strut apposition between stent types. Longer stent length is a well-described risk factor for restenosis following both BMS and DES placement (Goto K, et al. *Am J Cardiol* 2015;116(9):1351-1357).

18.3 Answer C. Inflammation plays a key role in the pathogenesis of coronary restenosis. Angioplasty-induced injury leads to deendothelialization of the vascular wall leading to localized platelet and fibrin deposition, which in turn promotes leukocyte and monocyte recruitment via expression of multiple surface adhesion molecules and release of chemokines. This inflammatory response promotes proliferation and migration of vascular smooth muscle cells and fibroblasts from the vessel media, leading to the development of the neointimal tissue that, when excessive, is ultimately responsible for restenosis. Unlike atherosclerotic plaque, which typically demonstrates complex features such as lipid pools, necrotic cores, fibrous caps, and often focal calcification, restenotic lesions usually exhibit more homogenous fibrohyperplastic morphology. For this reason, acute plaque rupture with thrombotic vessel occlusion is a much less common presentation with restenosis than atherosclerosis (Costa MA, et al. *Circulation* 2005;111(17):2257-2273). Although still poorly understood, genetic susceptibility appears to play a role in the development of restenosis and may ultimately allow for individually targeted antirestenosis therapy (Takahashi M. *Arterioscler Thromb Vasc Biol* 2009;29:1407-1408).

18.4 Answer A. A wide variety of animal models have been created to assess the pathophysiology, prevention, and treatment of restenosis. Animal models have provided valuable insights regarding the potential safety, efficacy, and mechanism of action of perspective antirestenosis therapies; however, these models are also associated with limitations in their ability to replicate human atherosclerosis and restenosis. The histologic appearance and composition of restenotic and atherosclerotic lesions found in humans differ to varying degrees from that found in all animal models. Likewise, myriad metabolic, physiologic, and hemodynamic differences between animals and humans can affect response to therapeutic agents, and there are numerous examples therapies that have inhibited neointimal hyperplasia in animals but failed to demonstrate efficacy in human clinical trials. While various animal models have been developed, no single model can replicate all features of human restenosis. For example, even though smooth muscle cell proliferation and migration from media to intima is a prominent feature of all animal models of restenosis, the degree of neointima formation in response to arterial injury varies widely based on species, as many animals (including mice, pigs, and dogs) rarely form more than a thin layer of hyperplastic tissue. Likewise, no model can replicate the complex phenotypes associated with clinical conditions that predispose to restenosis, such as diabetes or metabolic syndrome (Perkins LE. *Vet Pathol* 2010;47(1):58-76).

18.5 Answer D. ISAR DESIRE-3 was a randomized trial that compared the efficacy of PEB angioplasty, PES placement, and noncoated balloon angioplasty among 402 patients with in-stent restenosis following prior DES placement. At 6- to 8-month angiographic follow-up, patients who underwent PEB and PES demonstrated similar rates of angiographic restenosis (27% and 24%, respectively), while the angiographic restenosis rate among patients treated with balloon angioplasty was significantly greater at 57%. There were no significant differences among treatment groups in the frequency of death, MI, or stent thrombosis (Byrne RA, et al. *Lancet* 2013;381(9865):461–467).

In the PEPCAD China ISR study, 220 patients with in-stent restenosis following prior DES placement were randomized to PEB vs. PES, and at 9-month angiographic follow-up, the PEB group demonstrated similar late lumen loss and clinical event rates compared to the PES group (Xu B, et al. *JACC Cardiovasc Interv* 2014;7(2):204–211). Two randomized trials (RIBS IV and RIBS V), however, comparing the use of a second-generation (everolimus) DES to PEB angioplasty for the treatment of DES in-stent restenosis suggested clinical superiority of the everolimus stent over PEB angioplasty (Alfonso F, et al. *Am J Cardiol* 2016;117(4):546–554). A meta-analysis of 7,474 patients with DES in-stent restenosis enrolled in randomized or observational studies, however, demonstrated no significant differences in TLR rates between drug-eluting balloon and DES placement but significantly higher rates among those treated with standard balloon angioplasty. Other clinical end points including MI, stent thrombosis, and mortality were similar between the different treatment modalities (Goel SS, et al. *Catheter Cardiovasc Interv* 2016;87(6):1080–1091).

18.6 Answer E. Late loss is the key angiographic parameter used to quantitate the degree of intimal hyperplasia at the site of PCI between the time of the procedure and subsequent angiographic follow-up. Late loss within a stent is defined as the in-stent minimum lumen diameter immediately following stent placement minus the in-stent minimum lumen diameter on late follow-up angiography. In this example, late loss is calculated as:

3.40 − 2.98 = 0.42 mm.

18.7 Answer A. The amount of late loss following angioplasty can depend on the degree of acute gain achieved during the procedure. For example, using a stent that is oversized for a vessel may result in greater acute gain in luminal diameter than a properly sized stent but may trigger an exaggerated hyperplastic response resulting in excessive late loss. Late loss can be normalized for acute gain by using the late loss index, which is calculated as late loss divided by acute gain (Mauri L, et al. *Circulation* 2005;111(3):321–327). In this example, the late loss index can be calculated as:

$$\frac{\text{Late loss}}{\text{Acute gain}} = \frac{3.40 - 2.98}{3.40 - 1.08} = \frac{0.42}{2.32} = 0.18.$$

18.8 Answer D. Compared to stand-alone balloon angioplasty, stent implantation is associated with an exaggerated vascular smooth muscle cell proliferative response and, consequently, an increased degree of neointima formation. Stent placement, however, essentially eliminates long-term negative remodeling of the vessel wall, which typically more than compensates for the exaggerated proliferative response and results in the reduced frequency of restenosis observed with stenting compared to balloon angioplasty. Restenotic tissue obtained following balloon angioplasty demonstrates fewer smooth muscle cells and greater collagen deposition than tissue recovered from stents that have developed restenosis.

18.9 Answer C. Transplant arteriopathy affects about 50% of individuals who undergo orthotopic heart transplantation and represents a major cause of morbidity and mortality among transplant recipients. While transplant arteriopathy is often diffuse in nature and therefore not amenable to revascularization, PCI is associated with high procedural success rates when used to treat lesions that are more focal in nature. In-stent restenosis, however, occurs with greater frequency following treatment of transplant arteriopathy than following treatment of atherosclerotic disease. As with native vessel coronary disease, balloon angioplasty in the setting of transplant arteriopathy is associated with higher restenosis rates than BMS, and DES placement appears to result in lower recurrence rates than BMS placement. Nevertheless, as a result of continued disease progression outside of the treated segment, PCI has not been shown to ultimately increase longevity of transplanted hearts afflicted by coronary arteriopathy. Several medical therapies have been associated with reduced restenosis rates and improved graft survival following PCI for transplant arteriopathy, including higher antiproliferative immunosuppressant dosing, early reduction of steroid dosing, and use of statins.

18.10 Answer B. Microtubules are a fundamental component of the mitotic spindle apparatus and play essential roles in other cellular functions, including migration and growth factor signaling. The assembly and disassembly of microtubules within a cell are maintained in a well-regulated equilibrium. Paclitaxel produces its antiproliferative effects by stabilizing microtubules, thus shifting the dynamic balance toward assembly, which consequently interrupts cellular division. The "limus" class of drugs impairs vascular smooth muscle cell division by blocking cell cycle progression at the G1- to S-phase transition (Garg S, et al. *J Am Coll Cardiol* 2010;56(10 Suppl):S1–S42).

18.11 Answer C. Several randomized trials have demonstrated higher rates of late loss and/or target vessel failure following PES compared to EES placement (SPIRIT III, SPIRIT IV, and COMPARE trials); however, rates of angiographic and clinical restenosis appear similar between EES and SES (SORT OUT IV and RESET trials). Interestingly, while second-generation DES have brought about a reduction in the frequency of stent thrombosis, the second-generation ZES has been associated with greater late lumen loss and TLR rates than the first-generation SES (SORT OUT III and ENDEAVOR III trials). In a large meta-analysis of 76 randomized trials comparing BMS and multiple types of DES, TVR rates consistently were lower for all DES than BMS, but the magnitude of reduction varied between DES type, with EES, SES, and ZES-Resolute associated with lower TVR rates than PES and the non-Resolute iteration of ZES (Bangalore S, et al. *Circulation* 2012;125(23):2873–2891). In a study examining the clinical implications of drug release kinetics, ZES coated with a polymer that leads to a longer duration of drug elution was associated with a more favorable late lumen loss profile than a preparation with a shorter duration of release. Duration of $P2Y_{12}$ inhibitor use has not been associated with angiographic restenosis. The incidence of stent fractures has not decreased with the introduction of currently available second-generation DES (Goto K, et al. *Am J Cardiol* 2015;116(9):1351–1357).

18.12 Answer A. Frequency distribution curves are used to evaluate the immediate and late angiographic results of competing therapies in clinical trials of restenosis. The median acute luminal gain for each therapy can be determined by measuring the distance between the prestent and poststent curve for each stent on a horizontal line drawn at the 50% mark on the *Y* (cumulative frequency) axis. In the example, this distance is similar for Stents A and B. Late lumen loss can be determined by comparing the distance between the poststent and the 6-month follow-up curve for each stent, which in the example is greater for Stent B. The angiographic restenosis rate for each therapy can be determined by drawing a vertical line upward from the 50% diameter stenosis point on the *X* (percent diameter stenosis) axis. The point on the *Y*-axis that corresponds to where this vertical line intersects the 6-month follow-up curve for each stent reveals the percentage of individuals who had a ≤50% stenosis at 6-month follow-up. The frequency of angiographic restenosis for that particular stent is determined by subtracting this number from 100. In the example, the frequency of angiographic restenosis is approximately 10% for Stent A and 40% for Stent B. The frequency distribution curve does not contain information regarding stent length.

18.13 Answer A. Neoatherosclerosis within a stent is a process that has been observed late after BMS and DES implantation and is characterized by the same pathologic stigmata as de novo atherosclerosis, including the presence of lipid-laden macrophages, a thin fibrous cap, and a necrotic core (Finn AV, et al. *Circ Cardiovasc Interv* 2012;5(1):6–9). Compared to in-stent restenosis related to fibrointimal thickening, which tends to present clinically with progressive stable angina, neoatherosclerosis is more prone to plaque rupture and clinical presentation with an ACS or stent thrombosis. Neoatherosclerosis can often be differentiated from neointimal hyperplasia by OCT or IVUS imaging. For reasons that are incompletely understood, neoatherosclerosis tends to occur much earlier following DES compared to BMS implantation (Nakazawa G, et al. *J Am Coll Cardiol* 2011;57(11):1314–1322).

18.14 Answer B. In-stent restenosis occurs following BMS implantation typically within the first 6 months following stent implantation. After 6 months, serial angiographic follow-up studies have demonstrated a gradual spontaneous improvement in the degree of luminal narrowing within the stent (spontaneous regression) (Kimura T, et al. *N Engl J Med* 1996;334(9):561–566). Late stent recoil, while occasionally noted on serial IVUS imaging, is an uncommon occurrence. Patients presenting with restenosis early (within the first 3 months following stent implantation) have an increased risk of recurrent restenosis following repeat PCI compared to patients who present later (Klugherz BD, et al. *Am J Cardiol* 2000;85(12):1427–1431).

18.15 Answer D. While repeat PCI remains the most common treatment approach for symptomatic in-stent restenosis, other strategies including medical therapy or CABG should also be considered based on patient and lesion specific factors. The patient in this question presented with a non-STEMI related to severe in-stent restenosis of the LAD in the setting of multivessel CAD, diabetes mellitus, and reduced left ventricular systolic function. Because routine early invasive strategy is associated with a decreased incidence of major adverse cardiac events (MACE) compared to a conservative approach among patients presenting with ACS, medical management is not the preferred treatment option for this individual (Mehta SR, et al. *N Engl J Med* 2009;360(21):2165–2175). Regarding mode of revascularization, results from the randomized FREEDOM trial indicate that bypass surgery is associated with reduced rates of death and MI compared to DES placement among patients with diabetes and multivessel disease, such as the patient presented here (Farkouh ME, et al. *N Engl J Med* 2012;367(25):2375–2384).

18.16 Answer B. The patterns of in-stent restenosis demonstrated in the figure are (a) focal; (b) total occlusion; (c) diffuse proliferative, in which the restenotic lesion extends beyond the stent margin; and (d) diffuse intrastent. Mehran et al. devised a classification system for BMS restenosis based on the likelihood of late patency following repeat percutaneous intervention. In their analysis of 288 in-stent lesions treated with PCI, the focal pattern was associated with the lowest need for repeat revascularization (19%), followed by the diffuse intrastent (35%), diffuse proliferative (50%), and total occlusion (82%) patterns (Mehran R, et al. *Circulation* 1999;100(18):1872–1878). When in-stent restenosis occurs within a DES, the probability of recurrent restenosis following therapy is likewise significantly greater when the initial pattern of in-stent restenosis is diffuse rather than focal (Cosgrave J, et al. *J Am Coll Cardiol* 2006;47(12):2399–2404).

18.17 Answer D. Histologically, DES restenosis is more likely to demonstrate evidence of organized thrombus and fibrin deposition within the stent than BMS restenosis, which typically reveals a more homogenous hypercellular neointima. The tendency toward thrombus deposition within DES may reflect the lack of protective neointima that is nearly ubiquitous following BMS placement. While vascular inflammation plays a pivotal role in the pathogenesis of restenosis following both BMS and DES implantation, serum markers of inflammation, most notably CRP, appear predictive of BMS, but not DES, restenosis (Niccoli G, et al. *J Am Coll Cardiol* 2010;56(22):1783–1793). It is hypothesized that the high local concentrations of antiproliferative drug associated with DES placement may overcome the enhanced systemic inflammatory state reflected by elevated serum CRP levels that otherwise would predispose to restenosis. A localized allergic-type hypersensitivity reaction to stent materials (metal, polymer), evidenced by the finding of eosinophil infiltrates in restenotic tissue adjacent to stent struts following both bare metal and drug-eluting stenting, is also thought to play a potential role in the development of in-stent restenosis. Eosinophil infiltrates are not seen after stand-alone balloon angioplasty. Late development of neointimal hyperplasia 2 to 4 years following DES implantation has been observed in several studies employing serial angiography and IVUS. Despite this "catch-up" phenomenon, the degree of late intimal hyperplasia has not been sufficient to adversely affect the advantages of DES over BMS with respect to TLR rates (Dangas G, et al. *J Am Coll Cardiol* 2010;56(23):1897–1907).

18.18 Answer A. IVUS guidance, presumably by allowing for optimization of stent sizing, is associated with reductions in measures of restenosis following both BMS and DES placement. A meta-analysis of seven randomized trials (2,193 patients) comparing IVUS and angiographic guidance following BMS implantation demonstrated significant reductions in both angiographic restenosis and repeat revascularization associated with IVUS (Parise H, et al. *Am J Cardiol* 2011;107(3): 374–382). Likewise, a meta-analysis of eight randomized studies examining IVUS guidance following DES placement among 3,192 patients showed a significant reduction in ischemia-driven repeat TLR with IVUS compared to angiographic guidance (Elgendy IY, et al. *Circ Cardiovasc Interv* 2016;9(4):e003700).

18.19 Answer D. Randomized trial results show that the use of stents with thinner struts is associated with a significant reduction of angiographic and clinical restenosis (Pache J, et al. *J Am Coll Cardiol* 2003;41(8):1283–1288). Heparin coating has not been shown to affect the likelihood of subsequent in-stent restenosis; likewise, there is no evidence to suggest that the use of cobalt chromium stent platforms is related to higher rates of restenosis than stainless steel. In fact, because the composition of cobalt chromium allows for thinner strut thickness, these stents may be associated with less risk of restenosis. Stents with a coil design, such as the historical Gianturco-Roubin stent, are associated with significantly greater restenosis rates than slotted tubular stents (Lansky AJ, et al. *Circulation* 2000;102(12):1364–1368). Randomized studies have shown that gold coating is associated with higher rates of restenosis than identically designed stents that are not gold coated (Kastrati A, et al. *Circulation* 2000;101(21):2478–2483).

18.20 Answer D. While restenosis is nearly ubiquitous following balloon valvotomy for calcific aortic valve stenosis, it offers much more durable results and is often the procedure of choice for children and young adults with severe noncalcific congenital aortic stenosis. Balloon valvotomy is contraindicated for the treatment of subvalvular or supervalvular aortic stenosis. Pulmonary balloon valvotomy is often the procedure of choice for pulmonic valve stenosis and is associated with late restenosis rates well below 20% in several series. A lower echo score is associated with both lower procedural complication and restenosis rates following mitral balloon valvotomy (Warnes CA, et al. *J Am Coll Cardiol* 2008;52(23):e143–e263).

18.21 Answer B. Recurrent in-stent restenosis following multiple interventions is an uncommon problem but is still encountered in the era of DES. The ideal treatment approach, especially among patients with multiple layers of stent already present, is unknown. Techniques that do not involve placement of additional stents (i.e., brachytherapy and drug-eluting balloons) are not readily available in the United States at present. In a retrospective analysis of 276 patients with resistant in-stent restenosis, a high frequency of diabetes and chronic kidney disease (CKD) were identified. The majority of lesions were calcified, and while 77% of lesions were classified as focal in nature, the angiographic pattern (focal vs. diffuse) was not associated with the likelihood of multiple recurrent target lesion failure following repeat percutaneous intervention (Theodoropoulos K, et al. *Catheter Cardiovasc Interv* 2016;88(5):777–785).

18.22 Answer D. The likelihood of restenosis is significantly greater when PCI is performed to treat lesions located at the aorto-ostium or within the body of SVGs compared to lesions at the distal anastomosis (Platko W, et al. *J Am Coll Cardiol* 1989;14(7):1645–1650). This difference is likely a result of differences in plaque composition. Smaller trials have suggested that DES are superior to BMS for the prevention of restenosis following vein graft PCI (Brilakis ES, et al. *J Am Coll Cardiol* 2009;53(11):919–928) and that second-generation DES are associated with improved mortality rates following vein graft intervention compared to first-generation DES or BMS (Iqbal J, et al. *Circ Cardiovasc Interv* 2017;10:e004457).

18.23 Answer C. Intracoronary brachytherapy represented the first effective therapy for in-stent restenosis with documented efficacy for the treatment of both focal and diffuse in-stent restenosis within native vessels and SVGs. Because of better ease of use and superior outcomes for prevention of recurrent in-stent restenosis, DES placement has now replaced brachytherapy as first-line therapy for the treatment of in-stent restenosis within a BMS, and brachytherapy remains available only at limited locations in the United States. "Geographic mismatch," in which recurrent restenosis following brachytherapy or DES develops at the edge of the treated segment, can occur when either the brachytherapy catheter or DES fails to completely cover the length of the vessel segment injured by balloon predilation. Late aneurysm formation is a rare (<1% incidence) complication of both DES placement and brachytherapy.

18.24 Answer A. In the SAPPHIRE Trial, 334 patients with severe symptomatic or asymptomatic carotid stenosis who had features that placed them at increased surgical risk were randomized to undergo carotid stenting or endarterectomy. At 1 year, carotid stenting was noninferior to carotid endarterectomy with respect to the composite primary end point of stroke, MI, or death; however, repeat carotid revascularization occurred in fewer patients treated with stenting vs. endarterectomy (0.6% vs. 4.3%; $p = 0.04$) (Yadav J, et al. *N Engl J Med* 2004;351(15):1493–1501). In the randomized CREST trial, restenosis or reocclusion rates at 2 years were not significantly different among patients randomized to carotid stenting vs. endarterectomy (6.0% vs. 6.3%, respectively) (Lal BK, et al. *Lancet Neurol* 2012:11(9);755–763). The preferred treatment choice for carotid in-stent restenosis remains uncertain, especially for asymptomatic patients, and while repeat angioplasty or stenting is often performed in clinical practice, it remains uncertain if this approach is associated with better (or worse) clinical outcomes than medical therapy. Because restenosis is uncommon following carotid stenting and the use of aggressive postdilation following stent deployment is associated with an increased risk of procedural stroke, practice guidelines advocate avoiding the use of oversized balloons for this purpose. Balloon-expandable stents are not used for carotid bifurcation stenting given the superficial location of the carotid bifurcation with the possibility of the stent kinking or deformation if subjected to external trauma.

18.25 Answer D. Clinical and angiographic risk factors for in-stent restenosis following BMS placement include SVG location, ostial lesion location, female gender, nonsmoking status, diabetes mellitus, ACS, a lesion length >20 mm, smaller vessel diameter, prior PCI, multiple stents, and ACC/AHA type C lesion classification.

18.26 Answer D. Sirolimus (also known as rapamycin) was discovered in the 1970s and is a product of the bacteria *Streptomyces hygroscopicus*. It binds to and inhibits the mechanistic target of rapamycin (mTOR) protein, also known as the FK506-binding protein 12-rapamycin-associated protein 1 (FRAP1), which is highly conserved among eukaryotic cells. The mTOR protein functions as a serine/threonine protein kinase that is integral to cellular survival and growth. Blockade of mTOR ultimately results in cell-cycle arrest at the G_1/S phase. The "limus" drugs are thought to block restenosis by inhibiting vascular smooth muscle cell proliferation and migration and through their potent anti-inflammatory effects (Garg S, et al. *J Am Coll Cardiol* 2010;56(10 Suppl):S1–S42).

18.27 Answer C. Late stent fracture is more common than previously recognized and appears to represent an important risk factor for in-stent restenosis. In a meta-analysis of eight studies that included a total of <5,000 patients who underwent DES placement, the mean incidence of late stent fracture was 4.0%, with a range of 0.8% to 8.4% among the individual studies (Chakravarty T, et al. *Am J Cardiol* 2010;106(8):1075–1080). Compared to intact stents, stent fracture was associated with significantly increased incidences of angiographic in-stent restenosis (38.0% vs. 8.2%, $p < 0.0001$) and TLR (17.2% vs. 5.6%, $p < 0.0001$). Stent fracture was significantly more common in the RCA than in the LAD or LCx arteries, perhaps, resulting from a tendency toward greater tortuosity and dynamic torsion in the RCA. Longer stent length, overlapping stents, and stent overexpansion were also identified as risk factors for stent fracture. In a large Chinese database of 6,555 patients with 16,482 DES who underwent surveillance angiography, stent fracture was detected in 12% of patients and 22% of stents. Compared to nonfractured stents, stent fracture was associated with higher rates of in-stent restenosis (42.1% vs. 10.7%), TLR (24.8% vs. 6.6%) and definite stent thrombosis (4.6% vs. 1.0%) (Kan J, et al. *JACC Cardiovasc Interv* 2016;9(11):1115–1123).

18.28 Answer B. Randomized controlled clinical trials have compared PCB to standard balloon angioplasty among patients with symptomatic lower extremity peripheral arterial disease, and most have demonstrated significant reductions in both angiographic and clinical measures of restenosis with use of the paclitaxel-coated balloon. A dose-effect relationship has been demonstrated in which higher doses of paclitaxel are associated with lower degrees of late lumen loss (Katsanos K, et al. *J Endovasc Ther* 2016;23(2):356–370). Trials examining treatment of in-stent restenosis have likewise shown superiority of paclitaxel coated balloons over standard balloon angioplasty (Kinstner CM, et al. *JACC Cardiovasc Interv* 2016;9(13):1386; Krankenberg H, et al. *Circulation* 2015;132(23):2230–2236).

18.29 Answer C. The stent is symmetrically deployed and all of the stent struts appear well apposed to the adjacent intima/neointima; however, the stent is underexpanded relative to the size of the vessel. The stent was likely undersized when initially implanted; however, it is also possible that the stent was appropriately sized when it was deployed 5 months earlier, but the vessel underwent positive remodeling in the interim.

18.30 Answer A. In accordance with current guidelines, coarctation repair is indicated for symptomatic or asymptomatic individuals when the peak instantaneous pressure gradient is ≥20 mm Hg, or if collateral vessels are detected (Warnes CA, et al. *Circulation* 2008,118(23):e714–e833). Catheter-based therapy (angioplasty or stenting) is currently the procedure of choice for the treatment of recoarctation, although treatment should be individualized and directed by a heart team approach. Recoarctation is more common among children than adults following balloon angioplasty. One randomized trial compared covered and bare stents in 120 adolescent and adult patients with discrete coarctation lesions and reported no differences in the incidence of recoarctation or pseudoaneurysm at follow-up (Sohrabi B, et al. *JACC Cardiovasc Interv* 2014;7(4):416).

19 Orbital and Rotational Atherectomy, Cutting and Scoring Balloon Angioplasty, and Laser

Robert J. Applegate

QUESTIONS

19.1 Which of the following is TRUE with respect to rotational atherectomy and restenosis?

(A) When compared with balloon angioplasty in randomized clinical trials, restenosis is lower with rotational atherectomy
(B) No randomized clinical trial has shown reduced restenosis rates with rotational atherectomy
(C) Adjunctive use of rotational atherectomy before coronary stenting is associated with lower restenosis rates compared to the use of stenting alone
(D) Restenosis is lower with rotational atherectomy in small vessels compared to balloon angioplasty

19.2 A 75-year-old female with stage III chronic kidney disease (CKD) is admitted with progressive angina. Her biomarkers are not elevated, but she had transient ST-segment depression in the anterior precordial leads, with return to baseline after initiation of medical therapy. At catheterization, she is found to have a 90% stenosis in the mid-left anterior descending (LAD) coronary artery but, otherwise, diffuse moderate nonobstructive disease. The lesion is successfully crossed with a 0.014-in. guidewire, and predilation is attempted with a 2.5 × 15 mm noncompliant balloon. At 15 atmospheres (atm), there is a persistent waist in the balloon. Further attempts to "crack the lesion" using higher pressures are not successful (Fig. Q19-2A and B). An angiogram reveals that the lesion severity

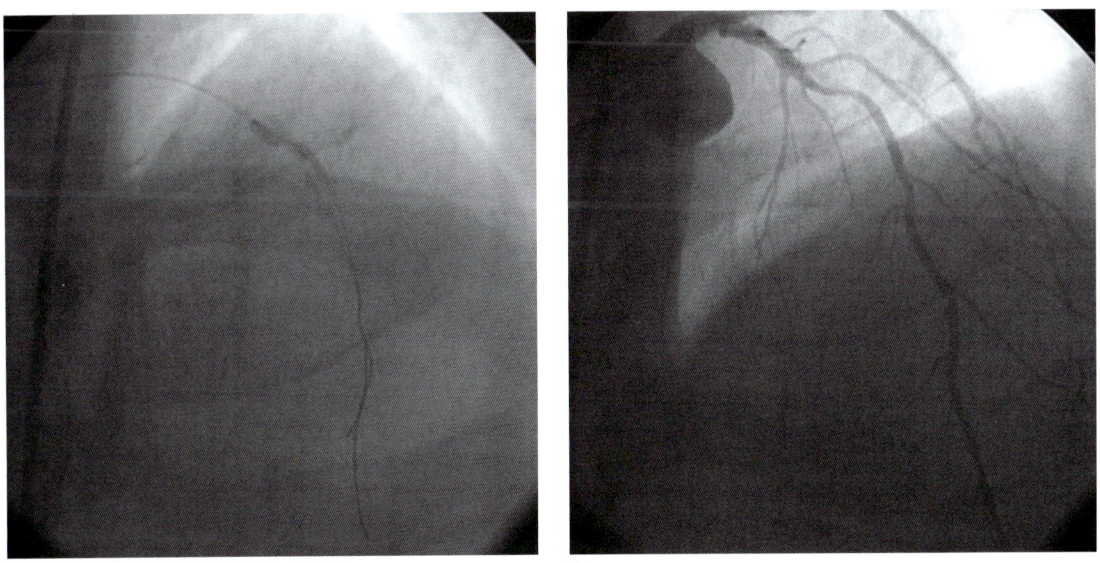

A B
Figure Q19-2

and reference segments are relatively unchanged. What would be the MOST optimal next strategy?

(A) Repeat attempts at predilation with a 3.0 × 15 mm noncompliant balloon
(B) Exchange the 0.014-in. guidewire for a Rotowire and perform rotational atherectomy with a 1.5-mm burr
(C) Repeat attempts at predilation using a 2.5 × 10 mm cutting balloon
(D) Stop the procedure and call for a consult for coronary artery bypass graft (CABG)

19.3 All of the following are clinical indications for the use of laser angioplasty, EXCEPT:

(A) Restenosis in 316L stainless steel stents
(B) Failed previous balloon angioplasty
(C) Long lesions
(D) Highly angulated entry and exit from the lesion

19.4 A 67-year-old male was admitted with progressive angina. His history was significant for a drug-eluting stent (DES) placement in a long, calcified mid-LAD stenosis with mild to moderate nonobstructive disease elsewhere 3 weeks prior to admission in the setting of unstable angina. Repeat catheterization revealed a significant new lesion 5 mm from the distal edge of the recently placed stent. Because the operators had difficulty with predilation using balloon angioplasty, they considered using cutting balloon angioplasty (CBA) for better lesion preparation. Which of the following is TRUE considering use of CBA?

(A) CBA is appropriate in lesions with angiographic calcification
(B) CBA may be used for high-pressure balloon-resistant lesions
(C) CBA is contraindicated in use distal to a recently implanted stent
(D) CBA is contraindicated for use in the presence of visible thrombus

19.5 Which of the following is MOST likely to lead to potential complications during rotational atherectomy?

(A) Wire bias
(B) Orthogonal displacement of friction
(C) Differential cutting
(D) Microparticulate debris <12 μm

19.6 The scoring balloon has been evaluated prior to DES placement and compared to either direct stenting or predilation with a conventional balloon. Compared to either direct stenting or a conventional balloon, the scoring balloon resulted in which of the following using percentage of cases achieving >5.0 mm^2 final minimal luminal diameter (ultrasound derived) after stenting?

(A) Similar percentage of cases
(B) Lower percentage of cases
(C) Higher percentage of cases

19.7 A 76-year-old man was evaluated for progressive angina. Outpatient nuclear stress testing revealed normal left ventricular function and a large reversible perfusion defect in the anterior and inferoapical walls of the left ventricle (LV). Cardiac catheterization revealed diffuse moderate to heavy calcification of the coronary arteries, with a focal severe stenosis in the proximal LAD coronary artery (Fig. Q19-7). Which of the following would allow the MOST flexible manner of lesion preparation for this lesion?

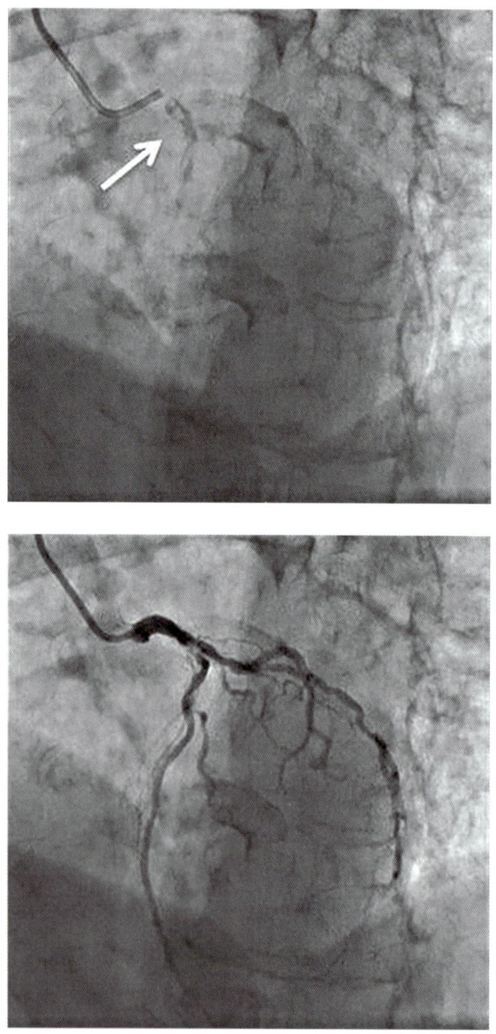

Figure Q19-7 (Courtesy of Robert Applegate.)

(A) Orbital atherectomy
(B) CBA
(C) Rotational atherectomy
(D) Laser atherectomy

19.8 A 64-year-old woman is admitted with progressive angina. Coronary angiography reveals a Medina 1-1-1 bifurcation lesion of the LAD and first diagonal vessels. The diagonal is a 2.7-mm vessel and its takeoff from the LAD is almost 90 degrees. The operators are considering a two-stent approach and wish to perform lesion preparation with guidewires in both vessels. Which of the following would not allow the operators to maintain two guidewires during lesion preparation?

(A) Rotational atherectomy
(B) Laser atherectomy
(C) CBA
(D) Scoring balloon angioplasty

19.9 Optimal technique for laser angioplasty includes all of the following techniques, EXCEPT:

(A) Coaxial guidewire positioning
(B) Use of frequent contrast injections to monitor progress of lasing
(C) Use of lasing cycles of 5 seconds on and 10 seconds off for up to 45 seconds
(D) Adjunctive stenting in appropriate-sized vessels

19.10 An 87-year-old female was admitted with unstable angina. Her history was significant for longstanding hypertension and stage III CKD. She had no prior cardiac history. The diagnostic coronary angiogram of her right coronary artery (RCA) is shown (Fig. Q19-10). Which of the following would be the MOST optimal device for lesion preparation in this patient?

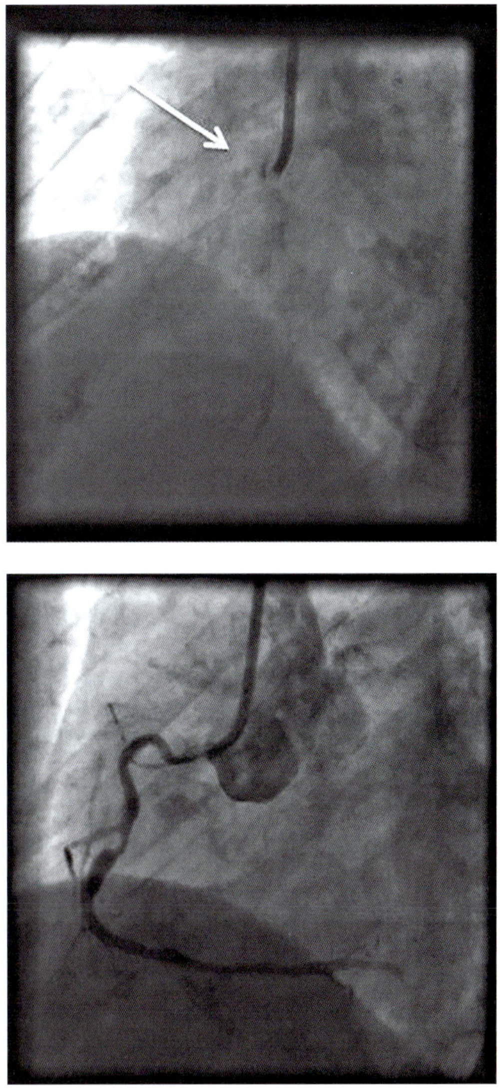

Figure Q19-10 (Courtesy of Robert Applegate.)

(A) Scoring balloon angioplasty
(B) Rotational atherectomy
(C) CBA
(D) Orbital atherectomy

19.11 Rotational atherectomy of a midcircumflex coronary artery lesion (Fig. Q19-11) is performed in a stepped fashion with 1.5- and 2.0-mm burrs. The result is shown. The MOST likely cause of this result after rotational atherectomy is:

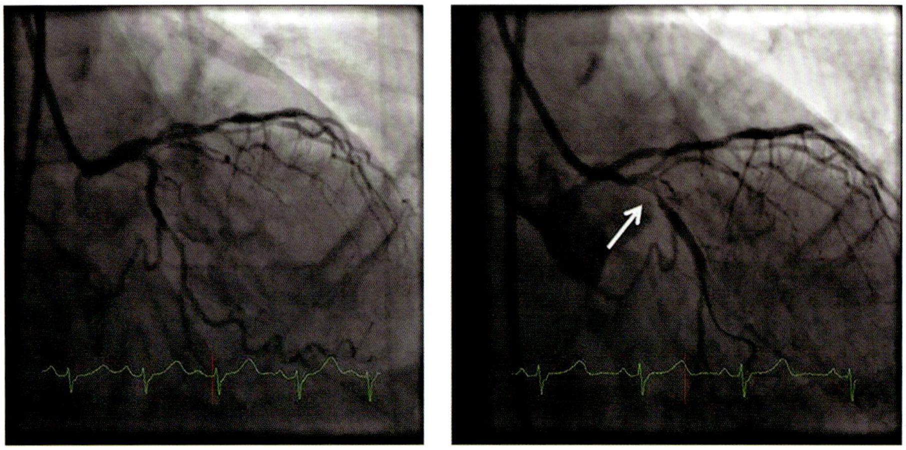

Figure Q19-11 (Courtesy of Robert Applegate.)

(A) Coronary vasospasm
(B) Guide catheter dissection
(C) Centrifugal displacement of friction
(D) Wire bias

19.12 A 69-year-old retired bank president is seen by his primary care provider for progressive angina and dyspnea on exertion. He has had long-standing hypertension and poorly controlled diabetes but has been otherwise active. A stress cardiolite study reveals a reversible large perfusion defect in the anterior wall. Cardiac catheterization is recommended, and a severe, heavily calcified stenosis is found in the proximal LAD coronary artery. Because of the calcification, it is decided to pretreat the lesion with rotational atherectomy. There is a 50% diameter residual stenosis after 1.25- and 1.75-mm burrs. What would be the MOST optimal next step?

(A) Upsize to a 2.15-mm burr and repeat rotational atherectomy
(B) Perform balloon angioplasty with a 3.0 × 20-mm noncompliant balloon
(C) Place a 3.0 × 23-mm cobalt chromium stent
(D) Place a 3.0 × 23-mm DES

19.13 Which of the following does NOT apply to orbital atherectomy?

(A) Differential ablation of inelastic material
(B) Effective clearing of thrombus
(C) Generation of particles sized <2 μm
(D) Treatment of heavily calcified lesions

19.14 A 72-year-old man develops progressive angina and undergoes a stress echocardiogram. He develops angina at 4 minutes and is noted to have inferior and lateral wall hypokinesis on echo. He undergoes elective cardiac catheterization and is found to have diffuse severe coronary calcification, with a significant and lengthy lesion in the midcircumflex coronary artery (Fig. Q19-14A and B). Rotational

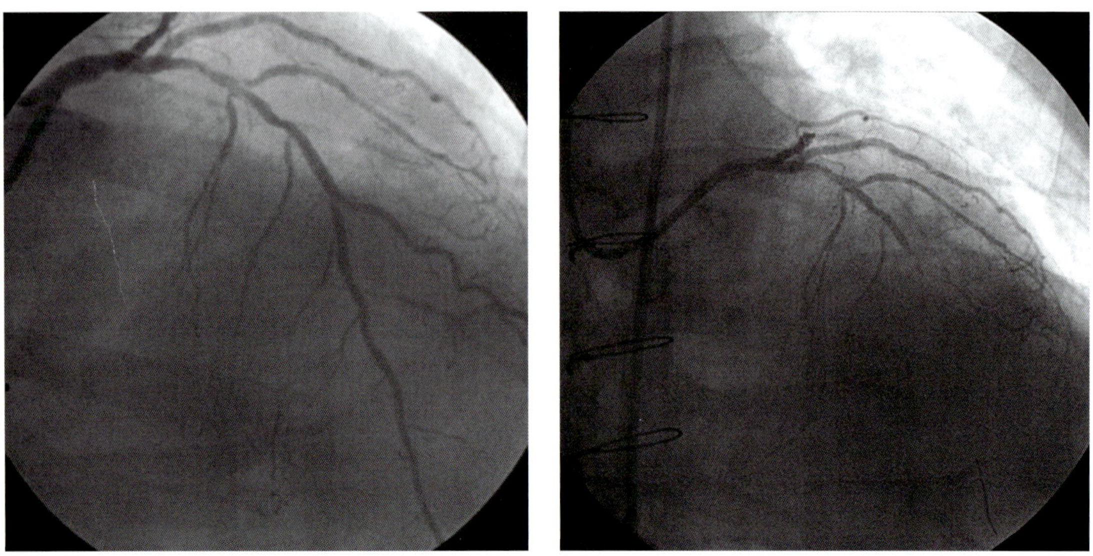

A B

Figure Q19-14

atherectomy is performed with a 1.25-mm burr without complications. Rotational atherectomy with a 1.75-mm burr is unsuccessful after multiple attempts and an angiogram is obtained. The patient develops chest pain, and it is noted that there is ST-segment elevation in the inferior leads. What should be the subsequent steps in this case?

(A) Wait a few minutes and then repeat rotational atherectomy
(B) Perform pericardiocentesis
(C) Administer intracoronary vasodilators and maintain adequate blood pressure with pressors as needed
(D) Perform high-pressure balloon angioplasty with an oversized balloon at the lesion site

19.15 Which of the following is a percutaneous coronary intervention (PCI) guideline class III recommendation for rotational atherectomy?

(A) Routine treatment of de novo or in-stent restenosis
(B) Inability to cross a lesion with a balloon catheter
(C) Long lesions
(D) Treatment of heavily calcified lesions

19.16 A 72-year-old diabetic man is admitted with recurrent chest pain during hemodialysis. Myocardial infarction (MI) is ruled out. A dobutamine echocardiogram reveals anterolateral hypokinesis at peak stress. Cardiac catheterization is advised, and significant stenosis is observed in the midportion of a heavily calcified LAD coronary artery. Rotational atherectomy of the LAD lesion was planned using a 1.5-mm burr prior to stent placement (Fig. Q19-16). The burr speed was set to 160,000 rotations per minute (rpm). The burr entered the lesion but met resistance each time the lesion was engaged with the burr. On the third pass marked deceleration was noted and the patient complained of chest pain. An angiogram was obtained. Which of the following is the BEST option for treatment of this patient at this time?

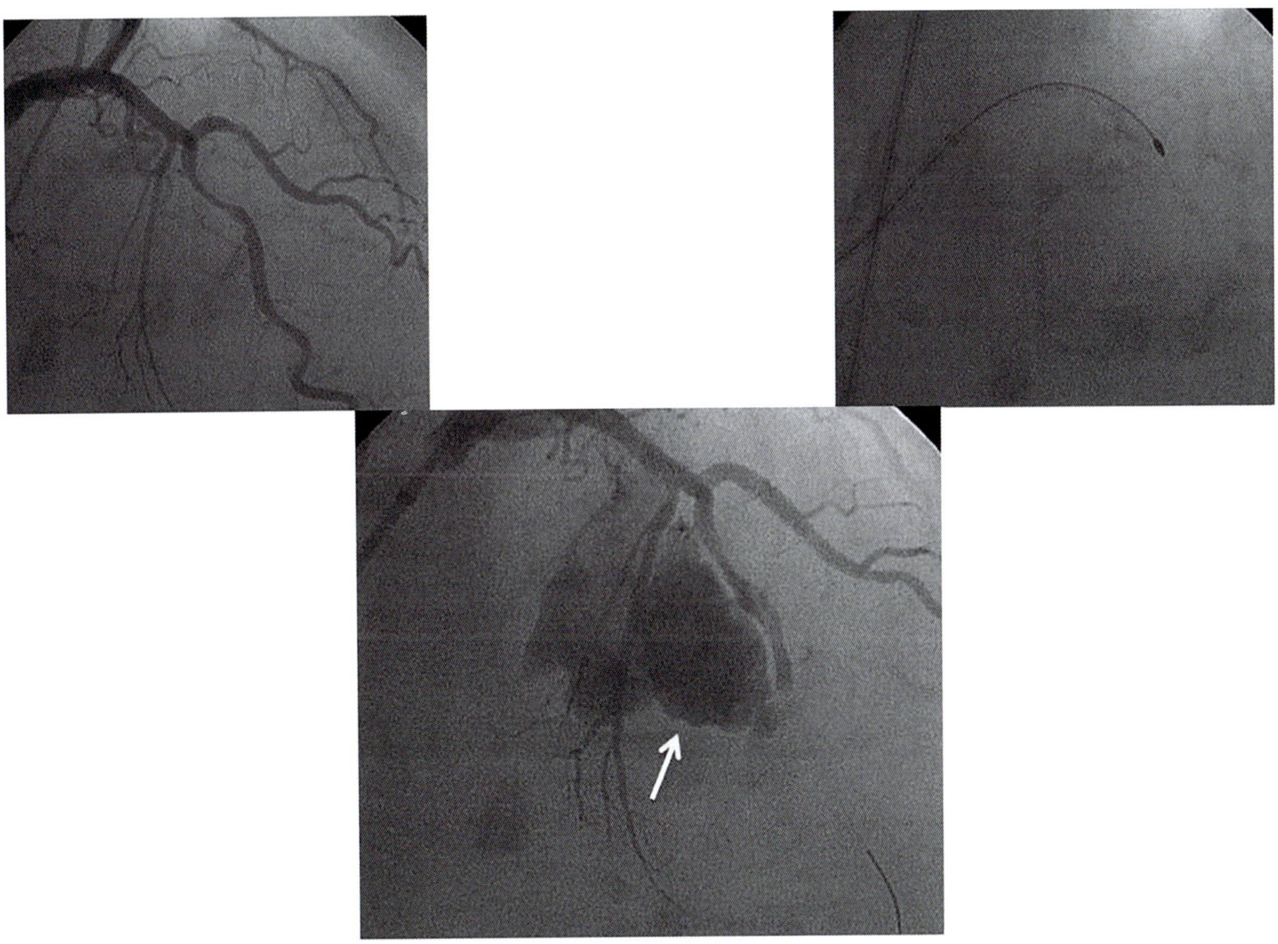

Figure Q19-16 (Courtesy of Robert Applegate.)

(A) Exchange the burr for an appropriately sized balloon and perform prolonged balloon inflations until the perforation is sealed
(B) Exchange the burr for an appropriately sized balloon and seal the perforation, prepare for immediate pericardiocentesis, and place a covered stent
(C) Upsize to a 2.25-mm burr and repeat atherectomy
(D) Place a bare metal stent (BMS) in the LAD

19.17 Which of the following would NOT be an accepted contraindication for use of orbital atherectomy?

(A) Severely angled lesion
(B) Angiographically visible thrombus
(C) Severely calcified coronary artery lesion
(D) Inability to pass a guidewire distal to the lesion

19.18 A 49-year-old woman is evaluated for progressive angina. Her medical history is significant for long-standing insulin-dependent diabetes mellitus, stage III CKD, and tobacco abuse. A nuclear perfusion study indicates a large perfusion defect in the inferior and inferolateral walls of the left ventricle. Coronary angiography reveals diffuse calcification of her coronary arteries and a focal high-grade stenosis in the midportion of a large dominant RCA. Initial attempts at passing a workhorse guidewire across the lesion are unsuccessful. After further efforts, a Fielder XT successfully crosses the lesion into the distal RCA. Which of the following would NOT be appropriate for use to prepare the lesion prior to stenting at this point in the procedure?

(A) Scoring balloon angioplasty
(B) Laser atherectomy
(C) Rotational atherectomy
(D) CBA

19.19 A 73-year-old male was admitted with progressive angina. His history was significant for tobacco abuse, hypertension, non-insulin-dependent diabetes mellitus, and stage III CKD. He had no prior cardiac history. Diagnostic coronary angiography revealed diffuse moderate disease of the coronary vasculature with diffuse narrowing of the mid RCA. PCI of the RCA was planned. The RCA was wired and predilated with a 2.5 × 12 mm and then 3.0 × 20-mm compliant balloons. A 3.0 × 38-mm DES was placed and dilated to 22 atm (Fig. Q19-19). There

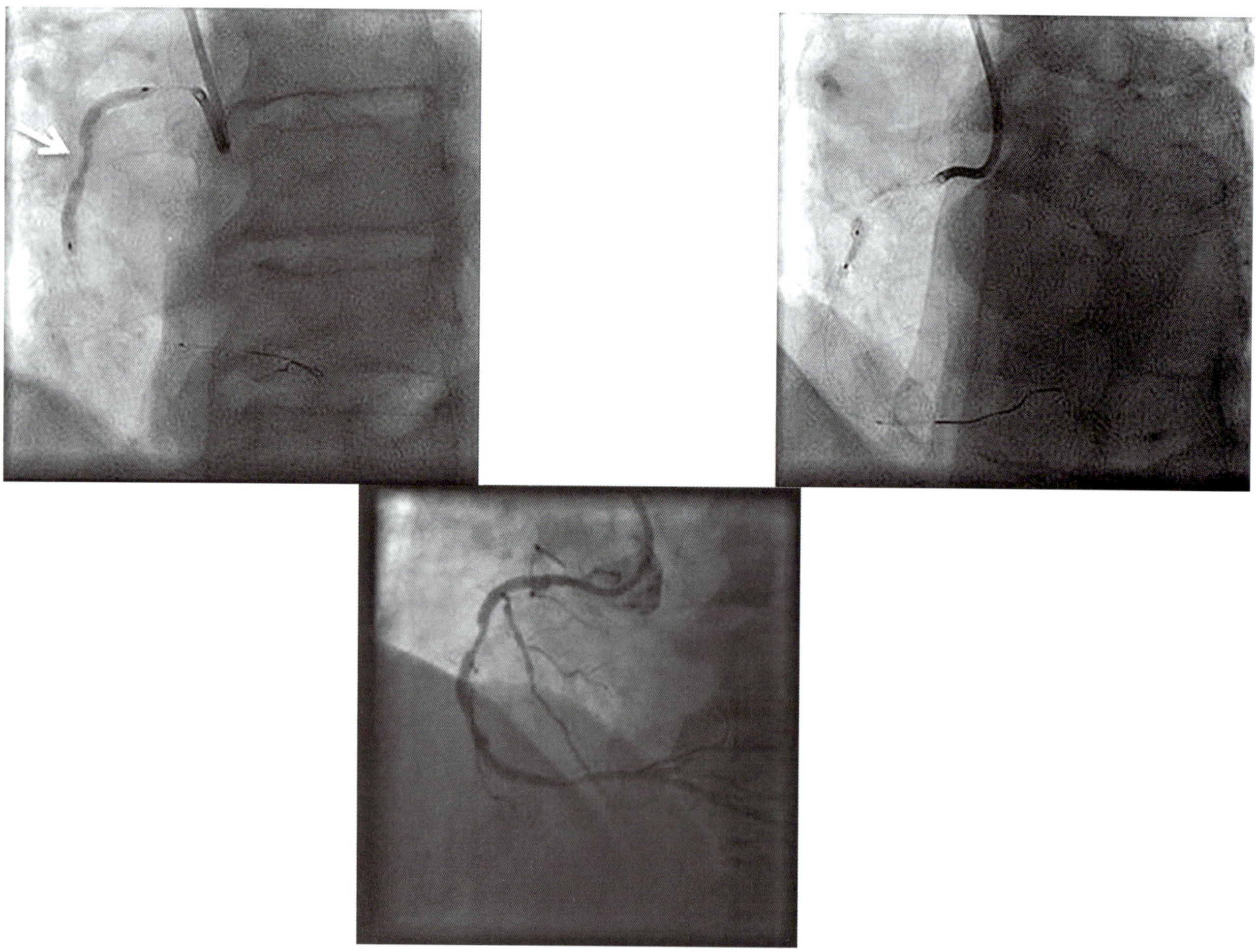

Figure Q19-19 (Courtesy of Robert Applegate.)

was severe narrowing of the midportion of the stent, which did not change after high-pressure balloon dilation with a 3.0 × 8 mm, then 2.5 × 8 noncompliant balloons to 24 atm. Which of the following would be the MOST optimal strategy for treating the underdeployed stent in this patient?

(A) Referral for CABG
(B) Rotational atherectomy
(C) Laser atherectomy
(D) Orbital atherectomy

19.20 Which of the following BEST describes the results of randomized clinical trials evaluating the outcomes of orbital atherectomy?

(A) Lower restenosis rates compared to rotational atherectomy
(B) Higher restenosis rates compared to rotational atherectomy
(C) Similar restenosis rates as rotational atherectomy
(D) There are no randomized trials to date evaluating outcomes of orbital atherectomy

ANSWERS AND EXPLANATIONS

19.1 Answer B. The Rotablator (Boston Scientific, Natick, MA) is an over the wire system that consists of a nickel-plated, diamond-coated brass burr attached to a drive shaft, which is driven by compressed gas and can achieve speeds up to 200,000 rpm. The 20- to 30-μm-sized diamond chips are located only on the front half of the olive-shaped burr. The burr and drive shaft are placed on a 0.09-in. guidewire with a floppy tip of 30 cm, which has a 0.21 olive at the joint between the flexible tip and the shaft of the guidewire to prevent the burr from advancing to the flexible tip of the guidewire. The reusable console can be adjusted to achieve burr speeds up to 200,000 rpm in the fully activated mode and speeds of 80,000 rpm when used in the Dynaglide mode (used for the purpose of removing the burr from the guide catheter). Much like a high-speed sander, the Rotablator burr ablates with the creation of microparticulate debris when the burr comes into contact with relatively inelastic tissue. Although rotational atherectomy has been used extensively in the past to debulk lesions, the STRATAS trial (Whitlow PL, et al. *Am J Cardiol* 2001;87(6):699–705) and the DART trial (Mauri L, et al. *Am Heart J* 2003;145(5):847–854) examined restenosis rates in a randomized fashion, comparing rotational atherectomy with balloon angioplasty. Neither study found a lower incidence of restenosis with rotational atherectomy.

19.2 Answer B. In the prestent era, rotational atherectomy was used to treat a variety of complex coronary artery lesions including lesions >20 mm in length, calcified lesions, and ostial and bifurcation disease. With the advent of intracoronary stents, in particular DES, use of rotational atherectomy fell dramatically. According to the 2011 update of the American College of Cardiology (ACC) and American Heart Association (AHA) guidelines for coronary interventions, rotational atherectomy is indicated for use in nondilatable lesions as debulking prior to placement of a stent (Levine GN, et al. *J Am Coll Cardiol* 2011;58(24):e44–e122). In this case, further attempts at predilation would be unhelpful. Cutting balloons have been used with limited success in calcified lesions but are also associated with higher potential rates of dissections, which would preclude use of rotational atherectomy. CABG with a left internal mammary artery (LIMA) is an acceptable alternative, but would not be preferred by most patients or interventionalists.

19.3 Answer D. The excimer laser coronary atherectomy system (ELCA) (Spectranetics, Colorado Springs, CO) consists of a multifiber catheter and a CVX-300 console that emits light at ultraviolet wavelengths of 308 nm. It is 0.014-in. guidewire compatible, available either as Rx or over the wire catheters. Catheters are available in sizes ranging from 0.9 to 2.0 mm (Rx configuration) and 0.9 mm in the over the wire configuration. Fluence (laser power) of 30 to 60 mJ/mm^2 are available for all catheters, while the 0.9 mm X-80 has the unique quality of being able to deliver fluence up to 80 mJ/mm^2. Lasers produce very high electromagnetic energy delivered through coaxial optical fibers bundled inside a coronary delivery catheter. The optimal lasing technique involves delivery of the tip of the laser catheter directly to the area of interest. Activation of the device produces a cone of laser energy, which extends no more than 50 μm beyond the tip of the catheter and leads to vaporization of plaque. The vaporization of organic material such as plaque is achieved by photochemical, photomechanical and photothermal effects. The laser beam does not interact with inorganic material, such as calcium or steel, which allows it to be used safely in the presence of a guidewire or stent. Use of laser angioplasty with highly angulated entry and exit from the lesion is associated with an increase in the incidence of perforation and is relatively contraindicated in this situation. Use of laser angioplasty for restenosis in 316L stainless steel stents, failed previous balloon angioplasty, or long lesions are all clinically accepted indications for its use. Thus, the correct answer is D.

19.4 Answer C. The Flextome Cutting Balloon Device (Boston Scientific, Minneapolis, MN) is a novel device that features atherotomes (microsurgical blades) longitudinally fixed to a balloon. The atherotomes measure 10 to 15 mm in length by 0.011- to 0.013-in. in height and 0.04- to 0.06-in. in width, depending on balloon diameter and length. Balloon sizes from 2.0 to 3.25 mm have three atherotomes, while those balloon sizes 3.5 to 4.0 have four atherotomes. These atherotomes are folded within the balloon material along its long axis in the deflated position and are slowly deployed over approximately 1 minute. This process creates controlled longitudinal incisions as a result of the deployment process. When the balloon is deflated, the atherotomes are folded within the balloon material to minimize the risk of trauma as the balloon is withdrawn from the coronary circulation. Because of the atherotomes, the balloons have a crossing profile that is larger than either compliant or noncompliant conventional balloons and may offer resistance during withdrawal. Based on the results of these three randomized clinical trials, CBA was not felt to be superior to simple balloon angioplasty and should be reserved for difficult to treat in-stent restenosis or ostial lesions of side branches. In a 2011 update of the PCI guidelines, CBA received a class IIB indication to avoid slippage-induced coronary artery trauma during PCI for in-stent restenosis or ostial lesions in the side branches (Level of Evidence C). It received a class III (no benefit) recommendation for routine PCI (Level of Evidence A) (Levine GN, et al. *J Am Coll Cardiol* 2011;58(24):e44–e122). The use of a cutting balloon distal to a recently implanted stent is relatively contraindicated for fear of having the device entangled (the atherotomes) with the stent on withdrawal from the lesion site. The cutting balloon is clinically used to treat lesions with mild to moderate calcification and for high-pressure balloon-resistant lesions. It is relatively contraindicated in the presence of angiographically visible thrombus due to fear of embolization of the thrombus.

19.5 Answer A. Wire bias refers to the position of the rotational atherectomy wire in an eccentric position within the coronary vessel. In spite of the relatively floppy nature of the rotational atherectomy wire, the physical strength of the wire in an eccentric position leads to ablation following the position of the wire. If the wire is eccentrically lying against the lesion, this may facilitate the effectiveness of rotational atherectomy. However, if it is against the normal vessel, this may create a track outside of the normal vessel lumen and may lead to local complications, including perforation. Both differential cutting and orthogonal displacement of friction are believed to represent principles that contribute to the effective use of rotational atherectomy. The small size of microparticulate debris allows the debris to pass through the distal coronary vasculature and minimizes plugging and vessel obstruction, although inadequate flushing of the vessel during atherectomy may still result in microvascular plugging.

19.6 Answer C. The AngioSculpt scoring balloon (Spectranetics, Colorado Springs, CO) is a novel balloon catheter consisting of a semicompliant balloon catheter around which three rectangular nitinol scoring wires are wrapped in a helical fashion. The balloon catheter can be expanded to 20 atm of pressure, allowing greater force to be applied focally compared to standard balloon angioplasty. The scoring balloon has the potential advantage over conventional balloons in restenotic lesions where "watermelon seeding" or slippage with conventional balloons may occur. With its helical cage design and square, rather than round, wire shape, the scoring balloon provides circumferential scoring and helps minimize slippage, locking the device within the lesion. The scoring balloon was used to treat the side branch of bifurcation lesions treated with a DES in 93 patients in the AGILITY trial (Weisz G, et al. *Catheter Cardiovasc Interv* 2013;82(3):352–359). The postscoring balloon dissection rate was 6.0% (2.1% after stenting), and the 9-month MACE rate was 5.4%. Guidelines for use of the scoring balloon were not included in the 2011 PCI ACC, AHA, and Society for Cardiovascular Angiography and Interventions (SCAI) guidelines (Levine GN, et al. *J Am Coll Cardiol* 2011;58(24):e44–e122). In an observational trial of 299 patients, ultrasound was used to assess DES placement (Cypher or Taxus) after direct stenting, predilatation with a conventional balloon, and after scoring balloon pretreatment. Use of the scoring balloon resulted in greater luminal gain and a higher percentage of lesions achieving a final stent diameter >5.0 mm^2 compared to either direct stenting or predilation with a conventional balloon (Costa JD Jr, et al. *Am J Cardiol* 2007;100(5):812–817). Thus, the correct answer is C.

19.7 Answer A. The orbital atherectomy system (OAS) (Cardiovascular Systems, Inc., St. Paul, MN) is an over the wire system with a single, eccentrically mounted diamond-coated crown. The crown orbits on the wire, rather than spins (as does rotational atherectomy), utilizing the mechanism of centrifugal force, which presses the crown against the lesion and results in differential sanding. The entire system consists of four components, including the device (orbital atherectomy device [OAD]), which is an over the wire sheath-covered drive shaft and crown; a guidewire; a reusable external pump system; and a lubricant solution. The OAD has a single crown size (1.25 mm) that can be used for all cases. The angiogram shows a moderately calcified lesion in an LAD that has a distal reference diameter of at least 3.25 mm. CBA could be used for lesion preparation prior to stenting; however, it can be difficult to cross a severely stenotic, calcified lesion with a cutting balloon. Rotational atherectomy would be appropriate to pretreat this lesion but may require more than one burr to achieve optimal lesion preparation. Similarly, laser atherectomy could be used in this case but is less ideal than either rotational or orbital atherectomy. The use of orbital atherectomy provides the most flexible device for lesion preparation since the extent of ablation can be achieved with a single crown by simply increasing the speed of orbit from 80,000 to 120,000 rpm.

19.8 Answer A. Scoring balloon angioplasty and CBA can both be used in the presence of a second guidewire, primarily in the pretreatment of a branch vessel lesion of a bifurcation stenosis. Laser atherectomy does not ablate inorganic material and thus can be used in the presence of a second guidewire (or metallic stents). Both rotational and orbital atherectomy ablate inelastic material, such as metal; thus, it is generally agreed that they should not be used in the presence of a second guidewire for fear of shearing it in half.

19.9 Answer B. In the excimer laser, rotational atherectomy, and balloon angioplasty comparison trial (ERBAC), excimer laser angioplasty was associated with both an increase in coronary complications, as well as higher restenosis rates compared with balloon angioplasty (Reifart N, et al. *Circulation* 1997;96(1):91-98). In that study, saline flushes were not used and may have been in large part responsible for the higher rates of local complications. Since that study, it has been appreciated that the laser light is scattered by contrast, which can lead to vessel dissection and perforation. Coaxial guidewire positioning, and use of lasing cycles of 5 seconds on and 10 seconds off for up to 45 seconds, are important strategies for successful lasing. Laser atherectomy is used to prepare a lesion for stenting in appropriately sized vessels.

19.10 Answer B. The angiogram reveals a very heavily calcified ostium of the RCA. Neither the scoring balloon nor the cutting balloon is likely to cross and/or adequately dilate this lesion given the extent of calcification. Orbital atherectomy would be an excellent choice for a heavily calcified lesion. However, the ostial location of the lesion makes its use problematic. Rotational atherectomy is well suited for a heavily calcified ostium of the RCA and prepares the lesion for subsequent stenting.

19.11 Answer D. In this case, wire bias resulted in rotational atherectomy of the "inner curve" of the bend in the midcircumflex, with a subintimal channel outside of the original coronary lumen. Wire bias represents the phenomenon of eccentric position of a guidewire "cutting the corner" of a tortuous vessel, with subsequent atherectomy within the vessel along this eccentrically positioned guidewire. Although coronary spasm and guide catheters may result in injury to the coronary circulation during rotational atherectomy, they are not likely to have caused this result. Centrifugal displacement of friction is one principle that allows movement of the burr over the guidewire with the minimal tolerances between burr lumen and guidewire size.

19.12 Answer D. Most experts agree that the optimal technique of using rotational atherectomy is to perform "facilitated" stenting: lesion preparation with rotational atherectomy aimed at achieving low burr-to-artery ratios, followed by intracoronary artery stenting. In the absence of a contraindication to prolonged use of dual antiplatelet therapy (DAPT), most experts would recommend use of a DES. In the ROTAXUS trial of 240 patients, late lumen loss was similar with or without rotational atherectomy prior to Taxus stent placement (Abdel-Wahab M, et al. *JACC Cardiovasc Interv* 2013;6(1):10-19). Therefore, the statement that rotational atherectomy reduces restenosis rates before use of DES is incorrect.

19.13 Answer B. The mechanism of action of orbital atherectomy is similar to that of rotational atherectomy: both ablate inelastic tissue but spare elastic tissue. Similar to rotational atherectomy, orbital atherectomy generates small particles that cross the capillaries and eventually are believed to end up in the reticuloendothelial systems of the liver and spleen. However, the size of particles generated during orbital atherectomy (<2 μm) are smaller than those of rotational atherectomy (5 to 12 μm). Treatment of heavily calcified lesions is the primary indication for use of orbital atherectomy. Orbital atherectomy is contraindicated for use in the presence of angiographically visible thrombus, as it will likely cause distal embolization and potential slow or no reflow.

19.14 Answer C. This patient has developed slow flow vs. no reflow as a result of the high microparticulate burden during multiple burr runs. This leads to microvascular obstruction and ischemia. Prevention of this phenomenon can be achieved with several strategies during rotational atherectomy. Lower burr speeds, short runs <45 to 60 seconds, applying Rotaglide lubricant, aggressive vasodilation with nitroglycerin or nitroprusside, and maintenance of blood pressure with short acting pressors, such as neosynephrine, have all been used to prevent or minimize slow flow. Continuation of rotational atherectomy without restoring adequate flow would compound the situation. Use of balloon angioplasty may be helpful in this situation to help relieve spasm but is usually achieved with low pressure inflations.

19.15 Answer A. Routine use of rotational atherectomy for de novo or restenotic lesions has not been shown to improve outcomes or reduce rates of restenosis. Thus, it was given a class III indication if used for this purpose (Levine GN, et al. *J Am Coll Cardiol* 2011;58(24):e44–e122). Inability to cross a lesion with a balloon, heavily calcified lesions, and long lesions are all clinically accepted indications for its use.

19.16 Answer B. This patient has developed a type III, free-flowing perforation at the lesion site in the mid-LAD coronary artery. This may have occurred as a result of ablation deep in the wall of the vessel, signaled by the deceleration of the burr. Although resistance is not uncommon during rotoblation, excessive forward pressure on the burr should be avoided to prevent situations like this. It is unlikely that attempts at prolonged balloon inflation alone would seal a type III perforation. Placement of a stent would not seal the perforation and could even make it worse. However, placement of a covered stent would seal the perforation. If bleeding is so severe that exchanging the balloon for the covered stent would lead to immediate tamponade, then a second guide can be positioned from an alternative access site and the covered stent placed from this guide, leaving the perforation unsealed for the time necessary to move the balloon back into the original guide.

19.17 Answer C. Similar to rotational atherectomy, use of orbital atherectomy in a severely angled lesion increases the likelihood of perforation. Angiographically visible thrombus is a relative contraindication for use of orbital atherectomy as it increases the risk of slow or no reflow. Orbital atherectomy is designed for use over a device specific guidewire, and it is recommended that the guidewire be positioned at least 10 cm distal to the lesion. The primary indication for orbital atherectomy is for treatment of a severely calcified coronary artery lesion.

19.18 Answer C. Both scoring balloon and CBA can be delivered over a 0.014-in. workhorse guidewire. However, in a lesion this difficult to cross with a guidewire alone, it is unlikely they would be effective here. Similarly, laser atherectomy is delivered over a standard 0.014-in. guidewire and would be appropriate for use here. Rotational and orbital atherectomy both require use of a device specific guidewire: 0.009-in. for rotational atherectomy and a 0.012-in. guidewire for orbital atherectomy. Thus, at this stage of the procedure, rotational atherectomy cannot be used until the 0.014-in. guidewire has been exchanged for the device specific 0.009-in. Rotowire.

19.19 Answer C. Failure to obtain stent expansion despite high-pressure balloon angioplasty with a noncompliant balloon is uncommon but is almost always due to calcific constraint of the stent. Use of rotational atherectomy would require first ablating the stent struts before the calcific portion of the lesion could be ablated. Depending on how much the stent was constrained, it might require a much larger burr than is typically used (2.38 or 2.50 mm), requiring a 9- or 10-Fr guide catheter. Orbital atherectomy is relatively contraindicated for use within stents. Laser atherectomy has been reported to be effective in this type of situation, likely by altering the calcific matrix constraining stent expansion since it does not ablate metal. An additional strategy is to inject contrast while lasing, which can expand the ablative radius of the laser—although this has been associated with an increased risk of vessel dissection. CABG would be an alternative consideration if the above failed.

19.20 Answer D. The data evaluating the clinical safety and efficacy of orbital atherectomy are derived from the ORBIT I and ORBIT II studies. There is no randomized controlled trial directly comparing rotational atherectomy with orbital atherectomy or any other device. The ORBIT I trial was a two-center prospective nonrandomized feasibility study in 50 patients (Parikh K, et al. *Catheter Cardiovasc Interv* 2013;81(7):1134–1139). Device success was 98% and procedural success was 94%. Major adverse events occurred in 4% in-hospital, 6% at 30 days, and in 8% at 6 months. The ORBIT II trial was a prospective multicenter nonblinded single-arm trial in 443 patients with severely calcified lesions (Chambers JW, et al. *JACC Cardiovasc Interv* 2014;7(5):510–518). Successful stent delivery after orbital atherectomy occurred in 97.7% of patients. The rates of slow flow and no reflow were very low, occurring in <1% of patients. In-hospital MI occurred in 0.7%, target vessel revascularization in 0.7%, and cardiac death in 0.2%.

20 Stents and Stent Thrombosis

Giuseppe Gargiulo and Marco Valgimigli

QUESTIONS

20.1 The first stent implanted in a human coronary artery was implanted in March 1986 by Jacques Puel in Toulouse (France) and was called the:

(A) Dotter stent
(B) Wallstent
(C) Palmaz-Schatz stent
(D) Igaki-Tamai stent
(E) Cypher stent

20.2 Although infrequent, stent thrombosis remains an important concern because of its sequelae, including myocardial infarction (MI) and death. Regarding mechanisms of very late stent thrombosis, occurring beyond 1 year after drug-eluting stent (DES) implantation, which of the following sentences reporting causes in descending order of frequency is CORRECT?

(A) Strut malapposition, neoatherosclerosis, uncovered struts, and stent underexpansion
(B) Stent underexpansion, strut malapposition, restenosis, and neoatherosclerosis
(C) Stent underexpansion, uncovered struts, evagination, and neoatherosclerosis
(D) Strut malapposition, neoatherosclerosis, uncovered struts, and bifurcation stenting
(E) Neoatherosclerosis, strut malapposition, restenosis, and stent underexpansion

20.3 A 52-year-old engineer is referred for a staged percutaneous coronary intervention (PCI) of an 80% stenosis of a large first obtuse marginal branch 6 weeks after primary PCI for acute anterior MI with thrombotic occlusion of the proximal left anterior descending (LAD) coronary artery. While providing informed consent for the procedure, the patient is interested in the key prerequisites or attributes for a coronary artery stent. All of the following are correct, EXCEPT:

(A) Tacking of intimal flaps and plaque coverage
(B) Prevention of elastic recoil by scaffolding of the arterial wall
(C) Facilitation of positive arterial remodeling
(D) Ability to fenestrate and access side branches
(E) Favorable deliverability due to a low profile and high flexibility

20.4 The use of covered stents is warranted in which of the following situations depicted in angiograms in Figure Q20-4A–E?

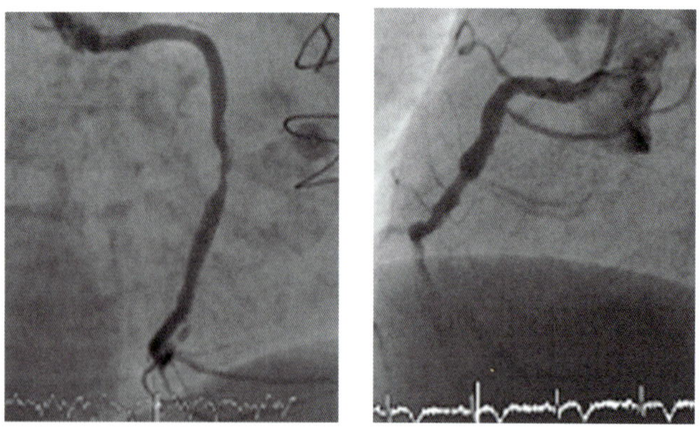

A B
Figure Q20-4

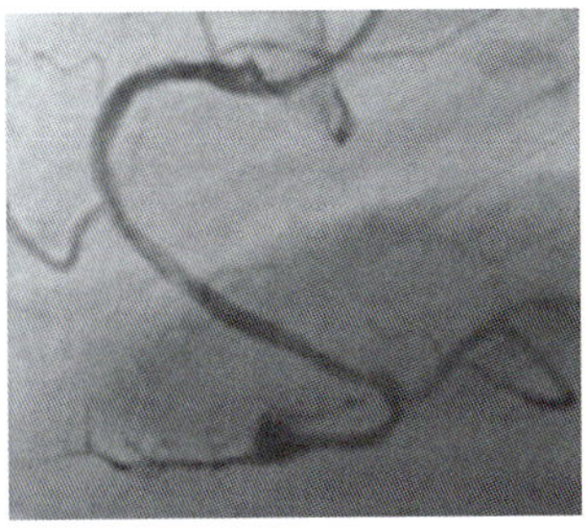

C

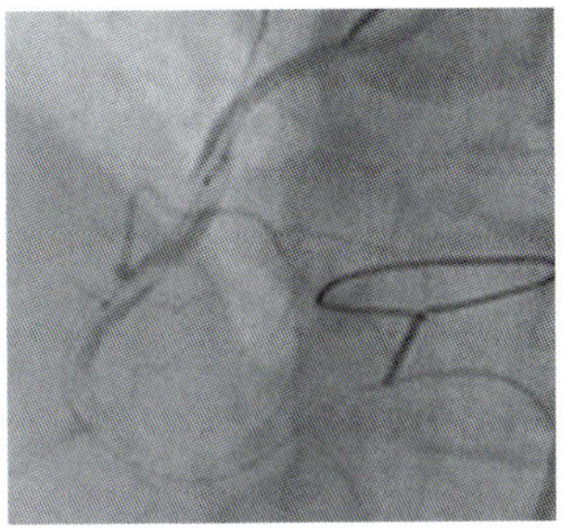

D

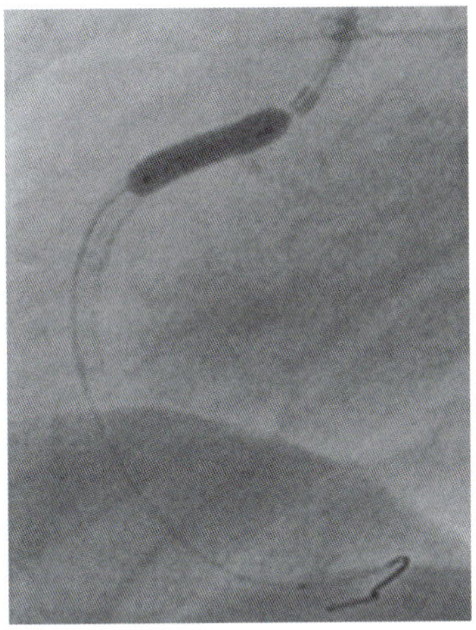

E

(A) Figure A
(B) Figure B
(C) Figure C
(D) Figure D
(E) Figure E

20.5 A 62-year-old nurse with a medical history remarkable for percutaneous transluminal angioplasty (PTA) and stenting of the left common femoral artery 2 years ago, active tobacco use, and a brother suffering an MI at the age of 48 is referred for coronary angiography due to exertional chest pain and evidence of ischemia during stress echocardiography. Since the peripheral vascular disease had been treated with a self-expanding stent, she wishes to know whether you will consider using a self-expanding stent to treat her coronary artery disease (CAD). All statements are correct, EXCEPT:

(A) Self-expanding stents are less prone to cause edge dissections
(B) Self-expanding stents have been associated with negative recoil due to continued outward radial force after deployment
(C) Self-expanding stents have a reduced rate of side branch occlusion and no reflow
(D) A concern of self-expanding stents is placement accuracy caused by foreshortening on expansion and sudden spring movements
(E) Self-expanding stents tend to have a better profile as compared to balloon-expandable stents

20.6 In patients with ST-segment elevation myocardial infarction (STEMI), which of the following statement regarding stent thrombosis is CORRECT?

(A) Stent thrombosis is not increased when radial access is used compared with femoral access
(B) Stent thrombosis is reduced in patients receiving bivalirudin compared with unfractionated heparin (UFH) during primary PCI
(C) To reduce the risk of stent thrombosis, bare metal stents (BMS) should be preferred to DES implantation
(D) STEMI patients have similar rates of stent thrombosis compared with stable patients
(E) The absorb bioresorbable vascular scaffold (BVS) has reduced rates of stent thrombosis compared with everolimus-eluting stents (EES)

20.7 A 57-year-old male with CAD and multiple PCI of all three coronary vessels is concerned about late consequences of BMS and DES. He inquires about fully BVS. BVS were developed to overcome the shortcomings of DES in PCI. Which statement is CORRECT?

(A) Device thrombosis is clearly lower in BVS compared with EES
(B) Device thrombosis seems to be higher in BVS compared with EES
(C) Mortality is similar in BVS compared with EES
(D) Target vessel failure seems to be lower in BVS compared with EES
(E) Statements B and C are correct

20.8 A 55-year-old man presents with stable angina and a single lesion on the midtract of his LAD artery. You decide to implant a bioresorbable scaffold. Which of the following procedural suggestions would be better to apply?

(A) Predilatation, correct scaffold sizing, and postdilatation with >1:1 noncompliant balloon (PSP score)
(B) Direct implantation of the scaffold
(C) Direct implantation of the scaffold and postdilatation
(D) Predilatation but not postdilatation
(E) Postdilatation to be performed with a 1:1 noncompliant balloon

20.9 Which statement regarding intravascular ultrasound (IVUS) is CORRECT?

(A) Routine use of IVUS to guide stent implantation has been shown to reduce mortality and the risk of MI
(B) IVUS is not an adequate tool to assess complete apposition of stent struts to the vessel wall
(C) A minimal stent area of >5 mm^2 is never considered satisfactory
(D) Routine use of IVUS reduces the risk of stent thrombosis
(E) IVUS allows for tissue characterization

20.10 Which statement is CORRECT regarding the percentages of complications associated with PCI (Fig. Q20-10)?

(A) A denotes in-hospital death, B denotes MI, C denotes emergency coronary artery bypass grafting (CABG), and D denotes stroke
(B) A denotes stroke, B denotes MI, C denotes emergency CABG, and D denotes in-hospital death
(C) A denotes in-hospital death, B denotes emergency CABG, C denotes MI, and D denotes stroke
(D) A denotes MI, B denotes severe access site complications, C denotes emergency CABG, and D denotes stroke
(E) A denotes stroke, B denotes emergency CABG, C denotes stroke, and D denotes MI

20.11 Which of the following is NOT a bioresorbable scaffold?

(A) Igaki–Tamai
(B) DESolve
(C) IDEAL
(D) Orsiro
(E) REVA

20.12 Dual antiplatelet therapy (DAPT) is recommended after coronary stent implantation in order to reduce ischemic complications. When deciding on the optimal duration of this therapy, which of the following could be a useful tool to help clinicians in the decision-making?

(A) DAPT score
(B) Thrombolysis in myocardial infarction (TIMI) risk score
(C) PRECISE-DAPT score
(D) SYNTAX score
(E) A and C are correct

20.13 Which of the following variables is NOT included in the DAPT score?

(A) Diabetes
(B) Peripheral arterial disease
(C) Previous MI
(D) Implantation of a TAXUS stent
(E) Vein graft stenting

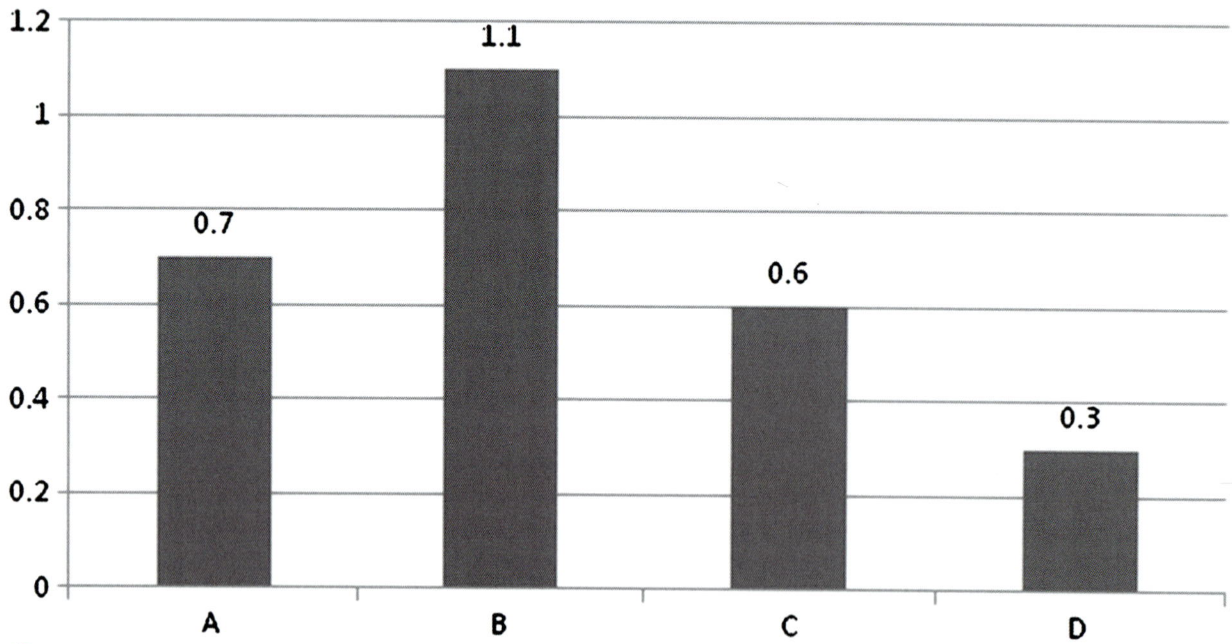

Figure Q20-10

20.14 A 72-year-old male with three-vessel CAD status post CABG 12 years ago presents with typical chest pain and a positive stress test. Coronary angiography shows a patent left internal mammary artery (LIMA) graft to the LAD, a chronic occlusion of the saphenous vein graft (SVG) to the circumflex in the setting of a 50% stenosis of the native circumflex, as well as a significant stenosis of the SVG to the chronically occluded right coronary artery (RCA). You decide to treat the SVG to the RCA with PCI. Which statement(s) is CORRECT?

(A) PCI of SVGs is associated with an increased risk of periprocedural MI
(B) There is no significant difference in the rate of restenosis requiring target lesion revascularization (TLR) for SVGs and native coronary arteries
(C) Compared with BMS, the use of DES has been associated with adverse clinical outcomes in the treatment of SVGs and should be discouraged
(D) Embolic protection devices reduce periprocedural MI in PCI for SVGs and their use is mandatory
(E) Statements A and C are correct

20.15 A 75-year-old female with a past medical history remarkable for MI of the inferior wall without revascularization complains of angina on moderate exertion and is found to have a left ventricular ejection fraction (LVEF) of 45% on transthoracic echocardiography (TTE). She is referred for coronary angiography. Based on the angiogram (Fig. Q20-15), which of the following statements is CORRECT?

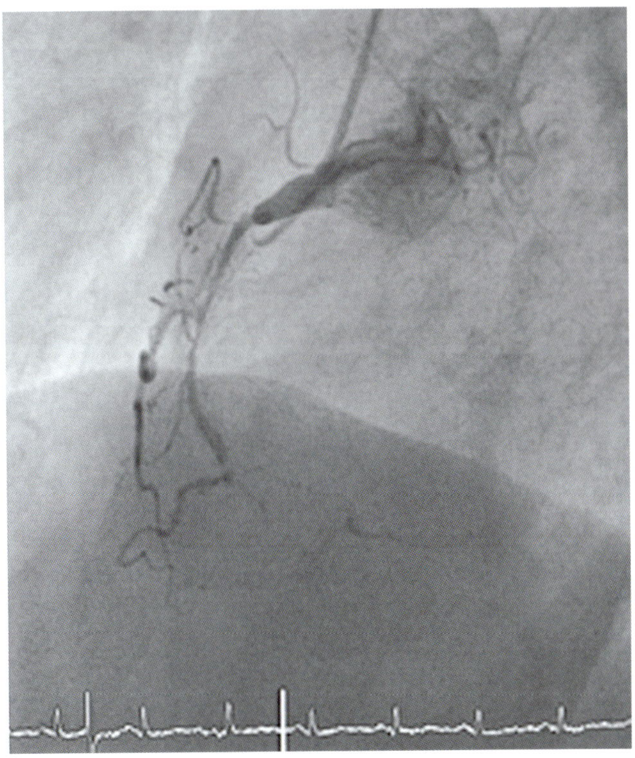

Figure Q20-15

(A) Treatment of the finding shown above may reduce symptoms and improve left ventricular function
(B) PCI in this setting has consistently been demonstrated to improve survival and should be performed in any case
(C) IVUS did not show to be useful in PCI of chronic total occlusions (CTOs)
(D) Randomized clinical trials demonstrate benefits of BMS over DES
(E) Lesions can be classified as CTOs when there is TIMI 0 to 1 flow within the occluded segment and an occlusion duration >1 month

20.16 What is the Medina classification of the bifurcation lesion shown in Figure Q20-16?

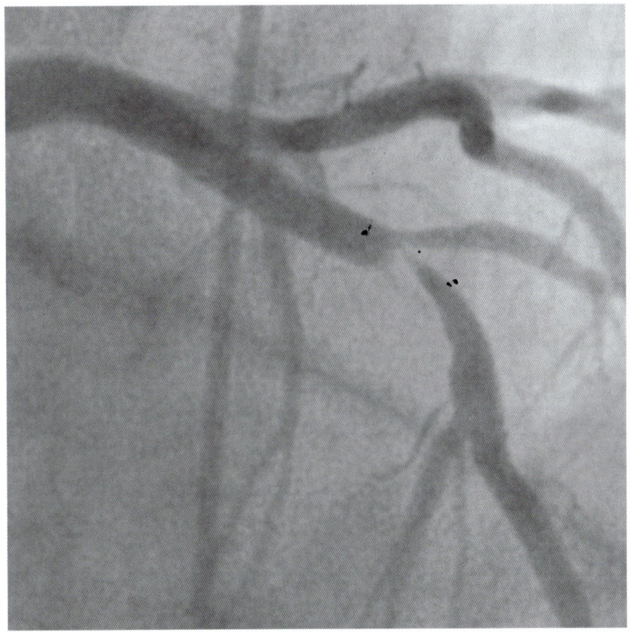

Figure Q20-16

(A) 1,1,1
(B) 0,1,1
(C) 1,0,1
(D) 0,0,1
(E) 1,1,0

20.17 Which of the following variables is the equivalent of two points in the DAPT score?

(A) Diabetes
(B) Current smoking
(C) Vein graft stenting
(D) History of chronic heart failure or LVEF < 30%
(E) C and D are correct

20.18 A 72-year-old patient with left main CAD with involvement of the proximal segments of both the LAD and left circumflex (LCx) coronary arteries asks you whether he should undergo CABG or PCI.

Regarding current evidence about PCI vs. CABG for the treatment of unprotected left main coronary artery disease, which of the following statements is NOT correct?

(A) At 5 years, there is equipoise of hard end points between PCI and CABG, but PCI suffers from an excess of repeat revascularization
(B) Target-vessel revascularization (TVR) is the main driver of different composite end points between PCI and CABG, but new statistical approaches may offer new insights in this comparison
(C) The EXCEL and NOBLE trials are the most recently published randomized trials comparing PCI vs. CABG for left main CAD
(D) The EXCEL trial compared PCI with SES vs. CABG in high-risk patients
(E) The NOBLE trial is an open-label, noninferiority trial, enrolling patients with left main CAD in northern Europe

20.19 Which of the following mechanisms may lead to the image shown in Figure Q20-19?

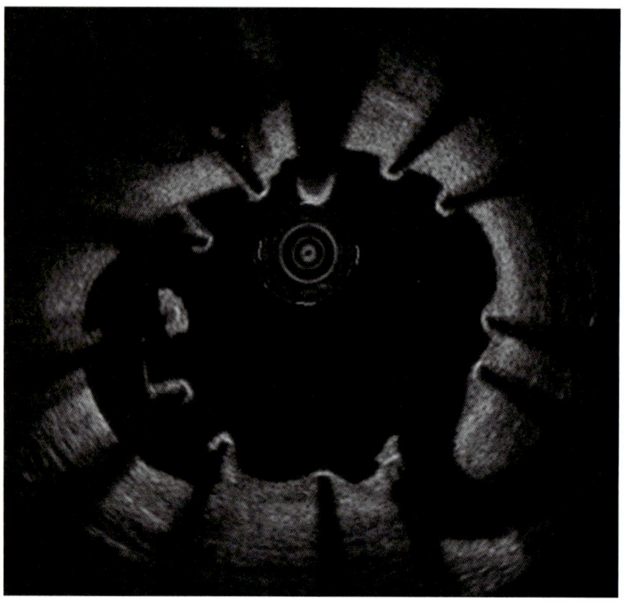

Figure Q20-19

(A) Positive arterial remodeling
(B) A decrease in plaque due to dissolution of jailed material
(C) Stent underexpansion
(D) Statements A, B, and C are correct
(E) None of the statements is correct

20.20 A 57-year-old patient with history of CAD and PCI of the RCA presents for repeat angiography according to a study protocol. He is asymptomatic and a stress test was inconclusive due to a left bundle branch block (LBBB). Which statement regarding the finding shown in Figure Q20-20A and B is CORRECT?

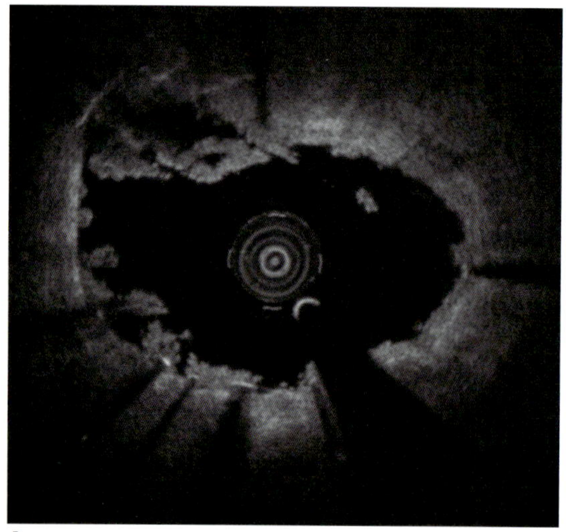

A

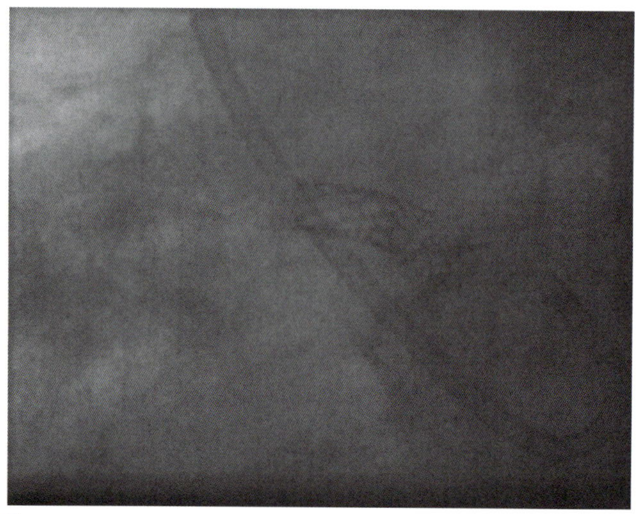

B

Figure Q20-20

(A) This finding is extremely frequent with BMS
(B) This angiographic finding is associated with a higher incidence of clinical adverse events
(C) The finding is positively correlated with stent length, stent overlap, and increasing duration after stent implantation
(D) This finding is more commonly observed in the RCA
(E) Statements B, C, and D are correct

20.21 After PCI of a significant stenosis in the mid-RCA of a 75-year-old female, you get the following result. Which of the following statements regarding the angiogram shown in Figure Q20-21 is most accurate?

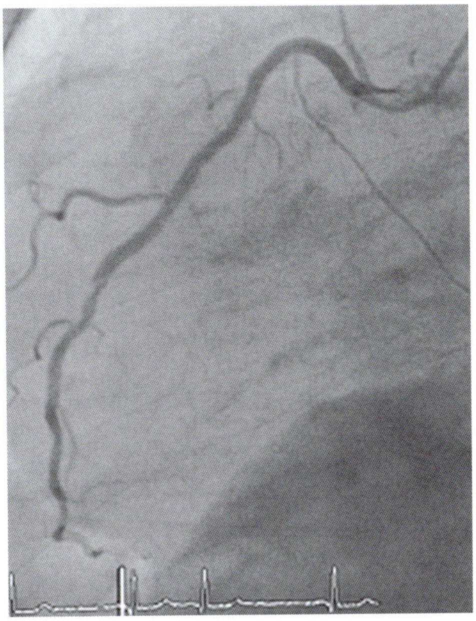

Figure Q20-21

(A) It is safe to leave this finding untreated
(B) It is safe to leave this finding untreated if glycoprotein (Gp) IIb/IIIa inhibitors are administered
(C) This finding can adequately be treated with balloon dilatation
(D) This finding is associated with an increased risk of early stent thrombosis
(E) This finding is caused by vasospasm

20.22 Which of the following images (Fig. Q20-22A–D) obtained with optical coherence tomography (OCT) or angiography after stenting is associated with the greatest risk of early stent thrombosis?

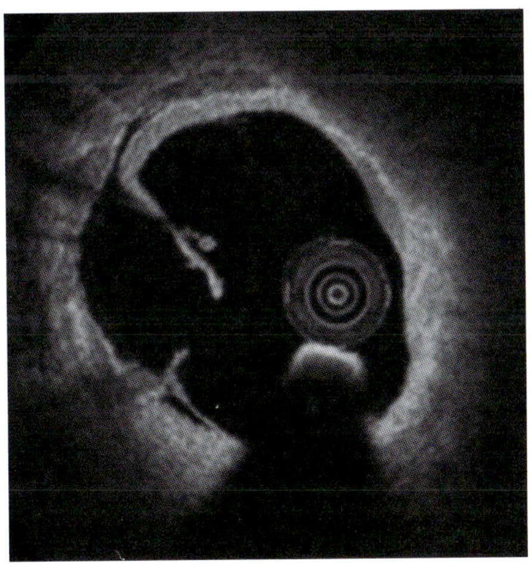

A

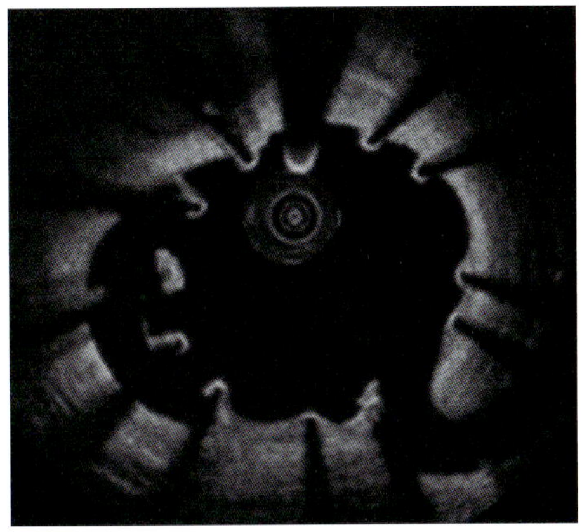

B

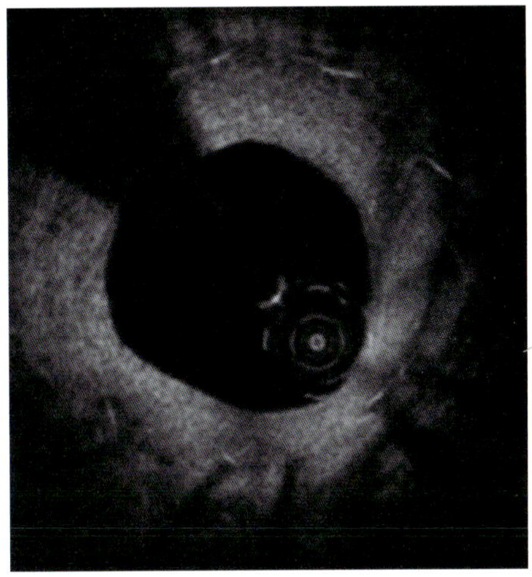

C

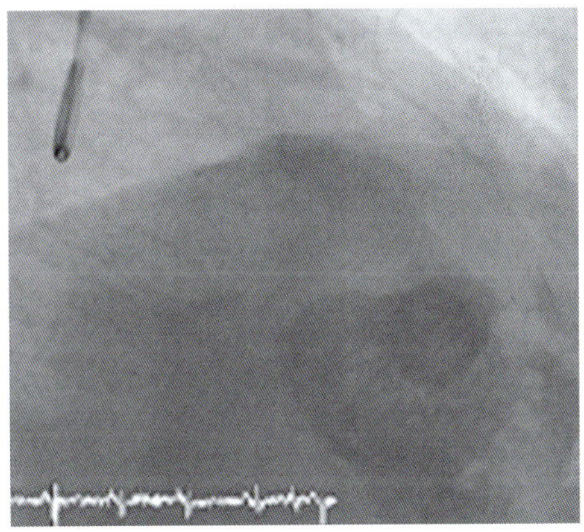

D

Figure Q20-22

(A) Figure A
(B) Figure B
(C) Figure C
(D) Figure D

Questions 20.23 through 20.26 refer to Academic Research Consortium (ARC) definitions of stent thrombosis. Match the following case vignettes with the appropriate term according to the ARC definition of stent thrombosis.

20.23 A 57-year-old male with STEMI 35 days after PCI with angiographically proven stent thrombosis.

(A) Definitive, primary, late stent thrombosis
(B) Definitive, primary, early stent thrombosis
(C) Definitive, secondary, late stent thrombosis
(D) Probable, primary, late stent thrombosis
(E) Probable, primary early stent thrombosis

20.24 A 45-year-old male with sudden cardiac arrest 20 days after PCI of a significant ostial LAD lesion.

(A) Definitive, secondary, early stent thrombosis
(B) Probable, primary, early stent thrombosis
(C) Probable, primary, late stent thrombosis
(D) Possible, primary, early stent thrombosis
(E) Possible, secondary, early stent thrombosis

20.25 A 78-year-old female with a history of PCI of a proximal RCA lesion 2 years ago and a new PCI of an in-stent restenosis 1 year ago presents to a primary care facility in cardiogenic shock with new ST-segment elevations in leads II, III, and aVF. She dies before transfer to the catheterization laboratory.

(A) Possible, secondary, very late stent thrombosis
(B) Possible, secondary, late stent thrombosis
(C) Probable, secondary, very late stent thrombosis
(D) Probable, primary, very late stent thrombosis
(E) Definite, secondary, late stent thrombosis

20.26 An 82-year-old female dying in a nursing home 18 months after implantation of a DES.

(A) Possible, primary, late stent thrombosis
(B) Possible, secondary, very late stent thrombosis
(C) Probable, primary, very late stent thrombosis
(D) Possible, primary, very late stent thrombosis
(E) Definite, primary, very late stent thrombosis

20.27 A 59-year-old patient with known CAD and stent placement to the proximal LAD 9 months ago presents to the emergency room with chest pain at rest and ST-segment elevations in leads V1 to V5. Coronary angiography shows the finding in Figure Q20-27. All of the following are risk factors for the event shown below, EXCEPT:

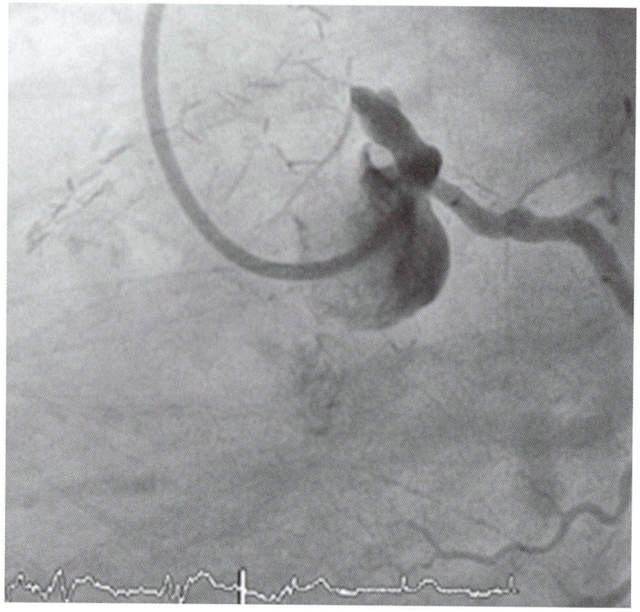

Figure Q20-27

(A) Insulin-dependent diabetes
(B) Impaired LVEF
(C) Renal failure
(D) Acute coronary syndrome (ACS) at the time of the index procedure
(E) Male gender

20.28 The PRECISE-DAPT score is a five-variable score. Which variables are included?

(A) Age, creatinine clearance, hemoglobin, white blood cell count, and previous spontaneous bleeding
(B) Age, peripheral arterial disease, hemoglobin, white blood cell count, and previous spontaneous bleeding
(C) Age, female gender, creatinine clearance, oral anticoagulation, and previous spontaneous bleeding
(D) Age, female gender, hemoglobin, oral anticoagulation, and previous spontaneous bleeding
(E) Age, female gender, oral anticoagulation, white blood cell count, and previous spontaneous bleeding

20.29 A 60-year-old man with diabetes and no other risk factors receives PCI with DES implantation due to stable CAD. Which of the following statements is INCORRECT?

(A) The presence of diabetes increases the risk of ischemic recurrences during follow-up
(B) A DAPT duration of at least 12 months should be recommended
(C) Regular physical activity should be recommended
(D) Optimal glycemic control should be recommended
(E) Adherence to therapies should be recommended

20.30 Which of the following statements is INCORRECT regarding current evidence on PCI for bifurcation lesions?

(A) A bifurcation coronary lesion is a lesion occurring at, or adjacent to, a significant division of a major epicardial coronary artery
(B) Coronary bifurcations are involved in 15% to 20% of all PCIs
(C) The preferred approach should be to use main vessel stenting with a proximal optimization technique and provisional side branch stenting
(D) MADS classification is an alternative to the Medina classification for anatomy of bifurcation lesions
(E) Stenting of the side branch is indicated during the provisional approach when side branch flow is compromised

20.31 Angiographic assessment of bifurcations has several limitations calling for a low threshold for use of IVUS or OCT. Which of the following statements is INCORRECT?

(A) OCT and IVUS may be of particular value in guiding bifurcation treatment due to high degree of angiographic ambiguity
(B) IVUS is recommended for left main bifurcation treatment and OCT may be used with the provision that aorto-ostial assessment is most often not possible
(C) IVUS may be superior to OCT in evaluation of the side branch ostium, stent positions, stent strut malapposition, wire position, and detection of thrombus
(D) Wire positions in-stent recrossing affect stent appositions and can be evaluated by OCT
(E) Accidental abluminal stent rewiring is a concern and may be ruled out by OCT

20.32 An 80-year-old woman with atrial fibrillation and chronic oral anticoagulation presents in the catheterization lab with stable inferior ischemia. You see a subocclusive stenosis of the mid-RCA and decide to treat with stent implantation. Which of the following is CORRECT?

(A) DES cannot be implanted in such patients
(B) The BioFreedom or Endeavor stents are considered a better option compared to BMS
(C) There is no increased risk of bleeding by prescribing DAPT together with oral anticoagulation
(D) Due to increased risk of bleeding, oral anticoagulation can be replaced with DAPT
(E) The patient will need oral anticoagulation and aspirin long-life

20.33 Which statement regarding the applicability of the ARC definition of stent thrombosis is CORRECT?

(A) Probable and possible stent thrombosis provides a high degree of sensitivity
(B) The combination of probable and possible stent thrombosis is suitable for the detection of safety signals
(C) Definite stent thrombosis provides a high specificity but may underestimate the true incidence of stent thrombosis
(D) The composite of definite and probable stent thrombosis is considered a reasonable balance of specificity and sensitivity
(E) All of the statements above are correct

20.34 A 52-year-old patient presents with chest pain at rest and inferior ST-segment elevations. Past medical history is significant for PCI of the proximal RCA 14 months ago. Coronary angiography shows a complete occlusion of the RCA; OCT reveals the finding depicted in Figure Q20-34. Which of the following mechanisms may have been associated with the occurrence of the event in question?

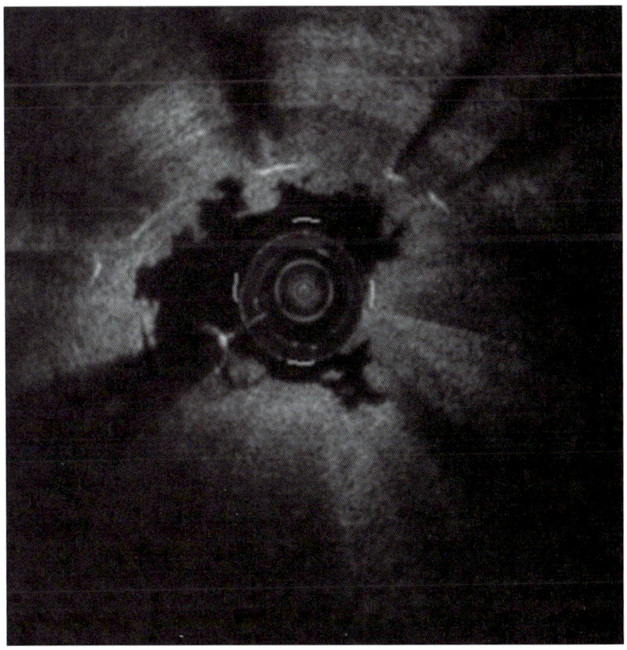

Figure Q20-34

(A) Delayed healing
(B) Chronic inflammation
(C) Hypersensitivity reactions
(D) Neoatherosclerosis
(E) All of the above

20.35 Which of the following statements with respect to histologic findings of thrombus aspirates of patients with very late stent thrombosis is CORRECT?

(A) They may show evidence of severe inflammation with eosinophilic infiltrates
(B) The eosinophilic infiltrates correlate with the amount of vessel remodeling
(C) Eosinophilic infiltrates are most commonly found in patients treated with SES
(D) Both sirolimus and paclitaxel have been shown to activate the coagulation cascade
(E) All of the statements above are correct

20.36 In a patient undergoing PCI, which of the following is NOT a characteristic of high bleeding risk?

(A) Advanced age
(B) Assumption of oral anticoagulation
(C) Chronic use of nonsteroidal anti-inflammatory drugs (NSAIDs)
(D) Diabetes
(E) Previous major bleeding

20.37 A 60-year-old man is going to receive PCI with stent implantation and asks to have information regarding the ischemic and bleeding risks. Which of the following sentences regarding 30-day outcomes is CORRECT?

(A) MI is more frequent and always associated with higher mortality than bleeding events
(B) MI, not bleeding, impacts prognosis
(C) Severe bleeding (i.e., Bleeding Academic Research Consortium [BARC] 3c) may be associated with higher risk of death compared to MI
(D) MI and minor bleeding are associated with the same risk of death
(E) Mortality is higher in patients experiencing a BARC 3b bleeding compared with MI

20.38 DAPT is generally recommended after PCI with stent implantation to reduce ischemic complications, including stent thrombosis and reinfarction. Which of the following is CORRECT?

(A) In case of complex PCI, but low risk of bleeding, the patient may benefit from a prolonged regimen of DAPT
(B) In patients at high bleeding risk, DAPT should be at least 6 months, even if PCI is performed for stable CAD
(C) The majority of ischemic events during follow-up are due to stent thrombosis
(D) Prolongation of DAPT over 12 months reduces stent thrombosis without increasing bleeding risk
(E) Patients with a history of MI do not benefit from an extended DAPT duration

20.39 Which of the following statements is NOT correct regarding the Nobori stent?

(A) The Nobori stent is a new-generation DES
(B) The Nobori stent has a bare metal platform with open cell
(C) The Nobori is a biolimus-eluting stent (BES)
(D) Stent thrombosis at 5 years in patients receiving the Nobori stent is dramatically high
(E) The coating process is the main difference between the Nobori and BioMatrix stents

20.40 Biolimus' peculiar chemical structure presents a modification at position 40 of the rapamycin ring that confers higher lipophilicity compared with sirolimus. The family of BES includes many stents, EXCEPT:

(A) BioMatrix
(B) Nobori
(C) AXXESS
(D) Xtent
(E) Orsiro

20.41 A 60-year-old patient with stable angina receives PCI with AXXESS implantation for a bifurcation lesion of the LAD artery and first diagonal. The AXXESS BES has several characteristics, EXCEPT:

(A) Nitinol platform
(B) Self-expanding
(C) Biodegradable polylactic acid (PLA) polymer
(D) Strut thickness 100 μm
(E) Conical shape

20.42 A 59-year-old patient with stable angina receives PCI with Orsiro implantation for a significant lesion of the LCx. Which of the following statements regarding this stent is FALSE?

(A) Orsiro is a cobalt chromium DES
(B) Orsiro has an ultrathin layer of 60 μm
(C) Orsiro platform includes a hybrid combination of passive (PROBIO) and active (PLLA) coatings
(D) PROBIO is a "nonactivating passive" biomaterial that blocks the electron transfer process on the stent surface
(E) The polymer compound carries and releases everolimus and is completely degradable

20.43 Regarding the clinical evidence available for the Orsiro stent, which of the following is FALSE?

(A) The BIOFLOW-I was the first-in-man study of Orsiro stent implantation
(B) The BIOFLOW-II trial showed the noninferiority of the Orsiro stent vs. the Xience stent
(C) The BIOSCIENCE trial enrolled 2,119 patients with STEMI
(D) The HATTRICK-OCT compared tissue coverage and apposition of Orsiro vs. Resolute
(E) Stent thrombosis was reduced in Orsiro vs. Nobori stents in the SORT OUT VII trial

20.44 Regarding the magnesium used in bioresorbable scaffolds, which of the following statement is FALSE?

(A) Biotronik has developed different absorbable magnesium scaffolds
(B) Magnesium is more electronegative than other metals used for implants
(C) Magnesium has showed antithrombotic properties
(D) AMS-1 was tested in the PROGRESS AMS first-in-man study
(E) The AMS-3 (DREAMS) is a sirolimus-eluting new-generation magnesium scaffold

20.45 Which of the following is FALSE regarding the SYNERGY stent?

(A) SYNERGY is a platinum-chromium EES
(B) SYNERGY is not a chromium-cobalt EES
(C) SYNERGY has the same structure as the XIENCE stent
(D) SYNERGY employs a fully biodegradable poly-lactic-co-glycolic acid (PLGA) polymer applied to the abluminal surface of the stent
(E) SYNERGY was investigated in the EVOLVE I, EVOLVE II, and BIO-RESORT TWENTE trials

20.46 Stent technology uses polymers as the interface between stent and vascular tissue, carriers of antiproliferative drugs, and controllers of drug release. Which of the following statement is CORRECT?

(A) Durable polymers used in first-generation DES were not associated with any complications
(B) Biodegradable polymers allow drug elution by particle dissolution while durable polymers use drug diffusion or matrix degradation
(C) Nonpolymeric DES systems incorporate alternative technologies, such as reservoirs, surface modifications, and nanoparticles to carry and control the release of antiproliferative drugs
(D) The Promus stent is a biodegradable polymer DES
(E) BMS, durable polymer DES, and biodegradable polymer DES showed similar safety and efficacy

20.47 A 75-year-old patient has recently received PCI with BMS implantation. During a visit, he expresses some concerns about the selection of the stent and the clinical events during long-term follow-up. Which of the following statements is CORRECT?

(A) A BVS is more appropriate than BMS and DES in any case
(B) A paclitaxel-eluting stent (PES) would have provided lower risk of death and stent thrombosis
(C) At 6 years, contemporary BMS have shown similar composite outcomes compared with contemporary DES
(D) The stent selection was inappropriate due to risks of death that emerge with BMS
(E) There are no data comparing long-term outcomes of BMS vs. DES

20.48 Different DES incorporate and elute different antiproliferative drugs. Most of the current DES use limus-related drugs, such as sirolimus, everolimus, Biolimus A9, zotarolimus and Novolimus, which bind to the intracellular receptor FKBP-12 and inhibit the mammalian target of rapamycin (mTOR)—blocking the cell cycle of the smooth muscle cell. Which of the following stent/drug associations is CORRECT?

(A) Endeavor–Sirolimus
(B) Orsiro–Paclitaxel
(C) DESyne–Novolimus
(D) Resolute Integrity–Paclitaxel
(E) Promus Element–Biolimus

ANSWERS AND EXPLANATIONS

20.1 Answer B. After Charles Dotter had implanted the first vascular stent in a canine popliteal artery in 1968, the first coronary stent was a self-expanding stent called Wallstent. Jacques Puel implanted Wallstent for the very first time in 1986 in the LAD artery of a 63-year-old patient presenting with restenosis after plain balloon angioplasty. The Palmaz–Schatz stent was the first balloon-expandable (tubular-slotted) stent; it was implanted for the first time in December 1987 in São Paolo, Brazil. The Igaki–Tamai stent consisted of poly-L-lactic acid and was the first fully bioabsorbable stent. The sirolimus-eluting Cypher stent was the first DES approved by the U.S. Food and Drug Administration (FDA) in 2002.

20.2 Answer A. In a recent study (Taniwaki M, et al. *Circulation* 2016;133(7):650–660), 64 patients were investigated at the time point of very late stent thrombosis as part of an international OCT registry. A total of 38 early- and 20 newer-generation DES were suitable for analysis. Very late stent thrombosis occurred at a median of 4.7 years (interquartile range, 3.1 to 7.5 years). An underlying putative cause by OCT was identified in 98% of cases. The most frequent findings were strut malapposition (34.5%), neoatherosclerosis (27.6%), uncovered struts (12.1%), and stent underexpansion (6.9%). Uncovered and malapposed struts were more frequent in thrombosed compared with nonthrombosed regions (ratio of percentages, 8.26; 95% confidence interval, 6.82 to 10.04; $p < 0.001$ and 13.03; 95% confidence interval, 10.13 to 16.93; $p < 0.001$, respectively). The maximal length of malapposed or uncovered struts (3.40 mm; 95% confidence interval, 2.55 to 4.25; vs. 1.29 mm; 95% confidence interval, 0.81 to 1.77; $p < 0.001$), but not the maximal or average axial malapposition distance, was greater in thrombosed compared with nonthrombosed segments. The associations of both uncovered and malapposed struts with thrombus were consistent among early- and newer-generation DES. Therefore, the leading associated findings in very late stent thrombosis patients in descending order were malapposition, neoatherosclerosis, uncovered struts, and stent underexpansion without differences between patients treated with early- and new-generation DES. The longitudinal extension of malapposed and uncovered stent was the most important correlate of thrombus formation in very late stent thrombosis.

20.3 Answer C. Key prerequisites of coronary artery stents are the sealing of coronary artery dissections by tacking of intimal flaps against the arterial wall and the prevention of elastic recoil after balloon angioplasty. Limited deformability is required for bifurcation stenting techniques, and a low profile and high flexibility facilitate stent placement in calcified and tortuous coronary arteries. Positive arterial remodeling is a rare adverse process observed with metallic DES that may lead to late-acquired stent malapposition and may be associated with an increased risk of late stent thrombosis.

20.4 Answer C. Figure C shows a perforation of a posterior descending coronary artery following plain balloon angioplasty. The use of covered stents is confined to the emergency treatment of coronary perforations or for the exclusion of giant coronary aneurysms (not shown) (Eshtehardi P, et al. *Circ Cardiovasc Interv* 2008;1(1):85–86). Figure A shows a significant stenosis of an SVG. It has been hypothesized that covered stents might decrease distal embolization by entrapping friable degenerated material and reduce neointimal hyperplasia. However, a randomized multicenter trial of 400 patients failed to show any advantage of a polytetrafluoroethylene (PTFE)-covered stent compared with a BMS in terms of percent diameter stenosis or major adverse cardiac events (MACE) at 8 months (Turco MA, et al. *Catheter Cardiovasc Interv* 2006;68(3):379–388). Figure B shows thrombotic occlusion of a RCA, Figure D illustrates a periprocedural coronary dissection, and Figure E demonstrates stent implantation in an ostial lesion.

20.5 Answer E. Whereas self-expanding stents and balloon-expandable stents had been used with similar frequency in the early days of coronary artery stenting, several drawbacks of self-expanding stents, such as less precise placement and negative recoil, have outweighed the potential advantages mentioned in statements B and D. Self-expanding stents have been associated with a lower incidence of edge dissections and side-branch occlusions (König A, et al. *Catheter Cardiovasc Interv* 2002;56(4):478–486). However, the mechanism of self-expanding stents is based on the shape memory of nitinol, an alloy of nickel and titanium, which continues to exert an outward radial force after release, leading to negative chronic recoil. In contrast to balloon-expandable stents, deliverability is dictated by the delivery sheath and strut dimensions rather than balloon profile. Self-expandable stents are currently being investigated in patients with bifurcation lesions, vulnerable plaques, and small-diameter vessels.

20.6 Answer A. The risk of stent thrombosis is not increased but similar when using a radial access compared with femoral access site (Vranckx P, et al. *Eur Heart J* 2017;38(14):1069–1080). The use of bivalirudin or Absorb BVS is not associated with a reduction of stent thrombosis; rather, this risk is similar or increased. STEMI patients are known to be at increased risk of ischemic complications, including stent thrombosis compared to stable patients. Several studies have clarified that DES have not increased risk of stent thrombosis compared with BMS, particularly new-generation DES, which seem to reduce this risk (Palmerini T, et al. *Lancet* 2012;379(9824):1393–1402).

20.7 Answer E. BVS theoretically leave no permanent implant and allow for restoration of vessel function. In the Amsterdam Investigator-Initiated Absorb Strategy All-Comers Trial (AIDA), BVS was compared with the EES metallic stent in a patient population that reflects that seen in routine clinical practice. Recently, an early report of the data was published as recommended by the data and safety monitoring board due to safety concerns (Wykrzykowska JJ, et al. *N Engl J Med* 2017;376(24):2319–2328). In this study, 1,845 patients undergoing PCI were randomly assigned to receive either a BVS (924 patients) or a metallic EES (921 patients). The primary end point was target vessel failure (a composite of cardiac death, target vessel MI, or TVR). In this preliminary report, there was no significant difference in the rate of target vessel failure between the patients who received a BVS and the patients who received a metallic stent. The BVS was associated with a higher incidence of device thrombosis than the metallic stent through 2 years of follow-up. Additionally, a recent meta-analysis investigated the comparative effectiveness of the FDA-approved Absorb BVS vs. metallic EES in patients undergoing PCI at longest available follow-up. The study included seven trials (ABSORB II, ABSORB III, ABSORB China, ABSORB Japan, EVERBIO II, TROFI II, AIDA) and 5,583 patients were randomized to receive either the study Absorb BVS (n = 3,261) or EES (n = 2,322) at median follow-up of 2 years. Compared with metallic EES, risk of target lesion failure (9.6% vs. 7.2%, absolute risk difference [ARD] = +2.4%, relative risk [RR]: 1.32, 95% confidence interval [CI]: 1.10 to 1.59, number needed to harm [NNH] = 41, p = 0.003, I2 = 0%) and stent thrombosis (2.4% vs. 0.7%, ARD: +1.7%, RR: 3.15, 95% CI: 1.87 to 5.30, NNH = 60, p < 0.0001, I2 = 0%) were both significantly higher with BVS. The increased risk for ST associated with BVS was concordant across the early (<30 days), late (30 days to 1 year), and very late (>1 year) periods. There were no significant differences in all-cause or cardiovascular mortality between groups (Sorrentino S, et al. *J Am Coll Cardiol* 2017;69(25):3055–3066). Similarly, a further meta-analysis including five of those trials showed that compared with EES, the use of Absorb BVS was associated with a higher rate of device thrombosis and a trend toward a higher risk of target lesion failure and that very late device thrombosis occurred in 1.4% of the patients (the majority of these events occurred in the absence of DAPT) (Collet C, et al. *Eur Heart J* 2017;38(33):2559–2566. doi: 10.1093/eurheartj/ehx155).

20.8 Answer A. The PSP score has recently been generated and validated into the GHOST-EU registry, which included all-comer patients treated with BVS. PSP was shown to predict 1 year, device-oriented composite end point (DoCE) composed of cardiac death, target-vessel MI, and clinically driven TLR. Furthermore, no patient with a maximum PSP-1 score had scaffold thrombosis, compared to those with a nonmaximum PSP-1 score (Ortega-Paz L, et al. *Eurointervention* 2017;12(17):2110–2117). The correct sizing was defined as the following:

- Implantation of a 2.5-mm diameter scaffold in a vessel with a proximal/distal reference vessel diameter ≥2.5 mm and <2.75 mm
- Implantation of a 3.0-mm diameter scaffold in a vessel with a proximal/distal reference vessel diameter ≥2.75 mm and <3.25 mm
- Implantation of a 3.5-mm diameter scaffold in a vessel with a proximal/distal reference vessel diameter ≥3.25 mm and ≤3.75 mm
- If proximal and distal reference vessel diameter differed, mean value was used.

Postdilatation was optimal when performed with a noncompliant balloon of larger diameter than the scaffold, up to a maximum of 0.5 mm.

20.9 Answer E. Routine IVUS-guided PCI in the pre–DES era has been shown to improve angiographic minimum lumen diameter and reduce angiographic restenosis and the rate of repeat revascularization in a meta-analysis. However, no effect on death and MI was appreciated during a follow-up period of 6 months to 2.5 years (Parise H, et al. *Am J Cardiol* 2011;107(3):374–382). A minimal stent area of >5 mm^2 is generally considered satisfactory. Although IVUS can reliably assess stent apposition, there is not large evidence from a prospective study proving that routine use of IVUS reduces the incidence of stent thrombosis. IVUS is able to assess tissue characteristics of underlying plaques (virtual histology).

20.10 Answer A. An analysis from the ACC/National Cardiovascular Data Registry, which included 558,273 PCIs performed between 2001 and 2004, reported an in-hospital mortality of 0.7%, a rate of MI of 1.1%, the need for emergency CABG in 0.6%, and stroke ranging from 0.1% to 0.3% during the in-hospital period.

20.11 Answer D. While the Orsiro stent is a biodegradable polymer SES, the Igaki–Tamai (the first fully bioresorbable stent to be implanted in humans), the DESolve (a PLLA-based polymer scaffold coated with the myolimus mounted on a rapid exchange balloon catheter delivery system; Elixir Medical Corporation), the REVA (a tyrosine poly carbonate stent that is both resorbable and radio-opaque after chemical modification of tyrosine to incorporate iodine molecules; Boston Scientific), and the IDEAL (biodegradable stent consisting of a backbone of polyanhydride ester based on salicylic acid and adipic acid anhydride and a coating of sirolimus; Bioabsorbable Therapeutics, Inc.) are bioresorbable scaffolds.

20.12 Answer E. TIMI risk score is a prognostic score estimating mortality in ACS patients, while SYNTAX score is an angiographic score estimating severity and complexity of coronary disease. Recently, the DAPT score and the PRECISE-DAPT score have been generated in larger populations of PCI patients to help decision-making on the optimal duration of the DAPT after stent implantation (Yeh RW, et al. *JAMA* 2016;315(16):1735–1749; Costa F, et al. *Lancet* 2017;389(10073):1025–1034).

20.13 Answer B. Diabetes, prior MI, PES stent implantation, and PCI stenting of vein graft are predictors of ischemic events and were included in the DAPT score. Peripheral arterial disease emerged to be a predictor of both ischemic and bleeding events in DAPT and was not entered in the DAPT score.

Table A20-13 DAPT score

Variable	Points
Age ≥ 75 y	−2
Age 65–74 y	−1
Age < 65 y	0
Current smoking	1
Diabetes mellitus	1
MI at presentation	1
Prior PCI or prior MI	1
Paclitaxel-eluting stent	1
Stent diameter < 3 mm	1
CHF or LVEF < 30%	2
Vein graft stenting	2
TOTAL SCORE RANGE	**From −2 to 10**

Abbreviations: CHF, chronic heart failure; DAPT, dual antiplatelet therapy; LVEF, left ventricular ejection fraction; MI, myocardial infarction; PCI, percutaneous coronary intervention.

20.14 Answer A. PCI for SVGs is associated with suboptimal results due to high rates of periprocedural MI and high rates of restenosis requiring TLR (Savage MP, et al. *N Engl J Med* 1997;337(11):740–747). Embolic protection devices reduce periprocedural MIs in PCI for SVGs and are recommended when technically feasible. In contrast to lesions in native vessels, there is lower evidence investigating the potential benefits of DES over BMS in SVGs. However, the majority of them demonstrate DES superiority (Aggarwal V, et al. *J Am Coll Cardiol* 2014;64(17):1825–1836; Wiisanen ME, et al. *JACC Cardiovasc Interv* 2010;3(12):1262–1273; Alam M, et al. *Clin Cardiol* 2012;35(5):291–296).

20.15 Answer A. The angiographic picture shows a CTO of the mid- to distal RCA. Lesions can be classified as CTOs when there is TIMI 0 flow within the occluded segment and an occlusion duration >3 months. CTO recanalization is generally indicated in patients with symptoms and evidence of ischemia, and viability should be confirmed in case of patients with prior Q-wave MI. DES should be preferred to BMS.

IVUS can be used for the identification of the proximal cap in stumpless CTOs, for wire redirection in cases of subintimal wire entry, to monitor the course of the retrograde wire course during retrograde procedures, and for optimization of stent placement, especially in complex CTOs (Sianos G, et al. *EuroIntervention* 2012;8(1):139–145; Galassi AR, et al. *Eur Heart J* 2016;37(35):2692–2700).

20.16 Answer B. The Medina classification of bifurcation lesions indicates the presence or absence of stenosis at the site of bifurcation as 1 or 0 in three segments. The first digit indicates the proximal main vessel, the second digit the distal main vessel, and the third digit the side branch. The stenosis shown in Figure A20-16 involves the distal segment of the main vessel and the side branch (0,1,1).

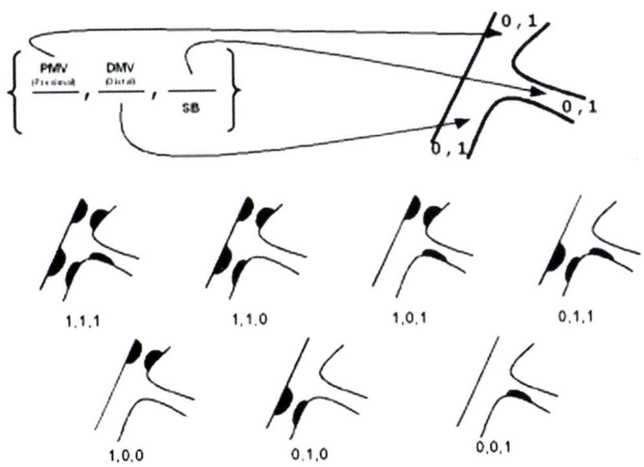

Figure A20-16

20.17 Answer E. Both vein graft stenting and heart failure attributes two points, while one point is attributed in case of diabetes, current smoking, previous MI or PCI, MI at presentation, implantation of PES, and stent diameter <3 mm. Regarding age, 0 is attributed to <65 years, −1 to from 65 to 74 years, and −2 points if age is ≥75 years (see Table A20-13).

20.18 Answer D. At 5 years, PCI and CABG were found to be associated with similar rates of death, MI, and stroke, but TVR was significantly higher in PCI-treated patients (Gargiulo G, et al. *Int J Cardiol* 2015;195:79–81). In a recent analysis from the DELTA registry, a large, multicenter registry of unprotected left main coronary artery disease, the impact of different computing methods for composite end points other than time-to-event statistics were investigated. In particular, the time-to-event, Andersen–Gill, win ratio, competing risk, and weighted composite endpoint computing methods were applied and compared. Incorporating the clinical relevance of the individual outcomes resulted in sensibly different findings as compared with the conventional TTE approach. Indeed, the TTE approach resulted in similar MACE when TVR was excluded (death or MI or cerebrovascular accident) between PCI and CABG, but advantage of CABG over PCI with MACE included TVR. When using the weighted composite endpoint computing method, which assigns a weight to each event based on its severity, PCI and CABG were no longer significantly different with respect to the composite of death, MI, cerebrovascular accident, or TVR at a median of 3 years (Capodanno D, et al. *JACC Cardiovasc Interv* 2016;9(22):2280–2288).

The EXCEL trial has recently randomly assigned 1,905 eligible patients with left main coronary artery disease of low or intermediate anatomical complexity to undergo either PCI with fluoropolymer-based cobalt-chromium EES (PCI group, 948 patients) or CABG (CABG group, 957 patients). Anatomic complexity was assessed at the sites and defined by a Synergy between Percutaneous Coronary Intervention with Taxus and Cardiac Surgery (SYNTAX) score of 32 or lower. Overall, it demonstrated that in patients with left main coronary artery disease and low or intermediate SYNTAX scores by site assessment, PCI with EES was noninferior to CABG with respect to the rate of the composite end point of death, stroke, or MI at 3 years (Stone GW, et al. *N Engl J Med* 2016;375(23):2223–2235).

The NOBLE trial is a prospective, randomized, open-label, noninferiority trial, in which patients with left main coronary artery disease were enrolled in 36 centers in northern Europe and randomized 1:1 to treatment with PCI or CABG. In this trial, 1,201 patients were randomly assigned, 598 to PCI and 603 to CABG, and 592 in each group entered analysis by intention to treat. At 5 years, noninferiority was not met for major adverse cardiovascular and cerebrovascular events (MACCE) (composite of all-cause mortality, nonprocedural MI, any repeat coronary revascularization, and stroke) and CABG was significantly better than PCI. This finding was driven by significant increase of nonprocedural MI and any revascularization in the PCI group, but all-cause mortality was similar (Mäkikallio T, et al. *Lancet* 2016;388(10061):2743–2752).

20.19 Answer D. The cross-sectional OCT image shows incomplete stent apposition at follow-up, which may be the result of positive arterial remodeling, a decrease in plaque due to dissolution of jailed material (i.e., thrombus) at the time of stent implantation, or stent underexpansion (Cook S, et al. *Circulation* 2007;115(18):2426–2434).

20.20 Answer E. The image is an example of a stent fracture as a late complication of stent implantation with an incidence ranging from 1% to 29% in randomized, observational, and autopsy studies (Lee MS, et al. *Catheter Cardiovasc Interv* 2007;69(3):387–394; Aoki J, et al. *Catheter Cardiovasc Interv*

;69(3):380–386; Lee SH, et al. *Am J Cardiol* 2007;100(4):627–630; Nakazawa G, et al. *J Am Coll Cardiol* 2009;54(21):1924–1931). Stent fractures have predominantly been reported with Cypher stents, whereas stent fractures with TAXUS stents and other stents appear to be less frequent. The risk of stent fracture has been correlated with several mechanical factors and lesions characteristics, such as lesion location in the RCA, severely tortuous vessels, long/overlapping stents, and stent implantation duration (Nakazawa G, et al. *J Am Coll Cardiol* 2009;54(21):1924–1931). Approximately three-quarters of patients with a stent fracture will present with in-stent restenosis. Some will present with stent thrombosis (Aoki J, et al. *Catheter Cardiovasc Interv* 2007;69(3):380–386).

20.21 Answer D. The image shows a distal edge dissection. Residual dissections after PCI may cause early stent thrombosis. Whereas it is acceptable to leave mild luminal haziness untreated, intraluminal linear dissection increases the risk of abrupt closure (Cutlip DE, et al. *Circulation* 2001;103(15):1967–1971) (Table A20-21).

Table A20-21 National Heart, Lung and Blood Institute's classification system of coronary dissection

Type	Description	Rate of Acute Closure (%)
A	Mild luminal haziness	0
B	Intraluminal linear dissection	3
C	Extraluminal contrast dye staining or extraluminal cap (with persistence of dye after dye clearance)	10
D	Spiral dissection	30
E	Dissection with filling defects	9
F	Dissection with limited or no flow	69

20.22 Answer A. Figures A through C are OCT images. Figure A shows a dissection of the intima just distal to the stent edge (no stent struts visible). Figure B illustrates strut malapposition between 7 and 11 o'clock. Figure C shows stent struts covered by neointimal hyperplasia, consistent with in-stent restenosis. Figure D, plain fluoroscopy performed without contrast, shows a long-stented segment involving the proximal, mid, and distal segment of the LAD. Both incomplete stent apposition and stent length have been associated with stent thrombosis. An IVUS study showed that incomplete stent apposition was more frequent (77% vs. 12%; $p < 0.001$) and maximal incomplete stent apposition area was larger (8.3 ± 7.5 mm² vs. 4.0 ± 3.8 mm²; $p = 0.03$) in patients with very late stent thrombosis compared with 144 controls (Cook S, et al. *Circulation* 2007;115(18):2426–2434). In a consecutive cohort of 3,145 patients treated with DES, stent lengths ≥31.5 mm were associated with higher rates of ST (4.0% vs. 0.7%, $p < 0.001$), death (5.2% vs. 3.0%, $p = 0.005$), and MI (2.4% vs. 0.7%, $p = 0.001$) at 3 years, as compared with stent length < 31.5 mm (Suh J, et al. *JACC Cardiovasc Interv* 2010;3(4):383–389). Nevertheless, intraluminal dissection portends the highest risk for early stent thrombosis.

For Answers 20.23 through 20.26, refer to Table A20-23.

Table A20-23 The definition of stent thrombosis according to the Academic Research Consortium

Definite stent thrombosis
Either angiographic or postmortem evidence of thrombotic stent occlusion in the presence of symptoms consistent with an acute myocardial infarction

Probable stent thrombosis
Any unexplained death within 30 days of stent implantation, or any myocardial infarction in the territory of the implanted stent irrespective of time

Possible stent thrombosis
Any unexplained death beyond 30 d until the end of follow-up

Early stent thrombosis: ≤1 mo
≤1 day: acute stent thrombosis
>1 day: subacute stent thrombosis

Late stent thrombosis: >1 mo up to 1 y

Very late stent thrombosis: >1 y

Primary stent thrombosis
Stent thrombosis without intercurrent target lesion revascularization

Secondary stent thrombosis
Stent thrombosis following intercurrent target lesion revascularization

20.23 Answer A.

20.24 Answer B.

20.25 Answer C.

20.26 Answer D.

20.27 Answer E. Several patient- and lesion-related risk factors for stent thrombosis have been identified. Diabetes has been identified as an independent predictor of stent thrombosis in numerous studies. In a registry of more than 15,000 patients treated with SES, diabetes mellitus was associated with a two- to threefold increased risk of stent thrombosis

(OR 2.76, 95% CI 1.71 to 4.29; $p < 0.0001$) (Urban P, et al. *Circulation* 2006;113(11):1434–1441). It also emerged as an independent predictor of early stent thrombosis in a large two-institutional cohort of patients treated with DES (HR: 1.96; 95% CI: 1.18 to 3.28) (Daemen J, et al. *Lancet* 2007;369(9562):667–678). In both the cited studies, ACS at the time of the index procedure was a predictor for stent thrombosis. Impaired LVEF was found to increase the risk of stent thrombosis (HR, 1.09; 95% CI, 1.05 to 1.36; $p < 0.001$ for each 10% decrease) in a prospective observational cohort study with 2,229 patients undergoing SES or PES implantation. The same study reported an increased risk of stent thrombosis in patients with renal failure (HR, 6.49; 95% CI, 2.60 to 16.15; $p < 0.001$) (Iakovou I, et al. *JAMA* 2005;293(17):2126–2130). No gender difference in the occurrence of stent thrombosis has been clearly reported.

20.28 Answer A. The PRECISE-DAPT score (age, creatinine clearance, hemoglobin, white blood cell count, and previous spontaneous bleeding) is a simple five-item risk score, which provides a standardized tool for the prediction of out-of-hospital bleeding during DAPT. In the context of a comprehensive clinical evaluation process, this tool can support clinical decision-making for treatment duration. A total of 14,963 patients treated with DAPT after coronary stenting, largely consisting of aspirin and clopidogrel and without indication to oral anticoagulation, were pooled at a single-patient level from eight multicenter randomized clinical trials with independent adjudication of events. Using the Cox proportional hazards regression, predictors of out-of-hospital TIMI major or minor bleeding stratified by trial were identified, and a numerical bleeding risk score was developed. The predictive performance of this novel score was assessed in the derivation cohort and validated in patients treated with PCI from the PLATO trial (n = 8,595) and BernPCI registry (n = 6,172). The novel score was assessed within patients randomized to different DAPT durations (n = 10,081) to identify the effect on bleeding and ischemia of a long (12 to 24 months) or short (3 to 6 months) treatment in relation to baseline bleeding risk. (See the answer to Question 20.12.)

20.29 Answer B. Although the presence of diabetes emerged as an independent predictor of MACE after implantation of a DES, 3 to 6 months of DAPT showed to be noninferior to 12 months DAPT in a large individual patient meta-analysis from randomized clinical trials. DAPT prolongation did not reduce the risk of MACE but increased the risk of bleeding among patients with stents with and without diabetes (Gargiulo G, et al. *Br Med J* 2016;355:i5483). Regular physical activity, optimal glycemic control, and adherence to therapies should be recommended in diabetic patients.

20.30 Answer D. A bifurcation coronary lesion is a lesion occurring at, or adjacent to, a significant division of a major epicardial coronary artery. A "significant" side branch is most often arbitrarily defined based upon the subjective judgment of the operator. Coronary bifurcations are involved in 15% to 20% of all PCIs and remain one of the most challenging lesions in interventional cardiology in terms of procedural success rate as well as long-term cardiac events.

The European Bifurcation Club (EBC) released recently its 11th consensus document pointing to the fact that there is a multitude of strategies and approaches to bifurcation stenting within the provisional strategy and in the different two-stent strategies (Lassen JF, et al. *EuroIntervention* 2016;12(1):38–46). The main EBC recommendation for PCI of bifurcation lesions remains to use main vessel stenting with a proximal optimization technique and provisional side-branch stenting as a preferred approach. A simple description of bifurcation lesions, stenosis quantification, and PCI techniques is not straightforward. Consensus was reached by promoting a simplified and universal classification of bifurcation lesions, the Medina classification, and an accurate definition of each of the various techniques used in bifurcation stenting combined with a precise classification system to facilitate the description, the MADS classification (Louvard Y, et al. *Catheter Cardiovasc Interv* 2008;71(2):175–183). The MADS classification is a systematic description of bifurcation stenting techniques grouped in families and is based on two principles: (1) the final position of the stent(s) (one to three stents) in the bifurcation and (2) the implantation order. The position of the first implanted stent in a bifurcation corresponds to a given strategy out of four (MADS): M begins with a stent in the proximal part of the main vessel; A begins with a stent in the main vessel across the side branch; D defines a double stent implantation, whether simultaneously or not; and S consists of a stent implantation in the side branch first. The two classifications are strongly recommended because they have provided the valuable opportunity to standardize reports, to allow comparisons between studies, and to facilitate interpretation of published results.

Stenting of the side branch is indicated during the provisional approach: (1) when side-branch flow is compromised, (2) in the presence of a major side-branch dissection; or (3) when the side branch is significantly diseased and large enough to lead to significant residual ischemia.

20.31 Answer C. All the statements are correct except C because OCT may be superior to IVUS in evaluation of the side branch ostium, stent positions, stent strut malapposition, wire position, and detection of thrombus (Lassen JF, et al. *EuroIntervention* 2016;12(1):38–46).

20.32 Answer B. DES can be considered in patients with high bleeding risk; in particular, the BioFreedom stent and the Endeavor stent have been found to offer superior efficacy and safety compared with BMS in the LEADERS-FREE and ZEUS trials, respectively (Urban P, et al. *N Engl J Med* 2015;373(21):2038–2047; Ariotti S, et al. *J Am Coll Cardiol Interv* 2016;9(5):426–436).

20.33 Answer E. Whereas definite stent thrombosis may underestimate the true incidence of stent thrombosis, the combination of probable and possible stent thrombosis provides a high sensitivity suitable for the detection of safety signals. The composite of definite and probable stent thrombosis is considered a reasonable balance of specificity and sensitivity and is therefore frequently used as an end point in clinical trials.

20.34 Answer E. The OCT image shows stent struts covered by thrombotic debris consistent with the diagnosis of very late stent thrombosis. Several underlying pathophysiologic mechanisms have been suggested and are summarized in statements A through D. In autopsy studies, incomplete reendothelialization and persistent fibrin deposition indicated delayed healing (Joner M, et al. *J Am Coll Cardiol* 2006;48(1):193–202). Histologic examination of thrombus aspirates revealed severe inflammation with eosinophilic infiltrates, which correlated with the amount of incomplete stent apposition (Cook S, et al. *Circulation* 2009;120(5):391–399). In a registry of 5,783 patients, 17 patients with hypersensitivity symptoms probably or certainly related to DES were found, of which four patients had died of coronary stent thrombosis. Poor intimal healing and neoatherosclerosis have been reported as mechanisms of very late stent thrombosis (Nakazawa G, et al. *J Am Coll Cardiol* 2011;57(11):1314–1322; Taniwaki M, et al. *Circulation* 2016;133(7):650–660).

20.35 Answer E. In histologic examination of thrombus aspirates, severe inflammation with eosinophilic infiltrates was demonstrated, which correlated with the extent of incomplete stent apposition. This finding was particularly evident in patients with SES (Cook S, et al. *Circulation* 2009;120(5):391–399). Sirolimus and paclitaxel both activate the coagulation cascade by increasing endothelial tissue factor expression, which is a receptor of factor VII (Steffel J, et al. *Circulation* 2005;112(13):2002–2011; Stähli BE, et al. *Circ Res* 2006;99(2):149–155).

20.36 Answer D. Advanced age, oral anticoagulation, use of NSAIDs, and history of bleeding are known risk factors for bleeding and were inclusion criteria for "high bleeding risk" in both the LEADERS-FREE and ZEUS trials. Diabetes mellitus is not generally recognized as high bleeding risk factor (see the answer to 20.32).

20.37 Answer C. Bleeding is known to impact on prognosis. In a recent study, in patients treated with antiplatelet therapy after ACS, both MI and bleeding significantly impacted mortality with similar time dependency. Although BARC 2 and 3a bleeding were less prognostic for death than MI, the risk of mortality was equivalent between BARC 3b bleeding and MI and was higher following BARC 3c bleeding (Valgimigli M, et al. *Eur Heart J* 2017;38(11):804–810).

20.38 Answer A. Alongside other established clinical risk factors, procedural complexity is an important parameter to take into account in tailoring upfront duration of DAPT. In a recent meta-analysis of six randomized trials of DAPT regimens, compared with short-term DAPT, long-term DAPT yielded significant reductions in MACE in the complex PCI group vs. the noncomplex PCI group and the magnitude of the benefit with long-term DAPT was progressively greater per increase in procedural complexity (Giustino G, et al. *J Am Coll Cardiol* 2016;68(17):1851–1864). On the other hand, patients at high bleeding risk may benefit from a shorter DAPT duration, even 1 month, and particularly if it was elective PCI (LEADERS-FREE and ZEUS trials). Stent thrombosis during follow-up is not frequent, and the DAPT trial has shown that the majority of MI events during follow-up were nonstent related. This trial also showed that DAPT prolongation was effective in reducing stent thrombosis and composite events but at the cost of increased risk of bleeding (Mauri L, et al. *N Engl J Med* 2014;371(23):2155–2166). Several data have shown that patients with prior MI have increased ischemic risk and benefit from DAPT prolongation (Bonaca MP, et al. *N Engl J Med* 2015;372(19):1791–1800; Udell JA, et al. *Eur Heart J* 2016;37(4):390–399).

20.39 Answer D. Nobori stent is a new-generation Biolimus A9–eluting stent consisting of (1) a bare metal platform with open cell, quadrature link design, and strut thickness of 120 μm and (2) abluminal coating with biodegradable PLA as drug carrier, Parylene C as a primer coating and biolimus at a dose of 15.6 μg/mm stent length. Recently, the 5-year follow-up of the NOBORI 2 study (a prospective, multicenter, observational registry evaluating the safety and the efficacy of Nobori among 3,067 patients recruited at 125 international sites) showed that definite/probable stent thrombosis was 1.1%, of which 0.6% was very late stent thrombosis, which is in line with other stents (Danzi GB, et al. *Heart* 2017;103(2):111–116). The main difference between Nobori and BioMatrix BES is related to a different coating process, which is based on chemical vapor deposition for Nobori while on automated autopipette for BioMatrix stent.

20.40 Answer E. The BES family includes all the stents except the Orsiro, which is a new-generation SES.

20.41 Answer D. The AXXESS stent is a self-expanding bifurcation-dedicated device. It was Conformité Européene (CE) marked in 2010. It has a nitinol (nickel–titanium alloy) platform with a conical shape (flared distal diameter) and a strut thickness of 160 μm. It is specially designed to conform to the anatomy at the level of the bifurcation carina (up to an angle of 70 degrees) and can accommodate vessels of 3.0 to 4.25 mm diameter, but a specific version has been designed for left main bifurcation lesions allowing for larger diameters (up to 4.75 mm).

20.42 Answer E. The Orsiro stent consists of an ultrathin (60 μm) cobalt–chromium alloy platform with a hybrid combination of passive (PROBIO) and active (PLLA) coatings. This polymer compound carries and releases sirolimus and is completely degradable during a period of 12 to 24 months.

20.43 Answer C. The BIOFLOW-I was a prospective first-in-man study including 30 patients with significant single de novo lesion in one coronary artery (with a reference vessel diameter between 2.5 and 3.5 mm and lesion length ≤22 mm) treated with Orsiro stent in two centers in Romania. At 1 year, the composite of MACE (cardiac death, ischemia-driven TLR, and target-vessel MI) was 10% and there were no stent thrombosis events (Hamon M, et al. *EuroIntervention* 2013;8(9): 1006–1011).

The multicenter randomized BIOFLOW-II trial established the noninferiority of the Orsiro vs. Xience stent in 452 patients with stable or unstable CAD. The primary end point was late lumen loss (LLL) at 9 months, which was 0.10 ± 0.32 mm vs. 0.11 ± 0.29 mm, respectively (noninferiority $p < 0.0001$). There was similar target lesion failure at 1 year without cases of stent thrombosis, and these findings were consistent at 2 years and in subgroups of patients with diabetes or small vessel disease (Windecker S, et al. *Circ Cardiovasc Interv* 2015;8(2):e001441).

The BIOSCIENCE multicenter randomized trial proved the noninferiority of the Orsiro vs. the Xience in a broad population of 2,119 patients with stable CAD or ACS. There were no differences in the primary end point (target lesion failure) at 12 months (6.5% vs. 6.6%; noninferiority $p < 0.0004$) and in-stent thrombosis (0.9% vs. 0.4%; $p = 0.16$) (Pilgrim T, et al. *Lancet* 2014;384(9960):2111–2122).

The HATTRICK-OCT prospective multicenter study included 44 ACS patients randomized to Orsiro vs. the Resolute zotarolimus-eluting stent and compared tissue coverage and apposition by OCT after 3 months. The rates of uncovered and malapposed struts were significantly reduced in the Orsiro group (Karjalainen PP, et al. *Circ J* 2015;79(2):360–367).

The SORT OUT VII compared the safety and efficacy of the Orsiro with Nobori stent in all-comer patients ($n = 2{,}525$), showing noninferiority for the primary end point (target lesion failure) at 1 year and lower definite stent thrombosis in the Orsiro group (0.4% vs. 1.2%; $p = 0.03$) (Jensen LO, et al. *Circ Cardiovasc Interv* 2016;9(7). pii:e003610).

20.44 Answer E. Biotronik has developed different absorbable magnesium scaffolds including AMS 1, AMS 2, AMS 3 (DREAMS 1G), and the most recent DREAMS 2G. Magnesium is a mineral with an essential role for human physiology (i.e., bone metabolism, immune functions, muscle and nerve function, and heart rhythm). It is also a biocompatible metal with unique electrochemical properties. Indeed, it is more electronegative than other metals used for implants and has also shown antithrombotic properties in vivo. While AMS 1 and 2 are not eluting scaffolds, the AMS-3/DREAMS 1G is a paclitaxel-eluting scaffold that was tested in the BIOSOLVE I trial, and the DREAMS 2G is a sirolimus-eluting scaffold that was investigated in the BIOSOLVE II trial (Haude M, et al. *Lancet* 2013;381(9869):836–844; Haude M, et al. *Lancet* 2016;387(10013):31–39; Haude M, et al. *Eur Heart J* 2016;37(35):2701–2709).

20.45 Answer C. SYNERGY is a platinum-chromium EES like the PROMUS stent but different from the XIENCE, which is a chromium-cobalt EES. SYNERGY employs a fully biodegradable PLGA polymer applied to the abluminal surface of the stent and was investigated in the EVOLVE I, EVOLVE II, and BIO-RESORT TWENTE trials (Meredith IT, et al. *J Am Coll Cardiol* 2012; 59(15):1362–1370; Lam MK, et al. *Am Heart J* 2014;167(4):445–451; Kereiakes DJ, et al. *Circ Cardiovasc Interv* 2015;8(4). pii:e002372).

20.46 Answer C. Durable polymers used in first-generation DES (Cypher and Taxus) were thick and their permanent presence has been correlated with inflammatory responses and local toxicity in preclinical analysis. They have been associated with mechanical complications (such as polymer delamination leading to stent expansion issues) and nonuniform coating, which resulted in abnormal drug distribution. Therefore, clinical research has focused on investigating new drug carrier systems. Biodegradable polymers allow drug elution by drug diffusion or matrix degradation while durable polymers use particle dissolution. The Promus (EES), Xience (EES), and Resolute (ZES) stents are not biodegradable polymer DES, but a durable polymer DES. These stents, compared with first-generation DES, incorporate more biocompatible materials, such as acrylic and fluoropolymers, but also change the metallic alloy on their platform (from stainless steel to cobalt or platinum-chromium), reaching thinner struts and lower crossing profiles to tackle more challenging anatomies. BMS, durable polymer DES, and biodegradable polymer DES were compared in a network meta-analysis investigating the outcomes of 258,544 patient-years of follow-up enrolled in 126 randomized trials. This study showed that the newer-generation durable polymer DES (Resolute-ZES, cobalt-chromium EES, and platinum-chromium EES) were the most efficacious stents in terms of reduced rates of TVR, and the cobalt-chromium EES were the safest with a significant reduction of stent thrombosis, MI, and death compared with BMS (Bangalore S, et al. *Br Med J* 2013;347:f6625).

20.47 Answer C. BVS have showed some concerns, particularly in unselected patients and should be considered in selected cases. PES has not demonstrated to reduce death or stent thrombosis. The recent Norwegian Coronary Stent Trial (NORSTENT) randomly assigned 9,013 patients who had stable or unstable CAD to undergo PCI with the implantation of either contemporary DES or BMS. There were no significant differences in the composite outcome of death from any cause and nonfatal spontaneous MI, but rates of repeat revascularization were lower in the group receiving DES (Bønaa KH, et al. *N Engl J Med* 2016;375(13):1242–1252).

20.48 Answer C. DESyne is a new-generation cobalt-chromium DES-eluting Novolimus. The Endeavor and Promus are EES, Orsiro is a SES, and Resolute Integrity is a ZES.

21 Drug-Eluting Stents and Local Drug Delivery for the Prevention of Restenosis

Samuel E. Horr and Leslie Cho

QUESTIONS

21.1 Stents eluting drugs of the "limus" family reduce the incidence of in-stent restenosis. The main effect of the drugs is on:

(A) Elastic recoil
(B) Arterial remodeling
(C) Smooth muscle cell proliferation/migration
(D) Extracellular matrix production

21.2 Which of the following is TRUE regarding everolimus (Fig. Q21-2)?

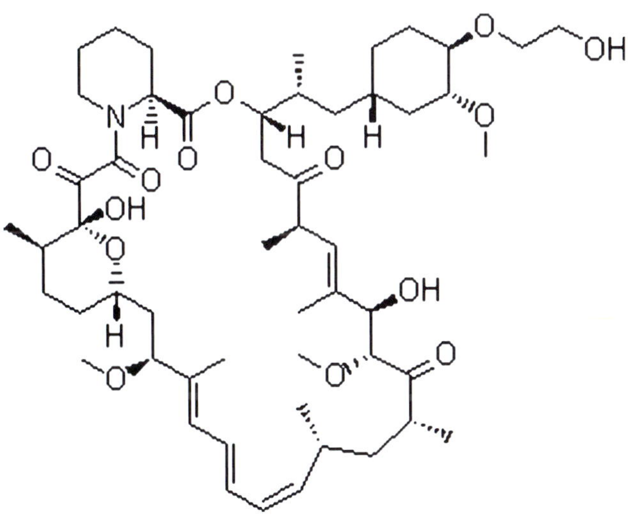

Figure Q21-2 (From *Nat Rev Drug Discov* 2009;8:535–536.)

(A) It inhibits microtubule assembly
(B) It has been tested as an immunosuppressive agent that prevents the cell from entering the M phase (cell division)
(C) It binds to an intracellular protein, FKBP-12, resulting in an inhibitory complex formation and inhibition of mTOR kinase activity and has been developed for the treatment of advanced renal cell carcinoma
(D) It affects the cell cycle at multiple phases in a dose-dependent fashion

21.3 Which of the following statements concerning paclitaxel is correct?

(A) At low doses, apoptosis is induced
(B) It was discovered in a crude extract from the bark of a Pacific yew
(C) It induces disassembly of microtubules
(D) It inhibits FKBP-12 similar to sirolimus and everolimus

21.4 Which of the following statements regarding drug-eluting stent (DES) platforms is CORRECT?

(A) The sirolimus-eluting (Cypher) stent is composed of a cobalt–chromium (CoCr) stent, coated with nonerodable polymers
(B) Polymers are long-chain molecules, form a reservoir, and facilitate controlled and prolonged drug delivery
(C) Paclitaxel can only be used in combination with a polymer-based stent platform
(D) Drugs cannot be released from a stent without a polymer coating

21.5 Polymeric materials coated on stents:

(A) Allow a controlled and sustained release of agents
(B) Increase the radiopacity of the stent
(C) Are nontoxic and reduce inflammation
(D) Enhance the radial strength of a stent

21.6 The first randomized comparison of a sirolimus-eluting stent (SES) with a standard bare metal stent (BMS) showed a reduced occurrence of significant in-stent restenosis after 6 months to:

(A) 20%
(B) 15%
(C) 10%
(D) <5%

21.7 A 49-year-old patient was treated with percutaneous coronary intervention (PCI) and BMS implantation in the setting of an acute coronary syndrome (ACS). Seven months later, he complains of recurrent chest pain during minor exertion. The invasive evaluation shows the following (Fig. Q21-7):

For the treatment of this patient with an in-stent restenosis following BMS implantation:

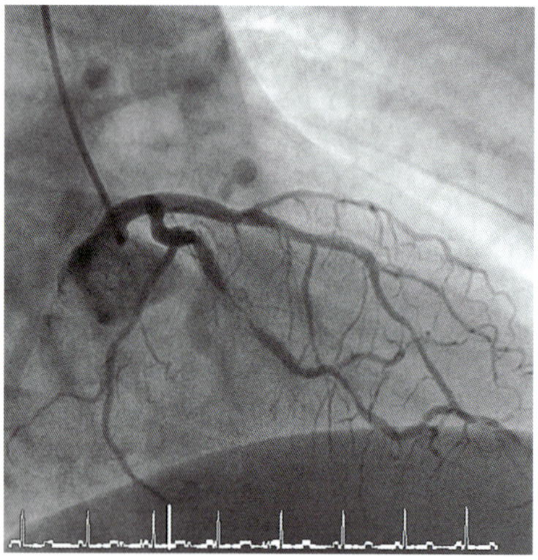

Figure Q21-7

(A) Paclitaxel-eluting stent (PES) implantation appears to be superior to SES implantation
(B) Simple balloon angioplasty is the best option and superior to drug-coated balloon dilatation
(C) A treatment with β-radiation has been shown to be inferior to balloon angioplasty
(D) Treatment with DES is superior to simple balloon angioplasty

21.8 Experimental models of stent implantation in human coronary arteries show:

(A) That the deployment of sirolimus- or paclitaxel-eluting DES is associated with an increase in neointimal thickness at 28 days in comparison with BMS
(B) A delayed healing process is also observed with the newer-generation DES (e.g., everolimus) in comparison with BMS
(C) Always a greater inflammatory reaction after DES implantation in comparison with BMS within 28 days
(D) Complete healing after BMS implantation within 2 to 4 months

21.9 A 45-year-old patient suffers from a stent thrombosis 2.5 years after DES implantation in the left anterior descending (LAD) artery (Fig. Q21-9). Which of the following statements is INCORRECT?

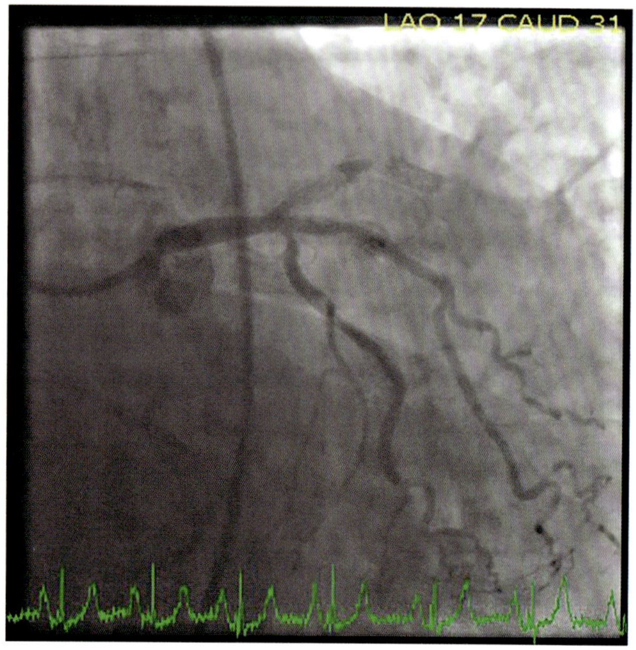

Figure Q21-9 (Courtesy of Leslie Cho.)

(A) Inadequate stent expansion and apposition are procedural risk factors for stent thrombosis
(B) Is rare (1% per year)
(C) Elective PCI carries a higher risk of stent thrombosis than PCI in the setting of a myocardial infarction (MI)
(D) Carries a high morbidity and mortality

21.10 Which of the following agents are used in coronary stent platforms?

(A) Everolimus
(B) Biolimus
(C) Zotarolimus
(D) Sirolimus
(E) Paclitaxel
(F) Novolimus
(G) Myolimus
(H) All of the above

21.11 The SIRTAX trial, a randomized, controlled, single-blind study comparing SES with PES in about 1,000 all-comer patients, favors treatment with an SES because of:

(A) A lower incidence of cardiac death
(B) Fewer major adverse cardiac events (MACE), primarily by decreasing rates of clinical and angiographic restenosis
(C) A lower incidence of stent thrombosis
(D) Better acute gain and higher success of stent implantation

21.12 Current data suggest that a late loss of more than _______ triggers a target lesion revascularization (TLR).

(A) 0.2 to 0.3 mm
(B) 0.5 to 0.6 mm
(C) 0.9 to 1.0 mm
(D) 1.2 to 1.3 mm

21.13 The assessment of coronary endothelial function 6 months after SES implantation compared with BMS, assessed with bicycle exercise as a physiologic stimulus (Fig. Q21-13), revealed that:

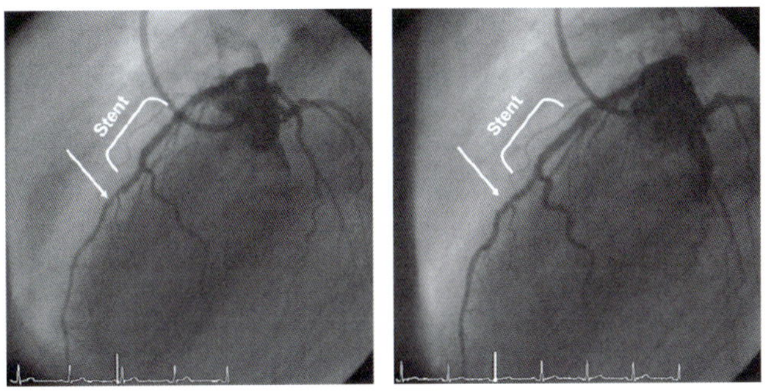

Figure Q21-13

(A) Implantation of either a BMS or an SES affects physiologic response to exercise proximal and distal to the stent
(B) Implantation of a BMS does affect physiologic response to exercise proximal and distal to the stent, while implantation of an SES does not affect the response
(C) Implantation of a BMS does not affect physiologic response to exercise proximal and distal to the stent, while implantation of an SES does affect the response
(D) Neither implantation of a BMS or an SES affects physiologic response to exercise proximal and distal to the stent

21.14 What are possible advantages of biodegradable DES using a pure polymer platform

(A) Reduced neoatherosclerosis compared to stainless steel or a cobalt-chromium stent platform
(B) Improved radial force in comparison with a stainless steel or a cobalt-chromium stent platform
(C) Reduced deformability of the stent
(D) Improved radiopacity

21.15 The sirolimus-(Cypher) and the everolimus-eluting (Xience) stent platforms share the following characteristics:

(A) Stainless steel stent
(B) Release of drug within 28 days: ≥80%
(C) Strut thickness of 130 to 140 μm
(D) Polymer thickness of 12 to 16 μm

21.16 A 59-year-old patient is referred from another hospital due to an acute anterior ST-elevation myocardial infarction (STEMI) 7 years after SES implantation. The repeat angiography shows the following (Fig. Q21-16):

Based on the published data, which interventional treatment would be recommended to treat this lesion?

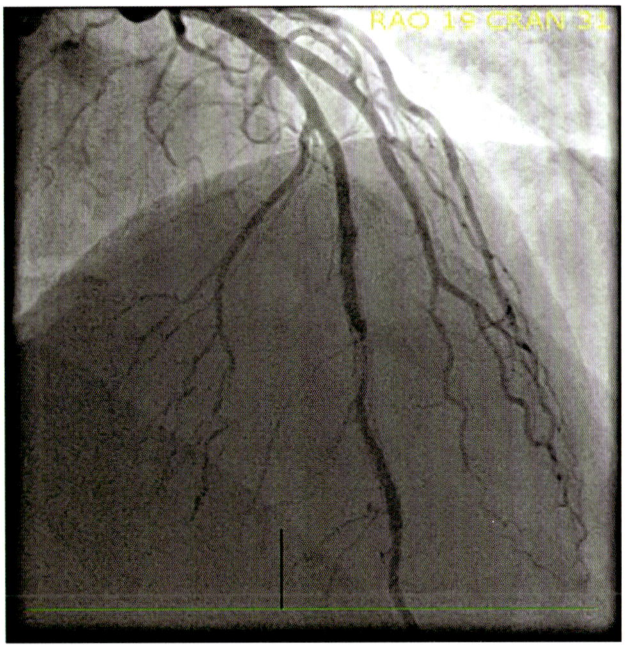

Figure Q21-16 (Courtesy of Leslie Cho.)

(A) Balloon angioplasty has equivalent results to DES and BMS
(B) DES is superior to balloon angioplasty
(C) Brachytherapy is the first-line treatment
(D) BMS is superior to balloon angioplasty

21.17 A 55-year-old patient presents with acute chest pain and 2-mm ST elevation in the inferior leads. The ostial right coronary artery (RCA) is totally occluded due to a thrombus (Fig. Q21-17A). After aspiration of thrombus, balloon dilatation, and everolimus-eluting stent (EES) implantation, the vessel is open with normal thrombolysis in myocardial infarction (TIMI) flow (Fig. Q21-17B). The

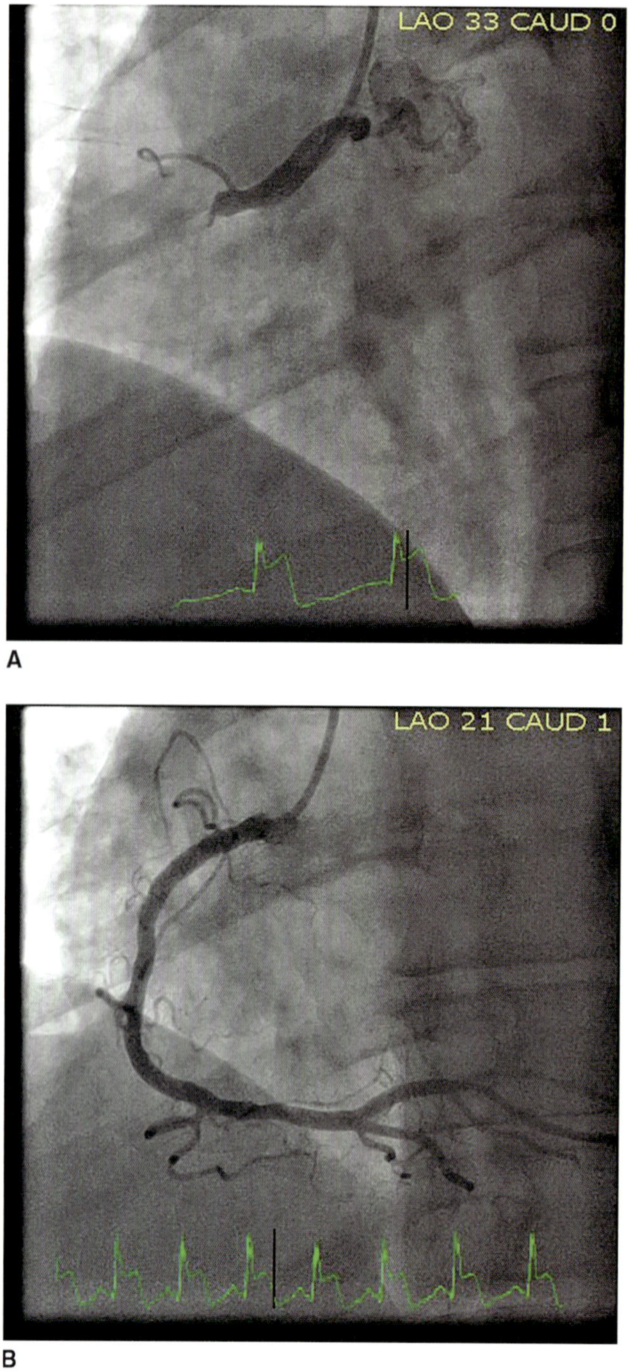

Figure Q21-17 (Courtesy of Leslie Cho.)

left coronary system shows diffuse CAD with no significant stenosis. Six weeks later, the patient presents again with acute chest pain and ST elevation in the inferior leads. What is the most probable cause for the recurrent symptoms?

(A) Severe in-stent restenosis
(B) Vasospasm of the RCA
(C) Allergic reaction to medication
(D) Stent thrombosis

21.18 The patient is brought to the catheterization laboratory, and the invasive evaluation shows a thrombotic occlusion of the ostium of the RCA (Fig. Q21-18). What are the possible causes for this presentation?

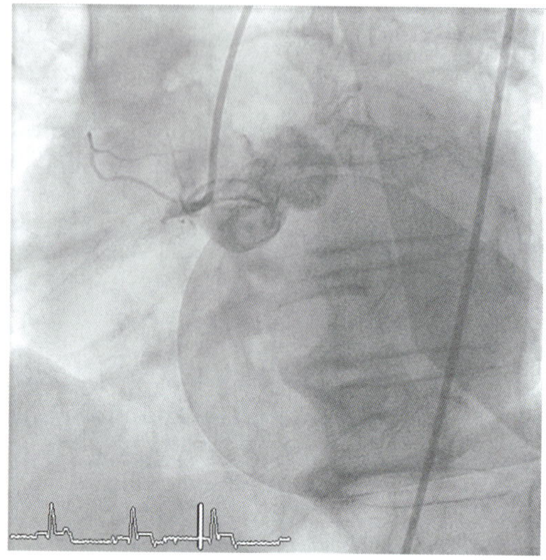

Figure Q21-18

(A) Stent fracture not recognized during the first intervention
(B) Hyporesponsiveness to dual antiplatelet treatment (DAPT)
(C) Rupture of the thin neointima
(D) Noncompliance to drug intake with discontinuation of DAPT
(E) Stent malapposition
(F) All of the above

21.19 An optical coherence tomography (OCT) performed after initial stent deployment is shown in Figure Q21-19. What is your interpretation?

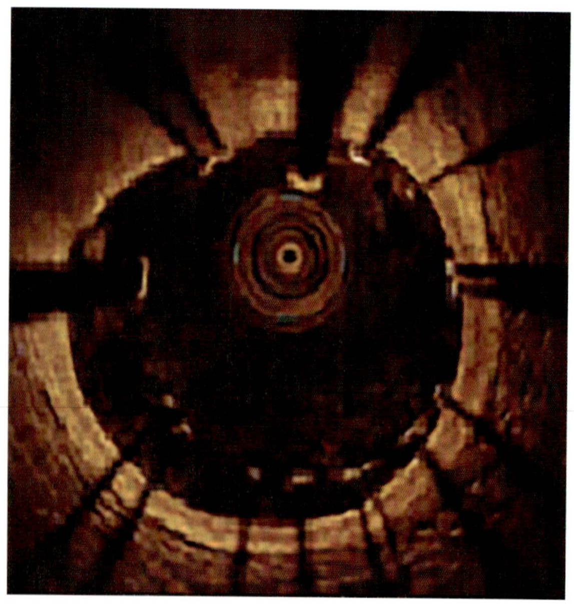

Figure Q21-19 (Courtesy of Leslie Cho.)

(A) Well-apposed and expanded stent
(B) Stent underexpansion
(C) Stent fracture
(D) Malapposition

21.20 In the SPIRIT II, III, and IV trials, Xience EES stents showed ________ rates of target lesion failure and ________ rates of all-cause mortality at 3 years compared to the TAXUS PES stent.

(A) Equivalent, equivalent
(B) Lower, equivalent
(C) Lower, lower
(D) Equivalent, lower

21.21 A 69-year-old female patient was successfully treated with acute PCI and single BMS implantation for an anterior MI 6 months ago. Otherwise, the coronaries were normal. An echocardiographic follow-up exam reveals a mildly reduced left ventricular ejection fraction (LVEF). A treadmill stress test demonstrates ST-segment depression and mild chest discomfort after six metabolic equivalents (METs). The patient is examined invasively, including with OCT. What is your interpretation of the image (Fig. Q21-21)?

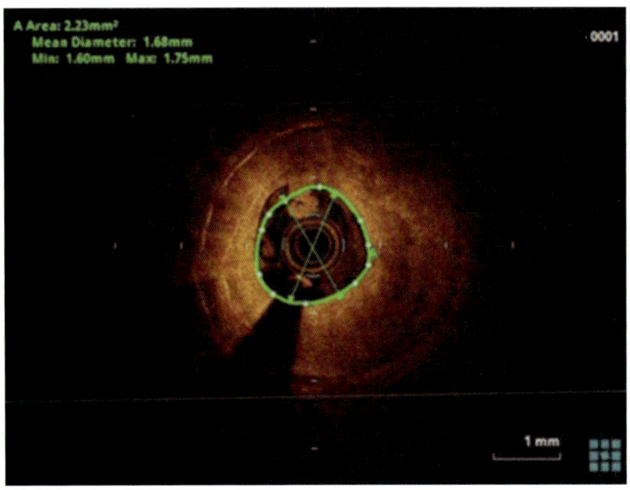

Figure Q21-21 (Courtesy of Leslie Cho.)

(A) Optimal result with a thin layer of neointima
(B) Restenosis due to excessive formation of neointima
(C) Single-stent fractures with formation of thrombus
(D) Stent underexpansion with thrombotic material in the vessel lumen

21.22 A randomized comparison of the everolimus-eluting Xience stent (EES) with the zotarolimus-eluting Resolute stent (ZES) has demonstrated in an all-comer patient population, including 2,300 patients:

(A) Clinically indicated TLR was >5% in both groups
(B) Resolute ZES was found to be noninferior to EES with respect to the primary clinical end point of target lesion failure
(C) The mean in-stent diameter restenosis was significantly higher in the ZES than in the EES group
(D) The rate of overall stent thrombosis was higher in the EES than in the ZES group

21.23 Comparisons between the Xience (CoCr EES) and the PROMUS Element (platinum-chromium [PtCr] EES) demonstrated which of the following results at 2 years?

(A) Higher target lesion failure in the Xience stent with similar mortality and stent thrombosis outcomes between the two stents
(B) Higher target lesion failure in the PROMUS stent with similar mortality and stent thrombosis outcomes between the two stents
(C) Higher late stent thrombosis rates in the Xience stent with similar mortality and target lesion failure rates between the two stents
(D) Higher late stent thrombosis rates in the PROMUS stent with similar mortality and target lesion failure rates between the two stents
(E) Similar rates of target lesion failure, stent thrombosis, and mortality between the two stents

21.24 Bioabsorbable polymers, such as in the SYNERGY stent, were created in part to decrease the risk of late/very late stent thrombosis and improve stent healing. Compared to the durable polymer stent PROMUS, rates of stent thrombosis at 2 years in patients treated with the SYNERGY stent were:

(A) Lower
(B) Higher
(C) Equivalent

21.25 Poly-L-lactic acid (PLLA):

(A) Is metabolized via the Krebs cycle over a period of 12 to 18 months
(B) Is the most frequently used polymer for the current generation of biodegradable stents
(C) Is in use for resorbable sutures and different implants
(D) Is radiopaque and provides as much radial force as a metallic stent
(E) Is phagocytosed by macrophages
(F) All but E are correct
(G) A, B, and C are correct
(H) All but D are correct

21.26 The bioresorbable vascular scaffold (BVS) stent technology was developed to address which of the following limitations of current metallic stents?

(A) Decreasing radial strength over time
(B) Limited radiopacity
(C) Prevention of late vessel remodeling
(D) Poor deliverability of antiproliferative drugs

21.27 In trials comparing the BVS stent ABSORB with current generation DES, which of the following concerns has been raised?

(A) Increased rates of bleeding
(B) Increased rates of stent thrombosis
(C) Longer hospital stay
(D) Higher target lesion failure

ANSWERS AND EXPLANATIONS

21.1 **Answer C.** The main effect of antiproliferative drugs is on the inhibition of smooth muscle cell proliferation and migration by interfering with the cell cycle (Adelman SJ. *Curr Pharm Des* 2010;16(36):4002–4011) (Fig. A21-1A). The radial force of a stent inhibits a potential elastic recoil of the vessel (Windecker S, et al. *Heart* 2000;83(4):481–490) (Fig. A21-1B). As a side effect, positive arterial remodeling resulting in late malapposition of the stent might be induced by the implantation of a DES (Vorpahl M, et al. *Minerva Cardioangiol* 2009;57(5):621–628).

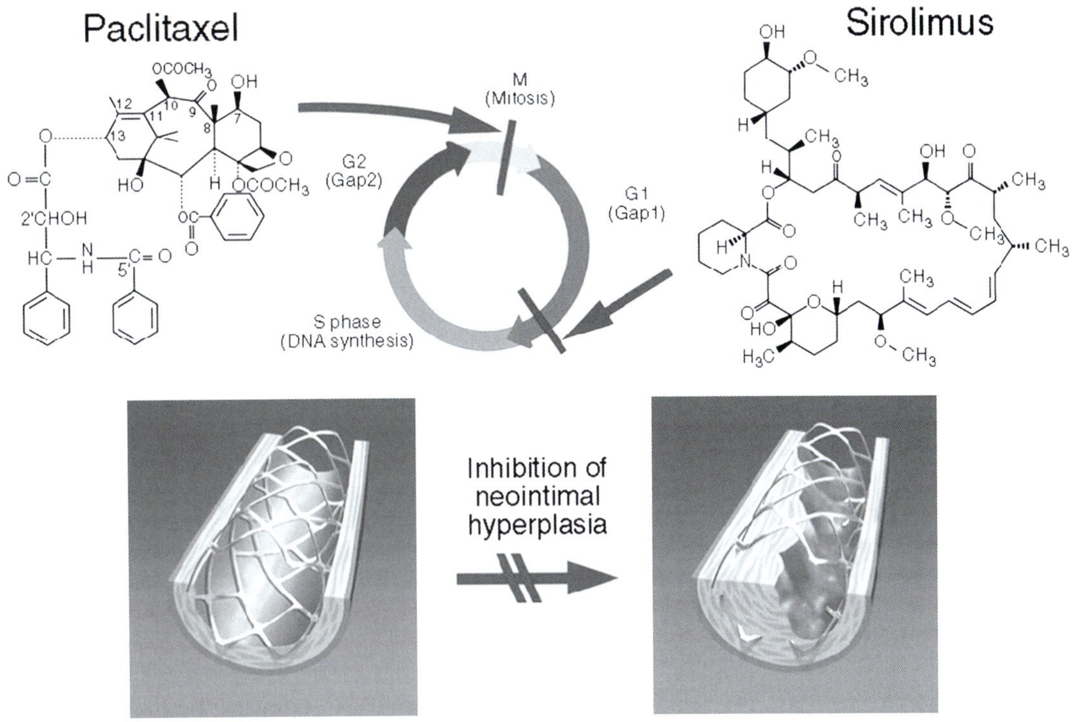

A

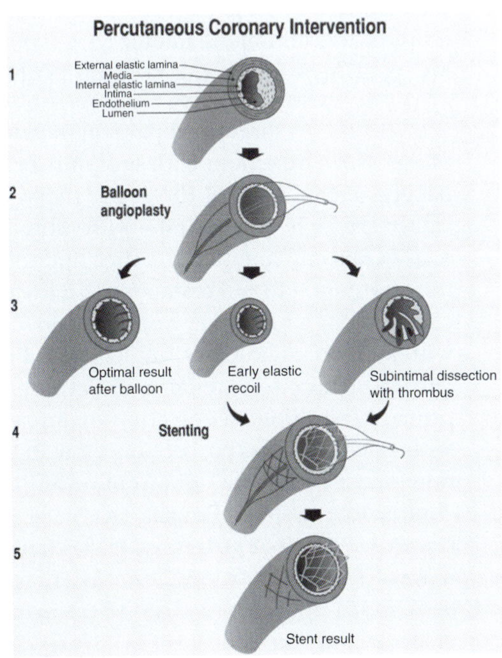

B

Figure A21-1

21.2 Answer C. Developed primarily as immunosuppressant inhibiting the expression of hypoxia-inducible factor (e.g., HIF-1) and reducing the expression of vascular endothelial growth factor, it was found to be useful in the prevention of coronary restenosis (Eisen HJ, et al. *N Engl J Med* 2003;349(9):847–858). Everolimus binds to FKBP12, forming a complex that inhibits mTOR kinase activity, and reduces the activity of the downstream effectors S6 ribosomal protein kinase (S6K1) and eukaryotic elongation factor 4E-binding protein (4EBP). Everolimus has been shown to inhibit cell proliferation and angiogenesis, with the latter mediated by inhibition of hypoxia-inducible factor 1a (HIF1a) expression.

21.3 Answer B. Paclitaxel promotes the polymerization of tubulin and does not induce the disassembly of microtubules like other antimicrotubule agents like colchicine (Rowinsky EK, et al. *N Engl J Med* 1995;332(15):1004–1014). At high doses, paclitaxel promotes apoptosis and is cytostatic at low doses. In 1962, on an excursion in Washington State, USDA botanist Arthur Barclay collected bark and other samples from the Pacific yew tree. Two years later, Monroe E. Wall, Ph.D., and Mansukh Wani, Ph.D., who were under contract to NCI at the Research Triangle Institute in North Carolina, discovered that extracts from the Pacific yew were toxic to living cells. Dr. Wall and his colleagues then isolated the most cytotoxic compound from the bark of the tree and called it paclitaxel.

21.4 Answer B. The sirolimus-eluting Cypher stent was the first DES tested in a randomized clinical trial (Fig. A21-4) and is composed of stainless steel. For drug release, two nonerodable polymers were used: polyethylene-co-vinyl acetate (PEVA) and poly *n*-butyl methacrylate (PBMA). A drug-free coat of PBMA is also applied to the stent surface to control drug release. Only some specific drugs can be loaded directly onto metallic surfaces (e.g., biolimus, prostacyclin, paclitaxel) (Sousa JE, et al. *Circulation* 2003;107(17):2274–2279).

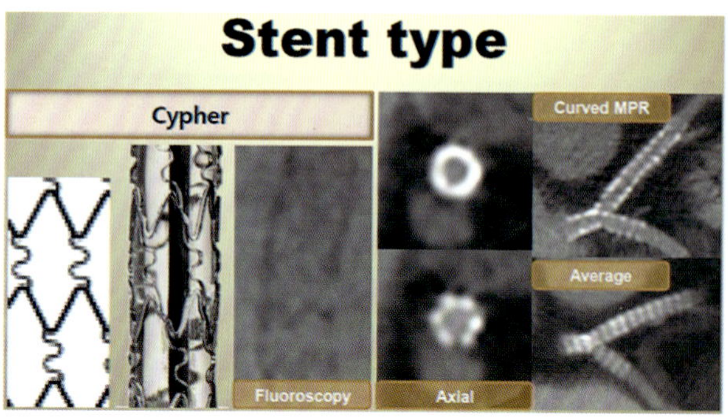

Figure A21-4 (Courtesy of Leslie Cho.)

21.5 Answer A. A polymer is a natural or man-made high molecular weight organic compound, consisting of many repeating simpler chemical units or molecules called monomers (Fig. A21-5). Natural examples of polymers are proteins (polymer of amino acids) and cellulose (polymer of sugar molecules).

Polymers bind and release drugs from a coronary stent, serve therefore as a drug reservoir, and may induce inflammation in the vessel wall (hypersensitivity reaction) (Kavanagh CA, et al. *Pharmacol Ther* 2004;102(1):1–15).

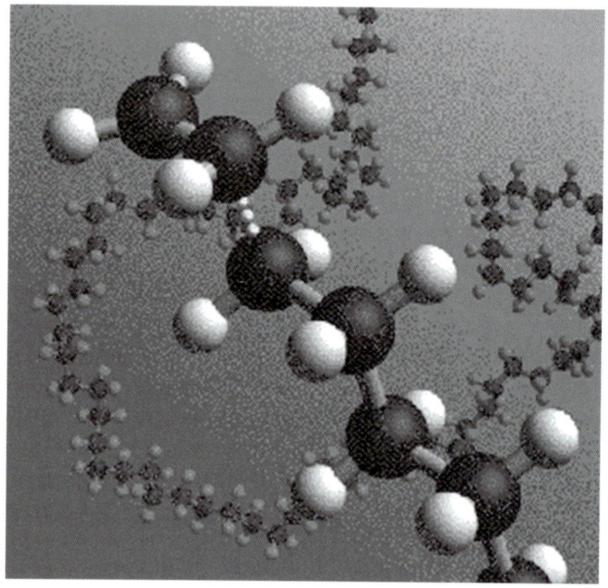

Figure A21-5 (Example of synthetic polymer: PVC [a polymer of vinyl chloride].)

21.6 Answer D. None of the patients in the sirolimus-stent group, as compared with 26.6% of those in the standard stent group, had restenosis of 50% or more of the luminal diameter ($p < 0.001$) (Morice MC, et al. *N Engl J Med* 2002;346(23):1773–1780).

21.7 Answer D. A direct comparison of balloon angioplasty with a treatment with sirolimus- (Cypher) and paclitaxel-eluting (TAXUS) stent showed a significantly lower restenosis rate with either stent (Fig. A21-7). SES implantation may be superior to PES for the treatment of BMS restenosis. β-Radiation significantly reduced in-stent restenosis in comparison with balloon angioplasty, but its use is limited with current generation stents. A direct comparison of primary transluminal coronary angioplasty (PTCA) with paclitaxel-coated balloon vs. a PES implantation for the treatment of in-stent restenosis showed comparable results (Dangas GD, et al. *J Am Coll Cardiol* 2010;56(23):1897–1907; Scheller B, et al. *N Engl J Med* 2006;355(2):2113–2124; Kastrati A, et al. *JAMA* 2005;293(2):165–171; Unverdorben M, et al. *Circulation* 2009;119(23):2986–2994).

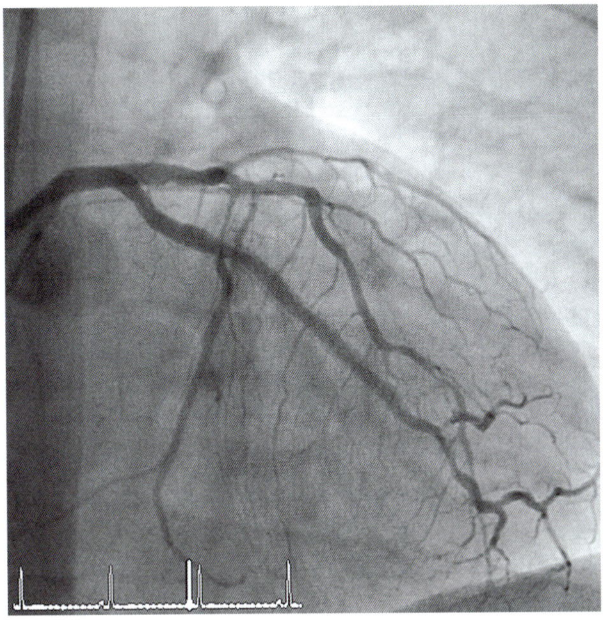

Figure A21-7 After PTCA and DES implantation.

21.8 Answer B. Complete re-endothelialization is usually achieved within 1 month after BMS implantation. After DES implantation, even for second-generation DES (e.g., EES), the healing process is prolonged (Soucy NV, et al. *EuroIntervention* 2010;6:630–637).

21.9 Answer C. Several factors have been associated with the risk of late stent thrombosis. Hypersensitivity to drug coating and polymer and incomplete endothelialization are device-related risk factors for stent thrombosis. Procedural factors, such as inadequate stent expansion and apposition, result in higher rates of stent thrombosis. Patient and lesion factors, such as diabetes, impaired left ventricular function, malignancy, MI, long lesions, and bifurcation lesions, raise the risk for stent thrombosis. The rate of late stent thrombosis is <1% per year with the first-generation DES (Farb A, et al. *Circulation* 2003;108(14):1701–1706; Holmes DR Jr, et al. *J Am Coll Cardiol* 2010;56(17):1357–1365; Wenaweser P, et al. *J Am Coll Cardiol* 2008;52(14):1134–1140).

21.10 Answer H. All of the agents listed are in clinical use on coronary stent platforms (Garg S, et al. *Nat Rev Cardiol* 2013;10(5):248–260).

21.11 Answer B. The SIRTAX trial demonstrated fewer MACE with sirolimus, primarily by decreasing rates of clinical and angiographic restenosis (Fig. A21-11) (Windecker S, et al. *N Engl J Med* 2005;353(7):653–662).

21.12 Answer B. The late loss is minimal lumen diameter at follow-up minus the postprocedural minimal lumen diameter at baseline. Current data suggest that a late loss of 0.5 to 0.6 mm triggers a TLR (Ellis SG, et al. *J Am Coll Cardiol* 2005;45(8):1193–2000).

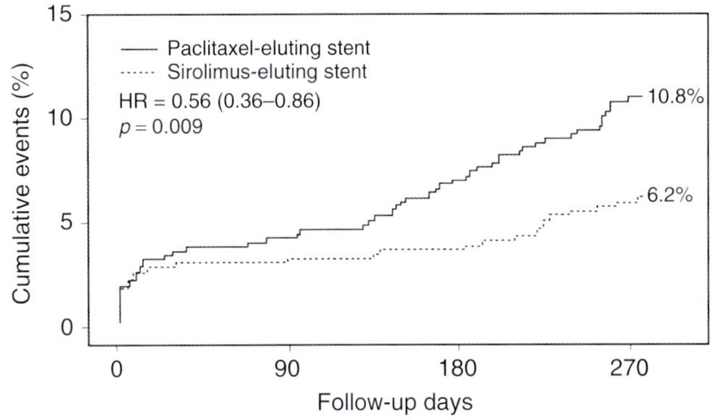

Figure A21-11 Primary end point: composite of cardiac death, myocardial infarction, and target lesion revascularization.

21.13 Answer C. Implantation of a BMS does not affect physiologic response to exercise proximal and distal to the stent. However, SES or PES is associated with exercise-induced paradoxic coronary vasoconstriction of the adjacent vessel segments, although vasodilatory response to nitroglycerin is maintained (Togni M, et al. *J Am Coll Cardiol* 2005;46(2):231–236; Togni M, et al. *Int J Cardiol* 2007;120(2):212–220).

21.14 Answer A. As there is no radiopacity of a polymer stent, radiopaque markers need to be added to the stent. The radial force of a pure polymer stent is clearly inferior to a stainless steel or a CoCr stent. The reduced deformability of a polymer stent might be a disadvantage with respect to deliverability of the stent (Di Mario C, et al. *Lancet* 2008;371(9616):873–874; Garg S, et al. *J Am Coll Cardiol* 2010;56(10 Suppl):S43–S78). The biodegradable polymer stents seemed theoretically attractive because its polymer degrades and eliminates itself from the body leaving the permanent metallic stent without polymer, which would facilitate reendothelialization and reduce neoatherosclerosis.

21.15 Answer B. Cypher is a stainless steel stent with a strut thickness of 140 μm and a polymer thickness of 12.6 μm. The Endeavor and Xience V stents are CoCr stents with reduced strut and polymer thickness (91/81 μm as well as 4.1/7.6 μm, respectively). The drug-polymer matrix on the Cypher stent allows a sirolimus release resulting in elution of 80% of drug within the first 30 days after DES implantation. Similarly the Endeavor and Xience V stents allows elution of 80% of drug within the first 30 days *Circ Cardiovasc Interv* 2016;9(6):e002943. (Garg S, et al. *J Am Coll Cardiol* 2010;56(10 Suppl):S43–S78).

21.16 Answer B. In the ISAR-DESIRE trial, treatment of in-stent restenosis with a SES or PES was superior to balloon angioplasty alone. For the treatment of in-stent restenosis, both a new SES and PES implantation were associated with comparable degree of efficacy and safety in ISAR-DESIRE 2. For the treatment with second-generation DES, no sufficient clinical data are available so far. Both SES and PES were found to be superior to brachytherapy in the treatment of single-layer in-stent restenosis in the TAXUS V ISR and SISR trials (Mehilli J, et al. *J Am Coll Cardiol* 2010;55(24):2710–2716).

21.17 Answer D. In-stent restenosis rarely induces an acute MI. A restenosis after DES implantation is usually not earlier than several months after the implantation observed. Vasospasm is unlikely as the patient suffers from diffuse CAD and the treated lesion was at the ostium of the RCA. Stent thrombosis is therefore the most likely diagnosis.

21.18 Answer F. All the mentioned answers are correct. The phenomenon of stent thrombosis is associated with a number of procedural, blood, and patient factors (Holmes DR Jr, et al. *J Am Coll Cardiol* 2010;56(17):1357–1365).

21.19 Answer D. The OCT images show a malapposed stent, which is a known risk factor for stent thrombosis. Here are examples of well-apposed and malapposed stents by OCT and IVUS (Fig. A21-19).

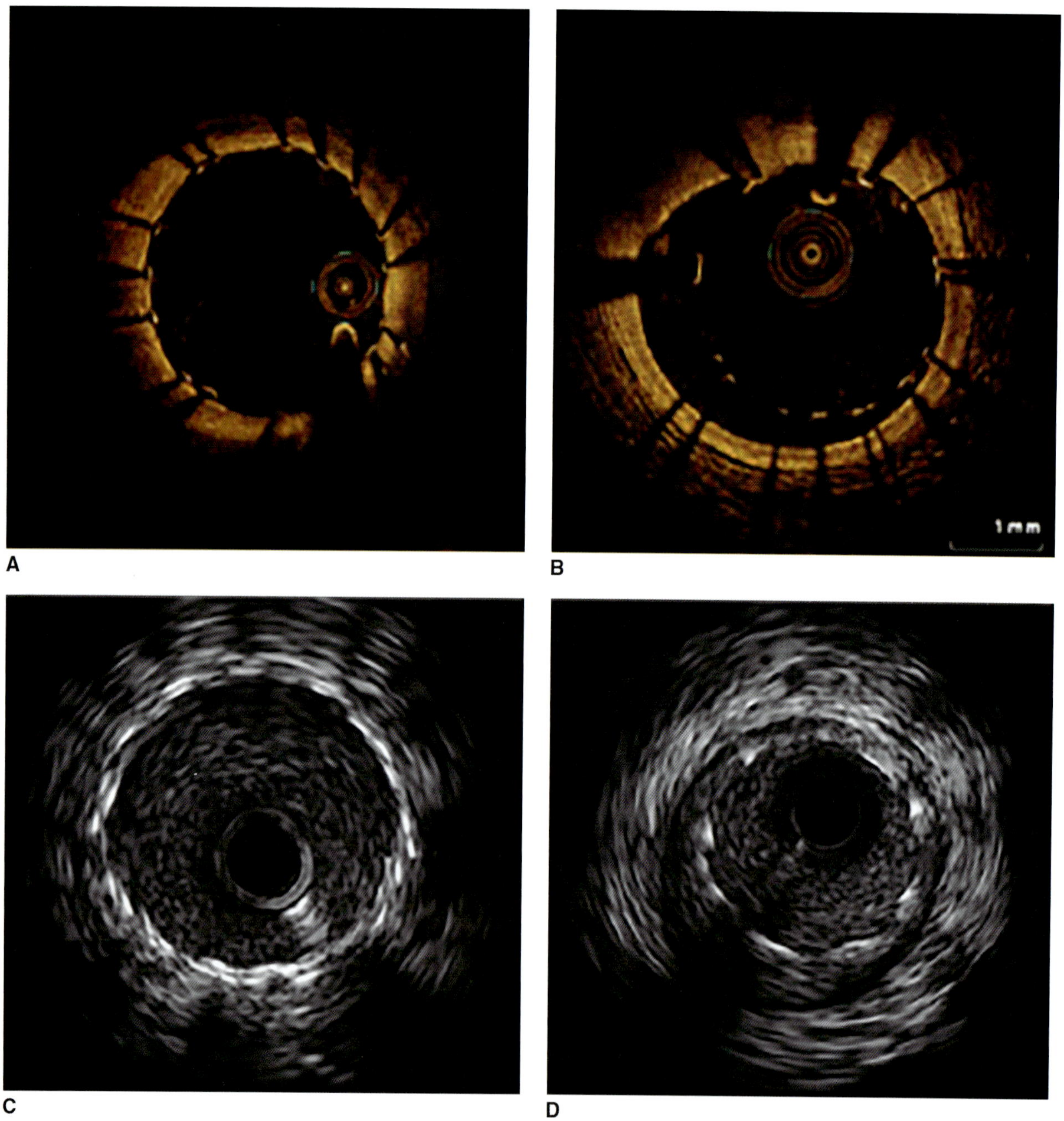

Figure A21-19 (With permission from Koganti S, et al. *Radcliffe Cardiol* 2016;11(1):11–16. © 2016 Radcliffe Cardiology.)

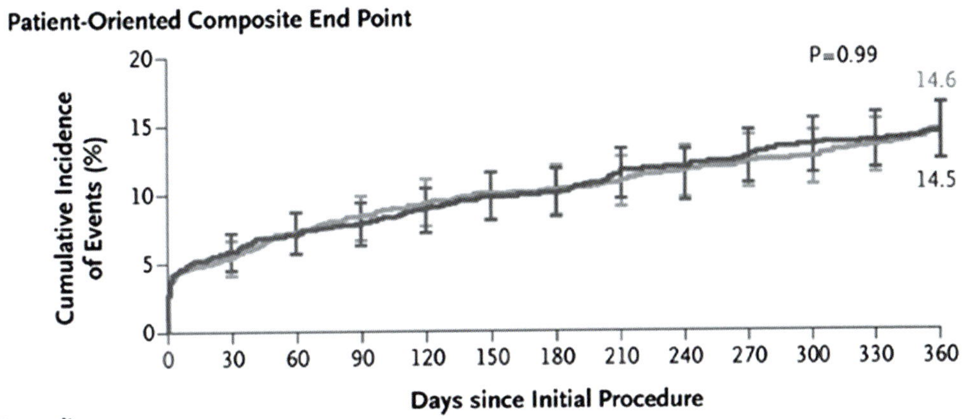

Zotarolimus

No. of patients	1140	1109	1070	1049	1037	1025	1019	1014	1003	995	987	984	966
No. of events	30	32	21	12	12	6	4	7	8	8	3	9	11
Cumulative incidence (%)	2.6	5.4	7.3	8.4	9.4	10.0	10.3	10.9	11.6	12.4	12.6	13.4	14.6

Everolimus

No. of patients	1152	1119	1076	1059	1051	1040	1029	1024	1003	996	987	977	963
No. of events	28	20	15	8	11	11	3	15	6	8	9	4	6
Cumulative incidence (%)	2.8	5.9	7.2	7.9	8.9	9.9	10.1	11.4	12.0	12.7	13.5	13.8	14.5

Figure A21-22

21.20 Answer C. Combined date from the SPIRIT trials showed lower rates of target lesion failure, all-cause mortality, MI, stent thrombosis, and TLR at 3 years with the Xience EES compared to the TAXUS PES stent (Dangas GD, et al. *JACC Cardiovasc Interv* 2013;6(9):914–922).

21.21 Answer B. The OCT image shows significant in-stent restenosis due to excessive formation of neointima.

21.22 Answer B. This large randomized clinical trial including mainly off-label patients showed equal effectiveness of both stent types with no difference with respect to target lesion failure, overall rate of stent thrombosis, or in-stent diameter restenosis with a TLR rate of 3.4% and 3.9%, respectively (Fig. A21-22) (Serruys PW, et al. *N Engl J Med* 2010;363(2):136–146).

21.23 Answer E. Two-year outcomes in the PLATINUM trial showed similar rates of target lesion failure, stent thrombosis, all-cause mortality, and MI between the two stent groups. This trial led to the approval of the PROMUS Element stent (Stone GW, et al. *J Am Coll Cardiol* 2011;57(16):1700–1708).

21.24 Answer C. EVOLVE II randomized 1,684 patients to receive either the SYNERGY or PROMUS stents. Despite the theoretical advantage, rates of definite and probably stent thrombosis were low in both groups <1% with statistically equivalent rates in the SYNERGY (n = 3, 0.4%) and PROMUS (n = 6, 0.8%) groups (p = 0.31) (Kereiakes DJ, et al. *Circ Cardiovasc Interv* 2015;8(4). pii: e002372).

21.25 Answer H. The most frequently used polymers for bioresorbable stents are aliphatic polyesters, such as PLLA, poly(glycolic acid) (PGA), and poly(ε-caprolactone) (PCL) (Bittl JA. *Circulation* 2010;122(22):2236–2238). PLLA is radiolucent.

21.26 Answer C. Bioabsorbable EES, or BVS, is made up of two layers of a biodegradable polymer: one that contains the immunosuppressant drug everolimus and the other forming a longer-lasting backbone. Over time, the body breaks down and absorbs the polymer, ultimately leaving nothing behind (Fig. A21-26A,B). Choices A and B are limitations of current BVS. Metallic stents prevent vasomotion and are associated with the development of neoatherosclerosis (Garg S, et al. *J Am Coll Cardiol* 2010;56(10 Suppl):S43–S78; Serruys PW, et al. *Lancet* 2009;373(9667):897–910).

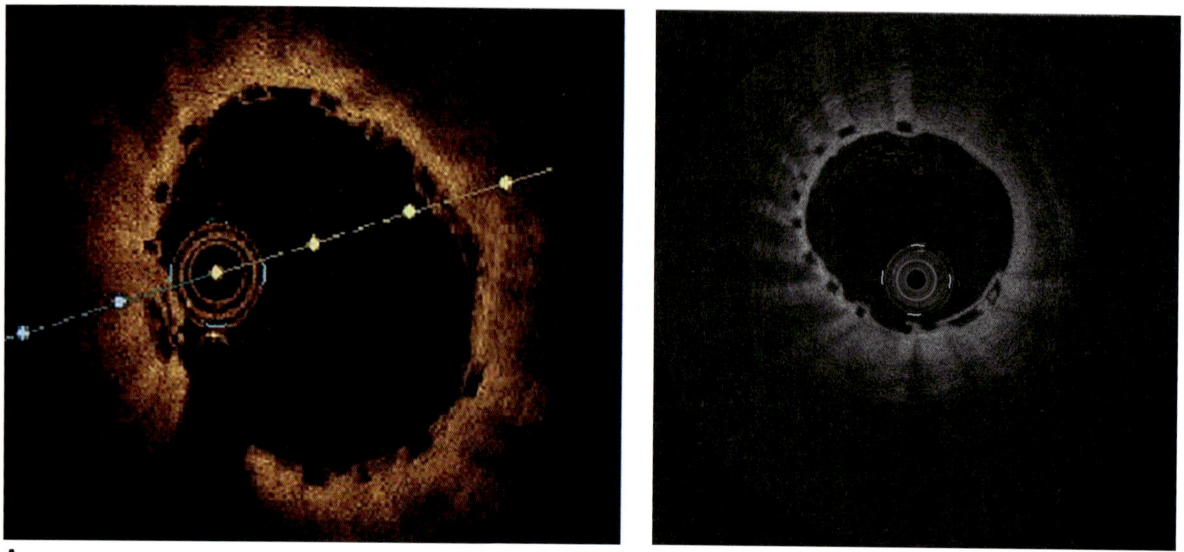

Figure A21-26 A: Example of an OCT of a newly implanted BVS showing well-apposed struts. (Courtesy of Leslie Cho.) B: Example of a 6-month follow-up OCT image of a BVS stent showing complete coverage of the stent struts.

21.27 **Answer B.** ABSORB is the only currently FDA-approved BVS. It was originally studied in the ABORB I, II, and III trials (Ellis SG, et al. *N Engl J Med* 2015;373(20):1905–9015). The stent met its noninferiority end points when compared to the current second-generation stent XIENCE, leading to FDA approval. Several meta-analyses raised the concern for higher stent thrombosis rates. In the AIDA study, rates of stent thrombosis were statistically higher in the ABSORB group (3.5% vs. 0.9%, $p < 0.001$) at 2 years. Rates of target lesion failure, cardiac death, and TLR did not differ between the groups. Long-term data beyond 2 years are pending. Newer-generation BVS is currently undergoing investigations and may address some of the limitations of the current generation BVS platforms (Mukherjee. *N Engl J Med* 2017;376:2388–2389).

22 Percutaneous Interventions in Aortocoronary Saphenous Vein Grafts

Stephane Noble and Marco Roffi

QUESTIONS

22.1 Which statement about the historical background of surgical revascularization in humans is TRUE?

(A) Coronary artery bypass grafting (CABG) using saphenous vein grafts (SVGs) was first performed in the 1960s
(B) SVGs were used as bypass conduits earlier than the internal mammary artery (IMA)
(C) The first venous bypass grafting was performed in the 1950s
(D) The first conduit used was the IMA
(E) A and D are true

22.2 Which statement is TRUE?

(A) Percutaneous coronary intervention (PCI) in vein grafts represents more than 15% of all PCI in the United States
(B) 95% of vein grafts are patent at 1 year
(C) Patency of vein grafts is influenced by the diameter of the recipient vessel
(D) 60% of vein grafts are patent at 10 years
(E) C and D are true

22.3 Which of the following morphologic features is the least representative for vein graft atherosclerosis (Fig. Q22-3)?

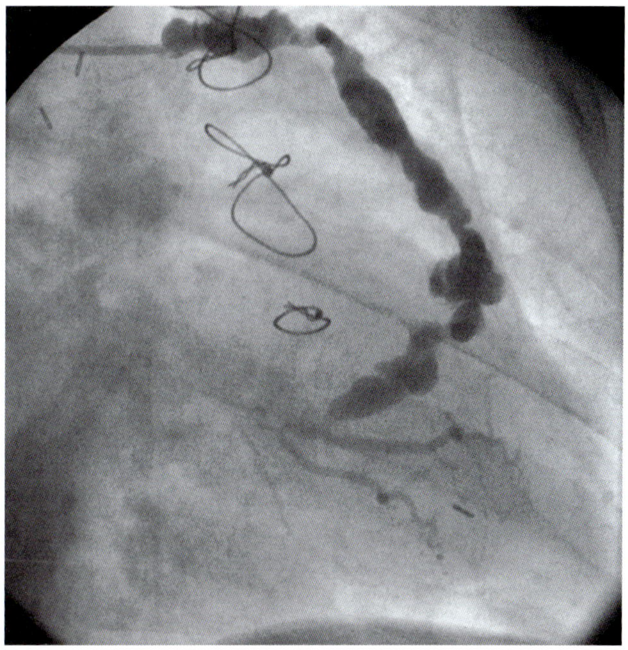

Figure Q22-3 Massively degenerated SVG to a marginal branch of the LCx. The extension of the disease is such that PCI does not appear to be a reasonable option.

(A) Neointimal hyperplasia
(B) Atherosclerotic plaque with highly developed fibrous cap
(C) Thrombosis
(D) Absent or mild calcification
(E) Diffuse involvement

22.4 A 75-year-old woman presented with an acute coronary syndrome (ACS) and dynamic ST-segment depression in the lateral leads. She underwent CABG 4 months earlier (left internal mammary artery [LIMA] to left anterior descending [LAD], right internal mammary artery [RIMA] to the right coronary artery [RCA], sequential SVG to the first diagonal branch and to the first obtuse marginal branch of the left circumflex [LCx]). Her preoperative left ventricular ejection fraction (LVEF) was 30%. Coronary angiography demonstrated an occlusion of the SVG to the diagonal branch and marginal branch. Which statement about SVG occlusion within the first 6 months after surgery is TRUE?

(A) Female gender is a significant predictor of early SVG graft occlusion
(B) Dyslipidemia reduces 6-month vein graft patency
(C) Optimal graft flow at the end of surgery has a protective effect against graft occlusion
(D) Preoperative congestive heart failure is a significant predictor of early SVG occlusion
(E) C and D are correct

22.5 A 74-year-old gentleman presents with angina (Canadian Cardiovascular Society [CCS] Class III) 7 years following CABG performed in an emergency situation with an SVG to the RCA (whose proximal segment was severely calcified and chronically occluded), an SVG to the first marginal, and an SVG to the LAD in the presence of a calcified subtotal left main trunk (LMT) stenosis. Three years prior to current presentation, intermediate lesions of the SVG to the LAD and SVG to the RCA were seen on a coronary angiogram but treated conservatively, while a PCI with a drug-eluting stent (DES) implantation of the SVG to the marginal branch was performed to treat a critical lesion. Current angiogram shows that the SVG to the first marginal is patent, the SVG to the RCA is occluded, and the SVG to the LAD has an extensive disease. Which of the following statements is the most appropriate?

(A) SVG atherosclerosis remains the primary cause of graft failure and the presence of SVG lesions is the most important predictor of subsequent SVG failure
(B) Sealing of intermediate lesions with DES implantation is safe, but it is not associated with a significant reduction of cardiac events at 3-year follow-up
(C) Reoperation for CABG is preferred for patients with extensively diseased or occluded bypass grafts, reduced left ventricle function, multiple total occlusions of native coronary arteries, and absence of patent arterial grafts
(D) The IMA grafts, if available, are the conduit of choice for redo CABG
(E) All of the above

22.6 A 68-year-old diabetic man presented with ACS and dynamic ST depression in leads V4 to V6. Eight months earlier, he underwent quadruple bypass (LIMA to LAD, vein to diagonal branch, jump graft to the LCx, and vein to RCA). The likely cause of ischemia is:

(A) A stenosis at the proximal anastomosis due to aorto-ostial disease
(B) A midgraft stenosis of an SVG conduit due to neointimal hyperplasia
(C) A subacute thrombotic SVG occlusion
(D) A stenosis at the distal anastomosis site
(E) B and D

22.7 Which statement about SVG atherosclerosis is FALSE?

(A) Lipid handling of SVG endothelium is characterized by fast lipolysis, less active lipid synthesis, and low lipid uptake
(B) Late thrombotic occlusion occurs rarely in old degenerated SVG with advanced atherosclerotic plaque formation
(C) SVG atherosclerosis tends to be diffuse with plaque having little evidence of calcification
(D) Compared to the native vessel atherosclerotic process, SVG atherosclerosis is less rapidly progressive
(E) Within the first year following vein graft implantation, the vein wall is thickened by the neointimal growth because of the hemodynamic pressure load from the veins being exposed to arterial pressure

22.8 Which of the following factors influence long-term SVG patency?

(A) Native-vessel diameter distal to the anastomotic site
(B) Cigarette smoking
(C) Hyperlipidemia
(D) Severity of native-vessel atherosclerosis proximal to the anastomotic site
(E) All of the above

22.9 One of your referring general practitioners asks you which of the following strategies is NOT associated with improved outcomes among patients post-CABG:

(A) Antiplatelet therapy
(B) Routine coronary angiogram 1 year post surgery
(C) Lipid-lowering therapy
(D) The use of arterial grafts
(E) Smoking cessation

22.10 The same general practitioner challenges you on the antithrombotic therapy in patients who have undergone CABG. Which one of his statements is NOT correct?

(A) Aspirin alone has been reported to improve vein graft patency and mortality
(B) Clopidogrel is the lifelong alternative for patients who are aspirin intolerant after CABG
(C) Dual antiplatelet therapy (DAPT) (aspirin and clopidogrel) has no influence on arterial graft patency
(D) DAPT (aspirin and clopidogrel) should be resumed after CABG to 12-month treatment duration after ACS
(E) DAPT post-CABG is recommended for 6 and 12 months in stable CAD and ACS patients, respectively

22.11 You are starting an elective PCI of an aorto-ostial long-segment stenosis in a patient with a 7-year-old vein graft (Fig. Q22-11). Which of the following complications should be of LEAST concern in this setting?

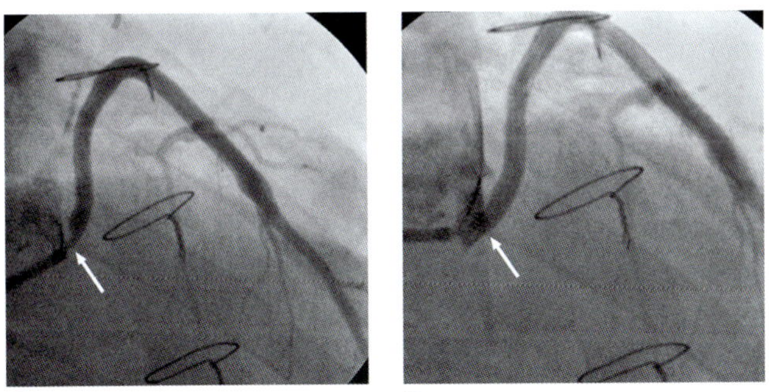

Figure Q22-11 An aorto-ostial lesion (*arrow*) of an SVG to the LAD is demonstrated in panel A. Panel B shows the result following stenting.

(A) Dissection
(B) Distal embolization
(C) No-reflow
(D) Abrupt closure
(E) Proximal anastomosis rupture

22.12 A 77-year-old man underwent stent implantation without emboli protection of a long segment involving the ostial portion of a 15-year-old SVG conduit (Fig. Q22-12) and suffered a periprocedural myocardial infarction (MI) following prolonged no-reflow. The antithrombotic regimen included aspirin, clopidogrel, and unfractionated heparin (UFH). What should have been done differently?

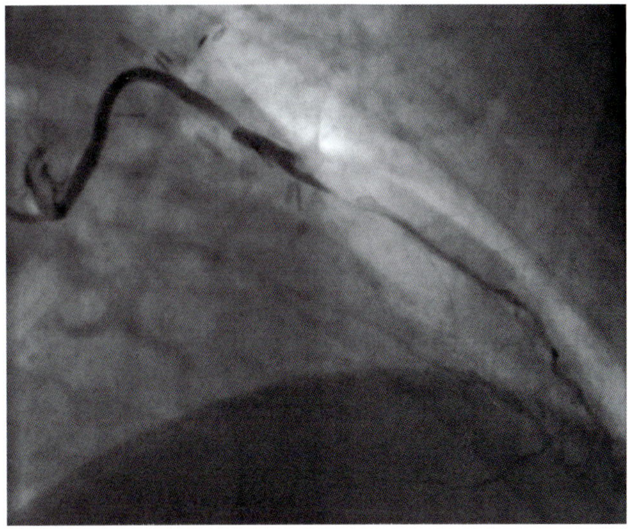

Figure Q22-12 Long stenosis involving the mid- and distal portion of the SVG to the diagonal branch (15-year-old vein conduit).

(A) The use of a filter as an embolic protection device would have reduced the risk of periprocedural MI
(B) The use of glycoprotein (GP) IIb/IIIa inhibitors would have reduced the risk of periprocedural MI
(C) The combination of a filter and GP IIb/IIIa inhibitors would have reduced the risk of periprocedural MI
(D) The use of bivalirudin instead of UFH would have reduced the risk of periprocedural MI
(E) The use of ticagrelor instead of clopidogrel would have reduced the risk of periprocedural MI

22.13 A 62-year-old gentleman underwent quadruple bypass (LIMA to the LAD and first diagonal branch, SVG to the second obtuse marginal branch, and SVG to the posterolateral branch of the RCA). On postoperative day 2, he developed ST-elevation myocardial infarction (STEMI) in the lateral leads. Coronary angiogram (Fig. Q22-13) showed an ostial lesion (arrow) associated with a suspected thrombus in the SVG. You plan to perform a PCI of the SVG. Which answer is correct?

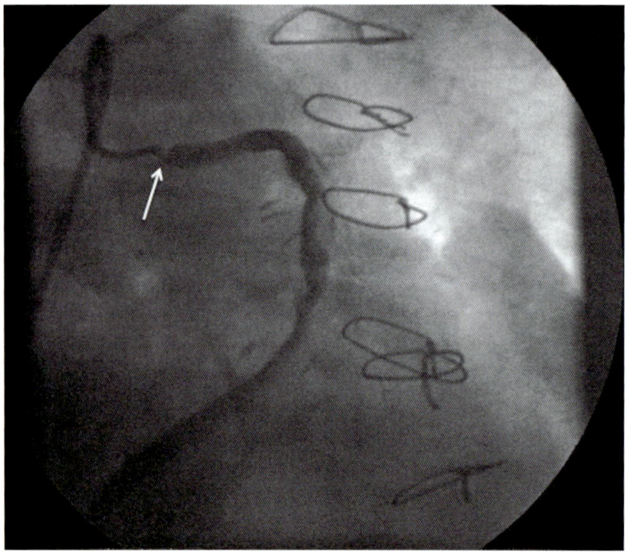

Figure Q22-13 Aorto-ostial SVG lesion (*arrow*) associated with a suspected thrombus in a 2-day-old SVG to the posterolateral branch of the RCA.

(A) Disruption of fresh thrombus may lead to no-reflow
(B) Use of embolic protection devices in SVG PCI is associated with a significant reduction in a 30-day major adverse cardiac events (MACE)
(C) In addition to distal embolization, suture rupture at the aortic anastomosis site is a concern, and the intervention should be done after agreement with the surgical colleague
(D) Direct stenting may be associated with a reduction in the volume of atheroembolic debris
(E) All of the above

22.14 A 78-year-old woman experienced a malaise. She presented 6 hours later to the emergency room because of ongoing typical chest pain and shortness of breath. She had previous pacemaker implantation, and the electrocardiogram (ECG) showed a left bundle branch block (LBBB). She underwent double bypass 10 years earlier (SVG to LAD and SVG to RCA). Which of the following statements is NOT correct?

(A) SVG to the LAD has worse patency rate than SVG to the RCA or LCx
(B) Smoking is a risk factor for early and late graft thrombosis
(C) Diameter of the recipient artery by angiography is highly predictive of SVG patency
(D) The presence of intermediate SVG lesions is a predictor of subsequent graft failure and cardiovascular events
(E) All of the above

22.15 In the patient detailed in Question 22.14, two DES were implanted in the SVG to the LAD 2 years prior to current presentation. Clopidogrel was stopped 15 days prior to this event. At the time of angiography (Fig. Q22-15), 8 hours after symptom onset, the patient still had chest pain. SVG to RCA is patent, and the native LCx shows only nonsignificant lesions. Proximal native LAD is chronically occluded with heavy calcification. What is your diagnosis and treatment strategy?

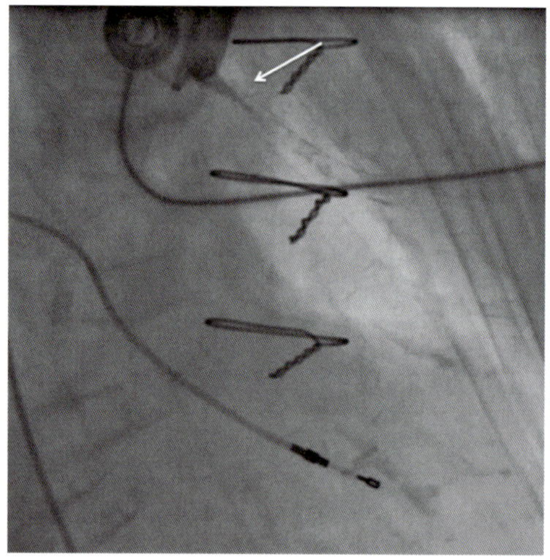

Figure Q22-15 Proximal SVG to LAD occlusion 2 years after DES implantation.

(A) Acute anterior MI following SVG to LAD occlusion, medical management
(B) Acute anterior MI following SVG to LAD occlusion, attempt SVG PCI
(C) Acute anterior MI following SVG to LAD occlusion, attempt native LAD recanalization
(D) Chronic SVG to LAD occlusion, medical management
(E) Chronic SVG to LAD occlusion, attempt native LAD recanalization

22.16 A 71-year-old diabetic man underwent emergent surgical revascularization 13 years earlier with SVGs to the LCx and RCA (LAD was free of significant lesions). Two years prior to current presentation, PCI of the proximal portion of the SVG to the RCA was performed with implantation of a DES. At that time, LVEF was 45%. The patient is now admitted for progressive shortness of breath, pulmonary edema, mild upper abdominal pain, and diffuse ST depression in the anterior leads. Troponin I was 10 UI/L (100 times the upper limit of normal) at presentation but declined 4 hours later. LVEF was 35%. At day 2, coronary angiography showed occlusion of the SVG to the RCA (suspected to be subacute), a severely diffused disease SVG to the LCx in the presence of a proximal LCx occlusion and a diffusely infiltrated left main stem (degree of stenosis estimated at 70%) involving the bifurcation, and a long proximal severe LAD lesion. The native RCA was occluded but was collateralized from the LAD. LVEF was now 35% in the presence of hypokinesia. Cardiac positron emission tomography (PET) showed viability of the entire left ventricle with the exception of a small area of transmural necrosis in the RCA territory. What treatment should be proposed to the patient?

(A) Recanalization of the SVG to the RCA that was stented 2 years earlier and PCI of the SVG to the LCx
(B) PCI of the left main stem and LAD with DES
(C) Optimal medical treatment and implantable cardioverter–defibrillator (ICD) implantation
(D) Redo surgery
(E) A and B

22.17 Which of the following statements about redo CABG is the most appropriate?

(A) Redo surgery carries a higher mortality rate than the first CABG
(B) Redo surgery carries a higher morbidity rate than the first CABG
(C) Redo surgery is associated with reduction of SVG patency as compared with initial surgery
(D) Redo surgery conveys less relief from angina than the first CABG
(E) All of the above

22.18 A 70-year-old man presented with angina CCS Class II. He underwent surgical revascularization 10 years previously (LIMA to the LAD, SVG to the RCA, and SVG to the second obtuse marginal of the LCx). Coronary angiography (Fig. Q22-18) showed a focal ostial lesion of the SVG to obtuse marginal. Which one of the following statements is CORRECT?

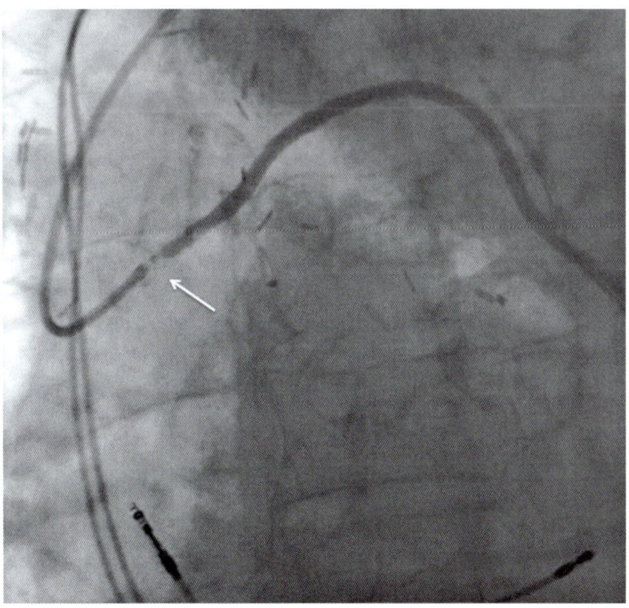

Figure Q22-18 Coronary angiography 10 years postsurgical revascularization showing an ostial lesion on an SVG to the marginal branch of the LCx (*arrow*).

(A) PCI of this ostial SVG lesion carries a high risk of vessel rupture
(B) Distal embolization rates of ostial SVG lesions PCI are similar to interventions at the level of the body of the graft.
(C) Primary stenting is contraindicated in SVG PCI
(D) DES should be preferred over bare metal stents (BMS) in SVG PCI

22.19 A 67-year-old man treated for hypertension and dyslipidemia underwent surgical revascularization (LIMA to LAD, SVG to RCA, and SVG to an obtuse marginal branch of the LCx) for three-vessel coronary artery disease (CAD) with focal proximal RCA stenosis, an ostial lesion of the left main stem, and normal LVEF. At postoperative day 2, the patient became dependent to inotropic agents and developed diffuse ST-segment depression on ECG as well as a mild rise of cardiac biomarkers beyond what was expected following CABG. Urgent coronary angiography was performed. The SVG to the marginal branch and to the RCA are demonstrated in Figure Q22-19. Injection of the native coronary arteries demonstrated, in addition to the preoperative findings, a diffuse luminal narrowing of all three vessels. What statement regarding this case is INCORRECT?

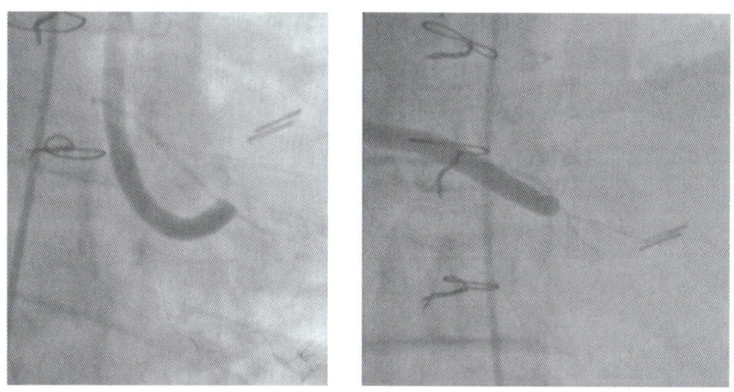

Figure Q22-19 Two SVGs anastomosed to a spastic marginal branch of the LCx (panel A) and a spastic distal RCA (panel B).

(A) In patients immediately post-CABG, urgent coronary angiography should be performed when medium-size or large perioperative MI is suspected
(B) Perioperative MI is not associated with increased risk of subsequent congestive heart failure and adverse long-term outcomes
(C) In this case, inotropic support should be discontinued if needed following insertion of an intra-aortic balloon pump (IABP)
(D) Whenever possible, nitroglycerine perfusion should be started
(E) All of the above

22.20 An 84-year-old man underwent surgical revascularization (SVG to the LAD, SVG to the obtuse marginal branch of the LCx) for two-vessel coronary disease 8 years earlier. He presents now with angina on exertion (CCS Class II) despite optimal medical therapy. Coronary angiography shows a stenosis on the proximal portion of the SVG to the obtuse marginal branch (Fig. Q22-20). Which statement is correct?

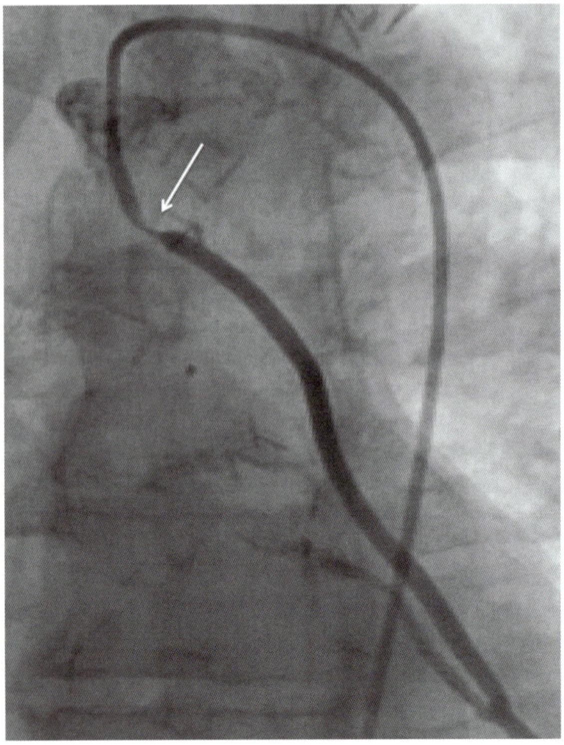

Figure Q22-20 Proximal lesion (*arrow*) on an 8-year-old SVG to the obtuse marginal branch in a patient presenting with angina (CCS Class II).

(A) PCI of SVG using newer-generation DES is associated with similar outcomes than DES-based PCI of native coronary arteries
(B) Covered stents do reduce periprocedural MI during SVG PCI because they prevent distal embolization
(C) Implantation of DES in SVG lesions is associated with a lower risk of repeat revascularization than with BMS
(D) There is an increase in mortality rate after DES compared with BMS implantation in SVG PCI
(E) None of the above

22.21 A 64-year-old patient presented with angina on exertion 5 years after having undergone CABG (LIMA to LAD and SVG to RCA). Coronary angiogram showed a significant lesion in the midportion of the SVG, and PCI was performed using a DES. Which statement about DES use in SVG PCI is INCORRECT?

(A) Compared with BMS, DES use is associated with reduced target lesion revascularization (TLR) and target vessel revascularization (TVR)
(B) Evidence suggests increased rates of MI and mortality with DES compared with BMS
(C) There is no evidence of an increased stent thrombosis rate associated with DES implantation compared with BMS implantation
(D) The superiority of DES compared with BMS was demonstrated in randomized controlled trials
(E) Compared to PCI of native coronary arteries using DES, PCI in SVG with DES are associated with worse long-term outcomes

22.22 A 71-year-old patient anticoagulated for chronic atrial fibrillation presented with unstable angina 12 years post-CABG (SVG to LAD and SVG to the obtuse marginal branch of the LCx). You plan to perform a coronary angiogram and the patient is asking you if a transradial approach would be an option for him. Which statement about transradial approach compared with the transfemoral one for SVG angiography is INCORRECT?

(A) Transradial approach is associated with higher rate of crossover
(B) Right radial access is preferred over left radial access in all post-CABG patients
(C) Transradial approach is associated with longer procedure and fluoroscopy time
(D) Transradial approach is associated with more contrast use
(E) Transradial approach provides greater patient satisfaction

22.23 A 70-year-old diabetic patient underwent surgery for a three-vessel CAD (LIMA to LAD, SVG to LCx, and SVG to RCA). Four years later, coronary angiography was performed because of worsening dyspnea on exertion. This showed an ostial lesion on the SVG to the LCx that was treated by PCI using a filter emboli protection device (Fig. Q22-23). What statement is correct concerning the use of embolic protection device in SVG interventions?

(A) In the SAFER trial, a study comparing the use of emboli protection vs. no protection device, primary composite end point (death, MI, emergency CABG, and TLR) was reduced by approximately 40% at 30 days
(B) In restenotic lesions, routine use of embolic protection device is needed since the neointimal proliferation makes distal embolization likely

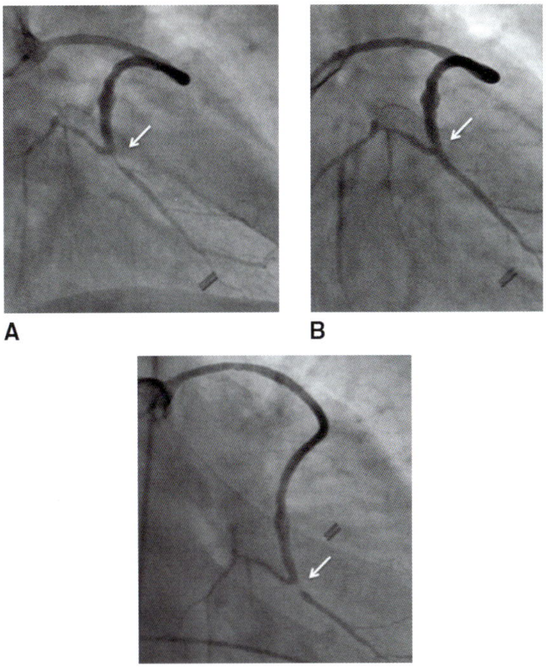

A B C

Figure Q22-23 A: Twelve years post-SVG to the obtuse marginal branch, presence of a severe lesion involving the distal anastomosis (*arrow*). B: Result post-PCI with a 2.5- × 12-mm BMS. C: Angiographic control at 6 months because of recurrent angina showing severe in-stent restenosis.

(C) The use of emboli protection devices is not required if primary stenting is performed because this decreases the risk of distal embolization
(D) The use of emboli protection devices is not required if ticagrelor is administered because this agent decreases the risk of distal embolization
(E) None of the above

22.24 A 63-year-old obese woman underwent CABG (LIMA to LAD, SVG to RCA, and SVG to the first obtuse marginal of the LCx) for a three-vessel disease. Fourteen days post surgery, she developed transient ST-segment elevation in the lateral leads and cardiac enzyme elevation. The angiogram is shown in Figure Q22-24. Which statements apply in general for early SVG failure?

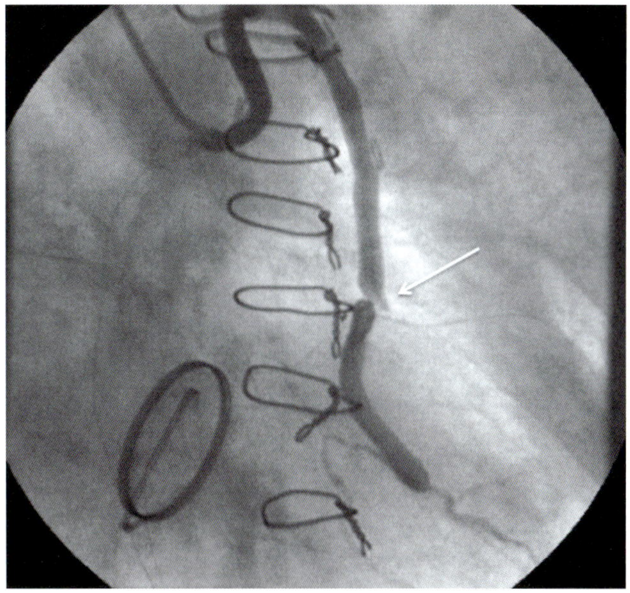

Figure Q22-24 Early SVG failure resulting from clips (*arrow*) compromising flow in the SVG.

(A) It may result from a technical (surgical) issue
(B) It may result from nonlaminar flow patterns secondary to SVG–coronary artery mismatch
(C) It may result from venous varicosities
(D) It may result from compromised outflow from distal CAD
(E) All of the above

22.25 Important breakthrough(s) in SVG PCI has/have been:

(A) GP IIb/IIIa receptor antagonist
(B) Embolic protection device
(C) Covered stent
(D) DES
(E) B and D

ANSWERS AND EXPLANATIONS

22.1 Answer E. The first successful aortocoronary SVG was implanted by Garrett and colleagues in May 1967 (Garrett HE, et al. *JAMA* 1973;223(7):792-794), and the technique was subsequently refined and brought to success by René Favaloro, an Argentinean cardiac surgeon working at the Cleveland Clinic Foundation in Cleveland, Ohio.

The IMA was the first conduit used as a coronary bypass graft in humans. In 1946, Arthur Vineberg from Canada implanted the LIMA within the anterior myocardium to improve myocardial blood supply through the intramyocardial vascular sinusoids. During several years, this Vineberg procedure was the most successful surgical therapy of angina. On May 2, 1960, R. Goetz and his team in New York performed the first successful CABG performing an anastomosis of the RIMA to the right coronary. V. Kolesov was the first to show long-term patency of the LIMA on the LAD artery (Chaikhouni A. *Heart Views* 2010;11(1):31-37).

22.2 Answer E. PCI in vein grafts represents 6% of all PCI in the United States according to national cardiovascular data registry (Brilakis ES, et al. *JACC Cardiovasc Interv* 2011;4(8):844-850; Dehmer GJ, et al. *J Am Coll Cardiol* 2012;60(20):2017-2031).

A major limitation of SVG as conduits for CABG is the atherosclerosis developing in the vein grafts. Historically, the perioperative and 10-year SVG occlusion rates were 10% and 50%, respectively (Morrison DA, et al. *J Am Coll Cardiol* 2002;40(11):1951-1954). Additional data from a multicentric cohort of 1,074 patients with angiographic assessment at 1 week and 1, 3, 6, and 10 years reported that 95% of SVGs were patent at 7 to 10 days. Furthermore, early patency was associated with a 76% 6-year patency rate and 68% 10-year patency. The overall 10-year SVG patency rate was 61%. The strongest long-term predictors of SVG graft patency were grafting into the LAD coronary artery and grafting into a vessel that is at least 2.0 mm in diameter (Goldman S, et al. *J Am Coll Cardiol* 2004;44(11):2149-2156).

22.3 Answer B. Three distinct and temporally separated pathophysiologic processes are observed in SVG disease: subacute thrombosis (usually occurring within <1 month of surgery), neointimal hyperplasia (between 1 month and 1 year post-CABG), and vein graft atherosclerosis (usually clinically relevant >3 years after surgery). Morphologically, vein graft lesions tend to be diffuse, concentric, and friable with a poorly developed or absent fibrous cap. SVG atherosclerosis is often rapidly progressive and associated with greater numbers of foam and inflammatory cells. Severe calcifications are rare (Motwani JG, et al. *Circulation* 1998;97(9):916-931).

22.4 Answer E. Optimal graft flow as assessed at the end of surgery has a protective effect against graft occlusion. Good flow conditions are observed in patients with large-diameter target vessels, lack of significant native disease distal to the anastomosis, and several run-off branches. Since SVG lack side branches, any process resulting in decreased flow may precipitate thrombosis. Significant predictors of SVG attrition or occlusion at 6 months after surgery in a study on 200 patients (Yun KL, et al. *J Thorac Cardiovasc Surg* 2005;129(3):496-503) included congestive heart failure, grafting to diagonal arteries, larger vein graft size, and poor runoff. Hypertension, gender, dyslipidemia, and previous MI did not affect early graft patency (Cataldo G, et al. *Circulation* 1993;88(5 Pt 2):II93-II98). Accordingly, graft attrition during the first postoperative year results principally from early thrombotic occlusion related to rheologic and technical issues rather than from vein graft atherosclerosis.

22.5 Answer E. SVG atherosclerosis is the primary cause of graft failure years after the index surgery. The presence of SVG lesions is the most important predictor of subsequent SVG failure. Sealing of intermediate lesions with DES implantation appears to be safe but not associated with a significant reduction of cardiac events at 3-year follow-up. Indeed, 125 patients with intermediate SVG lesions were randomized between DES implantation and medical treatment. There were no 30-day events related to the target SVG. At a median follow-up of 3.4 years, the MACE rate related to the target SVG was not different between both groups (15% in the DES group vs. 20% in the medical treatment group, $p = 0.33$) (Rodés-Cabau J, et al. *Circ Cardiovasc Interv* 2016;9(11). pii: e004336).

According to the 2014 European Society of Cardiology (ESC) and European Association for Cardio-Thoracic Surgery (EACTS) guidelines on revascularization, reoperation for CABG is preferred for patients with extensively diseased or occluded bypass graft, reduced left ventricular function, several total occlusion of native coronary arteries, and absence of patent arterial grafts. Internal mammary grafts, if available, are the conduit of choice for redo CABG (Windecker S, et al. *Eur Heart J* 2014;35(37):2541–2619).

22.6 Answer E. While within the first month after surgery thrombosis is the main mechanism of SVG disease, between 1 month and 1 year post surgery, ischemia in the territory supplied by an SVG is most often due to lesions at the distal perianastomotic site or midgraft stenosis caused by neointimal hyperplasia. Neointimal hyperplasia, defined as proliferation of smooth muscle cells and accumulation of extracellular matrix in the intimal compartment, is the characteristic adaptive mechanism of venous conduits to systemic blood pressure. This process represents the foundation for later development of graft atherosclerosis. Graft occlusion due to subacute thrombosis and lesions at the proximal anastomotic site less frequently cause ischemia between 1 month and 1 year after CABG.

22.7 Answer D. Although the fundamental processes of atherosclerosis in native coronary vessels and in vein grafts are similar, there are several temporal, histologic, and metabolic differences between the two pathologies. Lipid handling by SVG endothelium is characterized by slower lipolysis, more active lipid synthesis, and higher lipid uptake than in the native coronary arteries. From a histologic point of view, SVG atherosclerosis is characterized by the presence of a larger number of foam and inflammatory cells. SVG atherosclerotic involvement is diffuse, and lesions are friable with a poorly developed fibrous cap and little evidence of calcification (Motwani JG, et al. *Circulation* 1998;97(9):916–931).

A more recent analysis confirmed the more rapid atherosclerotic lesion progression in vein grafts compared with native coronary arteries. Within the first year following vein grafts implantation, the vein wall is thickened by the neointimal growth, which most probably occurs since the veins are exposed to arterial pressure (10-fold higher than venous pressure) (Yazdani SK, et al. *JACC Cardiovasc Interv* 2012;5(6):666–674).

22.8 Answer E. A number of morphologic factors have been associated with reduced vein graft patency. It has been described for a long time that 1-year vein graft patency was significantly lower if the native grafted vessel was <1.5 mm compared to grafted vessels with a diameter >1.5 mm (Roth JA, et al. *Ann Thorac Surg* 1979;28(2):176–183). More recently, Goldman et al. confirmed that the diameter of the recipient artery by angiography is highly predictive of SVG patency (grafting of a vessel >2 mm in diameter) has an 88% 10-year patency rate compared with an artery ≤2 mm, which has 55% 10-year patency rate ($p < 0.001$) (Goldman S, et al. *J Am Coll Cardiol* 2004;44(11):2149–2156). The severity of native-vessel atherosclerosis proximal to the anastomotic site influences the flow in the vein graft. Interestingly, a study with 164 patients showed that the occlusion rate of bypass grafts at 1 year were twice as high when bypass grafts were implanted on a stenosis with preserved fractional flow reserve (FFR) values compared with bypass grafts implanted on functionally significant lesions. Of note, the FFR assessment remained undisclosed before CABG and the decision for CABG was based on surgeons' best evaluation of stenosis severity (Botman CJ, et al. *Ann Thorac Surg* 2007;83(6):2093–2097).

Cigarette smoking is an important predictor of recurrent angina during the first year after surgery and of poor long-term clinical outcome. The evidence implicating hyperlipidemia as a key risk factor in the development of vein graft atherosclerosis is as consistent and strong as it is for native coronary disease.

22.9 Answer B. Aspirin has been shown to increase short- and midterm vein graft patency. Cessation of smoking is a highly effective strategy in preventing atherosclerosis. Accordingly, it has been shown that persistent smokers had more than twice the risk of suffering MI or requiring redo surgery at 1 year following CABG compared with patients who quit smoking at the time of surgery (Voors AA, et al. *Circulation* 1996;93(1):42–47). Several trials have shown a clear-cut benefit for aggressive lipid-lowering therapy in the post-CABG setting. Similarly, the use of arterial grafts has been a major breakthrough in bypass surgery due to the better long-term patency compared with SVG.

Routine follow-up angiography post-CABG is not recommended because it has never been shown to improve long-term patency rates. Indeed, in a randomized trial, medical therapy sealing of intermediate lesions with DES implantation was not associated with a significant reduction of cardiac events in a 3-year follow-up (Rodés-Cabau J, et al. *Circ Cardiovasc Interv* 2016;9(11). pii: e004336).

22.10 Answer E. Aspirin alone has been reported to improve vein graft patency and mortality (Mangano DT. *N Engl J Med* 2002;347(17):1309–1317).

After CABG, clopidogrel is a reasonable alternative for patients who are aspirin intolerant. It is reasonable to continue it indefinitely according to the scientific statement on secondary prevention after CABG (Kulik A, et al. *Circulation* 2015;131(10):927–964).

In patients who undergo CABG for non-ST-segment elevation ACS, the CURE study has demonstrated that the combination of aspirin and clopidogrel, 75 mg/day for 9 to 12 months, is superior to aspirin alone (Fox KAA, et al. *Circulation* 2004;110(10):1202–1208). Nevertheless, that benefit was only observed in the preoperative phase, while no additional benefit for clopidogrel was demonstrated after CABG. A meta-analysis of five randomized controlled trials (958 patients) comparing DAPT to antiplatelet monotherapy post-CABG suggested that DAPT was associated with a significantly lower SVG occlusion rate at 1 year compared with antiplatelet monotherapy (Nocerino AG, et al. *Am J Cardiol* 2013;112(10):1576–1579). However, given the limited data available and the low risk of thrombotic events after CABG in stable patients, there is insufficient evidence to generally recommend DAPT postoperatively to reduce SVG occlusion in this patient subset. In patients with ACS, DAPT should be resumed after surgery to complete 12 months of DAPT (Levine GN, et al. *J Am Coll Cardiol* 2016;68(10):1082–1115).

22.11 Answer E. Suture line rupture is of concern only in the early phase after surgery. Characteristic complications of PCI in degenerated SVG include distal embolization, no-reflow, dissection, and abrupt closure. Overall, SVG PCI is associated with significantly worse outcomes compared to interventions in the native coronary circulation (Table A22-11) (Roffi M, et al. *Circulation* 2002;106(24):3063–3067).

22.12 Answer A. Mechanical emboli protection is based on the concept of either interposing a filter device between the lesion treated and the distal vasculature supplied by the graft or interrupting the flow—by either proximal or distal balloon occlusion—and then aspirating the blood column with the debris as a prevention of distal embolization.

Filter-based emboli protection—the Spider (ev3., MN, USA), the FilterWire (Boston Scientific, MA, USA), or the Emboshield (Abbott Vascular, IL, USA)—allows blood flow throughout the procedure, but particles smaller than the pore size (usually 100 μm) may reach the distal vasculature.The distal occlusion device is the GuardWire (Medtronic Vascular, Santa Rosa, CA). It is a 0.014 in. guidewire with a distal balloon that is inflated in order to stop antegrade flow, and subsequently, at the end of the intervention, the blood column within the vein graft is aspirated with a thrombectomy catheter before restoring antegrade flow. Distal balloon occlusive devices should not be used for aorto-ostial vein graft lesions since a lack of antegrade flow during distal occlusion may lead to debris embolization into the ascending aorta and the brain. The proximal occlusion device (Proxis, St. Jude, MN, USA) is no longer available. Indeed, the occlusion devices in contrast to the filters can be cumbersome to use and blood flow interruption may be poorly tolerated, especially when the myocardium supplied by the graft is large.

The benefit of emboli protection in SVG PCI was demonstrated in a randomized controlled trial (the SAFER trial) using the distal balloon occlusion GuardWire device (Baim DS, et al. *Circulation* 2002;105(11):1285–1290). Subsequently, the use of a filter device (FilterWire, Boston Scientific, MA, USA) proved to be noninferior to distal balloon

Table A22-11 Event rates in SVG PCI (compared to PCI in native vessels)

	Grafts PCI (N = 627)	Native PCI (N = 13,158)	p
30-day events (%)			
Death	2.1	1.0	0.006
MI	13.1	7.7	<0.001
Urgent revascularization	2.6	3.6	0.15
Death/MI	14.0	8.2	<0.001
Death/MI/urgent revascularization	15.2	10.0	<0.001
6-month events (%)			
Death	4.7	2.0	<0.001
MI	18.3	9.4	<0.001
Revascularization	24.5	19.1	0.003
Death/MI	20.4	10.6	<0.001
Death/MI/revascularization	37.1	25.4	<0.001

Abbreviations: MI, myocardial infarction; PCI, percutaneous coronary intervention.

occlusion for reducing periprocedural MI in a randomized trial involving 651 patients (Fig. A22-12) (Stone GW, et al. *Circulation* 2003;108(5):548–553). Indeed, flow occlusive devices allow for more complete retrieval of small particles suspended in the blood column at the time of intervention, but they have the disadvantages of inducing ischemia and of poor visualization of the lesion. Anastomotic lesions are not suitable for any of the currently available embolic protection devices. Finally, the proximal occlusion device was assessed in the PROXIMAL trial (Mauri L, et al. *J Am Coll Cardiol* 2007;50(15):1442–1449), which was a multicenter, prospective randomized trial comparing proximal balloon occlusion vs. distal protection with either a balloon occlusion or a FilterWire. The primary composite end point (death, MI, TVR) at 30 days by intention-to-treat analysis occurred in 9.2% of the proximal protection group and 10% of the distal protection group ($p = 0.0061$ for noninferiority).

The use of GP IIb/IIIa inhibitors in SVG interventions is not useful (see answer to Question 22.18). Similarly, currently, there are no data to prefer ticagrelor over clopidogrel in patients undergoing SVG PCI. Of note, the TiCAB study, randomizing aspirin alone vs. ticagrelor 90 mg twice daily post-CABG, is ongoing and will assess the 1-year major cardiovascular events (de Waha A, et al. *Am Heart J* 2016;179:69–76). Finally, no randomized data on bivalirudin in SVG PCI are available. In a retrospective study, administration of bivalirudin as a single antithrombotic agent (54 patients) vs. heparin alone (60 patients) in the context of SVG PCI with a distal protection device was described as clinically safe and associated with a trend toward fewer in-hospital non–Q-wave MI, repeat revascularization, overall vascular complications, and significantly fewer major creatine kinase-MB (CKMB) increases compared with heparin. The bivalirudin group also showed a trend toward fewer MACE at 1-month clinical follow-up (Rha SW, et al. *Am J Cardiol* 2005;96(1):67–70).

22.13 Answer E. Recurrent ischemia early after surgical revascularization with SVG is usually caused by acute SVG thrombosis. Stenosis at proximal or distal anastomosis may exist. Disruption of fresh thrombus at the time of PCI may lead to no-reflow from embolization of platelet aggregates and intense microvascular constriction following the release of soluble mediators of vasoconstrictions (serotonin, thromboxane A2). Risk factors for distal embolization include angiographically visible thrombus, intervention in ACS, plaque ulceration, and SVG degeneration.

In the SAFER (Saphenous vein graft Angioplasty Free of Emboli Randomized) trial in which the GuardWire distal protection device was tested against a control group, the primary end point (death, MI, emergency bypass or TLR by 30 days) occurred in 16.0% in the control group and in 9.6% in the distal protection device arm. It corresponds to a 42% relative reduction in the primary end point mainly driven by the reduction in MI (8.6% vs. 14.7%, $p = 0.008$) (Baim DS, et al. *Circulation* 2002;105(11):1285–1290). There is some nonrandomized evidence that direct stenting of SVG (i.e., without predilatation) may be associated with a reduction in the volume of atheroembolic debris.

22.14 Answer A. In a series of 1,074 patients, it has been suggested that the location of SVG anastomosis predicted 10-year SVG patency with a corresponding rate of 69%, 58%, and 56% for the LAD, LCx, and RCA, respectively (Goldman S, et al. *J Am Coll Cardiol* 2004;44(11):2149–2156). The same analysis showed that the diameter of the recipient artery was highly predictive of SVG patency (grafted vessel >2 mm in diameter had an 88% 10-year patency rate compared with only 55% for a grafted vessel ≤2 mm) ($p < 0.001$) (see also answer to Question 22.8).

The presence of nonobstructive SVG lesions has been recently identified as a predictor of graft failure

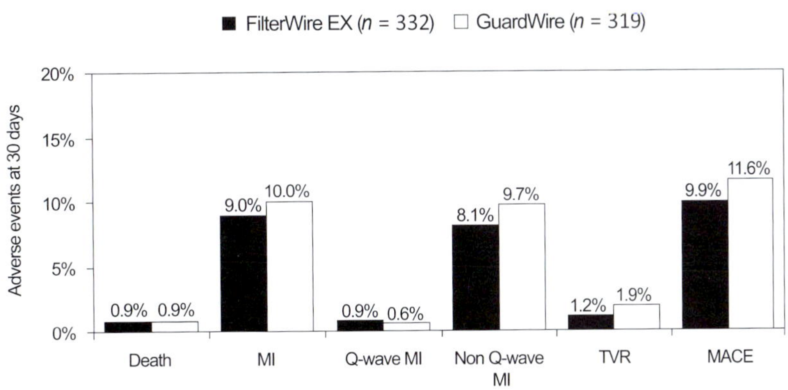

Figure A22-12 MACE (death, MI, and TVR) at 30 days among 651 patients undergoing SVG PCI randomized to a filter emboli protection (FilterWire EX, Boston Scientific, Natick, MA) or to distal balloon occlusion (PercuSurge GuardWire, Medtronic, Minneapolis, MN). For all end points, no statistically significant difference was observed.

and cardiovascular events (Rodés-Cabau J, et al. *Circ Cardiovasc Interv* 2016;9(11). pii: e004336).

22.15 Answer B. Two weeks after clopidogrel cessation and according to the clinical presentation and coronary angiography, a very late DES thrombosis in the SVG to the LAD is the most likely diagnosis. The native LAD is occluded in its midportion and not suitable for PCI (chronically occluded and heavily calcified). Medical management was not selected in the context of ongoing ischemia (chest pain). PCI of SVG was successfully performed. A BMW wire was easily advanced across the thrombus burden, and thromboaspiration brought large volume of atheroembolic debris. Intragraft administration of verapamil was performed before balloon dilatation to improve flow in this SVG with no-reflow. Flow then increased from thrombolysis in myocardial infarction (TIMI) 1 to TIMI 3 (Fig. A22-15). However, it is important to underscore that, with the exception of an acute MI in the presence of a native circulation nonaccessible to revascularization, recanalization of an occluded SVG is generally not recommended due to high risk of distal embolization with no-reflow phenomenon.

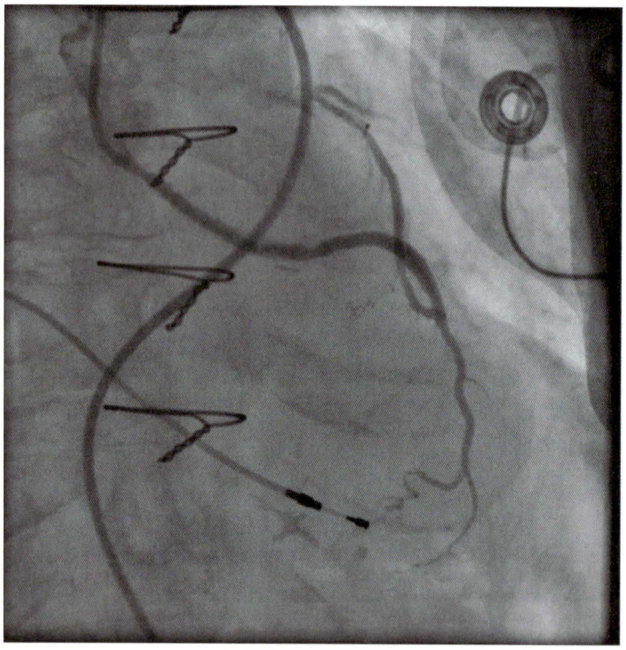

Figure A22-15 SVG to LAD postcatheter thromboaspiration and balloon angioplasty.

22.16 Answer D. PCI of the native vessels or of the grafts is a viable option if the lesions are suitable. In this patient, based on the fact that he is diabetic, has a moderately severe depressed left ventricular function, has advanced SVG disease to the LCx, and has a complex left main–LAD lesion and a largely viable RCA territory, redo CABG should be considered. This is also because no IMA grafting was previously performed. The use of LIMA has been associated with improved long-term graft patency and survival. In addition, in the SYNTAX (SYNergy between percutaneous coronary intervention with TAXus and cardiac surgery) trial (Banning AP, et al. *J Am Coll Cardiol* 2010;55(11):1067–1075), diabetic patients with a high SYNTAX score (i.e., complex anatomy like in this case) randomized to surgery had a survival benefit compared to those allocated to DES. However, these data should be interpreted cautiously with respect to our patient because the SYNTAX trial excluded patients with previous cardiac surgery.

22.17 Answer E. As compared with the first surgery, redo CABG is associated with higher mortality rate (3% vs. 7%) and higher rate of perioperative MI (4% vs. 11.5%). In addition, redo surgery is less efficacious in relieving angina, and the patency rate of venous conduits is decreased (Motwani JG, et al. *Circulation* 1998;97(9):916–931).

22.18 Answer D. PCI of ostial SVG lesions can be safely performed a few months after CABG. Early following surgery, the risk of suture line disruption and severe hemorrhagic complications is higher, and balloon sizing should be conservative.

The SAFER trial (Baim DS, et al. *Circulation* 2002;105(11):1285–1290), which randomized patients undergoing SVG PCI to emboli protection with distal balloon occlusion or no protection, and the FIRE trial (Halkin A, et al. *Am Heart J* 2006;151(4):915.e1–e7), which randomized emboli protection with filter vs. distal balloon occlusion in the same patient population, showed a dramatic reduction in no-reflow and its clinical sequelae with the use of embolic protection devices but no difference between different emboli protection strategies.

Administration of GP IIb/IIIa receptor antagonists in nonrandomized trials has been associated with increased MACE risk in patients undergoing SVG PCI, potentially because of biased patient selection (Coolong A, et al. *Circulation* 2008;117(6):790–797). A meta-analysis of five randomized trials of GP IIb/IIIa inhibitors also failed to show improved outcome in 627 patients undergoing SVG PCI (Roffi M, et al. *Circulation* 2002;106(24):3063–3067). At 30 days, MI or TVR occurred in 16.5% of patients treated with GP IIb/IIIa inhibitors vs. 12.6% in the placebo group.

Given the propensity of SVG atheroma to embolize, primary stenting without predilatation should be the preferred option whenever possible. Most of the time, postdilatation can be avoided when the correct stent size is used and implantation is performed at high pressure. When high-pressure postdilatation is required because of insufficient stent expansion, it should be performed with an embolic protection device in place, as this step carries the highest risk of all for distal embolization.

In the first DES study in SVG, the RRISC (Reduction of Restenosis in Saphenous vein grafts with Cypher Sirolimus-Eluting Stent) trial, which randomized the Cypher stent (Cordis, Warren, NJ) with a BMS in 75 patients, reported reduced 6-month angiographic restenosis and TLR (Vermeersch P, et al. *J Am Coll Cardiol* 2006;48(12):2423–2431). Surprisingly, in the long-term follow-up (median follow-up of 32 months), DES were associated with higher long-term mortality than BMS (10/38 patients (26%) in the DES arm vs. 0/37 patients (0%) in the BMS arm, $p < 0.001$), but obviously, the trial was not powered to address mortality. However, the rates of MI and TVR were not different (18% and 34% after DES vs. 5% and 38% after BMS, $p = 0.15$ and $p = 0.74$, respectively) (Vermeersch P, et al. *J Am Coll Cardiol* 2007;50(3):261–267).

The second randomized study with DES in SVG was the SOS (Stenting of Saphenous Vein Grafts) trial, which compared a paclitaxel-eluting stent (TAXUS, Boston Scientific, Natick, MA) to a similar BMS in 80 patients. At 1.5-year follow-up, PES had lower rate of TLR (5% vs. 28%, $p = 0.003$) and target-vessel failure than BMS (22% vs. 46%, $p = 0.03$) and similar mortality rate (12% vs. 5%, $p = 0.27$) (Brilakis ES, et al. *J Am Coll Cardiol* 2009;53(11):919–928). At a median follow-up of 35 months, use of PES was associated with better outcome than BMS with lower incidence of MI and TVR. All-cause mortality and cardiac mortality was not different in both groups (Brilakis ES, et al. *JACC Cardiovasc Interv* 2011;4(2):176–182).

In the largest randomized trial, ISAR-CABG (is Drug-Eluting-Stenting Associated with Improved Results in Coronary Artery Bypass Grafts), which randomized 610 patients (307 BMS, 303 DES), there were no differences in terms of death, MI, or stent thrombosis (Mehilli J, et al. *Lancet* 2011;378(9796):1071–1078).

In the SCAAR (Swedish Coronary Angiography and Angioplasty Registry) registry, which is a cohort of 3,063 SVG PCIs, the incidence of death was lower among patients who received DES with a mean follow-up of 3 years and 4 months. When adjusted for baseline characteristics, the restenosis rate was significantly lower after DES than BMS (risk ratio: 0.83, $p = 0.019$) (Frobert O, et al. *Am Heart J* 2012;164(1):87–93).

Finally, in the very large Medicare-Linked National Cardiovascular Data Registry CathPCI with 49,325 patients older than 65 years of age undergoing SVG PCI, the risk of death, MI, and urgent revascularization following DES or BMS implantation was comparable at 3 years (Brennan JM, et al. *Catheter Cardiovasc Interv* 2016;87(1):43–49).

In summary, implantation of DES in SVG lesions is associated with a lower risk of restenosis than with BMS. In addition, except for the first randomized trial, which was clearly underpowered and raised concerns about long-term mortality following DES implantation, the other trials showed either no differences or significant advantage of DES over BMS.

22.19 Answer B. Urgent coronary angiography post-CABG should be performed when a sizable perioperative MI is suspected. This allows for a differentiation between graft-related ischemic events and other causes of myocardial damage, such as prolonged extracorporeal circulation, and for a minimization of the ischemic time. In the presence of acute ST-segment elevation on ECG corresponding to a coronary territory, rise of cardiac biomarkers, and hemodynamic instability or sustained ventricular arrhythmia, a sudden graft occlusion should be suspected. Perioperative MI is associated with increased risk of subsequent congestive heart failure and short- as well as long-term adverse outcomes (Steuer J, et al. *Eur Heart J* 2002;23(15):1219–1227). Emergency PCI—either by treating the graft (e.g., in the presence of an anastomosis stenosis) or by approaching the native vessel supplied by the occluded graft—is an alternative to redo surgery for acute graft occlusion. The choice between percutaneous and surgical revascularization should be made by the heart team on a case-by-case basis based on the nature of the graft dysfunction, the territory affected, and the patency status of the corresponding native vessel. In the case presented, ischemia was secondary to diffuse spasm of the native coronary vessel, likely induced by inotropes. A conservative treatment was the preferred option, allowing for a discontinuation of inotrope agents and subsequent introduction of vasodilators. The clinical course was uneventful.

22.20 Answer C. Although partially explained by the increased prevalence of high-risk characteristics among the patients undergoing graft intervention, it has been demonstrated that SVG PCI is associated with worse outcomes compared with interventions of the native circulation (Roffi M, et al. *Circulation* 2002;106(24):3063–3067). The Symbiot trial (Turco MA, et al. *Catheter Cardiovasc Interv* 2006;68(3):379–388) showed that covered stents have a higher binary in-stent restenosis rate than BMS with no difference in MACE. Therefore, the hypothesis that covered stents may reduce periprocedural complications by potentially preventing distal embolization and reduce restenosis by serving as a possible barrier to cell migration has been invalidated.

Implantation of DES in SVG lesions is associated with a lower risk of repeat revascularization than with BMS. In the SCAAR (Swedish Coronary Angiography and Angioplasty Registry) registry, the crude analysis showed no significant difference between BMS and DES for restenosis at 1 and 3 years (12.5% and 22.0% for BMS, 7.5% and 20% after DES at 1 and 3 years, respectively). When the analysis was adjusted for baseline characteristics, including a propensity score for receiving a DES, the restenosis rate was significantly lower with DES than BMS (RR 0.83, CI 0.70 to 0.97, $p = 0.019$) (Frobert O, et al. *Am Heart J* 2012;164(1):87–93). See also the answer to Question 22.18.

22.21 Answer B. The DELAYED RRISC (Vermeersch P, et al. *J Am Coll Cardiol* 2007;50(3):261–267) study, a prospective, randomized trial of DES vs. BMS in SVG lesions in 75 patients, showed at a median follow-up of 32 months that DES use was not associated with a reduction in repeat revascularization procedures. Moreover, higher mortality was observed with DES implantation. However, the study was small and massively underpowered to address mortality. In addition, most fatal adverse outcomes were neither cardiac nor procedure related. Finally, this observation was not replicated in other randomized trials (see answer to Question 22.18) and in two meta-analyses. Accordingly, the DELAYED RRISC study included only 75 patients and obviously did not provide sufficient power to detect true effects in terms of repeat revascularization, morbidity, or mortality. The first meta-analysis (Paradis JM, et al. *Circ Cardiovasc Interv* 2010;3(6):565–576) using Bayesian methods addressing DES and BMS use in SVG PCI included 25 studies (three randomized studies and 22 nonrandomized studies, for a total of 5,755 patients) and concluded that DES use in SVG PCI was associated with improved TLR and TVR rates up to 30 months in the absence of increased rates of mortality, MI, or stent thrombosis. The second meta-analysis published thus far (Wiisanen ME, et al. *JACC Cardiovasc Interv* 2010;3(12):1262–1273) included 23 studies (four randomized and 19 nonrandomized studies), and the median follow-up was 18 months. DES use was associated with improved mortality, MACE, TLR, and TVR, and there was no evidence of increased risk of MI or stent thrombosis.

Compared to PCI of native coronary arteries, PCI in SVG has impaired long-term clinical outcomes (Brilakis ES, et al. *JACC Cardiovasc Interv* 2010;3(7):742–750).

22.22 Answer B. Transradial approach in SVG angiogram was assessed in the RADIAL-CABG trial, which is a randomized trial comparing transradial and transfemoral approaches in 64 patients per group. Transradial access was associated with more contrast volume (mean 171 ± 72 mL vs. 147 ± 39 mL, $p < 0.01$), longer procedure (34.2 ± 14.7 min vs. 21.9 ± 6.8 min, $p < 0.01$) as well as fluoroscopy time, greater patient and operator radiation exposure, higher crossover rate (17% vs. 0%, $p < 0.01$), but greater patient satisfaction according to a questionnaire. Of note, a fellow performed all procedures first; and after two to three attempts without success, a senior operator took over. All procedures by transradial approach were performed using the left radial artery (Michael TT, et al. *JACC Cardiovasc Interv* 2013;6(11):1138–1144). The right radial approach in the case described is not a good option since the LIMA was grafted to the LAD and selectively cannulating the LIMA from the right radial access is highly challenging, although feasible.

22.23 Answer A. The SAFER trial (Baim DS, et al. *Circulation* 2002;105(11):1285–1290) randomized patients undergoing SVG PCI to emboli protection vs. no protection and showed a dramatic improvement in the outcomes and a clear cost-effectiveness. Indeed, there was a 42% relative reduction in the primary end point, mainly driven by the reduction in MI (8.6% vs. 14.7%, $p = 0.008$). In restenotic lesions in SVG, routine use of embolic protection device is not needed since the neointimal proliferation makes distal embolization unlikely. See also the answer to Question 22.12.

22.24 Answer E. Early SVG failure may result from any process that contributes to flow reduction or thrombosis, such as prethrombotic states, surgical issues—such as constrictive sutures or clips (as in this case), severe stenosis at the distal anastomosis site, and graft kinking or overstretching—nonlaminar flow patterns secondary to SVG coronary artery mismatch, compromised outflow from distal CAD, and venous varicosities (Thielmann M, et al. *Eur J Cardiothorac Surg* 2006;30(1):117–125). The diameter of the recipient artery (>2 mm) is highly predictive of the 10-year patency rate of the corresponding vein graft (Goldman S, et al. *J Am Coll Cardiol* 2004;44(11):2149–2156).

22.25 Answer E. A summary of the efficacy of different strategies for SVG interventions is demonstrated in Table A22-25. GP IIb/IIIa inhibitors showed no benefit in SVG interventions (Roffi M, et al. *Circulation* 2002;106(24):3063–3067). (See the answer to Question 22.18.) Mechanical emboli protection is based on the concept of interposing a device between the lesion treated and the distal vasculature supplied by the graft as a prevention of distal embolization. The use of embolic protection devices has been a major breakthrough in SVG PCI because they are associated with a significant reduction in 30-day MACE, mainly related to a reduction in periprocedural MI. (See the answers to Questions 22.18 and 22.23 and refer to Figures Q22-24 and A22-25A,B). The Symbiot trial (Turco MA, et al. *Catheter Cardiovasc Interv* 2006;68(3):379-388) showed that covered stents have a higher binary in-stent restenosis rate than BMS with no difference in MACE. The use of DES reduced target lesion failure and improved long-term outcomes (see Questions 22.18 and 22.21).

Table A22-25 Efficacy of different treatment strategies in PCI of SVG

Therapy	Efficacy	Comments
Stents	Likely	Not prospectively addressed in large-scale randomized trials Majority of SVG PCIs performed are stent-based
Covered stents	Failed	Lack of efficacy demonstrated in a randomized trial Preliminary data on new-generation covered stents promising
DES	Effective	Three randomized trials showed better outcome after DES compared to BMS. The first trial raised concerns for increase mortality with DES at 33 years, but the two others did not reproduce this concern. Large registry also showed no increased mortality after DES implantation in SVG compared to BMS.
Glycoprotein IIb/IIIa inhibitors	Failed	Not recommended
Emboli protection devices	Highly effective	Efficacy in terms of MACE reduction demonstrated in randomized trials Distal balloon occlusion and filter devices equally effective
Ultrasound thrombolysis	Failed	Tested in a randomized trial
Atherectomy devices	Unknown	Insufficient safety and/or efficacy data

Abbreviations: BMS, bare metal stent; DES, drug-eluting stent; MACE, major adverse cardiac events; PCI, percutaneous coronary intervention; SVG, saphenous vein graft.

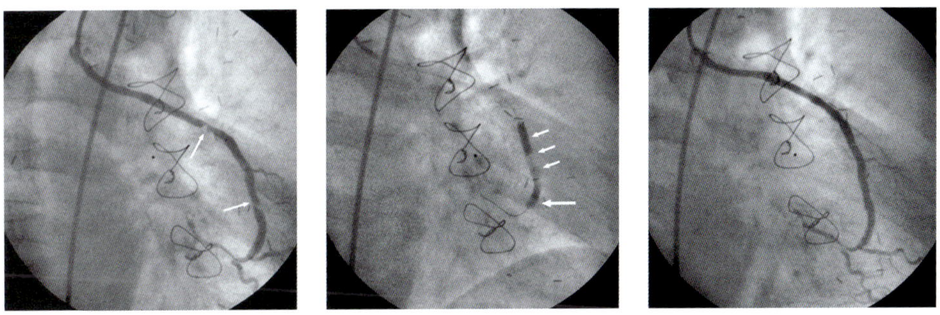

A

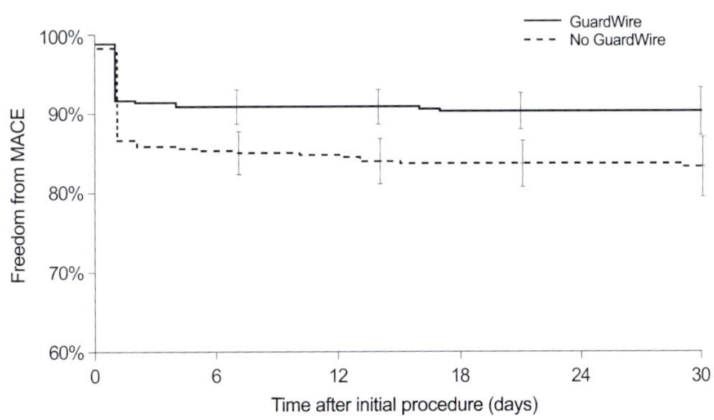

B

Figure A22-25 A: The use of a distal balloon occlusive emboli protection system (PercuSurge GuardWire, Medtronic, Minneapolis, MN) is demonstrated. Panel A shows two significant lesions (*arrows*) in the mid- to distal portion of an SVG to the marginal branch of the LCx. In panel B, the distal balloon is inflated (*large arrow*) and the graft occluded. The no-flow state is documented by the stagnant column of contrast media (*small arrows*). Panel C demonstrates final result following stent and retrieval of the distal protection. B: Freedom from MACE (i.e., death, MI, emergent bypass surgery, or TVR) at 1 month among 800 patients undergoing SVG PCI randomized to distal balloon occlusion (PercuSurge GuardWire, Medtronic, Minneapolis, MN) vs. conventional guidewire. The event rate was 9.6% in the GuardWire group and 16.5% in the control group, and the difference was statistically significant ($p = 0.004$).

23 Vascular Closure and Devices

Kashish Goel and Abhiram Prasad

QUESTIONS

23.1 An 82-year-old male presented with acute left-sided heart failure and was admitted to the cardiac intensive care unit. Transthoracic echocardiogram (TTE) revealed severe aortic stenosis and an ejection fraction (EF) of 25% (changed from 55% 2 years previously). The patient is sent to the catheterization laboratory for balloon aortic valvuloplasty and coronary angiography. A 12-Fr sheath is placed for valvuloplasty and the patient tolerated the procedure well. What type of closure device should be used in this patient?

(A) Angio-Seal
(B) One Perclose ProGlide device prior to 12-Fr sheath insertion
(C) Two Perclose ProGlide devices after 12-Fr sheath insertion
(D) Two Perclose ProGlide devices prior to 12-Fr sheath insertion
(E) Mynx

23.2 Manta, a new collagen anchor/vascular plug, is currently in clinical trials for use in large-bore access. What is the largest sheath size that may be sealed with this closure device?

(A) Up to 14 Fr size
(B) Up to 20 Fr size
(C) Up to 25 Fr size
(D) Up to 10 Fr size

23.3 A patient undergoes percutaneous coronary intervention (PCI) of the proximal left anterior descending (LAD) artery for non–ST-elevation myocardial infarction (NSTEMI) via right femoral access. A 6-Fr Angio-Seal device is placed at the end of procedure with good hemostasis. The patient presents again to the hospital 1 week later with worsening chest pain. Which of the following statements regarding Angio-Seal is TRUE?

(A) Right femoral access can be obtained safely without imaging guidance
(B) Same access site should not be used within 30 days of placing an Angio-Seal device
(C) Same access site can be used 1 cm proximal to the original site using angiographic/ultrasound imaging
(D) Ultrasound or angiographic imaging is not helpful in examining the Angio-Seal device site during reaccess

23.4 Vascular closure devices are commonly used after femoral PCI to achieve hemostasis. A recent study evaluated the postapproval use of the Mynx device compared with other vascular closure devices for the primary end point of access site bleeding, access site hematoma, retroperitoneal bleeding, or any vascular complication requiring intervention. The rate of primary end point with the Mynx device compared to other closure devices was:

(A) Similar
(B) Increased
(C) Decreased
(D) None of the above

23.5 A patient undergoes transradial catheterization using a 6-Fr sheath. PCI is performed to the mid-right coronary artery (RCA) without any complications. At the end of procedure, the sheath is removed and a band is placed with good hemostasis. One hour later, you are called to the patient's room. Significant swelling of the right hand is noted with increased tenderness at the site of puncture. Urgent ultrasound is performed and shows the following. What is the next best step? (Fig. Q23-5).

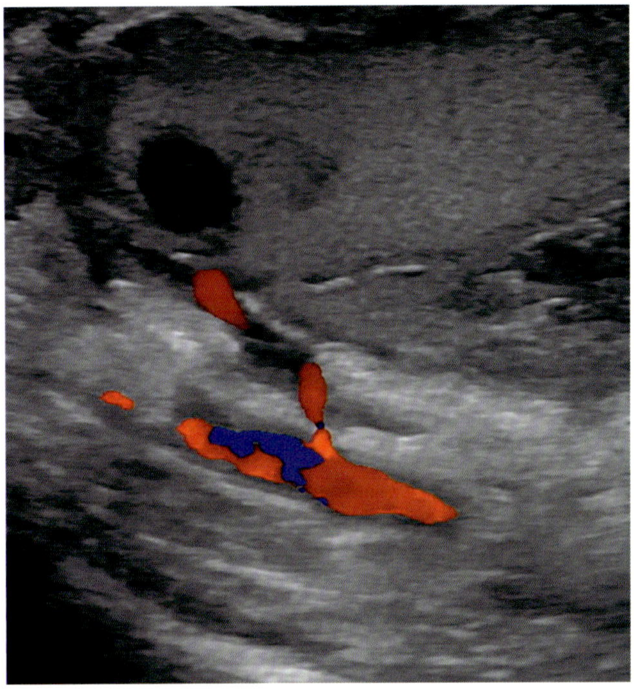

Figure Q23-5 (Courtesy of Kashish Goel and Abhiram Prasad.)

(A) Deploy a closure device
(B) ACE wrap and compression
(C) Apply two hemostasis bands
(D) Hand/vascular surgery consult
(E) Thrombin injection

23.6 An 88-year-old female undergoes transcatheter aortic valve replacement (TAVR) for severe symptomatic aortic stenosis via the right transfemoral route. The valve deployment was good, and the right femoral access site was closed using two Perclose ProGlide sutures with hemostasis. In the recovery area, the patient's right foot is noted to be cool, and there is discoloration of the right lower leg. Physical exam reveals impalpable popliteal, dorsalis pedis, or posterior tibial pulses. There is a small hematoma at the access site. She also has loss of sensation to the midfoot dorsum. Motor exam is normal, and calf compartments are soft. Which is the most likely cause for the patient's presentation?

(A) Severe stenosis at the suture site
(B) Dissection with acute thrombotic occlusion
(C) Retroperitoneal bleed
(D) Distal embolization
(E) Perforation

23.7 A 63-year-old female presents for an urgent catheterization in the setting of diffuse T-wave inversions in the anterior leads. The right radial approach is used, and during initial access, resistance was encountered with the wire. Radial angiogram was performed and demonstrated the following. Which of the following is the next best step in the management of this complication? (Fig. Q23-7).

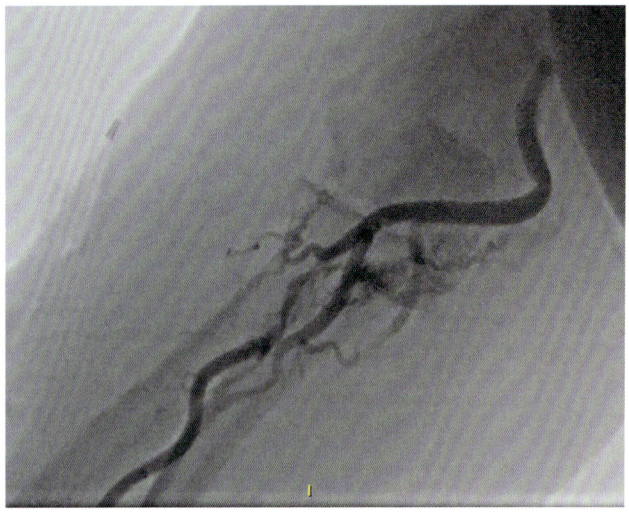

Figure Q23-7 (Courtesy of Kashish Goel and Abhiram Prasad.)

(A) Remove the sheath and proceed to left radial or femoral access
(B) Place a long sheath covering this area
(C) Stop the procedure and call for urgent hand surgery consult
(D) ACE wrap and compression after aborting the procedure

23.8 The proven benefits of vascular closure devices include all of the following, EXCEPT:

(A) Reduced risk of vascular complications
(B) Faster hemostasis
(C) Shorter duration of bed rest
(D) Improved patient comfort

23.9 Match the mechanism of closure with a device:

1. Utilizes a nitinol clip to close the arteriotomy site
2. Suture-mediated closure
3. Mechanical seal by sandwiching the arteriotomy between a bioabsorbable anchor and the collagen sponge

4. Balloon catheter that initiates hemostasis and ensures the precise placement of procoagulant (a flowable mixture of thrombin, collagen, and diluent) at the puncture site in the entire tissue tract
5. Polyethylglycol sealant delivered to the surface of the arteriotomy

(A) Angio-Seal
(B) Duett
(C) Mynx
(D) Perclose
(E) StarClose

23.10 Which of the following is not bioresorbable?

(A) Angio-Seal
(B) Duett
(C) Mynx
(D) Perclose
(E) VasoSeal

23.11 A 68-year-old diabetic man underwent PCI and uneventful closure of his femoral access site with a Perclose device. Two weeks later, he noted redness and swelling at the access site with drainage of serosanguineous material. Figure Q23-11 was taken at the time of exploration of his groin and most likely represents which of the following?

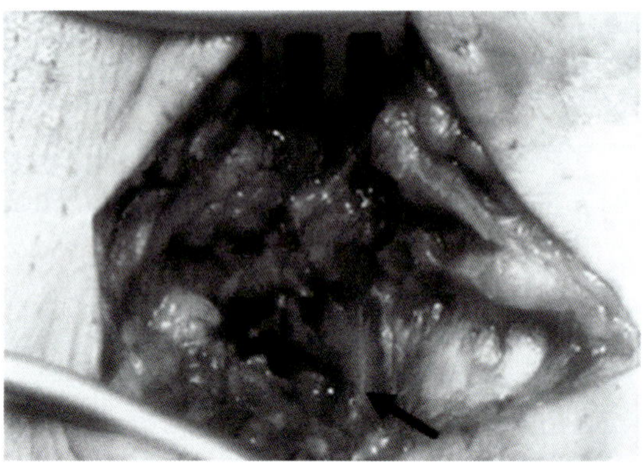

Figure Q23-11

(A) Generalized sepsis
(B) Mycotic pseudoaneurysm
(C) Carbuncle
(D) Infective endocarditis
(E) Femoral endarteritis

23.12 A 55-year-old man undergoes uncomplicated cardiac catheterization and PCI of the RCA. Aspirin, clopidogrel, and bivalirudin were administered during the case. A femoral angiogram is obtained through the procedural sheath in anticipation of the use of a closure device (Fig. Q23-12). What is the most optimal next step?

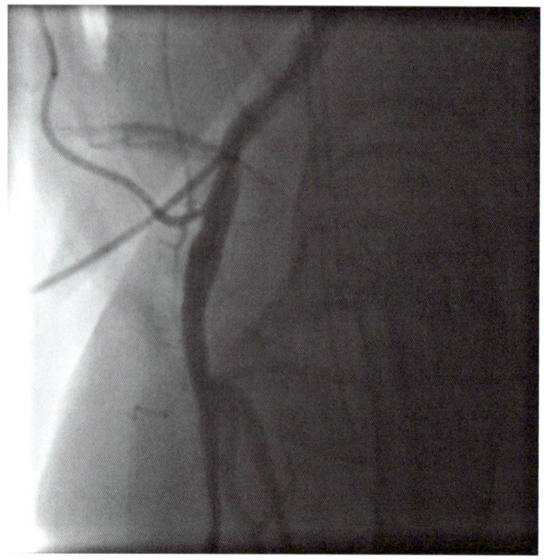

Figure Q23-12

(A) Place a FemoStop and pull the sheath
(B) Obtain an abdominal computed tomography (CT) scan and call vascular surgery
(C) Place an Angio-Seal device
(D) Wait 2 hours, and then pull the sheath and apply manual compression

23.13 A 65-year-old woman undergoes elective uncomplicated cardiac catheterization and PCI of the LAD. Aspirin, clopidogrel, and heparin were administered during the case. A femoral angiogram is obtained through the procedural sheath in anticipation of use of a closure device (Fig. Q23-13). What closure device should be chosen in this case?

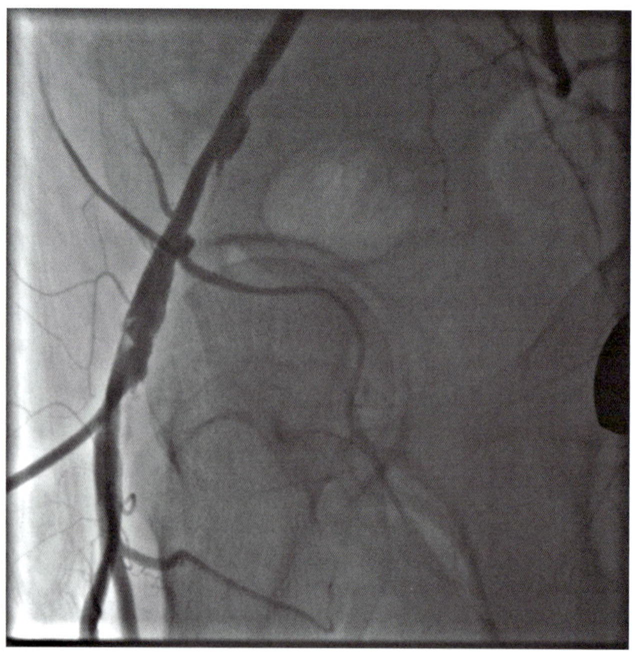

Figure Q23-13

(A) Angio-Seal
(B) Perclose
(C) Mynx
(D) StarClose
(E) None of the above

23.14 A 48-year-old man undergoes uncomplicated cardiac catheterization and PCI of the LAD after a non-STEMI. Aspirin, prasugrel, and bivalirudin were administered during the case. Since the initial femoral access was achieved with a single anterior wall stick, the operator placed a closure device without apparent complication. The patient complained of pain and swelling at the access site throughout the night. A pulsatile mass was found in the groin the following morning. Which of the following likely corresponds to this case?

(A) Arteriovenous fistulae (AVF)
(B) Hematoma
(C) Pseudoaneurysm
(D) Limb ischemia

23.15 A 45-year-old woman undergoes diagnostic catheterization after having a positive stress test for atypical chest pain. She is found to have mild luminal irregularities, and the cardiologist decides to use a closure device for the femoral access. The patient is obese, so he elects to place a buddy wire in the event he does not get complete closure with an Angio-Seal device. The patient complains of immediate leg pain and is found to be pulseless and have pain, pallor, and paresthesia of her right leg. A sheath is inserted over the buddy wire, and the following angiogram is obtained. What should you do next? (Fig. Q23-15).

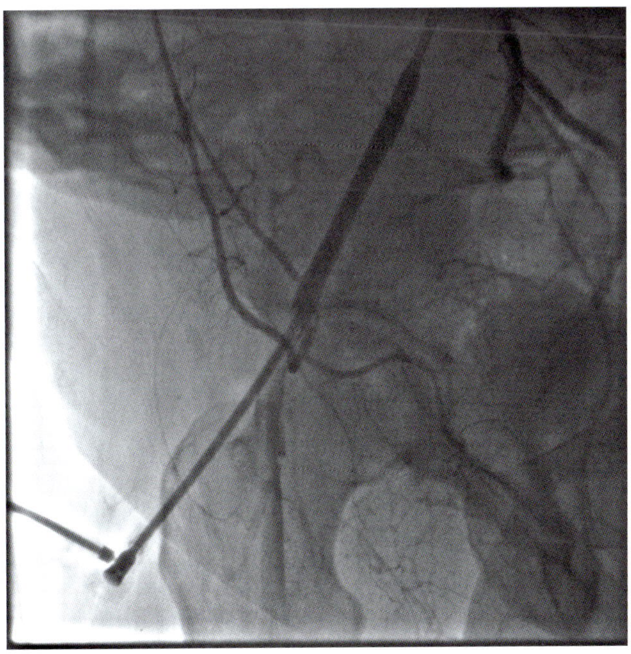

Figure Q23-15

(A) Urgent surgery consult or urgent percutaneous peripheral vascular intervention
(B) Intravenous (IV) heparin and glycoprotein (GP) IIb/IIIa inhibitor
(C) IV fibrinolytic therapy
(D) Give pain pills for relief

23.16 A 67-year-old woman is admitted to the hospital with NSTEMI. Cardiac catheterization is performed revealing diffuse three-vessel coronary artery disease (CAD). At the end of the procedure, she appears to be uncomfortable and complains of vague abdominal discomfort. The angiogram in Figure Q23-16 is obtained. What should be the next step?

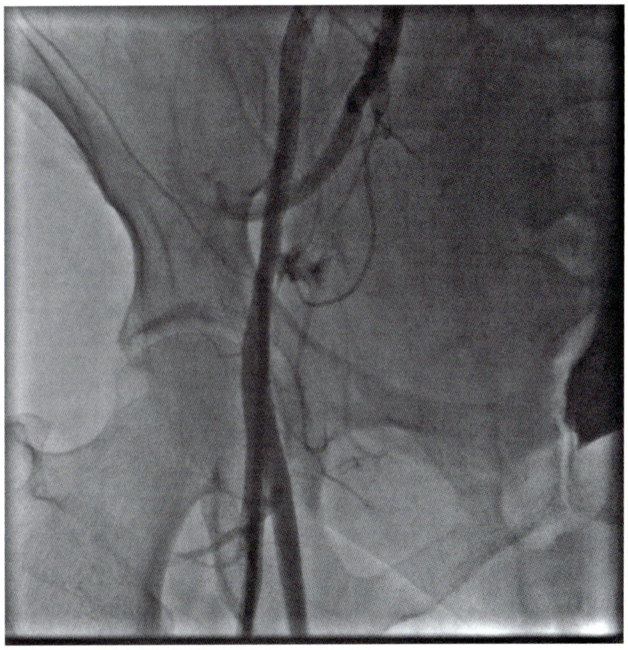

Figure Q23-16

(A) Place a closure device
(B) Pull the sheath in the lab and apply manual compression
(C) Gain contralateral access and perform balloon angioplasty
(D) Continue anticoagulation in preparation for coronary artery bypass graft (CABG)

23.17 What are the distinguishing characteristic features upon physical examination of a femoral artery pseudoaneurysm as compared to a hematoma?

(A) Pulsatile groin mass and bruit
(B) Pain and audible bruit
(C) Groin mass
(D) Continuous groin pain and neuralgia

23.18 An 81-year-old patient undergoes an urgent catheterization for acute myocardial infarction (MI). She is found on angiogram to have 100% occlusion of the LAD artery. She has a successful PCI to LAD with 3.0 × 33-mm drug-eluting stent (DES) and 3.0 × 28-mm DES with heparin and abciximab. She is allergic to latex. She is unable to keep her leg still. Can you use Angio-Seal?

(A) Yes, Angio-Seal can be used in patients with latex allergy
(B) No, Angio-Seal cannot be used in patients with latex allergy
(C) Only manual pressure should be applied to patients with latex allergy
(D) No, only Perclose can be used in patients with latex allergy

23.19 The following devices are approved for use outside of the common femoral artery:

(A) Angio-Seal
(B) StarClose
(C) Perclose
(D) Mynx
(E) None of the above

23.20 Which of the following has been associated with acute vessel closure at the time of device deployment?

(A) Angio-Seal
(B) StarClose
(C) Perclose
(D) Mynx
(E) All of the above

ANSWERS AND EXPLANATIONS

23.1 Answer D. Sheaths above 10 Fr cannot be closed with one Perclose, Angio-Seal, or Mynx device. Vascular closure in this scenario may be performed by deploying two Perclose ProGlide sutures in a "preclose" fashion prior to insertion of the large sheath. This approach may also be used for TAVR and circulatory support devices. A novel device, Manta, is being tested in clinical trials, which may be deployed after sheath removal; however, it is currently not approved in the United States.

23.2 Answer C. The Manta vascular closure device is a novel, collagen plug-based device designed for large-bore procedures requiring devices up to 19 Fr (true outer diameter profiles up to 24.5 Fr). The first prospective feasibility study in 50 patients reported a 94% success rate at hemostasis and one major complication requiring vascular surgery (Van Mieghem NM, et al. *JACC Cardiovasc Interv* 2017;10(6):613–619). Larger prospective studies and clinical trials comparing this with other devices are required.

23.3 Answer C. The instruction for use for the Angio-Seal device states that *"if repuncture at the same location of previous Angio-Seal device use is necessary in ≤90 days, re-entry 1 cm proximal to the previous access site can be performed safely. Before considering Angio-Seal use, a femoral angiogram of the site is indicated."* Applegate et al. studied the restick issue with Angio-Seal and found that restick can occur safely within 1 to 7 days of Angio-Seal (Applegate RJ, et al. *Catheter Cardiovasc Interv* 2003;58(2):181–184). In this study, the femoral angiogram taken at the time of the initial Angio-Seal deployment was reviewed, and the second access was attempted 1 cm above or below the initial access site (while staying within the common femoral artery). If the initial puncture was high, then the second stick was made 1 cm below. Ultrasound imaging may be a useful adjunct.

23.4 Answer B. A postapproval surveillance study using the National Cardiovascular Data Registry (NCDR) CathPCI Registry reported that use of the Mynx device was associated with a significantly increased risk of any vascular complications (1.2% vs. 0.8%; relative risk, 1.59), access-site bleeding (0.4% vs. 0.3%; relative risk, 1.34), and transfusion (1.8% vs. 1.5%; relative risk, 1.23) (Resnic FS, et al. *N Engl J Med* 2017;376(6):526–535).

23.5 Answer D. This image shows a pseudoaneurysm, an infrequent complication of transradial catheterization. A size <1 cm can usually be managed conservatively. Thrombin injection is not recommended for radial artery pseudoaneurysms. Pseudoaneurysms >2 cm generally require surgical intervention. Hand/vascular surgery consult would be indicated for this patient to guide management.

23.6 Answer B. The most likely explanation for the acute limb ischemia in the patient is acute dissection with thrombotic occlusion. This patient will require urgent imaging (computed tomography angiography [CTA] or peripheral angiogram) followed by intervention (surgical or percutaneous). Stenosis can happen with cinching of an artery with two sutures. However, those patients do not present with acute limb ischemia. They usually present with claudication and are diagnosed as a late complication. Retroperitoneal bleed presents with hemodynamic instability and is unlikely just acute limb ischemia. Similarly, a significant arterial perforation would present with a large hematoma and hemodynamic instability. Distal embolization is possible with large-bore sheaths and presents with ischemia in distal territories. This patient has ischemia of the entire leg, which is less likely from distal embolization. Based on a meta-analysis of 31 studies, ischemic complications occurred in 0.3% of the patients who had vascular closure devices (Biancari F, et al. *Am Heart J* 2010;159(4):518–531).

23.7 Answer B. This image shows a radial artery perforation. The best next step is to cross the perforation with a 0.014-in. wire and place a long sheath, resulting in tamponade of the vessel. Reangiogram should be performed after the procedure is completed. The perforation generally seals with this approach. Removing the sheath without compression will lead to a hematoma and potential risk for compartment syndrome. A vascular surgery consult is required if there is evidence of progressive hematoma or concerns of compartment syndrome.

23.8 Answer A. Vascular closure devices have some obvious advantages. The time spent by catheterization laboratory staff in manually compressing the puncture site is reduced, which in turn improves patient flow in busy catheterization laboratories. Other proven benefits include the reduction in time to hemostasis, earlier ambulation of patients, and earlier discharge for some patients. Small studies comparing patient satisfaction after management of the access site indicate that closure devices enhance patient comfort. A rigorously performed systematic review and meta-analysis of first-generation devices suggested that vascular closure devices may actually increase the risk of hematoma and pseudoaneurysm (Koreny M, et al. *JAMA* 2004;291(3):350–357). The scientific statement from the American Heart Association (AHA) on vascular closure devices gave a class III recommendation for routinely using closure devices for the specific purpose of reducing vascular complications (Patel MR, et al. *Circulation* 2010;122(18):1882–1893).

23.9 Answers. **1-E** StarClose, **2-D** Perclose, **3-A** Angio-Seal, **4-B** Duett, and **5-C** Mynx.

23.10 Answer D. All of the devices listed except for Perclose undergo breakdown and eventually resorption by the body. Perclose utilizes a nonbiodegradable suture, similar to the suture that is used to directly close the artery by surgeons. Perclose did offer a biodegradable suture at one point, but the product was withdrawn from the market because of issues with suture breakage.

23.11 Answer B. Sohail et al. reviewed all cases of closure device–related infection seen in their institution and searched the English language medical literature for all previously published reports (Sohail MR, et al. *Mayo Clin Proc* 2005;80(8):1011–1015). They identified 46 cases from the medical literature and six cases from their institutional database. Diabetes mellitus and obesity were the most common comorbidities. The median incubation period from device insertion to presentation with access-site infection was 8 days (with a range of 2 to 29 days). The most common presenting symptoms were pain, erythema, fever, swelling, and purulent drainage at the access site. Mycotic pseudoaneurysm was the most common complication (22 cases). *Staphylococcus aureus* was responsible for most of the infections (75%). The mortality rate was 6% (three patients). This suggests that infection associated with closure device placement is uncommon, but is an extremely serious complication. Morbidity is high, and aggressive medical and surgical interventions are required to achieve cure.

23.12 Answer D. The femoral angiogram indicates that the access site is above the inferior epigastric artery and likely within the external iliac artery. Several recent retrospective observational studies have identified a "high stick" such as this as associated with an increase in the incidence of retroperitoneal hemorrhage. Moreover, these studies found an association with closure device use and an increase in the likelihood of a retroperitoneal hemorrhage, although there was not complete consensus on this point. However, in the study of Tiroch et al., (Tiroch KA, et al. *Am J Cardiol* 2008;102(11):1473–1376) the absolute rate of a retroperitoneal hemorrhage after a "high stick" was only about 4%. At this point in time, watchful waiting would be indicated, unless there was active concern about retroperitoneal hemorrhage and avoidance of a closure device. Pulling the sheath in an actively anticoagulated patient in the absence of a complication may not be the wisest course of action, even if a FemoStop is applied.

23.13 Answer E. Appropriate use of all the closure devices relies on review of the femoral angiogram prior to use of a closure device. Each of the information for use instructions indicates that the device can be used for closure of access within the common femoral artery, of an appropriately sized vessel (4 to 6 mm depending on the device), and with the absence of significant atherosclerotic disease at the access site. This patient has evidence of severe atherosclerosis at the access site with a vessel diameter at the access site of only 2 mm. Thus, none of the currently available devices, including the extravascular closure devices, are approved for use in this patient.

23.14 Answer C. The patient's symptoms and findings are consistent with a pseudoaneurysm. The angiogram not only reveals a pseudoaneurysm (Fig. A23-14) but indicates that the access site was likely in the femoral bifurcation. A "low stick" is associated with an increase in the risk of both pseudoaneurysm and AVF. Moreover, there is no evidence that closure device use decreases this risk. Usually, ultrasound imaging of the access site can help make the diagnosis. Thrombin injection can be performed at the same time if technically feasible.

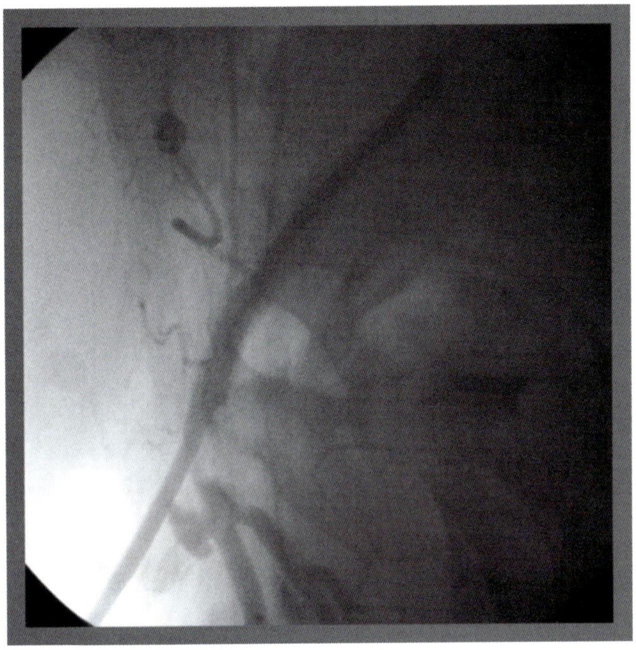

Figure A23-14

23.15 Answer A. She has acute femoral artery thrombosis. There is an approximately 1% to 2% risk of major complication from vascular closure device. Acute femoral artery thrombosis requires urgent intervention (Koreny M, et al. *JAMA* 2004;291(3):350–357).

23.16 Answer C. This patient has developed a retroperitoneal hemorrhage with extravasation of contrast from the access site in the external iliac artery. Closure devices have been associated with a higher rate of retroperitoneal bleeding in cases of "high sticks" and are not recommended for use in this situation. Manual compression is unlikely to achieve hemostasis this deep into the pelvis, and pulling the sheath may exacerbate the situation. Given the compression of the bladder, this patient has an active retroperitoneal bleed and needs to be urgently treated with endovascular rescue using contralateral access to tamponade the bleeding and potentially place a covered stent or taken for urgent surgery.

23.17 Answer A. A hematoma is associated with a groin mass, but there should not be an audible bruit. Patients with preexisting atherosclerotic disease may have a preexisting bruit, which decreases the specificity of these combined physical examination findings. A pseudoaneurysm can be diagnosed on physical examination by pulsatile mass and audible bruit. Many are asymptomatic. A groin mass associated with a bruit should prompt imaging of the groin with ultrasound to investigate whether a pseudoaneurysm is present and to guide management.

23.18 Answer A. Angio-Seal is comprised of a polylactic-glycolic acid anchor, bioresorbable collagen suture, and bovine collagen extravascular sponge. Although patients with a beef allergy may experience a mild inflammatory reaction to the collagen in Angio-Seal, this device can be used safely in patients with latex allergy.

23.19 Answer E. While each of the devices listed have been used in access sites outside of the common femoral artery, none of these devices are approved for use in this location. This would be considered an "off-label" use of a closure device and should be monitored closely at each institution until definitive studies confirm the safety of this strategy.

23.20 Answer E. All of the closure devices listed have been reported to be associated with acute vessel closure at the time of device deployment. Fortunately, the incidence of this potentially devastating complication has decreased dramatically since the introduction of closure devices in 1994, occurring in <0.1% of cases in most series.

24 Management of Intraprocedural and Postprocedural Complications

Saurav Chatterjee

QUESTIONS

24.1 A 72-year-old man with a prior history of coronary artery bypass grafting (CABG) and known low ejection fraction (EF) of 30% was admitted with mild atypical chest pain and dyspnea at rest. He was diuresed overnight and referred for a diagnostic angiogram. However, while being prepped on the table, he started feeling short of breath, and his oxygen saturation dropped to 90%. The saturation improved to 95% with 3-L/min supplemental oxygen. What should be done next?

(A) Proceed with the diagnostic left heart catheterization
(B) Cancel the procedure
(C) Get an echocardiogram
(D) Perform a right heart catheterization
(E) Increase supplemental oxygen to 5 L/min

24.2 A 38-year-old previously healthy woman presents to the emergency room with severe chest pain and an electrocardiogram (ECG) showing ST-segment elevation. An emergent coronary angiogram was performed and revealed moderate diffuse stenosis in the left anterior descending (LAD) artery and thrombolysis in myocardial infarction (TIMI) III flow with no significant coronary artery disease (CAD) noted in the other epicardial coronary arteries. Intravascular ultrasound (IVUS) of the LAD was performed (Fig. Q24-2). What is the diagnosis based on Figure Q24-2?

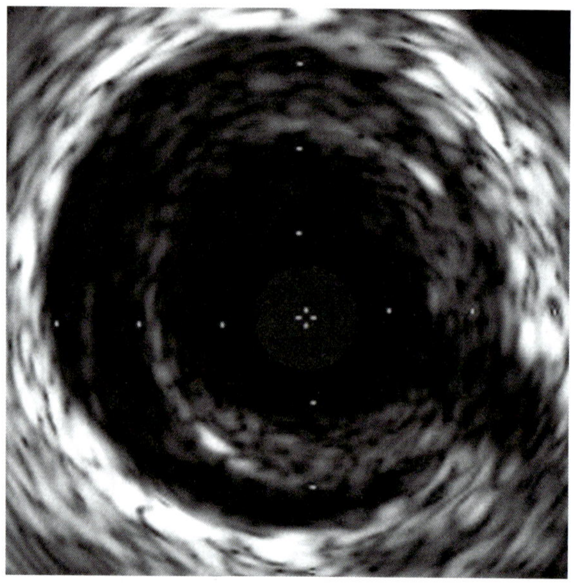

Figure Q24-2

(A) Pericarditis
(B) Plaque rupture leading to ST-segment elevation myocardial infarction (STEMI)
(C) Coronary artery dissection
(D) Moderate nonobstructive CAD

24.3 A 65-year-old male with a mildly positive stress test presents for a cardiac catheterization. During preprocedural workup, the patient mentions a history of generalized swelling after contrast administration during a computed tomography (CT) scan a few years prior, which required medications for treatment and overnight hospital stay. What should be done?

(A) Proceed with the catheterization; chances of a repeat reaction are low
(B) Reschedule the patient after prescribing premedication to be taken before procedure
(C) Administer intravenous (IV) diphenhydramine and proceed
(D) Administer steroids orally, and wait for an hour before proceeding

24.4 An 86-year-old patient with hypertension, diabetes mellitus, hyperlipidemia, chronic renal insufficiency, and previous CABG in 2000 with saphenous vein graft (SVG) to the LAD, SVG to the posterior descending artery (PDA), and SVG to the left circumflex (LCx) presents to your office with 4 weeks of exertional chest pain. He undergoes stress thallium, which shows left ventricular (LV) dilatation and possible anterior ischemia. His EF is 55% on the stress test.

He is taken to catheterization laboratory. His native arteries are occluded, and his SVG to PDA and SVG to LCx are also occluded. His SVG to LAD has severe 95% hazy lesion. SVG to LAD provides collateral flow to the right coronary artery (RCA), as well as to the LCx. He is evaluated by the surgeons and turned down for surgery. You decide to proceed with percutaneous coronary intervention (PCI) to SVG to LAD. Given the high-risk nature of his lesions, you decide to use the device that is shown in Figure Q24-4. How much blood is pumped from the LV to the aorta by the system above?

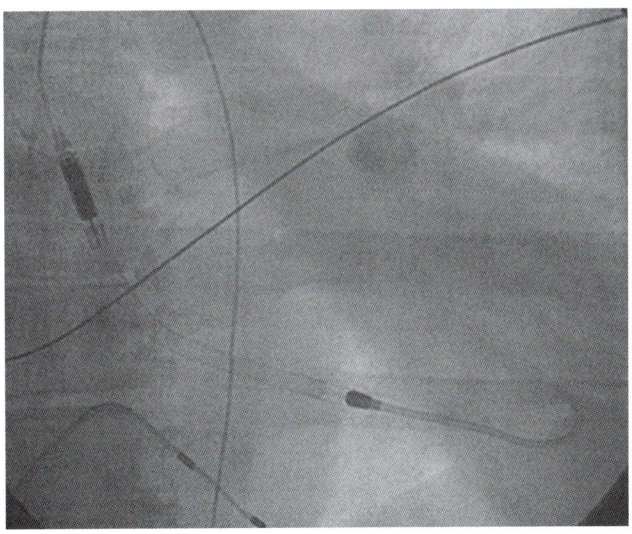

Figure Q24-4

(A) 2.0 L/min
(B) 2.5 L/min
(C) 3.0 L/min
(D) 3.5 L/min

24.5 During the above procedure of the SVG to LAD, the patient has no reflow, and he goes into ventricular fibrillation and cardiac arrest. He is resuscitated with defibrillation. Then, after repeated pharmacologic intervention, his SVG to LAD has TIMI 2 flow, and he is taken to the intensive care unit, intubated, and on two pressors. He recovers after several days, and his EF is now 15% to 20%. He and his family are upset that this happened and are threatening legal recourse. They claim that it was the device that made him have complications. Based on trial data, what is known about the device in Figure Q24-4?

(A) There has not been a study of nonemergent high-risk PCI patients using the Impella device
(B) There was a study of nonemergent high-risk PCI patients using Impella, and it showed significant reduction of major adverse cardiac events (MACE) with the Impella device
(C) There was a study of nonemergent high-risk PCI patients using Impella, and it showed higher risk of complications and MACE with the Impella device
(D) There was a study of nonemergent high-risk PCI patients using Impella, and there was no difference between intra-aortic balloon pump (IABP) and Impella

24.6 For the same patient, his Impella flow just prior to his clinical decompensation fell to 1.0 L/min. The following waveform was seen on the controller screen. What was the most likely reason for the reduction in flow (Fig. Q24-6)?

(A) Aortic placement of the cannula
(B) Ventricular placement of the cannula
(C) Pump thrombosis
(D) Electrical malfunction

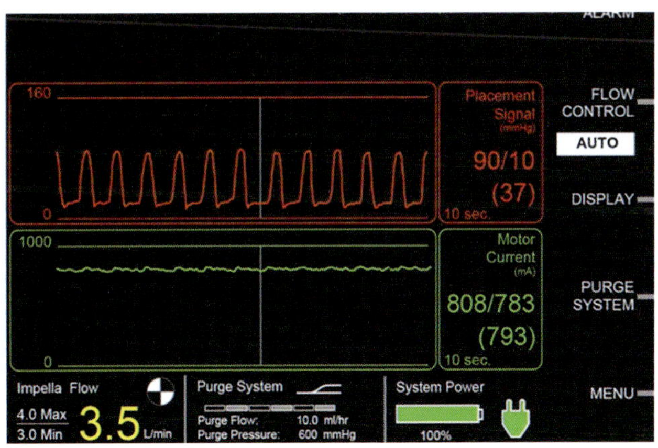

Figure Q24-6 (Courtesy of Saurav Chatterjee.)

24.7 During the selective cannulation of the left main coronary ostium, the blood pressure (BP) waveform, as seen in Figure Q24-7, was recorded. Which of the following is the most likely explanation for the waveform?

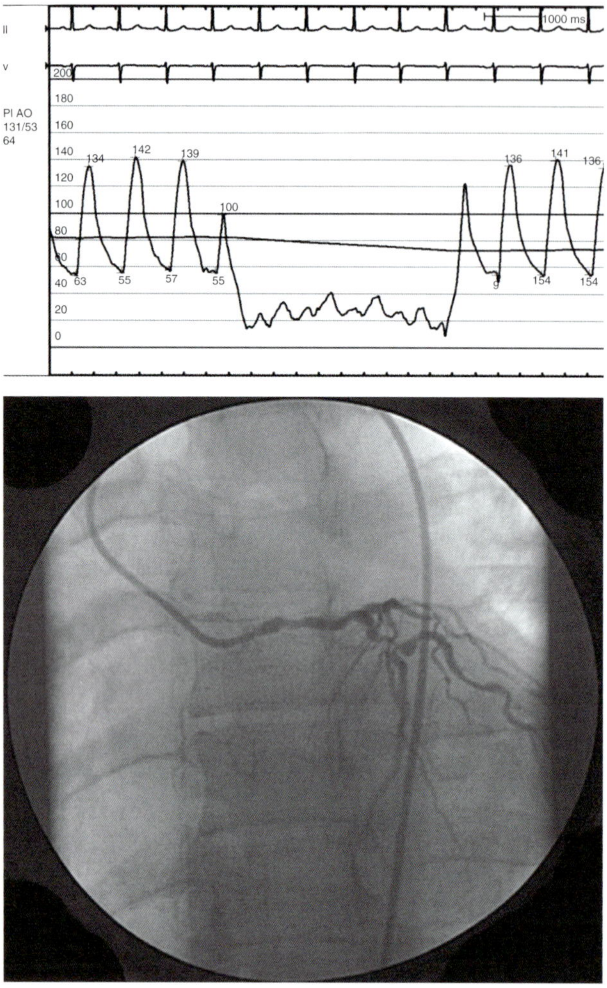

Figure Q24-7

(A) The pressure waveform indicates that the catheter tip prolapsed into the LV
(B) The pressure transducer contains air
(C) There is catheter kink
(D) The catheter is up against the vessel wall
(E) The catheter is engaged into a diseased left main artery

24.8 A 67-year-old retired lawyer with diabetes mellitus, hyperlipidemia, and hypertension presents to you for a second opinion. He underwent cardiac catheterization for increasing exertional chest pain and was found to have a chronically occluded moderate-size RCA, 50% LAD stenosis, and a mild LCx lesion. He underwent PCI to RCA and had 2.5 × 28-mm, 2.5 × 33-mm, and 2.25 × 28-mm bare metal stents (BMS) placed. Drug-eluting stents (DES) were not used because of the patient's history of gastric ulcers. Immediately after the intervention, the patient started complaining of chest pain and had inferior ST elevation. He underwent immediate catheterization and was found to have an occluded RCA. However, the artery could not be successfully opened. In the stent era, all factors have been correlated with abrupt vessel closure, EXCEPT:

(A) Stent length
(B) Small vessel diameter
(C) Poor distal runoff
(D) Excessive tortuosity
(E) Unstable angina

24.9 A 51-year-old woman presents to you for elective PCI to the LCx for exertional chest pain. Her creatinine is 1.4 and her glomerular filtration rate (GFR) is 45 mL/min/1.73 m^2. What intervention is most likely to reduce her risk of contrast-induced nephropathy?

(A) Sodium bicarbonate
(B) *N*-acetylcysteine
(C) Iso-osmolar contrast media
(D) IV saline started before procedure and continued 12 hours post
(E) Fenoldopam

24.10 A 45-year-old obese, female patient with diabetes who was hypercholesterolemic, hypertensive, and a heavy (two-packs-a-day) smoker with NSTEMI is referred for elective PCI of the LAD. She is planned for radial access PCI. Which anticoagulation regimen would minimize her risk of bleeding complications?

(A) Unfractionated heparin (UFH)
(B) Bivalirudin
(C) Low molecular weight heparin (LMWH)
(D) Fondaparinux
(E) None of the above

24.11 A 75-year-old patient traveled 4 hours by car to get to the hospital for a 7 AM first case, elective, complex, multilesion, multivessel coronary intervention. Although the angioplasty procedure was difficult to perform because of lack of adequate guide support, finally after trying several guide catheters, an Amplatz no. 3 guide catheter was found to give a good guide support to deliver three long Taxus stents. At the end of the procedure, the operator informed the patient that he was successful in opening all the blockages. The catheterization laboratory staff moved the patient to the recovery room. The patient was asymptomatic without any complaint and had normal vital signs. Later, the recovery room registered nurse (RN) noticed that the patient became progressively lethargic and less responsive. The physician in charge was notified. After obtaining the vital signs, which were noted to be unchanged, the most appropriate action at this time should be:

(A) Have the RN check the patient's ECG and his vital signs again
(B) Give the patient naloxone (Narcan)
(C) Perform a screening neurologic examination or obtain an urgent neurology consult

(D) Check the patient's complete blood count (CBC), blood sugar, blood urea nitrogen, and creatinine level

24.12 The patient mentioned in the preceding text recovers and is discharged without any residual deficits. He has filed a formal complaint against you to the hospital. The chief of staff's office would like to know about periprocedural stroke during coronary interventions. Which of the following statements is correct?

(A) Periprocedural stroke occurs approximately 0.5%
(B) Patients who suffer a stroke have an increased in-hospital mortality of 37%
(C) Patients who suffer a stroke have an increased 1-year mortality of 56%
(D) It is mostly embolic and not hemorrhagic stroke
(E) All of the above

24.13 You are asked to examine a 65-year-old heavy smoker with a strong family history of CAD and history of multivessel PCI with left-sided stroke for cardiology evaluation. His past medical history is notable for PCI to a heavily calcified ostial LAD and mid-LCx 8 months ago. Recently, he has been under treatment for methicillin-resistant *Staphylococcus aureus* bacteremia following a right below-knee amputation for gangrene. At baseline, he has an abnormal ECG with nonspecific ST changes in the precordial leads. The two-dimensional (2D) echocardiogram demonstrated moderate aortic insufficiency with multiple large vegetations on the aortic valve. He is examined by the cardiothoracic surgeons who would like to operate on him. They would like to visualize his coronary anatomy first and then ask for your opinion. The most appropriate action at this time is:

(A) Because of high risk of embolization with left heart catheterization, he should undergo cardiac CT to assess patency of ostial LAD and mid-LCx stents
(B) Send the patient for emergency heart surgery without cardiac angiogram
(C) Perform left-sided cardiac catheterization to visualize coronary anatomy
(D) Transfer the patient to the neurointensive care unit for stroke management and treat endocarditis medically

24.14 A 75-year-old morbidly obese patient (378 lb, 5 ft 5 in. tall) is referred from an outside hospital for angioplasty and stenting of a large proximal dominant RCA lesion. She has an infected skin lesion in the right groin beneath a large abdominal pannus. The operator decides to cannulate the left groin instead, and after multiple sticks, he is finally able to cannulate the left leg artery and to place a 7-Fr arterial introducer. The angioplasty procedure is successful using a 3.5 × 33-mm Cypher stent to the RCA with heparin and the glycoprotein (GP) IIb/IIIa inhibitor eptifibatide (Integrilin). Following the angioplasty procedure, all equipment is removed from the patient's heart. At the end of the procedure, the activated clotting time (ACT) is measured at 287 seconds. The operator decides to close the left groin artery entry site with an 8-Fr Angio-Seal device. Before doing so, he performs a peripheral angiogram using the introducing sheath to inject dye. The angiogram shows that the introducer was placed in the proximal profunda femoris artery too close to its bifurcation. The operator elects to place the Fem Stop instead. The Fem Stop is successfully applied and the patient is moved to the recovery room. In the recovery room, the RN notices that the patient's BP has dropped from 130/90 to 96/70, and her pulse has increased from 68 to 78 beats per minute (bpm). The physician is notified, and he orders an increase in IV fluids to 200 mL/h for 1 hour. The patient's BP normalizes, but an hour later, it drops again. This time, it measures 90/68, with a pulse of 90 bpm. Soon after that, the patient starts to complain that the Fem Stop causes her to have left groin pain. The physician comes and adjusts the Fem Stop. He examines the groin and it appears normal. The IV fluids are increased and the systolic BP returns to 102/70 mm Hg. After a while, the patient again starts complaining of being uncomfortable in bed with the Fem Stop compressing her groin, and she becomes diaphoretic, her BP drops to 75/50, and her heart rate (HR) slows down to 45 bpm. The physician is notified. The most appropriate initial response at this time should be:

(A) Loosen or reposition the Fem Stop, and give the patient a pain medication with sedation for comfort
(B) Send the patient for CT scan
(C) Send the patient to vascular laboratory for ultrasound
(D) Order patient's CBC, and type and cross
(E) Remove Fem Stop and apply direct manual pressure on the artery entry site
(F) Continue rapid fluid infusion to expand the volume
(G) Stop GP IIb/IIIa inhibitors
(H) Consult a vascular surgeon to consider surgery
(I) A, B, and C are correct
(J) D, E, F, and G are correct
(K) A–H are correct

24.15 The patient mentioned in the preceding text does well with manual pressure and goes upstairs to the telemetry floor. In 3 hours, you are called to see the patient because she has developed pulselessness, pain, pallor, and paresthesia of her left leg. What is the best way to treat this patient at this time?

(A) Start IV heparin and careful clinical monitoring
(B) Start IV heparin, GP IIb/IIIa inhibitor, and careful monitoring
(C) IV fibrinolytic therapy
(D) Urgent peripheral vascular surgery consultation or urgent percutaneous peripheral vascular intervention

24.16 Complication of groin hematoma may lead to sensory or motor neurologic deficit by compressing the surrounding nerves. Which nerves are most commonly affected by groin hematoma?

(A) Femoral and sciatic nerves
(B) Sciatic, femoral, and lateral cutaneous nerves
(C) Femoral and lateral cutaneous nerves

24.17 The most common cause of procedurally related retroperitoneal (RP) hematoma includes:

(A) Spontaneous RP venous bleeding triggered by aggressive anticoagulant therapy
(B) Arterial bleed caused by a back wall puncture of the femoral artery distal to the origin of the superficial iliac artery circumflex
(C) Arterial bleeding caused by a back wall puncture of the femoral artery proximal to the origin of the deep iliac artery circumflex

24.18 A 54-year-old woman is transferred to the medical center from an outside hospital for an elective angioplasty of an RCA artery lesion. Three days before admission, the patient suffered an acute inferior wall MI, which was successfully treated with IV tissue plasminogen activator (tPA). On the day of the procedure, the patient was asymptomatic, but she was quite anxious about the upcoming coronary angioplasty. The 80% lesion in the proximal RCA was opened with a 3.5 × 23-mm stent. The final angiogram showed a widely patent RCA, normal left coronary system, and EF of 50% with moderate inferior wall hypokinesia. The right groin entry site was successfully closed with a Perclose device after angiogram was taken (Fig. Q24-18).

The patient was transferred to the recovery unit, and within 45 minutes, she began to complain of right groin and right flank pain, which improved when she adjusted her position. Thirty minutes later, her BP and pulse, which previously read 130/70 and 70, respectively, measured 100/60 and 80. Fluids were administered, and her BP improved, but she continued to complain about the right lower abdominal quadrant pain. The physician was called. He examined the groin and found no evidence of bleeding and hematoma.

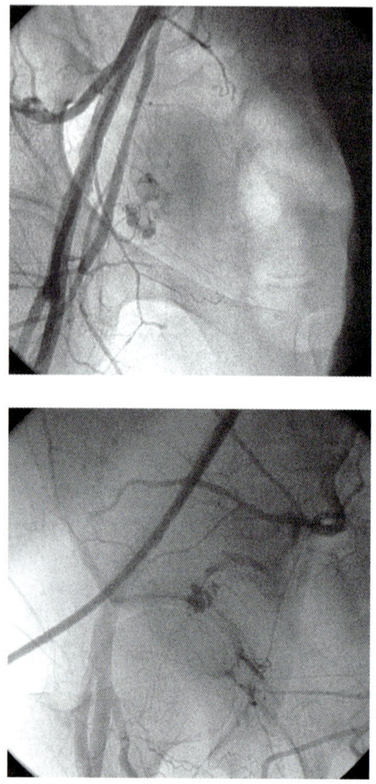

Figure Q24-18

Bowel sounds were weak but present. He reassured the patient and returned to the catheterization laboratory. Fifteen minutes later, her BP dropped again to 76 mm Hg with a pulse of 60 bpm. The patient became slightly diaphoretic and restless, complaining of increasing abdominal discomfort. Soon thereafter, her BP dropped to 60/40, HR was 45 bpm, and the patient began to retch but could not vomit. The most likely diagnostic explanation of this patient's problem is:

(A) The patient is allergic to IV pyelogram dye
(B) The patient has femoral artery dissection
(C) The patient has spontaneous RP bleed
(D) The patient has adverse reaction to midazolam (Versed) and fentanyl
(E) The patient has arterial external iliac artery perforation with RP dye extravasation

24.19 The best treatment for a patient who, during the PCI, suffers an accidental large right iliac artery laceration is:

(A) Aggressive fluid and blood replacement therapy
(B) Emergency consultation from vascular surgery
(C) Immediate percutaneous intervention using contralateral approach to block bleeding from the iliac artery by inflating properly sized angioplasty balloon followed by placing a covered stent to seal the vessel wall
(D) Manual pressure

24.20 Match each of the following figures to a diagnosis (Fig. Q24-20[1–6]):

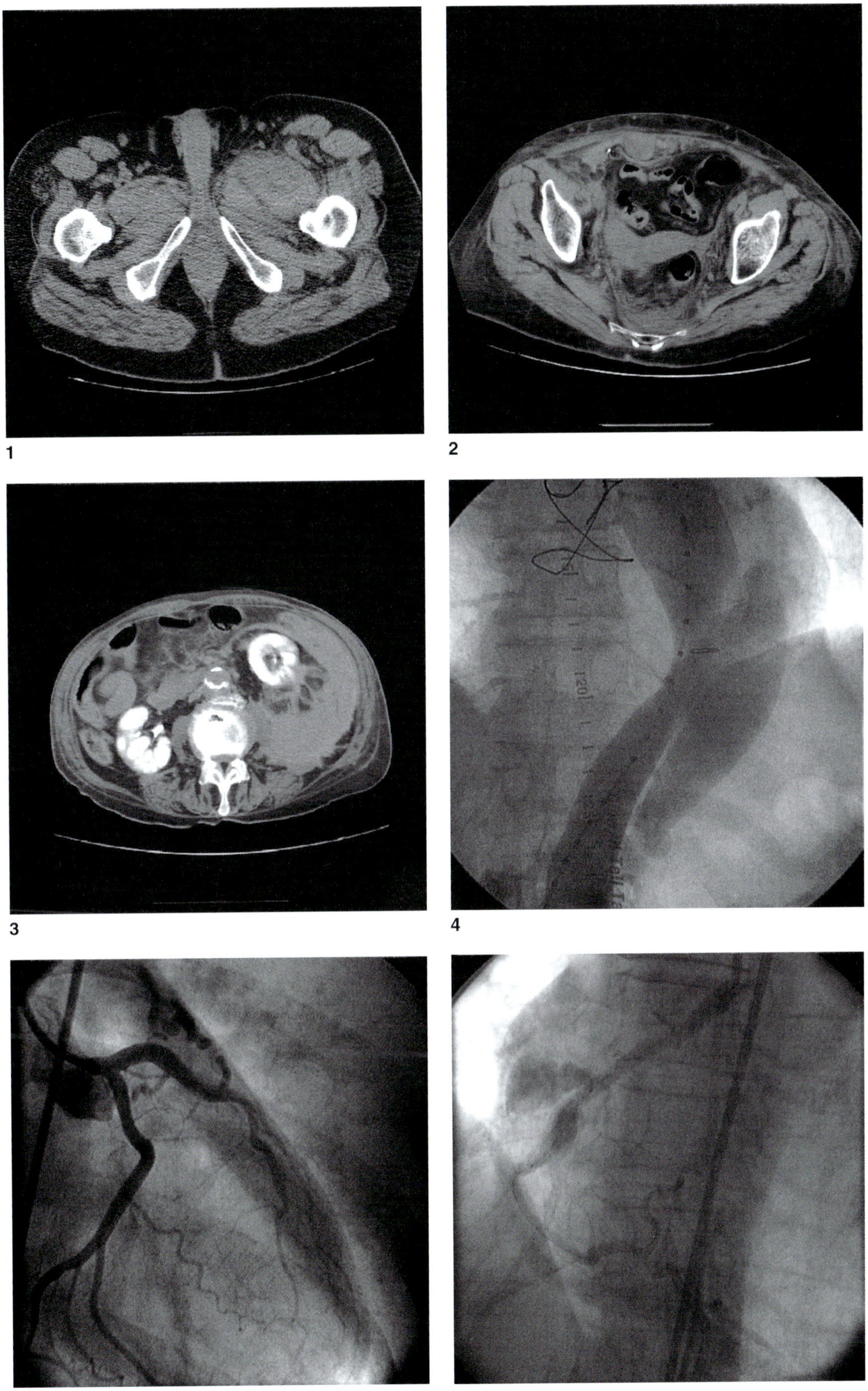

Figure Q24-20

(A) RP hematoma
(B) Thigh hematoma
(C) Rectus muscle hematoma
(D) Aortic dissection
(E) Coronary atrioventricular (AV) malformation
(F) Coronary perforation

24.21 A 63-year-old morbidly obese woman presents to your office for follow-up. She underwent successful PCI to the RCA, which was complicated by the development of a femoral artery pseudoaneurysm. On initial duplex, it measured 2.5 cm. It was treated with ultrasound-guided thrombin injection. She underwent a repeat duplex study 2 months later, and the pseudoaneurysm remains unchanged. She is asymptomatic. What are the appropriate management at this time?

(A) Ultrasound-guided compression of the neck of the pseudoaneurysm
(B) Injection of the cavity of the pseudoaneurysm with procoagulant or embolization coils
(C) Surgery
(D) Conservative management with good BP control and repeat ultrasound in 2 months

24.22 The angiogram in Figure Q24-22 demonstrates which of the following abnormalities?

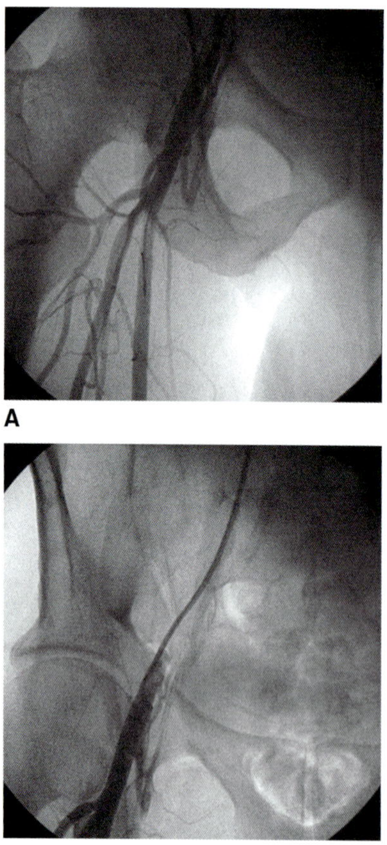

A

B

Figure Q24-22

(A) Iliac artery lesion
(B) Femoral artery dissection
(C) Postprocedural AV fistula
(D) Right groin mass
(E) Congenital AV malformation

24.23 A 75-year-old woman with hypertension and hyperlipidemia was admitted to an outside hospital for an anterior wall MI 4 days ago. She was given thrombolytic therapy and was doing well until this morning when she developed shortness of breath. She has been transferred to your hospital, and a diagnostic angiogram was performed via radial access. The coronary angiogram showed TIMI 3 flow in the LAD with an 85% proximal lesion and residual thrombus. An LV angiogram was performed with a Tiger catheter, and the interventionist missed a pressure dampening prior to the LV injection (Fig. Q24-23). The best course of action for the patient is to have:

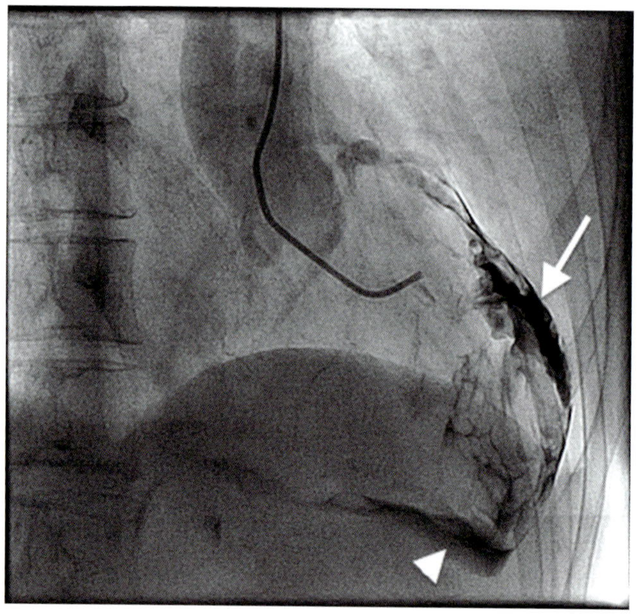

Figure Q24-23 (With permission from Frizzell JD, et al. *JACC Cardiovasc Interv* 2014;7(12):1456–1457.)

(A) Percutaneous transluminal coronary angioplasty (PTCA) plus stent of the residual LAD lesion
(B) Intracoronary thrombolysis, followed by PTCA plus stent of the LAD lesion
(C) AngioJet procedure, followed by PTCA plus stent of the LAD lesion
(D) Immediate Doppler echocardiogram and heart surgery

24.24 The incidence of coronary perforation during coronary intervention is low. These preprocedural and postprocedural angiograms (Fig. Q24-24) demonstrate:

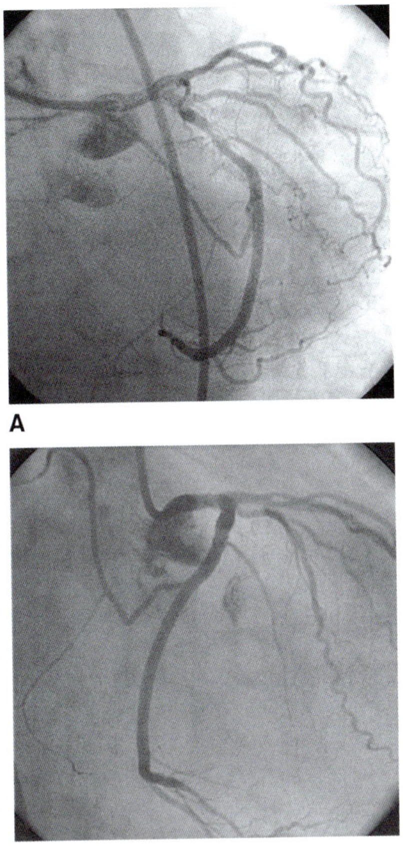

A

B

Figure Q24-24

(A) Type I coronary perforation
(B) Type II coronary perforation
(C) Type III coronary perforation

24.25 Which of the following options is NOT a correct choice to treat coronary perforation?

(A) Prolonged inflation of the balloon across the perforation
(B) Reverse anticoagulation, giving protamine 1 mg IV for each 100 units of heparin
(C) Reverse anticoagulation, giving protamine 0.1 mg SC for each 1,000 units of heparin
(D) Use of covered stent
(E) Use of coils to embolize leaking branch
(F) Pericardiocentesis

24.26 If a severe reaction to dye occurs, with which of the initial concentrations of IV epinephrine can hypotension be reversed before it is diluted further?

(A) 1 mL of 1:1,000 epinephrine
(B) 1 mL of 1:100,000 epinephrine
(C) 1 mL of 1:10,000 epinephrine

24.27 A 68-year-old man with history of CABG 10 years ago presents with chest pain. He is noted to have nonspecific ST changes, but his initial troponin is 2.0 ng/mL. He is brought to the cardiac catheterization laboratory. His angiograms are presented in Figure Q24-27. He undergoes PCI to a diseased SVG with an embolic protection device. During the procedure after stent deployment, he has severe chest pain with ST elevation. An angiogram at that time is shown. What would you do next?

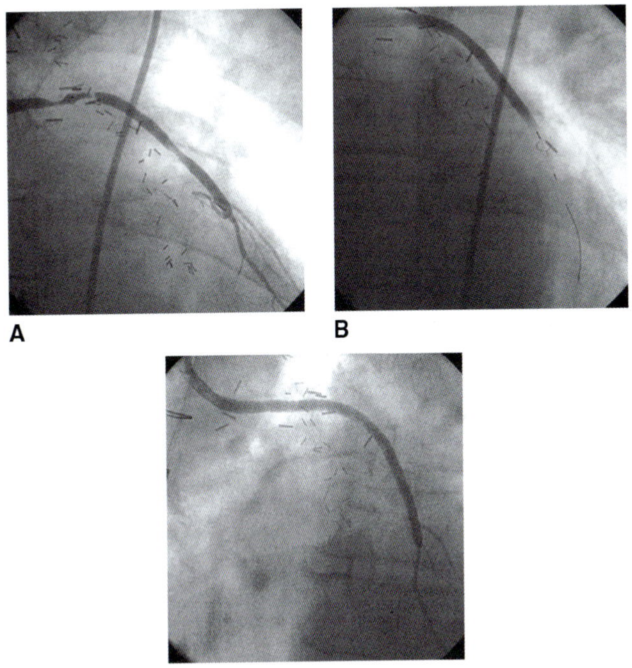

A B C

Figure Q24-27

(A) Capture and remove the filter device because it did not adequately capture the debris
(B) Capture and remove the filter device because it is full of debris
(C) Give intracoronary nitroglycerin (IC NTG)
(D) IVUS of the stent site because there might be a dissection

24.28 Which is not a treatment of no-reflow during SVG PCI?

(A) Adenosine
(B) Nitroprusside
(C) Streptokinase
(D) Verapamil

24.29 A 90-year-old male with multiple comorbidities and severe symptomatic aortic stenosis underwent transcatheter aortic valve replacement (TAVR).

Post valve deployment, the patient had desaturation and was found to have pulmonary edema on chest x-ray. A TTE revealed the following image (Fig. Q24-29). What has this complication been associated with?

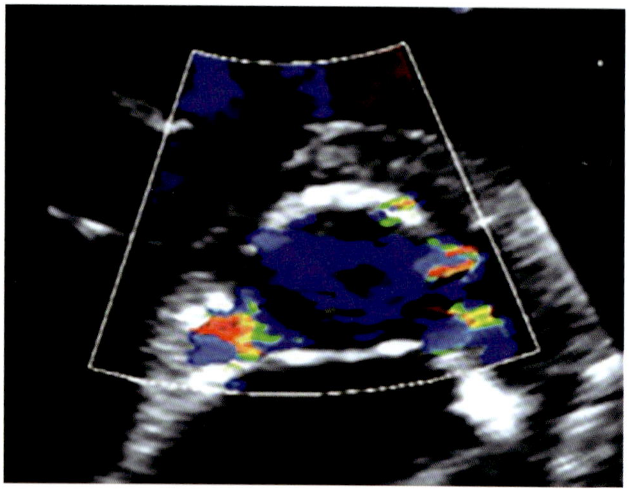
Figure Q24-29 (Courtesy of Saurav Chatterjee.)

(A) Mortality
(B) Heart failure
(C) Anemia
(D) Endocarditis
(E) All of the above

24.30 A 51-year-old man with chronic lung disease comes to your emergency room with severe chest pain for 2 hours. His past medical history is unremarkable except for hyperlipidemia. He is found to have ST elevation in the anterior leads and is taken to the catheterization laboratory, where he undergoes successful PCI to the mid/distal LAD with a 3.0 × 28 DES, heparin, and abciximab (ReoPro). His EF is 50%. He does well and is transferred to the cardiac care unit. Two hours later, he becomes very short of breath and hypoxemic. He has hemoptysis, goes into respiratory distress, and is intubated. His chest x-ray shows alveolar infiltrates. What is the most likely cause of his shortness of breath?

(A) Pulmonary hemorrhage
(B) Congestive heart failure
(C) LV rupture
(D) Papillary muscle rupture
(E) Aortic dissection

ANSWERS AND EXPLANATIONS

24.1 Answer D. Performing a right heart catheterization, while not routine in contemporary practice, may provide important insights especially where there may be concern for impending pulmonary edema with administration of contrast or keeping the patient supine on the procedure table. A pulmonary capillary wedge pressure (PCWP) >25 mm Hg and a systolic blood pressure <100 mm Hg may be used to decide to defer a diagnostic catheterization. If the catheterization is considered imperative, then improving hemodynamics with IV diuretics, supplemental oxygen, and arterial vasodilator like NTG should be considered. A cardiac index <2.2 before an intervention may lead the operator to decide on using hemodynamic support.

24.2 Answer C. IVUS shows a dissection of the LAD. This was a spiral dissection that started in the proximal LAD and extended down to the distal portion.

24.3 Answer B. Premedication is recommended in patients with prior severe reaction to contrast (this patient had angioedema). A commonly used protocol is to administer prednisone 50 mg orally 13, 7, and 1 hour prior to contrast administration, diphenhydramine 50 mg IV or oral 1 hour before contrast use, and famotidine 40 mg before starting the procedure.

24.4 Answer B. The figure is that of an Impella device that is placed across the aortic valve through a femoral artery site to pump blood from the LV into the ascending aorta at 2.5 L/min. The newer Impella CP can generate up to 3.5 to 4 L/min of flow, and the surgically implantable Impella 5.0 can provide 5.0 L/min.

24.5 Answer D. PROTECT II was a randomized, multicenter trial comparing the Impella system with an IABP in patients undergoing nonemergent high-risk PCIs. The primary end points were the composite rate of 10 major adverse events, including death, MI, stroke, or repeat revascularization within 20 to 40 days after the procedure; secondary end points were maximum chronic left ventricular pressure overload (CPO) decrease from baseline and the rate of in-hospital major events between the Impella and IABP. The company stopped the trial after the data safety, and monitoring committee reviewed partial trial data because they felt that the study could not reach the primary end point. The available data showed no difference between IABP and Impella.

24.6 Answer B. The tracing shows ventricularization of the pressure tracing, which is consistent with ventricular position of the cannula (too far in). The controller screen usually provides a warning: "Impella position in the ventricle." Aortic placement can be determined with an arterial tracing. Pump thrombosis usually does not happen frequently as the purge fluid contains heparin. Electrical malfunction is rare.

24.7 Answer E. There is an ostial left main coronary trunk stenosis with no reflux of dye.

24.8 Answer D. In the stent era, unstable angina, bailout stenting, small-vessel diameter, long lesions, large plaque volume, residual uncovered dissection, slow flow or poor distal runoff, and suboptimal final procedural lumen have all been associated with abrupt vessel closure. Excessive tortuosity is a risk factor for abrupt vessel closure during balloon angioplasty but not stent thrombosis.

24.9 Answer D. IV saline hydration is the only validated measure shown in trials to reduce the risk of contrast-induced nephropathy. In this regard, 0.9% saline has been proven to be superior to 0.45% saline.

24.10 Answer E. The recent MATRIX trial has shown that the bleeding reduction advantage of bivalirudin over other anticoagulants is mitigated with the use of radial access route (Valgimigli M, et al. *N Engl J Med* 2015;373(11):997-1009).

24.11 Answer C. Strokes are rare but devastating complications of cardiac interventions. The interventionalist should be familiar with potential etiologies, preventive strategies, and treatments for catheterization-related stroke and should develop the routine habit of speaking with the patient directly at the end of the procedure. If the patient is less alert, has slurred speech, or has visual, sensory, or motor symptoms, there should be a low threshold for performing a screening neurologic examination or obtaining an emergent stroke neurology consult. For most hemispheric events, an urgent carotid angiogram and neurovascular rescue should be considered (Sandoval AE, et al. *Cathet Cardiovasc Diagn* 1998;44(4):412–414).

24.12 Answer E. Stroke related to contemporary PCI is associated with substantial increased mortality. Patients who suffer procedural stroke tend to be older, have lower LVEF and more diabetes, and experience a higher rate of intraprocedural complications necessitating emergency use of IABP. The in-hospital mortality and 1-year mortality are substantially higher in patients with stroke (Fuchs S, et al. *Circulation* 2002;106(1):86–91).

24.13 Answer C. The question of central nervous system embolic risk arises when it is necessary to perform catheterization on a patient with endocarditis of left-sided (aortic or mitral) heart valves. Although echo appearance of these vegetations looks friable and they can embolize spontaneously, left heart catheterization can be done safely in these patients. In a series of 35 patients with active endocarditis who had left heart catheterization, none had catheterization-induced embolic events. Patency is difficult to visualize with heavily calcified arteries with cardiac CT (Welton DE, et al. *Am J Cardiol* 1979;44(7):1306–1310).

24.14 Answer J. Occult bleeding at the arterial entry site is the cause of this patient's hypotension. The patient needs to be stabilized first before being sent to CT scan or vascular laboratory (Farouque HM et al. *J Am Coll Cardiol* 2005;45(3):363–368).

24.15 Answer D. This patient has acute femoral artery thrombosis. This is an emergency case that needs immediate surgery or peripheral vascular intervention.

24.16 Answer C. Nerve complications following cardiac catheterization through the femoral route are rare. Although femoral nerve is most likely to be affected, lateral cutaneous nerve can also be affected (Butler R, et al. *Catheter Cardiovasc Interv* 2002;56(1):69–71).

24.17 Answer C. Arterial back wall puncture is the most common cause of RP hematoma (Witz M, et al. *Eur J Vasc Endovasc Surg* 1999;18(4):364–365).

24.18 Answer E. The angiogram shows external iliac artery perforation with dye extravasation.

24.19 Answer C. Bleeding from the lacerated iliac artery could be fatal within a matter of minutes without catheter-based control of large bleeding. Therefore, immediate contralateral access with going "up and over" the iliac bifurcation and balloon inflation to stop bleeding is essential. After achieving temporary hemostasis, a vascular surgeon may be consulted, but due to logistics and comparable outcomes, treatment with a covered stent is appropriate.

24.20 Answer. A-2, B-3, C-1, D-4, E-5, F-6.

24.21 Answer C. This aneurysm has been treated in the past and still persists after 2 months. Therefore, it should be operated (Kent KC, et al. *J Vasc Surg* 1993;17:125–131, discussion 131–133; Samal AK. *Catheter Cardiovasc Interv* 2001;53(2):259–263; and Taylor BS, et al. *J Vasc Surg* 1999;30(6):1052–1059).

24.22 Answer C. An AV fistula is noted in the figure. Small AV fistulas are often monitored with ultrasound imaging. Indications for intervention are lack of spontaneous closure, increase in fistula size, and/or the development of symptoms.

24.23 Answer D. The LV angiogram demonstrates impending LV rupture (high anterior wall) with dye staining the fistula track in the LV wall. Echocardiography showed moderate pericardial effusion. The patient had an emergency surgery.

24.24 Answer B. The angiographic appearance of coronary perforations could be classified as type I—extraluminal crater without extravasation, type II—pericardial and myocardial blush, and type III—dye extravasation (Ellis SG, et al. *Circulation* 1994;90(6):2725–2730).

24.25 Answer B. The current dose of protamine is 1 mg for each 100 units of heparin (Fejka M, et al. *Am J Cardiol* 2002;90(11):1183–1186).

24.26 Answer C. Epinephrine of 0.5 to 1.0 mL of 1:10,000 administered intravenously over several minutes should be considered. This may be repeated at intervals of 5 to 10 minutes, preferably with cardiac monitoring because adverse effects of IV epinephrine may occur. In the setting of profound hypotension, a continuous infusion of epinephrine (5 to 15 μg/min) titrated to effect may be administered. If IV access cannot be obtained immediately, epinephrine (3 to 5 mL of 1:10,000 dilution of epinephrine) can be delivered through the endotracheal tube.

24.27 **Answer B.** The filter device is full of debris. Although it is possible that distal embolization occurred, if there was good apposition of the filter to the vessel wall throughout the case, it is less likely. Therefore, at this point, you can wire with another wire and capture and remove the emboli filter device. After the removal of filter wire, the angiogram shown in the figure was taken.

24.28 **Answer C.** Common agents for treatment of no-reflow encountered during graft intervention and STEMI include adenosine, nitroprusside, verapamil, and often empirically GP IIb/IIIa receptor antagonists with prolonged infusion. Thrombolytics have no role in treatment of no-reflow.

24.29 **Answer E.** Paravalvular leak (PVL), especially of moderate to severe degree post TAVR, has been prognostic of adverse outcomes including mortality, heart failure, anemia, endocarditis, and poor valve hemodynamics.

24.30 **Answer A.** Pulmonary alveolar hemorrhage has been rarely reported during the use of abciximab. This can present with any or all of the following in close association with ReoPro administration: hypoxemia, alveolar infiltrates on chest x-ray, hemoptysis, or an unexplained drop in hemoglobin.

25 Qualitative and Quantitative Angiography

Sorin J. Brener

QUESTIONS

25.1 Characteristics of type non-C lesions, as defined by American College of Cardiology (ACC) and American Heart Association (AHA) criteria, include all the following, EXCEPT:

(A) Length > 20 mm
(B) Ostial location
(C) Moderate calcification
(D) Eccentric nature

25.2 The incidence of definite stent thrombosis of everolimus-eluting stents (EES) is:

(A) Similar to other drug-eluting stents (DES)
(B) Lower than all other DES and bare metal stents (BMS)
(C) Similar to other second-generation DES
(D) Higher than paclitaxel-eluting stents (PES)

25.3 Predictive factors for stent thrombosis include all the following, EXCEPT:

(A) Diabetes mellitus
(B) Chronic kidney disease (CKD)
(C) Reduced ejection fraction (EF)
(D) Stent placement in setting of acute coronary syndrome (ACS)

25.4 Which of the following cases is expected to have the highest complication rate?

(A) Coronary perforation type II
(B) Coronary perforation type I
(C) Coronary perforation type III
(D) Coronary aneurysm

25.5 Stent thrombosis that occurs between 6 and 12 hours after a procedure is defined as:

(A) Hyperacute
(B) Acute
(C) Late
(D) Subacute

25.6 The SYNTAX score evaluates the:

(A) Number of diseased vessels
(B) Volume of plaque
(C) Complexity and extent of coronary lesions
(D) Impact of comorbidities on outcome of revascularization

25.7 All of the following are limitations of the thrombolysis in myocardial infarction (TIMI) flow classification, EXCEPT:

(A) Good correlation with mortality for ST-segment elevation myocardial infarction (STEMI) patients
(B) Flow in reference artery(ies) may not be totally normal
(C) Categorical nature
(D) It does not evaluate myocardial perfusion

25.8 Which of the following describe the correct landmarks for TIMI frame count (TFC) assessment in the left anterior descending (LAD) and left circumflex (LCx) arteries, respectively?

(A) LAD—last septal perforator
(B) LAD—last diagonal branch
(C) LCx—the most distal bifurcation of the segment with the longest total distance that includes the culprit lesion for the LCx
(D) LCx—end of most distal obtuse marginal branch

25.9 Advantages of corrected TFC (CTFC) over TIMI flow grades include:

(A) Lower interobserver variability
(B) Continuous nature
(C) Relationship with clinical outcomes
(D) All of the above

25.10 Choose the combination of values associated with the lowest risk for mortality after STEMI (Table Q25-10):

Table Q25-10

	TIMI Flow Grade	TIMI Myocardial Perfusion Grade
A	3	2
B	2	2
C	3	3
D	3	0/1

TIMI, thrombolysis in myocardial infarction.

(A) A
(B) B
(C) C
(D) D

25.11 Which of the following can lead to erroneous quantitative coronary angiography evaluation of coronary stenoses?

(A) Analyzing systolic frames
(B) Analyzing end-diastolic frames
(C) Analyzing two orthogonal views
(D) None of the above

25.12 Late luminal loss after DES implantation:

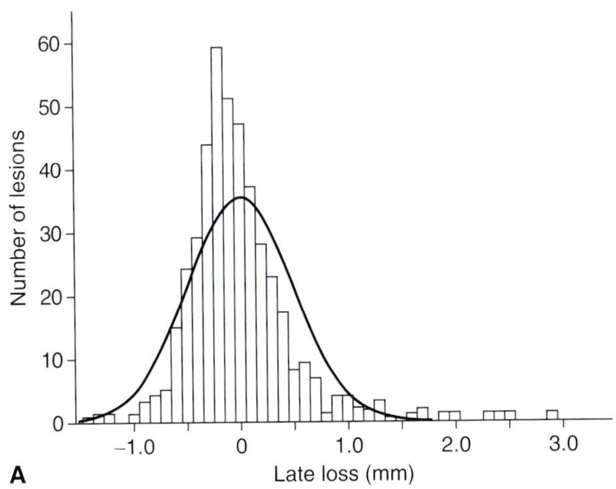

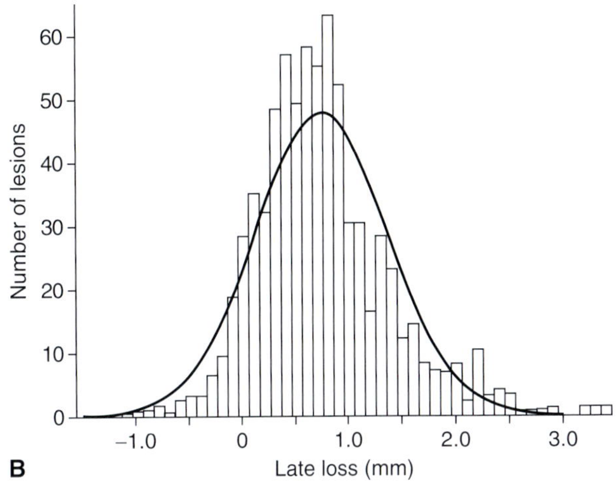

Figure Q25-12

(A) Is defined as the difference in minimal luminal diameter between postpercutaneous coronary intervention (PCI) and follow-up angiograms and shows the distribution depicted in Figure Q25-12A
(B) Does not differ from the distribution observed for BMS
(C) Is defined as the difference in luminal diameter between baseline and follow-up angiograms and shows the distribution depicted in Figure Q25-12B
(D) Is defined as the change in minimal luminal diameter that occurs immediately after PCI

25.13 Bioresorbable vascular scaffolds (BVS) are:

(A) Stronger than metallic stents
(B) Devices eluting sirolimus
(C) Thinner than EES
(D) Invisible on cine angiography except for the two edge markers

25.14 The TIMI myocardial perfusion (TMP) grade evaluates the quality of:

(A) Epicardial flow
(B) Myocardial flow
(C) Epicardial and myocardial flow
(D) Neither

25.15 Determination of the reference diameter in this right coronary artery (RCA) lesion (Fig. Q25-15) is best done at:

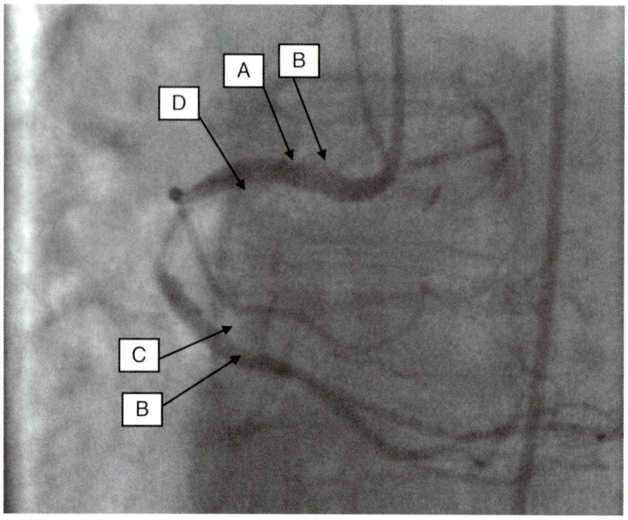

Figure Q25-15

(A) Point A (10 mm proximal to the lesion)
(B) Points B (two 10-mm segments without irregularities proximal and distal to the lesion)
(C) Point C (10 mm distal to the lesion)
(D) Point D (proximal shoulder of the lesion)

25.16 The residual SYNTAX score is defined as the:

(A) SYNTAX score after revascularization
(B) Difference between SYNTAX score before and after revascularization
(C) Addition of clinical parameters to the angiographic SYNTAX score
(D) Product of age × creatinine × EF

25.17 Compared with patients without progression of coronary artery disease (CAD), those who show angiographic progression by quantitative coronary analysis have:

(A) Smaller plaque volume at baseline intravascular ultrasound (IVUS) examination but significantly increased plaque volume over time
(B) Larger plaque volume at baseline IVUS examination without a significant increase in plaque volume over time
(C) Both greater plaque volume at baseline IVUS and significantly higher increases in plaque volume over time
(D) None of the above

25.18 The Medina classification of bifurcation lesions is based on the severity and location of the lesion in the proximal and distal segments of the parent vessel and the ostium of the side branch. Which of the bifurcations represented in Figure Q25-18A–D are "true bifurcation lesions"?

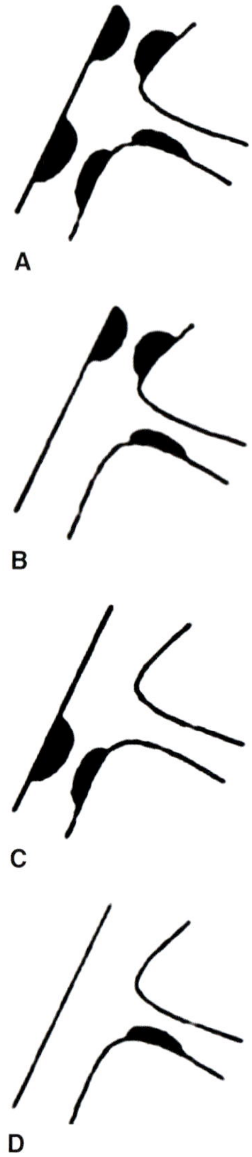

Figure Q25-18

(A) A
(B) C
(C) D
(D) A and B

25.19 Which of the following pair of values is typical of TFCs in noninfarct arteries after reperfusion and in arteries examined during elective angiography?

(A) 45 and 28
(B) 35 and 28
(C) 21 and 21
(D) 31 and 21

25.20 Intraprocedural stent thrombosis:

(A) Is defined as persistent vessel closure during PCI
(B) Is defined as transient or permanent thrombus formation during PCI
(C) Correlates with the occurrence of stent thrombosis and death after PCI
(D) Answers B and C

ANSWERS AND EXPLANATIONS

25.1 Answer A. The relation of lesion morphology to angioplasty outcome has been known for many years. The more complex the morphology, the less favorable the initial (and later) results of coronary angioplasty. Diffuse (>20 mm length), excessive tortuosity of proximal segment, extremely angulated segments (>90 degrees), total occlusion >3 months duration, inability to protect major side branches, and degenerated vein grafts with friable lesions are all characteristics of type C lesions (Ryan TJ, et al. *J Am Coll Cardiol* 1988;12(2):529-545; Myler RK, et al. *J Am Coll Cardiol* 1992;19(7):1641-1652).

25.2 Answer B. EES use a fluoropolymer to contain and elute everolimus. This polymer is thromboresistant (Liu TY, et al. *Polym Adv Technol* 2005;16(5):413-419). In a network meta-analysis of 49 randomized clinical trials including 50,844 patients, Palmerini et al. found that EES have the lowest rate of definite stent thrombosis at all time points compared to all other stents, including BMS (Palmerini T, et al. *Lancet* 2012;379(9824):1393-1402).

25.3 Answer C. An analysis of nearly 19,000 patients stented between 1998 and 2011 demonstrated that, using BMS as reference, first-generation DES, diabetes mellitus, current smoking, prior myocardial infarction (MI), presentation with STEMI, complex lesion morphology, and increasing residual stenosis were independently associated with higher rates of definite stent thrombosis up to 3 years from procedure (Tada T, et al. *JACC Cardiovasc Interv* 2013;6(12):1267-1274). Other analysis suggested additional factors, such as CKD, complex lesion morphology, and premature discontinuation of dual antiplatelet therapy (DAPT) (Park DW, et al. *Am J Cardiol* 2006;98(3):352-356).

25.4 Answer C. Coronary perforation during PCI occurs very infrequently. In contrast with type I (fully contained) and type II (limited extravasation) that rarely develop tamponade or result in ischemia, type III perforations (brisk extravasation) are associated with a high incidence of dramatic complications, including abrupt tamponade, need for urgent bypass surgery, and a high mortality (up to 19% in the original multicenter report that evaluated this complication) (Ellis SG, et al. *Circulation* 1994;90(6):2725-2730).

25.5 Answer B. The Academic Research Consortium recommends temporal categories of acute stent thrombosis (0 to 24 hours after implantation), subacute stent thrombosis (>24 hours to 30 days after implantation), late stent thrombosis (31 days to 1 year), and very late (>1 year) stent thrombosis. The purpose of this classification is to create consensus definitions for DES study end points to distinguish likely differences in the contribution of the various pathophysiologic processes during each of these intervals. Acute or subacute (0 to 30 days) is frequently replaced by the term early stent thrombosis in numerous clinical trials (Cutlip DE, et al. *Circulation* 2007;115(17):2344-2351).

25.6 Answer C. The SYNTAX score is an angiographic score that quantifies the extent and complexity of coronary lesions based on location, lesion length, presence of thrombus, total occlusion or calcification, presence of branches, and tortuosity. It assists in selecting the method of revascularization and correlates with outcome, particularly for PCI-treated patients (Serruys PW, et al. *N Engl J Med* 2009;360(10):961-972). Patients with scores of ≤32 tend to do as well with PCI as with coronary bypass surgery, while those with high scores are better served by surgery.

25.7 Answer A. Almost two decades ago, the GUSTO trial demonstrated that the more rapid the restoration of flow through the infarct-related artery, the better the preservation of left ventricular systolic function and the survival (GUSTO Angiographic Investigators. *N Engl J Med* 1993;329(22):1615-1622). Using the CTFC, in which the number of frames required for contrast material to reach standardized distal landmarks is counted, the TIMI group investigators demonstrated that acute MI slows flow not only in the culprit artery but also in the nonculprit ones by up to 45%. Although it improved postpercutaneous transluminal coronary angioplasty (PTCA), both culprit and nonculprit artery flows were still 45% slower than normal (Gibson CM, et al. *J Am Coll Cardiol* 1999;34(4):974-982). The categorical, rather than continuous, nature of the TIMI flow classification clearly limits its statistical power in clinical trials. The TMP grade is used to characterize the filling and clearance of the microcirculation, serving as an index of myocardial reperfusion (Gibson CM, et al. *Circulation* 2000;101(2):125–130).

25.8 Answer C. Two of the limitations of the TIMI flow grade are its subjective and categorical nature. The TFC was created to overcome those deficiencies and standardize the assessment of coronary flow. It consists of a simple, continuous measure of coronary flow in which the number of cine frames required for contrast material to reach standard distal coronary landmarks is determined. The first frame used for TIMI frame counting is the first frame in which the dye fully enters the artery. This occurs when three criteria are met: (1) a column of nearly full or fully concentrated contrast agent must extend across the entire width of the origin of the artery; (2) contrast agent must touch both borders of the origin of the artery; and (3) there must be antegrade motion to the contrast agent. If the LAD is subselectively engaged and the LCx is the culprit vessel, the TFC begins when the contrast agent first touches both borders at the origin of the LCx. The same rule holds for subselective engagement of the LCx. The last frame is counted or included as one of the frames and is defined as the frame when contrast material first enters the distal landmark point. The standard distal landmarks are the first branch of the posterolateral artery for the RCA, the most distal bifurcation of the segment with the longest total distance that includes the culprit lesion for the LCx, and the distal bifurcation ("moustache" or "fork") in the LAD. Proper planning is essential for counting the number of cine frames required to first opacify the distal artery, particularly the LAD. The TFC of the LAD and circumflex arteries is often assessed best in either the right or left anterior oblique (LAO) views with caudal angulation, and the RCA often is assessed best in the LAO projection with steep cranial angulation. Since the LAD is a longer artery, its frame counts are divided by 1.7 to derive the CTFC (Gibson CM, et al. *Circulation* 1996;93(5):879–888).

25.9 Answer D. There is modest agreement between an angiographic core laboratory and clinical centers in the assessment of TIMI grade 2 flow, which may limit the broad clinical applicability of this measure. In addition, a categorical variable—such as TIMI flow grade—limits its statistical power and sensitivity. For example, even if two interventions result in TIMI grade 3 flow, there may be a difference in contrast agent velocity between the two interventions when analyzed as a continuous variable with the CTFC. Despite high rates of TIMI grade 3 flow reported in the literature, only a third of patients with an open artery actually achieve flow that is truly within the normal range (CTFC ≤ 27). In contrast to the conventional TIMI flow grade system, the CTFC is a simple, reproducible, objective, and quantitative index of coronary flow that allows standardization of TIMI flow grades and facilitates comparisons of angiographic end points between trials (Gibson CM, et al. *Circulation* 1996;93(5):879–888).

25.10 Answer C. Impaired myocardial perfusion, as assessed with the TMP grade, is associated with a higher mortality after administration of thrombolytic drugs, independent of flow in the epicardial artery. Gibson et al. reported mortality being lowest in patients with TMP grade 3 (2.0%), intermediate with TMP grade 2 (4.4%), and highest with TMP grades 0 and 1 (6.0%; three-way $p < 0.05$). Even among patients with TIMI grade 3 flow in the epicardial artery, the TMP grades allowed further risk stratification of 30-day mortality: 0.7% for TMP grade 3, 2.9% for TMP grade 2, and 5.0% for TMP grade 0 or 1. Patients with both normal epicardial flow (TIMI grade 3 flow) and normal tissue level perfusion (TMP grade 3) have an extremely low risk of mortality (Gibson CM, et al. *Circulation* 2000;101(2):125–130).

25.11 Answer A. There are many potential sources of error in the quantitative assessment of coronary arteries. Among others, frame selection is associated with substantial interobserver variability: the end-diastolic frame showing the stenosis with most clarity and severity should be used (Herrington DM, et al. *Catheter Cardiovasc Diagn* 1993;29(4):314–321).

25.12 Answer A. The pattern of late lumen loss after DES implantation follows a peculiar behavior that differs from lesions treated with conventional stents. The distribution of late loss of DES is largely skewed to the left (i.e., most patients exhibit small amounts of late loss). In contrast, the pattern of late angiographic observed after bare stent implantation follows an almost Gaussian distribution (Lemos PA, et al. *Circulation* 2004;110(20):3199–3205).

25.13 Answer D. In the case of the ABSORB scaffold, BVS are made of polylactate acid and elute everolimus; it is the only BVS approved for use in the United States. The scaffold lacks metal and thus is invisible on x-ray imaging (Serruys PW, et al. *J Am Coll Cardiol* 2016;67(7):766–776).

25.14 Answer B. There are two important methods for the determination of TMP grade: the densitometric method (evaluates the maximal density of contrast in the region of interest) and the kinetic method (evaluates the speed of entry and exit of contrast in the area of interest). While epicardial flow is necessary for myocardial perfusion, it is not sufficient. Patients may experience TIMI 3 flow in the infarct artery with poor myocardial perfusion due to dysfunction of the microcirculation or distal embolization of plaque and thrombus after reperfusion. Conversely, patients may have suboptimal TIMI flow (usually TIMI 2) in the infarct artery with excellent myocardial perfusion. Rarely, even collateral flow may be sufficient to provide adequate myocardial perfusion (TMP grade 2 or 3) (Ito H, et al. *Circulation* 1996;93(2):223–228; Gibson CM, et al. *Circulation* 2002;105(16):1909–1913; van't Hof AW, et al. *Circulation* 1998;97(23):2302–2306).

25.15 Answer B. There are two methods to estimate reference diameter at the point of maximal stenosis. The interpolation method uses a second-order polynomial equation to estimate the reference diameter by tracking the arterial contour proximal and distal to the lesion. A second method uses an arithmetic average of the diameter of two 10-mm segments without obvious irregularities located equidistantly from the maximal stenosis (Hermiller JB, et al. *Catheter Cardiovasc Diagn* 1992;25(2):110–131; Reimers B, et al. *Catheter Cardiovasc Diagn* 1997;40(4):343–347).

25.16 Answer A. In general, the more complete the revascularization, the lower the incidence of clinical ischemic events is. To quantify the extent and complexity of residual, untreated CAD, the residual SYNTAX (rSS) score was designed. It is calculated as the SYNTAX score (SS) after revascularization is performed. Among 2,686 patients from the ACUITY trial, 40% had rSS = 0. The 30-day and 1-year rate of ischemic events was significantly higher in the incomplete revascularization group compared with the complete revascularization group, especially in those with high rSS. By multivariable analysis, rSS was a strong independent predictor of all ischemic outcomes at 1 year, including all-cause mortality (hazard ratio, 1.05; 95% confidence interval, 1.02 to 1.09, $p = 0.006$) (Généreux P, et al. *J Am Coll Cardiol* 2012;59(24):2165–2174).

25.17 Answer C. The relationships between atherosclerosis progression (or regression) as assessed by quantitative coronary analysis and IVUS were evaluated in a substudy of the Avasimibe and Progression of Coronary Lesions Assessed by Intravascular Ultrasound (A-PLUS) trial, a multicenter placebo-controlled study of the acyl coenzyme A: cholesterol acyltransferase enzyme inhibitor avasimibe. Although there was no correlation between changes in quantitative coronary analysis measures and changes in plaque volume on IVUS as continuous variables, patients with angiographic progression had both greater plaque volume at baseline on IVUS and significantly higher increases in plaque volume over time compared with patients without angiographic progression (Berry C, et al. *Circulation* 2007;115(14):1851–1857).

25.18 Answer A. Type 1,1,1 is the most common cause of bifurcation lesions (45%) and is associated with the highest rate of branch compromise during PCI (15% to 20%) (Medina A, et al. *Rev Esp Cardiol* 2006;59(2):183).

25.19 Answer D. During the analysis of infarct-artery flow in reperfusion studies with fibrinolytic agents, it was observed that the flow in noninfarct arteries was slower (higher TFC) than the flow observed in patients undergoing elective angiography. This important observation strengthens the current paradigm claiming that during an ACS, systemic activation of platelets occurs and marked secretion of vasoactive substances leads to diffuse slowing of coronary flow (Gibson CM, et al. *Circulation* 1996;93(5):879–888; Gibson CM, et al. *J Am Coll Cardiol* 1999;34(4):974–982).

25.20 Answer D. Intraprocedural stent thrombosis (IPST) is a recently described complication of PCI. Its diagnosis entails frame-by-frame review of cine angiograms in the quantitative coronary analysis laboratory. IPST is defined as new or increasing thrombus in a treated lesion and can be transient or permanent. In a detailed analysis from ACUITY and HORIZONS AMI, major adverse ischemic events were markedly higher in patients with IPST vs. those without IPST, including mortality at 30 days (12.9% vs. 1.4%, $p < 0.0001$) and 1 year (12.9% vs. 3.1%, $p < 0.0001$). Out-of-lab Academic Research Consortium definite or probable stent thrombosis also occurred significantly more often among IPST patients at 30 days (17.4% vs. 1.8%, $p < 0.0001$) and 1 year (19.9% vs. 2.7%, $p < 0.0001$). IPST was a significant independent predictor of 1-year mortality (hazard ratio, 3.86; 95% confidence interval, 1.66 to 9.00, $p = 0.002$) (Brener SJ, et al. *JACC Cardiovasc Interv* 2013;6(1):36–43).

26 Intracoronary Doppler and Pressure Monitoring

Morton J. Kern, Arnold H. Seto, Katherine Yu and Sonia Samtani

QUESTIONS

26.1 Which of the following best states the rationale for use of in-laboratory coronary physiology to assess the significance of a stenosis?

(A) The use of stress testing has low specificity and sensitivity
(B) The angiogram cannot provide enough information to determine flow for lesions 40% to 70% narrowed
(C) Chest pain syndromes are unreliable
(D) Coronary artery disease (CAD) is diffuse, obscuring the degree of atherosclerosis
(E) Intravascular ultrasound (IVUS) imaging shows plaque distribution and flow limitations

26.2 You have performed both fractional flow reserve (FFR) and coronary flow reserve (CFR) on an intermediate 60% diameter narrowing in the left anterior descending (LAD) artery in a patient with hyperlipidemia. CFR was 1.7 and FFR was 0.88. What is the most likely explanation?

(A) The FFR overestimated lesion severity
(B) The FFR underestimated lesion severity
(C) There is an inadequate response to pharmacologic hyperemia
(D) There is an impairment of the microcirculation
(E) The lesion is physiologically significant

26.3 A 42-year-old woman has chest pain syndrome and is evaluated for CAD and microvascular angina. This patient has a family history of CAD, migraine headaches, and treated hyperlipidemia. Coronary angiography shows a 40% eccentric right coronary artery (RCA) plaque. The results of her physiologic studies are shown below in Figure Q26-3. Based on these findings, what can be concluded?

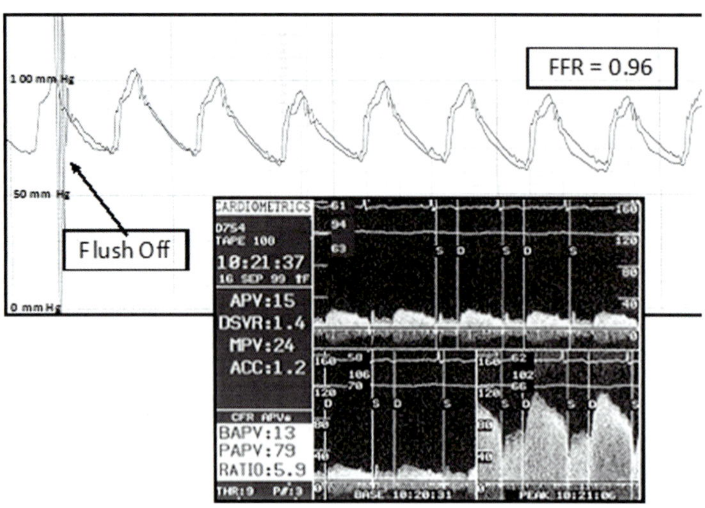

Figure Q26-3

(A) This patient has significant microvascular disease, which accounts for chest pain
(B) This patient has significant epicardial coronary disease, which accounts for chest pain
(C) This patient has impaired CFR and normal FFR
(D) This patient has combined abnormalities of CFR and FFR
(E) This patient has a noncardiac cause of chest pain

26.4 FFR is an invasive measurement of hemodynamic significance for epicardial coronary stenosis. An FFR of <0.75 has been best validated against which of the following noninvasive tests of ischemia?

(A) Exercise electrocardiogram (ECG)
(B) Stress echocardiography
(C) Myocardial perfusion imaging (SPECT)
(D) Ischemia by any of the above tests with resolution of the stress test result following percutaneous coronary intervention (PCI)

26.5 A patient has multivessel CAD in a right dominant system, with a 50% diameter stenosis mid-LAD, 50% mid-left circumflex (LCx), and 50% mid-RCA. Which of the vessels is LEAST likely to have a positive FFR?

(A) LAD
(B) RCA
(C) LCx
(D) They are equally likely to have a positive FFR

26.6 A patient undergoes FFR assessment of an intermediate lesion using intravenous (IV) adenosine. Which of the following points is the best place to measure FFR (Fig. Q26-6)?

(A) A
(B) B
(C) C
(D) None of the above

26.7 A 65-year-old woman has a RCA stent placed for acute inferior ST-elevation myocardial infarction (STEMI). She has a LAD lesion of 60% on angiography. She returns 4 weeks later for evaluation of the LAD and on stress testing demonstrates hypertension (200/105), dyspnea, nonsustained ventricular tachycardia (VT) (four to six beats), and 2 mm ST-segment depression (left ventricular hypertrophy [LVH] on EKG at rest). Radionuclide perfusion images are normal. Repeat angiography shows the RCA stent to be patent, normal LV function, and a 60% LAD lesion in one view. What is the best way to approach this patient?

(A) Place LAD stent
(B) IVUS and place LAD stent if cross-section area (CSA) is <4 mm^2
(C) Stop procedure and repeat stress test
(D) FFR and place stent if abnormal
(E) Obtain true lateral image of LAD lesion then stent

26.8 A 75-year-old man with progressive angina and positive stress testing undergoes catheterization and is found to have multivessel CAD: LAD 60%, LCx 80%, and RCA 90% with normal LV systolic function. Which of the following correctly states the case for the use of coronary physiology in this setting?

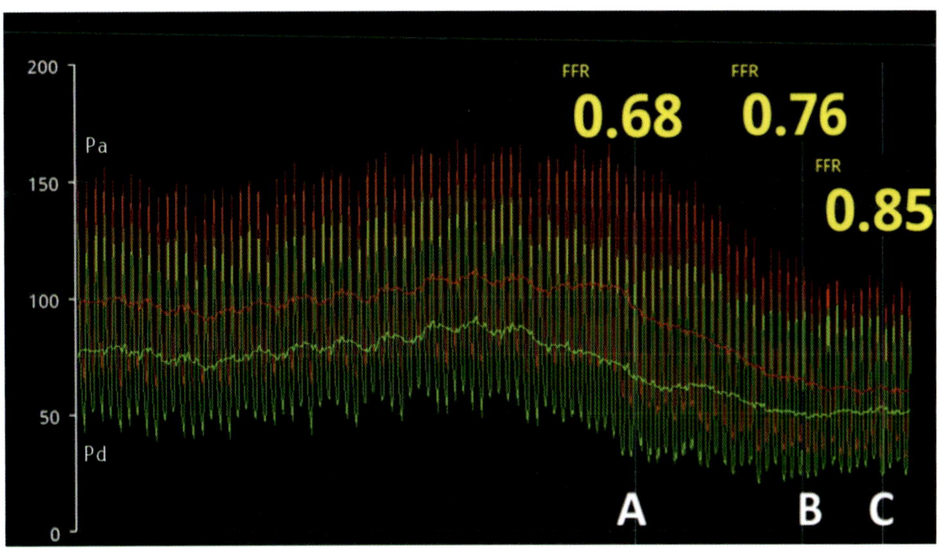

Figure Q26-6 (Adapted with permission from Kern MJ, et al. *JACC Cardiovasc Interv* 2015;8(8):1028–1030.)

(A) FFR of all vessels is unnecessary. Proceed to coronary artery bypass grafting (CABG)
(B) FFR of all vessels provides information useful to the surgeon alone
(C) FFR of the LAD alone is sufficient to assist in deciding between revascularization by PCI or CABG
(D) FFR of the LAD is not reliable in three-vessel (3V) CAD
(E) IVUS is preferable to FFR in patients with 3V CAD

26.9 An 81-year-old woman has an acute STEMI and comes to the emergency department (ED). She has a blood pressure (BP) of 90/60 mm Hg, a heart rate (HR) of 95 beats per minute (bpm), clear lungs, elevated neck veins, and distant heart sounds. The EKG shows 2-mm ST-segment elevation in leads II, III, and aVF. The patient develops a brief run of nonsustained VT, but the chest pain abates and the ST segments are substantially reduced. In the catheterization laboratory, the LAD has a 65% narrowing, the LCx is nondominant and unobstructed, and the RCA has a 50% hazy-appearing lesion. Which of the following is an appropriate use of FFR?

(A) FFR of the RCA to determine necessity to stent
(B) FFR of the LAD only to determine necessity to stent at this time or in near the future
(C) FFR of both the RCA and LAD to determine necessity to stent both in this sitting
(D) FFR of both the RCA and LAD to determine necessity to stent both at another time
(E) FFR should not be used in STEMI regardless of vessel assessed

26.10 A 42-year-old man with multiple CAD risk factors has a positive exercise Cardiolite perfusion imaging study with reversible anterior perfusion. He has had minor atypical chest pain. EKG shows LVH without repolarization abnormalities. At coronary angiography, the RCA is normal. The LCx has minimal lumen irregularities. The LAD has two narrowings: lesion 1 (55%) is proximal to the first septal and lesion 2 (60%) is 25 mm more distal at the second diagonal branch. What is the best use of FFR to treat this patient?

(A) FFR across lesion 1 only and then treat if FFR is abnormal; defer treatment of lesion 2
(B) FFR across both lesions 1 and 2; treat both lesions 1 and 2
(C) FFR across both lesions 1 and 2 with pullback; treat only the lesion with the biggest gradient
(D) FFR across only lesion 2; treat lesion 2 and defer treatment of lesion 1
(E) FFR across both lesions 1 and 2 with pullback; treat the lesion with the greatest gradient and then repeat FFR across the remaining lesion
(F) Do not use FFR for serial lesions

26.11 A 79-year-old man has atypical chest pain with exertional dyspnea. He has no CAD risk factors, medical problems, or significant past surgical or medical history. A maximal exercise Cardiolite perfusion study is negative. Because of persistent chest pain at rest without EKG abnormalities, coronary angiography was performed and demonstrated a 50% LAD lesion and no other evidence of CAD. FFR is 0.88. Treatment with PCI is deferred. Acetylsalicylic acid (ASA), beta-blockers, angiotensin-converting enzyme (ACE) inhibitors, and statins are prescribed. What is the expected major adverse cardiovascular event (MACE) rate for this patient over the next 2 years?

(A) <1% per year
(B) 4%—the same as any patient with CAD
(C) 10%—twice the rate of patients with CAD
(D) Unpredictable because CAD is highly variable
(E) Acute myocardial infarction (MI) can be expected because this is an intermediate lesion that will predictably progress

26.12 A 60-year-old woman with diabetes mellitus has atypical chest pain and an equivocal stress echo examination. She smokes one pack of cigarettes a day. Her EKG is normal and her weight is 285 lb. She is 5 ft 2 in. tall. Angiography (below) shows that she has an intermediate stenosis. Which is the best way to treat this lesion (Fig. Q26-12)?

(A) Rotablator
(B) Crush stenting
(C) Plain old balloon angioplasty
(D) Determine CFR for individual branches
(E) Determine FFR for individual branches
(F) CABG

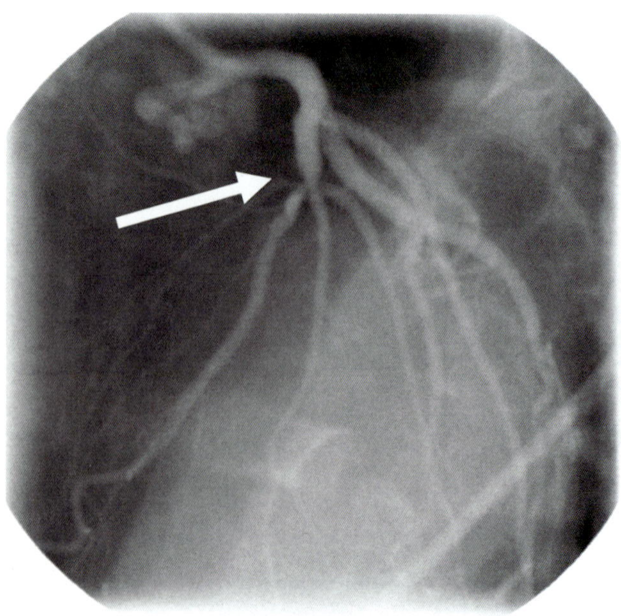

Figure Q26-12

26.13 A 56-year-old gentleman presents with chest discomfort that lasted for 30 minutes after running 1.5 miles. He undergoes exercise nuclear stress testing during which he achieves 11 metabolic equivalents (METS), and nuclear images show no reversibility, but there is a concern for transient ischemic dilation. Thus, he undergoes cardiac catheterization. Cardiac catheterization shows a smooth, tapering intermediate stenosis in the mid-LAD. You insert the pressure wire with some difficulty and notice two new stenoses in the proximal LAD. What is the immediate next step to ensure an accurate FFR measurement?

(A) Injection of intracoronary nitroglycerine, 200 mcg
(B) Injection of intracoronary adenosine, 200 mcg
(C) Pullback and removal of the pressure wire
(D) Use of a pressure catheter over a workhorse guidewire

26.14 A 76-year-old veteran presents for cardiac catheterization after having an abnormal treadmill stress test where she made 4 METS and had 1.5 mm ST depressions in the lateral leads. During her angiogram, she is noted to have a 70% lesion, which is concerning for ischemia in her RCA. You decide to perform an FFR. Due to a history of chronic lung disease, you elect to use intracoronary (IC) rather than IV adenosine. What would the appropriate IC adenosine dose for an RCA FFR be?

(A) 10 to 20 mcg
(B) 60 to 100 mcg
(C) 140 mcg/kg
(D) 200 mcg

26.15 A 61-year-old man has intermediately severe LAD and FFR is measured. During pullback across the lesion, the FFR changes from abnormal to normal as shown below. What would you do to assure this is a correct value (Fig. Q26-15)?

(A) Repeat pullback with higher adenosine dose
(B) Check IV infusion pump for delivery of adenosine
(C) Use side hole guide catheter and repeat pullback
(D) Change to 8-Fr guide catheter for better signal fidelity
(E) Continue IV adenosine and remove guide catheter from ostium

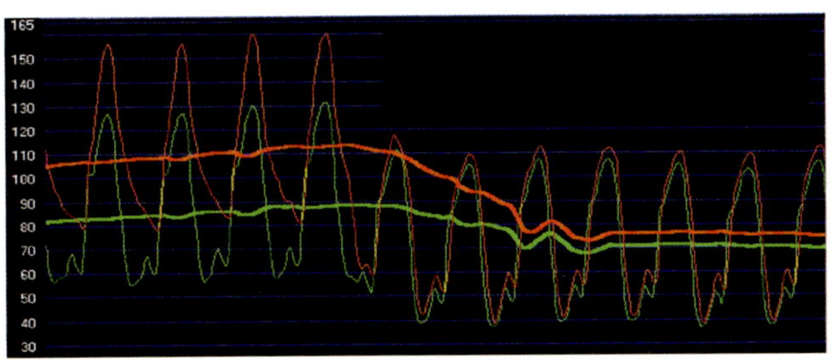

Figure Q26-15

26.16 A 67-year-old man with diabetes, angina, and a normal nuclear was found to have a proximal LAD stenosis with an FFR of 0.67. Following successful stenting, the FFR is still abnormal (FFR is 0.76). What is the best way to assess the final result of stenting in this patient (Fig. Q26-16)?

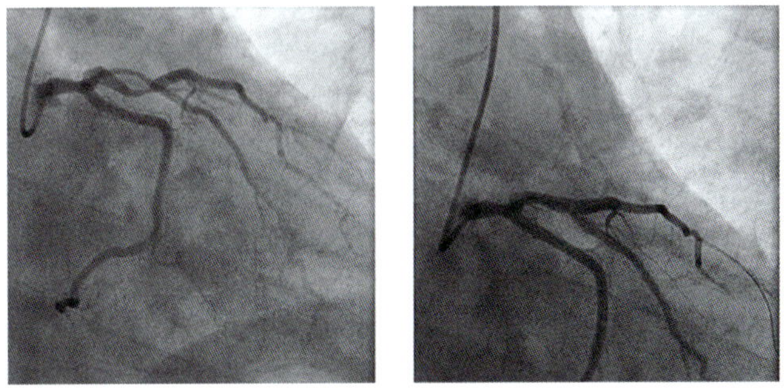

Figure Q26-16 (Courtesy of Arnold Seto.)

(A) IVUS
(B) CFR
(C) FFR during a wire pullback
(D) SPECT scanning
(E) Relative coronary flow reserve (RCFR)

26.17 A patient with stable angina undergoes coronary angiography and is found to have a single RCA stenosis of 60%. FFR is measured and is <0.80. What could be best said about revascularization with PCI?

(A) PCI is not indicated until medical therapy fails
(B) PCI will decrease the need for subsequent urgent revascularization
(C) PCI will reduce progression of disease
(D) PCI will reduce mortality

26.18 A patient without diabetes mellitus presents with unstable angina and is found to have an 80% LAD, 50% RCA, and 50% LCx stenosis. The operator is considering multivessel PCI. Compared with angiography-guided therapy, routine measurement of FFR during PCI in multivessel disease results in (Fig. Q26-18):

(A) Increased risk of periprocedural MI
(B) Increased time of procedure
(C) Shifting more patients toward CABG
(D) Decreased number of stents

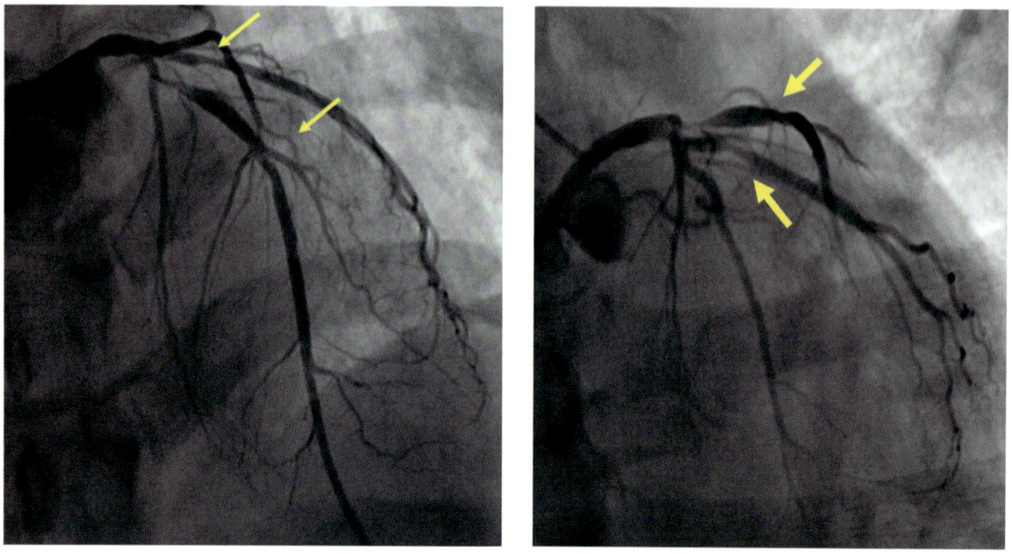

Figure Q26-18 (Courtesy of Morton Kern.)

26.19 A 55-year-old woman with advanced knee osteoarthritis presents with chest pain with exertion. She does not have any known classic CAD risk factors. EKG is normal. Which noninvasive test would simultaneously provide the most precise information about her coronary anatomy while also identifying lesions that cause ischemia?

(A) Exercise ECG
(B) Coronary computed tomography angiography (CTA)
(C) Coronary CT angiography with FFR
(D) Dobutamine stress echocardiogram
(E) Radionuclide dual isotope myocardial perfusion imaging

26.20 A patient asks you about the risk and benefits of PCI for stable angina in her case of a 60% LAD stenosis. Her risk of death, myocardial infarction, or revascularization without PCI would be highest in which of the following cases?

(A) FFR 0.65
(B) FFR 0.71
(C) FFR 0.78
(D) Her risk of MACE is the same as the FFR is positive in each of the above choices.

26.21 In which of the following situations can FFR absolutely not be used?

(A) Serial lesions
(B) Bifurcation lesions
(C) Acute MI, infarct-related vessel
(D) Saphenous vein grafts
(E) Acute MI, non–infarct-related vessel

26.22 All of the following patients would benefit from avoiding FFR with IV adenosine by using an instantaneous wave-free ratio (iFR) measurement, EXCEPT:

(A) Patient with 50% LAD stenosis, chronic obstructive pulmonary disease (COPD), and active wheezing on theophylline
(B) Patient with a 60% LAD stenosis taking Aggrenox (aspirin/dipyridamole) with a history of stroke
(C) Patient with a 40% stenosis and 2:1 heart block
(D) Patient with a 50% LAD stenosis with resting P_d/P_a of 0.93 and a poor ECG tracing

26.23 An intermediate RCA stenosis is being assessed with a pressure wire. The patient has a baseline 2:1 atrioventricular heart block and you are concerned about using IV or IC adenosine. Which of the following measurements would sufficiently assure you with at least 75% accuracy that the patient has a hemodynamically significant stenosis compared with hyperemic FFR of $\leq$0.80?

(A) A resting P_d/P_a of 0.86
(B) An iFR of 0.88
(C) A contrast FFR of 0.83
(D) Any of the above
(E) None of the above

26.24 An elderly patient with stable angina is found to have an intermediate stenosis in the LAD and a FFR of 0.70. PCI is successfully performed. Her risk of death, MI, or urgent revascularization following PCI is best described as which of the following?

(A) Similar to the risk of patients with an FFR > 0.80
(B) Similar to the risk of patients with an FFR < 0.80 treated with optimal medical therapy alone
(C) Her risk is minimal as her CAD has been resolved
(D) Higher than the risk with optimal medical therapy, due to the risk of stent thrombosis
(E) Unchanged

26.25 A patient presents with chest pain and a troponin of 0.4 ng/mL. She is found to have multivessel CAD with a distal left main stenosis that appears to be 60% in one view and 30% on another. There is a distal 50% LAD and mid-RCA 60% stenosis, but no evident disease in the LCx. What should be done next?

(A) Referral for CABG for left main stenosis.
(B) FFR measurement of the left main into the LAD, proximal to the distal stenosis
(C) FFR measurement of the left main into the LCx
(D) Medical therapy
(E) Stenting of LAD stenosis, measurement of left main stenosis with FFR

ANSWERS AND EXPLANATIONS

26.1 Answer B. Stress testing has a highly variable sensitivity and specificity depending on the test, the study population, and incidence of CAD. However, the rationale for in-laboratory physiology is that the angiogram for intermediate lesions cannot predict which lesions will or will not produce ischemia by whatever measures are used for testing. It is also true that chest pain syndromes are not specific, but the patient still must have a coronary narrowing to require further testing. IVUS shows diffuse disease and distribution, but does not directly give a picture of flow responses in a single cross-sectional image. Coronary angiography produces a silhouette image and can neither identify intraluminal detail nor provide the angiographer with information about the characteristics of the vessel wall. Diffuse disease as well as angiographic artifacts of contrast streaming, image foreshortening, or calcification complicate accurate identification of both the normal and diseased vessel segments. Bifurcation or ostial lesion locations may be obscured by overlapping branch segments. Even with numerous angiographic angulations to reveal the lesion in its best view, the physiologic significance of a coronary stenosis, especially for an intermediately severe luminal narrowing (approximately 40% to 70% diameter narrowing), cannot be accurately determined.

26.2 Answer D. Assuming that FFR and CFR was correctly performed, the FFR accurately reflects the ischemic potential of the narrowing. The CFR reflects the status of both the conduit and the microvascular bed. Therefore, the CFR is not lesion specific, and in the presence of a near-normal FFR, microvascular disease is likely the explanation. For the assessment of an epicardial stenosis, FFR is a measurement of lesion significance that, unlike CFR, has low variability and high reproducibility and is relatively unaffected by changes in hemodynamics.

26.3 Answer E. The chest pain complaint is associated with a completely normal FFR (0.96, top panel) and normal CFR (ratio 5.9 shown on lower IC Doppler tracing). The Doppler panel shows continuous flow at top half of signals and the bottom two panels show basal flow on left and peak hyperemic flow on right. The ratio of average peak velocity (APV) at baseline (BAPV = 13 cm/s) to peak (PAPV 79 cm/s) produces the CFR ration (ratio = 5.9). This patient has no epicardial obstruction and no abnormalities of the microvasculature.

26.4 Answer D. In a seminal study, Piljs et al. established FFR as a potential gold standard for coronary ischemia. FFR was compared against a battery of three noninvasive tests—exercise ECG, stress echo, and myocardial perfusion imaging—which were required to resolve following successful PCI. In all 21 patients with FFR < 0.75, ischemia could be shown by at least one positive test. The overall sensitivity, specificity, positive and negative predictive values, and accuracy of FFR were 88%, 100%, 100%, 88%, and 93%, respectively.

26.5 Answer C. The likelihood of a positive FFR depends on the amount of viable subtended myocardium. Smaller myocardial territories, such as the LCx or diagonal, are less likely to have a positive FFR for the same diameter stenosis, while LAD stenoses are more likely to have a positive FFR. Similarly, distal lesions are less likely to have a positive FFR than a proximal vessel stenosis. Finally, areas of prior infarction are less likely to manifest hyperemia and thus are less likely to have a low FFR given the same degree of stenosis.

26.6 Answer A. Point A represents the lowest ratio of P_d/P_a during the entire period of hyperemia and the point selected by most FFR machines. This value represents the point of maximal hyperemia and thus the point of lowest resistance in the microcirculation. Although prior recommendations suggested waiting until a stable hyperemic phase had been achieved, a truly stable hyperemic value often cannot be sustained for more than 1 minute with intravenous adenosine, and often generates a value significantly higher than the lowest P_d/P_a. Because of variable responses to adenosine, even within the same individual, the most reproducible value of FFR has been found to be the *lowest* P_d/P_a and is the current recommended value to be used.

26.7 Answer D. FFR and stent if abnormal. The FFR turned out to be 0.89 twice with 50 and 60 mcg IC adenosine. The correlation between radionuclide stress and FFR is good. ST-segment changes on exercise tolerance test (ETT) with an abnormal resting EKG are unreliable. VT is not specific in this setting, and symptoms of dyspnea with uncontrolled hypertension are likewise not specific for ischemia.

26.8 Answer C. FFR is useful to identify, which vessels have hemodynamically significant lesions. If FFR of the LAD is abnormal, CABG is favored over PCI for revascularization given the excellent outcomes with internal mammary grafts. If FFR of the LAD is normal, multivessel PCI of the LCx and RCA is preferred. FFR can be used in multivessel disease and it is superior to IVUS for physiologic decisions. IVUS is mainly indicated for anatomic information.

26.9 Answer B. The FFR of the RCA is unnecessary and may be misleading. The RCA lesion is hazy and recently had spontaneous reperfusion as shown by the VT- and ST-segment reductions after STEMI. This lesion should be treated. More importantly, acute FFR physiology data are neither available nor validated in the dynamic environment of acute coronary syndrome (ACS). As for the LAD, FFR would be helpful to see whether PCI of the 65% lesion is needed during this or a future procedure. Although nonculprit vessel PCI was previously restricted to patients in shock, more recent data suggest a clinical benefit in preventing recurrent MI, particularly when guided by FFR. Although concern previously existed that global microvascular dysfunction or vasoconstriction during STEMI precludes accurate FFR, in the absence of frank cardiogenic shock or vasopressor use, the accuracy of nonculprit lesion FFR has been validated.

26.10 Answer E. The achievement of the exact FFR of each individual lesion in a tandem stenosis is difficult in most clinical settings and can be obtained only with a coronary occlusion wedge pressure. For clinical purposes, conduct FFR across both lesions. Use the biggest hyperemic gradient to identify the lesion to treat first, then repeat FFR across the remaining lesion, and treat according to FFR thresholds. Deferring treatment when the FFR can confirm the lesion significance is inappropriate.

26.11 Answer B. Deferring PCI in patients with stable angina or atypical chest pain with normal FFR yields an excellent, low 2-year MACE. Fifteen-year results of the DEFER study of lesions with FFR > 0.75 have demonstrated that the rate of MACE does not significantly differ from the reference population. Patients with stable CAD have an event rate of 4% per year. MI has not been demonstrated in stable lesions undergoing FFR during follow-up.

26.12 Answer E. Because of the high-risk and complex lesion characteristics, determination of ischemic potential is needed. No percutaneous intervention is optimal for trifurcation lesions. CFR is not lesion specific. FFR for each branch will identify which, if any, narrowing needs to be treated. FFR for each branch in this patient was 0.90, 0.91, and 0.90. No intervention was performed. Gastroesophageal reflux disease (GERD) was treated successfully.

26.13 Answer A. Administration of IC nitroglycerin (100 to 300 mcg) prior to guidewire insertion is considered standard to ensure that the pressure wire or catheter measure the effects of a fixed coronary stenosis rather than spasm. Guidewire or catheter insertion can induce coronary spasm that is not resolved with adenosine administration. Pullback and removal of the guidewire can help resolve spasm or guidewire bias (pseudostenosis) but precludes measurement of FFR.

26.14 Answer B. 100 mcg is the optimal RCA IC adenosine dose according to a dose-response study, although it may be associated with transient AV block (Adjedj J, et al. *JACC Cardiovasc Interv* 2015;8(11):1422-1430). Lower doses may not provide sufficient hyperemia to ensure an accurate FFR assessment. Larger doses do not provide additional benefit and are more likely to cause AV block (Fig. A26-14).

Table 2. Hyperemic agents for FFR.

	Adenosine	Adenosine	Papaverine	NTP	Regadenoson
Route	IV	IC	IC	IC	IV
Dosage	140 mcg/kg/min	200 mcgLCA 100 mcgRCA	15 mcgLCA 10 mcgRCA	50–100 mcg	0.4 mg
Half Life	1–2 min	30–60 s	2 min	1–2 min	2–4 min (up to 30 min)
Time to Max Hyperemia	< 1–2 min	5–10 s	20–60 s	10–20 s	1–4 min
Advantage	GOLD STANDARD	Short action	Short action	Short action	IV bolus
Disadvantage	↓BP, chest burning	AV Block, ↓BP	Torsades, ↓BP	↓BP	↑HR, ?redose, long action

Figure A26-14 (From Kern M. *Cath Lab Digest* 2015;23(12).)

26.15 Answer E. This tracing shows that the guide catheter was pulled into the ostium and obstructed the opening, producing a damped ("ventricularized") pressure wave. This is not related to adenosine and should be repeated with the guide unseated. Even when obvious damping is not evident, routine guide disengagement has been demonstrated to measure a more accurate (lower) FFR due to more accurate aortic pressure measurement. Side hole guide catheters also result in suboptimal signal because of creation of a second pseudo gradient through the side hole into the ostium.

26.16 Answer C. FFR during a wire pullback will show the physiologic impact of the entire artery and any focal lesions, as well as the effect of flow immediately distal to stent. CFR will be abnormal in diffuse disease and in patients with diabetes and microvascular impairment. IVUS will show diffuse disease but not specific lesions in a diffusely diseased vessel. Although IVUS is useful to assess for stent expansion and apposition, it is less useful in determining the significance of other stenoses. As shown in the figure, IVUS demonstrates stenosis of the ostium, however, the hemodynamic significance of the stenosis is still unclear without FFR. SPECT scanning will likely be abnormal, but not helpful in diffuse disease. RCFR may be helpful, but not for diffuse disease. In this case, the FFR pullback revealed that the ostial LAD was significantly stenosed, which was not evident by angiography (Fig. A26-16).

26.17 Answer B. Based on the FAME2 results of 888 stable angina patients with coronary stenosis and FFR $\leq$ 0.80, PCI with optimal medical therapy was superior to optimal medical therapy alone and reduced the risk of the primary endpoint to the level of a comparator group with FFR > 0.80. The primary outcome was driven by urgent revascularization, though a landmark analysis suggests that death or MI would also be reduced.

26.18 Answer D. Based on the FAME study of 1,005 patients with multivessel disease, an FFR-guided revascularization strategy was superior to an angiographic revascularization strategy. FFR-guided revascularization reduced MACE and material costs, including a reduction in stents from an average of 2.7 to 1.9 stents per patient. More patients with multivessel disease were downgraded to two- or one-vessel disease with FFR and thus from CABG to PCI.

26.19 Answer C. Coronary CT with FFR. Coronary computed tomography angiography (CTA) is a noninvasive technique for the evaluation of CAD. The addition of noninvasive FFR using coronary CTA has high sensitivity and specificity for identifying ischemic lesions (sensitivity 85% to 90%, specificity 67% to 83%) and can be added to coronary CTA without additional radiation or medications. This has been shown in three pivotal trials (DISCOVER-FLOW, DeFACTO, and NXT). FFR is calculated by computational fluid dynamics to produce a 3-D model of blood flow and pressure fields in coronary arteries (Fig. A26-19).

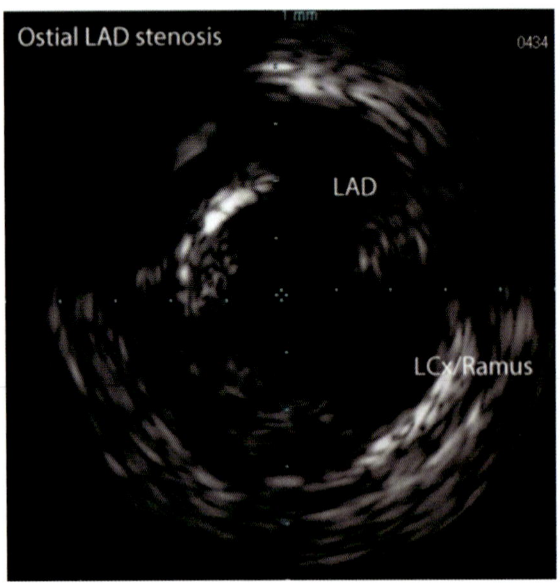

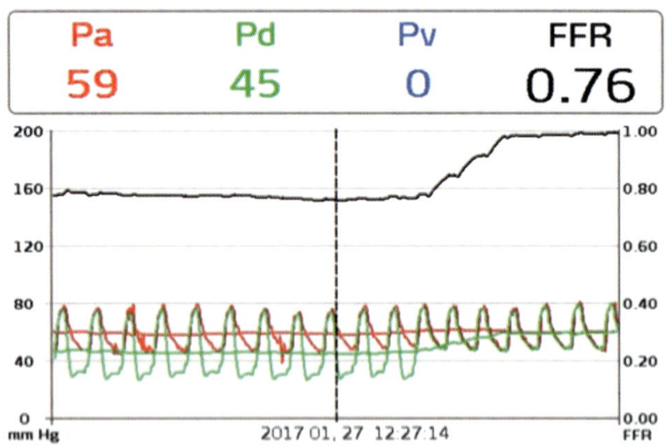

Figure A26-16 (Courtesy of Arnold Seto.)

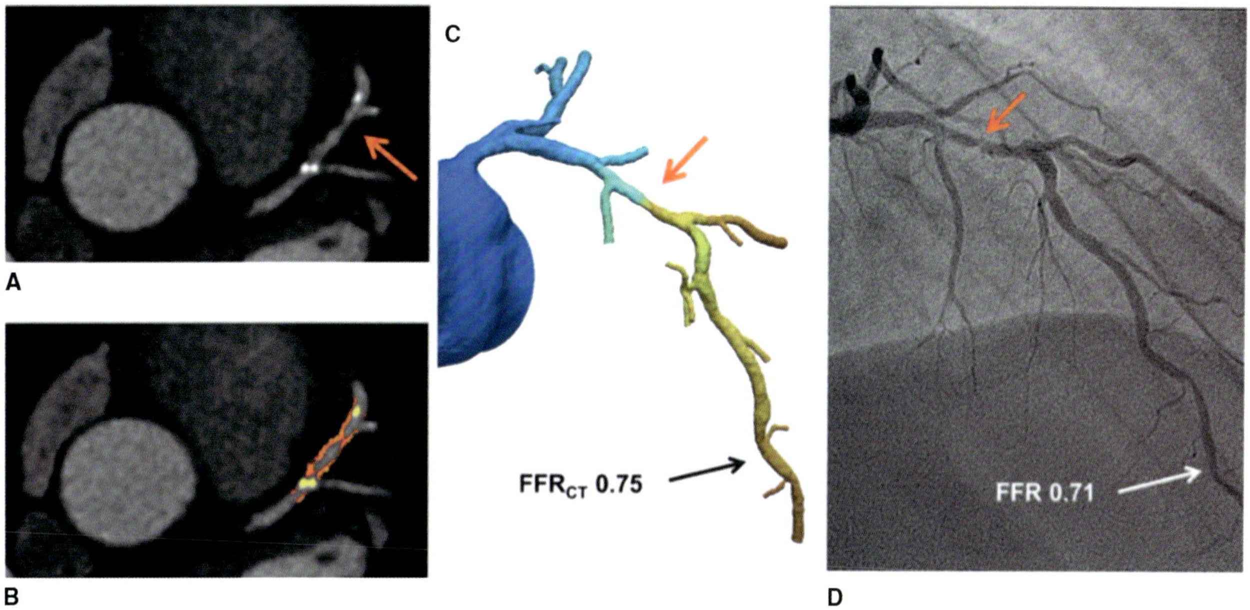

Figure A26-19 (With permission from Gaur S, et al. *Eur Heart J* 2016;37(15):1220–1227.)

26.20 Answer A. The risk of clinical events with a coronary stenosis depends on the degree of ischemia present. Based on patient-level outcome studies, the risk of an ischemic FFR is not dichotomous around 0.80, but rather resides on a continuum. The risk of a critical stenosis with FFR < 0.65 is higher than one with a borderline value of 0.75 to 0.80. As a result, borderline ischemic values can be compared with the risk of the revascularization strategy planned (i.e., bifurcation stenting, rotastenting) to develop the most appropriate clinical decision (Fig. A26-20).

26.21 Answer C. FFR cannot be used in the culprit infarct-related artery because the myocardial bed flow is dynamic and may recover and increase flow in the next few days, reducing a nonsignificant FFR. FFR is accurate in the nonculprit vessel during STEMI as recent data have suggested that complete revascularization in these patients is associated with better outcomes than culprit-vessel-only revascularization.

FFR can be used in the clinical circumstances listed, but it requires careful interpretation. FFR can be used to assess serial lesions in a stepwise

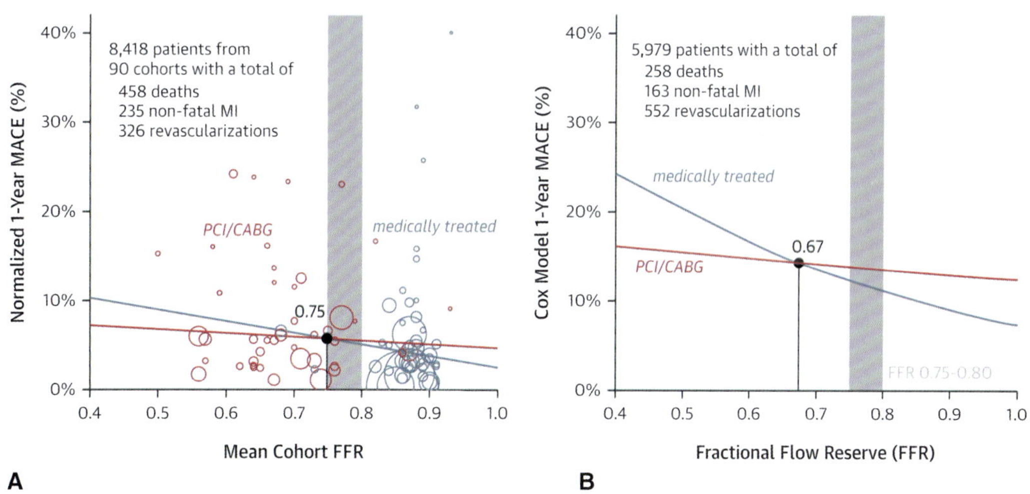

Figure A26-20 (With permission from Johnson NP, et al. *J Am Coll Cardiol* 2014;64(16):1641–1654.)

fashion. The FFR wire is advanced across each lesion into the distal vessel, hyperemia is induced, and the summed FFR is measured to determine the need for treatment. If the FFR is significant, then a pressure pullback is performed to determine which lesion to treat first; the lesion with the larger pressure step-up is treated first. Then the untreated lesion is evaluated by FFR, and if FFR is significant, revascularization is justified. FFR of side branch stenosis after main branch PCI can reduce unnecessary interventions and associated complications.

26.22 Answer D. Based on the DEFINE-FLAIR and iFR-SWEDEHEART studies, the iFR is noninferior to FFR in assessing the physiologic significance of coronary stenosis. The advantage of iFR is the avoidance of the need for adenosine hyperemia. Adenosine is most likely to cause adverse reactions in patients with active wheezing (bronchospasm), preexisting heart block, or those who are taking adenosine reuptake inhibitors, such as dipyridamole.

26.23 Answer D. Each of the measurements can be used as a surrogate for a hyperemic FFR, with varying degrees of accuracy depending on the threshold used. A resting P_d/P_a of <0.92 is the best cutoff for a FFR ≤ 0.80, with a value of 0.86 being well within the range of ischemia. Iodinated contrast (8 mL) injected into a coronary artery causes approximately 80% of the maximal hyperemia of adenosine, and a contrast-FFR value of <0.83 accurately predicts a FFR < 0.80. iFR < 0.89 is the best estimator of FFR < 0.80 but more importantly is backed by clinical outcome studies validating its value, independent of FFR as a reference standard.

26.24 Answer A. The FAME2 study randomized 888 patients with FFR ≤ 0.80 to PCI plus optimal medical therapy (OMT) or OMT alone. At 1 year, there was a 68% reduction in the composite endpoint of death, MI, or urgent revascularization with PCI, compared to OMT alone. The rate of the endpoint with PCI was similar to that with the reference population of FFR > 0.80. A landmark analysis excluding the first 7 days of periprocedural MI suggested that PCI may reduce death or MI, and not just urgent revascularization. These results stand in contrast with the COURAGE study, which suggested equivalence between OMT and PCI, albeit in a low-risk population.

26.25 Answer C. Angiographic assessment of the left main is particularly inaccurate due to angulation and the presence of a bifurcation. The risk of overestimating or underestimating a left main stenosis approaches 60%. IVUS or FFR assessment of the left main is important before committing to what may be a high-risk revascularization by PCI or CABG. In this case, FFR assessment is best performed into the nondiseased LCx artery. The LAD stenosis must be both very severe (FFR combined < 0.65) and proximal to cause any significant interaction with the left main FFR. Stenting of the LAD first, before measuring the left main stenosis, may lead to an unnecessary stent before CABG (Fig. A26-25).

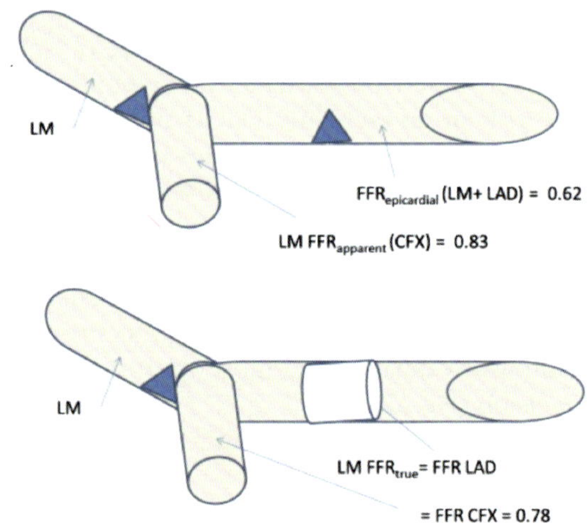

Figure A26-25 Diagram of left main (LM) segments, LAD and left circumflex (LCx) branches. In the circumstance of a LM and downstream LAD lesion, the LM FFR apparent (measured in the CFX) = 0.83, when FFR epicardial (LM + LAD) = 0.62. The clinical decision to treat becomes a difficult decision should the LAD be stented, and subsequently, it is recognized that the FFR true is now significant as is shown (bottom panel). The LM FFR without LAD or CFX disease can be assessed as LM FFR true = FFR LAD = FFR CFX = 0.78. (Courtesy of Morton Kern.)

27 Intravascular Ultrasound

Khaled M. Ziada

QUESTIONS

27.1 Following an intravascular ultrasound (IVUS) imaging of a moderately diseased coronary artery (Fig. Q27-1A), offline measurements are performed (Fig. Q27-1B). All of the following statements about these measurements are TRUE, EXCEPT:

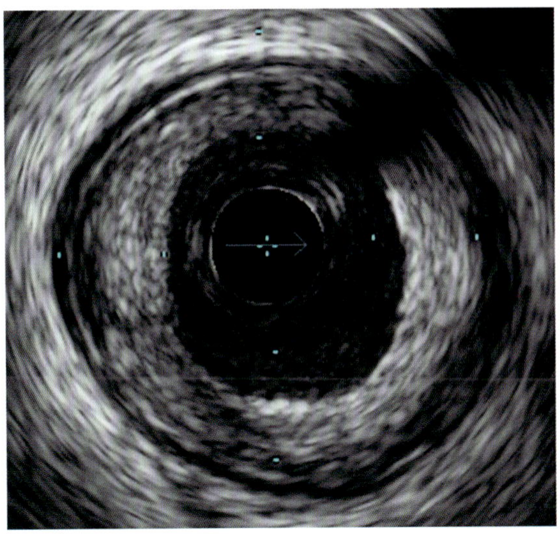

A

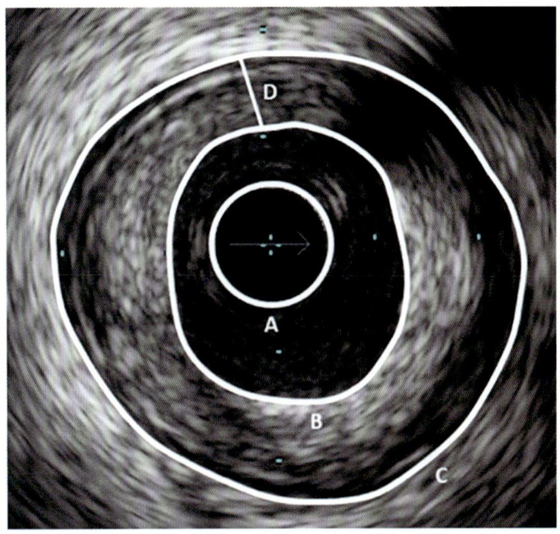

B

Figure Q27-1 (Courtesy of Khaled Ziada.)

(A) Line B traces the leading edge of the intima
(B) Line C traces the leading edge of the adventitia
(C) The difference between areas A and B represents the lumen area
(D) The difference between areas B and C represents the atheroma area
(E) Line D is the minimal atheroma thickness

27.2 Following difficult catheter engagement of a mildly diseased right coronary artery (RCA), a subsequent angiogram reveals an extensive dissection (Fig. Q27-2A). Emergent bailout stenting is planned, and a guiding catheter is advanced to engage the RCA. The angioplasty wire is passed to the distal vessel with some difficulty. An IVUS catheter is then advanced over the wire to confirm its position. Figures Q27-2B and Q27-2C are obtained from the mid- and proximal RCA. The next best course of action is as follows:

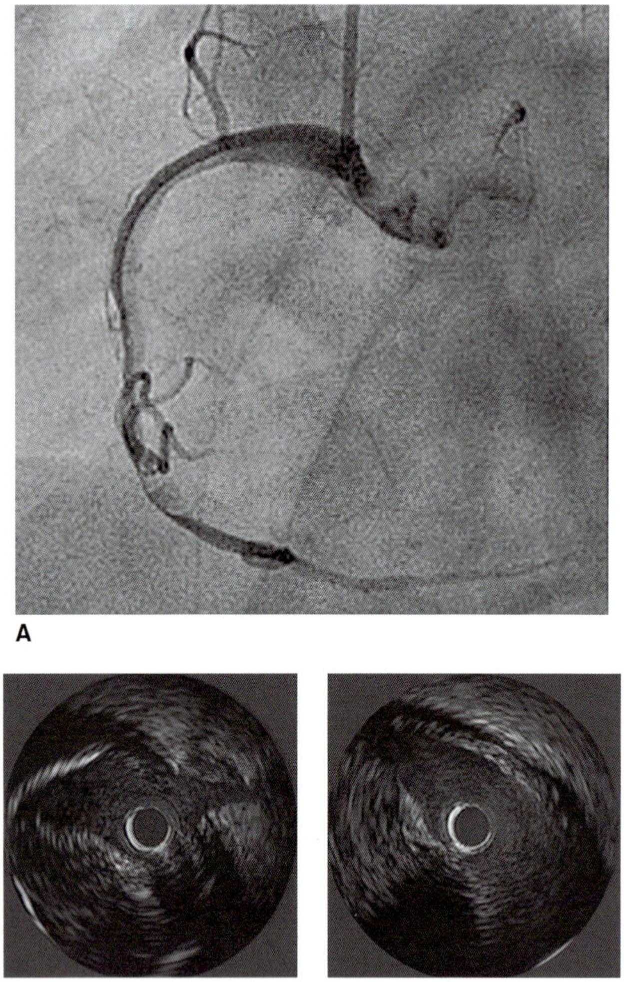

A B C

Figure Q27-2

(A) The wire should be removed and the procedure terminated
(B) The wire should remain in place; balloon angioplasty and stenting should follow
(C) The wire should be removed, and another attempt at passing it in the true lumen should be performed
(D) The wire should remain in place, but another wire should be used to access the true lumen

27.3 Virtual histology (VH) is a technical advancement that allows for better characterization of coronary plaque morphology compared to standard grayscale IVUS imaging. Which of the following statements is FALSE regarding IVUS-derived VH?

(A) VH technology is based on advanced frequency domain analysis of the radiofrequency backscatter of the ultrasound signals
(B) The color-coded display of the VH information allows for easier and faster interpretation of the information by operators
(C) Radiofrequency analysis is not reliable in distinguishing between lipid-laden plaque material and organizing thrombus
(D) The VH data superimposed on the cross-sectional image obtained by grayscale IVUS result in higher axial and lateral resolution

27.4 A physically active 66-year-old hypertensive patient is referred for coronary angiography because of typical angina precipitated by moderate exertion. Right coronary angiography showed a severe focal lesion in the mid segment. Left coronary angiography revealed moderate disease in a marginal branch of the circumflex artery, but more importantly, it also revealed ostial left main disease (Fig. Q27-4A). An IVUS imaging is then performed to better define the left main trunk disease. The minimal lumen area (MLA) in the left main trunk was measured to be 7.4 mm^2 (Fig. Q27-4B). What is the most appropriate next step?

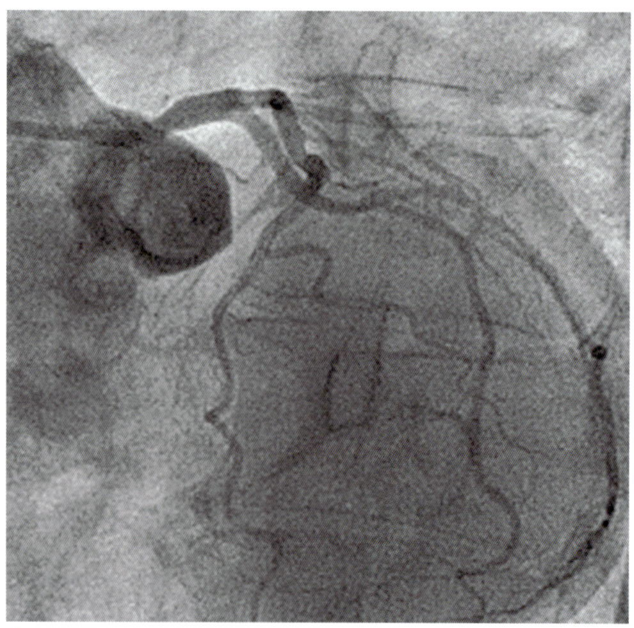

A

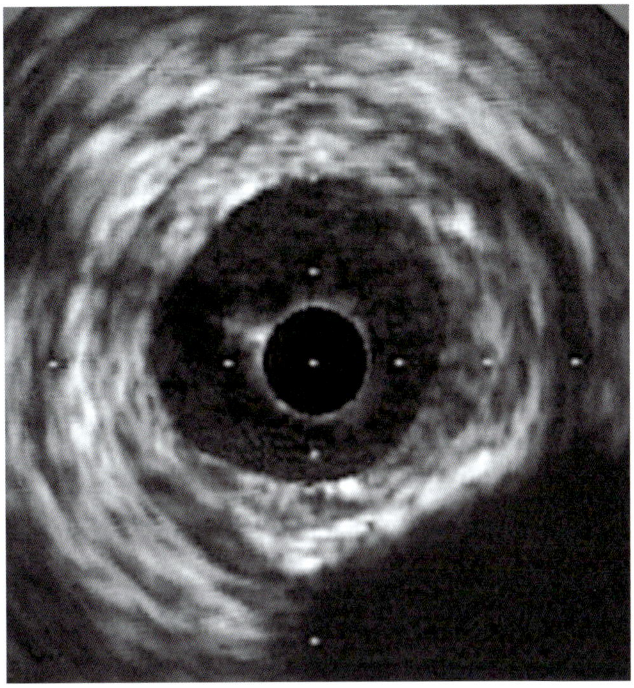

B

Figure Q27-4

(A) Measure fractional flow reserve (FFR) distal to the left main stenosis
(B) Place an intra-aortic balloon pump (IABP) and arrange for three-vessel bypass surgery
(C) Consider stenting of the right coronary lesion for symptom relief
(D) Reevaluate the patient with a pharmacologic nuclear stress test

27.5 Comparing an IVUS-guided to angiography-guided stent implantation strategies, which of the following statements is TRUE?

(A) Randomized trials comparing these strategies in all comers demonstrated a significant advantage of IVUS guidance in reducing the rate of repeat revascularization
(B) Retrospective studies and meta-analyses demonstrated IVUS-guided stenting is associated with improved clinical outcomes, driven by reduction in repeat procedures
(C) An angiography-guided strategy was associated with increased balloon utilization
(D) The risk of subsequent death and myocardial infarction (MI) is significantly reduced with the use of an IVUS-guided strategy in left anterior descending (LAD) artery stenting
(E) At 6 months, target vessel revascularization (TVR) is more frequent with the IVUS-guided strategy

27.6 A 70-year-old male patient with hypertension and hyperlipidemia presents with recurrent episodes of chest burning for several days. His electrocardiogram (ECG) reveals T-wave inversion in leads V_3 through V_6. His troponin I is 3.0, but the creatine kinase-MB (CK-MB) is not elevated. Coronary angiography is performed: the right coronary angiogram is unremarkable, and the left coronary angiogram is seen in Figure Q27-6A. IVUS imaging was then performed to better define the mid-LAD segment. Figures Q27-6B and C demonstrate the representative images from the LAD at the level of and just proximal to the diagonal bifurcation, respectively. Upon review of the angiogram and the IVUS images, which of the following statements would be considered CORRECT?

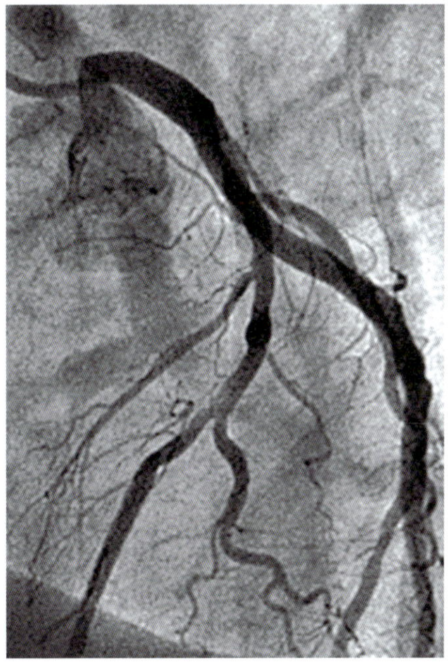

A

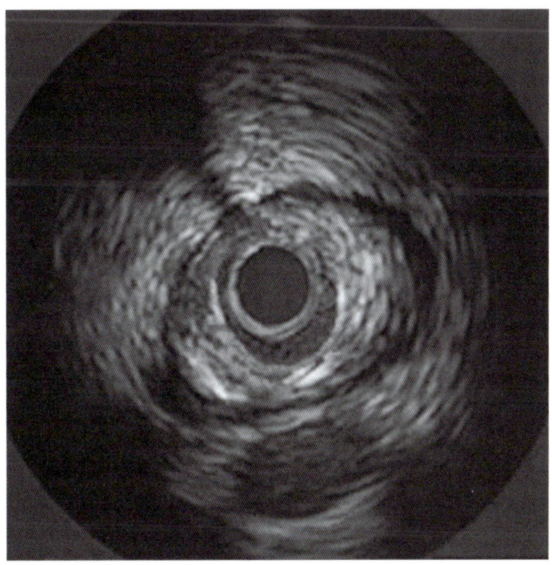

B

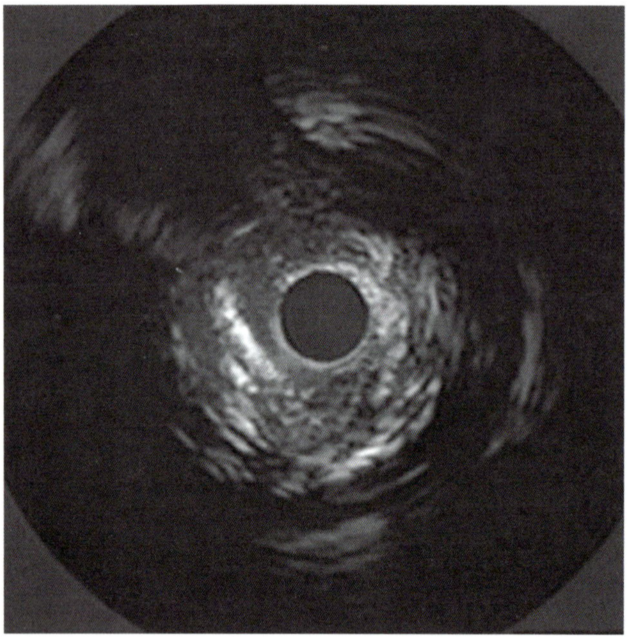

C

Figure Q27-6

(A) The haziness of the mid LAD is caused by heavy calcification
(B) In this case, IVUS imaging is associated with a significant risk of complications
(C) The clinical management of the patient will be influenced by the IVUS findings
(D) FFR in the distal LAD will likely be ≥0.85
(E) Following angiographic and ultrasound interrogation, there is no clear explanation for the patient's clinical syndrome

27.7 IVUS imaging has been the primary imaging modality used in coronary atherosclerosis progression-regression trials of statin therapy in the last decade. All of the following statements regarding these trials are TRUE, EXCEPT:

(A) IVUS measures of change in atheroma volume (total or percent atheroma volume [TAV or PAV]) were the primary efficacy end points of these studies
(B) The change in TAV or PAV was proportionate to the change in the low-density lipoprotein (LDL) cholesterol level
(C) These studies demonstrated an association between regression of disease and reduced adverse cardiac events
(D) There was a significant reduction in the IVUS measures of atheroma volume with intensive or very intensive lipid lowering
(E) There was evidence of progression in the IVUS measures of atheroma volume with moderate lipid lowering

27.8 Serial IVUS imaging of coronary lesions following balloon angioplasty and atherectomy improved our understanding of the mechanisms of acute lumen gain and subsequent restenosis. Regarding these mechanisms, the following statement is TRUE:

(A) At 6 months, the change in lumen area correlates more strongly with the change in the plaque area than with the change in the vessel area
(B) The serial changes in the minimal luminal diameter seen by angiography correlate with the changes seen by IVUS imaging
(C) At 1 month, the increase in vessel area is more significant in the nonrestenotic lesions compared with the restenotic lesions
(D) Between 24 hours and 1 month after balloon angioplasty, there is significant adaptive remodeling
(E) Between 1 and 6 months, constrictive remodeling was less significant in restenotic lesions than in nonrestenotic lesions

27.9 Figure Q27-9 represents a longitudinal section of a severe focal coronary stenosis. Which of the following measurements are needed to calculate the remodeling index?

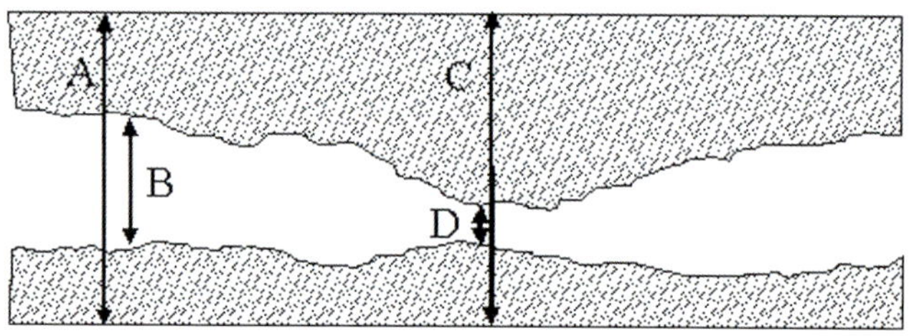

Figure Q27-9

(A) A and B
(B) C and D
(C) A and C
(D) B and D
(E) A to D

27.10 A 52-year-old patient presented with angina on moderate exertion. On the treadmill, he stopped after 5.5 minutes because of chest pressure and 2 mm ST depression. A diagnostic angiogram of the left coronary system (Fig. Q27-10A) revealed a tight lesion in the first obtuse marginal branch of the left circumflex artery (LCx). After deciding to proceed with percutaneous coronary intervention (PCI), a 6-Fr guiding catheter was selected. Catheter engagement was difficult, and the patient developed chest discomfort but was hemodynamically stable. Another angiogram was obtained just before passing the angioplasty wire (Fig. Q27-10B). IVUS imaging of the left main trunk was performed (Fig. Q27-10C). What is the most appropriate next step?

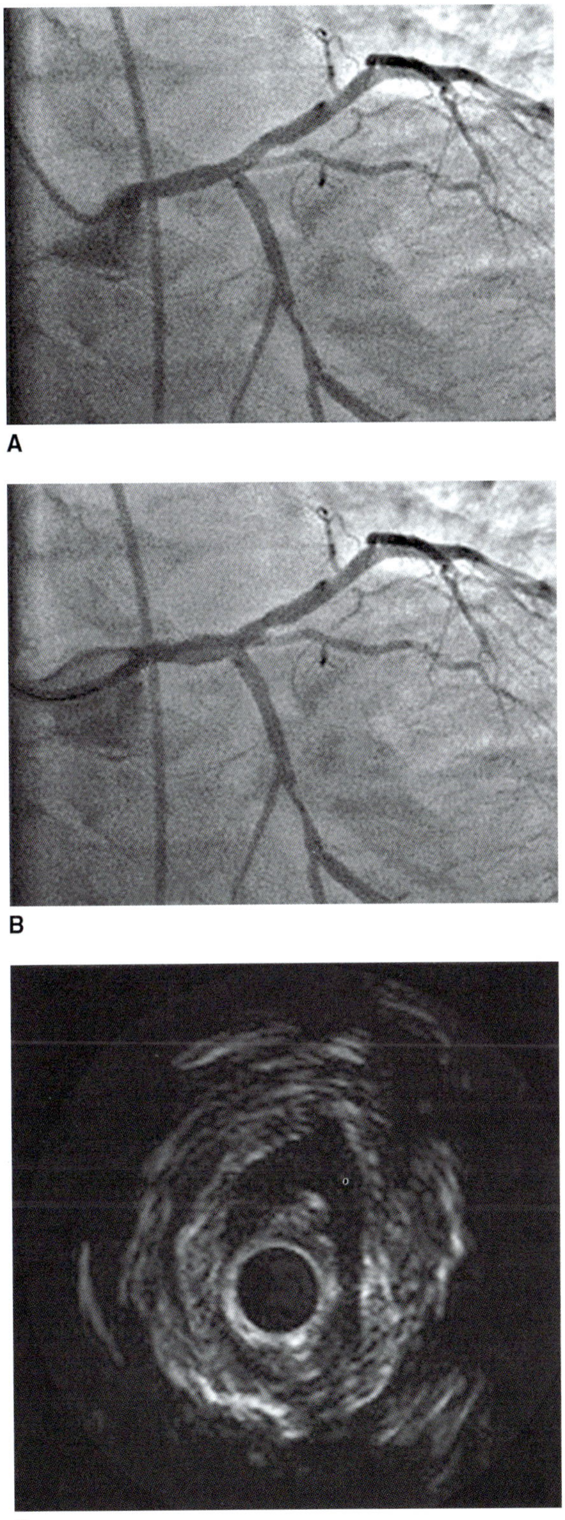

Figure Q27-10

(A) Abort the planned PCI, and schedule the patient to see a cardiac surgeon
(B) Abort the planned PCI, and consult with the cardiac surgeon in the laboratory
(C) Proceed with the planned PCI of the LCx artery
(D) Proceed with the planned PCI of the LCx artery after inserting an IABP

27.11 All of the following applications of IVUS imaging are appropriate, EXCEPT:

(A) Assessment of an angiographically hazy segment in the marginal branch of the LCx after balloon angioplasty
(B) Measurement of the minimum lumen area and the adequacy of strut apposition after stenting the mid RCA
(C) Evaluation of an ostial LAD lesion considered for directional atherectomy
(D) Confirmation of the presence of atherosclerotic coronary disease in a patient with atypical symptoms whose angiograms reveal minimal disease
(E) Evaluation of a 30-40% ostial left main coronary artery lesion in a patient with Class 1 angina

27.12 Which of the following images (Fig. Q27-12A, B, C, or D) is obtained from the saphenous vein graft (SVG) of a patient presenting with chest pain for the first time 5 years after his bypass surgery?

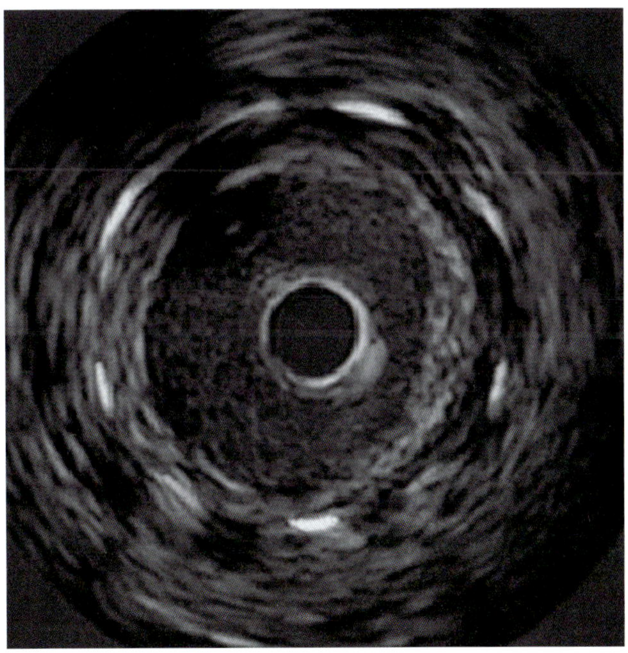

A

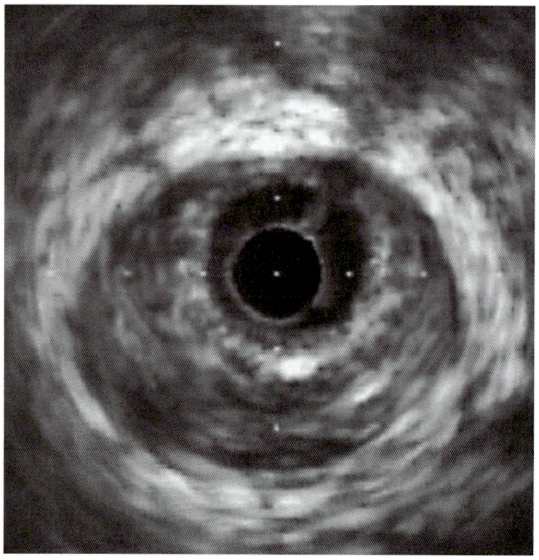

B

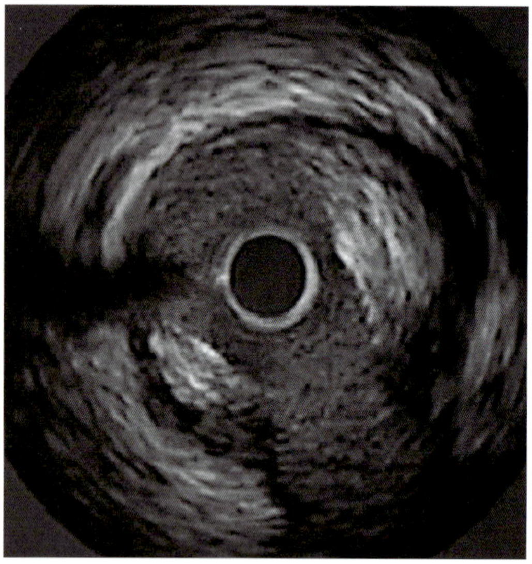

C

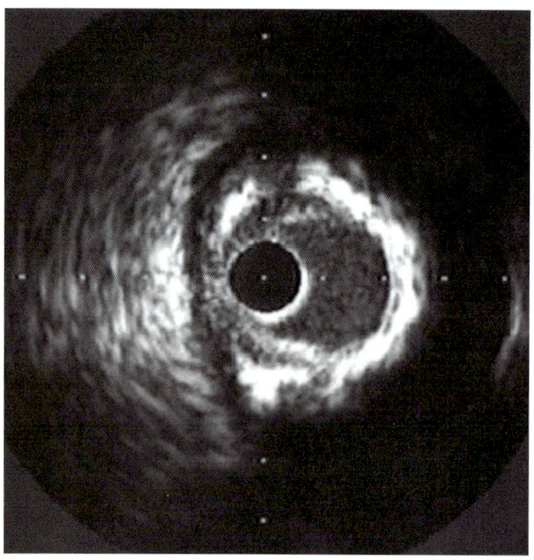

D

Figure Q27-12

27.13 A patient with typical angina is referred for coronary angiography after a nuclear stress test reveals an anterior reversible perfusion defect. The LAD angiograms reveal a 50% to 60% diameter stenosis in the mid segment (Fig. Q27-13A,B), though the other vessels contain only mild irregularities. An IVUS examination of the LAD is performed. The bottom left figure shows the section with the narrowest lumen (Fig. Q27-13C). The middle and right IVUS images represent more proximal LAD (Fig. Q27-13D and E, respectively). Which of the following conclusions about this patient is TRUE?

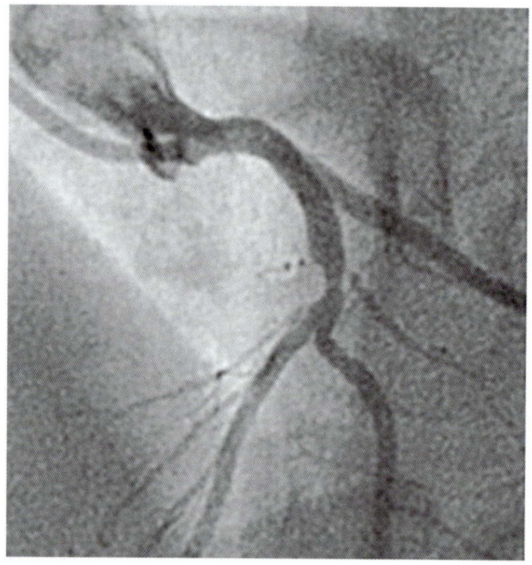

A

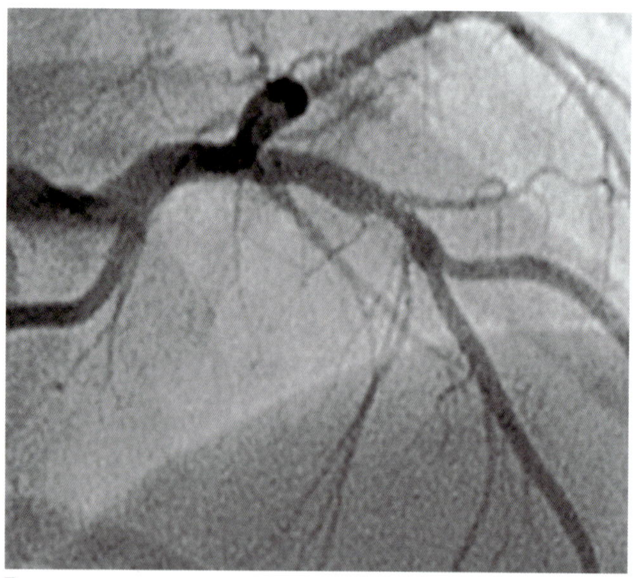

B

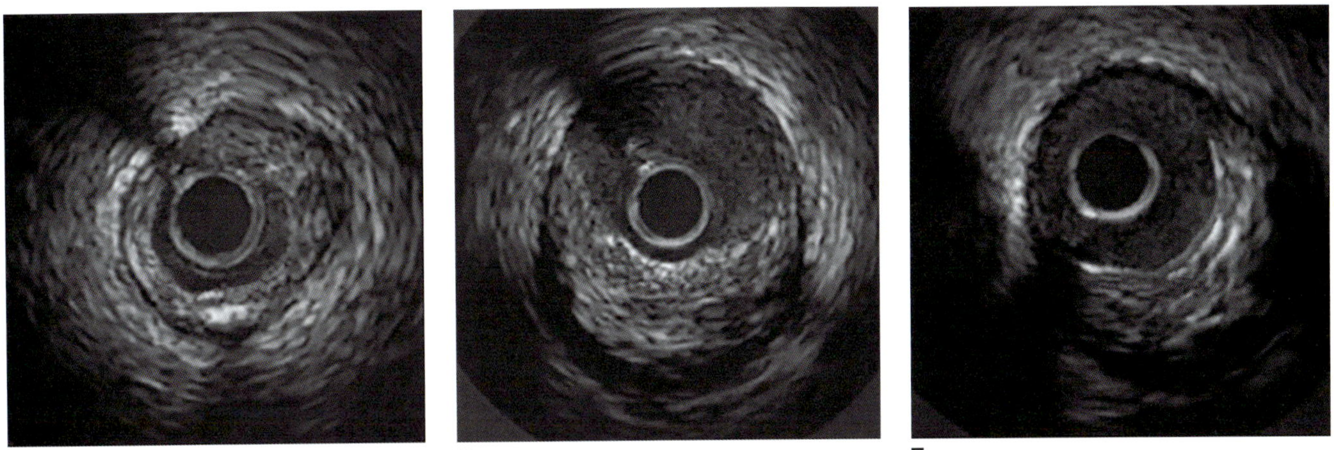

C D E

Figure Q27-13

(A) IVUS imaging did not explain the discrepancy between the angiogram and the result of the stress test
(B) The IVUS images explain why the stress test result was false positive
(C) An FFR of 0.70 would confirm the findings of the IVUS images
(D) The IVUS images are inconclusive because of the proximity of the diagonal branch

27.14 A patient is referred for PCI of a severe proximal LAD lesion. IVUS imaging is performed to evaluate the lesion and plan the intervention. A representative image from the diseased segment is shown in Figure Q27-14. On evaluating this lesion, which of the following statements would be considered TRUE?

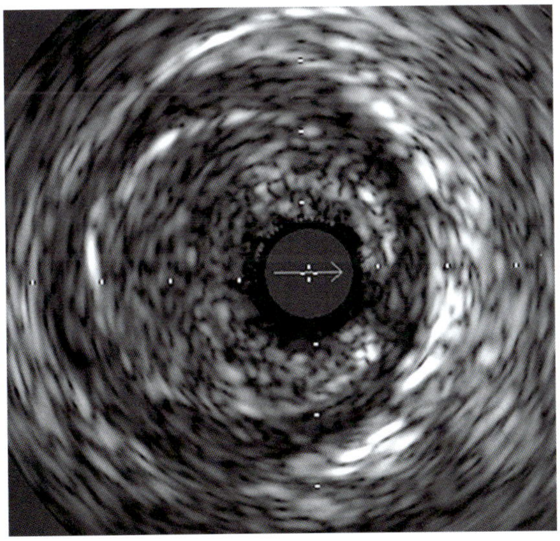

Figure Q27-14 (Courtesy of Khaled Ziada.)

(A) Directional atherectomy before stenting will result in greater acute lumen gain compared with direct stenting
(B) Adequate stent expansion cannot be achieved without pretreatment with rotational atherectomy
(C) IVUS imaging is reasonable to rule out the possibility of intraluminal thrombus prior to stenting
(D) Debulking using directional or rotational atherectomy will reduce the risk of repeat procedures

27.15 All of the following statements regarding in-stent restenosis are CORRECT, EXCEPT:

(A) Late lumen loss correlates strongly with tissue growth inside the stent
(B) Late lumen loss measured by IVUS correlates with angiographic late loss
(C) Negative remodeling is a major determinant of in-stent restenosis
(D) Late lumen loss is usually uniformly distributed along the stented segment
(E) Late lumen loss distal to the edge of the stent is most likely because of negative remodeling

27.16 IVUS imaging can be used to assess angiographically mild nonculprit lesions in patients undergoing coronary angiography for acute coronary syndromes (ACS). Figure Q27-16 represents four different nonculprit lesions assessed by IVUS with VH analysis. Assuming these lesions were not treated, which is more likely to result in an adverse cardiac event in the ensuing few years?

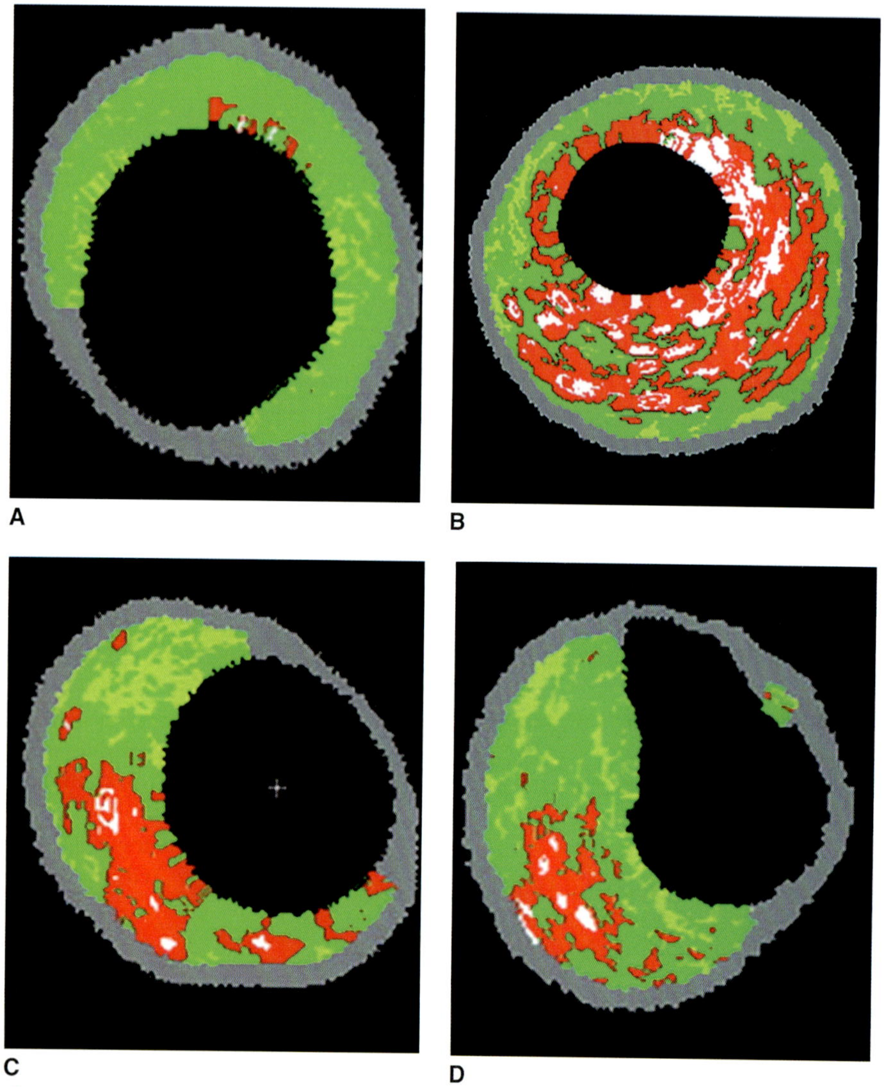

Figure Q27-16

(A) Figure Q27-16A
(B) Figure Q27-16B
(C) Figure Q27-16C
(D) Figure Q27-16D

27.17 A 59-year-old patient presents with typical angina 8 months after undergoing primary angioplasty using a 33-mm long drug-eluting stent (DES) in the mid LAD in the setting of an acute anterolateral MI. A nuclear scan reveals reversible ischemia in addition to a small scar in the anterolateral and apical regions. The RCA and LCx are free of significant obstructions. The LAD angiogram is shown in Figure Q27-17A. IVUS imaging is performed; the

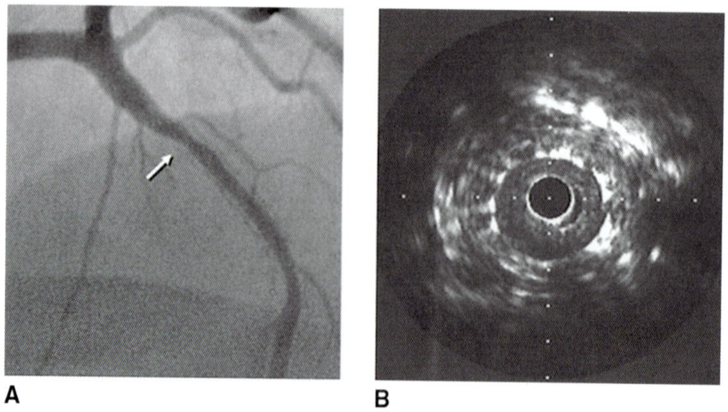

Figure Q27-17

image in Figure Q27-17B is obtained from the proximal stent segment (see arrow). Which of the following statements is TRUE regarding the IVUS findings?

(A) Drug-eluting in-stent restenosis is focal in approximately 50% of cases
(B) Intimal hyperplasia is the only explanation of this stent failure
(C) With DES of that length, IVUS-defined underexpansion is rare
(D) The mechanism of diameter stenosis is not related to the stent length

27.18 IVUS imaging is frequently used to assess the results of high-pressure stent deployment. Which of the following images of coronary stents is the LEAST likely to need the use of a larger balloon and/or higher inflation pressure (Fig. Q27-18A, B, C or D)?

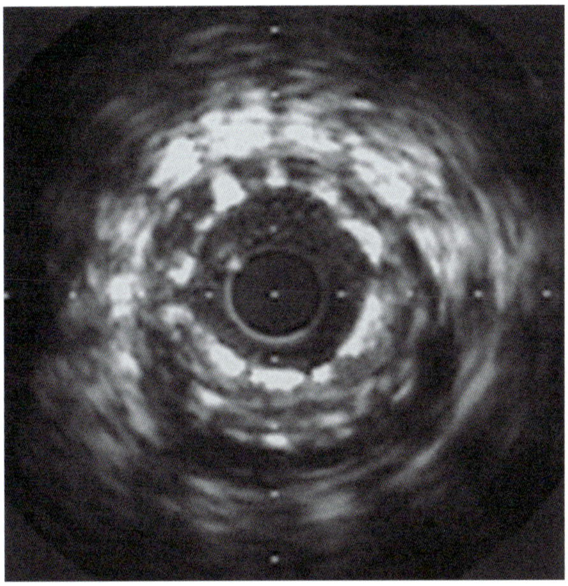

A

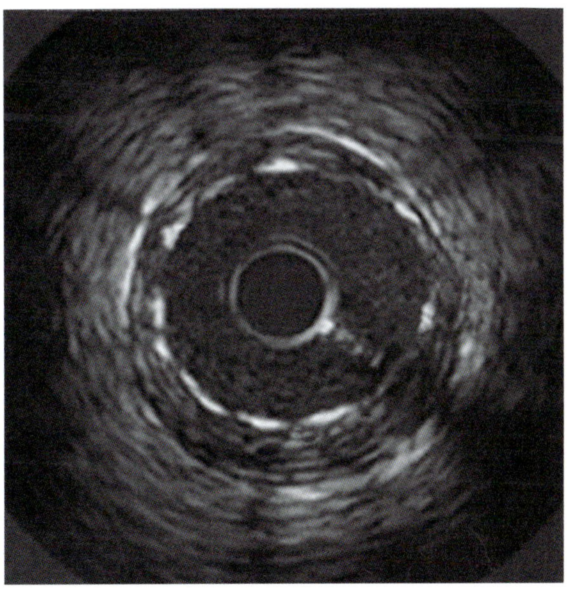

B

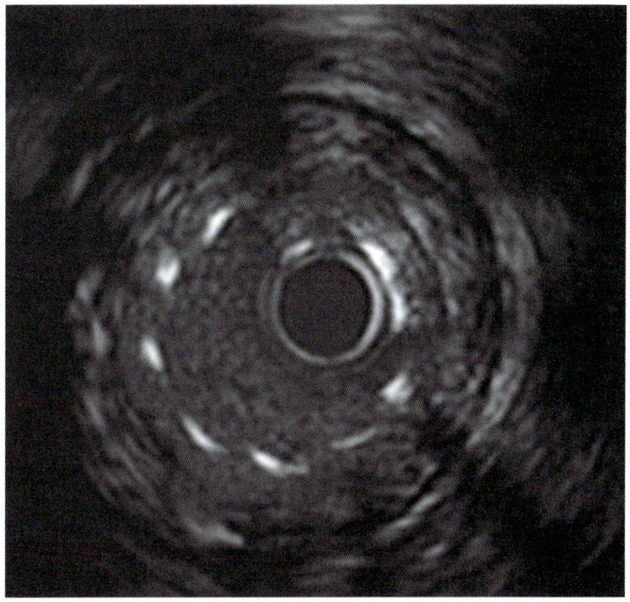

C

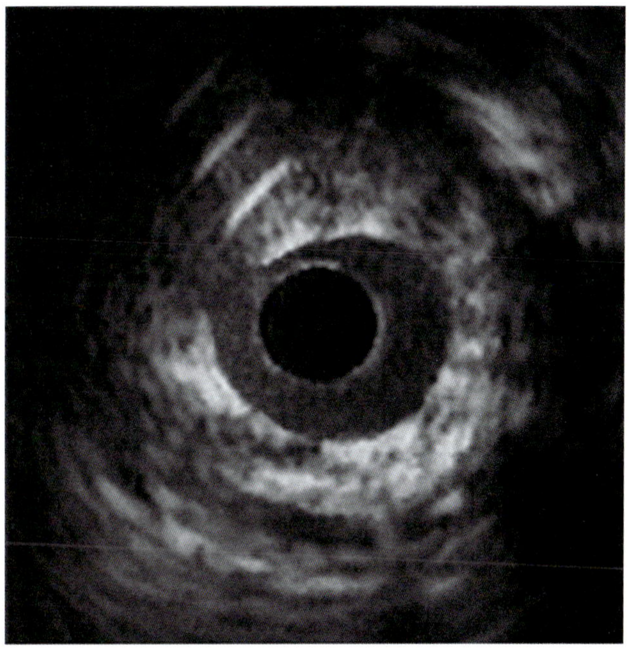

D

Figure Q27-18

27.19 Which of the following IVUS findings is NOT associated with very late stent thrombosis after DES implantation?

(A) Longer stented segment
(B) Incomplete strut apposition
(C) Smaller reference segment vessel area
(D) Larger in-stent segment vessel area

27.20 A middle-aged hypertensive patient presents with atypical chest pain that is precipitated by effort and sometimes occurs at rest. Coronary angiography reveals slight luminal irregularities in the RCA and LCx arteries. A cranial projection shows an indeterminate lesion in the mid-distal LAD (Fig. Q27-20A).

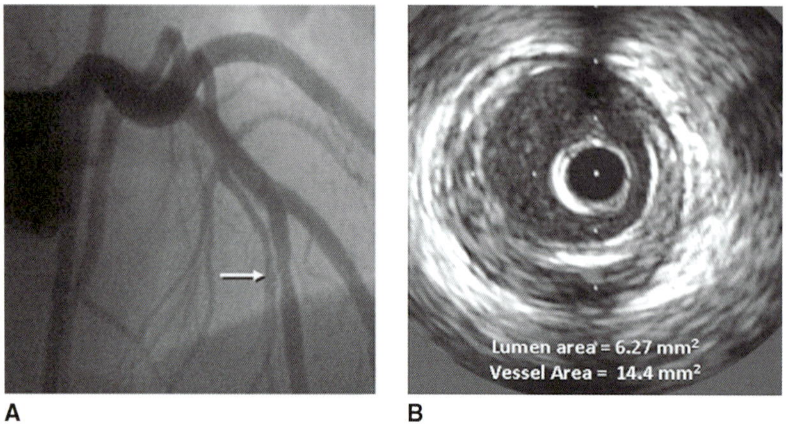

Figure Q27-20

IVUS imaging is performed to evaluate the significance of the lesion, and a representative image of the minimum lumen area is shown (Fig. Q27-20B). Which of the following statements is most accurate?

(A) IVUS findings suggest statin therapy is the most appropriate course of action
(B) The angiogram did not reveal the true severity of the lesion due to heavy calcification
(C) FFR across this lesion is most likely to be <0.75
(D) PCI on this lesion will reduce the risk of death or MI

27.21 IVUS imaging in complex cases of chronic total occlusion (CTO) PCI can help with all of the following, EXCEPT:

(A) Identifying true from false lumen
(B) Defining the extent of dissection flaps
(C) Identifying the ambiguous ostium of an occluded vessel to help direct wiring
(D) Facilitate stent sizing since angiographic reference measurement often overestimates the size of the vessel

27.22 A 54-year-old female with history of smoking and hypertension presents with typical angina and a high-risk stress test result. She is referred to coronary angiography, where she is found to have a single severe stenosis (Fig. Q27-22). She undergoes IVUS-guided stenting; angiograms and IVUS images at various steps of the procedure are shown here.

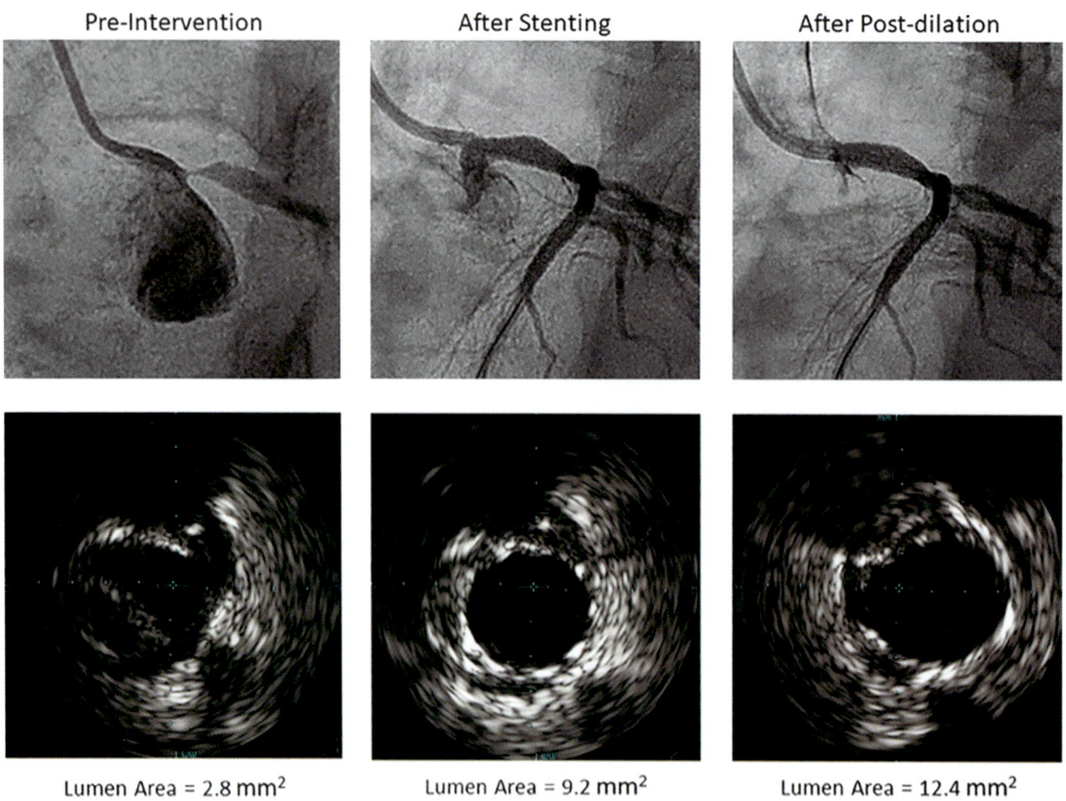

Figure Q27-22 (Courtesy of Khaled Ziada.)

Use of IVUS imaging in this setting is associated with all of the following, EXCEPT:

(A) Improved angiographic result
(B) Reduced need for repeat procedures
(C) Reduced risk of death or MI
(D) Reduced balloon utilization
(E) Reduced stent thrombosis

27.23 Compared to optical coherence tomography (OCT), IVUS imaging is associated with all of the following, EXCEPT:

(A) Lower resolution
(B) Lower penetration
(C) Better ability to define external elastic membrane (EEM) area
(D) Lower ability to define intraluminal thrombus
(E) Lower ability to define endothelial strut coverage

ANSWERS AND EXPLANATIONS

27.1 Answer C. As a general rule, the measurements on IVUS images are performed from the leading edge of an echo-dense layer to the leading edge of another echo-dense layer. The lumen area is defined as the area bound by the leading edge of the intima or the interface between the echo-dense intima and the echolucent blood elements in the lumen (line B on Fig. Q27-1B). The vessel area is the area bound by the EEM that can be identified as the interface between the leading edge of the echo-dense adventitia and the echo-lucent medial layer (line C on Fig. Q27-1B). Line A traces the acoustic artifact of the ultrasound catheter itself. Since the catheter is within the boundaries of the lumen, that tracing is not used for any clinical measurement. The difference between the lumen and EEM areas (lines B and C, respectively) represents the atheroma area. In fact, this area includes the atheroma and the thickness of the media. This has traditionally been accepted to avoid the inaccurate tracing around the trailing edge of the atheroma. In addition, the thickness of the medial layer is relatively unchanged by the presence or severity of disease. The minimum thickness of the atheroma can be measured (line D on Fig. Q27-1B) (Mintz GS, et al. *J Am Coll Cardiol* 2001;37(5):1478–1492; Ziada KM, et al. *Curr Probl Cardiol* 1999;24(9):541–566).

27.2 Answer B. In extensive coronary artery dissections, it is challenging to distinguish between the true and the false lumens. Usually, this is the first and most important step in bailout stenting, which is intended to restore flow in the true lumen and obliterate the false channel. Passage of the angioplasty wire in a side branch and/or injecting contrast through the distal tip of an over-the-wire balloon are some of the maneuvers used to confirm the position of the wire. However, this does not exclude the possibility of "fenestration" (i.e., that the wire passed from the false to the true lumen). IVUS imaging can assist in confirming the position of the wire before stenting. The two important features of the true lumen are the trilaminar appearance of the wall and the presence of side branches. Figure A27-2A shows a side branch (arrow) in continuity with the vessel lumen that is surrounding the IVUS catheter, confirming the catheter is in a true lumen. Figure A27-2B reveals the characteristic trilaminar appearance (arrows) of the true lumen with an intra-arterial wall hematoma (asterisk) seen in the false lumen. These findings confirm the true lumen position of the wire, and proceeding with PTCA/stenting would be the appropriate next step.

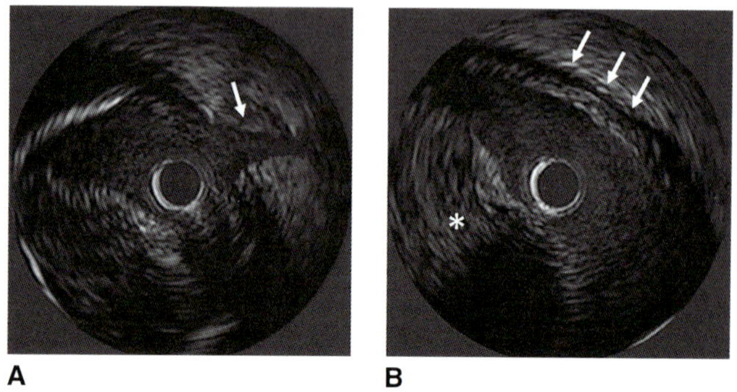

Figure A27-2

27.3 Answer D. IVUS-derived VH depends on advanced analysis of the radiofrequency backscatter of the ultrasound signal, using a larger number of parameters. Rather than just using the signal amplitude to define a shade of gray for each reflected line, this method utilizes a more complex mathematical autoregressive model to calculate the frequency spectrum from the region of interest (i.e., the coronary plaque) (Nair A, et al. *Circulation* 2002;106(17):2200–2206). The complex mathematical calculations do not lend themselves to quick interpretation by clinicians, hence the development of a simplified color-coded display (Fig. A27-3). Despite the improvement in differentiation between various tissue components of plaques, radiofrequency analysis remains unreliable in distinguishing between organizing thrombus and lipidic or soft plaques. The VH data provide incremental information from a more advanced analysis of the radiofrequency backscatter but do not directly influence the image resolution of the ultrasound image.

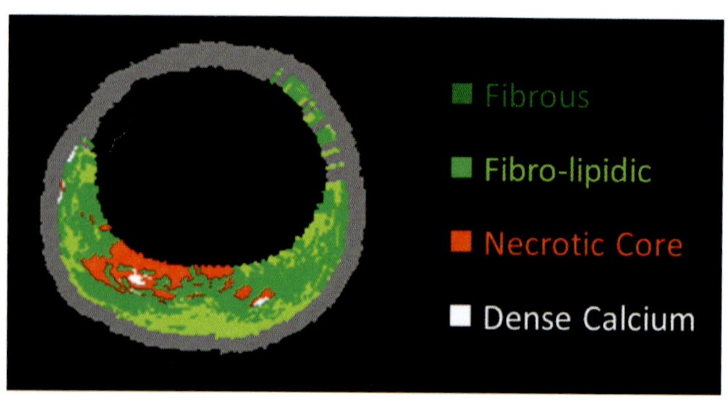

Figure A27-3

27.4 Answer C. In the absence of a reference segment to compare with, defining the severity of ostial left main trunk lesions can be difficult. In addition to the angiographic appearance, the absence of backflow of contrast into the aortic cusp when the catheter is engaged is a worrisome sign that significant ostial stenosis is present. An additional clue is the pressure waveform, which is "ventricularized" or shows "dampening" if the catheter is obstructing flow into the ostial left main trunk. However, pressure dampening can occur in the absence of a severe obstruction if the catheter tip is directed toward and makes contact with the arterial wall. In most cases of suspected left main lesions, an adjunctive modality is utilized to assess stenosis severity. This can be achieved by using a pressure wire and calculating the FFR or by IVUS imaging. Several studies have demonstrated the predictive value of the measurements obtained through either modality. An FFR $\geq$ 0.75 (or the more contemporary 0.80 threshold) predicts a low risk of death or cardiac events in the ensuing 2 to 3 years on medical therapy alone. Similarly, when an IVUS left main lumen area $\geq$5.9 mm^2 is correlated with an FFR $\geq$ 0.75, both measures strongly predict an event-free survival over a 3-year period. Given the stable clinical presentation and the lumen area exceeding 7 mm^2, placing a balloon pump and sending the patient to surgery for multivessel bypass would not provide any clinical benefit. FFR measurement in equivocal left main stenosis is appropriate and very useful in guiding therapy, but it would be redundant to perform both IVUS imaging and FFR measurement. With the availability of adjunctive modalities, such as the pressure wire and IVUS imaging, the decision about hemodynamic significance of such lesions can be made in the catheterization laboratory (Bech GJ, et al. *Heart* 2001;86(5):547–552; Jasti V, et al. *Circulation* 2004;110(18):2831–2836).

27.5 Answer B. There are few randomized trials that examined the role of IVUS guidance of stenting in comparison to the standard angiography-guided approaches. The majority of studies examining all comers demonstrated a trend favoring the IVUS-guided strategy in reducing the need for repeat revascularization, but most did not reach threshold of statistical significance. The IVUS-XPL randomized clinical trial (Hong SJ, et al. *JAMA* 2015;314(20):2155–2163) demonstrated a statistically significant advantage for IVUS guidance in reducing adverse events, but it was focused on long lesions only. However, retrospective studies and meta-analyses demonstrated that, in aggregate, an IVUS-guided strategy leads to larger acute lumen gain, less diameter reduction at follow-up, less angiographic restenosis, and less need for repeat revascularization (Parise H, et al. *Am J Cardiol* 2011;107(3):374–382; Jang JS, et al. *JACC Cardiovasc Interv* 2014;7(3):233–243; Witzenbichler B, et al. *Circulation* 2014;129(4):463–470). There is no conclusive evidence in any of the studies that the non-left main IVUS-guided strategy reduces the risk of the combined end point of death and MI. In most studies, the IVUS-guided approach was associated with increased utilization of balloons and number of balloon inflations.

27.6 Answer C. Clinical, ECG, and laboratory evidence confirm this patient sustained a non–ST-segment elevation myocardial infarction (STEMI), probably a few days before presentation. The angiograms reveal an area of haziness in the mid-LAD at the level of a diagonal bifurcation, although diameter reduction compared with the adjacent segments is not significant (Fig. A27-6A). Haziness could be the result of calcification of the arterial wall, but an important differential diagnosis for haziness in this context would be plaque rupture and/or overlying intraluminal thrombosis. Another possibility is an eccentric lesion that is more severe than what the angiogram reveals in this projection. In these situations, IVUS imaging can be very helpful in making the diagnosis. The risk of complications is small, with transient spasm being the most common. Typically, this can be avoided by intracoronary injection of nitroglycerin prior to advancing the IVUS catheter into the artery.

IVUS imaging revealed significant plaque burden with minimal calcification proximal to the diagonal bifurcation (Fig. A27-6B). The MLA (white border) was 3.4 mm^2, likely representing a hemodynamically severe stenosis. At the level of the bifurcation (Fig. A27-6C), there is evidence of plaque rupture, with flow communication (curved arrow) between the true LAD lumen and the ulcerated plaque "underneath" the fibrocalcific cap (arrow). On the basis of these findings, percutaneous or surgical revascularization would be more appropriate than medical therapy. In acute MI patients, the utility of FFR is not well studied, and with an area of 3.4 mm^2, the likelihood of FFR < 0.80 is over 85% (Takagi A, et al. *Circulation* 1999;100(3):250–255; Ziada KM, et al. *Curr Probl Cardiol* 1999;24(9):541–566) (Fig. A27-6A–C).

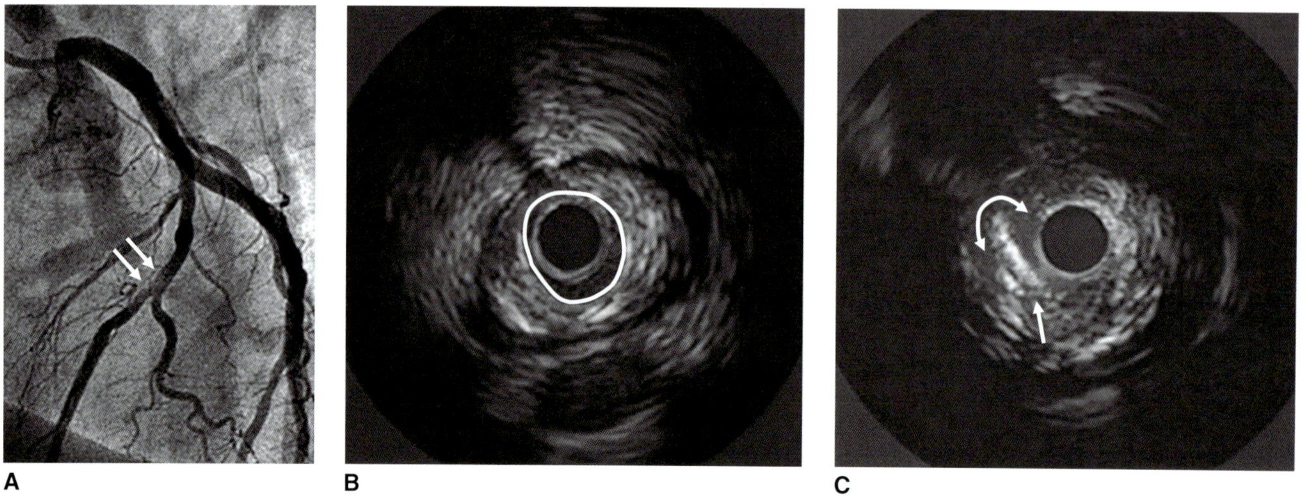

Figure A27-6

27.7 Answer C. In the REVERSAL trial, patients were randomly assigned to receive a moderate lipid-lowering therapy of pravastatin 40 mg/daily vs. a more intensive regimen of atorvastatin 80 mg/daily. An IVUS assessment of an angiographically mildly diseased coronary segment was performed upon enrollment and after 18 months. The primary end point of the study was the percentage change in TAV, which was computed as

$$\frac{\text{TAV}(\text{follow-up}) - \text{TAV}(\text{baseline})}{\text{TAV}(\text{baseline})} \times 100$$

The TAV was calculated as the sum of differences between EEM and lumen areas across all evaluable slices in the target segment. In the ASTEROID trial, a cohort of patients received 40 mg of rosuvastatin with IVUS imaging performed at baseline and after 24 months. The main metric examined in the study was the percent atheroma volume (PAV), which was computed as:

$$\frac{\sum(\text{EEM}_{\text{CSA}} - \text{LUMEN}_{\text{CSA}})}{\sum \text{EEM}_{\text{CSA}}} \times 100$$

where EEM_{CSA} is the EEM cross-sectional area and $\text{LUMEN}_{\text{CSA}}$ is the lumen cross-sectional area.

The primary end point of the study was the change in PAV, which was computed as the difference between PAV at follow-up imaging and PAV at baseline imaging.

In the moderate lipid-lowering (pravastatin) group, there was a positive change in the TAV, indicating net progression compared with baseline. In the intensive lipid-lowering (atorvastatin) arm, there was no evidence of progression in TAV compared with baseline. These findings suggested that intensive lipid lowering could result in arrest of disease progression. In the very intensive lipid-lowering (rosuvastatin) group, there was a significant reduction in PAV after 24 months of therapy, indicating regression of disease. Across all groups, there was a linear correlation between the change in measures of atheroma volume and the magnitude of reduction in LDL cholesterol. These studies were powered on the basis of the expected change in atheroma volume and did not enroll enough patients to detect differences in clinical outcomes (Nissen SE, et al. *JAMA* 2004;291(9):1071–1080; Nissen SE, et al. *JAMA* 2006;295(13):1556–1565).

27.8 Answer D. The serial ultrasound restenosis (SURE) study assessed patients who underwent coronary balloon angioplasty or atherectomy by serial angiographic and ultrasound examinations performed at preintervention, postintervention, 24-hour, 1-month, and 6-month follow-up. The serial examination of the treated lesion sites provided important insight into the remodeling responses and the mechanisms of late lumen loss or restenosis. Typically, lesions treated with balloon angioplasty or atherectomy undergo a biphasic remodeling response: A significant increase in vessel area between 24 hours and 1 month (adaptive remodeling) followed by a significant decrease (constrictive remodeling) between 1 and 6 months. At any point of time, the change in the vessel area (remodeling) was the most important determinant of the resultant lumen area. This correlation was much stronger than the correlation between changes in lumen area and those in plaque area. As for the mechanism of restenosis, the early adaptive remodeling response of the vessel was not different between lesions that did and did not develop restenosis, which meant that there was no apparent difference in vessel area at the 1-month time point. However, the constrictive remodeling response (between 1 and 6 months) was more significant in lesions that eventually developed restenosis compared with those that ended with a favorable outcome. In this study, IVUS imaging revealed a significant increase in lumen diameter between 24 hours and 1 month, which could not be identified by quantitative angiography (Kimura T, et al. *Circulation* 1997;96(2):475-483).

27.9 Answer C. As initially described by Glagov et al. in a necropsy study, arterial remodeling is the expansion of the EEM of the arterial wall at sites of atherosclerosis to accommodate atheroma volume and preserve lumen size. Stenoses develop when the ability of the artery to remodel is overcome by the progressive enlargement of the atheroma. This is known as positive or adaptive remodeling. Another form of arterial remodeling known as negative (or constrictive) remodeling is the local shrinkage of the vessel size at the site of disease, which has been implicated in stenotic atherosclerotic lesions and restenosis after balloon angioplasty. The IVUS investigators examining the phenomenon of remodeling compare the lesion of interest with a proximal reference segment free of disease and express a "remodeling index," which is calculated as the ratio of the EEM cross-sectional area at the lesion site to the EEM cross-sectional area at the proximal reference site. A remodeling index of >1.05 is consistent with positive remodeling, <0.95 is consistent with negative remodeling, and 0.95 to 1.05 is consistent with absence of remodeling. A positively remodeled atheroma is usually larger in size and more likely to present with unstable coronary syndromes (Schoenhagen P, et al. *Circulation* 2000;101(6):598-603; Schoenhagen P, et al. *J Am Coll Cardiol* 2001;38(2):297-306).

27.10 Answer B. This is a case of left main trunk dissection on engagement with a guiding catheter. The clue to the diagnosis was the change in the angiographic appearance of the left main trunk after the difficult engagement. IVUS imaging was used to confirm the diagnosis. There are two false channels in Figure A27-10 (arrows) and a developing intramural hematoma (asterisk), with the IVUS catheter artifact seen in the true lumen of the vessel. The false channels in cases of dissection and/or plaque rupture can be better visualized with saline or contrast injection while imaging, as this accentuates the difference in echo density between the lumen and the arterial wall structures. In addition, the injected fluid can be seen traveling from the true to the false lumen in real time. The left main coronary dissection requires urgent management. If the patient is hemodynamically stable or can be stabilized with the help of an IABP, then urgent coronary bypass surgery is probably the treatment of choice. If the patient is considered too unstable (e.g., severe ongoing ischemia, hypotension, and/or life-threatening ventricular arrhythmia), emergent stenting of the left main is an acceptable alternative. In either situation, the cardiac surgeon needs to be notified as soon as the diagnosis is made in the catheterization laboratory. Any elective PCI should be aborted and the situation should be managed immediately. A balloon pump would be helpful to support the patient's hemodynamics on the way to the surgery suite or if stenting of the left main trunk is considered, but not to support PCI of the circumflex artery.

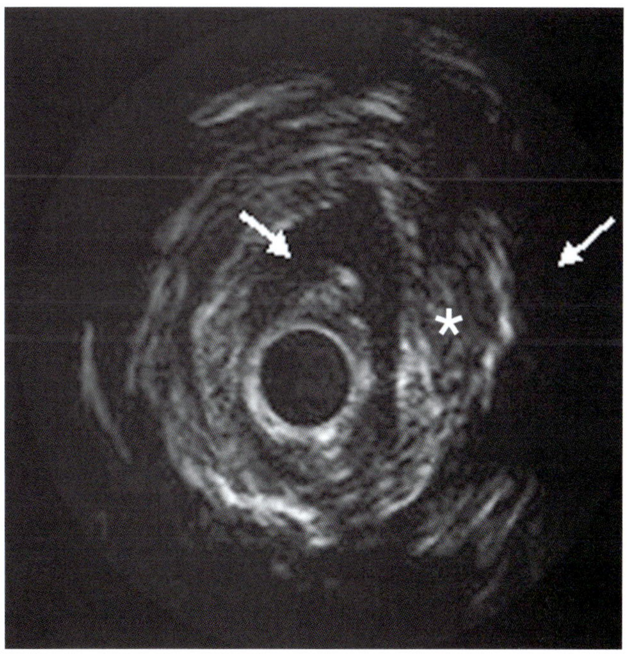

Figure A27-10

27.11 Answer D. IVUS imaging provides a detailed tomographic perspective of both the lumen and the wall of the artery. The IVUS findings frequently clarify and/or complement our understanding of the luminal silhouettes provided by contrast angiography. The American College of Cardiology (ACC)/American Heart Association (AHA) guidelines outline the clinical situations in which there is reasonable evidence for the benefit of IVUS imaging. These include assessment of the adequacy of stent deployment (measurement of the minimal in-stent lumen area and evaluating strut apposition), assessment of a suboptimal angiographic result after PCI, determination of the mechanism of restenosis to enable appropriate management, evaluation of coronary anatomy at a location difficult to image angiographically, and the preinterventional assessment of the coronary calcium extent and distribution in which use of an atherectomy device is contemplated. IVUS imaging may also be considered in the assessment of coronary atherosclerosis in patients with both characteristic angina and positive functional study without a clear angiographic lesion. IVUS is also the gold standard for the accurate identification and quantification of cardiac allograft vasculopathy or transplant coronary disease. There is no role for IVUS when an angiographic diagnosis is clear and there is no planned intervention (Smith SC Jr, et al. *Circulation* 2006;113(1):156–175).

27.12 Answer B. Figure Q27-12A shows the struts of a slotted-tube stent, which are seen as bright ultrasound reflections around the circumference of the artery. The presence of a layer of echolucent tissue (distinct from the speckle of blood elements in lumen) is evidence of intimal hyperplasia within the boundaries of the stent, thereby indicating that this stent has been implanted in this artery in a prior procedure. In this section, the intimal hyperplasia appears nonobstructive. Figure Q27-12B is obtained from a tight stenosis in a 5-year-old vein graft. The atheroma is heterogeneous in density but mostly echolucent. Vein graft lesions are typically echolucent in appearance and represent mixtures of lipid pools, collagen, and thrombotic material. In these lesions, heavy calcification is rare. The minimum lumen diameter is <2 mm. Figure Q27-12C is obtained from a native coronary artery at a bifurcation point. There is mild-to-moderate degree of atherosclerosis. The branch arising from the imaged vessel can be identified by following the continuity of the speckle of the blood elements around the IVUS catheter into the branch with an interruption of the layers of the wall (in the 5 o'clock direction). In this image, the wire artifact and its shadow are very apparent (in the 9 o'clock direction). Figure Q27-12D is obtained from a heavily calcified segment of a coronary artery. The arc of calcification occupies approximately three quadrants of the section and is seen as a bright echo with a shadow caused by the inability of the ultrasound beams to penetrate the tissue. Although this is not uncommon to see in native coronary arteries with advanced atherosclerosis, this degree of calcification does not typically develop in vein graft lesions (Motwani JG, et al. *Circulation* 1998;97(9):916–931).

27.13 Answer C. This is a case of a diffusely diseased LAD, in which the more severe segmental stenosis (shown in Fig. Q27-13C, left) is superimposed on moderate and diffuse disease (shown in Fig. Q27-13D and E, middle and right, respectively). Coronary angiograms are traditionally interpreted in a segmental fashion, where the least stenosed segment is assumed to be the "normal" reference to which the other segments are compared. In the presence of diffuse disease, this segmental approach to interpretation results in underestimation of stenosis severity. Another problem with angiographic interpretation is the projection of usually complex lumen shapes within stenosed segments onto a two-dimensional screen. Angiographers compensate by obtaining orthogonal views, but the choice of those projections is still arbitrary. Therefore, it is conceivable that the projection that would be perfectly perpendicular to the minimum lumen diameter may not be obtained. In this case, IVUS imaging did demonstrate a severe stenosis in the midvessel with a minimum lumen diameter of <2 mm and an area of <4 mm^2. These measurements indicate a hemodynamically significant stenosis that is likely to cause ischemia on a stress test. This minimum lumen area by IVUS has a good correlation with an FFR of <0.75, which explains why the stress test was positive, despite the apparently "moderate" narrowing on angiography. The degree of narrowing in a bifurcation lesion can be difficult to angiographically assess, but that does not apply to a tomographic imaging modality such as IVUS. The branching point of the diagonal branch is not seen in any of the images shown here. In all the three images, the interruption of the circumference of the arterial wall is caused by the shadow of the wire artifact (Takagi A, et al. *Circulation* 1999;100(3):250–255; Ziada KM, et al. *Curr Probl Cardiol* 1999;24(9):541–566).

27.14 Answer A. The IVUS image shows an echolucent plaque with small areas of echogenicity, suggesting a primarily lipidic or necrotic core composition. These lesions, when located in proximal vessels, were considered ideal for directional atherectomy, although it is not commonly used currently. Aggressive atherectomy, guided by repeat IVUS, results in significant debulking and improved stent expansion and acute lumen gain; however, there has been no evidence of reduction in restenosis with this approach. Pretreatment with rotational atherectomy has not been shown to improve acute or late outcomes. It remains useful in heavily calcified lesions where stents cannot be delivered or adequately expanded. IVUS imaging is not a reliable tool for identification of intracoronary thrombus. The echogenic characteristics of thrombus are similar to heterogeneous plaque. In certain situations, a thrombus can be identified in the context of an acute MI and when it is located within the lumen (Kim YH, et al. *Am Heart J* 2004;148(4):663-669; Stankovic G, et al. *Am J Cardiol* 2004;93(8):953-958).

27.15 Answer C. In-stent restenosis is a result of neointimal hyperplasia within the boundaries of the stented segment. Neointimal growth is uniformly distributed throughout the stent. Late lumen loss within the stented segments is directly proportional to the degree of neointimal hyperplasia. Slotted-tube stents abolish the negative remodeling response that is the primary driver of restenosis following balloon angioplasty. Therefore, the correlation between late loss and negative remodeling (shrinkage of the vessel area) is very weak in the stented segment. However, negative remodeling is more apparent in the few millimeters of the artery just distal to the edge of the stent and is the primary mechanism of late loss in this region of the artery. These changes are seen equally in native coronaries and SVGs, as well as in lesions treated with one or two stents. IVUS late lumen loss was found to correlate with, but was consistently smaller than, angiographic late lumen loss (Hoffmann R, et al. *Circulation* 1996;94(6):1247-1254).

27.16 Answer B. In the PROSPECT trial, approximately 700 ACS patients underwent angiography and revascularization if needed. Three-vessel IVUS imaging and VH analysis were performed. Patients who developed events over the ensuing 3 years underwent repeat angiography and imaging. Adverse events were related to an originally nonculprit lesion in 11.6% of patients. Lesion characteristics that predicted development of future events included plaque burden ≥70%, MLA ≤ 4 mm^2, and thin-cap fibroatheroma (TCFA) on IVUS-derived VH. The presence of more than one feature increased the risk of future events (Fig. A27-16).

The VH images demonstrate a variety of plaque types. (A) is a fibrotic plaque consisting mainly of fibrotic plaque (dark green) with <10% necrotic core (red) and <10% dense calcification (white). (B) and (C) are TCFAs characterized by the presence of >10% confluent necrotic core (red) and >30 degrees of the necrotic core abutting the lumen. (B) is more likely to cause future events because the plaque burden is larger and the lumen is smaller. (D) is a thick-cap fibroatheroma, which contains >10% necrotic core (red), but that is separated from the lumen by a thicker fibrotic layer (green) (Stone GW, et al. *N Engl J Med* 2011;364(3):226-235).

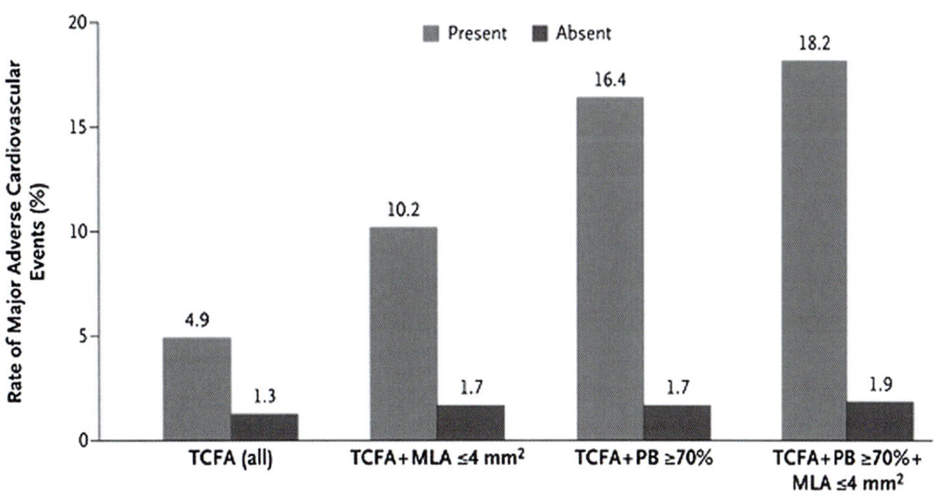

Figure A27-16

27.17 Answer A. This patient developed angina due to drug-eluting in-stent restenosis. IVUS imaging provided significant insight into mechanisms and patterns of DES restenosis. Although late loss is frequently diffusely distributed, significant intimal hyperplasia leading to >50% diameter reduction is focal in about half the cases. In the IVUS image shown, there are two mechanisms of restenosis: an underexpansion at the time of stent implantation and intimal hyperplasia that developed over time (Fig. A27-17A).

Underexpansion is defined as a procedural result with minimal stent area <5 mm^2, which is the area bound by the dashed black circle (Fig. A27-17B). The stent could have been better expanded or a larger stent may have been used given the size of the vessel (bound by the solid white circle). Selecting a smaller stent or accepting a smaller minimal lumen diameter is not uncommon in primary PCI because of the increased vessel tone that affects the angiographic reference size and can lead to underestimation of the true diameter. Intimal hyperplasia is significant when it occupies >50% of the stent area (area bound between the dashed black circle and the inner solid black circle demarcating the intimal leading edge). In restenosis of longer stents, underexpansion is seen in more than one third of cases, and the mechanism of diameter reduction is frequently a combination of underexpansion and intimal hyperplasia, as shown here. In shorter stents (≤28 mm), restenosis is primarily driven by intimal hyperplasia alone (Kang SJ, et al. *Circ Cardiovasc Interv* 2011;4(1):9–14).

27.18 Answer B. Following high-pressure stenting, a small postprocedure minimum in-stent lumen area is the most important predictor of TVR. IVUS criteria for optimal stent deployment emphasize achieving the largest possible in-stent lumen area. Increasing the in-stent lumen area usually requires larger balloons and/or higher inflation pressures; however, that would be limited by the reference vessel size. Panels A and D of the figure depict stents with relatively small lumen areas, which predispose a high risk of stent thrombosis on the short term and restenosis on the long term. Panels C depict a stent with gross mal-apposition of struts. Historically, such degrees of mal-apposition were commonly observed before routine use of high-pressure inflations and were considered a precipitating factor for stent thrombosis. In all three situations, operators typically resort to higher inflation pressures and/or balloon oversizing. Panel B depicts a well-expanded and well-opposed stent struts with a minimum area exceeding 7 mm^2. Even with bare metal stents (BMS), such lumen areas are associated with TVR rates in the single digits (da Jaegere P, et al. *Eur Heart J* 1998;19(8):1214–1223; Goldberg SL, et al. *J Am Coll Cardiol* 1994;24(4):996–1003; Ziada KM, et al. *Am Heart J* 2001;141(5):823–831).

27.19 Answer C. IVUS findings in DES patients presenting with very late stent thrombosis provide useful insights into the possible mechanisms of this serious clinical problem. IVUS findings in 13 DES patients with very late thrombosis were compared to 144 control DES patients who underwent imaging and had no documented stent thrombosis. Patients with very late stent thrombosis had

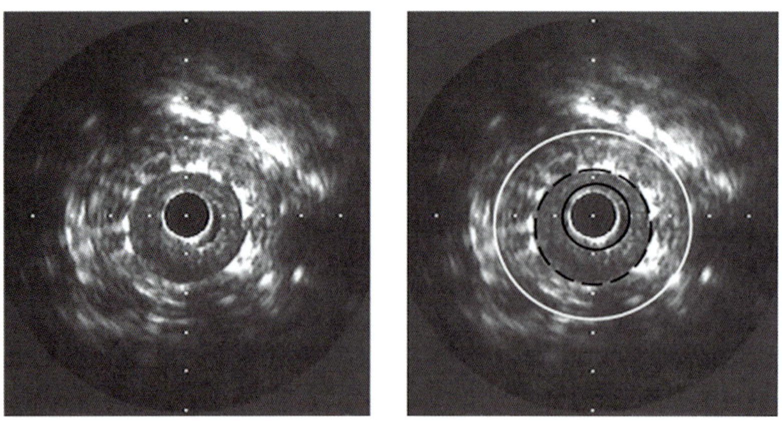

A B

Figure A27-17

longer stents, more overlapping stents, and more stents per lesion. The prevalence of incomplete strut apposition was 77% in the thrombosis group compared with 12% in the control group. There was no difference in reference segment vessel area, but the in-stent vessel area was significantly larger in the thrombosis group, indicating more positive remodeling (Cook S, et al. *Circulation* 2007;115(18):2426–2434). The high prevalence of incomplete strut apposition in stented segments presenting with late and very late thrombosis was confirmed in another small retrospective study that included 23 DES patients (Lee CW, et al. *J Am Coll Cardiol* 2010;55(18):1936–1942). The role of strut mal-apposition vs. that of a small in-stent lumen area remains debatable. In another small retrospective IVUS study, 15 patients with thrombosis and 45 control patients were examined. There was no difference in the prevalence of mal-apposition. However, stent area was significantly smaller in those who developed stent thrombosis (4.3 ± 1.6 mm^2 vs. 6.2 ± 1.9 mm^2, $p < 0.001$) compared to the matched controls. Additionally, severe reference segment disease was more common in the stent thrombosis group (Fujii K, et al. *J Am Coll Cardiol* 2005;45(7):995–998).

27.20 Answer A. When an intermediate lesion is encountered, further assessment of the lesion can be accomplished either by functional assessment using pressure or flow measurements or by morphologic delineation using IVUS imaging. FFR cutoff values of 0.75 to 0.80 have been correlated with short- and long-term clinical data; lesions with an FFR > 0.80 are associated with favorable clinical outcomes with no need for revascularization. The cutoff values for IVUS measurements that identify hemodynamically significant lesions have mostly been determined by correlation with FFR. In a study of 51 lesions in 42 stable patients, the IVUS measurements that maximized the sensitivity and specificity of the correlation with IVUS were minimum lumen area <3.0 mm^2 and area stenosis >60%. The combination of both criteria (lumen area <3.0 mm^2 and area stenosis >60%) had 100% sensitivity and specificity (Takagi A, et al. *Circulation* 1999;100(3):250–255) for identifying significant lesions. In another study of 53 lesions, a minimal luminal area $\leq$4 mm^2 and an area stenosis >70% were the best indicators of hemodynamic significance, as determined by an FFR < 0.75 (Briguori C, et al. *Am J Cardiol* 2001;87(2):136–141). Retrospective analysis of 1-year clinical outcomes after deferring PCI (357 intermediate lesions in 300 patients), the only independent predictors of an event (death, MI, or target lesion revascularization) were IVUS minimum lumen area and area stenosis. In lesions with a minimum area $\geq$4.0 mm^2, the event rate was acceptably low to allow reasonably safe deferral of PCI (Abizaid AS, et al. *Circulation* 1999;100(3):256–261). Other datasets suggest that a cutoff lumen area of 4 mm^2 has a very high specificity when correlated with an FFR threshold of 0.80, whereas the association between FFR and IVUS-derived lumen area <4 mm^2 can be quite variable (Ben Dor I, et al. *Cardiovasc Revasc Med* 2012;13(3):177–182). In this example, IVUS interrogation of this lesion reveals an eccentric heterogeneous plaque with minimal calcification. The lumen area and the area stenosis are consistent with a hemodynamically nonsignificant lesion that requires no revascularization but does warrant secondary prevention with statin therapy.

27.21 Answer D. In complex CTO PCI, it is sometimes difficult to define all variables needed for decision making using angiography alone. Vessels are typically diffusely and heavily diseased, dissections can occur with use of stiff wires and the distal cap of the occluded segment is commonly difficult to penetrate, leading to creation of false channels and dissection flaps. Advancing a low-profile IVUS catheter over the wire can help the operator determine whether the wire is in the true or false lumen, the extent of the dissection and potentially facilitate the reentry into the true lumen by allowing the visualization of both lumens with the flap in between. Additionally, IVUS imaging in a branching point can facilitate the localization of an ambiguous ostium of an occluded vessel (flush occlusions). In fact, in certain circumstances, this can even facilitate identification of the wire course into the occluded branch by examining the far field of the image. Typically, reference segments are underestimated by angiographic assessments due to distal vessel under filling and diffuse disease. IVUS imaging typically results in selection of a larger stent diameter than would have been using angiography alone.

27.22 Answer D. Recent evidence suggests a strong association between use of IVUS to guide stenting of the left main trunk and improved clinical outcomes, including reduction in overall mortality, need for revascularization, and stent thrombosis. Most of the data are derived from retrospective analyses, but those have been consistent and groups were propensity matched (Park SJ, et al. *Circ Cardiovasc Interv* 2009;2(3):167–177; de la Torre Hernandez JM, et al. *JACC Cardiovasc Interv* 2014;7(3):244–254; Andell P, et al. *Circ Cardiovasc Interv* 2017;10(5). pii: e004813). The improvement in clinical outcomes is probably driven by the reduced risk of restenosis and stent thrombosis, which is facilitated by IVUS imaging due to the larger stent lumen area and reduced risk of strut malapposition. IVUS imaging frequently results in additional use of larger balloons to achieve a larger MLA, as was the case here (center and left panels demonstrate improved angiographic and ultrasound size of lumen with use of a larger postdilation balloon).

27.23 **Answer B.** There is little debate that the higher resolution of OCT has some advantages over IVUS imaging: (1) improved spatial resolution (20 to 40 μm) that allows better definition of TCFA and dissection flaps and (2) diagnosis of intraluminal thrombus. The higher resolution also allows for the identification of very thin layers of neointima covering stent struts, which have opened a potential area of research related to timing of strut coverage and the potential role in determining the duration of dual antiplatelet therapy. However, there are certain advantages to IVUS imaging that remain relevant despite its lower resolution. The use of light waves in OCT imaging does not allow penetration and imaging of the full thickness of the arterial wall (i.e., OCT provides exquisite resolution but only of the luminal 1 to 2 mm of the wall). Thus, deeper structures that can influence the strategy and result of an interventional procedure (such as deep calcification and/or dense fibrous plaques) may not be adequately visualized with OCT. The better penetration of IVUS imaging allows measurement of the EEM, which in turn allows measurement of plaque thickness and volume—measures of plaque burden that have been shown to define future risk of clinical events in the PROSPECT trial. These measurements are also essential for study of phenomena such as remodeling, disease progression, and/or response to therapeutic interventions.

28 Approach to Patients with Hemodynamic Compromise

Zoran S. Nedeljkovic and Alice K. Jacobs

QUESTIONS

28.1 In performing transjugular endomyocardial biopsy, which of the following patients is at highest risk of hemodynamic deterioration in the event of cardiac perforation?

(A) A 30-year-old man undergoing routine biopsy 12 months following cardiac transplantation with a left ventricular ejection fraction (LVEF) of 60%

(B) A 22-year-old woman with HIV, idiopathic dilated cardiomyopathy, and normal right ventricular size and systolic function

(C) A 58-year-old man with severe biventricular enlargement and dysfunction and LVEF of 20%

(D) A 60-year-old man with severely increased left ventricular (LV) wall thickness and LVEF of 55%

28.2 A 36-year-old man undergoes diagnostic coronary and LV angiography for evaluation of chest pain. His cardiac examination is notable for the presence of a mid-peaking systolic ejection murmur, best heard at the left sternal border without radiation. His lungs are clear to auscultation. His electrocardiogram (ECG) shows left ventricular hypertrophy with secondary repolarization abnormalities. His coronary angiogram demonstrates normal left and right coronary arteries, and LV angiography reveals normal systolic function. A simultaneous LV and femoral arterial pressure tracing is shown below (Fig. Q28-2).

The procedure was uneventful, but later during recovery, the patient complains of chest pain and light-headedness. On physical examination, his

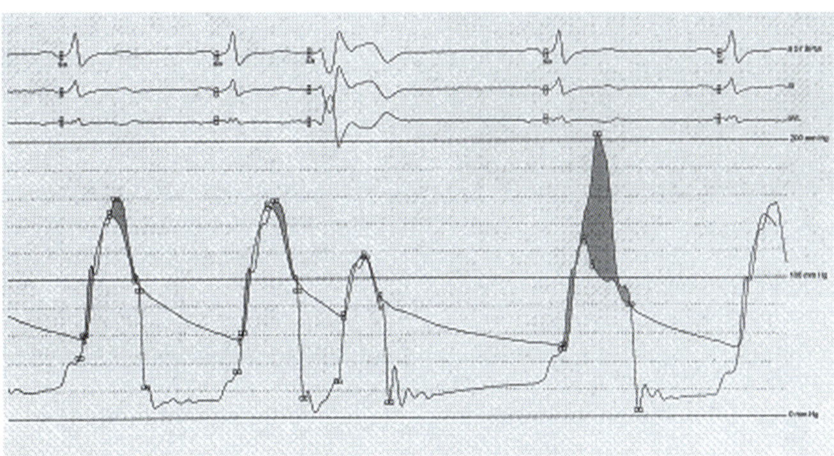

Figure Q28-2

blood pressure is 70/50 mm Hg with a heart rate of 88 beats per minute (bpm). He appears diaphoretic, and his extremities are cool. In addition to administration of intravenous (IV) fluids, which of the following should be administered?

(A) Atropine
(B) Dopamine
(C) Dobutamine
(D) Phenylephrine

28.3 A 66-year-old woman with a history of hypertension and hyperlipidemia undergoes diagnostic coronary angiography for an abnormal exercise stress test. The patient receives standard premedication for the procedure, including midazolam and fentanyl. The catheter is advanced around the aortic arch without difficulty, and the left main coronary is engaged. The initial single-frame cineangiogram of her left coronary artery is shown below (Fig. Q28-3).

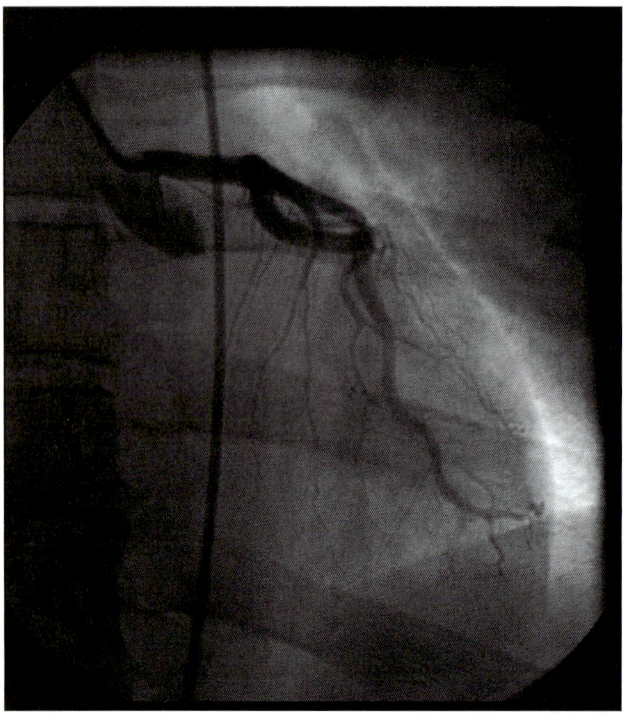

Figure Q28-3

The patient suddenly complains of shortness of breath and chest pain. Physical examination is notable for a blood pressure of 82/50 mm Hg, a heart rate of 94 bpm, a respiratory rate of 24 per minute, and an oxygen saturation of 92%. Cardiac examination reveals no murmurs or gallops, and her lungs demonstrate diffuse inspiratory and expiratory wheezing. Which of the following should be done next?

(A) Switch to a lower osmolar iodinated contrast agent
(B) Repeat left coronary angiography to exclude dissection of the left main coronary artery
(C) Administer diphenhydramine, antihistamines, and epinephrine
(D) Administer flumazenil to reverse the effects of the benzodiazepine

28.4 Which of the following hemodynamic profiles is most consistent with cardiogenic shock secondary to inferior wall myocardial infarction (MI) with right ventricular involvement (Table Q28-4)?

(Note: Table has the answer choices.)

Table Q28-4

RA	RV	PA	PCWP	Ao	CO	SVR
3	20/3	20/8	7	88/56	3.2	1590
15	35/14	36/15	15	85/60	3.0	1800
2	22/3	24/8	8	82/40	7.2	600
15	50/18	52/28	30	90/62	2.9	1550

Abbreviations: Ao, aortic pressure measured in mm Hg; CO, cardiac output expressed in liters/minute; PA, pulmonary arterial; PCWP, pulmonary capillary wedge pressure; RA, right atrial; RV, right ventricular; SVR, systemic vascular resistance in dynes-s-cm^{-5}.

28.5 A 50-year-old man presents to the hospital with worsening substernal chest discomfort that began 3 hours ago while shoveling snow. He has no significant past medical history and takes no medications. His risk factors for cardiovascular disease include current tobacco use and a family history of premature coronary artery disease (CAD). On arrival to the emergency room, his blood pressure is 100/70 mm Hg and heart rate is 84 bpm. His lung fields are clear to auscultation and percussion, and cardiovascular examination is notable for normal heart sounds and no audible murmurs. His ECG shows 2 mm of ST-segment elevation in leads II, III, and aVF, with 1-mm ST depression in leads V1 to V3.

He is taken to the cardiac catheterization laboratory for emergency percutaneous revascularization. Angiography of the left coronary artery is normal. A single-frame cineangiogram of the right coronary artery before and after dilation of the stenosis with a 2.5-mm balloon is shown below (Fig. Q28-5A,B).

The patient subsequently complains of nausea and vomits. The hemodynamic tracing from the monitor is shown below (Fig. Q28-5C).

Which of the following would you do next?

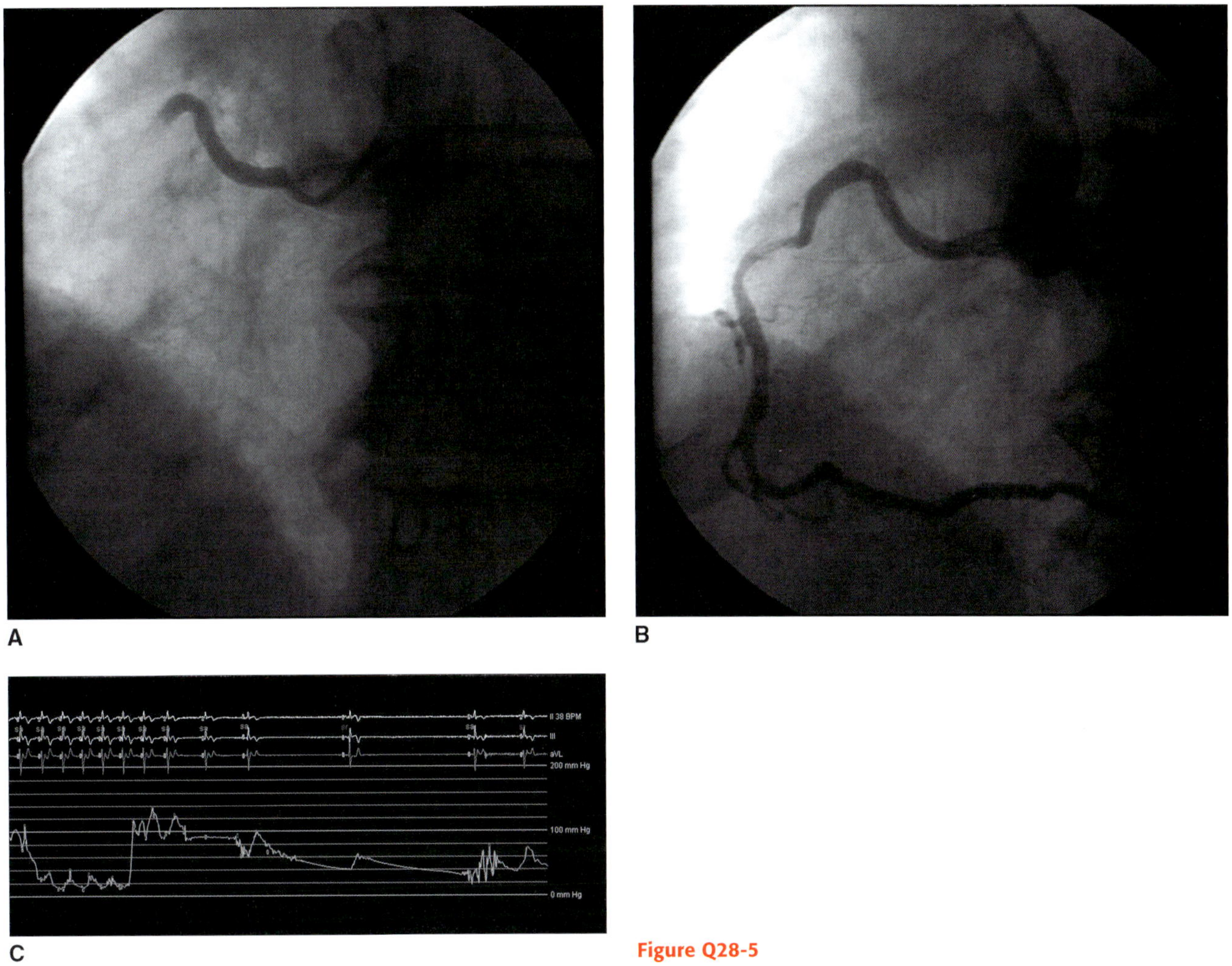

Figure Q28-5

(A) Reinflation of the angioplasty balloon in the proximal segment of the coronary artery and preparation for emergency pericardiocentesis
(B) Administration of atropine and IV fluids
(C) Insertion of a temporary transvenous pacemaker
(D) Administration of dopamine

28.6 Which of the following is associated with the greatest risk of coronary perforation during percutaneous coronary intervention (PCI)?

(A) Rotational atherectomy of a stenosis in the mid-portion of a tortuous right coronary artery
(B) Balloon angioplasty of a densely calcified proximal left anterior descending (LAD) artery stenosis using a high-pressure balloon
(C) Stent placement in a stenosis in the proximal right coronary artery following failed fibrinolysis for an acute inferior wall MI
(D) Stent placement in a stenosis in the mid-portion of a saphenous vein graft (SVG) to the obtuse marginal branch

28.7 A 68-year-old woman is undergoing rotational atherectomy of an angulated lesion in the mid-right coronary artery with a 1.5-mm burr. Her blood pressure suddenly drops to 70/30 mm Hg, and angiography demonstrates contrast extravasation into the pericardial space. In preparation for emergency pericardiocentesis for cardiac tamponade, protamine sulfate should be given if which of the following antithrombotic agents was used during PCI?

(A) Heparin
(B) Enoxaparin
(C) Bivalirudin
(D) Lepirudin

28.8 A 59-year-old man presents to the hospital with chest pain and is found to have anterior T-wave inversions and an elevated cardiac troponin. He is treated with aspirin, prasugrel, and unfractionated heparin (UFH). He is taken to the cardiac catheterization laboratory, and following angiography of the left coronary artery, he complains of severe chest pain with evidence of ST-segment elevation on the monitor. His blood pressure is 80/40 mm Hg with a heart rate of 90 bpm. A single-frame cineangiogram of the left coronary artery in the right anterior oblique (RAO) projection with caudal angulation is shown below (Fig. Q28-8).

Which of the following should be done next?

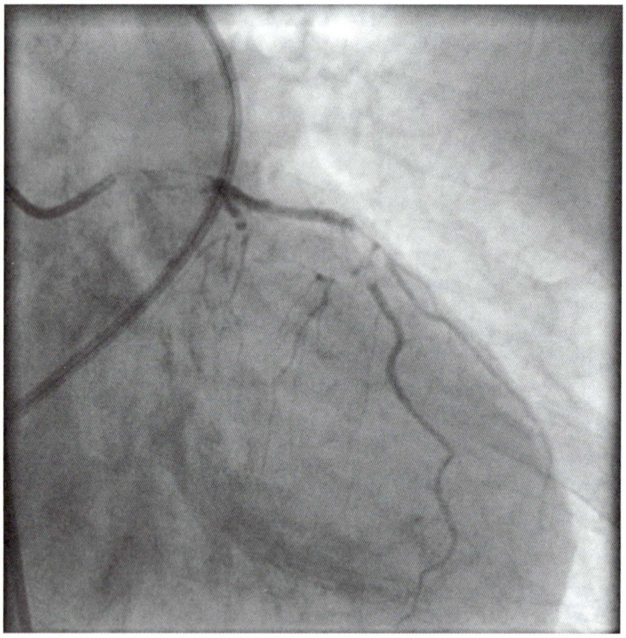

Figure Q28-8

(A) Insertion of an intra-aortic balloon pump (IABP)
(B) Emergent coronary artery bypass graft (CABG) surgery for dissection of the left main coronary artery
(C) Administration of 100% oxygen
(D) Administration of bivalirudin and preparation for emergency PCI of the left main and LAD arteries

28.9 A 54-year-old man undergoes rescue angioplasty following unsuccessful reperfusion with fibrinolytic therapy for an acute anterior wall MI. Coronary angiography reveals thrombotic occlusion of the proximal LAD artery with no other significant epicardial coronary disease. Following initial balloon inflation across the stenosis in the proximal LAD artery, there is restoration of antegrade flow. The ECG and arterial pressure from the guiding catheter are shown below (Fig. Q28-9).

Which of the following should be done next?

(A) Administration of bolus and infusion of amiodarone
(B) Administration of bolus and infusion of lidocaine
(C) Observation
(D) Direct-current cardioversion

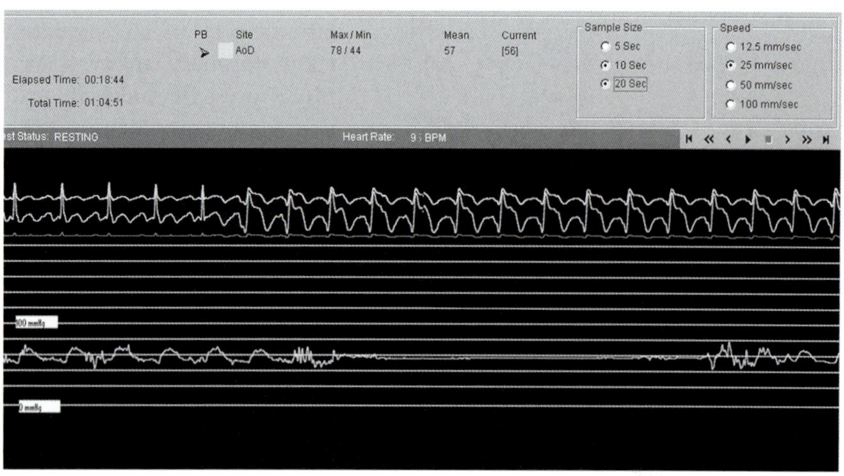

Figure Q28-9

28.10 A 68-year-old woman with a past history of well-controlled hypertension presents to the hospital with several days of intermittent substernal chest pressure and shortness of breath. On arrival to the emergency room, her blood pressure is 90/70 mm Hg, heart rate is 105 bpm, and respiratory rate is 26 breaths per minute. She is diaphoretic and in visible respiratory distress. Cardiovascular examination is notable for a jugular venous pressure of 8 cm, rales at the bases of both lung fields, and a 3/6 harsh systolic murmur at the left sternal border. Her extremities are cool. Her ECG reveals sinus tachycardia with 2 mm ST-segment elevation in leads V1 to V4 and 1 mm ST-segment depression in leads II, III, and aVF. Her baseline complete blood count, serum electrolytes, and renal function are normal.

She is given aspirin and heparin and undergoes endotracheal intubation for airway support. She is taken to the cardiac catheterization laboratory for emergency angiography. Single-frame cineangiogram in the left anterior oblique (LAO)-cranial projection of her left coronary and LV angiogram are shown below. The next most appropriate course of action would be (Fig. Q28-10A,B):

(A) Administration of bivalirudin followed by primary PCI of the LAD artery
(B) Insertion of an IABP followed by primary PCI of the LAD artery
(C) Primary PCI of the LAD artery and referral for emergency cardiac surgery
(D) Insertion of an IABP and referral for emergency cardiac surgery

28.11 A 70-year-old man is transferred to a tertiary hospital with cardiogenic shock secondary to an anterior wall MI. He presented to the referring hospital with several days of intermittent chest discomfort that became persistent over the last 12 hours. His ECG showed anterior ST elevation in leads V1 to V4, with Q waves in those leads. He is treated with aspirin and UFH, and dopamine is titrated to 5 mcg/kg/min.

On arrival to the catheterization laboratory, his blood pressure is 90/60 mm Hg and heart rate is 100 bpm. A grade 3 systolic murmur is heard over the left sternal border and rales are heard over the lower lung fields.

What is the most appropriate sequence of events to be performed in the catheterization laboratory?

(A) Coronary angiography followed by PCI
(B) Coronary angiography followed by bypass surgery
(C) Right heart catheterization followed by coronary angiography
(D) No cardiac catheterization as presentation is beyond the window of myocardial salvage

28.12 A 49-year-old woman undergoes diagnostic cardiac catheterization via the right femoral artery for evaluation of chest pain and an abnormal stress test. Coronary angiography reveals nonobstructive CAD. The 5-Fr arterial sheath is removed in the laboratory, and manual pressure is applied to achieve hemostasis. She is transferred to the recovery area and, after 45 minutes, develops nausea with an urge

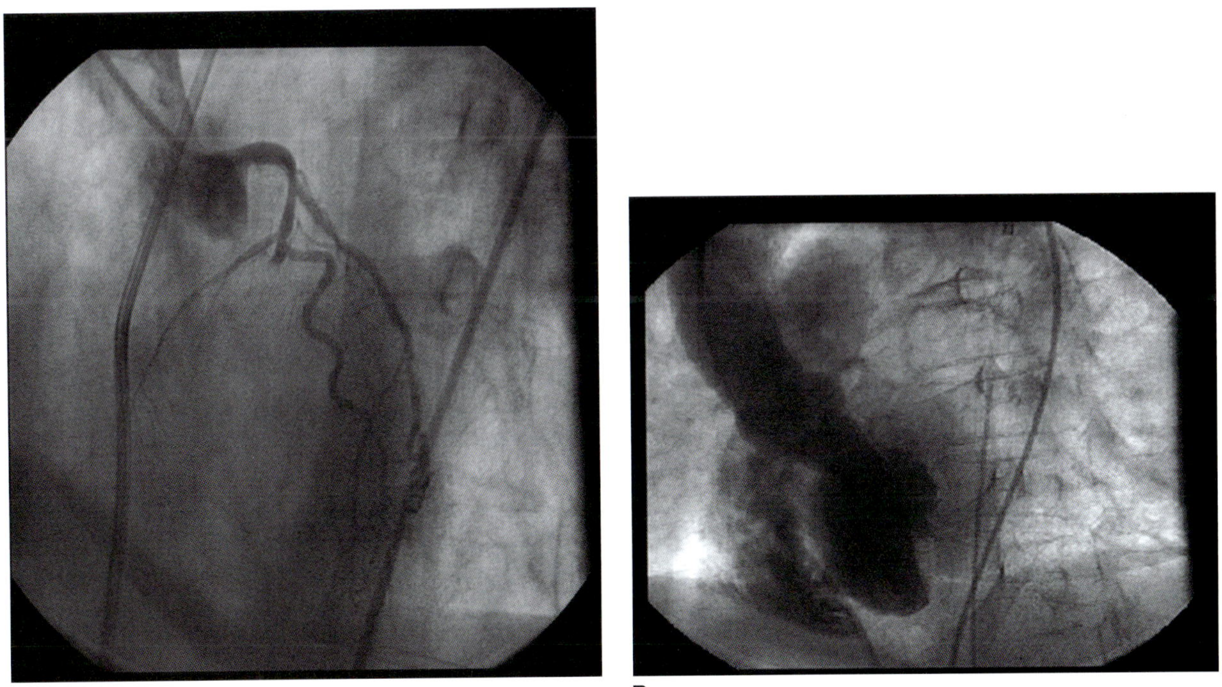

A B

Figure Q28-10

to vomit. Her blood pressure is 80/40 mm Hg, and her heart rate is 60 bpm. On examination, there is a small amount of blood saturating the dressing over the femoral arteriotomy, but no hematoma. She is brought back into the laboratory, and angiography of the right femoral artery is performed via the contralateral approach (pictured below) (Fig. Q28-12).

What would be the most rapid means of achieving hemostasis in this patient?

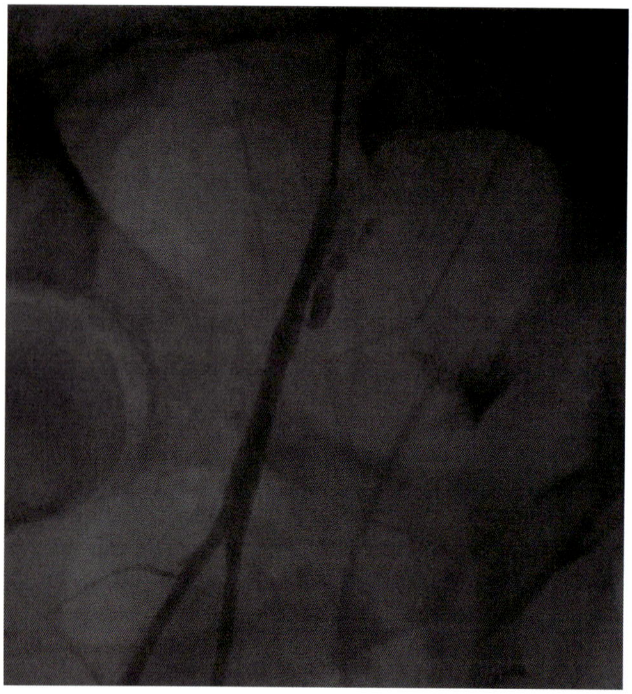

Figure Q28-12

(A) Surgical consultation for operative repair
(B) Prolonged manual pressure of the right femoral arteriotomy
(C) A trial of balloon occlusion with insertion of a covered stent if bleeding persists
(D) Transfusion of packed red blood cells and platelets

28.13 A 40-year-old woman undergoes LV angiography for evaluation of severe mitral insufficiency secondary to degenerative mitral valve disease, prior to coronary angiography. Following injection of radiographic contrast material at a rate of 15 mL/s for a total of 45 mL, she develops bradycardia associated with nausea and vomiting. What should be done next?

(A) Administer IV steroid and antihistamine
(B) Abort further angiography
(C) Switch to low-osmolar contrast agent
(D) Insert temporary transvenous pacemaker prior to further angiography

28.14 A 52-year-old man presents to the emergency department with 3 days of intermittent chest discomfort and progressively increasing fatigue and shortness of breath. Prior to being brought to the hospital, he had a near syncopal episode. Four weeks prior, he underwent minimally invasive bioprosthetic aortic valve replacement for a stenotic bicuspid aortic valve. On examination, his blood pressure is 90/60 mm Hg, and auscultation reveals clear lung fields and no audible murmur. His ECG is shown below (Fig. Q28-14).

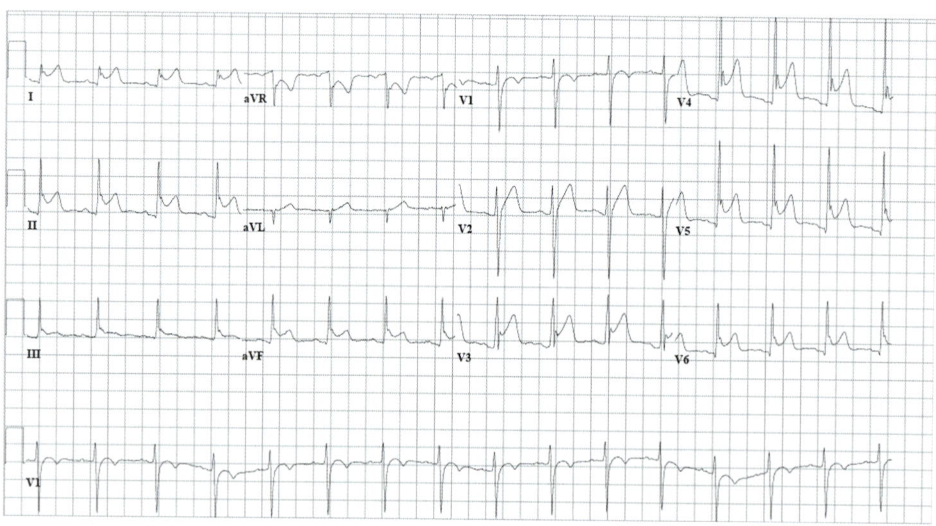

Figure Q28-14

IV fluids are administered. What should be the next step in his management?

(A) Administer aspirin and UFH, and perform urgent coronary angiography
(B) Echocardiography
(C) Insertion of temporary transvenous pacemaker
(D) Prescribe colchicine, a nonsteroidal anti-inflammatory drug, and discharge from emergency department

28.15 Benefits of the left atrium-to-femoral artery bypass (TandemHeart) percutaneous circulatory assist device include all of the following, EXCEPT:

(A) Decrease in pulmonary capillary wedge pressure (PCWP)
(B) Increase in myocardial oxygen demand
(C) Increase in mean arterial pressure
(D) Increase in cardiac output

28.16 A 68-year-old woman with hypertension undergoes cardiac catheterization for unstable angina. Coronary angiography demonstrated mild disease of the LAD and left circumflex (LCx) arteries. There were serial lesions in the mid and distal right coronary artery (pictured below) (Fig. Q28-16A).

The patient was pretreated with aspirin and clopidogrel, and bivalirudin was used for

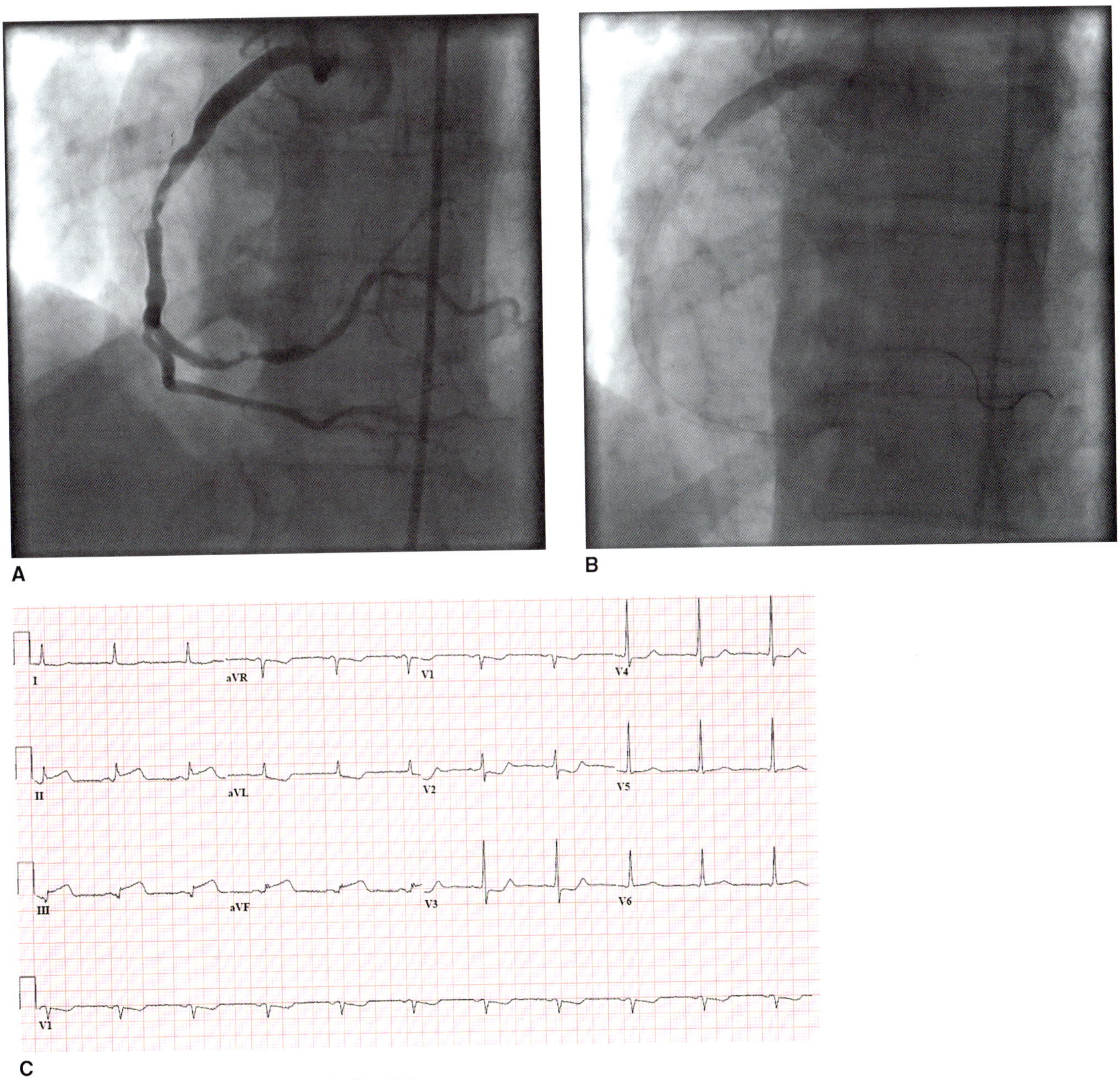

Figure Q28-16 (Courtesy of Zoran Nedeljkovic.)

anticoagulation. Following stent placement across both lesions, thrombolysis in myocardial infarction (TIMI) grade 1 flow was observed that was associated with chest pain. The angiogram is pictured below with the 12-lead ECG (Fig. Q28-16B,C).

Which of the following is the next best step in the management of this condition?

(A) Administration of intracoronary (IC) fibrinolytic therapy
(B) Administration of systemic glycoprotein (GP) IIb/IIIa inhibitor
(C) Administration of IC sodium nitroprusside
(D) Continued observation

28.17 A patient is undergoing PCI of a calcified stenosis in the mid-right coronary artery. The lesion is predilated with a 2.5-mm semicompliant balloon, which fails to expand at the site of the narrowing. The balloon is exchanged for a 2.75-mm semicompliant balloon. Following dilation of the balloon, the following arterial pressure tracing is observed (Fig. Q28-17).

Which of the following adverse events should be suspected?

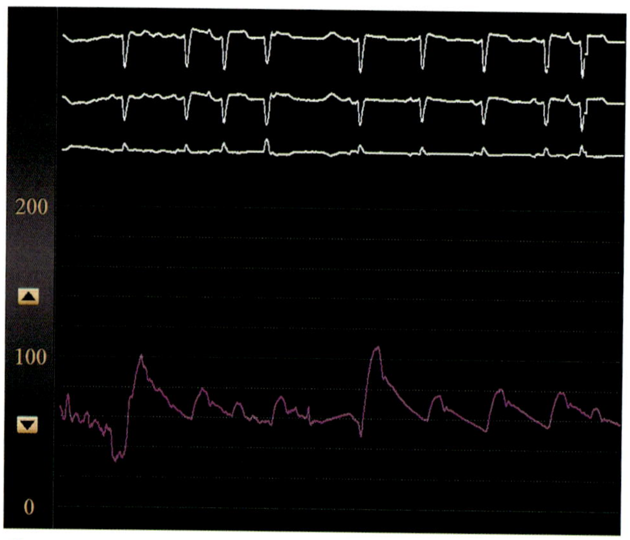

Figure Q28-17 (Courtesy of Zoran Nedeljkovic.)

(A) Abrupt vessel closure
(B) Coronary perforation
(C) Coronary dissection
(D) Distal coronary embolization

28.18 Infusion of isoproterenol can be administered in the emergency treatment of which of the following conditions?

(A) Hypotension related to anaphylactic shock
(B) Drug-induced torsades de pointes
(C) Hypotension after weaning from cardiopulmonary bypass
(D) Hypotension during therapeutic hypothermia

28.19 A 58-year-old man with a history of stage 3 HIV-associated Hodgkin's lymphoma, and recently completed treatment with AVD (doxorubicin, vinblastine, and dacarbazine), is admitted to the hospital with dyspnea. Echocardiography demonstrates a moderately dilated left ventricular cavity with global systolic dysfunction and a calculated LVEF of 18%. There was moderate left atrial dilation with moderate (2 to 3+) mitral regurgitation.

The cumulative dose of doxorubicin was 496 mg/m^2, and anthracycline-induced cardiotoxicity is suspected. He is referred to undergo diagnostic right and left heart catheterization for further evaluation.

The hemodynamic tracing below demonstrates a central aortic pressure of 70/55 mm Hg (mean 61 mm Hg) and a pulmonary artery pressure of 43/23 mm Hg (mean 31 mm Hg). The systemic oxygen saturation is 96% on ambient room air (Fig. Q28-19).

Which of the following values is most consistent with the clinical scenario?

(A) A PCWP of 8 mm Hg
(B) A systemic vascular resistance of 700 dynes-s-cm^5
(C) A pulmonary arterial saturation of 41%
(D) A pulmonary vascular resistance of 400 dynes-s-cm^5

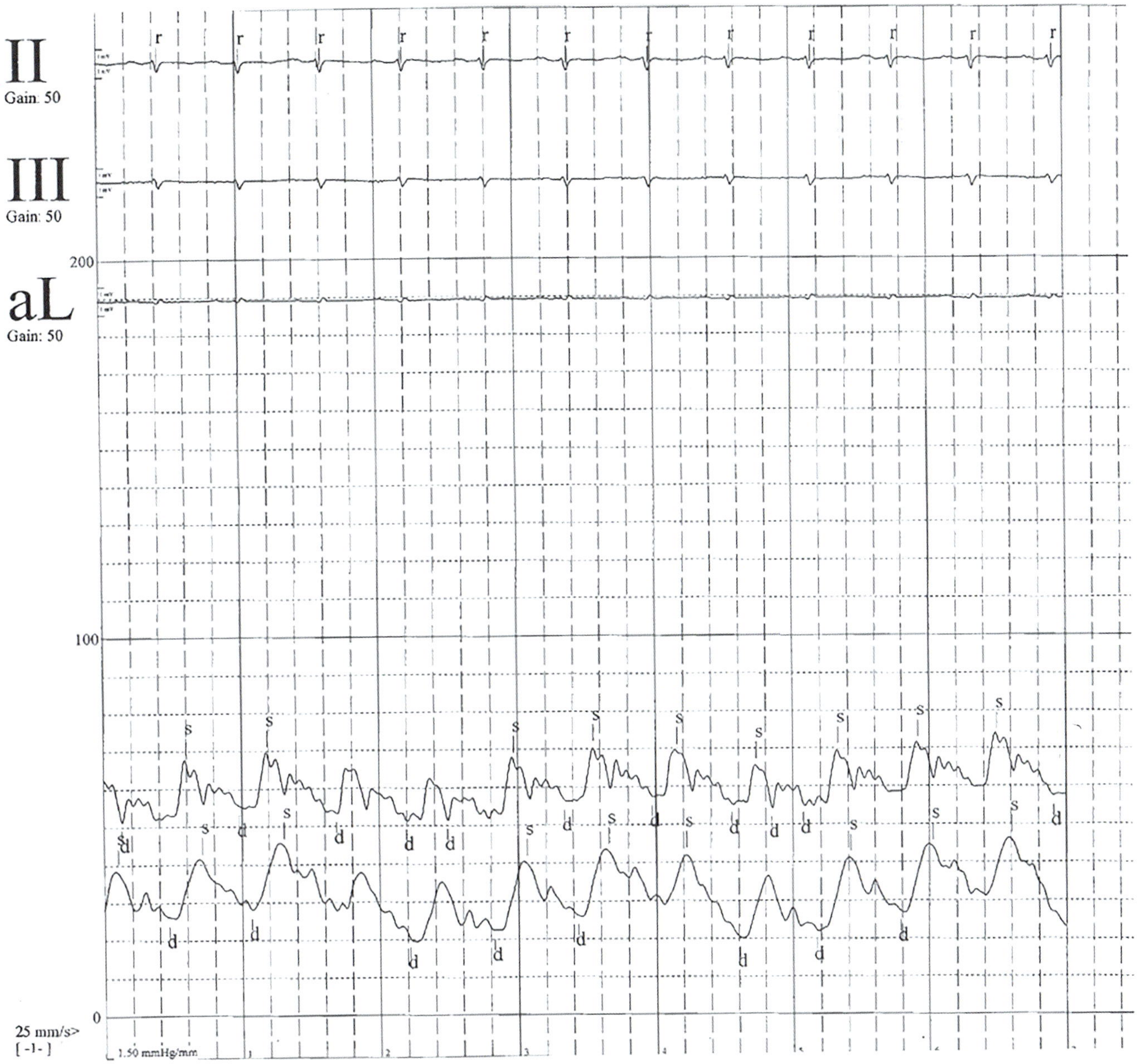

Figure Q28-19 (Courtesy of Zoran Nedeljkovic.)

28.20 A 42-year-old man with a history of stage IIIB/IV adenocarcinoma of the lung presents to the emergency department with symptoms of shortness of breath and dizziness within the past 24 hours. His blood pressure is 92/68 mm Hg and heart rate is 103 bpm with an oxygen saturation of 98% while breathing ambient room air. A chest x-ray demonstrates a markedly enlarged cardiac silhouette with patchy consolidation of the right lower lung field. A bedside ultrasound of the heart demonstrates a large pericardial effusion. Two liters of isotonic saline is administered IV.

He is taken to the catheterization laboratory to undergo right heart catheterization and pericardiocentesis. Simultaneous measurement of the right atrial (orange) and intrapericardial (white) pressure is shown below (Fig. Q28-20).

Which of the following was most likely observed?

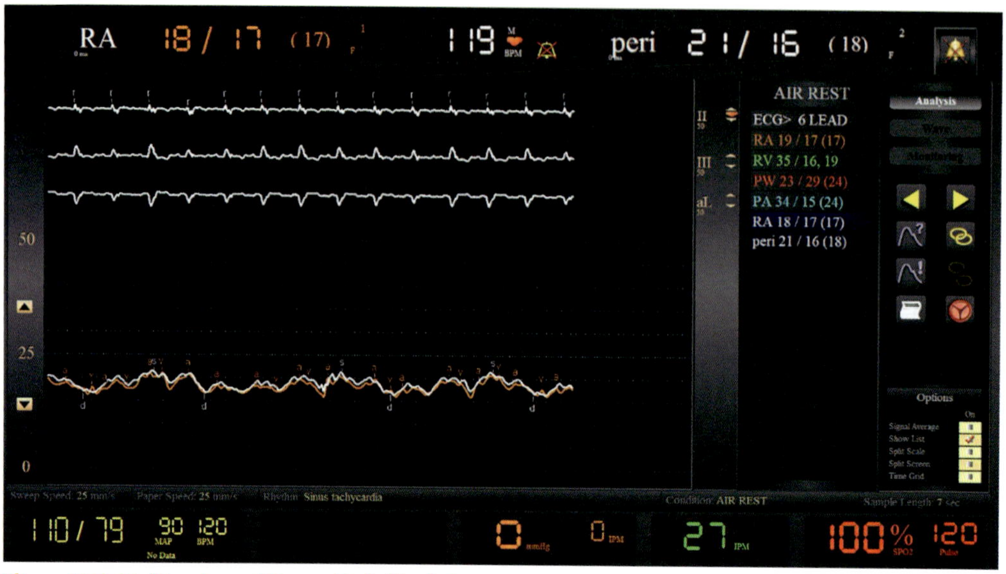

Figure Q28-20 (Courtesy of Zoran Nedeljkovic.)

(A) Right atrial inversion on echocardiography
(B) Left atrial inversion on echocardiography
(C) Normal respirophasic variation in the inferior vena cava (IVC) on echocardiography
(D) A pulsus paradoxus of 8 mm Hg

28.21 A 71-year-old woman with a history of prior St. Jude's mechanical aortic valve replacement for aortic stenosis presents to the hospital with several days of progressively worsening shortness of breath with minimal activity. She is awoken with severe shortness of breath, for which emergency medical services are summoned. In the emergency department, she is afebrile with a blood pressure of 100/60 mm Hg and a heart rate of 94 bpm. The oxygen saturation is 93% with 4 L of supplemental oxygen delivered via nasal cannula. She is in respiratory distress with rales at the bases of both lung fields. There is a mechanical second heart sound with a grade 2 systolic ejection murmur. The ECG demonstrates sinus rhythm with left bundle-branch block (LBBB), unchanged from prior. The international normalized ratio (INR) is 1.9.

The single-frame cineangiogram of the aortic valve in diastole (left) and systole (right) is shown below (Fig. Q28-21).

Which of the following should be considered next in the management?

(A) Weight-based low molecular weight heparin (LMWH) with oral anticoagulation
(B) Systemic UFH
(C) Systemic UFH, followed by fibrinolysis
(D) Emergent aortic valve replacement

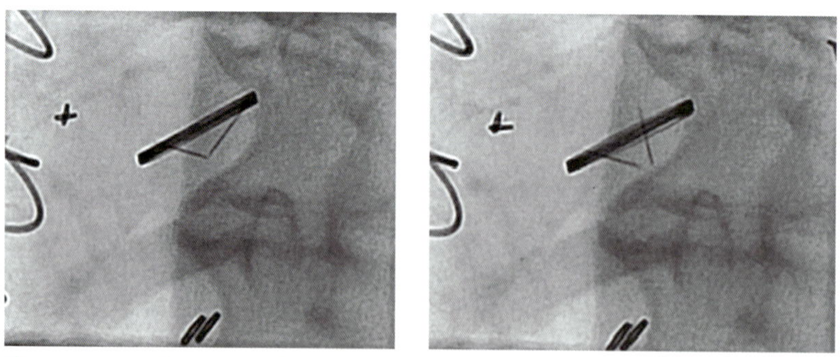

Figure Q28-21 (Courtesy of Zoran Nedeljkovic.)

ANSWERS AND EXPLANATIONS

28.1 Answer C. Serious complications associated with right ventricular endomyocardial biopsy include chamber perforation and pericardial tamponade, supraventricular and ventricular arrhythmias, complete atrioventricular (AV) block (especially in the presence of LBBB), and pulmonary embolism (Cooper LT, et al. *Circulation* 2007;116(19):2216–2233). The risk of such major complications are reported at <1% (Holzmann M, et al. *Circulation* 2008;118(17):1722–1728). Potential factors that may increase the risk of complications include right ventricular chamber enlargement, elevated right ventricular filling pressure, thrombocytopenia, or anticoagulation. Prior cardiac surgery that involved excision of the pericardium may have a lower risk of tamponade in the event a perforation were to occur.

28.2 Answer D. The hemodynamic tracing demonstrates a typical finding in patients with hypertrophic obstructive cardiomyopathy and LV outflow obstruction. There is no LV outflow tract gradient at rest, but following a premature ventricular beat, there is augmentation of LV contractility and the outflow tract obstruction, which leads to a significant systolic pressure gradient and a narrowing of the pulse pressure (Brockenbrough-Braunwald sign). Following the procedure, he develops signs and symptoms of acute LV outflow obstruction that should initially be managed by bed rest and administration of IV fluids to augment preload. Refractory hypotension should be managed with IV phenylephrine (a pure α-agonist, vasoconstrictor). Dopamine and dobutamine should not be given as any inotropic agent may worsen the outflow tract obstruction and exacerbate hypotension. Atropine can be used for situations associated with increased vagal tone, but would not be appropriate in the acute management in this setting.

28.3 Answer C. Reactions to iodinated contrast media occur in <1% of patients but may occur in 17% to 35% of patients with a prior contrast reaction (Levine GN, et al. *Ann Intern Med* 2003;139(2):123–136). Common clinical manifestations can range from mild (pruritus and urticaria) to serious (bronchospasm and angioedema) to life-threatening (shock). These manifestations are due to release of histamine from direct degranulation of tissue mast cells and circulating basophils and are anaphylactoid reactions in contrast to IgE-mediated true allergic reactions. Acute management of anaphylactoid contrast reactions in the catheterization laboratory includes administration of IV antihistamines (both anti-H_1 and anti-H_2) and corticosteroids (although the latter do not work immediately). Severe reactions that lead to respiratory and hemodynamic compromise should be treated with epinephrine (Goss JE, et al. *Cathet Cardiovasc Diagn* 1995;34(2):99–104).

28.4 Answer B. Right atrial pressure is elevated with a mildly elevated PCWP and systemic vascular resistance (SVR) and a low cardiac output. In **A**, filling pressures are all low and SVR is elevated, consistent with hypovolemic shock. In **C**, filling pressures are also low, but cardiac output is elevated and SVR is low, consistent with sepsis. In **D**, pulmonary capillary wedge pressure (PCWP) is elevated, cardiac output is relatively low, and SVR is elevated, consistent with cardiogenic shock. This contrasts with shock secondary to predominant right ventricular involvement, where the PCWP is only mildly elevated.

28.5 Answer B. Nausea and vomiting, often associated with hypotension and bradycardia, are common with MI, particularly with inferior wall infarction. Hypotension and bradycardia are attributed to direct activation of parasympathetic/vagal reflex pathways or left ventricular stretch receptors (Bezold-Jarisch reflex) that lead to bradycardia and peripheral vasodilation and are usually transient. Treatment includes administration of atropine and IV fluids. The Bezold-Jarisch reflex commonly occurs, as in this case, following reperfusion of the infarct artery in a patient with an inferior MI.

28.6 Answer A. Coronary artery perforation is an infrequent occurrence following PCI. Perforations during PCI can occur as a result of guidewire manipulation ("wire exit") or improper sizing of the balloon. Elderly patients and women appear to be at increased risk. However, PCI following fibrinolytic therapy and PCI of a SVG are not associated with increased risk of perforation. In a prospective study of the incidence of coronary artery perforation in the early 1990s, use of newer devices to treat coronary lesions by cutting or ablating tissue (atherectomy, laser) was associated with an increased incidence of perforation compared to balloon angioplasty alone (Ellis SG, et al. *Circulation* 1994;90(6):2725-2730). These investigators defined a scheme for classifying coronary artery perforations into one of three groups: extraluminal crater without extravasation (type 1), pericardial or myocardial blush without contrast extravasation (type 2), or extravasation through frank (≥1 mm) perforation (type 3). Type 1 and type 2 perforations can usually be managed with prolonged balloon inflations and reversal of anticoagulation. Type 3 perforations are usually associated with a higher incidence of adverse events (i.e., death, MI, tamponade, or emergency cardiac surgery).

Prolonged balloon inflations may not be well tolerated, and perfusion balloons have been used in this setting to seal off the perforation and maintain adequate distal perfusion. Heparin anticoagulation is usually reversed with protamine and pericardial tamponade is treated with pericardiocentesis. Polytetrafluoroethylene (PTFE)-covered stents are an alternative in the nonsurgical management of coronary artery perforations, with promising results (Briguori C, et al. *Circulation* 2000;102(25): 3028-3031). If these measures fail, emergency surgery is needed.

28.7 Answer A. Protamine sulfate is given intravenously to neutralize the anticoagulant effect of heparin. The usual dose is 1 mg of protamine sulfate for each 100 units of heparin (UFH). Protamine is not as effective in neutralizing the effect of low molecular weight heparin (LMWH), such as enoxaparin. Direct thrombin inhibitors (bivalirudin or lepirudin) and glycoprotein (GP) IIb/IIIa inhibitors are not affected by protamine either. For procedures that are associated with an increased risk of perforation (i.e., rotational atherectomy), it may be prudent to avoid anticoagulants that cannot be reversed with protamine.

28.8 Answer C. Coronary air embolus is a preventable complication of cardiac catheterization. When it does occur, treatment is usually supportive with administration of 100% inhaled oxygen. If the chest pain or ischemia persist despite oxygen, an IABP and pressor support may be necessary, although the ischemia is usually transient. CABG surgery is not indicated.

28.9 Answer C. The initial portion of the ECG demonstrates sinus tachycardia with a rate of approximately 100 bpm. The arterial pressure is 78/44 mm Hg. The wide-complex rhythm that develops is an accelerated idioventricular rhythm (AIVR) that is often seen following successful pharmacologic or mechanical reperfusion in acute MI and is usually transient. Antiarrhythmic therapy is not indicated for AIVR. Likewise, electrical cardioversion is also not indicated.

28.10 Answer D. The patient is presenting with an acute anterior wall MI caused by thrombotic occlusion of the mid-LAD artery, complicated by rupture of the ventricular septum and cardiogenic shock. Percutaneous revascularization of the LAD artery should not be performed. This patient appears to be a surgical candidate and should have an IABP inserted, followed by emergency cardiac surgery and repair of the ventricular septum.

28.11 Answer C. The case illustrates a late presentation following an acute anterior wall infarction complicated by cardiogenic shock. Symptoms had been present for several days, and the ECG, as described, shows evolving changes of a transmural, Q-wave infarction. The finding of a systolic murmur should alert the examiner to the possibility of a mechanical complication, in this case ventricular septal rupture (VSR). When VSR is suspected, right heart catheterization and sampling of blood for oximetry should be performed prior to angiography to assess for the presence of a left-to-right shunt. Echocardiography or left ventricular angiography can also be performed to establish the diagnosis. If VSR is confirmed, coronary angiography can be performed prior to referral for cardiac surgery.

28.12 Answer C. Acute retroperitoneal (RP) bleeding should be suspected in any patient who develops unheralded hypotension following transfemoral catheterization, even in the absence of visible bleeding in the groin. Femoral angiography prior to sheath removal is helpful in identifying whether the arterial puncture is above the inguinal ligament, in which case manual compression may be inadequate in achieving hemostasis. Angiography performed via the contralateral femoral artery can be performed to establish the site of bleeding and to determine if it is suitable for percutaneous treatment. In this case, angiography confirmed suspected bleeding in the retroperitoneal space and identified contrast extravasation from the external iliac artery. Although vascular surgery can be performed to repair the site of bleeding, a trial of balloon occlusion, followed by insertion of a covered stent, would deliver more immediate treatment and avoid higher morbidity associated with surgery. Manual pressure will likely be ineffective on its own with the location of bleeding above the femoral head. Transfusion of packed red blood cells may be needed, but would depend on the initial hemoglobin and how quickly the bleeding is arrested.

28.13 Answer C. Side effects related to IV contrast agents may include bradycardia, hypotension, nausea, and vomiting. These are related to the tonicity of the agent used and occur much more frequently when high-osmolar contrast agents are used, as compared to the newer, lower-osmolar contrast agents. These effects do not represent allergic reactions and should not be treated with steroids and/or antihistamines. The effect is usually transient, and the procedure can be continued.

28.14 Answer B. The ECG shows characteristic findings of acute pericarditis (diffuse, concave ST-segment elevation, and PR-segment depression). Pericardial inflammation and effusion can develop several days to weeks following cardiac surgery as part of the postpericardiotomy syndrome. Associated chest pain is pleuritic in nature, and a pericardial friction rub may be present on exam. The minimally invasive cardiac surgical technique may also be associated with more incomplete exposure and drainage of the pericardial space, as compared with the traditional full sternotomy incision. An echocardiogram should be obtained to assess for the presence of pericardial fluid and to further assess if features consistent with tamponade are present. The history and the ECG are not consistent with an acute coronary syndrome, so anticoagulation and urgent angiography are not appropriate at this stage. While nonsteroidal anti-inflammatory agents are part of the management of uncomplicated pericarditis, this patient's recent cardiac surgery and current hypotension require further investigation.

28.15 Answer B. The left atrium-to-femoral artery bypass (TandemHeart) is one of three commercially available platforms for providing temporary circulatory support. Others include the Impella catheter-mounted, intraluminal, axial pump, and venoarterial extracorporeal membrane oxygenation (VA-ECMO). The left atrium-to-femoral artery bypass system involves insertion of a transseptal cannula into the left atrium, with a separate cannula inserted in the femoral artery. Blood is then pumped via a continuous-flow centrifugal pump of 3.5 to 4.0 L/min, serving to augment the cardiac output, coronary, and end organ perfusion. Advantages of this system include unloading of the left ventricle with decreases in the PCWP. Decompression of the left ventricle allows for a more favorable balance of oxygen supply and demand, resulting in a decrease in myocardial oxygen demand.

28.16 Answer C. The no-reflow phenomenon represents an impairment in the coronary microcirculation following restoration of epicardial coronary blood flow, which is associated with less than TIMI grade 3 flow (Rezkalla SH, et al. *JACC Cardiovasc Interv* 2017;10(3):215–223). Normal flow can often be achieved with administration of IC vasodilating drugs, including sodium nitroprusside. This can be administered via the guiding catheter, or more directly to the distal coronary bed via the angioplasty balloon catheter. Additional agents, including adenosine and calcium channel blockers, have also been used in this setting. For refractory symptoms or ischemia that do not respond to pharmacologic intervention, an IABP may be used.

28.17 Answer B. Calcified lesions may fail to expand following dilation with a semicompliant balloon. Furthermore, unrestricted expansion of the semicompliant balloon on either side of the calcified lesion may lead to overdilation and coronary dissection or perforation. Coronary perforation may lead to pericardial tamponade and result in hemodynamic compromise. A characteristic finding related to pericardial tamponade is a pulsus paradoxus (>10 mm Hg decrease in systolic blood pressure with inspiration), which is demonstrated on the arterial tracing.

28.18 Answer B. Isoproterenol is a nonselective beta ($\beta_2 > \beta_1$) adrenergic receptor agonist used in the treatment of bradyarrhythmias. Torsades de pointes is a ventricular arrhythmia, usually precipitated by drugs that prolong the QT interval. It is more common with electrolyte disorders (hypokalemia and hypomagnesemia) and bradycardia. Isoproterenol infusion is used in the treatment of torsades de pointes by accelerating the heart rate and shortening the QT interval.

28.19 Answer C. Severe systemic hypotension is present with a narrow pulse pressure, consistent with a low cardiac output/index, and a wide systemic arterial–mixed venous oxygen difference (normal mixed venous oxygen saturation 65% to 75%). Although the PCWP is not provided in the summary, there is no reason to suspect elevated pulmonary vascular resistance and a high transpulmonary gradient, particularly with moderate mitral regurgitation. Cardiogenic shock is associated with an elevated, not decreased, SVR.

28.20 Answer A. The hemodynamic tracing demonstrates findings consistent with pericardial tamponade. With the pericardial pressure exceeding the mean right atrial pressure, there is likely transient right atrial inversion on echocardiography. IV fluids are initially given to optimize intracardiac filling, and the IVC is usually dilated with blunted respirophasic variation. As the mean PCPW is 24 mm Hg, left atrial inversion was likely not observed. A pulsus paradoxus >10 mm Hg is usually observed with cardiac tamponade.

28.21 Answer D. Prosthetic valve thrombosis (PVT) should be suspected in a patient with a history of mechanical valve replacement and abrupt onset of symptoms, especially in the setting of inadequate anticoagulation. The 2014 American Heart Association (AHA) and American College of Cardiology (ACC) Valvular Heart Disease Guideline (Nishimura RA, et al. *J Am Coll Cardiol* 2014;63(22):e57–e185) recommends echocardiography (transthoracic and transesophageal) for the initial evaluation of the hemodynamic severity of the valve dysfunction, valve leaflet motion, and thrombus size. Fluoroscopy overcomes limitations related to mechanical valve imaging by ultrasound and allows accurate assessment of the degree of leaflet opening and closing. The guideline assigns a Class I recommendation for emergency surgery in patients with a thrombosed left-sided prosthetic valve and New York Heart Association (NYHA) Class III or IV symptoms, as the patient described in the clinical vignette. Furthermore, the guideline assigns a Class IIa recommendation for recent onset (<14 days) of NYHA Class I or II symptoms and a small thrombus (<0.8 cm^2). Larger thrombi are associated with greater thrombolysis-related embolic complications.

29 Peripheral Interventional Procedures

Devin Patel and Mark Robbins

QUESTIONS

29.1 Which of the following patients is NOT an appropriate candidate for carotid artery stenting according to the SAPPHIRE trial criteria?

(A) An 82-year-old woman with a recent history of transient ischemic attack (TIA), poorly controlled hypertension, and a 60% stenosis of the internal carotid artery (ICA)
(B) A 72-year-old man with a history of myocardial infarction (MI) 3 weeks ago and an 80% stenosis of the right ICA
(C) A 60-year-old diabetic man with a history of cerebrovascular accident 6 weeks ago resulting in residual upper left extremity paresis with a 90% left ICA stenosis
(D) An asymptomatic 85-year-old man with severe emphysematous lung disease, New York Heart Association (NYHA) Class III congestive heart failure (CHF), and bilateral 80% stenosis of the ICAs

29.2 All of the following are complications of carotid artery stenting, EXCEPT:

(A) Stroke
(B) Hypotension/bradycardia
(C) MI
(D) Hyperperfusion syndrome
(E) All of the above

29.3 A 72-year-old diabetic male presents to clinic for evaluation of a recent TIA where he lost sensation in his right lower leg for 1 hour. Computed tomography angiography (CTA) shows a 90% stenosis in his left ICA. Which of the following is TRUE regarding options for revascularization of his carotid artery?

(A) His 2-year mortality is lower if he undergoes carotid artery stenting compared to carotid endarterectomy
(B) He would have had more mortality benefit from carotid artery stenting than carotid endarterectomy if he had been asymptomatic when his carotid artery stenosis was discovered
(C) His risk of periprocedural MI is lower if he undergoes carotid artery stenting than carotid endarterectomy
(D) His risk of periprocedural stroke is lower if he undergoes carotid artery stenting than carotid endarterectomy
(E) Neither carotid artery stenting nor carotid endarterectomy will decrease his risk of stroke or mortality

29.4 Which of the following statements regarding symptomatic peripheral arterial disease (PAD) is INCORRECT?

(A) Most patients participating in formal exercise rehabilitation programs have been shown to double their symptom-free walking period
(B) Because of their high rate of comorbid cardiovascular disease and vascular events, all patients with PAD should be considered to have coronary artery disease (CAD) until proved otherwise and initiated on drug therapy until their low-density lipoprotein C (LDL-C) levels are reduced to <100 mg/dL
(C) The presence of low ankle–brachial indices (ABIs) in hypertensive patients is a predictor of increased mortality
(D) The U.S. Food and Drug Administration (FDA) has approved both pentoxifylline and clopidogrel for the treatment of intermittent claudication

29.5 All of the following are TRUE regarding the diagnosis of PAD, EXCEPT:

(A) Resting ABI should be done in the initial workup of a patient with symptoms of PAD
(B) Toe-brachial index (TBI) testing should be performed if a symptomatic patient has an ABI of ≥1.6
(C) Exercise treadmill ABI testing is indicated if a symptomatic patient has an ABI of 1.1 and symptoms cannot be otherwise explained
(D) Resting ABI testing is reasonable in asymptomatic elderly (>65 years old) patients
(E) A TBI of 0.9 is considered abnormal and warrants revascularization consideration

29.6 The angiogram in Figure Q29-6 is that of a 65-year-old man who has a history of poorly controlled diabetes, hypertension, as well as tobacco abuse and who complains of claudication symptoms after walking approximately 100 ft. His symptoms have been stable for more than 3 years, and he denies rest pain or chronic, nonhealing wound infections. Which of the following statements regarding this patient's future management is INCORRECT?

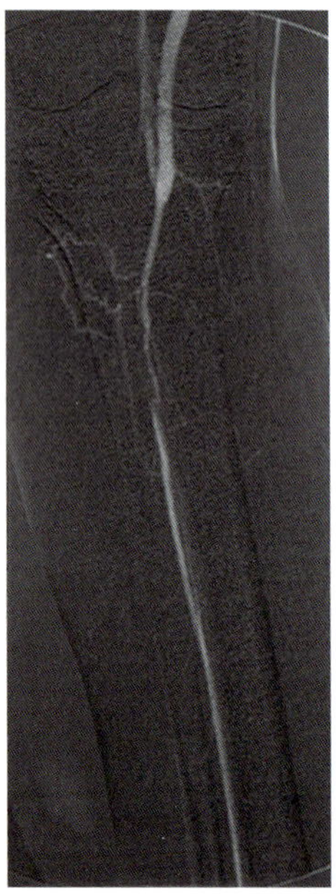

Figure Q29-6

(A) The patient should be counseled on risk factor modification, including smoking cessation, and should be referred to a formal exercise rehabilitation program
(B) Because of the high rate of complications during infrapopliteal interventions, including thrombosis and perforation, angioplasty of these lesions is contraindicated
(C) The indications for endovascular intervention of these lesions include critical limb ischemia, rest pain, nonhealing wounds, or limb salvage
(D) Long-term patency rates for infrapopliteal interventions are not as favorable as those for iliac or femoral procedures

29.7 Which of the following regarding the medical management of PAD is FALSE?

(A) Treatment with statin medications is indicated in all patients with PAD
(B) Pentoxifylline is effective in symptomatic management of PAD
(C) Cilostazol has been shown to increase walking distance in patients with PAD
(D) Aggressive risk factor management with blood pressure and diabetes should be done to reduce risk of major adverse cardiac events (MACE)
(E) Pharmacotherapy should be used to assist PAD patients with smoking cessation

29.8 Which of the following would favor surgical over endovascular revascularization of chronic limb ischemia?

(A) A single lesion in the left common femoral artery
(B) Prior coronary artery bypass graft (CABG) using a saphenous vein graft (SVG)
(C) Discrete multilevel disease in a patient with significant rest pain
(D) A patient with chronic ischemic heart disease with recent percutaneous coronary intervention (PCI)
(E) A patient with NYHA Class IV heart failure

29.9 A 65-year-old female presents to clinic for evaluation of claudication. She has severe intermittent claudication (Rutherford stage 3). Lower extremity CTA reveals a 10-cm-long 80% stenosis in her left superficial femoral artery (SFA) with target-vessel diameter of 4.5 mm. Balloon angioplasty is planned. Which of the following is TRUE regarding the use of a paclitaxel-coated balloon?

(A) Use of a paclitaxel-coated balloon will result in increased immediate primary vessel patency
(B) Use of a paclitaxel-coated balloon will result in increased 1-year primary vessel patency
(C) Use of a paclitaxel-coated balloon will result in decreased periprocedural major complications (i.e., death, amputation, and bleeding)
(D) Use of a paclitaxel-coated balloon will result in higher resting ABI at 1 year
(E) Use of a paclitaxel-coated balloon will result in improved functional status at 1 year

29.10 All of the following are indications for renal arteriography, EXCEPT:

(A) Onset of hypertension in an individual younger than 30 or older than 55 years or rapidly accelerating hypertension in a previously well-controlled patient
(B) Azotemia after the initiation of an angiotensin-converting enzyme (ACE) inhibitor
(C) Asymmetric kidney size as documented by noninvasive imaging in association with an unexplained elevation in creatinine (>1.5 mg/dL)
(D) The finding of an abdominal bruit on physical examination
(E) Following the completion of a diagnostic left heart catheterization in a patient with severe coronary atherosclerosis with normal renal function

29.11 A 54-year-old male with long-standing hypertension is evaluated for progressively difficult to control hypertension. He has been treated with multiple blood pressure regimens with failure to obtain adequate control. He has been admitted three times in the last year for pulmonary edema and has had multiple admissions for acute or chronic systolic heart failure. He has been intolerant of medical therapy due to side effects. A CTA is done and is notable for unilateral renal artery stenosis. Which of his characteristics make him a less desirable candidate for renal artery revascularization?

(A) Long-standing nature of hypertension
(B) Multiple prior failed regimens
(C) Intolerance of medical therapy
(D) Recurrent pulmonary edema
(E) Systolic heart failure

29.12 All of the following are TRUE regarding surgical abdominal aortic aneurysm (AAA), EXCEPT:

(A) Sexual history should be documented prior to surgery due to possible increase in sexual dysfunction after aneurysm repair
(B) CTA should be done to characterize the aneurysm's location and structural features
(C) Assessment of mesenteric arteries should be done to ensure abdominal visceral perfusion
(D) Patients should continue preoperative statin therapy after repair is completed
(E) Patients with a noninflammatory aneurysm are at a higher risk of perioperative mortality

29.13 Which of the following regarding treatment of asymptomatic AAA is TRUE?

(A) There is a marked increase in the rupture rate of aneurysms over 5.5 cm in size
(B) For a given size aneurysm, male patients have a higher rate of rupture than do female patients
(C) For a given size aneurysm, rate of aortic aneurysms expansions does not affect risk of rupture
(D) Patient with AAA should be started on aspirin and statin to decrease rate of aneurysm rupture
(E) Moderately strenuous activities should be avoided in patients with AAAs <5.5 cm in size due to risk of rupture

29.14 A 75-year-old woman with long-standing uncontrolled hypertension presents to the clinic for the management of resistant hypertension. She has been compliant with her antihypertensive regimen of lisinopril, carvedilol, chlorthalidone, and amlodipine. She has undergone workup for secondary causes of hypertension with no secondary etiology found. Her blood pressure in clinic is 165/95, which is consistent with her home readings. Which of the following is TRUE regarding possible renal denervation for this patient?

(A) Renal denervation will provide improved blood pressure control compared to medical therapy alone
(B) Renal denervation will provide decreased 6-month mortality compared to medical therapy alone
(C) The risk of major periprocedural complications from renal denervation is under 2%
(D) The patient is more likely to benefit from renal denervation due to her advanced age

29.15 Which of the following is TRUE regarding revascularization in patients with resistant hypertension from renal artery stenosis secondary to fibromuscular dysplasia?

(A) Percutaneous balloon angioplasty results in superior blood pressure control as compared to surgical revascularization
(B) Hypertension cure rates (defined as controlled blood pressure without treatment) are >80% with both balloon angioplasty and surgical revascularization
(C) Older patients are more likely than are younger patients to be cured of hypertension with revascularization of renal artery stenosis secondary to fibromuscular dysplasia
(D) The periprocedural mortality rate for balloon angioplasty is approximately 1%

29.16 A 65-year-old diabetic man with a history of hypertension, hypercholesterolemia, and heavy tobacco use presents to his local emergency department complaining of increasing lower abdominal pain over the past 3 weeks. During his physical examination, a tender, pulsatile mass is detected in the lower abdomen with an associated systolic murmur. High-resolution computed tomography (CT) scan reveals an infrarenal AAA with a maximal diameter of 6 cm without evidence of rupture or leak. Which of the following statements regarding the management of this patient's condition is TRUE?

(A) Current data regarding the long-term efficacy of endovascular aneurysm repair (EVAR) indicate that this patient would likely have a significantly reduced long-term all-cause mortality if he underwent EVAR as opposed to open surgical repair
(B) There is no long-term follow-up with EVAR, and hence EVAR should not be considered in a person at this age. Open surgical repair is the preferred modality of treatment
(C) The CT was unwarranted. An abdominal angiogram should have been the diagnostic modality of choice in preparation for EVAR
(D) Cardiac complications are the most common serious perioperative complication of EVAR and the most common cause of late death
(E) If records from the patient's primary care physician revealed that the AAA was actually discovered the previous year and was 5.5 cm in maximal diameter at that time (<0.5 cm/year), a reasonable management strategy would include aggressive medical management of the patient's hypertension, counseling for smoking cessation, and a repeat CT scan in 6 months to evaluate the AAA's dimensions

29.17 Which of the following is NOT typically noted as a complication of AAA endovascular repair?

(A) Leaking of blood into the aneurysmal sac from either the proximal or distal sites of endograft attachment
(B) Accumulation of blood in the aneurysmal sac due to retrograde blood flow from patent lumbar or inferior mesenteric arteries (IMAs)
(C) Increased graft porosity resulting in slow permeation of blood across the endograft into the aneurysmal sac
(D) Renal, mesenteric, or iliac artery ischemia
(E) Spinal cord ischemia (SCI)

29.18 A 75-year-old man with a history of poorly controlled hypertension, PAD, chronic obstructive pulmonary disease (COPD), and a 60-pack per year history of tobacco abuse presents to his primary care physician's office noting development of dizziness, blurred vision, and gait instability after chopping wood. The patient's wife states that he had difficulty with his speech and appeared to be disoriented the previous week when he was helping their son move. The patient's neurologic examination is unremarkable, with the exception of diminished radial pulse in the right upper extremity. Which of the following statements regarding this patient is TRUE?

(A) A noncontrast head CT would be the most informative diagnostic test and would likely reveal the etiology of the patient's symptoms
(B) The patient should be immediately transferred to the nearest emergency department for urgent neurologic evaluation and thrombolytic therapy
(C) After ordering a sedimentation rate and prescribing a course of oral steroid therapy, the patient should be referred to ophthalmology for an urgent slit lamp examination
(D) After obtaining a baseline electrocardiogram (ECG), complete blood count, basic metabolic panel, and coagulation studies (i.e., prothrombin time and activated partial thromboplastin time), the patient should be referred for an arch aortogram as soon as possible
(E) The patient should undergo a transthoracic echocardiogram (TTE) with agitated saline to rule out a patent foramen ovale (PFO)

29.19 Which of the following does the angiogram in Figure Q29-19 show?

(A) Right-sided aortic arch
(B) Retroesophageal right subclavian

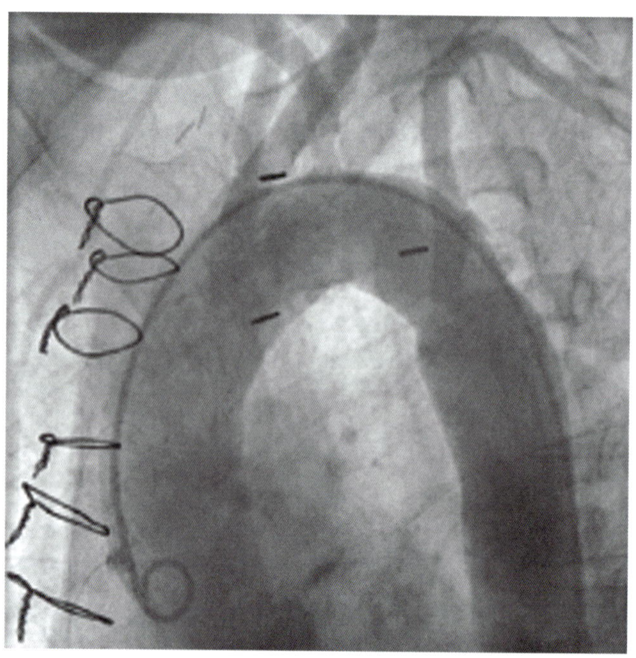

Figure Q29-19

(C) Anomalous origin of the left vertebral
(D) Normal aortic arch

29.20 A 26-year-old woman presents with low-grade fever over the past 6 to 8 weeks associated with weight loss, malaise, and nocturnal diaphoresis. The patient also notes that her right arm has become painful and "crampy" over the same time course. In addition, the patient states that since the previous week, her vision seemed to have become blurred, and she is now concerned that she may be losing her sight altogether. Remarkable findings on examination include a temperature of 38°C, blood pressure 185/100, the presence of a left infraclavicular bruit, and a diminished right radial pulse. The angiogram in Figure Q29-20 is of this patient. Which of the following statements regarding this patient's condition is TRUE?

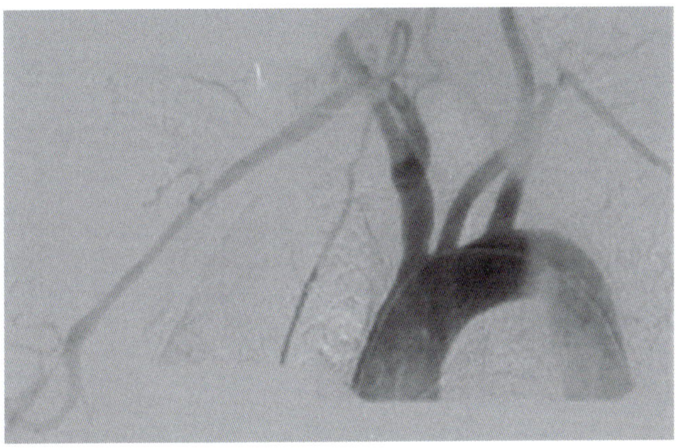

Figure Q29-20

(A) After obtaining a sedimentation rate, venereal disease research lab (VDRL) test, rheumatoid factor, antinuclear antibody, coagulation studies, and baseline blood chemistries, the patient should undergo urgent cerebral and aortic arch angiography for possible intervention
(B) Immediate, aggressive control of the patient's hypertension should be avoided in this situation
(C) Treatment for this condition should consist of high-dose glucocorticoids and cyclophosphamide
(D) Primary angioplasty offers a higher rate of cure for this condition
(E) Regardless of the mode of treatment, the patient faces a low relapse rate

29.21 Which of the following does the angiogram in Figure Q29-21 show?

(A) Superior mesenteric artery (SMA)
(B) Inferior mesenteric artery IMA

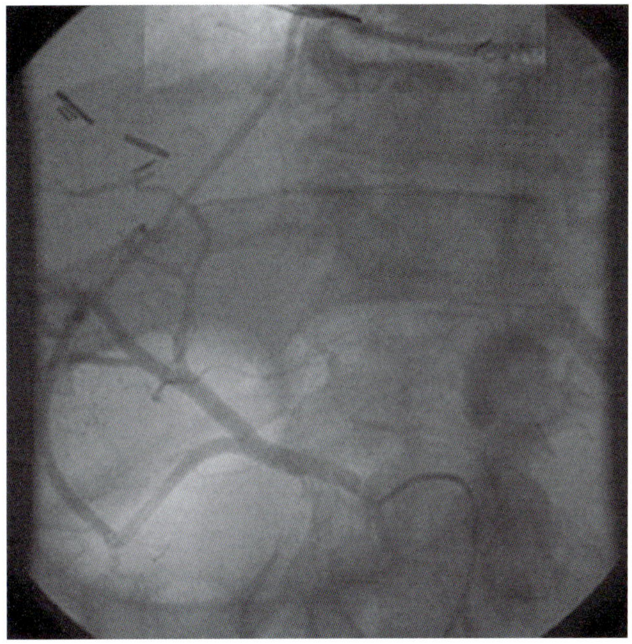

Figure Q29-21

(C) Hepatic and in situ right gastroepiploic graft to posterior descending branch of the right coronary artery the PDA
(D) Splenic artery
(E) Left gastric and in situ right gastroepiploic graft to PDA

29.22 A 73-year-old male patient who had treatment of his right SFA with balloon angioplasty 4 years ago and subsequent stenting 2 years ago has the following angiogram (Fig. Q29-22A–C). Which of the following is TRUE?

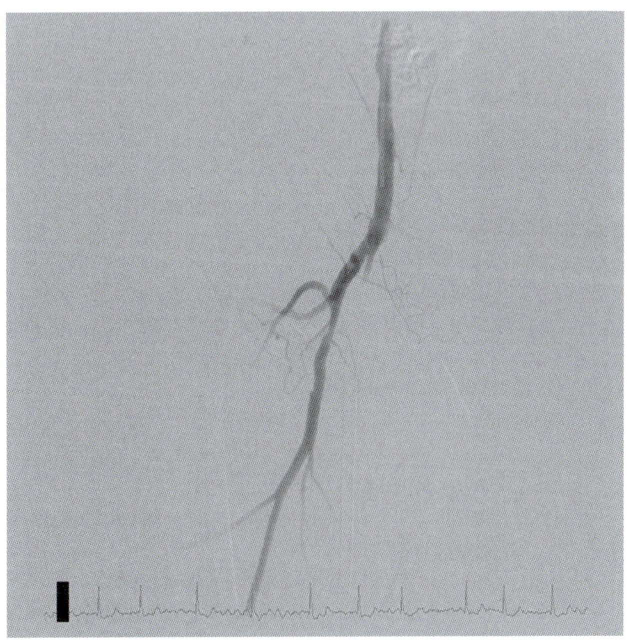

A
Figure Q29-22

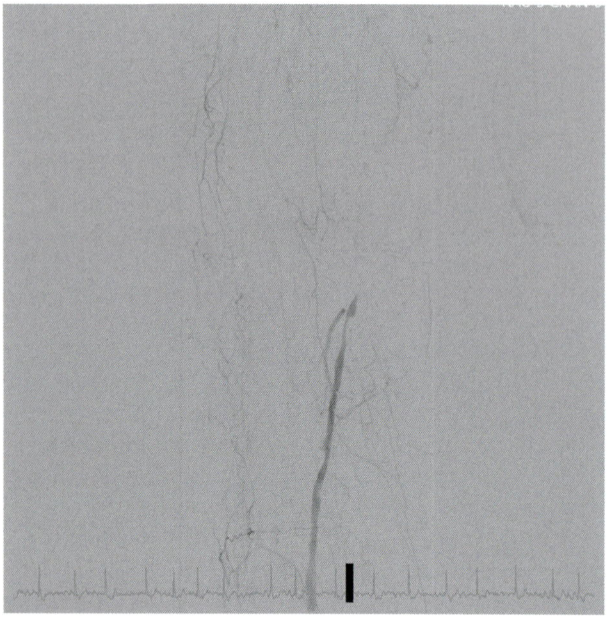

B

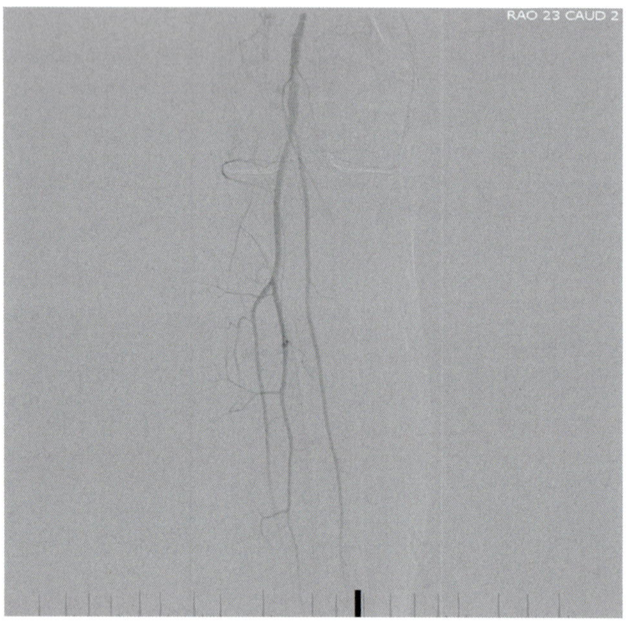

C

Figure Q29-22

(A) This is a Trans-Atlantic Inter-Society Consensus (TASC) B lesion, and endovascular repair is a reasonable option for the patient if he has a high surgical risk
(B) This is a TASC C lesion, and endovascular repair is a reasonable option if the patient has a high surgical risk
(C) This is a TASC D lesion, and surgical option is clearly preferred
(D) This is a TASC B lesion. However, neither surgical nor endovascular options are viable given the poor distal runoff

29.23 Figure Q29-23 is classic for:

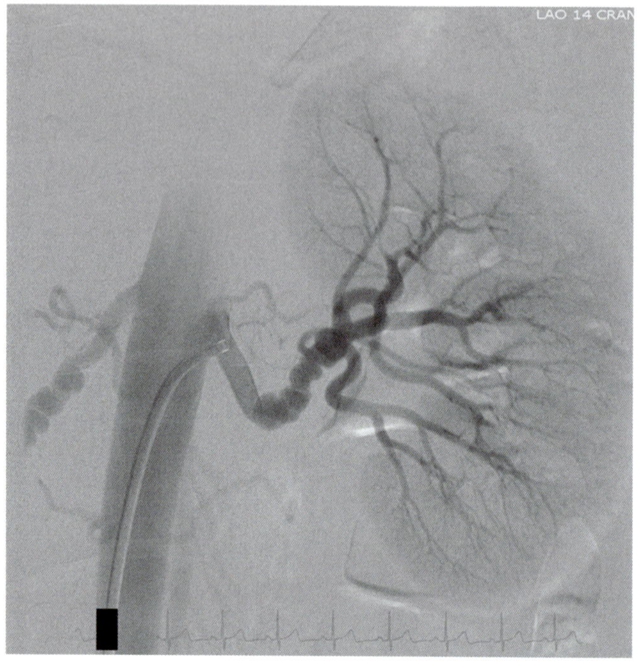

Figure Q29-23

(A) Fibromuscular dysplasia (FMD)
(B) Atherosclerotic renovascular disease
(C) Posttransplantation stenosis
(D) Neurofibromatosis

29.24 All of the following can be concluded from the CREST trial among patients with symptomatic or asymptomatic carotid stenosis, EXCEPT:

(A) Risk of the primary outcome of stroke, MI, or death is not significantly different in the group undergoing carotid artery stenting and the group undergoing carotid endarterectomy
(B) During the periprocedural period, there was a higher risk of minor stroke with stenting and a higher risk of MI with endarterectomy
(C) After the periprocedural period, the incidence of ipsilateral stroke was similar with carotid artery stenting and with carotid endarterectomy
(D) The risk of ipsilateral stroke was higher with stenting during the periprocedural period and continues to increase after the periprocedural period

29.25 The angiogram in Figure Q29-25 was performed after an unsuccessful attempt to place a large 14-Fr sheath in the left common femoral artery. The most important finding is:

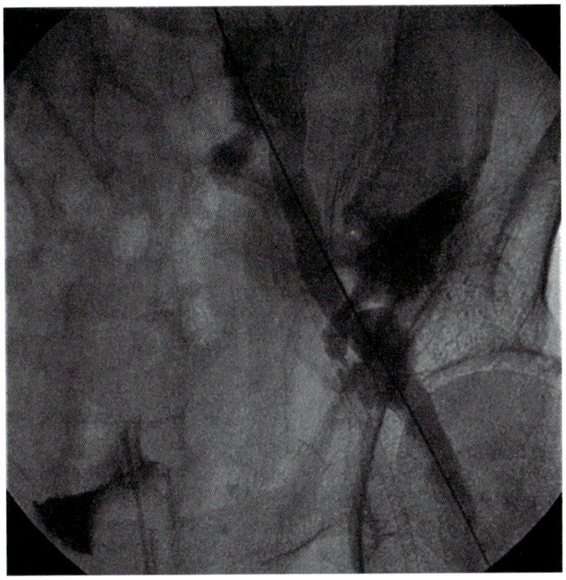

Figure Q29-25

(A) A severely diseased left external iliac artery
(B) Critical internal iliac artery stenosis that needs immediate intervention
(C) Small perforation that can be dealt with by placement of a larger sheath in the ipsilateral side
(D) Large perforation that needs immediate stenting from the ipsilateral side
(E) Large perforation that needs immediate balloon occlusion from contralateral side

ANSWERS AND EXPLANATIONS

29.1 Answer C. Several large registries and one randomized clinical trial have demonstrated that the outcomes following carotid artery stenting compare favorably with the traditional surgical carotid endarterectomy in select high-risk populations. The SAPPHIRE trial (Yadav JS, et al. *N Engl J Med* 2004;351(15):1493–1501) randomized 334 patients with symptomatic (>50% stenosis) or asymptomatic (>80% stenosis) carotid disease, traditionally considered at high risk for surgical intervention, to percutaneous carotid intervention with nitinol stents in conjunction with embolic protection devices (EPD) vs. conventional carotid endarterectomy. The results demonstrated the noninferiority of carotid artery stenting as well as a 39% reduction in the primary end point of a composite of death, stroke, and MI within 30 days. Additionally, patients randomized to carotid artery stenting enjoyed lower rates of target-vessel revascularization (TVR) and a shorter hospital stay, as well as a significantly greater 1-year event-free survival (88% vs. 79%, $p = 0.048$). On the basis of the balance of evidence, the FDA has approved elective carotid artery stenting only in the "high-risk" populations with symptoms listed subsequently. Although trials evaluating lower-risk populations are currently ongoing, only patients meeting one or more of the following criteria are deemed candidates for carotid artery stenting.

Clinical: Age >80 years, CHF III to IV, known severe left ventricular dysfunction (ejection fraction [EF] < 30%), open heart surgery needed within 6 weeks, recent MI (>24 hours and <4 weeks), unstable angina (Canadian Cardiovascular Society [CCS] Class III/IV), severe pulmonary disease, and contralateral laryngeal nerve palsy.

Anatomic: Previous carotid endarterectomy with recurrent stenosis, high cervical lesions or lesions below the clavicle, contralateral carotid occlusion, radiation therapy to the neck, prior radical neck surgery, and severe tandem lesions (Yadav JS, et al. *N Engl J Med* 2004;351(15):1493–1501).

Further, although age >80 years was a criterion for SAPPHIRE, a recent meta-analysis concluded that stenting for symptomatic carotid stenosis should be avoided in older patients (age ≥70 years) but might be as safe as endarterectomy in younger patients (Carotid Stenting Trialists' Collaboration, et al. *Lancet* 2010;376(9746):1062–1073). The patient in choice C does not meet any high-risk criteria.

29.2 Answer E. Data obtained from the high-risk carotid stenting registries indicate that the 30-day incidence of stroke post carotid artery stenting approaches 3%. The primary mechanism of procedure-related stroke is thought to be the distal embolization of atheromatous debris dislodged during the procedure. In addition, manipulation of wires, catheters, and guides in the aortic arch and common carotid artery are not protected by EPD and are frequently responsible for strokes outside the territory of the treated carotid artery.

Distention of the carotid sinus mechanoreceptors by angioplasty and stenting may activate the vasomotor center of the medulla through cranial nerve IX. Subsequent vagal activation results in peripheral vasodilatation with hypotension and bradycardia. This phenomenon is relatively common and occurs in up to 40% of the procedures involving internal carotid lesions. Interestingly, in the restenotic lesions after endarterectomy, this reflex is typically not encountered. Supportive therapy with intravenous (IV) fluids, atropine, pseudoephedrine (60 mg oral twice daily), and, infrequently, dopamine is needed to counter hypotension and bradycardia.

The incidence of MI within 30 days of carotid stenting in the high-risk cohort of patients in the SAPPHIRE trial was 1.9%, which was significantly lower than that seen after carotid endarterectomy in that trial (Yadav JS, et al. *N Engl J Med* 2004;351(15):1493–1501).

In a response to carotid occlusive disease and chronically decreasing cerebral perfusion pressures, the cerebral vessels may undergo a compensatory vasodilatation in an effort to maintain adequate blood flow to the brain. Following intervention to the carotid artery, there is a sudden concomitant increase in blood flow to the dilated vasculature, and the net effect can be hyperperfusion to the brain with resultant edema. Presenting symptoms can include a throbbing, retro-orbital headache that lateralizes to the side of the intervention, nausea, vomiting, visual changes, focal motor deficits, and even seizures. Increased flow velocities by transcranial Doppler in symptomatic patients even in the absence of any significant findings on CT imaging are suggestive of hyperperfusion. Aggressive control of blood pressure is necessary to prevent this complication (Abou-Chebl A, et al. *J Am Coll Cardiol* 2004;43(9):1596–1601).

29.3 Answer C. Carotid endarterectomy has been shown to be an effective treatment for carotid artery stenosis. Carotid artery stenting has recently been an attractive alternative to carotid endarterectomy. Previous trials had conflicting results regarding the efficacy of carotid stenting compared to carotid endarterectomy. The CREST trial was designed to compare outcomes of carotid artery stenting to those of carotid endarterectomy with symptomatic or asymptomatic carotid artery stenosis (Brott TG, et al. *N Engl J Med* 2010;363(1):11–23).

A total of 2,522 patients with asymptomatic or symptomatic carotid artery stenosis were included in this study. Patients were randomized to carotid endarterectomy or carotid artery stenting and followed for a medium of 2.5 years. The primary end point was a composite of stroke, MI, and mortality in the periprocedural period or ipsilateral stroke within 4 years. There was no significant difference in the 4-year rate of primary end point in the two groups (7.2% for carotid stenting and 6.8% for carotid endarterectomy). This finding was true, independent of whether a patient was asymptomatic or symptomatic.

Differences were identified in rates of periprocedural adverse events. While there was no difference in the rate of death between the two groups (0.7% for stenting and 0.3% for endarterectomy), patients who underwent stenting had a higher rate of stroke (4.1% vs. 2.3%) while patients who underwent endarterectomy had a higher rate of MI (2.3% vs. 1.1%).

29.4 Answer D. Participation in a formal exercise rehabilitation program results in a significant improvement in the time to claudication pain and the time to maximal pain as demonstrated by Gardner and Poehlman in their meta-analysis of 33 trials evaluating walking distances in patients with PAD before and after rehabilitation. Program characteristics that were noted to correlate to increased pain-free distances were exercise duration >30 minutes per session, participation in at least three sessions per week, walking as a mode of exercise, and the use of near-maximal claudication pain as an end point, with participation in the program of >6 months. The only independent predictors of increased walking distances were the use of the claudication end point, program length, and mode of exercise ($p = 0.001$) (Gardner AW, et al. *JAMA* 1995;274(12):975–980).

On the basis of the results of numerous studies detailing the elevated crude rates of coronary heart disease in patients with PAD, the current National Cholesterol Education Program/Adult Treatment Panel III recommendations consider PAD as a coronary heart disease risk equivalent and advise that the goal LDL-C be lowered to <100 mg/dL with consideration of drug therapy in addition to lifestyle modifications to achieve this goal (Grundy SM, et al. *Circulation* 2004;110(2):227–239). The heart protection study prospectively randomized 20,536 patients with CAD, diabetes mellitus, or PAD to either simvastatin 40 mg once daily vs. placebo and reported a reduction in all-cause mortality of 13% ($p = 0.0003$), major vascular events by 24%, coronary death by 18%, and nonfatal or fatal stroke by 25%. Most strikingly, the reduction in the event rates was also observed in the subgroups of patients without known coronary disease, including those with diabetes, cerebrovascular disease, and PAD (Shepherd J, et al. *Lancet* 2002;360(9346):1623–1630).

Abnormal ABIs (<0.9), as a noninvasive diagnostic tool for PAD, have been shown to be associated with other traditional cardiovascular risk factors as well as more than a threefold increase in coronary heart disease and cardiovascular disease mortality. In a prospective cohort study of 1,537 patients with systolic hypertension, 25.5% of participants recorded an ABI of <0.9. Abnormal ABI was statistically associated with the presence of other typical CAD risk factors. After 1- to 2-year follow-up, the presence of an abnormal ABI had an increased age–sex adjusted relative risk of mortality because of coronary heart disease of 3.8 (95% CI, 2.1 to 6.9), cardiovascular disease of 3.7 (95% CI, 1.8 to 7.7), and total mortality of 4.1 (95% CI, 2 to 8.3) (Newman AB, et al. *JAMA* 1993;270(4):487–489).

Currently, the only FDA-approved medications labeled for the purpose of relief of claudication because of PAD are pentoxifylline and cilostazol. Cilostazol, a type III phosphodiesterase inhibitor with direct action on the platelets and vascular smooth muscle, functions as a potent antiplatelet agent as well as vasodilator. A meta-analysis of eight randomized, placebo-controlled trials encompassing 2,702 patients with moderate to severe claudication demonstrated that cilostazol increased maximal and pain-free walking distances by 50% and 67%, respectively (Thompson PD, et al. *Am J Cardiol* 2002;90(12):1314–1319). Pentoxifylline, known to function by reducing the red blood cell viscosity, was shown to increase the pain-free walking distance by a mean of 29.4 m (95% CI, 13.0 to 45.9 m), and the absolute claudication distance by a mean of 48.4 m (95% CI, 18.3 to 78.6 m) in a total of 612 patients with moderate, claudication symptoms at baseline (Hood SC, et al. *CMAJ* 1996;155(8):1053–1059). Another study, however, indicated that cilostazol was more effective than pentoxifylline for increasing pain-free walking distances, but was associated with a greater incidence of side effects, such as diarrhea and headache (Dawson DL, et al. *Am J Med* 2000;109(7):523–530).

29.5 Answer E. History and physical examination can suggest a diagnosis of PAD. Presence of claudication, impaired walking function, ischemic rest pain, abnormal lower extremity pulse exam, vascular bruit, or nonhealing lower extremity ulcers all suggest PAD. Patients at increased risk for PAD include elderly (>65), those with known atherosclerotic disease, those with risk factors for atherosclerosis and aged 50 to 64, and those under the age of 50 with diabetes and with one additional risk factor for atherosclerosis. Patients' symptoms or physical exam suggestive of PAD should undergo diagnostic testing for PAD (Class I recommendation), while diagnostic testing is reasonable in those at increased risk of PAD (Class IIa recommendation).

Resting ABI is the initial test of choice per American Heart Association (AHA) Guidelines (Gerhard-Herman MD, et al. *Circulation* 2016;CIR.0000000000000470). The ABI is calculated by dividing the highest dorsalis pedis pressure or posterior tibial pressure by the highest right or left arm pressures. The normal range for ABI is 1.00 to 1.40. Diagnosis of peripheral vascular disease is confirmed in patients with symptoms of PAD and an ABI <0.9. In patients who are symptomatic without alternative diagnosis of symptoms but have an ABI in the normal range, additional examination with exercise ABI can be performed to induce limb ischemia. An ABI of >1.40 suggests a noncompressible artery, and alterative diagnostic testing must be used to further investigate the presence of PAD. Toe-brachial index can be used in this case. A toe-brachial index >0.70 is considered normal, while a toe-brachial index <0.70 suggests the presence of PAD.

29.6 Answer B. Given that the long-term patency rates following infrapopliteal angioplasty are inferior to that of the larger vessels above the knee, percutaneous transluminal angioplasty (PTA) should be reserved for situations of acute limb ischemia (ALI) or nonhealing wounds or for limb salvage in patients who are not surgical candidates. Medical therapy with antiplatelet agents, such as aspirin, clopidogrel, or cilostazol, should be the first line of therapy. In addition to participation in a formal exercise rehabilitation program, risk factor modification including the aggressive management of diabetes and the cessation of tobacco use is also essential. Although the rate of progression to eventual limb loss or severe ischemia is 2% per year, diabetic patients with claudication symptoms have a greater likelihood of progressing to rest pain, developing gangrene, and eventual limb loss. Smokers also have increased rates of disease progression and have a 20% risk of limb loss if they continue to smoke (Hirsch AT, et al. *J Am Coll Cardiol* 2006;47(6):1239–1312).

Although vessel perforation or thrombosis can occur during any interventional procedure involving a lower extremity vessel, the complication rate of PTA in the infrapopliteal vascular bed is not prohibitively high and, as noted in the preceding text, has clear indications. In a recent study evaluating the efficacy of below-the-knee stent-supported angioplasty to establish inline arterial flow in 82 patients with critical limb ischemia (68%) or lifestyle-limiting claudication (32%), the technical success rate was 94% for de novo lesions, and there were no major adverse events, such as death, MI, or limb loss reported. In addition, there was a significant increase (p = 0.0001) in the ABIs of both the groups following intervention, as well as a subjective improvement in wound healing and decreased rest pain (Feiring AJ, et al. *J Am Coll Cardiol* 2004;44(12):2307–2314). Treating below-the-knee critical limb ischemia with a drug-eluting stent (DES) may also be an effective and safe means of preventing major amputation and relieving symptoms (Feiring AJ, et al. *J Am Coll Cardiol* 2010;55(15):1580–1589).

29.7 Answer B. Numerous medical therapies have been studied for the management of PAD. Risk factor modification is indicated in all patients with PAD. Smoking cessation is recommended for all patients with PAD and should be advised at each visit. Pharmacologic therapy with varenicline, bupropion, and/or nicotine replacement should be provided to patients who smoke, and referral to a smoking cessation program can also be recommended (Class I recommendation). Comorbid conditions such as diabetes or hypertension should also be addressed to reduce the risk of MI, stroke, heart failure, or cardiovascular death. Additionally, supervised exercise programs have been shown to be safe, improve functional status, and reduce limb symptoms. These programs should take place at a medical facility, be supervised by a health care provider, be performed for 30 to 45 minutes three times per week at a minimum of 12 weeks, and entail a warm-up and cool down period with intermittent walking for moderate-to-maximal claudication. This can be considered as a treatment option prior to revascularization.

Statin medications have been shown to decrease major adverse cardiovascular and cerebrovascular events (MACCE) (HR 0.53; 95% CI, 0.28 to 0.99), mortality (HR 0.49; 95% CI, 0.24 to 0.97), and major amputation or death (HR 0.53; 95% CI, 0.35 to 0.98) and are recommended for all patients with PAD (Westin GG, et al. *J Am Coll Cardiol* 2014;63(7):682–690). Cilostazol has been shown to improve PAD symptoms and increase walking distance in patients with claudication. Pentoxifylline, iron chelation with ethylenediaminetetraacetic acid, or B-complex vitamin supplementation to lower homocysteine levels have been shown to be mostly ineffective in the treatment of claudication and are not recommended. The available data indicate that the benefit of pentoxifylline is marginal, particularly in light of more effective therapies such as cilostazol.

29.8 Answer A. Revascularization in chronic limb ischemia is aimed at decreasing limb pain and improving wound healing. Endovascular revascularization has been shown to be an effective alternative to surgical revascularization in all comers and is an attractive option in certain patients. Patients with high surgical risk, including those with significant comorbidities such as coronary ischemia, cardiomyopathy, heart failure, lung disease, or renal dysfunction, should be assessed for endovascular revascularization prior to surgical revascularization. Additionally, endovascular revascularization is favored in patients without suitable vasculature for bypass graft such as those who have undergone prior SVG for CABG. Staged intervention with endovascular treatment prior to surgical revascularization is also favored in patients with significant symptoms at rest when surgical revascularization would otherwise be delayed.

Certain characteristics, however, still favor surgical therapy. Endovascular treatment can be complex with a high failure rate in certain anatomical scenarios. Lesions involving the common femoral artery at the origin of the deep femoral artery, long segmental lesions involving the popliteal or infrapopliteal artery, diffuse disease at multiple vascular levels, and densely calcified lesions are all technically difficult, and endovascular repair has poor durability.

29.9 Answer B. Balloon angioplasty has been shown to effectively restore blood flow in patients with atherosclerotic disease in the femoral or popliteal arteries. Restenosis and neointimal hyperplasia, however, are common and occur in approximately 60% of patients within 1 year (Rocha-Singh KJ, et al. *Cathet Cardiovasc Interv* 2007;69(6):910–919). As such, adjunctive stenting is commonly performed to prevent vascular recoil and reduce restenosis rates but has been prone to fracture. To further reduce rates of restenosis, DES has been used and shown to have an antiproliferative effect on the artery wall. Drug-eluting balloons (DEB) were then tested in the LEVANT 2 trial (Rosenfield K, et al. *N Engl J Med* 2015;373(2):145–153).

A total of 476 patients with claudication or rest pain and angiographically significant atherosclerotic lesions were randomized in a 2:1 ratio to paclitaxel-coated balloon vs. standard angioplasty and followed for 12 months. The primary end point was freedom from restenosis or repeat revascularization of the target lesion at 12 months. The primary safety end point was a perioperative death and 12-month limb-related death, amputation, and reintervention.

Both groups had similar rates of immediate success (88.9% in drug-coated balloon and 86.8% with standard angiography). There was no significant difference in the rate of periprocedural complications. At 12 months, patient who underwent angioplasty with paclitaxel-coated balloons had a higher rate of primary patency than did patients who underwent angioplasty with standard balloons (65.2% vs. 52.6%). There was no significant difference in resting ABI or quality of life at 1-year follow-up.

29.10 Answer E. The vast majority of renal artery stenoses are because of either atherosclerotic disease or FMD; it is estimated to be present in up to 5% of hypertensive patients. In addition, renal artery stenosis may be noted in up to 30% to 40% of patients with documented atherosclerosis of other vascular beds (Safian RD, et al. *N Engl J Med* 2001;344(6):431–442). Atherosclerotic renal disease (>90% of renal artery stenoses) typically involves the ostium or proximal third of the renal artery, progresses with age, and is known to be associated with hypertension and renal insufficiency (Safian RD, et al. *N Engl J Med* 2001;344(6):431–442). FMD (<10% of renal artery stenoses) is most commonly found in women aged 15 to 50 years and involves the distal two-thirds of the vessel with a characteristic "string of beads" appearance on angiography (Slovut DP, et al. *N Engl J Med* 2004;350(18):1862–1871). In addition to the preceding indications, other indications for renal arteriography include azotemia without clear etiology in a patient with evidence of atherosclerotic disease in other vascular beds, malignant hypertension refractory to the addition of three or more antihypertensive medications, or unexplained renal failure. Although it is generally a safe and well-tolerated procedure, renal arteriography should only be considered for patients in whom the operator has strong clinical suspicion of renovascular disease. Although uncommon, complications of renal arteriography include atheroembolism, renal artery ostial trauma, dissection, and contrast nephrotoxicity. Performing routine angiography of the renal vasculature in a patient without one of the preceding indications is not recommended.

29.11 Answer A. Unilateral renal artery stenosis is a common finding in the elderly but is often an incidental finding rather than the primary cause of a patient's hypertension. There are numerous clinical clues that suggest a patient would benefit from treatment of renal artery stenosis. A strong predictor of drop in blood pressure after renal revascularization is the duration of blood pressure elevation. Patients with a shorter duration of hypertension prior to revascularization are more likely to benefit from revascularization than those with longstanding hypertension. Additionally, patients who have failed multiple prior blood pressure regimens or are intolerant of medical regimens are more likely to benefit from renal revascularization. Renovascular hypertension can cause acute rises in blood pressure leading to recurrent flash pulmonary edema or refractory heart failure. Younger patients or patients with confirmed severe FMD also benefit from revascularization over medical therapy alone.

29.12 Answer E. Appropriate preoperative workup and risk stratification are needed prior to surgical AAA repair. Baseline medical risk should be assessed with particular attention to cardiac, pulmonary, and renal disease. Patients should be continued on their preoperative cardiovascular medications at the time of surgery including aspirin, beta-blockers, and statin. Sexual history should also be assessed as there is a high prevalence of preexisting sexual dysfunction in AAA patients and AAA repair can result in autonomic nerve injury and compromise blood supply to the pelvic region. Additionally, as patients with AAAs have a high prevalence of coexisting vascular disease, coexisting aneurysms should be identified by clinical exam or imaging. Those with symptoms of peripheral vascular disease should be screened with ABI. Globally, consideration of risk benefit should be considered, particularly in morbidly obese patients, those with major medical comorbidities, and limited life expectancy.

Prior to surgery, abdominal anatomy should be defined. CTA is the initial test of choice to define the location of the aneurysm and features of the aneurysm. Inflammatory aneurysms can be identified based on their adherence to adjacent structure and thickening of the aneurysm wall, which aids in risk stratification as they have a significantly higher perioperative mortality rate than do noninflammatory aneurysms (Pennell RC, et al. *J Vasc Surg* 1985;2(6):859-869). Additionally, preoperative CTA can identify other anatomical structures that may alter repair. Specifically, abdominal vasculature should be assessed with particular emphasis on the SMA to assure patency of the vessel. If there is significant stenosis, it may require repair at the time of AAA due to loss of the IMA.

29.13 Answer A. Risk of rupture guides management strategy for asymptomatic AAAs, as AAA repair can be procedurally complex. Medical treatment is recommended in those where the risk of rupture is small, while surgical treatment is recommended for those patients with a high risk of rupture who are appropriate surgical candidates. The risk of rupture is based on multiple factors; however, size of aneurysm and rate of aneurysm expansion guide therapy. The risk of AAA rupture increases significantly above 5.5 cm. As such, multiple randomized controlled trials have compared surgical repair vs. observation for AAAs < 5.5 cm in diameter and have shown that risk of rupture does not exceed the risk of surgical repair in this population. Rapidly expanding AAAs have also been shown to have an increased rate of rupture. As such, surgical repair is recommended for AAAs that expand by >5 mm in 6 months or 10 mm in 1 year. Gender has also been shown to affect risk of rupture. Female patients have a higher rate of rupture than do male patients; however, they also have higher mortality rate during AAA repair. As such, the recommendations for AAA repair are independent of gender.

For those patients in whom observation is recommended, risk modification and reassessment of aneurysm size should be done. As the natural history of AAA is progressive expansion, many patients will ultimately require aneurysm repair. No therapies have been shown to reduce rate of expansion or rupture; however, medical therapies are aimed at reducing comorbid medical conditions. Patients should be started on aspirin and a statin as AAA is considered a CAD risk equivalence. Exercise is recommended for patients with an AAA as it will decrease overall cardiovascular morbidity and mortality. Moderately strenuous activities do not precipitate AAA rupture and will decrease perioperative risk.

29.14 Answer C. The autonomic nervous system, particularly the sympathetic nervous system, has been shown to play a role in resistant hypertension. As such, surgical sympathectomy through renal denervation has been studied in patients with resistant hypertension. Early observation studies, nonrandomized clinical trials, and nonblinded clinical trials showed large reductions in blood pressure in patients with resistant hypertension. As such, the SIMPLICITY HTN-3 trial was conducted to assess whether renal artery denervation improved blood pressure control over medical therapy alone in patients with resistant hypertension (Bhatt DL, et al. *N Engl J Med* 2014;370(15):1393–1401).

A total of 535 patients with resistant hypertension defined as an initial systolic blood pressure of 160 mm Hg on three or more blood medications, including a diuretic at maximally tolerated doses, were included in this study. Patients were assigned 2:1 to renal denervation vs. sham procedure and medical therapy. The primary end point of the study was mean change in office systolic blood pressure with a superiority margin of 5 mm Hg and ambulatory systolic blood pressure with a superiority margin of 2 mm Hg at 6 months with a primary safety endpoint composite of multiple major adverse events.

Both groups had a significant decrease in office blood pressure (14.13 for denervation group, 11.74 for sham procedure group) with no significant decrease with the prespecified superiority margin. Ambulatory blood pressure had similar results with a drop in systolic pressure of 6.75 mm Hg in the denervation group and 4.79 mm Hg in the sham group and no significant decrease with the prespecified superiority margin. Subset analysis showed no significant interaction effect of diabetes, sex, race, BMI, age, renal function, and medication changes. Renal denervation, however, was shown to be safe. The rate of major adverse events was low and not significantly different between groups (1.4% in the denervation procedure group and 0.6% in the sham procedure group).

Overall, the SIMPLICITY HTN-3 trial showed that while renal denervation was safe, it did not provide better blood pressure control than medical therapy alone.

29.15 Answer D. FMD is a nonatherosclerotic disease of small and medium-size arteries that often affects the renal arteries causing renal artery stenosis and resultant hypertension. Renal artery revascularization through either angioplasty or surgical reconstruction can be used to treat hypertensive patients with FMD. Numerous studies have assessed the blood pressure response and periprocedural complication rate of renovascular revascularization in FMD. Trinquart et al. published a meta-analysis reviewing 98 eligible articles that address surgical and percutaneous revascularization (Trinquart L, et al. *Hypertension* 2010;56(3):525–532).

Patients who underwent percutaneous revascularization had a technical success rate of 88.2%. The combined complication rate was 11.8% with a major complication rate of 5.3%. The periprocedural mortality rate was 0.9%.

Hypertension cure rates defined as controlled blood pressure without treatment were 45.7% for all definitions of hypertension. The likelihood of cure significantly decreased with increasing age.

Patients who underwent surgical revascularization had a combined complication rate of 16.9% with the majority defined as a major complication (15.4%) or a perioperative mortality of 1.2%. Hypertension cure rates with surgery were 57.5%.

29.16 Answer D. Preprocedural planning is the most critical component of a technically successful endovascular AAA repair. CT provides the backbone for evaluating patient candidacy. In addition to the indications of either an asymptomatic aneurysm of appropriate maximal diameter or a small aneurysm with features putting it at increased risk of rupture, patients being considered for EVAR must fulfill several anatomic criteria. These include (1) iliofemoral access vessels that will allow safe insertion and deployment of the device, adequate seal, and sufficient length to provide axial support for the graft and (2) an infrarenal aortic neck of adequate length, limited angulation, and appropriate diameter. These anatomic features, as well as the presence or absence of thrombus and calcium at each level, can be evaluated using CT. The short-term results in patients with AAA in the EVAR-1 trial, which randomized 1,082 patients aged 60 years and older with aneurysms >5.5 cm in diameter to either surgical or endovascular repair, showed a significant reduction in 30-day mortality in the endovascular repair group (1.6% vs. 4.7%, 0.33 0.15 to 0.74, $p = 0.007$) (Greenhalgh RM, et al. *Lancet* 2004;364(9437):843–848). However, long-term follow-up data from EVAR-1 revealed that 4 years after randomization, all-cause mortality between the groups was similar with that of the endovascular repair group experiencing higher overall rates of complication (17.6/100 person years vs. 3.3/100 person years; 95% CI, [3.5 to 6.8]; $p < 0.0001$) and needed reintervention (6.9/100 person years vs. 2.4/100 person years; 95% CI, 2.7 1.8 to 4.1; $p < 0.0001$) (EVAR Trial Participants. *Lancet* 2005;365(9478):2187–2192). Similar results were reported in the smaller Dutch Endovascular Aneurysm Management (DREAM) trial that randomized 351 patients with an aneurysm >5 cm to endovascular or open surgical repair. As in EVAR-1, there was a significant reduction in 30-day mortality in the endovascular group (1.2% vs. 4.6%; 95% CI, 0.1 to 4.2), but this difference was no longer significant at 6-month follow-up (Prinssen M, et al. *N Engl J Med* 2004;351(16):1607–1618). Although the recently published long-term follow-up results of the DREAM trial revealed a significant reduction in aneurysm-related mortality benefiting the endovascular group (2.1 vs. 5.7; 95% CI, −0.5 to 7.9), there was no significant difference in the cumulative survival between endovascular and open repair groups (89.7% vs. 89.6%). In contrast to the EVAR-1 trial, however, the rates of severe complication, aneurysm rupture, and reintervention were similar in both groups (Blankensteijn JD, et al. *N Engl J Med* 2005;352(23):2398–2405).

With longer follow-up now being achieved after EVAR, >97% 5-year and >94% 9-year rupture-free survival have been observed (Brewster DC, et al. *Ann Surg* 2006;244(3):426–438).

Although there are no randomized data to support the optimum time for aneurysmal repair, general expert opinion suggests that the larger the aneurysm, the greater the risk of rupture. Other independent risk factors for AAA rupture include COPD, hypertension, female gender, smoking, and symptoms including abdominal tenderness or back pain. Additionally, aneurysms that expand >0.6 cm in 1 year are at a high risk of rupture. Therefore, this patient would likely not do well with medical management and should be strongly considered for repair, either surgical or endovascular. Finally, cardiac complications are the most common serious perioperative complication of EVAR (Prinssen M, et al. *N Engl J Med* 2004;351(16):1607–1618) and the most common cause of late death (EVAR Trial Participants. *Lancet* 2005;365(9478):2179–2186).

29.17 Answer E. A dreaded complication, SCI is an infrequent complication of open surgical repair of a thoracic aortic aneurysm, although it can be seen following endovascular thoracic aortic repair as well. SCI is typically not a complication of AAA repair. The artery of Adamkiewicz is the largest anterior segmental medullary artery. When damaged or obstructed, it can result in anterior spinal artery syndrome, with loss of urinary and fecal continence (Wan IY, et al. *Eur J Cardiothorac Surg* 2001;19(2):203–213) and impaired motor function of the legs; sensory function is often preserved to a degree. Option A describes a type I endoleak, which can be because of undersizing of the stent, poor proximal or distal fixation, neck dilation, stent fracture or separation, or aneurysms with short, angulated necks. With rare exceptions, the presence of a type I endoleak requires immediate treatment that could include stenting at the location of the leak, further angioplasty of the graft, or open surgical repair. Option B describes a type II endoleak, which is considered a more benign complication with treatment typically reserved for cases where the aneurysmal sac continues to enlarge. Option C describes a type IV endoleak that is most commonly seen in conjunction with thin-walled Dacron grafts and is also not thought to be at high risk for causing significant clinical complications. Not mentioned in the preceding text is type III endoleak, which results from limb separation or fabric wear and may require the deployment of an additional cuff to adequately treat. As one might expect, embolization of thrombus or plaque debris during EVAR is a feared, but an unfortunate, reality that can result in ischemia of any distal vascular bed. Perforation and/or dissections of the iliac artery are fortunately decreasing in recent years partly because of increased flexibility and easier insertion of the delivery device (Drury D, et al. *Br J Surg* 2005;92(8):937–946).

29.18 Answer D. The group of symptoms described in the preceding text is referred to as the subclavian steal syndrome and can often be confused for TIA, stroke, migraine headache, intracranial mass, or temporal arteritis. The etiology of the symptom complex is vertebrobasilar insufficiency due to the presence of a proximal subclavian stenosis that results in retrograde blood flow in the ipsilateral vertebral artery. In addition to the symptoms mentioned in the preceding text, common presenting symptoms are that of upper extremity claudication, paresthesia, numbness, ataxia, confusion, diplopia, nystagmus, and visual symptoms. A rare but well-documented phenomenon is that of coronary steal due to retrograde blood flow in the ipsilateral internal mammary artery, thereby causing ischemia in the targeted coronary vascular bed. Indications for revascularization of the subclavian artery include symptomatic steal syndromes, disabling upper extremity weakness, vertebrobasilar insufficiency, preservation of flow to the in situ internal mammary grafts, or evidence of embolic phenomenon in the upper extremities thought secondary to the subclavian disease. The presence of subclavian disease in the absence of symptoms is not an indication for intervention and should be avoided. Although ultrasound and magnetic resonance angiography (MRA) can help diagnose this problem, angiography would be the most efficient and precise strategy to diagnose and treat the subclavian steal syndrome.

29.19 Answer A. There are many different variations of the right-sided aortic arch. The most commonly seen right-sided aortic arch has the left carotid as the first branch. The left subclavian is the last branch. The easiest way to understand

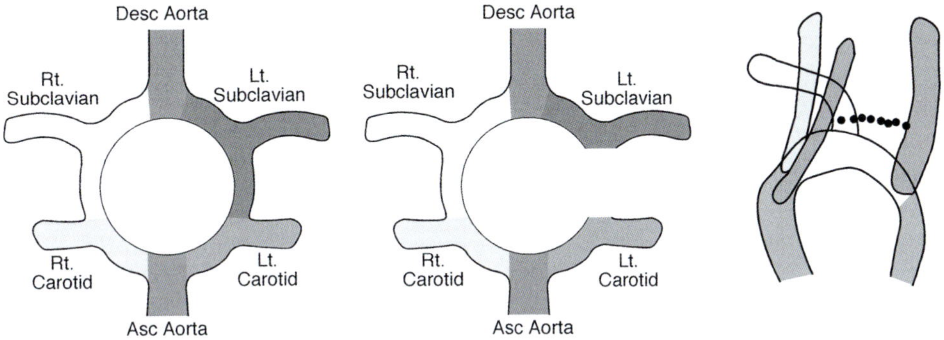

Figure A29-19

the right-sided aortic arch is to be familiar with embryology. As shown in Figure A29-19, normally, the segment between the right subclavian and the descending aorta disappears, but in right-sided arch that is most commonly encountered within adults, the segment between the left carotid and subclavian disappears.

29.20 Answer C. The clinical presentation in question is consistent with Takayasu's arteritis—a chronic, idiopathic disease that is characterized by inflammation of the aorta and its main branches. The disease affects almost exclusively female patients, is more common in Asian persons, and has a mean age presentation of 25 years. The symptoms at clinical presentation are because of limb or organ ischemia due to the progressive stenosis of involved arteries. In a prospective cohort study of 60 patients with confirmed Takayasu's arteritis after a mean follow-up of 5.3 years (Kerr GS, et al. *Ann Intern Med* 1994;120(11):919–929), it was reported that the most common presenting symptoms included arm claudication (63%); light-headedness (33%); visual changes (often bilateral); constitutional complaints, such as weight loss and fever; and, less commonly, chest pain and myalgias. Physical findings included carotid bruit (80%), diminished or absent radial pulse (53%), carotidynia (32%), visual aberration, and, less commonly, aortic insufficiency (due to aortic root inflammation and distention). Hypertension was noted in 33% of the patients at some point in their disease course and was highly associated with either unilateral or bilateral renal artery stenosis. Angiography demonstrated aortic lesions in 65% of these patients; 32% of these lesions involved the aortic arch and its branches, and 68% involved the aortic vasculature above and below the diaphragm. Interestingly, no patient was noted to have sole involvement of the abdominal aorta. Medical therapy usually consisted of oral steroids dosed at 1 mg/kg for up to 3 months with the addition of a cytotoxic agent, such as cyclophosphamide or azathioprine, if the steroid dose is unable to be weaned. Surgical treatment was indicated in patients with refractory hypertension due to renal artery stenosis, extremity ischemia, cerebrovascular ischemia, or critical (>70%) stenosis of at least three cerebral vessels, moderate or severe aortic regurgitation, or cardiac ischemia due to angiographically proven coronary artery stenosis. Angioplasty was less commonly performed and was most often employed in the revascularization of the subclavian and renal vessels. Approximately half of the interventions were successful on the first attempt, and only one-third were successful on the second attempt with restenosis being a common problem. In general, angioplasty is avoided during active inflammatory phase of the disease.

29.21 Answer C. Originating from the anterior portion of the aorta inferior to the aortic hiatus of the diaphragm, the celiac artery is a short arterial trunk that courses anteriorly and divides into three larger branches—the left gastric, the hepatic, and the splenic arteries (Fig. A29-21).

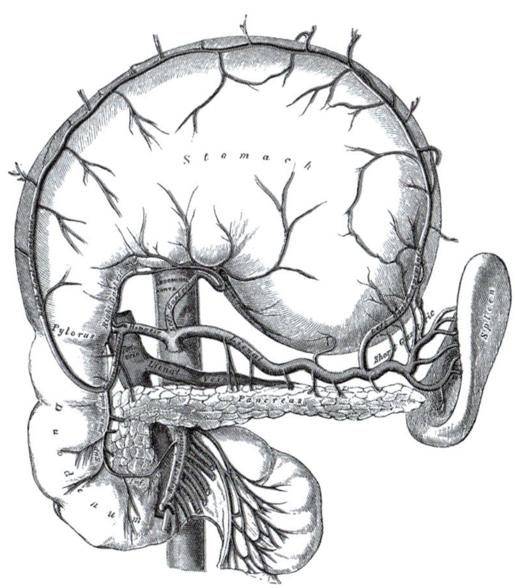

Figure A29-21

The smallest of the three vessels, the left gastric artery, courses superiorly and branches into numerous subdivisions to provide blood flow to portions of the esophagus and the cardiac portion of the stomach before passing along the lesser curvature of the stomach to the pylorus, where it commonly anastomoses with the right gastric artery.

The hepatic artery courses to the porta hepatis and branches into the right and left hepatic arteries, thereby supplying blood flow to both lobes of the liver.

Running along the greater curvature of the stomach, the right gastroepiploic artery anastomoses with the left gastroepiploic branch of the splenic artery and provides blood flow to both surfaces of the stomach. Given its large caliber and close proximity to the inferior aspect of the heart, the right gastroepiploic artery is amenable for grafting to the distal RCA and PDA as is seen in the preceding angiogram.

The SMA and IMA are large branches that arise from the aorta inferior to the celiac trunk and are not visualized in this angiogram.

29.22 Answer B. This patient has had two prior interventions (and the lesion is likely at least 15 cm in length). This makes it at least a TASC C lesion. However, there is no involvement of the popliteal artery. Hence, it is not a TASC D lesion. The distal runoff is good in all three vessels (i.e., the anterior tibial, peroneal, and posterior tibial are patent). For aortoiliac and femoral popliteal disease, endovascular repair is the recommended treatment of choice for type A lesions and is preferred for type B lesions, whereas open surgical repair is best suited for type D lesions. Type C lesions remain in a gray zone, with endovascular repair reserved for patients with a high surgical risk (Norgren L, et al. *Eur J Vasc Endovasc Surg* 2007;33(Suppl 1):S1-S75).

29.23 Answer A. FMD lesions typically show a beading pattern. With the most common subtype of FMD, medial fibroplasias, the dilated arterial segments are often larger in diameter than the original vessel. This is not the case with perimedial fibroplasias, in which the beads are up to, but not greater than, the caliber of the original vessel. In posttransplant renal artery stenosis, there could be a variety of reasons—faulty surgical technique, arterial injury during donor nephrectomy or perfusion preservation, chronic rejection, and atherosclerotic disease (Slovut DP, et al. *N Engl J Med* 2004;350(18):1862-1871).

29.24 Answer D. In the CREST trial, there were no significant differences in the estimated 4-year rates of primary end point between carotid artery stenting and carotid endarterectomy (7.2% and 6.8%, respectively; hazard ratio for stenting, 1.11; 95% CI, 0.81 to 1.51; $p = 0.51$). During the periprocedural period, the incidence of the primary end point was similar with carotid artery stenting and carotid endarterectomy (5.2% and 4.5%, respectively; hazard ratio for stenting, 1.18; 95% CI, 0.82 to 1.68; $p = 0.38$), although the rates of the individual end points differed between the stenting group and the endarterectomy group (death, 0.7% vs. 0.3%; $p = 0.18$; stroke, 4.1% vs. 2.3%; $p = 0.01$; MI, 1.1% vs. 2.3%; $p = 0.03$). After the periprocedural period, the incidence of ipsilateral stroke was similarly low with carotid artery stenting and with carotid endarterectomy (2.0% and 2.4%, respectively; $p = 0.85$). Note that the increased incidence was not in major strokes but in minor strokes (Brott TG, et al. *N Engl J Med* 2010;363(1):11-23).

29.25 Answer E. This was a significant perforation during attempted placement of a large arterial sheath. It is of critical importance to reverse anticoagulation and achieve contralateral access, followed by balloon occlusion from the contralateral side. This could be followed by treatment of a covered stent should there be inadequate results from the balloon treatment alone.

30 Cerebrovascular Interventions

Mehdi Shishehbor and Ankur Kalra

QUESTIONS

30.1 A 67-year-old Caucasian male presents to your office for evaluation. He states that he has had three episodes of transient ischemic attacks (TIAs) in the last year. His medical history is significant for hypertension and dyslipidemia. His laboratory evaluation shows evidence of left ventricular hypertrophy on his electrocardiogram (ECG), a creatinine of 1.3, and low-density lipoprotein (LDL) of 98 mg/dL. He is currently taking amlodipine for hypertension and simvastatin for dyslipidemia. He denies any history of coronary or peripheral vascular disease. Antiplatelet regimen for stroke prevention may include all of the following, EXCEPT:

(A) Aspirin monotherapy
(B) Aspirin and extended-release dipyridamole
(C) Clopidogrel monotherapy
(D) Aspirin and clopidogrel

30.2 The same patient above has a carotid Doppler ultrasound that demonstrates 50% stenoses in both the carotid arteries. All of the following are acceptable doses of statin therapy, EXCEPT:

(A) Atorvastatin 40 mg/day
(B) Rosuvastatin 20 mg/day
(C) Atorvastatin 80 mg/day
(D) Simvastatin 40 mg/day

30.3 A 73-year-old man presents with a history of frequent TIAs. His medical history is significant for prior myocardial infarction (MI), hypertension, and dyslipidemia. Baseline labs are unremarkable. A computed tomography (CT) angiogram was ordered by his primary care physician to assess for carotid stenosis. All the following may render carotid endarterectomy (CEA) difficult or not feasible, EXCEPT:

(A) Prior radiation to the neck or previous radical neck surgery
(B) Severe tandem lesion
(C) Aorto-ostial or proximal common carotid artery lesion
(D) Lesion location is distal cervical (C2 level and above)

30.4 A 59-year-old woman with a history of coronary artery disease (CAD) and prior left CEA presented with a history of two episodes of slurred speech and right-sided weakness. These episodes lasted for <1 hour, and the patient recovered completely. The patient's medications include aspirin, lisinopril, and atorvastatin. A carotid angiogram is shown in Figure Q30-4. The most appropriate option for the management of this patient is:

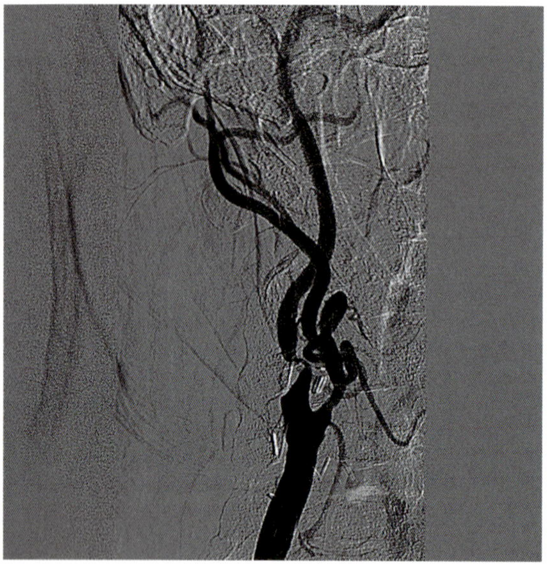

Figure Q30-4

(A) Repeating CEA
(B) Carotid artery stenting
(C) Adding clopidogrel to the current regimen
(D) Initiating warfarin

30.5 A 77-year-old woman presents with a history of an ischemic stroke 4 weeks ago. She has now completely recovered from the stroke and does not have any residual neurologic deficit. Her neurologist has ordered a magnetic resonance angiogram (MRA), which showed a type 3 aortic arch (Fig. Q30-5) and a severe 90% stenosis of the ostium of the internal carotid artery. MRA also revealed a moderate-size pedunculated thrombus in the left internal carotid artery. All of the following are considered high-risk factors during carotid artery stenting in her, but stenting is still considered feasible, EXCEPT in:

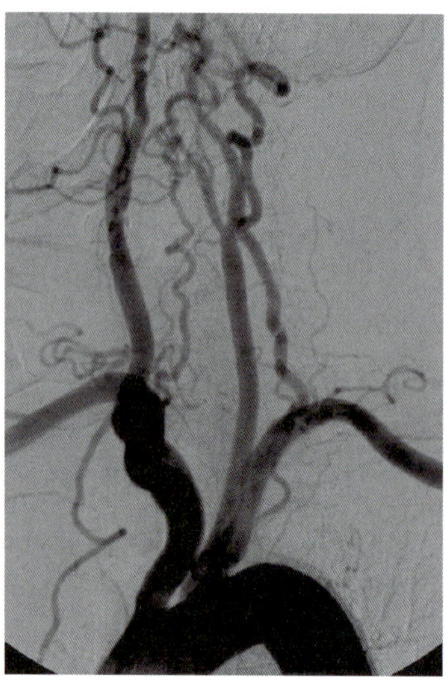

Figure Q30-5

(A) Age >75 years
(B) Type 3 aortic arch
(C) Pedunculated thrombus
(D) Stenosis involving the ostium of the internal carotid artery

30.6 CEA is not feasible in the same patient above due to prior radiation to the neck. Which of the following embolic protection devices is recommended during carotid artery stenting?

(A) Nav-6
(B) Acunet
(C) Angioguard
(D) Flow reversal (transcarotid arterial revascularization)

30.7 A 67-year-old man presents with episodes of dizziness and diplopia for the last 3 weeks. His past medical history is significant for diabetes and hypertension. Carotid and vertebral artery ultrasound is performed and reveals <30% stenosis of bilateral carotid arteries, a small diminutive left vertebral artery, and severe stenosis of the origin of a large dominant right vertebral artery. Subsequent angiography confirms a 90% ostial narrowing of a large right vertebral artery (Fig. Q30-7). In discussing with the patient his therapeutic options regarding his severe vertebral artery stenosis, all of the following are true, EXCEPT:

(A) The data are primarily limited to case series on the role of percutaneous intervention for vertebral artery stenosis
(B) Embolic events involving the brainstem can be life-threatening

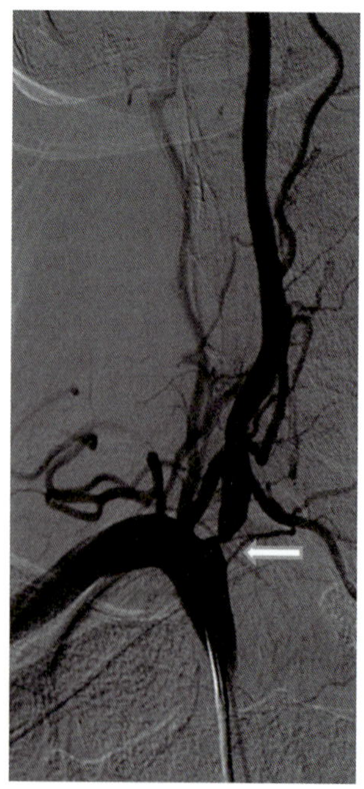

Figure Q30-7

(C) About 25% of patients with vertebrobasilar insufficiency have an associated significant carotid artery disease, the management of which may relieve the symptoms
(D) The risk of recurrent stroke in the acute phase of a vertebrobasilar TIA is low; however, the risk is high for recurrent cerebrovascular accident on longer-term follow-up

30.8 A 71-year-old gentleman undergoes carotid stenting for severe symptomatic right internal carotid artery stenosis. His blood pressure remains in the 80 to 90 mm Hg systolic range during the procedure. However, he remains asymptomatic. Which of the following is the next best step to treat intraprocedural hypotension?

(A) Fluid resuscitation
(B) Norepinephrine
(C) Dopamine
(D) Phenylephrine

30.9 A 67-year-old man with a history of hypertension, prior radiation to the neck in the context of thyroid cancer, and hyperlipidemia presented with recurrent short-lived episodes of visual loss in his left eye. His ECG shows normal sinus rhythm with left ventricular hypertrophy. A bilateral carotid duplex study was done, which was suggestive of total occlusion of the right internal carotid artery and severe stenosis of the left internal carotid artery. A carotid angiogram was done (Fig. Q30-9). What is the best route of action in the management of this patient?

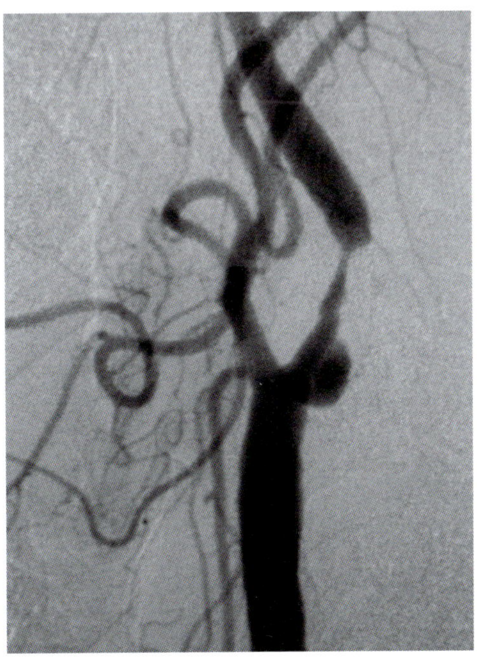

Figure Q30-9

(A) Proceed with carotid artery stenting
(B) Arrange a vascular surgery consultation for possible CEA
(C) Initiate anticoagulation with heparin followed by warfarin for 4 to 6 weeks with reevaluation with angiography at that time
(D) Initiate anticoagulation and plan reevaluation with angiography in 48 hours

30.10 A 61-year-old man was referred to interventional cardiology service for a second opinion on the management of a newly diagnosed carotid disease. The patient underwent, prior to his referral, a carotid duplex study to assess a bruit over the left carotid artery. This study was soon followed by an angiography by the local cardiology group (Fig. Q30-10). The patient has been experiencing occasional headache over the past 2 months. His blood pressure is 140/88 in your office. His total cholesterol is 220, and his LDL is 150. The patient was advised to consider undergoing CEA. What would be your recommendation to this patient at this point?

(A) The patient should undergo endarterectomy as he is at a low risk (<4%) for such procedure

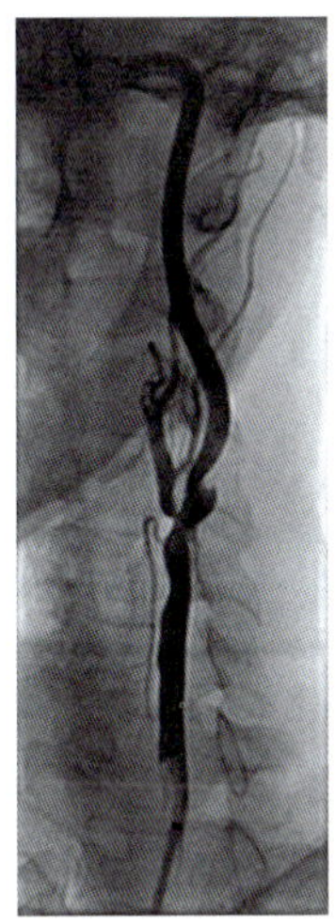

Figure Q30-10

(B) Proceed with carotid stenting with the use of a FilterWire to protect the distal circulation
(C) Initiate aspirin 162 mg oral (PO) once daily (QD), atorvastatin 80 mg PO nightly (QHS), and ramipril 2.5 mg PO QD
(D) Initiate aspirin 162 mg PO QD, clopidogrel 75 mg PO QD, atorvastatin 80 mg PO QHS, and ramipril 2.5 mg PO QD

30.11 Following postdilatation of a carotid stent, the same patient becomes acutely hemiparetic and aphasic. Figure Q30-11A–D shows the sequence of angiography, stenting, and postdilatation of the

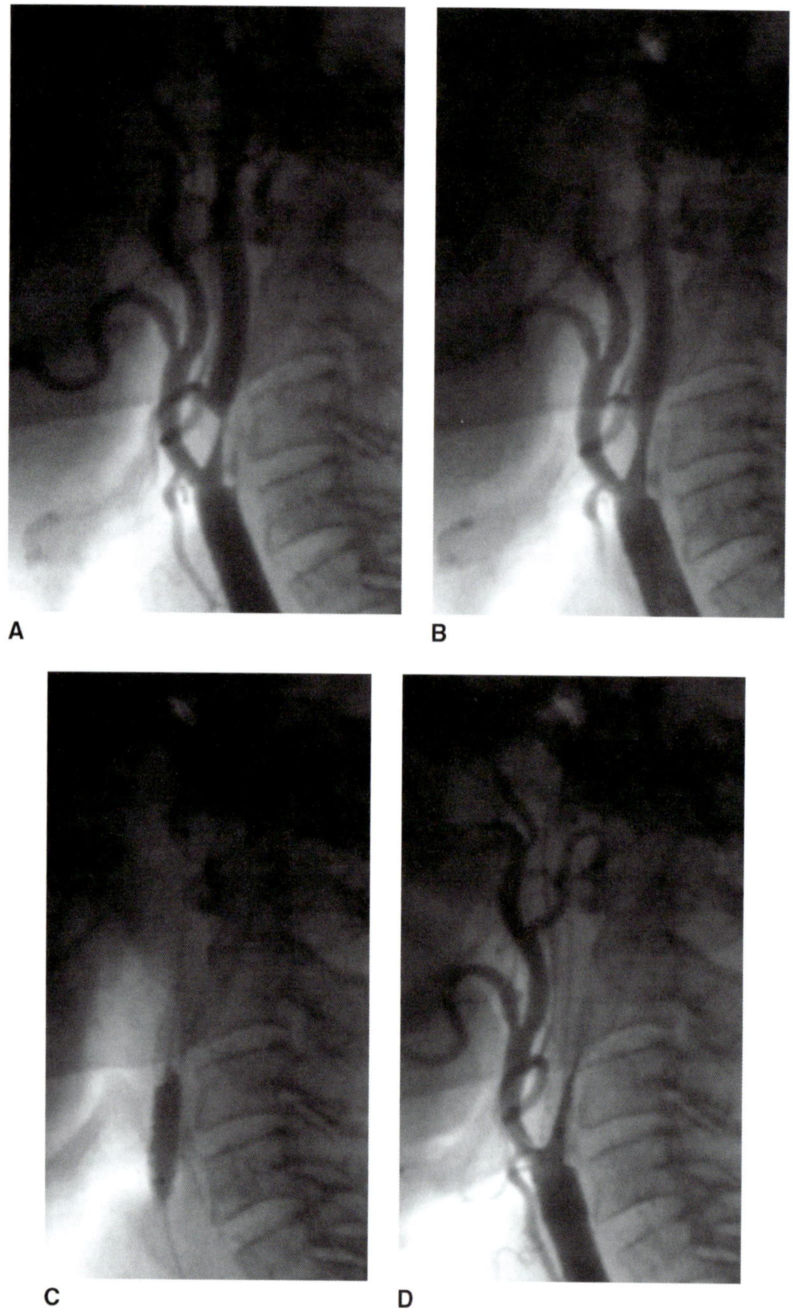

Figure Q30-11

stent. What should have been the best route of action prior to filter retrieval in this situation?

(A) Removal of the FilterWire
(B) Injection of intracarotid urokinase
(C) Use a larger balloon to further dilate the stent
(D) Angiography to confirm flow, and if no- or slow flow, use of an Export catheter to aspirate

30.12 A 69-year-old gentleman presents with unstable angina and coronary angiography reveals severe three-vessel obstructive CAD. A carotid ultrasound is ordered by the surgical team, which shows <50% stenosis in the right coronary artery (RCA) and 80% stenosis in the left internal carotid arteries. There is mild nonobstructive disease of bilateral vertebral arteries. In patients such as this individual with concomitant CAD and carotid disease, it is TRUE that:

(A) The risk of perioperative neurologic event following coronary artery bypass grafting (CABG) is about 9% for individuals with asymptomatic unilateral internal carotid artery disease with >50% stenosis
(B) Randomized clinical trials have confirmed that carotid stenting followed by CABG (staged) carries the lowest risk for perioperative neurologic events when compared with simultaneous CEA and CABG (combined)
(C) Retrospective reports showed little difference between the staged and the combined approaches for revascularization
(D) Asymptomatic >75% unilateral internal carotid artery stenosis carries a 14% risk of perioperative stroke in patients undergoing CABG

30.13 According to the North American Symptomatic Carotid Endarterectomy Trial (NASCET), when assessing carotid artery severity, all the following statements are TRUE, EXCEPT:

(A) Percent stenosis = (presumed normal segment diameter − diseased segment diameter)/presumed normal segment diameter × 100
(B) The normal segment is defined as the diameter of the segment just distal to the carotid bulb and not the carotid bulb itself or the poststenotic area distal to the lesion
(C) The normal segment is defined as the estimated diameter of the carotid bulb as it was prior to the atherosclerotic narrowing
(D) Percent of stenosis by the European Carotid Surgery Trial (ECST) is always more severe than the percent stenosis given by NASCET method

30.14 A 76-year-old diabetic with documented three-vessel disease underwent a carotid duplex study that was suggestive of total occlusion of bilateral internal carotid arteries. The surgeons are reluctant to proceed with CABG. Carotid angiogram confirmed total occlusion of the right and the left internal carotid arteries. What would be the best route of action in this patient?

(A) Bilateral CEA
(B) Unilateral CEA
(C) Bilateral carotid artery stenting
(D) Unilateral carotid artery stenting
(E) Abort plans for bypass surgery, and plan for high-risk percutaneous coronary intervention

30.15 A 68-year-old woman underwent carotid angiography for evaluation of recurrent TIAs. Angiography revealed an ulcerated stenosis with heavy plaque burden (Fig. Q30-15). What is the guideline recommendation for this patient for revascularization?

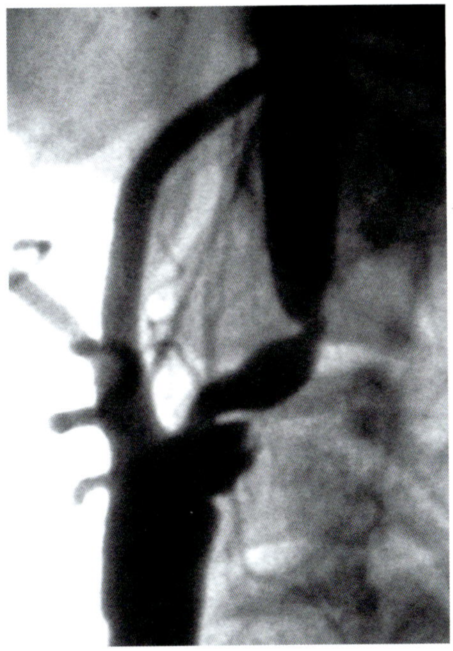

Figure Q30-15

(A) Stenting
(B) CEA
(C) Medical management
(D) Consider revascularization if the patient has a recurrent episode

30.16 The Carotid Revascularization Endarterectomy vs. Stenting Trial (CREST) randomly assigned patients with symptomatic or asymptomatic carotid stenosis to undergo carotid artery stenting or CEA. The primary composite end point was stroke, MI, or death from any cause during the periprocedural period or any ipsilateral stroke within 4 years after randomization. The study demonstrated that:

(A) The risk of the composite primary outcome of stroke, MI, or death did not differ significantly in the group undergoing carotid artery stenting and the group undergoing CEA
(B) The risk of the composite primary outcome of stroke, MI, or death was significantly higher in the group undergoing carotid artery stenting compared to the group undergoing CEA
(C) The risk of the composite primary outcome of stroke, MI, or death was significantly lower in the group undergoing carotid artery stenting and the group undergoing CEA
(D) The trial was stopped prematurely due to lack of funding

30.17 A major difference between coronary and cerebral arteries that interventionalists need to be aware of is that:

(A) Cerebral arteries have a thicker tunica media
(B) Cerebral arteries have no external elastic lamina
(C) Cerebral arteries have thick supportive adventitia
(D) Cerebral arteries have less tortuosity

30.18 A 53-year-old man with diabetes mellitus, hypertension, CAD, and cigarette smoking developed recurrent, crescendo left middle cerebral artery (MCA) TIAs despite treatment with clopidogrel. Carotid angiography (Fig. Q30-18) reveals:

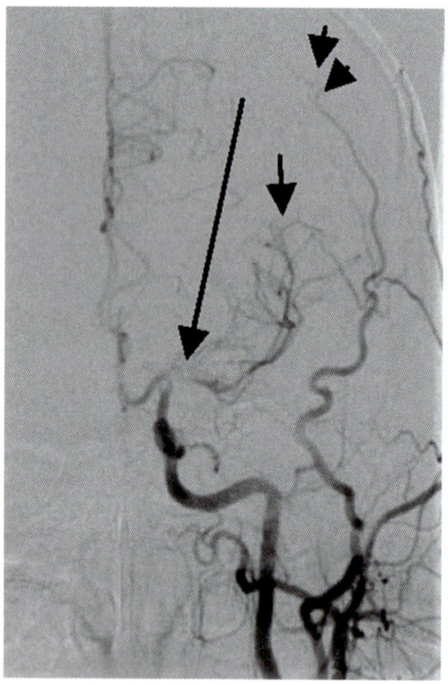

Figure Q30-18

(A) 90% left common carotid stenosis
(B) 90% left ostial internal carotid artery stenosis
(C) 90% left internal carotid artery terminus stenosis extending into the middle cerebral artery
(D) 90% left external carotid artery stenosis

30.19 A 71-year-old man presents with symptoms of dizziness and light-headedness for 3 weeks. The patient also gives history of a drop attack 4 days ago. An ultrasound study was suggestive of a severe stenosis in one of the blood vessels to the brain. An angiogram performed (Fig. Q30-19) shows:

(A) Severe stenosis of the proximal left vertebral artery
(B) Severe stenosis of the left carotid artery
(C) Severe stenosis of the right carotid artery
(D) Severe stenosis of the proximal right vertebral artery

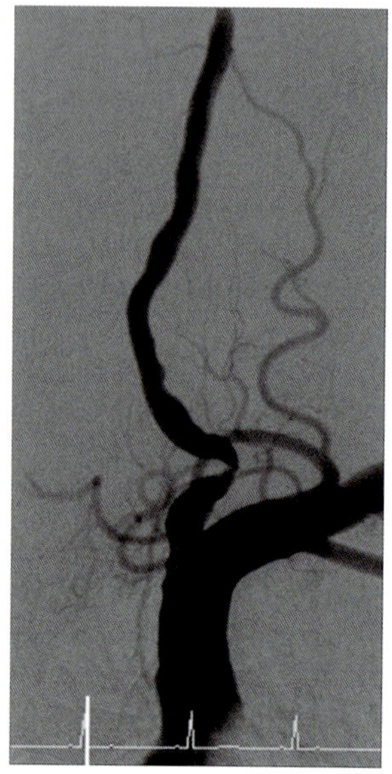

Figure Q30-19

30.20 Regarding training for carotid stenting, the Society for Cardiovascular Angiography and Interventions (SCAI), the Society for Vascular Medicine and Biology (SVMB), and the Society for Vascular Surgery (SVS) guidelines specify that:

(A) Operators perform a minimum of 30 supervised diagnostic cervicocerebral angiograms (at least 15 as a primary operator) and a minimum of 25 supervised carotid interventions (at least 13 as a primary operator) prior to performing carotid artery stenting independently
(B) Operators perform a minimum of 50 supervised diagnostic cervicocerebral angiograms (at least 25 as a primary operator) and a minimum of 45 supervised carotid interventions (at least 23 as a primary operator) prior to performing carotid artery stenting independently
(C) Operators perform a minimum of 100 supervised diagnostic cervicocerebral angiograms (at least 50 as a primary operator) and a minimum of 50 supervised carotid interventions (at least 26 as a primary operator) prior to performing carotid artery stenting independently
(D) Operators perform a minimum of 30 supervised diagnostic cervicocerebral angiograms (at least 5 as a primary operator) and a minimum of 25 supervised carotid interventions (at least 10 as primary operator) prior to performing carotid artery stenting independently

30.21 A 59-year-old man presents with vertigo and diplopia. As part of his evaluation, his neurologist orders ultrasound of both vertebrals, which reveals small occluded left vertebral. Doppler of the right vertebral (Fig. Q30-21) is suggestive of:

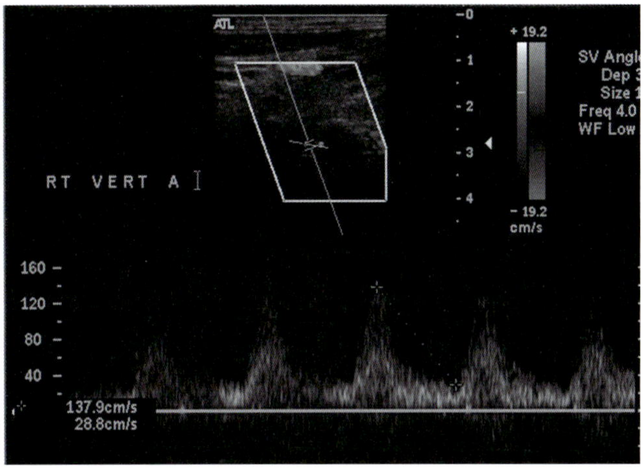

Figure Q30-21

(A) Normal flow in the right vertebral artery
(B) Severe stenosis of the right vertebral artery
(C) Moderate nonobstructive stenosis of the right vertebral artery
(D) Mild stenosis of the right vertebral artery

30.22 A 63-year-old man presents to your inpatient cardiology ward with unstable angina. Risk factors include hypertension and smoking history. On physical examination, he has a left carotid bruit, an S4 gallop, diminished dorsalis and posterior tibial pulses in the left leg, and absent dorsalis pedis in the right leg. Coronary angiography reveals 70% left main stenosis, severe (80%) mid-left anterior descending (LAD) artery stenosis, and 70% stenosis in the midportion of the RCA. Left ventriculography reveals mild systolic dysfunction with an estimated ejection fraction (EF) of 50% and left ventricular end-diastolic pressure (LVEDP) of 17 mm Hg. A carotid ultrasound is indicated prior to CABG based on all of the following, EXCEPT:

(A) Peripheral arterial disease
(B) Carotid bruit
(C) Age > 60 years
(D) Smoking history
(E) Left main stenosis

30.23 Current guidelines for carotid artery stenting in asymptomatic patients state all of the following, EXCEPT:

(A) The effectiveness of prophylactic carotid artery stenting in asymptomatic average surgical risk patients compared with medical therapy alone in highly selected patients is well established
(B) It is reasonable to choose carotid artery stenting over CEA when revascularization is indicated in patients with neck anatomy unfavorable for arterial surgery
(C) Selection of asymptomatic patients for carotid revascularization should be guided by an assessment of comorbid condition, life expectancy, and other individual factors
(D) All patients with carotid artery stenosis should receive statins

ANSWERS AND EXPLANATIONS

30.1 Answer D. The 2008 Update to the American Heart Association (AHA)/American Stroke Association (ASA) Recommendations for the Prevention of Stroke in Patients With Stroke and Transient Ischemic Attack recommends that aspirin (50 to 325 mg/day) monotherapy, the combination of aspirin and extended-release dipyridamole, and clopidogrel monotherapy are all acceptable options for initial therapy (Class I, Level of Evidence A) (Adams RJ, et al. *Stroke* 2008;39(5):1647-1652). Based on the ESPRIT trial, the combination of aspirin and extended-release dipyridamole is recommended over aspirin alone (Class I, Level of Evidence B). The efficacy of dual antiplatelet therapy (DAPT) with aspirin and clopidogrel was tested in the Management of Atherothrombosis with Clopidogrel in High-Risk Patients with Recent TIA or Ischemic Stroke (MATCH) trail. The MATCH trial did not show additional clinical value of adding aspirin to clopidogrel in high-risk patients with TIA or ischemic stroke, and the risk of life-threatening or major bleeding is increased with the combination of aspirin and clopidogrel (Diener HC, et al. *Lancet* 2004;364(9431):331-337).

30.2 Answer D. High-intensity statin therapy is indicated in patients with symptomatic carotid artery stenosis. Of all the options listed, simvastatin 40 mg/day is moderate in intensity, therefore not correct.

30.3 Answer B. CEA is generally technically challenging or not feasible in patients with prior radiations to the neck, prior neck surgery or ipsilateral CEA (the so-called hostile neck), or aorto-ostial or proximal common carotid disease. CEA is associated with higher risk in patients with restenosis following CEA, contralateral internal carotid artery occlusion, severe comorbidities, and contralateral laryngeal nerve palsy. Severe tandem lesions can be effectively treated with endarterectomy.

30.4 Answer B. The risk of a stroke is quite high in this patient with recurrent hemispheric TIA and a high-grade internal carotid artery disease (10% in the first year and about 30% in 5 years). Among the high-risk features for recurrent stroke are hemispheric TIA, recent TIA, increasing frequency of TIA, and high-grade carotid stenosis. The patient's anatomy is suitable for carotid artery stenting, which may be the best route of action in this scenario. Prior CEA in this patient increases the risk of complications with a second CEA but may also be considered, depending on local expertise. The use of clopidogrel or warfarin in addition to aspirin will offer the patients an inferior therapeutic intervention when compared to carotid artery revascularization. While patients with restenosis following CEA were not included in the NASCET and Asymptomatic Carotid Atherosclerosis Study (ACAS) trials, such history was a qualifying criterion for inclusion in the SAPPHIRE trial (Yadav JS, et al. *N Engl J Med* 2004;351(15):1493-1501), which focused on high-risk patients with severe carotid disease and showed that carotid artery stenting was noninferior to CEA.

30.5 Answer C. Presence of pedunculated thrombus is an absolute contraindication for both carotid stenting and endarterectomy, and neither should be attempted until thrombus is resolved. Older age and a type 3 arch may make the procedure technically challenging, but it is still feasible in experienced hands.

30.6 Answer D. Flow reversal (transcarotid arterial revascularization) is the recommended embolic protection strategy in comparison with the other listed options.

30.7 Answer D. The risk of recurrent stroke is extremely high in the acute phase (up to 7 days after the presenting symptoms); however, the risk of death and stroke is relatively low thereafter (Chambers BR, et al. *Cochrane Database Syst Rev* 2005;(4):CD001923).

30.8 Answer A. Although all are acceptable options to treat intraprocedural hypotension, the next best step is intravenous (IV) fluid resuscitation.

30.9 Answer C. Presence of pedunculated thrombus is an absolute contraindication for both carotid artery stenting and CEA (Bilkoo P, et al. *Curr Cardiol Rep* 2009;11(5):384-390). Anticoagulation should be initiated and a reassessment with angiography should be postponed for at least 4 to 6 weeks.

30.10 Answer A. While the efficacy of carotid artery stenting in the management of low-risk severe asymptomatic carotid atherosclerosis is under evaluation, CEA remains the standard of care in the management of patients with severe asymptomatic carotid artery disease who are at an acceptable surgical risk (<4%). The risk of stroke in this patient (with >60% stenosis) is 3.2% per year. In the ACAS trial, 1,659 patients with asymptomatic carotid stenosis of at least 60% were randomized to CEA vs. medical therapy (Walker MD, et al. *JAMA* 1995;273(18):1421–1428; Halliday A, et al. *Lancet* 2004;363(9420):1491–1502). The perioperative stroke or death reported in this study was 2.3%.

30.11 Answer D. No-reflow is a serious complication of carotid stenting. It is attributed to a large thrombus burden that overwhelms the FilterWire leading to stagnant forward circulation and essentially no flow distal to target lesion. Aspirating this thrombus column, while the FilterWire is in place, is the recommended strategy in this situation. Retrieving the FilterWire will release the thrombotic debris and result in distal embolization. The use of urokinase can further complicate this precarious situation with intracerebral bleeding. Larger balloon inflation will not resolve this complication and is likely to result in dislodgement of more thrombotic debris distally (Casserly IP, et al. *J Am Coll Cardiol* 2005;46(8):1466–1472; Raithel D. *Cardiovasc Surg (Torino)* 2005;46(3):261–265).

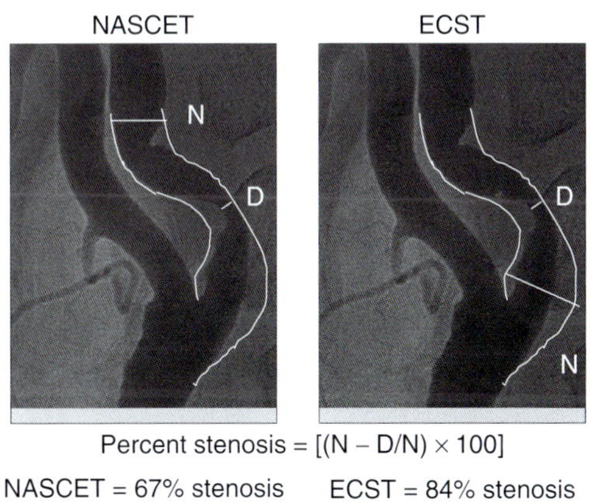

Figure A30-13

30.12 Answer C. Retrospective studies show little difference between staged and combined approaches for revascularization. There are no randomized trial data available to guide decision-making with regard to staged vs. combined approaches for CEA and CABG. The risk of a perioperative neurologic event following CABG is 9% in patients with asymptomatic bilateral (and not unilateral) carotid disease with >50% stenosis. Asymptomatic >75% unilateral internal carotid artery stenosis carries a <5% risk of perioperative stroke in patients undergoing CABG (Shishehbor MH, et al. *J Am Coll Cardiol* 2013;62(21):1948–1956; Venkatachalam S, et al. *Curr Opin Cardiol* 2011;26(6):480–487; Venkatachalam S, et al. *Ann Vasc Surg* 2012;26(1):125–140; Venkatachalam S, et al. *Heart* 2011;97(3):175–180).

30.13 Answer C. All the statements are accurate statements with the exception of C. In the European Carotid Surgery Trial (ECST), normal segment was defined as the estimated diameter of the carotid bulb as it was prior to the atherosclerotic narrowing (Fig. A30-13) (Gasecki AP, et al. *J Neurosurg* 1995;83(5):778–782; Warlow CP. *J Mal Vasc* 1993;18(3):198–201).

30.14 Answer E. In patients with total occlusion of bilateral carotid arteries, CABG poses an imminent risk for disabling stroke. The risk-benefit ratio is skewed toward significant risk for perioperative stroke. In such patients, bypass surgery may not be offered as a treatment option, and percutaneous revascularization with percutaneous coronary intervention may be pursued (Venkatachalam S, et al. *Curr Opin Cardiol* 2011;26(6):480–487).

30.15 Answer B. Carotid artery stenting is indicated for symptomatic patients at average or low risk of complications associated with endovascular intervention when the diameter of the lumen of the internal carotid artery is reduced by >70% as documented by noninvasive imaging, or >50% as documented by catheter angiography and the anticipated rate of periprocedural stroke or mortality is <6% and patient has high-risk feature for CEA. Patients at high risk for CEA are defined as having significant comorbidities and/or anatomic risk factors (i.e., recurrent stenosis and/or previous radical neck dissection) and would be poor candidates for CEA in the opinion of a surgeon. Significant comorbid conditions include but are not limited to:

- Congestive heart failure (CHF) Class III/IV
- Left ventricular ejection fraction (LVEF) < 30%
- Unstable angina
- Contralateral carotid occlusion
- Recent myocardial infarction (MI)
- Previous CEA with recurrent stenosis
- Prior radiation treatment to the neck
- Other conditions that were used to determine patients at high risk for CEA in the prior carotid artery stenting trials and studies, such as ARCHER, CABERNET, SAPPHIRE, BEACH, and MAVERIC II

Without any of the high-risk features, he would be a candidate for CEA.

30.16 Answer A. The CREST trial demonstrated that among patients with symptomatic or asymptomatic carotid stenosis, the risk of the composite primary outcome of stroke, MI, or death did not differ significantly in the group undergoing carotid artery stenting and the group undergoing CEA. During the periprocedural period, there was a higher risk of stroke with stenting and a higher risk of MI with endarterectomy, but overall risk was similar (Brott TG, et al. *N Engl J Med* 2010;363(1):11–23).

30.17 Answer B. There are major differences between the cerebral vessels and the coronary arteries or other muscular arteries. The cerebral vessels are histologically different: they have no external elastic lamina, and they have a thinner tunica media and trivial adventitia; this makes these vessels quite fragile. They also differ from the coronary arteries in being partly (i.e., the petrous and cavernous carotids) surrounded by bone or rigid and fibrous tissue (i.e., the dura mater). Combined with significant tortuosity in their proximal segments, this makes the navigation of endovascular devices to the intracranial vessels extremely difficult, if not impossible at times, which greatly increases the risk of vessel injury and perforation during endovascular therapy.

30.18 Answer C. An anteroposterior view of left common carotid angiogram shows a severe terminal internal carotid artery restenosis extending into the middle cerebral artery (long arrow). The stenosis was severely flow-limiting comparing the extent of middle cerebral artery filling (short arrow) with that of the occipital artery (double arrow). A 014-in. microwire was advanced into the inferior division of the left middle cerebral artery. A 2.0 × 9-mm balloon was advanced into the lesion and angioplasty was performed. An angiogram revealed significant lesion recoil with slow flow into the anterior cerebral artery. A 3.0 × 15-mm Wingspan stent was delivered. The patient's symptoms resolved, and at follow-up, he was asymptomatic.

30.19 Answer A. The angiogram shows severe stenosis of the left vertebral artery. This was treated with angioplasty and stenting and subsequent resolution of his symptoms.

30.20 Answer A. The SCAI/SVMB/SVS document (Rosenfield K, et al. *J Am Coll Cardiol* 2005;45(1): 165–174) specifies that new operators perform a minimum of 30 supervised diagnostic cervicocerebral angiograms (at least 15 as a primary operator) and a minimum of 25 supervised carotid interventions (at least 13 as a primary operator) prior to performing carotid artery stenting independently. Fewer studies required by the cardiology and vascular surgery organizations reflect their belief that previous experiences with coronary (minimum of 300 diagnostic coronary angiograms and 250 coronary interventions) and peripheral interventional procedures (minimum of 100 diagnostic peripheral angiograms and 50 peripheral interventions) are transferable to neurovascular interventions.

"Primary operator" means that the trainee is handling the catheter, guidewire, embolic protection device, balloon, and stent under the direct supervision of the mentoring physician. Furthermore, only one trainee can be considered the primary operator on any one carotid stenting procedure (American College of Cardiology Foundation, et al. *J Am Coll Cardiol* 2007;49(1):126–170).

30.21 Answer B. Normal peak systolic velocity (PSV) for the vertebral artery is approximately 20 to 60 cm/s. A focal PSV of >100 cm/s (as in this case) is indicative of a significant stenosis. Note that, due to asymmetry in vertebral artery diameter (present in >70% of normal individuals), there can be considerable difference in PSV between an individual's (normal) vertebral artery. A normal vertebral artery diameter on ultrasound is regarded as approximately 4 mm, with a tendency for the left vertebral artery to be usually larger than the right. The right vertebral duplex ultrasonography figure demonstrates PSVs of 137 cm/s with broadening of the spectral waveform suggestive of severe stenosis.

30.22 Answer C. In asymptomatic patients, there are no guidelines to support routine screening for carotid artery stenosis, except for some patients scheduled for CABG. Prior to CABG, carotid duplex screening is recommended in asymptomatic patients with age >65 years, left main coronary stenosis, peripheral arterial disease, history of smoking, history of TIA or stroke, or carotid bruit (American College of Cardiology Foundation, et al. *J Am Coll Cardiol* 2007;49(1):126–170).

30.23 Answer A. Prophylactic carotid artery stenting might be considered in highly selected patients with asymptomatic carotid stenosis (minimum 60% by angiography, 70% by validated Doppler ultrasound), but its effectiveness compared with medical therapy alone in this situation is not well established.

31 Valvuloplasty and Transcatheter Valve Repair and Replacement

Adnan K. Chhatriwalla and Paul Sorajja

QUESTIONS

31.1 A 79-year-old female presents to her local physician with 3 months of progressive shortness of breath and 1 week of substernal chest pressure while walking up two flights of stairs. Her past medical history is significant for diabetes mellitus, prior myocardial infarction (MI), and percutaneous coronary intervention (PCI). Echo/Doppler reveals significant aortic valve calcification with a peak instantaneous gradient of 4.2 m/s, no significant aortic regurgitation, and normal left ventricular (LV) function. Cardiac catheterization shows patent stents and no severe obstructive coronary artery disease (CAD). You are asked to consider the patient for transcatheter aortic valve replacement (TAVR). Which of the following statements are TRUE regarding TAVR in patients at intermediate risk for surgery?

(A) TAVR is a reasonable alternative to surgical aortic valve replacement (SAVR) in intermediate-risk patients
(B) The risk of disabling stroke is lower with TAVR compared to SAVR
(C) The durability of transcatheter valves is superior to surgical valves
(D) Results from randomized control trials of TAVR in patients at intermediate risk for surgery have not yet been reported

31.2 Which of the following statements is TRUE regarding the incidence of stroke related to TAVR?

(A) Embolic protection devices (EPD) have been shown to reduce the incidence of clinical stroke related to TAVR
(B) Dual antiplatelet therapy (DAPT) has been shown to reduce the incidence of clinical stroke related to TAVR
(C) Oral anticoagulation has been shown to reduce the incidence of clinical stroke related to TAVR
(D) The rate of disabling stroke with current generation TAVR devices is <5% at 30 days

31.3 A 60-year-old woman with prior mitral commissurotomy for rheumatic mitral stenosis is undergoing percutaneous mitral valvuloplasty. Following an Inoue 28-mm balloon dilation of the mitral valve, the left atrial mean pressure changes as shown in Figure Q31-3. The next most appropriate course of action is to:

(A) Remove the balloon and deem the procedure a success
(B) Upsize to a larger balloon for further dilation
(C) If the patient is hemodynamically unstable, place an intra-aortic balloon pump (IABP) and obtain urgent surgery consultation

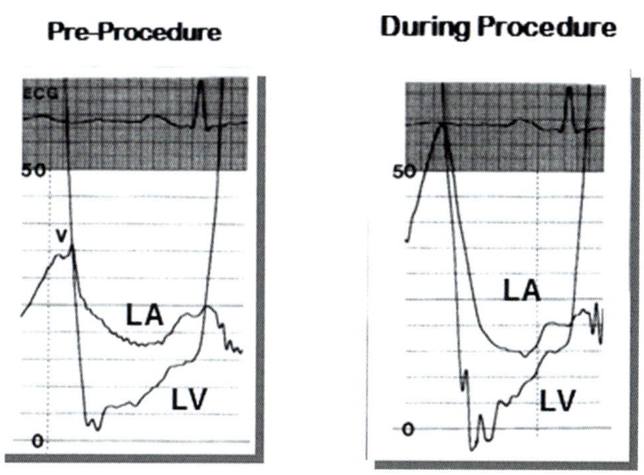

Figure Q31-3 The preprocedural left atrium and left ventricle tracings are compared to the postprocedural tracings.

(D) Hemodynamic support with phenylephrine
(E) Rezero the pressure transducer to ensure its accuracy

31.4 Which of the following characteristics of the rheumatic mitral valve is not considered in the Wilkins scoring system?

(A) Severity of mitral valve regurgitation
(B) Leaflet mobility
(C) Valvular thickening
(D) Valvular calcification
(E) Subvalvular thickening and fibrosis

31.5 A 40-year-old woman with a prior history of rheumatic fever as a child is experiencing progressive dyspnea with exertion. Echocardiogram is notable for moderate calcification of the mitral valve leaflets and severely reduced leaflet mobility with extensive valvular and subvalvular thickening. The mean mitral valve gradient is 12 mm Hg. The patient is referred for possible percutaneous balloon mitral valvuloplasty. She has had atrial fibrillation for at least 2 years. Based on the echocardiographic findings, you would suggest:

(A) Proceed with percutaneous mitral valvuloplasty
(B) Increase her diuretics and see her back in 4 to 5 weeks
(C) Add amiodarone and attempt direct current cardioversion (after transesophageal echocardiogram [TEE] is performed)
(D) Refer her for surgical mitral valve replacement
(E) Refer her for surgical mitral commissurotomy

31.6 In a patient with severe mitral stenosis, which one of the following is NOT an indication for balloon mitral valvuloplasty based on the current American College of Cardiology (ACC)/American Heart Association (AHA) valvular heart disease guidelines?

(A) Progressive dyspnea on exertion
(B) New-onset atrial fibrillation
(C) Evidence of hemodynamically significant mitral stenosis during exercise
(D) Pulmonary hypertension

31.7 A 55-year-old male presents to your office with severe right heart failure. Thirteen years ago, he had two-vessel coronary artery bypass grafting (CABG), a mitral valve replacement with a bileaflet mechanical mitral valve, and a tricuspid valve replacement with a porcine bioprosthesis. He has no angina but some dyspnea, and he has noted a progressive enlargement of his abdomen with peripheral edema above his ankles. You obtain an echocardiogram that includes the following (Fig. Q31-7). Based on the echo/Doppler above, you would suggest:

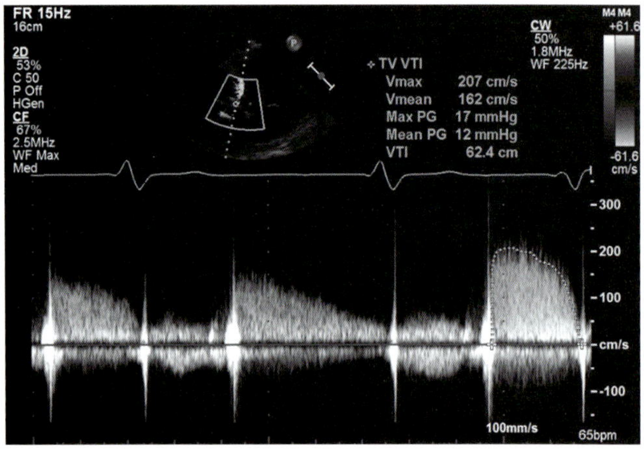

Figure Q31-7 A representative echo Doppler tracing through a prosthetic tricuspid valve replacement with mean gradient of 12 mm Hg.

(A) A cardiac magnetic resonance imaging (MRI) scan to better assess his right ventricular (RV) function, as echocardiography may be misleading in this situation
(B) A cardiac catheterization to assess his anatomy and hemodynamics and then the likely performance of percutaneous tricuspid valvuloplasty
(C) A cardiac catheterization to assess his anatomy and hemodynamics and referral for surgical tricuspid valve replacement
(D) An increase in his diuretics and an exercise sestamibi performed to determine if he has ongoing coronary ischemia

31.8 You are asked if a patient with mitral stenosis is a candidate for percutaneous mitral valvuloplasty. There is spontaneous echo contrast noted within the left atrium (LA) on TEE. Which of the following is TRUE regarding the presence of spontaneous left atrial contrast?

(A) It is most often associated with severe mitral regurgitation
(B) It is an indication of the need for immediate valvuloplasty or valve replacement
(C) It is often associated with a left atrial appendage (LAA) thrombus
(D) The presence of "smoke" in the LA contraindicates mitral valvuloplasty due to the high risk of embolic stroke
(E) It should be treated with long-term antiplatelet therapy

31.9 Which of the following is a valid statement regarding the results of a successful percutaneous balloon mitral valvuloplasty procedure?

(A) It allows for the cessation of antibiotic endocarditis prophylaxis
(B) A successful procedure can be defined as a postprocedural valve area >1.5 cm^2 with no more than 2+ mitral regurgitation
(C) A successful procedure prevents any recurrence of commissural fusion
(D) A successful procedure prevents early occurrence of atrial fibrillation
(E) Even with a low Wilkins score (<8), clinical restenosis is >50% at 10-year follow-up

31.10 An 80-year-old is referred to you for possible aortic valvuloplasty. He has chronic obstructive lung disease and has had a prior biventricular pacer with an implantable defibrillator placed due to congestive heart failure (CHF) and a left ventricular ejection fraction (LVEF) of 28%. The biventricular pacemaker has not improved his symptoms. His pulmonary function tests (PFTs) reveal moderate obstructive lung disease. His resting pO_2 is 91%. His estimated glomerular filtration rate (GFR) is 60 mL/min. He has been a heavy alcohol user in the past and knew about an aortic murmur for many years. Over the past few months, he has developed progressive symptoms of dyspnea and chest pressure. A cardiac catheterization in his local community revealed a 25 mm Hg mean aortic gradient with no aortic insufficiency and an aortic valve area (AVA) of 0.7 cm^2. He has no CAD. His brain natriuretic peptide (BNP) is elevated at 620 pg/mL.

He undergoes a second cardiac catheterization, during which time he is given intravenous (IV) dobutamine while simultaneously determining his cardiac output and valve gradient. The relevant hemodynamics of the aortic and LV pressures with graded doses of dobutamine are shown (Fig. Q31-10). Based on the hemodynamic result, he should be considered for which of the following?

(A) Aortic valve replacement
(B) Medical therapy only
(C) Balloon aortic valvuloplasty
(D) TEE to determine the AVA by planimetry

31.11 A 22-year-old college student is referred because of a murmur. On exam and by echocardiography, she has a classic doming pulmonary valve with a peak pulmonary valve gradient by echocardiography of 80 mm Hg. She is minimally symptomatic, but the decision is made to proceed with pulmonary valvuloplasty based on the hemodynamics. The procedure goes smoothly, but she becomes hypotensive immediately after the balloons are removed. The preprocedural and postprocedural right ventriculograms are shown (Fig. Q31-11). What is the most likely cause for hypotension in this setting?

(A) The pulmonary valve has ruptured and there is severe pulmonary regurgitation
(B) A ventricular septal defect (VSD) has been caused by the procedure
(C) Relief of the pulmonary valve stenosis has resulted in severe dynamic subpulmonic stenosis
(D) There is cardiac tamponade due to rupture of the pulmonary artery

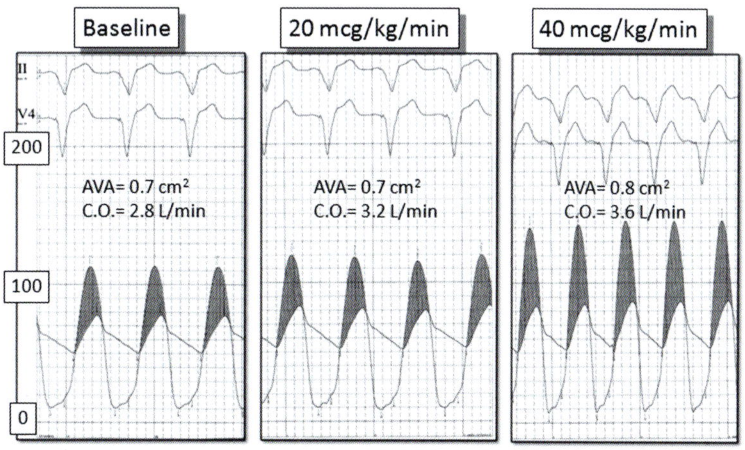

Figure Q31-10 Series of hemodynamic tracings comparing left ventricular and aortic pressures at baseline and with increasing doses of intravenous dobutamine in a patient with low-output low-gradient aortic stenosis. Valve areas calculated as indicated.

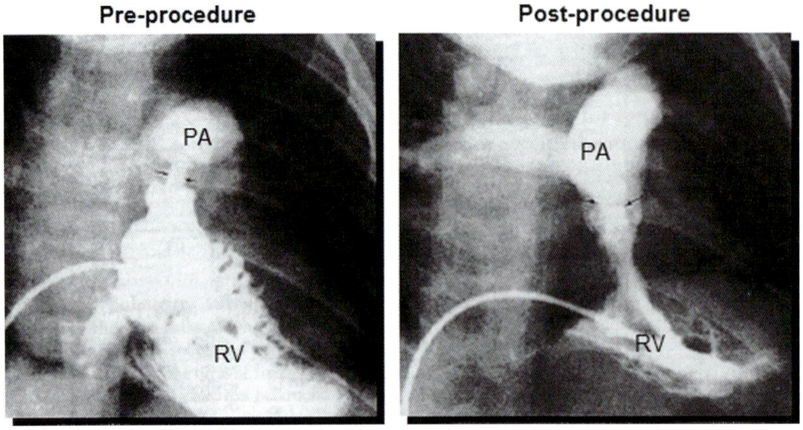

Figure Q31-11 The right ventricle (RV) angiogram before pulmonary valvuloplasty is shown on the left and the immediate postprocedural right RV angiogram on the right.

31.12 Which of the following is true regarding valve-in-valve (VIV) TAVR for the treatment of degenerated bioprosthetic valves?

(A) VIV TAVR is indicated for patients with bioprosthetic aortic stenosis and not for patients with bioprosthetic aortic regurgitation
(B) VIV TAVR is indicated for patients at either intermediate or high risk for redo SAVR
(C) The risk of coronary occlusion may be higher with VIV TAVR than with TAVR of a native aortic valve
(D) Outcomes following VIV TAVR are independent of the type or size of surgical bioprosthesis

31.13 You have just performed a second balloon inflation across a congenitally stenotic pulmonary valve using a single-balloon technique. The preprocedural and postprocedural pressure curves are obtained and are shown in Figure Q31-13. Based on the hemodynamics, the next most appropriate action would be to:

(A) Conclude the procedure is a success
(B) Upsize to a larger balloon to improve the valvular area
(C) Place an IABP and call for emergent pulmonary valve replacement
(D) Perform an emergent TEE to assess whether there is severe pulmonary regurgitation
(E) Add low-dose dobutamine for support given the drop in the right ventricle (RV) pressures

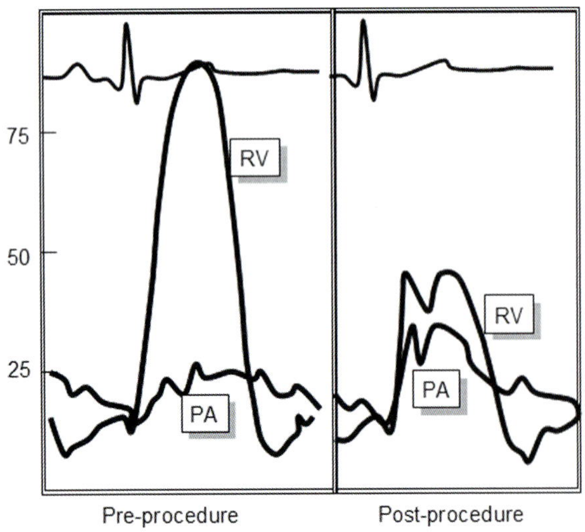

Figure Q31-13 The preprocedural right ventricle and pulmonary artery pressures are shown on the *left* and compared with the postprocedural pressures.

31.14 A 14-year-old Caucasian male sees you for consultation regarding a murmur. His local pediatric cardiologist had followed him for this. He has been feeling fine, except he notes some increased fatigue lately after an hour or so of pick-up basketball. He denies any chest pressure or presyncope. On exam, he has the murmur of aortic stenosis with mid-to-late peaking. You obtain an echocardiogram: his LV function is normal and the Doppler across his aortic valve reveals the following (Fig. Q31-14). What should be your next course of action?

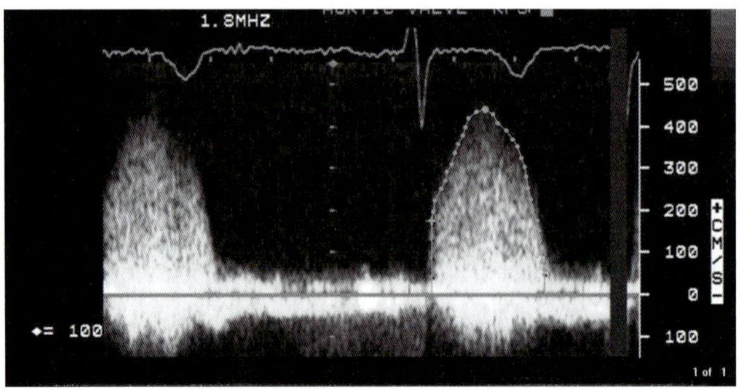

Figure Q31-14 Continuous wave Doppler signal through aortic valve showing peak velocity of 450 cm/s.

(A) He is asymptomatic clinically, and he needs no further studies
(B) He should be considered for balloon aortic valvuloplasty
(C) He should undergo a cardiac catheterization to confirm the aortic stenosis and evaluate his coronary arteries
(D) He should be started on beta-blockers and followed with an echocardiogram every 6 months
(E) He should be referred for surgical valve replacement

31.15 You are asked to see a 23-year-old woman who is 27 weeks pregnant. She has had little prenatal care. She has no known heart condition but is getting progressively short of breath as the pregnancy continues, now with New York Heart Association (NYHA) Class II CHF symptoms. She finally saw an internist who obtained an echocardiogram (Fig. Q31-15). On exam, she has a loud opening snap with an easy to discern diastolic rumble. She is in normal sinus rhythm. The mitral valve appears to move well, but there is evidence for thickening of the mitral valve and some calcium. The subvalvular apparatus looks mildly thickened. You decide she has a Wilkins score of 6. Mitral valve area is calculated at 1.2 cm^2, and no mitral regurgitation is evident by echo. Based on these data, your best therapeutic option in this situation is to use which of the following strategies?

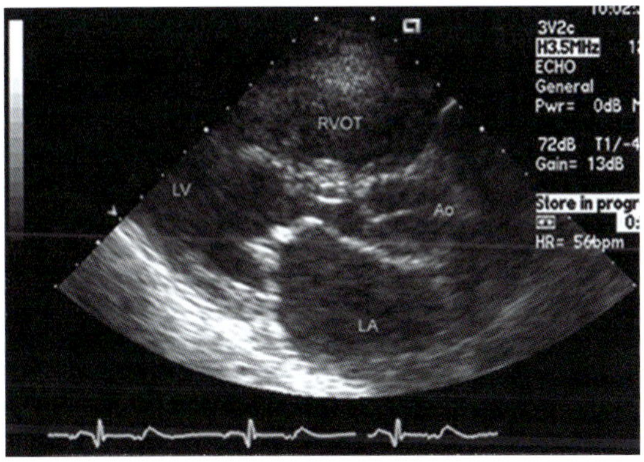

Figure Q31-15 Parasternal transthoracic echo image of a patient with mitral stenosis and mild leaflet calcification, moderate leaflet thickening, and mild thickening of the subvalvular apparatus.

(A) Medical management of heart failure with diuretics and beta-blockers
(B) Complete bed rest until she delivers the baby
(C) Consult cardiac surgery for mitral valve commissurotomy or replacement
(D) Consider balloon mitral valvuloplasty

31.16 An 86-year-old female with a history of hypertension, CAD, prior PCI, and stage IV chronic kidney disease (CKD) presents with NYHA Class III CHF symptoms. She has not had any symptoms of angina. On physical exam, she has a holosystolic murmur at the apex, radiating to the left axilla. There is no change in the murmur with inspiration. She appears euvolemic on physical exam. Echocardiography demonstrates hyperdynamic LV function with an EF of 70%. The mitral valve exhibits bileaflet prolapse, and severe mitral regurgitation is present. No other significant valvular heart disease is observed. Based on the patient's age and comorbidities, she is felt to be at prohibitive risk for surgical mitral valve repair or replacement.

Which of the following is TRUE regarding patients who were not candidates for mitral valve surgery who underwent transcatheter mitral valve repair in the EVEREST High-Risk Registry?

(A) No mortality difference was observed with transcatheter mitral valve repair
(B) Mortality at 1 year was $<10\%$ in patients undergoing transcatheter repair
(C) An initial improvement in NYHA Functional Class was observed at 1 and 6 months, but was no longer observed at 1 year
(D) Significant improvements in LV systolic and diastolic volumes were observed with transcatheter repair

31.17 Which of the following factors influences outcome in patients undergoing transcatheter paravalvular leak closure?

(A) Presence of hemolytic anemia
(B) Presence of CHF
(C) Type of valve (mechanical vs. bioprosthetic)
(D) Position of valve (mitral vs. aortic)

31.18 A 90-year-old female presents to the catheterization laboratory for balloon aortic valvuloplasty. She has severe aortic stenosis with preserved LV function and symptoms of dyspnea. You explain to her the most common complication from the procedure is:

(A) Aortic regurgitation
(B) Stroke
(C) Need for pacemaker implant
(D) Bleeding requiring transfusion
(E) Death

31.19 Which statement is TRUE regarding TAVR therapy as compared to medical therapy in patients at prohibitive risk for SAVR?

(A) There is a 1-year mortality improvement
(B) There is a 30-day mortality improvement
(C) Aortic valve regurgitation worsens over the course of the 1st year
(D) Hemolysis across the implanted valve worsens over the course of the 1st year

31.20 A variety of approaches have been evaluated for TAVR. All of the following are approaches to the aortic valve, EXCEPT:

(A) Antegrade following transseptal catheterization
(B) Retrograde from the subclavian artery
(C) Retrograde from the radial artery
(D) Antegrade via the LV apex
(E) Retrograde from the femoral artery

31.21 In the Endovascular Valve Edge-to-Edge Study (EVEREST) II of transcatheter mitral valve repair, patients were randomized in a 2:1 fashion to MitraClip transcatheter repair vs. surgical procedure. Results at 1 year suggested:

(A) Equivalent efficacy in reduction of mitral regurgitation at 1 year
(B) Similar rates of bleeding with either procedure
(C) Higher risk of endocarditis with a surgical approach
(D) Similar NYHA and quality-of-life indices at 1 year

31.22 In patients who are operable, but at high surgical risk due to comorbidities, TAVR confers:

(A) No improvement in quality-of-life measurements at 1 month as compared to SAVR
(B) A high rate of valve deterioration at the 1-year echocardiographic follow-up
(C) A lower risk for permanent pacemaker implant
(D) Improvement in NYHA Functional Class at 1 year similar to that seen in patients undergoing SAVR

31.23 The pulmonary angiogram in Figure Q31-23 reveals the results from percutaneous pulmonary valve replacement in a prior surgical RV to pulmonary artery conduit. Which of the following is not considered a potential complication from this procedure?

(A) Coronary artery compression
(B) Rupture of the pulmonary artery
(C) Compression of the aorta
(D) Tricuspid regurgitation

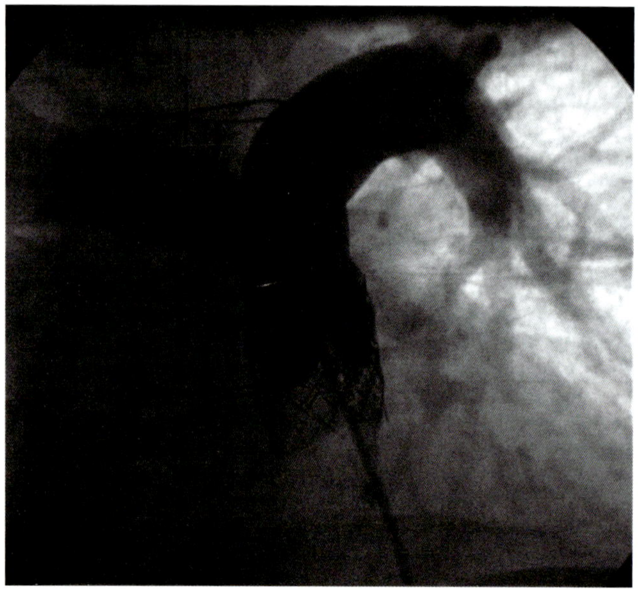

Figure Q31-23 Pulmonary angiogram with percutaneous pulmonary valve in place.

31.24 Which of the following is TRUE about balloon-expandable and self-expanding valves used for TAVR?

(A) Both technologies require rapid ventricular pacing at the time of valve deployment
(B) Balloon aortic valvuloplasty is a prerequisite to TAVR with both technologies
(C) Both technologies have demonstrated equivalent survival in randomized trials as compared to SAVR
(D) The rate of paravalvular aortic insufficiency is higher in patients treated with balloon-expandable valves

31.25 An 85-year-old male with severe aortic stenosis has had a gradual increase in exertional dyspnea for the last 3 months, consistent with NYHA Class III CHF. He has not had any symptoms of angina or syncope. He has diabetes mellitus and a history of CAD and prior CABG. On physical exam, he has a late-peaking systolic ejection murmur at the right upper sternal border. He appears euvolemic. Echocardiography demonstrates global LV dysfunction with a LVEF of 40%. The aortic valve is calcified, with limited excursion, and there is a mean gradient of 42 mm Hg across the aortic valve. No other significant valvular heart disease is present. The patient recently underwent coronary angiography, which demonstrated chronic total occlusions (CTO) of the native left anterior descending (LAD) and right coronary arteries with patent grafts to both. There is a 60% stenosis of the proximal left circumflex (LCx) artery and no bypass graft to the circumflex. Based on his age, comorbidities, and prior sternotomy, the patient is felt to be at high risk for SAVR and is referred for consideration of TAVR. Which of the following is TRUE regarding TAVR in high-risk surgical patients?

(A) TAVR is preferable to SAVR for patients at high surgical risk
(B) Choice of access site for TAVR does not impact patient outcomes
(C) A multidisciplinary heart team should collaborate to weigh treatment options and provide optimal care
(D) If TAVR is recommended, the patient will require PCI of the LCx artery at the time of the procedure

31.26 Which of the following represents the current guidelines in selecting patients for transcatheter paravalvular leak closure?

(A) Indicated for all patients with paravalvular regurgitation
(B) Treatment should be undertaken before patients have symptoms
(C) Paravalvular leak closure should be performed at experienced centers
(D) Anatomy is not an important factor in patient selection

31.27 Which of the following is TRUE regarding transcatheter mitral valve repair with MitraClip?

(A) By "cinching" the mitral valve annulus, MitraClip simulates the results of a surgical annuloplasty ring
(B) MitraClip therapy is not indicated for the treatment of patients with functional mitral regurgitation
(C) MitraClip therapy is indicated for the treatment of patients at intermediate or high risk for surgical mitral valve repair/replacement
(D) Asymptomatic patients with severe mitral regurgitation and pulmonary hypertension or atrial fibrillation may be considered for MitraClip therapy if they are at high surgical risk

31.28 A 64-year-old woman with severe mitral stenosis is seeing you 6 months following mitral valve replacement with a St. Jude bileaflet mitral valve. She initially did well after surgery, but now she has new anemia. She was seen by her family practice physician who found she had a hemoglobin of 7.5 mg/dL and a hematocrit of 24%. A haptoglobin was undetectable and the lactate dehydrogenase (LDH) was four times the upper limit of normal. On exam, she has a loud holosystolic murmur, and the echocardiogram confirms severe paravalvular mitral regurgitation. After being given iron, folate, and weekly erythropoietin, she continues to be anemic. All of the following are options to consider, EXCEPT:

(A) Continue anemia therapy until redo mechanical mitral valve replacement
(B) Continue anemia therapy until replacement of the mechanical mitral valve with a bioprosthetic mitral valve
(C) Immediate surgical repair of the paravalvular regurgitation
(D) Continue anemia therapy and withhold warfarin for 8 weeks to see if the paravalvular leak will close
(E) Attempt closure of the paravalvular leak with an occluder device now

31.29 A 40-year-old woman with severe mitral stenosis and an echocardiographic valve score of 7 is taken to the catheterization laboratory for percutaneous balloon mitral valvuloplasty. The procedure is going well, but just as the Inoue balloon catheter is placed in the LA, the patient becomes hypotensive.

The following 12-lead electrocardiogram (ECG) is obtained (Fig. Q31-29). Based on these data, the next appropriate action should be:

(A) Pericardiocentesis
(B) Protamine to reverse the effect of heparin
(C) Coronary angiography
(D) Immediate balloon mitral valvuloplasty

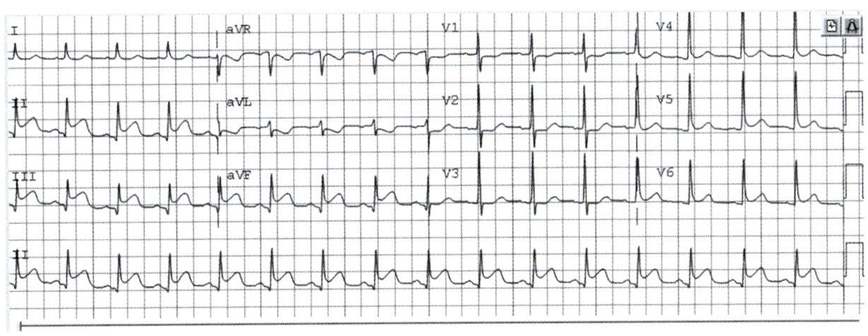

Figure Q31-29 Twelve-lead electrocardiogram showing acute inferior MI.

ANSWERS AND EXPLANATIONS

31.1 Answer A. The PARTNER II trial randomized patients with severe symptomatic aortic stenosis at intermediate surgical risk (STS score ≥4% and ≤8%) to SAVR or TAVR (Leon MB, et al. *N Engl J Med* 2016;374(17):1609–1620). There was no difference in all-cause death or disabling stroke between groups. Similarly, the SURTAVI study randomized patients with severe symptomatic aortic stenosis at intermediate surgical risk (STS score >3%) to SAVR or TAVR, with no difference in death or disabling stroke between groups (Reardon MJ, et al. *N Engl J Med* 2017;376(14):1321–1331). As a result, the 2017 Update of the ACC/AHA Guidelines for Management of Patients with Valvular Heart Disease recommends that TAVR is a reasonable alternative to SAVR for symptomatic patients with severe aortic stenosis and an intermediate surgical risk (Nishimura RA, et al. *Circulation* 2017;136(8):CIR.0000000000000503). While short-term durability of transcatheter valves appears excellent, and equivalent to the durability of surgical bioprosthesis, long-term durability of transcatheter valves is not yet known.

31.2 Answer D. While DAPT is often recommended following TAVR, its impact on stroke rates has not been evaluated. Research suggests that EPDs can decrease the number of embolic events seen on imaging studies (e.g., brain MRI), but no reduction in the rate of clinical stroke has been demonstrated to date (Haussig S, et al. *JAMA* 2016;316(6):592–601; Kapadia SR, et al. *J Am Coll Cardiol* 2017;69(4):367–377).

There is interest in the use of oral anticoagulation to reduce the risk of cerebrovascular events related to TAVR, and trials such as the GALILEO study (Windecker S, et al. *Am Heart J* 2017;184: 81–87) are currently underway to evaluate this issue. However, to date, oral anticoagulation has not been shown to reduce the incidence of stroke related to TAVR. Nevertheless, contemporary studies with current generation TAVR devices suggest that the rate of disabling stroke related to TAVR is <5% (Leon MB, et al. *N Engl J Med* 2016;374(17):1609–1620; Reardon MJ, et al. *N Engl J Med* 2017;376(14):1321–1331).

31.3 Answer C. This tracing clearly shows a large V wave within the atrial tracing consistent with severe mitral regurgitation as a complication of the balloon valvuloplasty procedure. Large V waves, however, may only reflect impaired LA compliance, thus the importance of comparing this to the preprocedural tracing. Mitral regurgitation during mitral valvuloplasty is a known complication, occurring in about 3% of patients. This is usually due to rupture of a chord in the heavily scarred subvalvular apparatus or to a tear in the leaflet itself. More than 2+ mitral regurgitation means that the procedure has been unsuccessful. One would not upsize the balloon diameter in the face of severe mitral regurgitation. Phenylephrine increases afterload on the LV and would increase the V wave in the LA tracing. While rezeroing of the transducer may be useful, it would not negate the presence of a V wave of this magnitude. Depending on the severity and baseline clinical status, the appropriate course would be to place an IABP and proceed to urgent surgery if the patient is hemodynamically compromised. Otherwise, elective surgery is indicated.

31.4 Answer A. Four characteristics are taken into account in the scoring system, with each given a 0- to 4-point value based on severity (Wilkins GT, et al. *Br Heart J* 1988;60(4):299–308).

(1) **Leaflet Mobility**
- (a) Highly mobile valve with only leaflet tip restriction
- (b) Midportion and base of leaflets with reduced mobility
- (c) Valve leaflets move forward in diastole mainly at the base
- (d) No or minimal forward movement of the leaflets in diastole

(2) **Valvular Thickening**
- (a) Leaflets minimally thickened (4 to 5 mm)
- (b) Mid-leaflet thickening, pronounced thickening of the margins
- (c) Thickening extends through the entire leaflets (5 to 6 mm)
- (d) Pronounced thickening of all leaflet tissue (>8 mm)

(3) **Subvalvular Thickening**
- (a) Minimal thickening of chordal structures just below the valve
- (b) Thickening of the chordae extending up to one-third of the chordal length
- (c) Thickening extending to the distal third of the chordae
- (d) Extensive thickening and shortening of all chordae extending down to the papillary muscles

(4) **Valvular Calcification**
  (a) A single area of increased echo brightness
  (b) Scattered areas of brightness confined to the leaflet margins
  (c) Brightness extending to the midportion of the leaflets
  (d) Extensive brightness throughout most of the leaflet tissue

A "0" score implies normal valve morphology. A total valve score of ≤8 implies a mobile valve readily amenable to percutaneous valvuloplasty. Progressively higher total valve scores result in less favorable results after valvuloplasty, both acutely and in the long term (Wang A, et al. *J Am Coll Cardiol* 2002;39(2):328–334). Neither mitral regurgitation severity nor MVA is a component of the valve score. In general, however, only those patients with <2+ mitral regurgitation are acceptable candidates for the procedure.

31.5 Answer D. Based on the echocardiographic description of moderate leaflet calcification, severely reduced leaflet mobility, and extensive valvular and subvalvular thickening, the patient's Wilkins score is in the range of 12 to 15, making it *unlikely* that balloon mitral valvuloplasty would be successful. Increasing diuretics may help in the short term, as might the return to normal sinus rhythm, if feasible. However, the patient is now symptomatic, and a surgical intervention is appropriate. The suitable valve morphology for a surgical commissurotomy is precisely the same as for balloon valvuloplasty, so that is not the best option for this patient. The appropriate option is surgical mitral valve replacement.

31.6 Answer D. The indications for balloon mitral valvuloplasty for mitral stenosis include the presence for severe mitral stenosis, which is defined as an MVA of ≤1.5 cm², the absence of an LA appendage thrombus, and <2+ mitral insufficiency (Nishimura RA, et al. *J Am Coll Cardiol* 2014;63(22):e57–e185).
Class I indication:

- Symptomatic mitral stenosis with favorable valvular anatomy and no contraindications

Class II indications:

- Asymptomatic, very severe mitral stenosis (MVA ≤ 1.0 cm²) with favorable valvular anatomy and no contraindications (IIa)
- Patients with significant symptoms and less favorable valve anatomy who are at high risk for surgery (IIb)
- Patients with new atrial fibrillation (IIb)
- Symptomatic patients with MVA > 1.5 cm² and evidence of hemodynamically significant mitral stenosis during exercise

Pulmonary hypertension is not an indication for balloon mitral valvuloplasty in the most recent guidelines for the management of patients with valvular heart disease (Nishimura RA, et al. *J Am Coll Cardiol* 2014;63(22):e57–e185).

31.7 Answer C. While a cardiac MRI does provide better information regarding RV mass and function, and RV dysfunction may be playing a role in his symptoms, a preserved RV by echocardiography is adequate to exclude this, and the important finding in the image shown is the presence of porcine tricuspid valve stenosis. The normal tricuspid valve area is about 10 cm² and any gradient over 2 mm Hg is considered abnormal, with severe tricuspid stenosis diagnosed when the mean gradient is >5 mm Hg. He clearly has severe tricuspid stenosis (mean gradient 12 mm Hg) with right heart failure due to degeneration of his bioprosthesis valve. In the tricuspid position, these valves can be expected to remain functional from 10 to 12 years. Degeneration usually results in both tricuspid regurgitation and stenosis. Balloon valvuloplasty of degenerated bioprosthetic valves is not recommended due to an extremely high risk of valvular tearing and valvular regurgitation. Given his clinical situation, redo tricuspid valve replacement is the best clinical option to resolve his situation.

31.8 Answer C. The implications of spontaneous echo contrast remain uncertain. It typically represents slow atrial flow, and while the phenomenon is clearly not circulating thrombi, it is often associated with a LAA or mural thrombus and a higher risk for embolization (Bernhardt P, et al. *J Am Coll Cardiol* 2005;45(11):1807–1812). There is no specific recommendation for anticoagulation based on this finding unless concomitant thrombus is visualized in the LA or LAA or the patient has intermittent or sustained atrial fibrillation. In that situation, warfarin therapy, not antiplatelet therapy, is recommended. Patients referred for percutaneous mitral valvuloplasty frequently have spontaneous left atrial contrast, and, if there is no evident atrial appendage thrombus, the patient can safely undergo the procedure.

31.9 Answer B. Based on the latest guidelines, patients with mitral valve stenosis do not require endocarditis prophylaxis, and the risk for endocarditis has not been shown to be reduced following mitral valvuloplasty. Successful mitral valvuloplasty should be attained in a high percentage of cases with suitable valve morphology (i.e., a Wilkins score of <8) (Wilkins GT, et al. *Br Heart J* 1988;60(4):299–308). While several definitions of success are possible, a common one defines success as a valve area >1.5 with no more than 2+ mitral regurgitation. Others have used a >50% increase in the baseline valve area or a >50% decrease in the valve gradient.

There are no data to suggest that mitral valve procedures reduce the risk of atrial fibrillation. Echocardiographic restenosis following balloon mitral valvuloplasty is more frequent than clinical symptoms of restenosis. By serial echocardiography at 5 years, 20% of patients have restenosis if the baseline echocardiographic score is <8, and 60% have restenosis if the baseline echocardiographic score is ≥8 (Wang A, et al. *J Am Coll Cardiol* 2002;39(2):328–334). Freedom from reintervention may be as high as 90% at 7 years in patients with suitable anatomy undergoing balloon mitral valvuloplasty, highlighting the importance of appropriate case selection (Ben Farhat M, et al. *Circulation* 1998;97(3):245–250).

31.10 Answer A. Low-gradient, low-output aortic stenosis is defined as a mean gradient <30 mm Hg and an AVA < 1.0 cm^2. In this case, the fundamental decision is whether his reduced aortic valve area is due to intrinsic valve disease (true stenosis) or due to his underlying cardiomyopathy (pseudostenosis). The Gorlin equation is unreliable at low outputs, and the valve area may appear severe in both instances. Using nitroprusside or dobutamine to increase the cardiac output provides a means to distinguish true stenosis from pseudostenosis. Using dobutamine in this situation increased his aortic valve gradient but changed his AVA trivially. His stroke volume increased by >20%, the definition of preserved contractile reserve. These data suggest that despite the low gradient, severe aortic valve stenosis is present, rather than reduced leaflet excursion due to the patient's underlying cardiomyopathy (Nishimura RA, et al. *Circulation* 2002;106(7):809–813). He would therefore benefit from AVR if he's an acceptable candidate otherwise.

Aortic valvuloplasty has been shown to provide only very limited symptomatic relief in patients with calcific aortic stenosis (Lieberman EB, et al. *J Am Coll Cardiol* 1995;26(6):1522–1528), should be considered only as a "bridge" to AVR (Class IIb indication) (Nishimura RA, et al. *Circulation* 2017;136(8): CIR.0000000000000503), and would not be the best choice in this situation. TEE is not necessary, as the findings of increased cardiac output, increased mean gradient, and lack of increase in AVA with dobutamine are sufficient to make the diagnosis of severe low-flow, low-gradient aortic stenosis in this patient.

31.11 Answer C. A classic domed pulmonary valve responds excellently to percutaneous balloon valvuloplasty techniques. On an average, the peak gradient can be expected to fall from about 90 to 29 mm Hg. The procedure has low risk, generally in the range of 1% to 2%, and complications include pulmonary edema (presumably from increasing flow to previously underperfused lungs), perforation of a cardiac chamber or vessel, high-grade atrioventricular (AV) block, pulmonary valve regurgitation, or the "suicide RV" shown in Figure Q31-11. Sudden relief of the pulmonary valve obstruction can produce transient dynamic RV outflow obstruction as shown in the postprocedural image. This is usually readily treated with IV beta-blockers, calcium blockers, and fluids. It is important not to give inotropic agents as these will worsen the dynamic obstruction.

31.12 Answer C. VIV TAVR is indicated for the treatment of degenerated aortic bioprosthesis with resultant aortic stenosis or regurgitation, in patients at *high* risk for redo SAVR. Acceptable short-term outcomes have been reported from the VIVID registry; however, outcomes following VIV TAVR are dependent on the size of the surgical bioprosthesis, as 1-year mortality was significantly higher in patients with small, as compared to intermediate or large, surgical valves (Dvir D, et al. *JAMA* 2014;312(2):162–170). Furthermore, the risk of coronary occlusion may be higher with VIV TAVR, as surgical valves are often placed in a supra-annular position and the leaflets or some surgical valves are exterior to the valve ring. Both of these factors increase the likelihood that a surgical valve leaflet fixed in the open position could obstruct a coronary artery.

31.13 Answer A. This tracing clearly shows a decrease in the gradient, which marks a successful procedure. A successful procedure is generally considered one in which the gradient has been reduced to <20 mm Hg. Pulmonary valvuloplasty has a success rate of over 90% and complications are rare (Rao PS. *Cathet Cardiovasc Diagn* 1997;40(4): 427–430). It is performed by using one or two balloons side by side to dilate to annular size of 1.2 to 1.4 times the measured annulus, as there is much elastic recoil in the pulmonary artery. The Inoue mitral valvuloplasty balloon has also been used with excellent results. Figure Q31-13 represents a successful result and no further action is needed.

31.14 Answer B. The echo/Doppler reveals a peak aortic velocity gradient of 4.5 m/s. This corresponds to a peak instantaneous aortic valve gradient of 81 mm Hg. The calculated valve area is 0.6 cm^2 by the continuity equation. Based on his activity level and early symptoms, he needs an intervention. While balloon aortic valvuloplasty has not proven to be an effective procedure in elderly patients, there are better data that it is useful in the adolescent age group. The success rate of valvuloplasty in this subset is high (90%) with a procedural mortality of <2% and an average reduction in the aortic gradient of about 60 (Mahle WT, et al. *J Pediatr* 2010;157(3):445–449). Progressive regurgitation or restenosis occurs in about half of patients by 8 to 9 years, though, and careful follow-up is warranted. Successful valvuloplasty in this age group allows deferral of surgical intervention to a later date and is particularly important in young women who wish to have children.

He does not need catheterization to confirm the diagnosis or for an evaluation of his CAD. If a percutaneous approach cannot be performed technically, he should consider surgical intervention. Surgery is usually done with a bioprosthetic valve (often an aortic homograft or his own pulmonary autograft as part of the Ross procedure), though young patients have earlier restenosis with bioprosthetic valves than older patients (Nishimura RA, et al. *Circulation* 2017;136(8):CIR.0000000000000503).

31.15 Answer A. During pregnancy, many hemodynamic changes occur, including a 25% increase in the red blood cell mass and a 30% to 50% increase in the blood volume. As a result, there is relative anemia. There is a reduction in systemic vascular resistance as well as pulmonary vascular resistance. The cardiac output increases until about the 32nd week of pregnancy where it levels out to 30% to 50% higher than prepregnancy. During the latter stages of pregnancy, the stroke volume declines and the cardiac output is maintained by an increase in the heart rate. In mitral stenosis, the increase in blood volume and stroke volume required markedly increases the mitral gradient. In the final trimester, the increasingly rapid heart rate also reduces diastolic time and further increases the mitral gradient. This can lead to progressive symptoms of heart failure. The use of angiotensin-converting enzyme (ACE) inhibitors is relatively contraindicated in pregnancy, though the risk is less in the last trimester. Complete bed rest has been used in the past, but patients become progressively deconditioned and its use is much less now.

Mitral valve intervention is a Class IIa indication for pregnant patients with severe mitral stenosis, defined as a mitral valve area ≤ 1.5 cm^2 with severe (NYHA Class III to IV) symptoms despite medical therapy with beta-blockers and diuretics (Nishimura RA, et al. *J Am Coll Cardiol* 2014;63(22):e57–185). Balloon mitral valvuloplasty can be performed safely during pregnancy and would be the procedure of choice in this patient if her symptoms worsened given the Wilkins score of 6. Surgical commissurotomy or valve replacement should be considered based on institutional experience in pregnant women with refractory and severe (NYHA Class IV) symptoms who are not anatomically suitable for balloon mitral valvuloplasty.

31.16 Answer D. The EVEREST II High-Risk Registry compared 78 patients with severe symptomatic mitral regurgitation who underwent transcatheter mitral valve repair with MitraClip to a matched historical control group. Patients who underwent transcatheter repair had a 1-year survival rate of 76% as compared to 55% in the control group. Furthermore, patients undergoing repair had early (1 month) as well as durable (12 months) improvements in NYHA functional status and significant improvements in LV systolic and diastolic volumes. However, the 1-year mortality in this high-risk cohort was 24% (Whitlow PL, et al. *J Am Coll Cardiol* 2012;59(2):130–139).

31.17 Answer A. In a retrospective study, 3-year survival following transcatheter paravalvular leak closure was 64.3%, and among survivors, 72% of patients with CHF symptoms at baseline demonstrated freedom from CHF symptoms or reoperation (Sorajja P, et al. *J Am Coll Cardiol* 2011;58(21):2218–2224). The severity of residual leak did not predict survival; however, it did predict freedom from death or reoperation. Hemolytic anemia was associated with poorer survival and increased need for reoperation. The belief is that in order to resolve hemolytic anemia, the paravalvular leak must be closed completely, and no residual leak can be present.

31.18 Answer D. A recent series reported that complications of aortic valvuloplasty occurred in 57% of patients, with serious adverse events in 15.6% and a procedural mortality of 1.6%. Vascular complications occurred in 6.9% of patients, moderate–severe aortic regurgitation in 1.3% of patients, stroke in 1.99%, pacemaker implant in 0.99%, and bleeding requiring transfusion in 17.6% (Ben-Dor I, et al. *JACC Cardiovasc Interv* 2010;3(11):1150–1156).

31.19 Answer A. Patients in the PARTNER trial who were not felt to be suitable candidates for SAVR due to comorbidities or technical aspects of surgery were randomized to medical therapy or TAVR (Leon MB, et al. *N Engl J Med* 2010;363(17):

1597-1607). Patients randomized to TAVR had a 1-year mortality of 30.7% compared with that of medically treated patients at 49.7%. However, there was slightly higher 30-day mortality with TAVR (5% vs. 2.8% for medically treated patients) due to procedural complications. Aortic regurgitation with moderate-to-severe paravalvular leak was noted in 11.8% of patients at 30 days and 10.5% at 1 year. Hemolysis from the valve was not reported.

31.20 Answer C. TAVR has been successfully performed by approaching the aortic valve retrograde via the iliofemoral vessels, via the ascending or descending aorta, or via the subclavian, axillary, or carotid arteries. TAVR can also be performed via an antegrade approach from the LA (transseptal approach) or via an LV puncture (LV apical approach using a mini-thoracotomy). While the sheath size requirement for TAVR continues to decrease, the smallest sheath is still a 14-Fr sheath—much too large to consider placement from the radial artery.

31.21 Answer D. The EVEREST II trial randomized 279 patients with 3+ to 4+ mitral regurgitation to transcatheter repair with the MitraClip device vs. surgical repair (Feldman T, et al. *N Engl J Med* 2011;364(15):1395-1406). The primary composite end point for efficacy of freedom from death, from surgery for mitral valve dysfunction, and from grade 3+ or 4+ mitral regurgitation at 12 months favored surgery (73% vs. 55%, $p = 0.007$) and was primarily driven by the difference in surgery for mitral valve dysfunction between groups (20% in the MitraClip arm vs. 2% in the surgical arm). The procedural safety end point, a composite that included death, major stroke, reoperation, urgent/emergency surgery, MI, renal failure, and blood transfusion, favored MitraClip with a 15% event rate vs. 48% for surgery at 30 days. This difference was primarily driven by the need for transfusion in 13% of patients randomized to MitraClip vs. 45% in patients randomized to surgery. While surgical repair clearly demonstrated better results in reduction of mitral regurgitation at 1 year (over half patients with MitraClip had 2+ to 4+ MR vs. 16% of surgical patients), quality-of-life scores were similar in the two groups. There was no difference in endocarditis between groups.

31.22 Answer D. In the PARTNER trial of high-risk patients, balloon-expandable TAVR was noninferior to SAVR for all-cause death at 30 days, 1 year, 2 years, and 5 years. There was no structural valve deterioration requiring repeat aortic valve replacement in either group (Leon MB, et al. *N Engl J Med* 2010;363(17):1597-1607). In the CoreValve US Pivotal Trial of high-risk patients, TAVR was associated with a 1-year mortality rate of 14.2% vs. 19.1% with SAVR (Smith CR, et al. *N Engl J Med* 2011;364(23):2187-2198). No significant differences in NYHA Functional Class at 1 year were observed between TAVR and SAVR in either study. However, in both studies, the rate of permanent pacemaker implantation was higher with TAVR. In both studies, quality-of-life measures favored TAVR at 1 month, but at 1 year, quality-of-life measurements were equivalent between TAVR and SAVR.

31.23 Answer D. Transcatheter pulmonary valve replacement is approved for patients with failed RV outflow conduits resulting in pulmonary valve regurgitation, pulmonary valve stenosis, or both. The procedure is associated with all of the complications listed, except for tricuspid regurgitation (Steinberg ZL, et al. *Heart* 2017;103:1455-1460).

31.24 Answer C. Rapid ventricular pacing at the time of valve deployment is typically required with balloon-expandable, but not self-expanding valves. Balloon aortic valvuloplasty is not a prerequisite, but can be performed prior to TAVR with either technology. Both balloon-expandable and self-expanding technologies have demonstrated equivalent survival in randomized trials as compared to SAVR (Adams DH, et al. *N Engl J Med* 2014;370(19):1790-1798; Leon MB, et al. *N Engl J Med* 2010;363(17):1597-1607; Leon MB, et al. *N Engl J Med* 2016;374(17):1609-1620; Reardon MJ, et al. *N Engl J Med* 2017;376(14):1321-1331). The rate of paravalvular aortic insufficiency is similar (approximately 5% incidence of moderate or severe paravalvular AI) in patients treated with balloon-expandable and self-expanding valves (Leon MB, et al. *N Engl J Med* 2016;374(17):1609-1620; Reardon MJ, et al. *N Engl J Med* 2017;376(14):1321-1331).

31.25 Answer C. Outcomes following TAVR are generally equivalent to outcomes following SAVR in high-risk patients (Leon MB, et al. *N Engl J Med* 2010;363(17):1597-1607; Smith CR, et al. *N Engl J Med* 2011;364(23):2187-2198). As such, both SAVR and TAVR are Class I indications for high-risk patients with severe, symptomatic aortic stenosis (Nishimura RA, et al. *Circulation* 2017;136(8): CIR.0000000000000503). Choice of access site does impact outcomes following TAVR, as patients undergoing transfemoral TAVR demonstrate a greater improvement in quality-of-life scores as compared to patients undergoing TAVR via alternative access routes (Arnold SV, et al. *JACC*

Cardiovasc Interv 2015;8(9):1207-1217). Optimal revascularization strategies for patients undergoing TAVR are not known. In this case, the patient has intermediate stenosis of the circumflex artery, and while revascularization could be considered, it is not required. The optimal timing of revascularization (i.e., before in the same setting or following TAVR) is not known.

31.26 Answer C. In the 2014 AHA/ACC Guideline for the Management of Patients with Valvular Heart Disease, transcatheter paravalvular leak closure is recommended as reasonable only for high-risk surgical patients with suitable anatomy and severe CHF symptoms or refractory hemolysis—when performed at centers with expertise (Class IIa recommendation) (Nishimura RA, et al. *J Am Coll Cardiol* 2014;63(22):e57-e185). Patients with a high risk of leaflet impingement or with defects involving greater than one-third of the annular ring would not be considered to have suitable anatomy for transcatheter closure.

31.27 Answer B. Transcatheter mitral valve repair with MitraClip simulates the results of the surgical edge-to-edge repair (Alfieri O, et al. *J Thorac Cardiovasc Surg* 2001;122(4):674-681) or "Alfieri stitch," but does not cinch the mitral annulus as a surgical annuloplasty ring does. MitraClip is approved only for the treatment of symptomatic patients with severe degenerative (or primary) mitral regurgitation who are at prohibitive surgical risk and not for functional mitral regurgitation (Nishimura RA, et al. *Circulation* 2017;136(8): CIR.0000000000000503). Pulmonary hypertension and atrial fibrillation are not indications for therapy, and the efficacy of transcatheter mitral valve repair with MitraClip for patients with functional (or secondary) mitral regurgitation is being evaluated in the COAPT trial.

31.28 Answer D. The paravalvular regurgitation likely represents dehiscence of a portion of the surgical ring from the mitral annulus. The hemolytic anemia is due to destruction of the red blood cells from the turbulence created through the paravalvular leak. While initial therapy with folate, iron, and erythropoietin may resolve the issue in patients with only mild hemolysis, this did not occur in the patient. Definitive repair may require surgical or transcatheter intervention, which should be considered only for high-risk surgical patients with suitable anatomy and severe CHF symptoms or refractory hemolysis when performed at centers with expertise (Nishimura RA, et al. *J Am Coll Cardiol* 2014;63(22):e57-e185). Withholding warfarin in this situation puts the patient at risk for thrombosis of the mechanical prosthetic valve; that strategy would not be appropriate.

31.29 Answer C. Complications following transseptal puncture and the insertion of a catheter in the LA are uncommon (<5%) in experienced centers. The immediate differential should include a vagal reaction, perforation of a cardiac structure with pericardial tamponade, bleeding from the access site, or a coronary embolus (either thrombus or air). If a vagal reaction had occurred, one would expect the heart rate to be lower. If a retroperitoneal or access site bleed had occurred, then one would expect a high heart rate. Proceeding with the procedure would not make sense until the cause of the hypotension has been discovered. In this instance, the ECG suggests acute inferoposterior myocardial injury, and coronary angiography would be appropriate to determine if there is a coronary embolus.

32 Adult Congenital Heart Disease

Mouhammad Fathallah and Richard A. Krasuski

QUESTIONS

32.1 A 26-year-old female presents to your clinic with palpitations. Over the last few years, she has noticed frequent pulmonary infections but otherwise feels "fine" and takes no medications. She has a strong family history of coronary heart disease. Her vitals are blood pressure (BP) 125/85, pulse 70, respiratory rate (RR) 15, and blood oxygen level (SpO_2) 98%. Her height, weight, and body surface area are 158 cm, 70 kg, and 1.72 m^2. On exam, she has a fixed, widely split S2 and a 2/6 systolic flow murmur heard best in the second left intercostal space. An electrocardiogram (ECG) demonstrates right atrial enlargement and right axis deviation. Transthoracic echocardiography (TTE) shows a dilated right atrium (RA) and right ventricular dilation with paradoxical motion of the ventricular septum. There is a 20-mm centrally located atrial septal defect (ASD) with a 10-mm rim of residual tissue around the defect. The pulmonary veins appear to drain normally. Right ventricular systolic pressure is estimated to be 35 mm Hg. The patient is brought to the catheterization laboratory for complete hemodynamic assessment. Precatheterization lab work demonstrates hemoglobin of 13.2 g/dL and hematocrit of 40%. The catheterization findings include:

RA mean: 8 mm Hg
Right ventricle (RV): 40/5 mm Hg
Pulmonary artery (PA): 40/10 mm Hg, PA mean: 20 mm Hg
Pulmonary capillary wedge pressure (PCWP) mean: 5 mm Hg
Ascending aorta: 120/80 mm Hg
Inferior vena cava (IVC) saturation: 78%
Superior vena cava (SVC) saturation: 70%
RA saturation: 92%
RV saturation: 90%
Main PA saturation: 89%
Aortic saturation: 99%

This patient's mixed venous saturation is:

(A) 70%
(B) 72%
(C) 74%
(D) 76%
(E) 78%

32.2 Calculate this patient's shunt flow and Q_P:Q_S, assuming oxygen consumption of 125 mL/min/m^2 while breathing room air.

(A) 5.0 L/min; 1.7:1
(B) 6.9 L/min; 1.7:1
(C) 7.2 L/min; 2.7:1
(D) 7.2 L/min; 3.0:1
(E) 7.6 L/min; 2.7:1

32.3 Percutaneous ASD closure in adults should be considered in all of the following circumstances, EXCEPT:

(A) Asymptomatic and otherwise unexplained RA enlargement
(B) Platypnea–orthodeoxia
(C) Q_P:Q_S > 1.5:1
(D) Chronic atrial tachyarrhythmia
(E) Left-to-right shunting and pulmonary arterial pressure 40% of systemic arterial pressure

32.4 A 67-year-old female is referred to your clinic after suffering a left middle cerebral artery (MCA) stroke resulting in motor deficits and memory problems. Since the stroke, she has had a number of transient ischemic attacks (TIAs) while on aspirin therapy. She has no other medical problems, and her age is her only atherosclerotic risk factor. Her neurologist found no embolic source after an extensive workup. Her transthoracic and subsequent intracardiac echocardiograms (ICEs) are shown in Figure Q32-4A and B. What is the most likely source of this patient's neurologic problems?

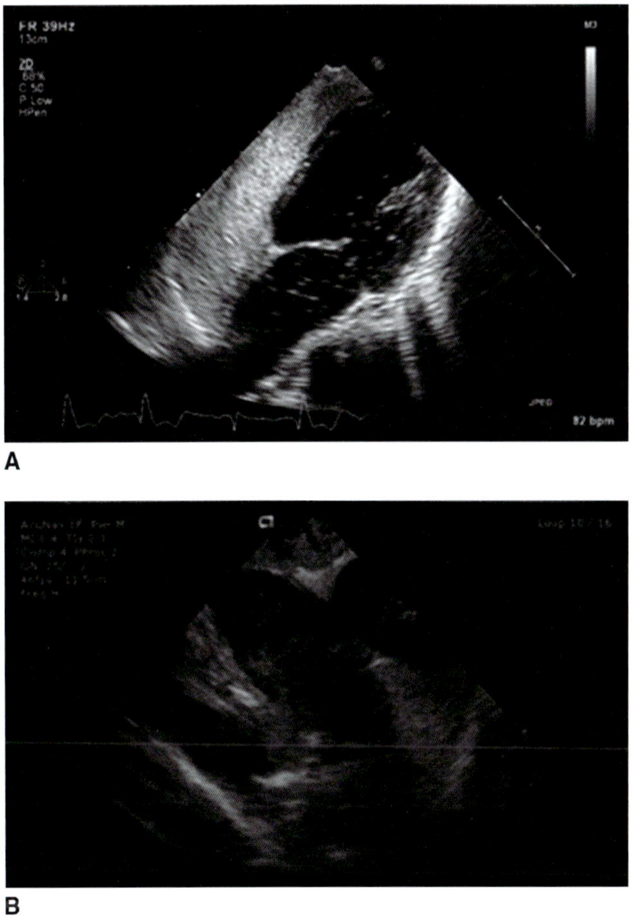

Figure Q32-4

(A) Unroofed coronary sinus
(B) Sinus venous ASD with partial anomalous venous return
(C) Pulmonary arteriovenous malformation
(D) Patent ductus arteriosus (PDA)
(E) Aortic atheroma

32.5 A patient referred to your clinic has a screening echocardiogram that reveals dilation of the coronary sinus. The person is otherwise doing well. The most likely associated finding will be:

(A) Tricuspid stenosis
(B) Tetralogy of Fallot (TOF)
(C) Primum ASD
(D) Persistent left-sided SVC
(E) Maternal alcohol ingestion

32.6 A 47-year-old male presents to your clinic with progressive shortness of breath. He notes that he "just doesn't have the stamina" that he used to and finds himself easily tired with his routine exercise. His vitals are BP 135/75, pulse 70, RR 15, and SpO_2 95%. His height, weight, and body surface area are 177 cm, 77 kg, and 1.94 m^2. There is a 2/6 systolic murmur heard best in the left infraclavicular space. He displayed no peripheral edema, and his distal pulses are 2/2 throughout. Lab work demonstrates hemoglobin of 14.5 g/dL and hematocrit of 42%. TTE demonstrates a normal RV, a mildly dilated left ventricle (LV) with normal function, an estimated RV systolic pressure of 75 mm Hg, and a 5-mm PDA with predominately left-to-right shunt flow. The patient is brought to the catheterization laboratory for complete hemodynamic assessment:

Mean RA: 11 mm Hg
RV: 76/5 mm Hg
PA: 90/20 mm Hg, PA mean: 45 mm Hg
PCWP mean: 10 mm Hg
Ascending aorta: 130/85 mm Hg
IVC saturation: 70%
SVC saturation: 68%
RA saturation: 66%
RV saturation: 65%
Mean PA saturation: 78%
Aortic saturation: 96%

Calculate this patient's shunt flow and Q_P:Q_S, assuming oxygen consumption of 125 mL/min/m^2 while breathing room air.

(A) 1.2 L/min; 1.5:1
(B) 2.2 L/min; 1.5:1
(C) 2.6 L/min; 1.7:1
(D) 2.8 L/min; 1.7:1
(E) 3.2 L/min; 1.9:1

32.7 This patient's pulmonary vascular resistance is:

(A) 3.7 Wood units
(B) 5.1 Wood units
(C) 7.6 Wood units
(D) 8.9 Wood units
(E) 11.1 Wood units

32.8 The next best step in management for this patient is:

(A) Clinical follow-up
(B) Clinical follow-up with endocarditis prophylaxis
(C) Percutaneous device closure
(D) Percutaneous device closure with endocarditis prophylaxis
(E) Surgical evaluation

32.9 A 40-year-old woman is referred to your office for increased shortness of breath and cyanosis. She has a history of complex congenital heart disease (CHD), including D-transposition of the great arteries, a large ventricular septal defect (VSD) with overriding tricuspid valve, and a mildly hypoplastic RV. She had regular cardiology follow-up until she lost her medical insurance at age 35. She has not been seen by a cardiologist since then. She notes that she has had chest pain "all her life," but recently experienced severe chest pain that sent her to the emergency department. An echocardiogram at that time revealed a left ventricular ejection fraction (LVEF) of 30% and a peripheral oxygen saturation of 80%. She has noticed that her fingers and toes are often blue or gray and she now becomes "winded" while doing household chores. She takes no medications and smokes about one pack per day. Her vitals are BP 80/50 (left arm), pulse 87, RR 20, and SpO_2 88% on 4 L of O_2. Her height, weight, and body surface area are 165 cm, 37 kg, and 1.35 m^2. On room air, her saturation dropped to 68% upon walking 50 ft. She has digital clubbing and moderate cyanosis. She has a prominent S2 with a 3/6 systolic murmur heard at the right upper sternal border. Imaging confirmed her congenital diagnosis and found her systemic ventricular EF to be 40%. Labs reveal hemoglobin of 19.8 g/dL and hematocrit of 60.0%. She is taken to the catheterization laboratory for complete hemodynamic assessment.

Mean RA: 7 mm Hg
RV: 109/4 mm Hg
PA: 102/32 mm Hg, PA mean: 59 mm Hg
PCWP mean: 18 mm Hg
IVC saturation: 70%
SVC saturation: 67%
RA saturation: 68%
RV (systemic ventricle) saturation: 81%
Aortic saturation: 80%
PV saturation: 96%
LV (pulmonary ventricle) saturation: 81%
Mean PA saturation: 79%

Calculate this patient's shunt flow, Q_P:Q_S, and pulmonary vascular resistance assuming oxygen consumption of 125 mL/m^2 while breathing room air.

(A) 1.3 L/min; 0.67:1; 11.0 Wood units
(B) 1.5 L/min; 0.71:1; 11.1 Wood units
(C) 1.8 L/min; 0.75:1; 11.5 Wood units
(D) 1.8 L/min; 0.67:1; 12.0 Wood units
(E) 2.0 L/min; 0.5:1; 12.5 Wood units

32.10 The patient above is administered 40 parts per million (ppm) of nitric oxide for 5 minutes. Her catheterization data now reveal:

PA: 89/26 mm Hg, Mean PA: 49 mm Hg
PCWP mean: 18 mm Hg
Aortic saturation: 92%
PA saturation: 93%

What is the next best step in management?

(A) Pulmonary vasodilator therapy
(B) Heart–lung transplantation
(C) Arterial switch with VSD closure
(D) Pulmonary artery banding
(E) Home oxygen therapy

32.11 The following statements regarding the Ebstein anomaly are TRUE, EXCEPT:

(A) ASD or patent foramen ovale (PFO) is usually present
(B) There is characteristic displacement of the septal and anterior leaflets into the RV
(C) ECG may reveal RA enlargement
(D) RV preload reserve is diminished
(E) 25% to 30% of these patients will have paroxysmal atrioventricular (AV) reentrant tachycardia

32.12 A 36-year-old male with TOF is referred to your office for progressive fatigue and palpitations. A palliative Blalock–Taussig shunt was placed at 6 months of age, and he underwent total correction at 2 years old with shunt takedown. When he was 21 years old, an RV-to-PA valved conduit was placed. His vitals are BP 130/80 (left arm), pulse 80, RR 15, and SpO_2 98% on room air. His height and weight are 170 cm and 64 kg. ECG is notable for paroxysmal atrial fibrillation. Echocardiography reveals mild LV dysfunction, moderate aortic insufficiency, and a moderately stenotic conduit. He is brought to the catheterization laboratory for further assessment, and his descending angiogram is shown (Fig. Q32-12). What is the most likely cause of his symptoms?

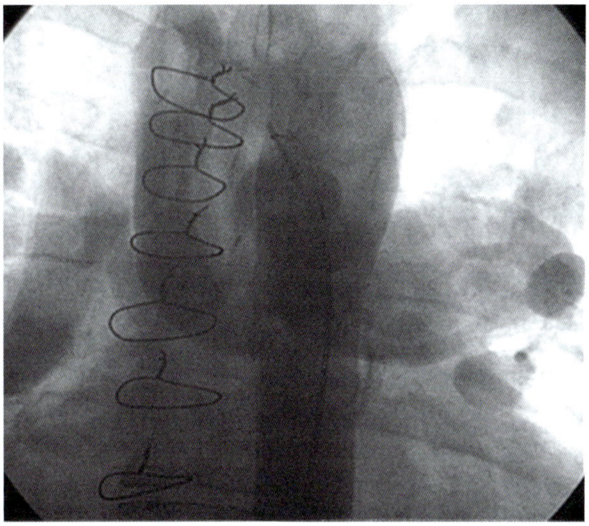

Figure Q32-12

(A) Free pulmonary insufficiency and right heart failure
(B) Pulmonary arteriovenous fistula (AVF)
(C) Residual Blalock-Taussig shunt flow
(D) Cameral fistula
(E) Aortopulmonary collaterals

32.13 Angiography is performed on a 21-year-old patient who presents with shortness of breath (Fig. Q32-13). What is the diagnosis?

(A) Pulmonary fistula draining into the RV
(B) Pulmonary fistula draining into the LV
(C) Venovenous collateral
(D) Coronary artery fistula draining into the RV
(E) Coronary artery fistula draining into the coronary sinus

32.14 You are seeing a 30-year-old gentleman with fairly complicated heart disease who presents with increasing abdominal distention. Through his mother and limited outside records, you learn that he had a Mustard repair of D-transposition of the great arteries as a child. He has not seen a cardiologist in over a decade and states that he has been feeling significantly tired lately. On examination, you note abdominal distention and likely ascites, as well as 2+ lower extremity edema. All of the following are possible causes of this problem, EXCEPT:

(A) Systolic failure of the systemic (morphologic right) ventricle
(B) Significant regurgitation of the systemic (morphologic tricuspid) AV valve
(C) Obstruction of the SVC limb of the systemic venous baffle
(D) Obstruction of the IVC limb of the systemic venous baffle

32.15 A 32-year-old female is referred to your clinic with a 6-month history of progressive dyspnea on exertion and fatigue. Her history is notable for multiple hospital admissions for pneumonia, and 3 months ago, she became increasingly short of breath after delivery of a healthy baby boy. Her echocardiogram showed a grossly dilated RV with

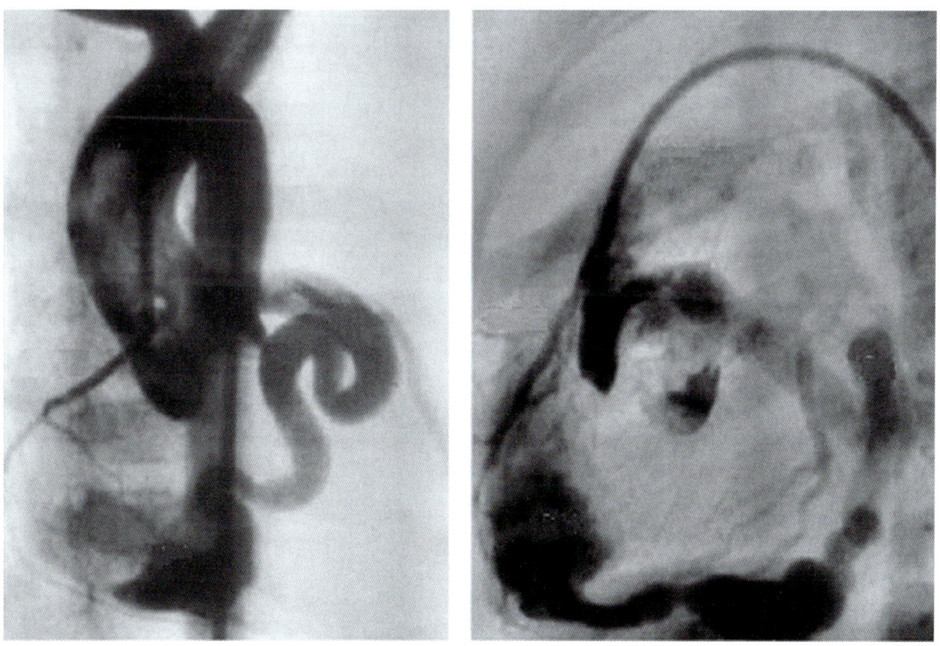

Figure Q32-13

mildly reduced function and RV systolic pressure of 85 mm Hg. Cardiac magnetic resonance imaging (MRI) is performed as part of her workup, and a portion is shown in Figure Q32-15. In addition to what is shown, the scan is notable for a hypoplastic right pulmonary valve and a large aortopulmonary collateral to the right PA. This constellation of findings is likely related to which syndrome?

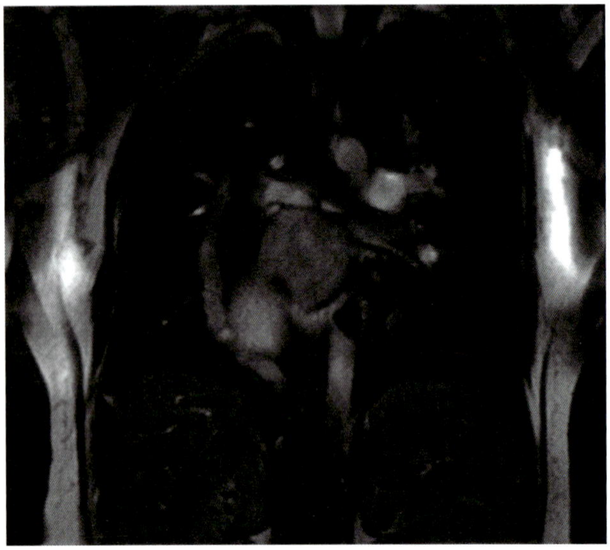

Figure Q32-15

(A) Noonan's syndrome
(B) Scimitar syndrome
(C) Holt-Oram syndrome
(D) Kartagener's syndrome
(E) Down's syndrome

32.16 A 53-year-old male is referred to your office for new-onset chest pain and exercise intolerance. He has a history of coarctation of the aorta that was surgically repaired at 3 years of age. He remembers having a cardiac catheterization procedure when he was a teenager but does not remember the results. He follows-up regularly with his primary care physician who treats his hypertension and dyslipidemia. His family history is notable for coronary artery disease (CAD). His vitals are BP 140/78 (right arm), 135/75 (left arm), and 120/60 (left leg), pulse 58, RR 12, and SpO_2 99%. His height and weight are 175 cm and 86 kg. On exam, he has a 2/6 systolic ejection murmur heard at the left upper sternal border and a 2/6 systolic ejection murmur heard over the left posterior thorax. TTE demonstrates normal ventricular function with trivial aortic insufficiency. Discrete narrowing of the descending aorta is noted. The patient is brought to the catheterization laboratory for complete hemodynamic assessment.

In which of the following situations is balloon angioplasty and/or stent placement not indicated?

(A) Significant aortopulmonary collateral flow
(B) Peak gradient of 25 mm Hg
(C) Long-segment coarctation
(D) Presence of bicuspid aortic valve
(E) Prior primary surgical repair with resection and end-to-end anastomosis

32.17 In addition to recoarctation and the need for transcatheter intervention, the following are possible late findings associated with aortic coarctation, EXCEPT:

(A) Cerebral aneurysm
(B) Elevated renin levels
(C) Premature coronary disease
(D) Aortic dissection
(E) Ventricular arrhythmia

32.18 Which of the following coronary artery anomalies is the most prevalent?

(A) Single coronary artery
(B) Origin of the left circumflex (LCx) coronary artery from the right coronary artery (RCA)
(C) Origin of the left anterior descending (LAD) coronary artery from the right coronary sinus
(D) Origin of the left main coronary artery from the right coronary sinus
(E) Origin of the left main coronary artery from the PA

32.19 A patient is found to have doming pulmonary valve stenosis on echocardiography with 1+ pulmonary regurgitation. After proper consenting, she is taken to the catheterization lab for formal hemodynamic assessment.

Mean RA: 13 mm Hg
RV: 85/7 mm Hg
PA: 34/22 mm Hg, Mean PA: 28 mm Hg
PCWP mean: 14 mm Hg
Ascending aorta: 130/80 mm Hg
Cardiac output (CO): 4.5 L/min

The next best step in management is:

(A) Immediate pulmonary balloon valvuloplasty
(B) Refer the patient for surgical valvotomy
(C) Follow-up echocardiogram in 3 to 6 months
(D) Follow-up catheterization in 1 year
(E) No further treatment is recommended

32.20 A patient with long-standing, severe pulmonary stenosis underwent successful balloon valvuloplasty. Right ventricular pressure suddenly rises to near systemic levels following the procedure. The most likely cause is:

(A) Valve leaflet avulsion
(B) Severe pulmonary insufficiency
(C) Puncture of the main PA
(D) Restenosis
(E) Infundibular spasm

32.21 A 43-year-old female with a history of TOF presents to your clinic with moderate chest discomfort, exercise intolerance, and fatigue. She had a palliative Blalock–Taussig shunt placed at 4 months of age and underwent a complete repair at 2 years old, including a VSD patch and a subpulmonary resection. She has been followed intermittently for the past two decades but does not report any other health conditions. ECG reveals a PR interval of 180 ms, QRS of 183 ms, and a QTc of 415 ms. Echocardiography reveals RV dilation, moderately decreased RV function, severe pulmonary insufficiency, moderate tricuspid valve regurgitation with a RV systolic pressure of 45 mm Hg, and a small residual VSD. She is sent for a cardiac MRI to better assess her anatomy.

Pulmonary valve peak velocity: 1.5 m/s
Pulmonary valve forward volume: 99 mL/beat
Pulmonary valve reverse volume: 38 mL/beat
Pulmonary valve regurgitant fraction: 39%
RV end-diastolic volume: 197 mL (113 mL/m^2)
RV end-systolic volume: 91 mL (52 mL/m^2)
RV stroke volume: 105 mL (60 mL/m^2)
Cardiac index: 6.5 L/min/m^2

All of the following are indications for pulmonary valve replacement in **this** patient, EXCEPT:

(A) Right ventricular dimensions on cardiac MRI
(B) Symptoms
(C) ECG findings
(D) Ventricular function on echocardiography
(E) Presence of residual VSD

32.22 A 22-year-old woman with complex CHD, including a single ventricle and transposition, is admitted for progressive hypoxia and fatigue. She has multiple prior surgical interventions, including a bidirectional Glenn procedure and then Fontan completion 10 years ago. At catheterization, the arterial oxygen saturation is 86% and the cardiac index is calculated to be 3.2 L/min/m^2. Hundred percent oxygen is administered and the arterial saturation increases to 90%. The following angiogram (Fig. Q32-22) suggests that the patient's hypoxia is most likely related to:

(A) Failure of the single ventricle and pulmonary edema
(B) Pulmonary arterial hypertension

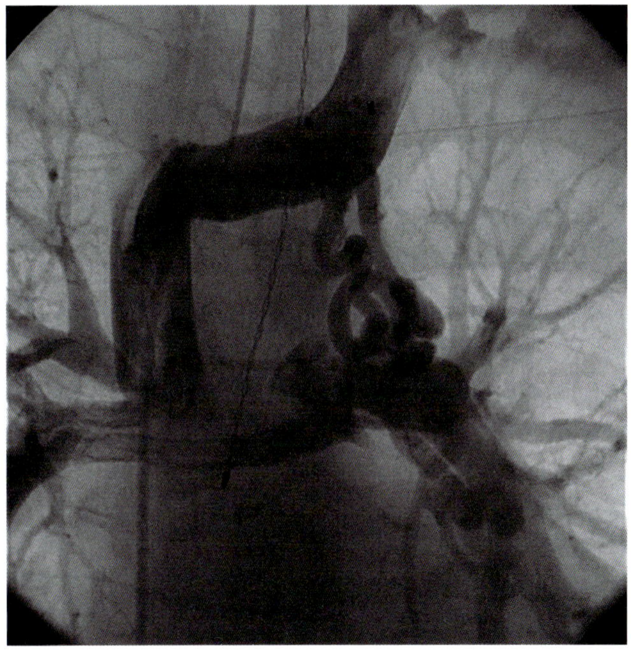

Figure Q32-22

(C) Venovenous collaterals
(D) A patent Fontan fenestration
(E) Pulmonary AV malformations

32.23 A 24-year-old patient presents to your office for chest pain, shortness of breath, and dizziness on exertion. An echocardiogram reveals subaortic stenosis. Your discussion with the patient includes the following statements, EXCEPT:

(A) This lesion is amenable to a transcatheter intervention
(B) This lesion is typically discrete
(C) This lesion can reform following surgical intervention
(D) Surgery is the most effective option for this patient
(E) This lesion can lead to aortic regurgitation that can progress over time

32.24 Subacute bacterial endocarditis prophylaxis should only be considered in which of the following situations?

(A) Cleft mitral valve
(B) TOF repair with a pericardial VSD patch and infundibular resection >10 years ago
(C) Percutaneous PFO closure 3 months ago
(D) Bicuspid aortic valve
(E) PDA occluder placed 1 year ago

32.25 For the lesion (arrow) demonstrated in this lateral projection angiogram (Fig. Q32-25) of a patient with TOF and previous surgical corrections, all of the following would be indications for a percutaneous intervention, EXCEPT?

(A) A flow discrepancy between lungs of 65:35 or greater
(B) The presence of concomitant valvular narrowing
(C) RV systolic pressure >50% systemic pressure
(D) A >50% luminal narrowing
(E) A gradient >30 mm Hg across the lesion

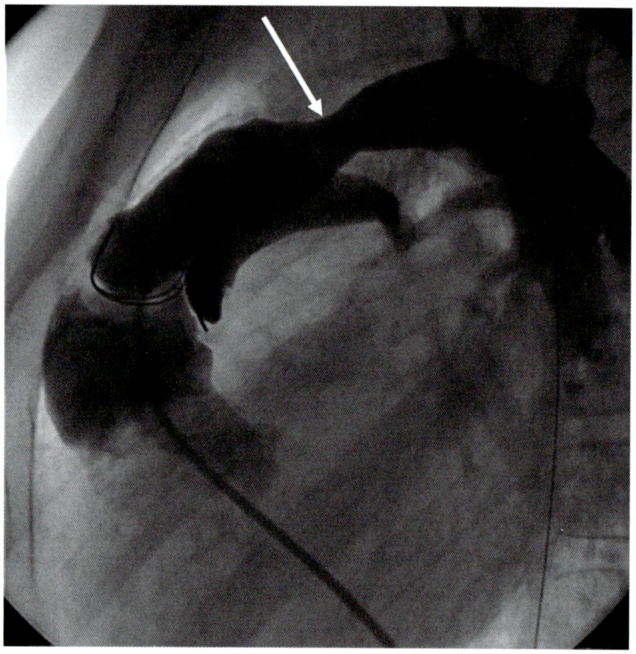

Figure Q32-25

ANSWERS AND EXPLANATIONS

32.1 Answer B. This patient has a secundum ASD with left-to-right atrial shunting. ASDs typically present with shortness of breath or palpitations in the adult population or are discovered incidentally on chest x-ray or echocardiography or during workup for stroke (from paradoxical embolization).

The first step in answering the question is to localize the shunt. This patient has an oxygen step-up at the level of the RA. A "positive" step-up in oxygen saturation at the atrial level must be ≥7% (absolute difference in mean saturation values). A "positive" step-up in oxygen saturation at the ventricular or pulmonary arterial levels must be ≥5% (Antman EM, et al. *Am J Cardiol* 1980;46(2): 265-271). The Fick method is used to calculate the pulmonary blood flow assuming oxygen consumption of the lungs to be 125 mL/min/m^2. But which systemic venous saturation do we use? The saturation in the IVC is typically higher than the saturation in the SVC (the kidney receives 25% of the cardiac output and consumes less oxygen than other organs), which is higher still than the saturation in the coronary sinus. The Flamm formula is used to estimate mixed venous saturation in this situation:

$$\text{MV\%} = \frac{(3 \times \text{SVC\%}) + \text{IVC\%}}{4} = \frac{(3 \times 70) + 78}{4} = 72\%$$

32.2 Answer E. Once the mixed venous saturation is estimated, the Fick method may be used to determine Q_P (pulmonary blood flow), Q_S (systemic blood flow) and Q_{Shunt} (shunt blood flow).

$$Q_P = \frac{O_2\text{ Consumption}}{(\text{PV} - \text{PA})O_2\text{ Content}}$$

$$\approx \frac{(125\,\text{mL/min/m}^2)(1.72\,\text{m}^2)}{(0.99-0.89)\left(\dfrac{13.2\,\text{g Hgb}}{100\,\text{mL blood}}\right)\left(\dfrac{1.36\,\text{mL }O_2}{\text{g Hgb}}\right)} = 12\,\text{L/min}$$

$$Q_S = \frac{O_2\text{ Consumption}}{(\text{SA} - \text{MV})O_2\text{ Content}}$$

$$\approx \frac{(125\,\text{mL/min/m}^2)(1.72\,\text{m}^2)}{(0.99-0.72)\left(\dfrac{13.2\,\text{g Hgb}}{100\,\text{mL blood}}\right)\left(\dfrac{1.36\,\text{mL }O_2}{\text{g Hgb}}\right)} = 4.4\,\text{L/min}$$

$$Q_{Shunt} = Q_P - Q_S = 12 - 4.4 = 7.6\,\text{L/min}$$

$$Q_P : Q_S = \frac{12}{4.4} = \frac{2.7}{1}$$

Or,

$$\frac{Q_P}{Q_S} = \frac{\dfrac{O_2\text{ Consumption}}{(\text{PV} - \text{PA})O_2\text{ Content}}}{\dfrac{O_2\text{ Consumption}}{(\text{SA} - \text{MV})O_2\text{ Content}}}$$

$$= \frac{(\text{SA} - \text{MV})O_2\text{ Content}}{(\text{PV} - \text{PA})O_2\text{ Content}} = \frac{0.99 - 0.72}{0.99 - 0.89} = \frac{0.27}{0.10} = \frac{2.7}{1}$$

32.3 Answer D. ASDs are among the most common adult congenital heart diseases encountered. In asymptomatic children, ASDs that are <6 mm in diameter are likely to close spontaneously within a few years. Closure is only pursued if symptoms develop or spontaneous closure does not occur during the follow-up period (Helgason H, et al. *Pediatr Cardiol* 1999;20(3):195-199). In adults, defects <5 mm with no evidence of right ventricular volume overload or paradoxical embolism are thought to present no additional risk and do not warrant closure. Small defects (<10 mm) may become symptomatic, but generally not until the fourth or fifth decade of life.

Hemodynamic studies have shown that the magnitude and direction of flow through an ASD depend on the size of the defect and the relative compliance of the ventricles. Large ASDs are said to be unrestrictive if the LA and RA pressures are equal. Initially, RV compliance is far greater than LV compliance, and the shunt flow tends to be left to right. If the RV dilates due to chronic volume overload, compliance will decrease and the magnitude of the shunt may decrease. However, insignificant shunts that did not lead to ventricular remodeling early may become problematic late in life if LV compliance decreases due to comorbidities such as hypertension, coronary disease, or left-sided valve disease.

According to the most recent guidelines, ASD closure is indicated when there is evidence of RA or RV enlargement (in the absence of prohibitive pulmonary arterial hypertension—pulmonary vascular resistance <5 Wood units), paradoxical embolism, or platypnea-orthodeoxia. Closure may be considered for net left-to-right shunting with pulmonary artery pressure <2/3 systemic pressure, pulmonary vascular resistance <2/3 systemic vascular resistance, or when responsive to pulmonary vasodilator therapy or following a successful balloon occlusion test (Warnes CA, et al. *Circulation* 2008;118(23):e714-e833). Furthermore, appropriate anatomy must be present for percutaneous closure. This includes one (or

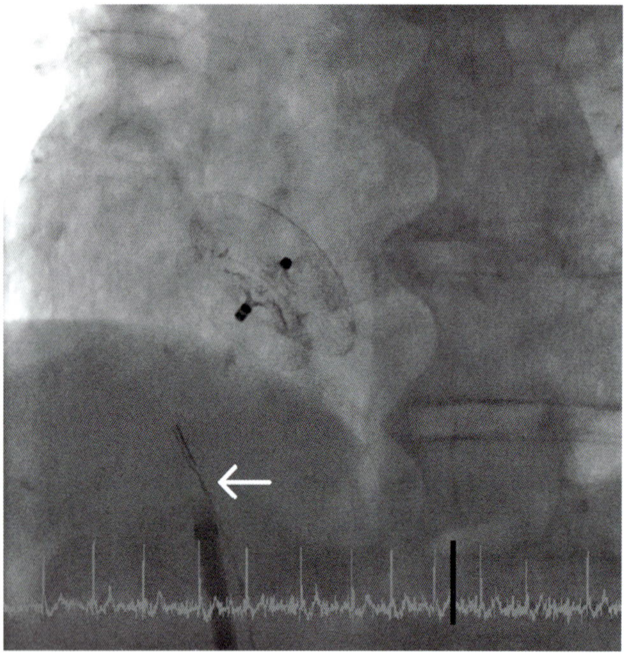

Figure A32-3

at most a few) defect(s) that are <4 cm in diameter located centrally in the atrial septum with at least a 4-mm rim of tissue surrounding the defect(s) to ensure proper seating of the occlusion device. Sinus venosus defects and primum septal defects are not amenable to percutaneous closure. Traditionally, a Q_P:Q_S ratio of >1.5:1 has been used to define a shunt that should be closed. While this definition may be useful in children and young adults, it may not be the best definition for adults with long-standing right ventricular volume overload and pulmonary overcirculation. The latter may increase right-sided pressures and decrease the shunt magnitude as discussed above, likely as a harbinger of Eisenmenger's syndrome (Krasuski RA. *Clev Clin J Med* 2007;74(2):137–147).

Medical management should be pursued for a patient with atrial tachyarrhythmia to restore sinus rhythm. If atrial fibrillation is present, anticoagulation should also be considered.

Figure A32-3 depicts an Amplatzer atrial septal occluder (St. Jude Medical; St. Paul, MN) on PA angiography. The arrow in the picture points to the AcuNav ultrasound catheter (Johnson & Johnson-Biosense Webster; Diamond Bar, CA) used to assist in device delivery. The delivery sheath filled with contrast sits in close proximity to the probe.

32.4 Answer C. PFO is thought to be a link between venous thrombus and arterial embolization. Serpiginous thrombi have even been captured in transit through the PFO tunnel. Both contrast echocardiograms in this case demonstrate right-to-left shunting. ICE demonstrates bubbles returning to the LA via the left upper pulmonary vein, not through the foramen tunnel (as would normally be seen with PFO). This suggests the presence of a pulmonary arteriovenous malformation. Pulmonary arteriovenous malformations are often congenital and associated with hereditary hemorrhagic telangiectasia (Rendu-Weber-Osler syndrome), but a small percentage of these are idiopathic (Pollak JS, et al. *J Vasc Interv Radiol* 2006;17(1):35–44). The majority of pulmonary arteriovenous malformations are "simple," where one or a few arteries from the same pulmonary segment feed the malformation. "Complex" lesions have multiple feeder vessels and may be diffuse. Pulmonary arteriovenous malformations can cause serious complications, such as stroke (as in this patient), brain abscess, life-threatening hemoptysis or hemothorax, and hypoxemic respiratory failure. Although the majority of pulmonary arteriovenous malformations remain stable in size, they do not seem to regress on their own, and some do actually enlarge slowly. The gold standard of treatment is embolotherapy when possible.

An unroofed coronary sinus defect is a rare lesion that could permit right-to-left shunting and paradoxical embolization, but would likely have been diagnosed by echocardiogram. An ASD could also permit transient right-to-left shunt and cause paradoxical embolization, but would be evident on echocardiography. A PDA could also cause paradoxical embolization in the setting of Eisenmenger's syndrome. Eisenmenger's syndrome would be highly unlikely in this patient, as they do not display any signs or symptoms of the disorder. Aortic atheroma is a

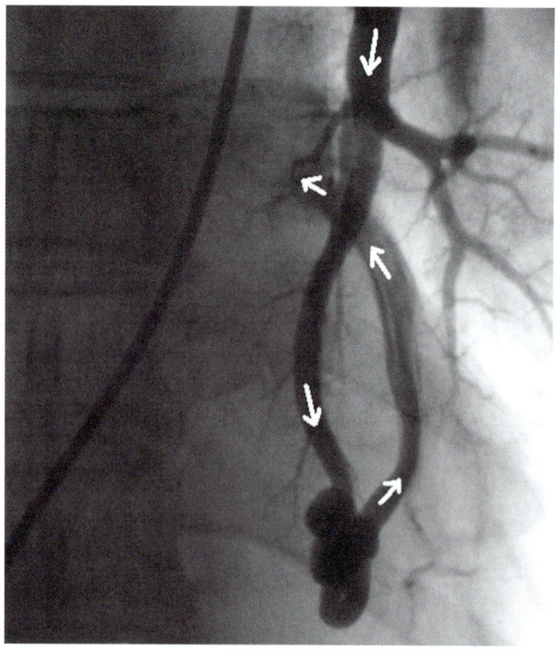

Figure A32-4

common source for embolization, especially during cardiac surgery, but this patient does not have risk factors for atheroma, making this choice less likely.

Figure A32-4 depicts a selective pulmonary angiogram demonstrating a pulmonary arteriovenous malformation, which then empties into the LA (arrows designate the path of blood through the arteriovenous malformation).

32.5 Answer D. Dilation of the coronary sinus should prompt the physician to consider the possibility of a persistent left-sided vena cava. The physiology of this finding is completely normal, and there are no clinical manifestations. Persistent left-sided vena cava may also be associated with TOF and other cyanotic cardiac defects, but this was not the case in this clinical scenario. Persistent left-sided vena cava becomes a consideration if patients are to undergo cardiac surgery or if they were to have a catheterization or pacemaker insertion with a venous approach from the left upper extremity.

32.6 Answer D. This patient has a PDA with left-to-right flow. Signs and symptoms supporting this diagnosis include dyspnea on exertion, widened pulse pressure, and a left subclavicular murmur (classically a continuous "machinery" murmur). Over time, chronic pulmonary volume overload will lead to remodeling of the pulmonary vasculature and increased pulmonary vascular resistance. This patient has elevated pulmonary artery pressure (mean PA, 45 mm Hg). Pulmonary arterial pressure will eventually reach or exceed systemic pressure, and flow through the shunt will become predominantly right to left, a condition known as Eisenmenger's syndrome. Body surface area was calculated using the Dubois method (Wang Y, et al. *J Clin Anesth* 1992;4(1):4-10):

$$\text{BSA}\left(\text{m}^2\right) = 0.007184 \times \text{weight}^{0.425}\left(\text{kg}\right) \times \text{height}^{0.725}\left(\text{cm}\right)$$

$$\text{BSA}\left(\text{m}^2\right) = 0.007184 \times 77^{0.425}\left(\text{kg}\right) \times 177^{0.725}\left(\text{cm}\right) = 1.94\,\text{m}^2$$

The first step in solving this problem is to localize the oxygen saturation step-up. Blood flow from the IVC, SVC, and coronary sinus mix in the RA. Each stream has different oxygen saturations, so measurements will vary depending on the sampling location in the atrium and the degree of mixing that occurs. A "positive" step-up in oxygen saturation between the systemic veins and the RA must be ≥7% (absolute difference in mean saturation values). As blood has more time to mix, saturation becomes more homogeneous, and a "positive" step-up in oxygen saturation between the RA and RV or RV and PA need only be ≥5% (Antman EM, et al. *Am J Cardiol* 1980;46(2):265-271). This patient has a 14% step-up in oxygen saturation between the RV and PA, consistent with a significant left-to-right shunt. The Fick method is used to calculate the pulmonary blood flow assuming oxygen consumption of the lungs to be 125 mL/m^2.

$$Q_P = \frac{O_2\ \text{Consumption}}{(\text{PV} - \text{PA})\,O_2\ \text{Content}} \approx \frac{\left(125\,\text{mL/min/m}^2\right)\left(1.94\,\text{m}^2\right)}{(0.96-0.78)\left(\dfrac{14.5\,\text{g Hgb}}{100\,\text{mL blood}}\right)\left(\dfrac{1.36\,\text{mL }O_2}{\text{g Hgb}}\right)} = 6.8\,\text{L/min}$$

If aortic saturation is ≥95%, it may safely be substituted for pulmonary venous saturation. If aortic saturation is <95%, right-to-left shunt must be ruled out with a hyperoxygen challenge. If right-to-left shunting is present, pulmonary venous oxygen saturation may be assumed to be 98% if there is no underlying pulmonary disease. The Fick method is also used to calculate systemic blood flow:

$$Q_S = \frac{O_2\ \text{Consumption}}{(\text{SA} - \text{MV})\,O_2\ \text{Content}} \approx \frac{\left(125\,\text{mL/min/ m}^2\right)\left(1.94\,\text{m}^2\right)}{(0.96-0.65)\left(\dfrac{14.5\,\text{g Hgb}}{100\,\text{mL blood}}\right)\left(\dfrac{1.36\,\text{mL }O_2}{\text{g Hgb}}\right)} = 4.0\,\text{L/min}$$

To determine systemic blood flow, the Fick method is used again, though with one important caveat. The mixed venous value must be obtained proximal to the shunt location (PA saturation is *not* mixed venous saturation in this instance). The shunt is located in the PA, so the RV saturation is used. If significant pulmonic regurgitation is present, it would be reasonable to use RA saturation instead.

Once Q_P and Q_S are known, shunt flow and Q_P:Q_S are easily calculated.

$$Q_{\text{Shunt}} = Q_P - Q_S = 6.8 - 4.0 = 2.8\,\text{L/min}$$

$$Q_P{:}Q_S = 6.8/4.0 = 1.7/1$$

Alternatively Q_P:Q_S may be quickly calculated as follows:

$$\frac{Q_P}{Q_S} = \frac{\dfrac{O_2\ \text{Consumption}}{(\text{PV}-\text{PA})\,O_2\ \text{Content}}}{\dfrac{O_2\ \text{Consumption}}{(\text{SA}-\text{MV})\,O_2\ \text{Content}}} = \frac{(\text{SA}-\text{MV})\,O_2\ \text{Content}}{(\text{PV}-\text{PA})\,O_2\ \text{Content}} = \frac{0.96-0.65}{0.96-0.78} = \frac{0.31}{0.18} = 1.7/1$$

32.7 Answer B. Pulmonary vascular resistance is calculated as follows:

$$PVR = \frac{\text{Mean PA Pressure} - \text{Pulmonary Venous Pressure } (\sim \text{PCWP})}{Q_P}$$

$$= \frac{45\text{mm Hg} - 10\text{mm Hg}}{6.8\text{L/min}}$$

$$= 5.1 \text{ Wood units}$$

32.8 Answer D. For patients with a small PDA and no evidence of left heart volume overload, clinical follow-up every 3 to 5 years is appropriate. Endocarditis prophylaxis is not recommended for patients with unrepaired PDA who are not cyanotic. Closure of a PDA is indicated if there is evidence of left atrial or LV enlargement, net left-to-right shunting, reversible pulmonary arterial hypertension, or history of endarteritis. This patient has multiple indications for closure of his PDA. He is symptomatic, has evidence of right ventricular enlargement, and is beginning to develop pulmonary arterial disease. Patients with indications for closure should be referred to an adult CHD specialist and evaluated for device closure. PDAs in adults tend to be highly calcified and present additional risk during surgical closure. Even if a patient is to undergo additional cardiac surgery, percutaneous PDA closure prior to surgery presents the lowest procedural risk to the patient. Endocarditis prophylaxis is indicated in this patient under two circumstances. He should receive prophylaxis for the first 6 months after repair if prosthetic materials are used (surgical or interventional repair). Second, he should receive prophylaxis if residual shunt is present adjacent to any prosthetic material. Asymptomatic patients should also be considered for device closure to prevent unavoidable pulmonary vascular disease and left heart enlargement. PDA closure is contraindicated for patients with clear pulmonary arterial hypertension and evidence of right-to-left shunting (Warnes CA, et al. *Circulation* 2008;118(23):e714–e833).

Figure A32-8 shows a lateral angiogram after delivery of an Amplatzer ductal occluder (St. Jude Medical; St. Paul, MN) as designated by the arrow.

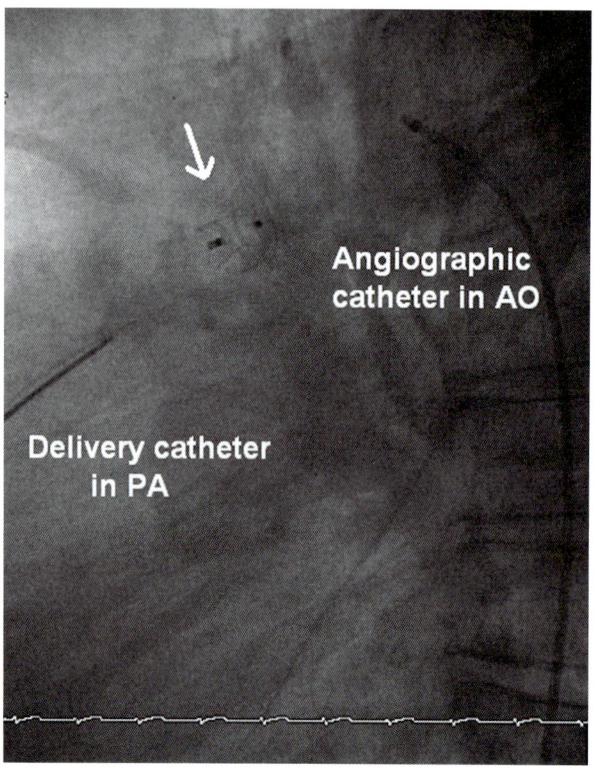

Figure A32-8

32.9 Answer B. Understanding the anatomy of this patient is the first step to understanding the solution. In dextrotransposition of the great arteries, there is AV concordance with ventriculoarterial discordance. In isolated dextrotransposition of the great arteries, the pulmonary and systemic circulations are completely separate. The presence of a communication (in this case a large VSD) between the two circulations is necessary for survival. This patient likely remained asymptomatic for much of her life as the shunt flow was predominantly systemic to pulmonary. Now, this patient has signs and symptoms of Eisenmenger's syndrome with pulmonary to systemic shunting. Once again, the Fick method is used to calculate pulmonary blood flow, systemic blood flow, and shunt flow.

$$Q_P = \frac{O_2 \text{ Consumption}}{(PV - PA)O_2 \text{ Content}}$$

$$\approx \frac{(125\text{mL/min/m}^2)(1.35\text{m}^2)}{(0.96 - 0.79)\left(\frac{19.8\text{g Hgb}}{100\text{mL blood}}\right)\left(\frac{1.36\text{mL } O_2}{\text{g Hgb}}\right)}$$

$$= 3.7\text{L/min}$$

$$Q_S = \frac{O_2 \text{ Consumption}}{(SA - MV)O_2 \text{ Content}}$$

$$\approx \frac{(125\text{mL/min/m}^2)(1.35\text{m}^2)}{(0.80 - 0.68)\left(\frac{19.8\text{g Hgb}}{100\text{mL blood}}\right)\left(\frac{1.36\text{mL } O_2}{\text{g Hgb}}\right)}$$

$$= 5.2\text{L/min}$$

$$Q_{Shunt} = Q_S - Q_P = 5.2 - 3.7 = 1.5\text{L/min}$$

$$Q_P : Q_S = 3.7/5.2 = 0.71/1$$

Alternatively, $Q_P:Q_S$ may be quickly calculated as follows:

$$\frac{Q_P}{Q_S} \approx \frac{\dfrac{O_2\ \text{Consumption}}{(PV - PA)O_2\ \text{Content}}}{\dfrac{O_2\ \text{Consumption}}{(SA - MV)O_2\ \text{Content}}}$$

$$= \frac{(SA - MV)O_2\ \text{Content}}{(PV - PA)O_2\ \text{Content}} = \frac{0.80 - 0.68}{0.96 - 0.79}$$

$$= \frac{0.12}{0.17} = \frac{0.71}{1}$$

Pulmonary vascular resistance is calculated as follows:

$$\text{PVR} = \frac{P_{\overline{PA}} - P_{\overline{PV}}}{Q_P}$$

$$= \frac{59\,\text{mm Hg} - 18\,\text{mm Hg}}{3.7\,\text{L/min}} = 11.1\ \text{Wood units}$$

32.10 Answer A. In general, pulmonary overcirculation from left to right shunts causes pulmonary vascular remodeling that leads to increased pulmonary vascular resistance and pulmonary arterial hypertension. Subpulmonary ventricular failure and increased right-sided pressures lead to reversal of the shunt and consequent cyanosis. Surgical or percutaneous correction of defects resulting in significant pulmonary overcirculation should take place as early as possible to prevent irreversible pulmonary vascular disease. Ideally, significant shunts from VSDs would be repaired prior to 2 years of life, while AV canal defects and conotruncal abnormalities (as in this case) would receive corrective surgery before 6 months of life (Newfeld EA, et al. *Am J Cardiol* 1974;34(1):75–82). Eisenmenger's syndrome is classified with other forms of pulmonary arterial hypertension according to the World Health Organization (WHO) based on similarities in clinical presentation, morphology, and response to treatments (Dana Point Classification). Although patients with Eisenmenger's syndrome have a longer life expectancy than those with idiopathic pulmonary arterial hypertension (77% survival vs. 35% survival at 3 years, untreated), the prognosis is still quite grim (Hopkins WE, et al. *J Heart Lung Transplant* 1996;15(1 Pt 1):100–105).

This patient demonstrated some reversibility of her pulmonary vascular disease and might benefit from selective pulmonary vasodilator therapy, such as endothelin antagonists, prostacyclin analogs, or phosphodiesterase 5 inhibitors (Beghetti M, et al. *Semin Respir Crit Care Med* 2009;30(4):421–428). Heart–lung transplant is performed in end-stage Eisenmenger's syndrome treatment. Late surgical correction with an arterial switch procedure and VSD closure after the development of pulmonary vascular disease would carry significant mortality risk now that pulmonary vascular disease has developed. Restricting flow to the pulmonary vascular bed with pulmonary artery banding has not been shown to alter the disease course. Administration of 100% oxygen to a patient with right-to-left shunting will not significantly improve systemic oxygen saturation. Furthermore, long-term oxygen therapy in Eisenmenger's syndrome has not been shown to improve symptoms, functional capacity, or survival (Sandoval J, et al. *Am J Respir Crit Care Med* 2001;164(9):1682–1687).

32.11 Answer B. Ebstein anomaly represents the most common congenital anomaly of the tricuspid valve. In Ebstein's, the anterior leaflet arises from the normal position on the tricuspid valve annulus. However, the septal and posterior leaflets are displaced into the RV to varying degrees. This results in the RV being divided into two chambers: an "atrialized RV" proximally and a functional RV that is of variable size distally. The anterior leaflet may be redundant, resulting in a "sail-like" appearance. Usually, an atrial level communication is present (either PFO or ASD) permitting right-to-left shunting. Ebstein morphology promotes atrial level right-to-left shunting by at least two mechanisms. Right ventricular outflow tract (RVOT) obstruction/poor RV filling caused by redundant valve leaflets, tricuspid valve regurgitation, RV failure, and increase in pulmonary vascular resistance all contribute to right-to-left shunting. Tricuspid valve leaflets are often elongated leading to atrial level shunting (Sommer RJ, et al. *Circulation* 2008;117(10):1340–1350). Patients with right-to-left shunting do not easily develop systemic venous congestion from right-sided heart failure compared to those with an intact septum, but the price paid is often exertional hypoxemia.

Management of Ebstein anomaly is driven by symptoms; asymptomatic patients require no specific therapy besides periodic monitoring. Accessory conduction pathways are present in up to 30% of these patients causing AV reciprocating tachycardia and may dictate medical management or catheter ablation (Cappato R, et al. *Circulation* 1996;94(3):376–383). Patients who present with exertional cyanosis secondary to atrial level shunting may benefit from percutaneous device closure. Temporary balloon occlusion of the defect may lead to elevation of RA pressure and a drop in cardiac output. In patients with favorable hemodynamics, these changes will be minimal and closure may be performed. If significant changes in RA pressure or cardiac output occur, the communication should be left patent (Agnoletti G, et al. *Heart* 2006;92(6): 827–831). Patients with severe symptoms requiring surgical management almost always present during childhood. Surgical management includes tricuspid valve repair (if possible) or replacement, shunt closure, ventricular plication, atrial reduction, and antiarrhythmic surgery. The bidirectional Glenn procedure has also been employed in these patients to unload the right heart (Dearani JA, et al. *Curr Opin Pediatr* 2009;21(5):565–572). Recent evidence suggests that prognosis of surgical management can be improved with aggressive preoperative treatment, antiarrhythmic, and vasoactive medications, along with comprehensive measures to reduce myocardial injury, decrease RV preload and afterload, and prevent myocardial edema (Luo M, et al. *Medicine (Baltimore)* 2017;96(1):e5627).

Figure A32-11 shows a right ventricular inflow view echocardiogram of a patient with Ebstein's anomaly. The arrow on the left points to an apically displaced posterior leaflet. The arrow on the right points to an elongated anterior leaflet that attaches to the valve annulus.

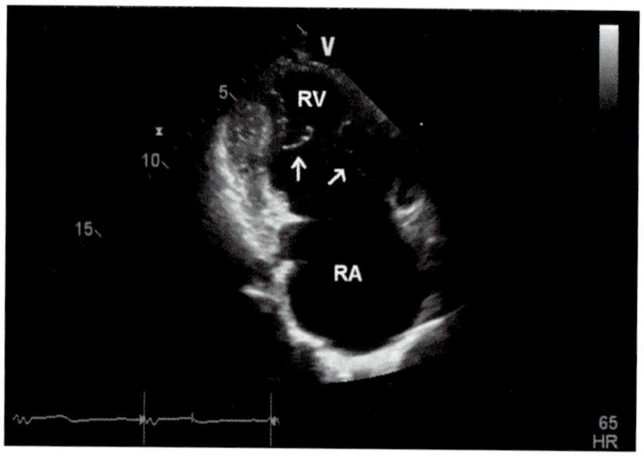

Figure A32-11

32.12 Answer E. TOF is characterized by pulmonic stenosis, VSD, right ventricular hypertrophy, and an overriding aortic valve—all of which are caused by anterior displacement of the conal septum. In the past, many centers employed palliative Blalock-Taussig shunts to augment pulmonary blood flow and then waited for some years to perform a "complete" repair. The complete repair consisted of pulmonary outflow tract resection usually with a transannular patch, VSD closure, and takedown of any surgically placed shunts. As operative techniques and patient management have improved, the complete repair is now performed as the initial procedure early in life. Relief of RVOT obstruction generally results in some degree of pulmonary insufficiency. Many late complications of surgically repaired TOF are a result of long-standing pulmonic insufficiency. The right heart dilates and eventually fails. Pulmonary valve repair or placement with a valved conduit is common, but necessitates frequent reoperations for valve replacements throughout life when a tissue valve is used. Percutaneous pulmonic valve implantation is also on the horizon and will undoubtedly have a positive impact in these patients. However, now that determinants of late outcomes after TOF repair have become more apparent, there has been a trend toward "valve-sparing" procedures during initial repair to prevent pulmonary insufficiency altogether.

Another frequent complication encountered in adults with TOF, particularly those with pulmonary atresia, is the formation of aortopulmonary collaterals. Initially, they develop in response to decreased pulmonary blood flow, but over time, this adaptation causes LV volume overload and pulmonary overcirculation. Collaterals can be singular or multiple and often follow a tortuous branched course. This patient has developed significant aortopulmonary collaterals as shown on the angiogram in the question, and these are likely the cause of his symptoms.

Percutaneous closure of collaterals is often undertaken to treat symptoms of pulmonary overcirculation and left heart volume overload. Collateral closure is also performed in preparation for open heart surgery, because collateral flow may compromise a bloodless field. The angiogram shows markedly decreased collateral flow after placement of vascular plugs in the collateral vessels (Fig. A32-12).

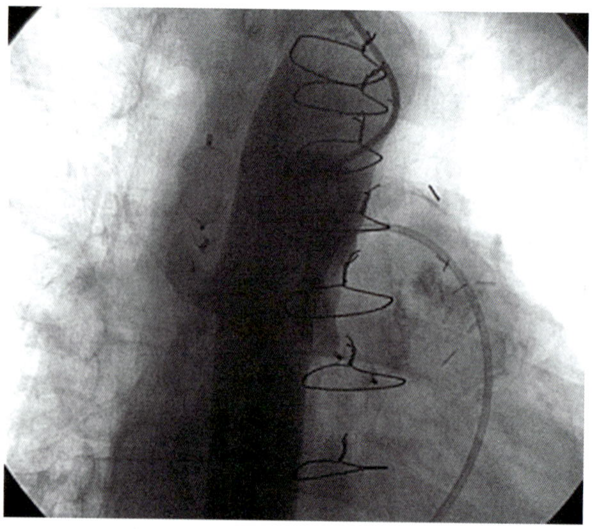
Figure A32-12

32.13 Answer D. This angiogram depicts a coronary artery fistula draining into the RV. These are also known as *coronary-cameral fistulae*, as they drain into a cardiac chamber. Most often, they are due to persistence of sinusoids that nourished the primitive myocardium in early embryogenesis. However, they can also be due to acquired causes such as trauma, invasive cardiac procedures, biopsies, or coronary angiography. Coronary fistulae most often originate from the RCA (55%), but may also originate from the left coronary artery (35%) or both (5%). The majority of coronary fistulae terminate on the right side of the heart (approximately 90%), most often in the RV (approximately 40%). Other termination locations include the right atrium, PAs, or left-sided structures. Cameral fistulae are typically small and do not affect myocardial oxygen supply. However, coronary steal may cause myocardial ischemia distal to the fistula and cause compensatory dilation proximal to the fistula. This may manifest as shortness of breath, angina, MI, arrhythmia, or thrombosis. Lesions tend to enlarge with age, and clinical symptoms have been reported in 63% of patients over the age of 20 (Liberthson RR, et al. *Circulation* 1979;59(5): 849–854). Excellent long-term outcomes have been demonstrated with surgical repair, but percutaneous closure has also been demonstrated to be safe and effective in addition to being less invasive.

32.14 Answer C. Transposition of the great arteries is an uncommon congenital heart lesion affecting approximately 20 out of 100,000 live births. There are associated lesions in the majority of patients, including VSD, subvalvular and valvular pulmonic stenosis, and aortic coarctation. Because there are essentially two separate circulations in these patients, a shunt (ASD, VSD, or PDA) needs to be present for infantile survival. Historically, the initial surgical repairs (Senning and Mustard procedures) involved building baffles (pathways) from the systemic venous circulation to the subpulmonic ventricle with pulmonary venous return routed back to the subaortic ventricle. The main complication seen as a result of this procedure is the eventual failure of the systemic (right) ventricle. Up to one-half of patients 15 to 18 years out from the surgery will have decreased systemic right ventricular function. Because the valve generally accompanies the morphologic ventricle, the tricuspid valve, which is ill-prepared to function under systemic demands, also becomes regurgitant (Kirjavainen M, et al. *J Thorac Cardiovasc Surg* 1999;117(3):488–495). Sinus node dysfunction is common in these patients and often requires pacemaker placement. The superior or inferior limb of the baffle can either become obstructed or develop leaking (the latter functioning like

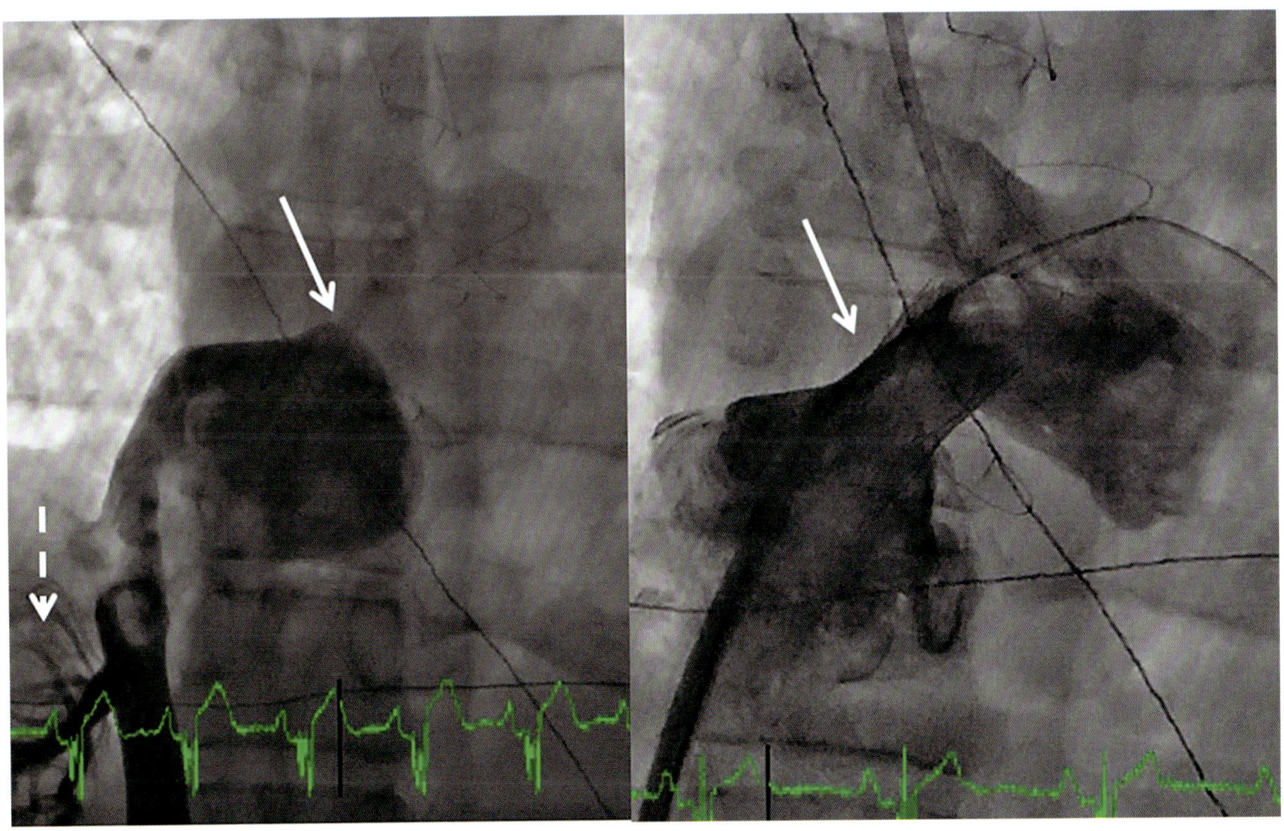

Figure A32-14

a secundum ASD). An *inferior vena caval baffle stenosis* (in the absence of good decompression by the azygos vein) can result in hepatic and lower extremity congestion. Figure A32-14 demonstrates an inferior baffle obstruction on IVC angiography (*arrow* on the left image), which was successfully treated with placement of a stent (*arrow* on the right image). Hepatic congestion is evidenced as reflux back to the hepatic veins (*dashed arrow*) during inferior vena caval angiography. A superior vena caval baffle obstruction would be expected to present with upper extremity swelling (often in the context of prior pacemaker lead placement though the superior limb of the baffle) and not hepatic or lower extremity congestion.

32.15 Answer B. Scimitar syndrome is a rare disorder characterized by hypoplasia of the right lung, anomalous right pulmonary venous drainage to the IVC, and aortopulmonary collateral flow to the right lung. The cardiac MRI image shows an anomalous pulmonary venous (on the left side of the image) draining to the base of the RA—the so-called scimitar vein for its appearance that mimics the look of a sword. Noonan's syndrome is an autosomal dominant disease notable for short stature, minor dysmorphic facial features, pulmonic stenosis, and hypertrophic cardiomyopathy. Kartagener's syndrome is a form of primary ciliary dyskinesia with coexistent situs inversus, sinusitis, and bronchiectasis. Holt–Oram syndrome is an autosomal dominant disorder notable for upper body limb deformities and ASDs. Down's syndrome is associated with many cardiovascular anomalies, but anomalous pulmonary venous drainage is not one.

32.16 Answer C. Coarctation of the aorta accounts for approximately 4% of all CHD, and more than 80% have additional cardiac anomalies, such as bicuspid aortic valve, aortic stenosis, ventricular defects, or complex cyanotic defects. Medical texts and review books frequently report the site of coarctation as either "preductal" or "postductal," but in reality, the vast majority are located opposite from the duct or "juxtaductal." Most patients with coarctation are diagnosed in infancy because of coexistent cardiac defects, but some remain asymptomatic into adulthood because of significant collateral flow. Patients with unoperated coarctation have a mean survival rate of 35 years owing to the high rate of cardiovascular complications that result from systemic hypertension. In adults, coarctation is usually diagnosed during the workup for secondary hypertension.

Management of coarctation combines both surgery and interventional strategies. Traditionally, surgical repair has been utilized for primary coarctation. Improved outcomes with newer generations of stents, conservative interventions with future planned hemodynamic reassessment and further stent expansion if necessary, as well as the use of recently approved covered stents have increased the number of primary coarctations that can be approached percutaneously.

Recoarctation is common following primary surgical repair, and most reinterventions are performed percutaneously. Indications for balloon angioplasty and/or stent placement include a gradient of 20 mm Hg or more (Warnes CA, et al. *Circulation* 2008;118(23):e714–e833) or a gradient <20 mm Hg with presence of significant collateral flow. Stent placement in a long-segment coarctation may be considered, but long-term studies of safety and efficacy are lacking and this may not be the best option. Bicuspid aortic valve is present in at least 50% of coarctation patients. Bicuspid aortic valve alone does not preclude balloon angioplasty or stent placement. The type of surgical repair does not appear to influence outcomes for balloon dilation or stent placement in patients with residual coarctation or recoarctation (Marshall AC, et al. *Am Heart J* 2000;139(6):1054–1060). The most often used surgical technique for isolated coarctation is resection with end-to-end anastomosis.

Figure A32-16 shows a BIB catheter (NuMed; Hopkinton, NY) inflation of a Genesis XD stent (Johnson & Johnson-Cordis Corp.; Warren, NJ) in the descending aorta at the site of recoarctation.

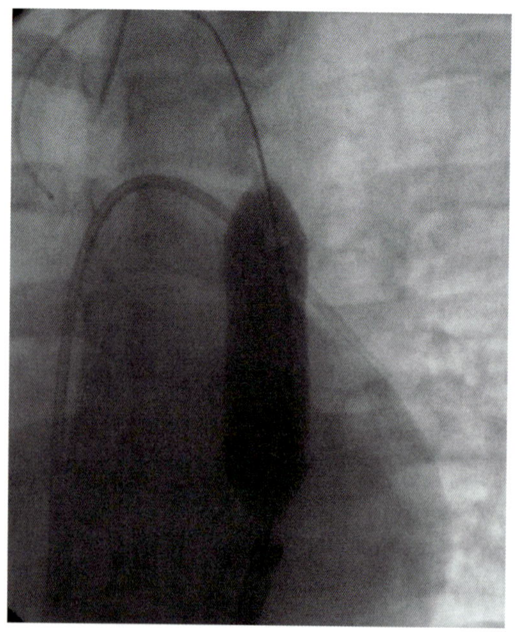

Figure A32-16

32.17 Answer E. The pathophysiology of hypertension in patients with coarctation of the aorta is multifactorial. One mechanism involves activation of the renin-angiotensin-aldosterone system as a result of decreased renal blood flow. This system does not always return to baseline after primary repair. Due to elevated systemic blood pressures, patients with aortic coarctation are predisposed to CAD and aortic dissection. Cerebral aneurysms have been reported in approximately 10% of adults with aortic coarctation, the rupture of which may be the presenting symptom for long-term asymptomatic patients (Connolly HM, et al. *Mayo Clin Proc* 2003;78(12):1491-1499). Development of ventricular arrhythmia is not associated with aortic coarctation.

32.18 Answer B. Origin of the LCx from the RCA is the most common congenital coronary anomaly. Single coronary arteries occur in approximately 5% to 15% of coronary anomalies and are seen in conditions such as truncus arteriosus, transposition of the great arteries, and TOF. Origin of the left main coronary artery from the right sinus of Valsalva carries important clinical significance as the course can lead between the ascending aorta and the main PA. This can result in compression of the artery with resultant sudden cardiac death. In fact, this is the second most common cause of death in young athletes after hypertrophic obstructive cardiomyopathy (HOCM). Origin of the left main coronary artery from the PA is also known as Bland-Garland-White syndrome; it is a very rare condition (Kayalar N, et al. *Congenit Heart Dis* 2009;4(4):239-251).

Figure A32-18 shows a right anterior oblique (RAO) angiographic image of an anomalous left main coronary artery (vessel on superior portion of the image), which originates from the right coronary cusp (the RCA is in the lower half of the image traveling downward) in this case and travels between the great vessels. This lesion has been associated with an increased risk of sudden death in children and young adults.

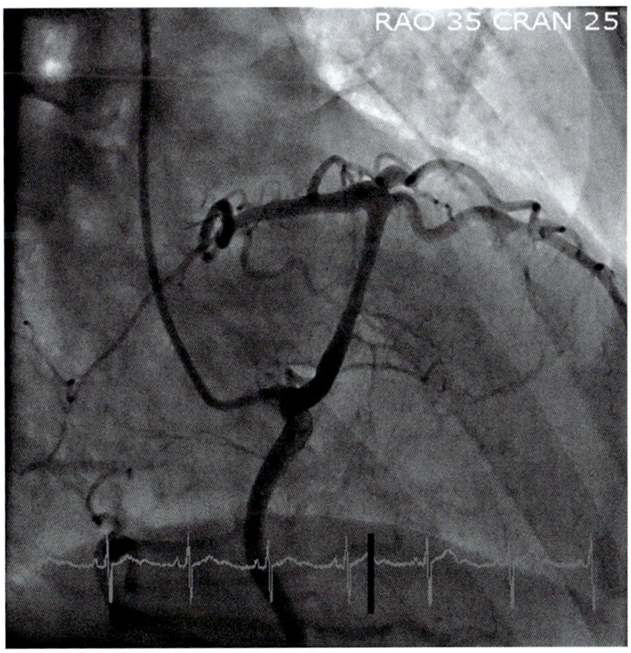

Figure A32-18

32.19 Answer A. This patient has a peak-to-peak pressure gradient of 51 mm Hg. Current guidelines recommend valvuloplasty in asymptomatic patients with a doming pulmonic valve and a peak-to-peak gradient >40 mm Hg and in symptomatic patients with a peak-to-peak gradient >30 mm Hg in the absence of moderate or worse pulmonary regurgitation. Asymptomatic patients with a peak-to-peak gradient <30 mm Hg may be safely observed as the natural history of mild pulmonic stenosis is typically benign and the stenosis rarely progresses. Patients with valvular pulmonic stenosis, right ventricular systolic pressure >80 mm Hg, and dysplastic valve morphology should be referred for surgical valvotomy (Bonow RO, et al. *Circulation* 2008;118(15);e523-e661; Warnes CA, et al. *Circulation* 2008;118(23):e714-e833). Other indications for surgical intervention include severe pulmonic stenosis with severe pulmonary regurgitation or an associated hypoplastic pulmonary annulus.

32.20 Answer E. The so-called suicide RV occurs when stenosis at the level of the valve is relieved and hypertrophied musculature along the infundibulum dynamically obstructs the RVOT. This only tends to occur when right ventricular pressures exceed 100 mm Hg (Thapar MK, et al. *Am Heart J* 1989;118(1):99-103) and when the intravascular volume is very low. Treatment usually includes IV fluids to expand intravascular volume, along with beta-blocker therapy to limit hypercontractility of the infundibular musculature. Pulmonary balloon valvuloplasty is a remarkably safe procedure with a very low complication rate. Other acute complications include ventricular ectopy, AV node block, and pulmonary regurgitation. The death rate has been estimated at 0.24% and major complication rate at 0.6% (Stanger P, et al. *Am J Cardiol* 1990;65(11):775-783). Transient systemic hypotension occurs during periods of balloon inflation along with bradycardia and premature ventricular contractions.

Figure A32-20 shows a lateral projection of an Inoue balloon (Toray Industries; Houston, TX) inflated in the RVOT and splitting the commissures of the valve (at central waist).

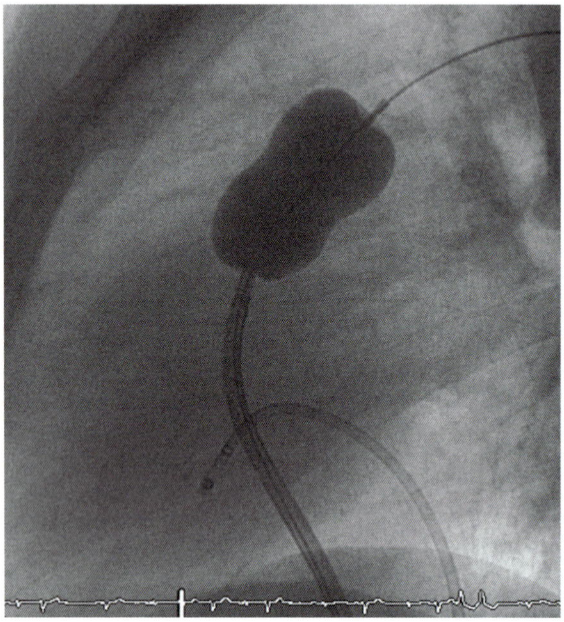

Figure A32-20

32.21 Answer A. There are a variety of anatomical and functional abnormalities associated with the heart after repair of TOF. Repair of the RVOT often compromises the integrity of the pulmonary valve apparatus leading to pulmonary valve insufficiency. It also causes conduction delay as a result of right bundle-branch block (RBBB). Chronic volume overload leads to right ventricular dilation, increased pulmonary insufficiency, and ventricular dysfunction. Right ventricular dysfunction promotes arrhythmia, fibrosis, RVOT aneurysm formation, LV dysfunction, and declining functional status. Ideally, valve replacement would take place prior to the onset of symptoms and before RV function begins to decline. This must be balanced with the expectation that a bioprosthetic valve has a median lifespan of 10 years and repeat surgeries will likely be necessary throughout the patient's life. Indications for valve replacement include symptoms of exercise intolerance or heart failure, QRS duration >180 ms, QRS prolongation >3.5 ms/year, sustained arrhythmia, right ventricular end-systolic volume >85 mL/m^2, right ventricular end-diastolic volume >170 mL/m^2, residual shunt defects, or residual right ventricular outflow tract obstruction (RVSP $\geq$ 2/3 systemic pressure) (Ammash NM, et al. *Congenit Heart Dis* 2007;2(6):386–403). Her RV volume indices (right ventricular end-diastolic volume, 113 mL/m^2, and right ventricular end-systolic volume, 52 mL/m^2) do not quite meet the criterion for surgery. However, it is important to mention that although a significant decrease in RV volumes occurs after valve replacement, improvement in RV function (ejection fraction) is unlikely, and it remains unknown whether pulmonary valve replacement improves survival in this population.

The development of transcatheter pulmonic valve technology has greatly advanced this field, and there appears to be a trend toward earlier intervention in patients with significant stenosis or regurgitation. Currently, transcatheter valves are only commercially approved for patients with conduits or (only recently) valve-in-valve interventions. The availability of larger and self-expanding prostheses will eventually bring this technology to patients with native RVOTs.

32.22 Answer C. Single ventricle physiology is marked by the obligation of one functional ventricle (either right or left) to generate sufficient cardiac output to traverse blood through both the systemic and pulmonary vasculatures. The stages of repair are dependent upon the complexity of the anatomy. In this patient's case, she underwent a Glenn procedure to route her superior vena caval circulation to the pulmonary arterial system and a lateral tunnel Fontal procedure to route the inferior vena caval flow to the pulmonary artery as well. The angiogram is an injection of the left innominate vein, which fills both PAs through the Glenn. Coming off the innominate are *venovenous* collaterals, which feed blood to the pulmonary veins, thus bypassing the lungs (a right-to-left shunt) and resulting in systemic hypoxemia. The lack of normalization of the oxygen saturation with supplemental oxygen is further indicative of right-to-left shunting being present. Venovenous collaterals are noted in 20% to 45% of patients undergoing cardiac catheterization after Glenn or Fontan operations. They usually form as a result of chronically elevated central venous pressure and when a significant pressure gradient occurs between the SVC and RA (Magee AG, et al. *J Am Coll Cardiol* 1998;32(2):502–508), and they carry a risk for paradoxical embolization. While all of the processes listed can result in hypoxia in patients with Fontan repair, only venovenous collaterals fit the image and clinical data. The collaterals were selectively cannulated (left panel of Fig. A32-22) and coiled (right panel of Fig. A32-22) with subsequent improvement in oxygen saturation. In some cases, the cardiac output may be dependent on right-to-left shunting, which functions as a "pop-off valve" for the

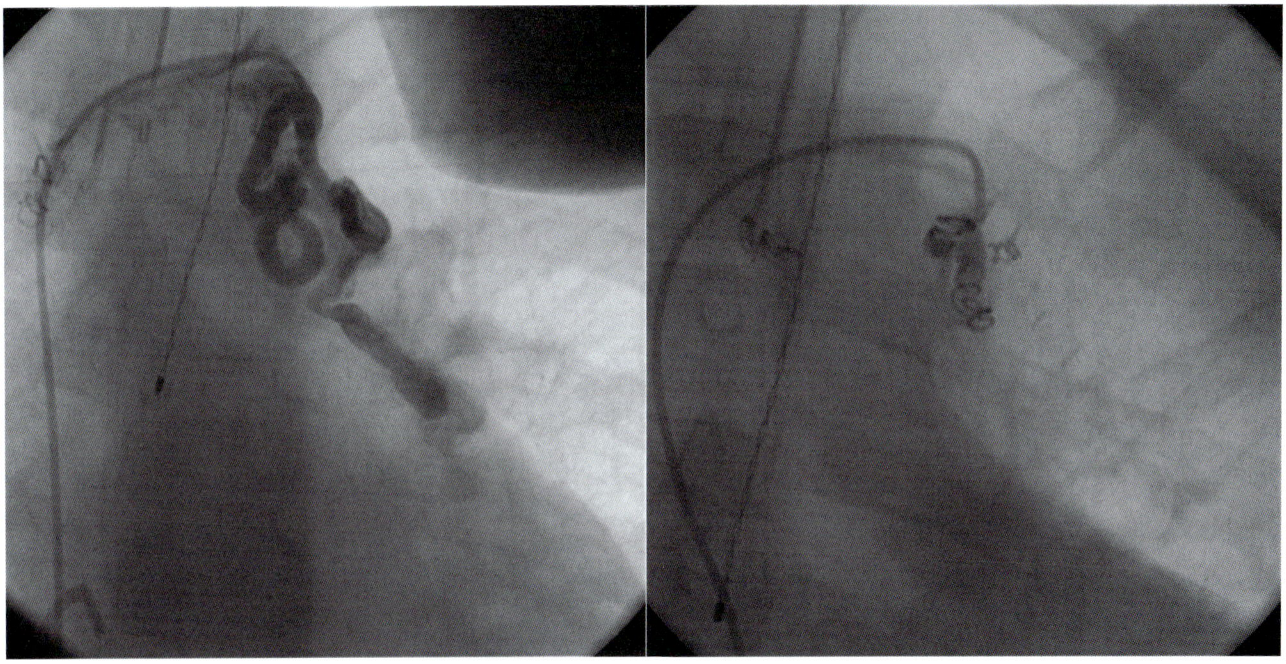

Figure A32-22

Fontan circuit and maintains cardiac output at the expense of hypoxia. Comprehensive hemodynamic data should ideally be collected prior to the intervention to ensure that the anomaly can be safely occluded. This may involve temporarily occluding the collateral with a balloon and reassessing hemodynamics. Failure of the systemic ventricle or regurgitation of either the aortic or AV valves is poorly tolerated in Fontan patients, as is pulmonary arterial hypertension. Even small increases in the pulmonary vascular resistance can result in serious consequences. Whether pulmonary vasodilators can help the latter is still under investigation. A fenestration in the Fontan circuit is often utilized to help patients through the initial perioperative period (again, working as a pop-off valve for the circuit). These can be maladaptive later on and can be successfully occluded using atrial septal occluder devices. While a patent fenestration is possible here, the angiogram does not demonstrate this finding.

32.23 **Answer A.** Subaortic stenosis is more common in men and can be difficult to differentiate from valvar aortic stenosis. Echocardiography, particularly transesophageal, is the best technique to evaluate this lesion. Surgical intervention is the standard approach as percutaneous techniques have been ineffective. Aortic insufficiency can develop secondary to thickening or impaired mobility of the valve leaflets and can worsen over time. Current guidelines recommend surgical intervention in subaortic stenosis for a peak instantaneous gradient of 50 mm Hg, a mean gradient of 30 mm Hg on echocardiography, or less if the LV end-systolic diameter is >50 mm, LVEF is <55%, or aortic regurgitation becomes progressive. Even with surgical resection, this lesion can recur (Warnes CA, et al. *Circulation* 2008;118(23):e714–e833).

32.24 **Answer C.** The most recent guidelines set forth by the ACC/AHA recommend subacute bacterial endocarditis (SBEs) prophylaxis for patients with implanted prosthetic materials; patients with a history of infective endocarditis; patients with unrepaired cyanotic CHD, including those with palliative shunts and conduits; patients with repaired CHD with residual defects adjacent to prosthetic material; or patients with completely repaired CHD with prosthetic material by surgery or cardiac catheterization for 6 months following the procedure (Nishumura RA, et al. *J Am Coll Cardiol* 2008;52(8):676–685).

32.25 **Answer B.** Pulmonary artery stenosis is common in patients with TOF and also occurs in patients with Williams or Alagille syndromes, following systemic to pulmonary shunts or after an arterial switch operation. In this pulmonary angiogram, a stenosis can be seen in the proximal right PA. Balloon angioplasty or stenting should be limited to appropriate anatomy, avoiding possible interference with pulmonic valve function and not impinging on the opposite branch vessel.

In children, stents should be avoided unless they are able to be dilated to the expected adult vessel size. Indications for an intervention include the presence of otherwise unexplained right ventricular systolic pressure elevation (usually at least 50% of the systemic pressure), a translesion gradient of at least 30 mm Hg, flow discrepancy to the distal pulmonary vascular bed (with >65% going to the opposite lung)—often quantified using nuclear perfusion scanning or cardiac MRI—and/or at least 50% luminal narrowing (Feltes TF, et al. *Circulation* 2011;123(22):2607-2652). The presence of concomitant valvular stenosis could confound assessment of lesion severity. Furthermore, the presence of concomitant lesions may favor a surgical over a transcatheter intervention. In this case, the patient was treated successfully with stenting (Fig. A32-25).

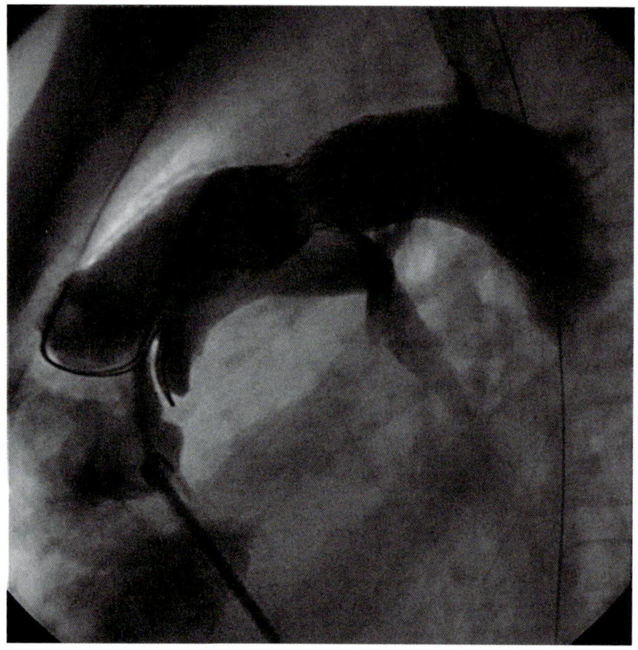

Figure A32-25

33 Patent Foramen Ovale and Atrial Septal Defect Closure

Hussam S. Suradi and Ziyad M. Hijazi

QUESTIONS

33.1 Figure Q33-1 shows a pictorial diagram of the heart with a patent foramen ovale (PFO) indicated with an arrow. Which of the following statements correctly identifies the additional anatomic structures?

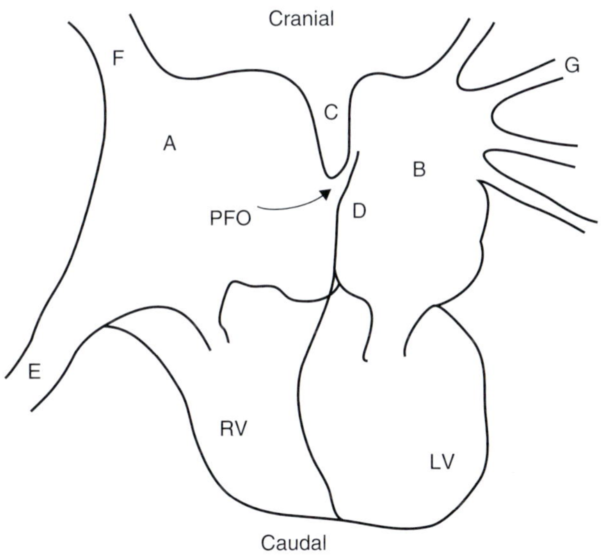

Figure Q33-1

(A) A = left atrium, C = septum secundum, G = inferior vena cava
(B) B = right atrium, A = left atrium, F = superior vena cava
(C) G = right upper pulmonary vein, D = septum secundum
(D) A = right atrium, B = left atrium, E = inferior vena cava
(E) A = right atrium, B = left atrium, G = left subclavian vein

33.2 Which of the following is a U.S. Food and Drug Administration (FDA)-approved indication for PFO closure?

(A) Cryptogenic stroke due to presumed paradoxical embolism
(B) Pulmonary hypertension
(C) Migraine headache
(D) Transient ischemic attack
(E) Orthodeoxia-platypnea syndrome

33.3 Which of the following statements about atrial septal aneurysm (ASA) is TRUE?

(A) The term ASA is used to describe a very floppy interatrial septum
(B) An ASA occurs where there is overabundant tissue in the septum primum
(C) The most widely accepted definition of an ASA is >15-mm excursion from left to right atrium on echocardiography
(D) The presence of an ASA in patients with patent foramen ovale and presumed embolic stroke appears to increase the risk of subsequent stroke
(E) All of the above are true

33.4 A 50-year-old man suffers an occipital stroke. His neurologic workup reveals no obvious cause for his stroke (cryptogenic). A transesophageal echocardiogram is completed to look for a cardiac source of embolism and reveals only a PFO with right-to-left shunting after injection of agitated saline. He is referred to you for percutaneous device closure of his PFO. In your discussion with the patient, which of the following statements is accurate?

(A) The CardioSEAL device is FDA-approved for PFO closure
(B) The Amplatzer septal occluder and Gore HELEX occluder are FDA-approved for PFO closure
(C) The Amplatzer PFO occluder is FDA-approved for PFO closure
(D) The Amplatzer multifenestrated septal occluder "cribriform" is FDA-approved for PFO closure

33.5 Cryptogenic stroke is defined as a brain infarction that is caused by:

(A) A definite cardioembolic source
(B) Large artery atherosclerosis
(C) Small artery disease
(D) All of the above
(E) None of the above

33.6 Percutaneous PFO closure is being considered for each of the patients below. For which of the following patients is percutaneous closure most reasonable?

(A) A 46-year-old man with lung cancer who suffers a stroke and has deep vein thrombosis in his right leg
(B) A 75-year-old man with recurrent transient ischemic attacks (TIAs), despite aspirin therapy. His transthoracic echocardiogram (TTE) shows mitral stenosis and a PFO
(C) A 42-year-old woman who suffers a stroke and has a PFO. Her workup reveals lupus and a positive anticardiolipin antibody
(D) A 45-year-old man who has had a presumed embolic stroke with no obvious risk factors for stroke. Magnetic resonance imaging (MRI) shows a recent as well as a remote infarct in two distinct areas. His transesophageal echocardiogram (TEE) shows a PFO and an atrial septal aneurysm

33.7 A 33-year-old woman with a PFO, migraine headaches, and a cryptogenic stroke comes to you for a second opinion about closure after being told by another physician not to have it done. You review her history and echocardiographic studies and are concerned about several high-risk features that, in your opinion, may warrant devise-based closure. Which of the following factors is NOT considered to increase the likelihood of recurrent stroke in patients with a presumed paradoxical embolism through a PFO?

(A) Large shunt
(B) Residual shunt after percutaneous closure
(C) Lipomatous septum secundum
(D) Prominent eustachian valve and right atrium strands
(E) Event occurring on warfarin anticoagulation

33.8 A patient is referred to you for percutaneous device closure of a PFO. During the procedure, the cine image reproduced in Figure Q33-8 is obtained. The figure illustrates which of the following findings and treatment strategies?

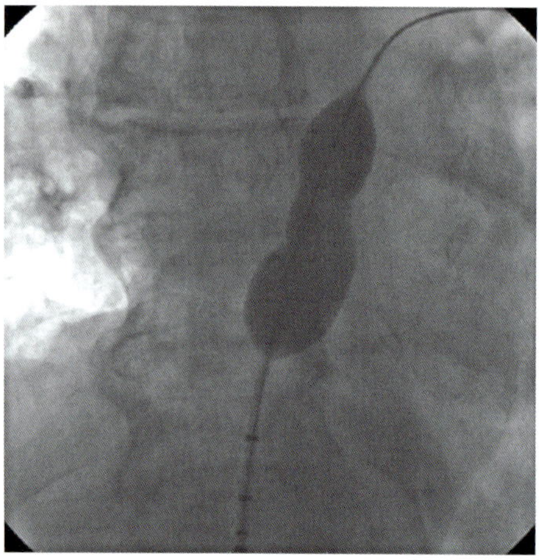

Figure Q33-8

(A) A sizing balloon is used to stretch and/or measure a long "tunnel"
(B) A sizing balloon is used to document the absence of a significant left-to-right shunting
(C) A percutaneous occluding device is being deployed by balloon inflation
(D) Pulmonary vein isolation is used to prevent atrial fibrillation before PFO closure

33.9 You are closing a PFO in a patient with a presumed paradoxical embolism. At the beginning of the procedure, you obtain the following echocardiographic image (Fig. Q33-9). Which of the following is TRUE about this image?

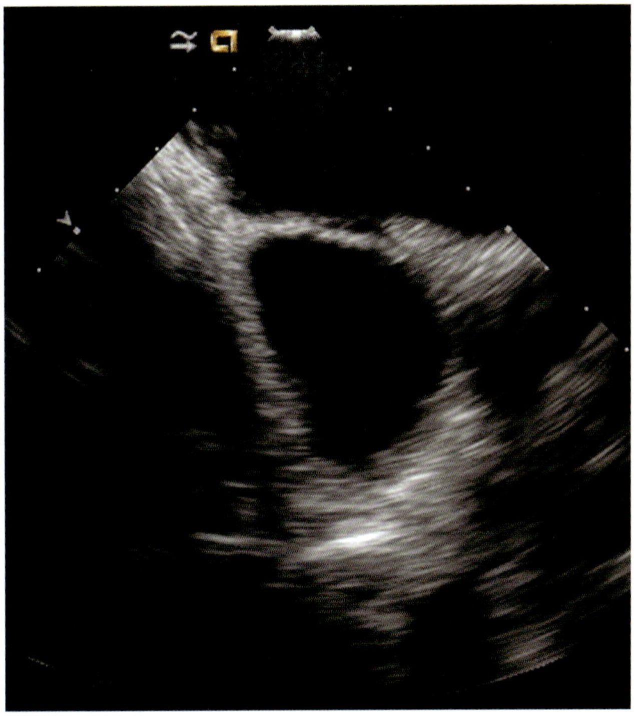

Figure Q33-9 (Courtesy of Hussam Suradi, MD.)

(A) It is an intracardiac echo (ICE) image with the right atrium on top, left atrium below, head to the right, and feet to the left
(B) It is an ICE image with the left atrium on top and right atrium below
(C) It is an ICE image with right atrium on top, left atrium below, head to left, and feet to right
(D) It is a transesophageal echocardiogram image with left atrium on top and right atrium below

33.10 All of the following indicate using ICE to guide atrial septal defect (ASD) closure as compared to TEE, except:

(A) Avoidance of general anesthesia
(B) Better visualization of the left atrium
(C) Less optimal visualization of the inferoposterior septum
(D) Shorter procedure time
(E) Additional echocardiographic personnel not necessary

33.11 Figure Q33-11A–C displays three images of closure devices. Which of the following statements correctly identifies one of the images?

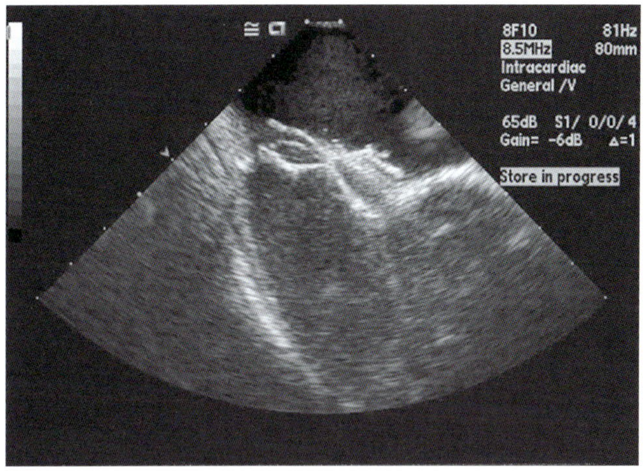

A

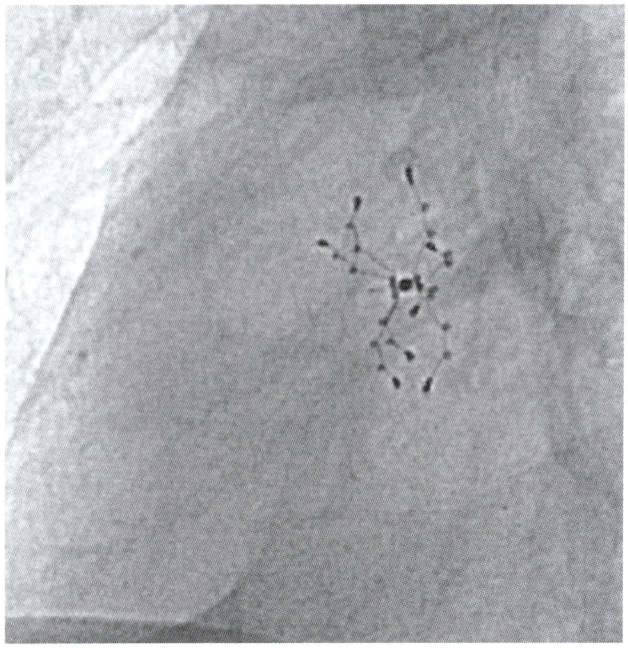

B

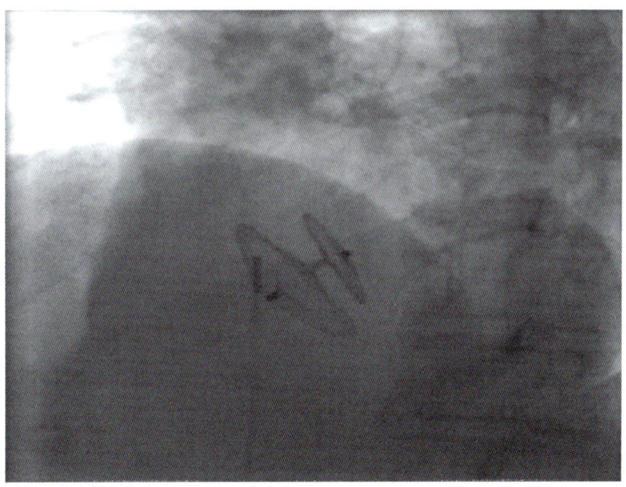

C

Figure Q33-11

(A) A = fluoroscopic image of a Gore HELEX device in a PFO
(B) B = fluoroscopic image of a CardioSEAL device deployed in a PFO
(C) C = fluoroscopic image of an Amplatzer atrial septal occluder device
(D) A = ICE image of an Amplatzer atrial septal occluder device

33.12 A 40-year-old woman suffers a cryptogenic stroke and is referred to you after a TTE with contrast injection demonstrates right-to-left shunting. You review her study noting that the bubbles enter the left atrium more than five heartbeats after their appearance in the right atrium. The most appropriate explanation for this finding is:

(A) Coexistent mitral stenosis
(B) Failure of the patient to provide a good Valsalva maneuver
(C) A pulmonary arterial-venous malformation (AVM)
(D) A persistent left superior vena cava

33.13 Figure Q33-13 illustrates the locations of various types of atrial septal defects. Which of the following statements correctly identifies these types?

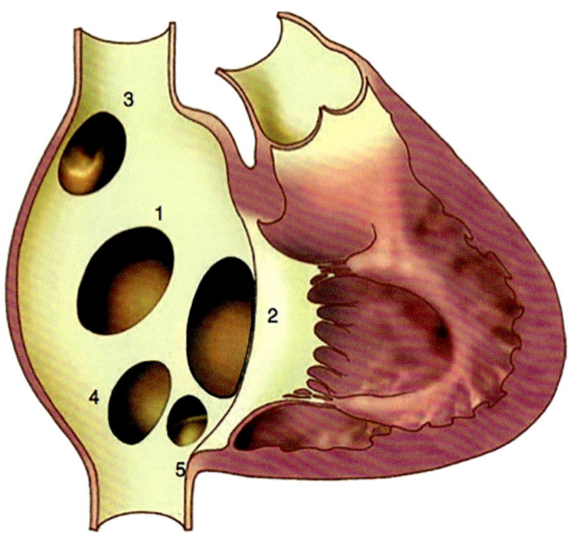

Figure Q33-13 (Courtesy of Hussam Suradi, MD.)

(A) (1) Secundum, (3) SVC sinus venosus, (5) coronary sinus
(B) (2) Secundum, (5) IVC sinus venosus, (4) coronary sinus
(C) (5) Secundum, (2) primum, (4) IVC sinus venosus
(D) (3) Secundum, (2) coronary sinus, (4) IVC sinus venosus

33.14 You are seeing a 27-year-old female who describes progressive fatigue over the past 5 months. She has a history of asthma treated with inhalers, though her pulmonary function tests and methacholine challenger were recently normal. On examination, she has a fixed split second heart sound and soft systolic ejection murmur over the left upper sternal border. Her lungs are clear and all her extremity pulses are equal and of normal intensity. All of the following would be expected to be present on her diagnostic studies except

(A) Right heart enlargement on echocardiography
(B) An rsR′ (incomplete bundle-branch block) pattern on an electrocardiogram
(C) Pulmonary hypertension on echocardiography
(D) Right-to-left shunt by bubble study on echocardiography
(E) Decreased pulmonary vascularity on chest x-ray

33.15 All of the following statements are consistent with the natural history of unrepaired ASD, except:

(A) Low prevalence of symptoms in the first three decades
(B) The majority of patients are symptomatic by the fifth decade
(C) Approximately 50% of patients develop pulmonary hypertension following the fourth decade and 20% develop atrial arrhythmias following the fifth decade
(D) Left ventricle (LV) dysfunction is unusual in patients older than 50 years
(E) In the sixth decade, mortality rate can approach 10%

33.16 A 19-year-old male college student suffers a TIA and is referred to you for workup by his neurologist who hears a heart murmur. You examine the patient and hear a soft systolic ejection murmur at the left upper sternal border with a fixed split S2. You suspect that he has an ASD and discuss the need for further imaging evaluation with a TEE to confirm the diagnosis and determine the type of ASD. Which of the following statements about ASDs and percutaneous closure is FALSE?

(A) Secundum ASDs are the most common type and are usually located in the septum secundum
(B) Sinus venosus ASDs are often associated with one or more anomalous pulmonary veins
(C) Septum primum ASDs may be associated with ventricular septal defects (VSDs)
(D) Most ASDs can now be closed percutaneously

33.17 A TEE on the patient in Question 33.16 confirms your suspicion that he has a septum secundum ASD. The anatomy appears favorable for percutaneous device closure with adequate rims on all sides. However, you explain to the patient that not all ASDs need to be closed. Current indications for ASD closure may include which of the following?

(A) Dyspnea
(B) Pulmonary hypertension
(C) Right-sided chamber enlargement
(D) Paradoxical embolism
(E) Q_P:Q_S > 1.5:1, even if asymptomatic
(F) All of the above

33.18 In order to obtain more information about the need for ASD closure on the patient in the above two questions, you decide to perform a right heart catheterization. On the basis of the oximetry measurements, you decide NOT to proceed with immediate closure of his defect. Which of the following measurements (see Table Q33-18) explains your hesitation?

Table Q33-18

	SVC Saturation (%)	IVC Saturation (%)	PA Saturation (%)	Aortic Saturation (%)
(A)	75	79	85	97
(B)	72	80	85	100
(C)	75	76	81	92
(D)	70	71	91	99

PA, pulmonary artery; IVC, inferior vena cava; SVC, superior vena cava.

33.19 A 50-year-old man presents with shortness of breath and paroxysmal atrial fibrillation. He has systolic ejection murmur at the left sternal border and fixed splitting of second heart sound. Echo showed secundum ASD with bidirectional shunting and evidence of a dilated right ventricle and atrium. Right ventricular systolic pressure is estimated at 70 mm Hg. He subsequently underwent heart catheterizations with the results below:

Saturations (%): IVC 70%; SVC 67%; RA 82%; RV 87%; PA 88%; PV 98%; aorta 92%
Pressures (mm Hg): PA 70/50 (56); FA 120/70; PCWP 10
Cardiac output: 6 L/min
Cardiac index: 3 L/min/m^2

What is the magnitude of the cardiovascular shunt, or Q_P/Q_S?

(A) 1.5:1
(B) 2:1
(C) 2.4:1
(D) 3:1
(E) 4:1

Abbreviations: FA, femoral artery; IVC, inferior vena cava; PA, pulmonary artery; PCWP, pulmonary capillary wedge pressure; PV, pulmonary vein; Q_P, pulmonary flow; Q_S, systemic flow; RA, right atrium; RV, right ventricle; SVC, superior vena cava

33.20 What is the next step in the management of the patient in the previous question?

(A) Proceed with percutaneous closure
(B) Referral for surgical repair of ASD
(C) Assessment of pulmonary vasoreactivity
(D) Medical therapy with diuretics

33.21 The patient underwent pulmonary vasoreactivity testing with inhaled nitric oxide and 100% oxygen. Hemodynamics were remeasured as defined below:

Pressures (mm Hg): PA pressure 40/20 (27); FA 115/80; PCWP 8
Cardiac output (L/min/m^2): 6.5
Cardiac index (L/min/m^2): 3.25

What is the next step in management?

(A) Abort procedure and recommend against ASD closure
(B) Proceed with percutaneous ASD closure if anatomically suitable
(C) Balloon occlusion testing of the ASD
(D) Place on vasodilator therapy and repeat hemodynamics in 3 months
(E) Refer for heart/lung transplant

Abbreviations: FA, femoral artery; PA, pulmonary artery; PCWP, pulmonary capillary wedge pressure

33.22 The ICE image (Fig. Q33-22) demonstrates which of the following?

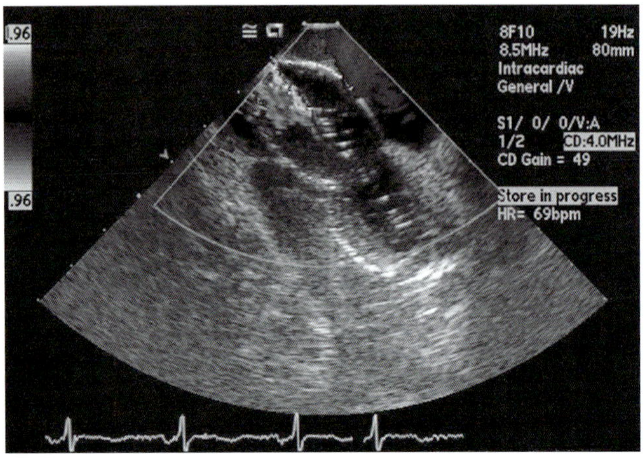

Figure Q33-22

(A) Balloon deployment of an Amplatzer atrial septal occlusion device
(B) Balloon sizing of an ASD
(C) Percutaneous balloon valvuloplasty for mitral stenosis
(D) Atrial septostomy to increase the ASD size before closure

33.23 A patient with a right-sided chamber enlargement and secundum ASD diagnosed on echo is referred for device closure. After placement of the ICE catheter to guide deployment, you obtain the image in Figure Q33-23. Which of the following statements best describes what you see?

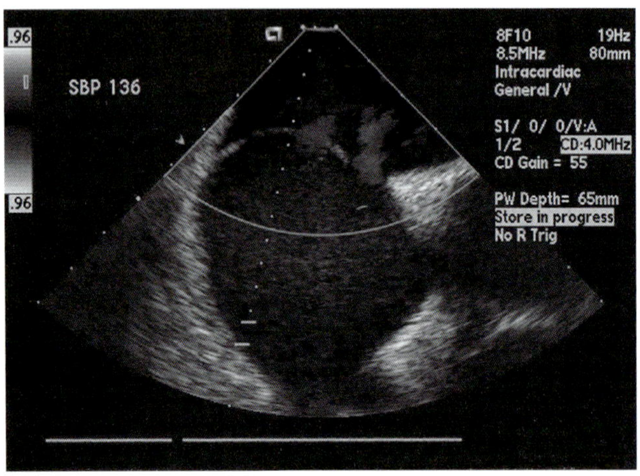

Figure Q33-23

(A) A septum primum defect with both an ASD and a VSD
(B) A fenestrated ASD that will require a surgically placed patch
(C) Echocardiographic reverberations from a bidirectional ASD
(D) Two discrete secundum defects that are potentially closable percutaneously

33.24 You are consenting a patient for device closure of an ASD. Which of the following complications (<30 days) and their incidence is INCORRECT for ASD device closure procedures?

(A) Perforation/Tamponade, <1%
(B) Stroke, <1%
(C) Device embolization, <1%
(D) Cardiac arrhythmia, approximately 5%
(E) Allergic reactions to nickel, approximately 5%
(F) Unsuccessful procedure, 2% to 3%

33.25 A 16-year-old teen has an incidentally discovered ASD and undergoes percutaneous device closure at your local children's hospital. He is subsequently lost to follow-up and is referred at age 29 to your hospital's adult congenital heart disease clinic. The cardiologist who sees the patient discusses the natural history of a successfully closed ASD. Which one of the following statements is TRUE in short-term and medium-term follow-up after percutaneous ASD closure?

(A) Most patients will not experience further enlargement or deterioration in right ventricular (RV) function
(B) Most patients will eventually require surgery to permanently close their defects
(C) Endocarditis prophylaxis and anticoagulation are required lifelong
(D) Pulmonary hypertension will return to normal over 1 to 3 months

33.26 A 42-year-old woman had her first episode of atrial fibrillation. Over the last year, she developed symptoms of fatigue and shortness of breath. Echo was performed and showed secundum ASD. Given her symptomatic status, percutaneous closure is planned using intracardiac echo guidance. What has to be judged after device positioning?

(A) Device position has to be stable
(B) Both disks should be opposed to the septum secundum
(C) Absence of residual shunt or additional defects
(D) Atrioventricular valve (AV) valve function
(E) All of the above

33.27 A 32-year-old woman has a large secundum ASD with dyspnea, right atrial (RA) and RV enlargement, and a 2.2:1 left-to-right shunt. LV function is normal. You bring her to the catheterization laboratory for percutaneous device closure under ICE and fluoroscopic guidance. Balloon sizing, until color flow ceases, demonstrates a diameter of 30 mm. You place, with some difficulty, a 30-mm diameter Amplatzer atrial septal occluder device. However, during the "push-pull," it easily pulls through the defect into the right atrium, and you decide to size up to a 32-mm diameter device. During the removal and reinsertion of the new device, you notice ST elevation in the inferior leads with premature ventricular contractions (PVCs) that resolve within 5 minutes. You attribute this to an air embolism and proceed with insertion of the 32-mm diameter device, which is successful. A follow-up echo 2 hours later demonstrates no LV wall motion abnormalities and telemetry shows no PVCs. However, 4 hours later, you are called to see her after the patient has repeated runs of non-sustained ventricular tachycardia (NSVT). Her BP is normal. Which of the following should you do?

(A) Call for a stat echo and make immediate arrangements for transfer to the catheterization laboratory for PCI
(B) Call for a stat echo, surgical consultation, and make immediate arrangements for transfer to the catheterization laboratory for device retrieval
(C) Call for a stat echo and perform a bedside emergent pericardiocentesis
(D) You are not concerned, as this likely represents continued effects of the air embolism

33.28 Which of the following tests can be used to detect a right-to-left shunt?

(A) Transthoracic echo with peripheral intravenous contrast (e.g., agitated saline microbubbles) injection
(B) Transesophageal echo with contrast injection
(C) Transcranial Doppler (power mode) ultrasonography with contrast injection
(D) Green dye indicator dilution curves
(E) Intracardiac echocardiography (ICE) with femoral venous contrast injection
(F) All of the above

33.29 Which of the following structural heart defects cannot be successfully closed with a percutaneous device?

(A) Secundum ASD
(B) Muscular VSD
(C) Postinfarction VSD
(D) Patent ductus arteriosus
(E) Sinus venosus ASD

ANSWERS AND EXPLANATIONS

33.1 Answer D. The foramen ovale is an interarterial communication defect present in up to 20% of normal adults. It is a small channel between the septum secundum (C) and septum primum (D) that may allow passage of blood or thrombotic emboli from the right atrium (A) to the left atrium (B) of the heart (paradoxical embolism).

33.2 Answer A. Currently, PFO closure is only FDA-approved to reduce the risk of recurrent ischemic stroke in patients predominantly between the ages of 18 and 60 who have had a cryptogenic stroke due to presumed paradoxical embolism. None of the other listed conditions are FDA-approved indications.

33.3 Answer E. An atrial septal aneurysm is a floppy interatrial septum resulting from overabundant tissue in the septum primum. A total septal excursion of >15 mm has been most widely accepted as the definition for this entity. If the septal excursion is less, it is generally referred to as a "redundant atrial septum." In patients with cryptogenic stroke and a patent foramen ovale, a concurrent atrial septal aneurysm appears to significantly increase the risk of future stroke.

33.4 Answer C. The Amplatzer PFO occluder is the only device approved by the FDA to reduce stroke risk for patients with prior cryptogenic stroke that's believed to be caused by a PFO-related paradoxical embolism.

33.5 Answer E. Cryptogenic stroke is defined as brain infarction that is not clearly attributable to a definite cardioembolism, large artery atherosclerosis, or small artery disease, despite extensive investigation.

33.6 Answer D. With a high-risk anatomy, this patient has evidence for recurrent paradoxical embolism. The other patients have other potential causes for stroke or accepted indications for chronic anticoagulation with warfarin.

33.7 Answer C. Lipomatous septum secundum has not been shown to be a factor for recurrent paradoxical embolism. All of the other characteristics have been associated with recurrent paradoxical embolism.

33.8 Answer A. The segment of overlap between septum primum and secundum may be discrete or have substantial overlap. In the latter case, the overlap segment or "tunnel" may be quite stiff, thereby preventing optimal deployment of certain devices. In this case, stretching or tearing of the tunnel with a balloon can facilitate device placement.

33.9 Answer A. This is a standard ICE image projection with the transducer in the right atrium (top of image) looking across the septum to the left atrium. It is oriented with the feet to the left and the head of the patient to the right.

33.10 Answer C. The main advantages of ICE over TEE for ASD closure include avoidance of general anesthesia, better visualization of the left atrium and posteroinferior part of the septum, shorter procedure times, and the ability of the interventionist to perform the procedure, as well as imaging, without the need for additional echocardiographic personnel.

33.11 Answer B. The figure in A is an ICE image of a deployed CardioSEAL device. Figure B is a fluoroscopic image of the same device. Figure C is a fluoroscopic image of an Amplatzer PFO occluder (note the thin connecting waist that differentiates this image from an ASD device).

33.12 Answer C. Although a Valsalva maneuver (or sniffing) can increase the detection of a PFO by increasing right atrium (relative to left atrium) pressure, most shunts will be visible because of normal respiratory variation within five cardiac cycles. Patients with a pulmonary AVM may have an extracardiac shunt that is only visible once the contrast has traversed the pulmonary circulation. These can also be a cause of paradoxical embolism and can be diagnosed by chest computed tomography and MRI.

33.13 Answer A. ASDs are relatively common, accounting for about 10% and 30% of all congenital heart diseases diagnosed in children and adults, respectively. There are four different types of ASDs that have different anatomical and clinical features ostium secundum, ostium primum, coronary sinus defects, and sinus venosus. (1) Secundum ASDs are the most common (75% of cases) and are usually located at the level of the fossa ovalis. (2) The primum ASD (15% to 20% of cases) is located in the inferior part of the atrial septum, near the crux of the heart, and is associated with atrioventricular septal defects. (3 and 4) The sinus venosus type (5% to 10% of cases) is located in the superior or inferior part of the septum, near the superior or inferior vena cavae entry to the right atrium. The superior part is usually associated with partial anomalous pulmonary venous drainage. (5) The uncommon coronary sinus septal defect (<1%) allows shunting across the ostium of the coronary sinus.

33.14 Answer E. The patient described in this case has an ASD. ASDs lead to right heart enlargement and an incomplete right bundle-branch block pattern on electrocardiography. Pulmonary hypertension can result from increased blood flow, and up to 10% of patients may develop Eisenmenger physiology if uncorrected. In this case, the chest x-ray would be expected to demonstrate increased lung vascularity.

33.15 Answer D. LV dysfunction is uncommon in younger patients, but the incidence is as high as 15% in patients older than 50 years. Most patients are asymptomatic in the first three decades of life, but after the age of 50, about 70% of patients are symptomatic. Pulmonary hypertension and atrial arrhythmias are also more prevalent after the fourth decade of life, and the annual mortality rate increases to 10% in the sixth decade.

33.16 Answer A. Secundum ASDs are the most common form of ASD (70%) and most can now be closed percutaneously (hence, D is true). Secundum ASDs are (paradoxically) located in the primum portion of the atrial septum. The ostium primum defects are associated with abnormalities of the endocardial cushion and may involve the upper portion of the ventricular septum (Fig. A33-16).

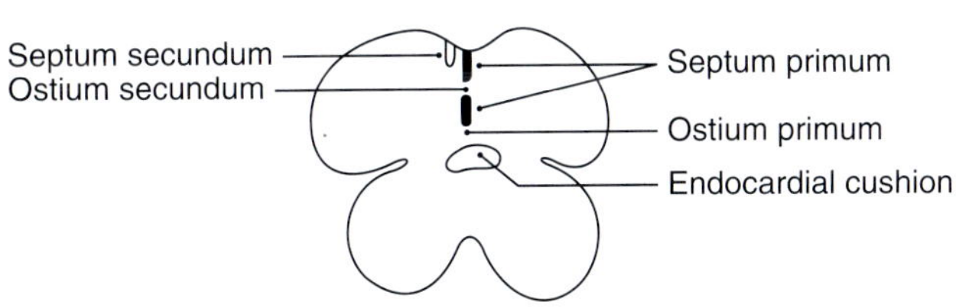

Figure A33-16

33.17 Answer F. All of these are reasonable indications for ASD closure in the presence of a significant left-to-right shunt. Traditionally, a $Q_P:Q_S$ ratio > 2 has been considered a cutoff for surgical closure in asymptomatic patients. However, it has been shown that percutaneous closure can increase peak oxygen consumption during exercise, even in some apparently asymptomatic patients with $Q_P:Q_S < 2$ (Giardini A, et al. *J Am Coll Cardiol* 2004;43(10):1886–1891).

33.18 Answer C. Patients A, B, and D all have significant left-to-right shunts ranging from 1.7 to 3.6. This was calculated using a mixed venous saturation of

$$\frac{3 \cdot \text{SVC} + \text{IVC}}{4}$$

and the shunt formula of

$$Q_P{:}Q_S = \frac{(\text{Aortic saturation} - \text{Mixed venous saturation})}{(\text{Aortic saturation} - \text{Pulmonary artery saturation})}$$

Patient C has systemic desaturation that can reflect associated lung disease or right-to-left shunting. In the latter se, the bidirectional shunt formula must be utilized. Eisenmenger syndrome (right heart failure leading to reversal of flow across the ASD) must be assessed to ensure that closure does not result in acute or progressive right heart failure.

33.19 Answer C.

$$Q_P/Q_S = \frac{\text{Pulmonic blood flow}}{\text{Systemic blood flow}}$$

Pulmonic blood flow =

$$\frac{O_2\ \text{consumption}}{\text{Pulmonary vein (PV) } O_2 \text{ content} - \text{Pulmonary artery (PA) } O_2 \text{ content}}$$

Systemic blood flow =

$$\frac{O_2\ \text{consumption}}{\text{Systemic arterial (SA) } O_2 \text{ content} - \text{Mixed venous (MV) } O_2 \text{ content}}$$

Oxygen content =

$$10\ \text{dL/L}\ (1.34\ \text{m/g} \times \text{Hgb g/dL} \times O_2\ \text{saturation})$$

Cancelling out the Hgb and correction factor:

$$Q_P/Q_S = \frac{\text{SA } O_2 \text{ saturation} - \text{MV } O_2 \text{ saturation}}{\text{PV } O_2 \text{ saturation} - \text{PA } O_2 \text{ saturation}}$$

Mixed venous saturation (Flamm equation) =

$$\frac{3 \cdot \text{SVC} + \text{IVC}}{4}$$

Substituting for the above:

$$Q_P/Q_S = (92 - 68)/(98 - 88) = 2.4:1$$

33.20 Answer C. Pulmonary arterial hypertension (PAH) is a rare but serious complication of unrepaired ASD, and the decision to close such defects in this patient population should be approached with caution and careful consideration. PAH is defined as a mean pulmonary arterial pressure of more than 25 mm Hg in the setting of normal left atrial pressure of <15 mm and a normal resting cardiac output corresponding to pulmonary vascular resistance (PVR) of more than 3 Wood units. ASD closure is indicated in all symptomatic patients with net left-to-right shunt and resting O_2 saturation of more than 92%. If there is a bidirectional shunt, then pulmonary vasodilator testing should be performed. If there is a net left-to-right shunt on vasodilation, or balloon test occlusion of the ASD shows a favorable response with a fall in mean pulmonary artery pressure and no drop in cardiac output or increase in right atrial pressure, then the ASD should be closed. In the absence of favorable response, ASD closure is contraindicated, and the patient should be placed on pulmonary vasodilators and reassessed in the cardiac catheterization lab after 6 months. Borderline cases may benefit from fenestrated ASD device closure, although no studies to document survival with this approach are available.

33.21 Answer B. Based on the patient's hemodynamic study, he had positive vasoreactivity response. A positive vasoreactivity response is defined as a reduction of mean pulmonary artery pressure (PAP) of >10 mm Hg with a resultant mean PAP of 40 mm Hg or less, without a fall in cardiac output. The degree of response to pulmonary vasodilators is thought to predict the likelihood that a patient's pulmonary vascular resistance (PVR) will fall once their intracardiac shunt is repaired. Therefore, in this case, it is safe to proceed with ASD closure.

33.22 Answer B. This ICE image shows a balloon inflated in a secundum ASD, which is an important part of percutaneous ASD closure. The balloon forces the defect into a circular configuration and is expanded until the color flow Doppler evidence of left-to-right shunting ceases. An atrial septal occluder is then chosen with a central diameter that is 1 to 2 mm greater than the waist measurement on the balloon or with a disc diameter that is >1.8 times the waist diameter.

33.23 Answer D. Secundum ASDs may have multiple defects or fenestrations. In some cases, these defects can be closed percutaneously by placing an ASD device in the largest fenestration (cribriform device) or by using multiple septal occluder devices. In the illustrated case, these two discrete defects were closed using two ASD devices placed in an overlapping or "sandwich" approach (Fig. A33-23).

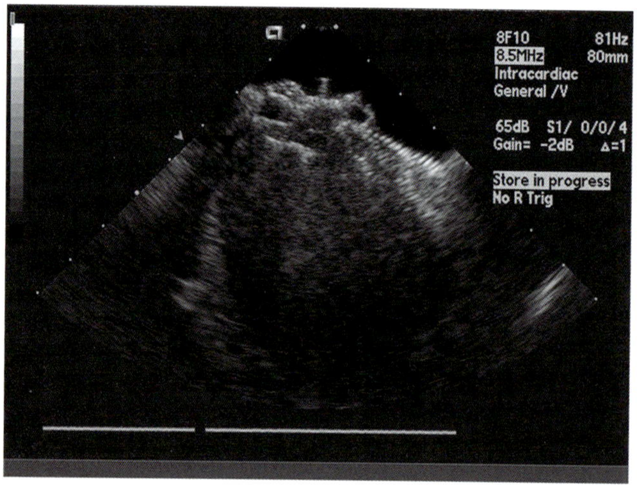

Figure A33-23

33.24 Answer E. Procedural success is more than 97%. Major complications are rare, but atrial arrhythmias occur in up to 5% of patients within the first month. Allergic reactions are usually related to concomitant medications (especially clopidogrel), and true allergies to the nickel contained in the device that is made of a nickel-titanium alloy (nitinol) are extremely rare (<1/1,000).

33.25 Answer A. In general, percutaneous closure of an ASD is a definitive therapy that eliminates the left-to-right shunt causing RV enlargement, pulmonary hypertension, and the stimulus to further RV hypertrophy. However, some patients with pulmonary hypertension will have developed permanent changes that prevent the pressure from returning to normal (fixed pulmonary hypertension). Antiplatelet medications are usually administered for 6 months following device closure, after which endothelialization reduces the risk of thrombus formation and infection. Anticoagulation is rarely necessary unless there is a separate indication, such as chronic AF.

33.26 Answer E. Stable device position, closure of the defect with no residual shunt, and lack of procedural complications are all part of the postprocedural assessment.

33.27 Answer B. Although air embolism can be a devastating complication, a small air embolism is usually well-tolerated, resolves rapidly, and has no lasting effects. The most likely explanation for the nonsustained ventricular tachycardia (NSVT) is that the device was not sufficiently oversized and embolized to the RV causing ectopy. This can be confirmed on echo and plans for device retrieval with a snare, and cardiac surgical backup is the most appropriate therapy. Perforation with tamponade can be ruled out by echo but would be unlikely without some hemodynamic compromise.

33.28 Answer F. Answer choices A, B, and C are the usual preprocedure methods utilized. ICE is often used during the procedure to confirm the shunt before closure. Indocyanine green dye dilution curves can also be used to assess cardiac output and to detect shunts. If dye is injected into the femoral vein, early appearance in a femoral artery sample due to bypass of the pulmonary circulation is evidence of a right-to-left shunt (Fig. A33-28) (Pepine CJ. *Diagnostic and therapeutic cardiac catheterization* 1994:388–390).

Because these calculations are somewhat cumbersome, this method has been replaced by imaging modalities with contrast injections. Currently, power mode transcranial Doppler and transesophageal echocardiogram are considered more sensitive than TTE, although the patient position, injection site, and the use of maneuvers (e.g.,

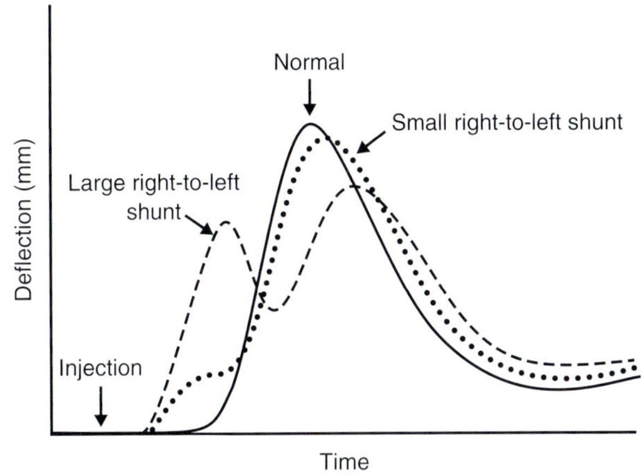

Figure A33-28

Valsalva and Mueller) affect the sensitivity and specificity of shunt detection (Spencer MP, et al. *J Neuroimaging* 2004;14(4):342–349; Telman G, et al. *J Neuroimaging* 2003;13(4):356–358).

33.29 Answer E. Sinus venosus defects are in the upper portion of the septum and are often associated with anomalous pulmonary vein drainage into the right atrium. The lack of a rim of tissue superiorly and the frequent need to baffle the anomalous pulmonary venous flow to the left atrium make these defects not suitable for currently available closure devices.

34 Percutaneous Balloon Pericardiotomy for Patients with Pericardial Effusion and Tamponade

Jay Thakkar and Jacqueline Saw

QUESTIONS

34.1 A 61-year-old woman with recent tricuspid valve repair presents with increasing dyspnea, orthopnea, and presyncope. The patient was hypotensive with distended jugular veins and distant heart sounds on physical examination. On the basis of the hemodynamic tracing from the right ventricle (RV) shown in Figure Q34-1, which of the following statements is INCORRECT?

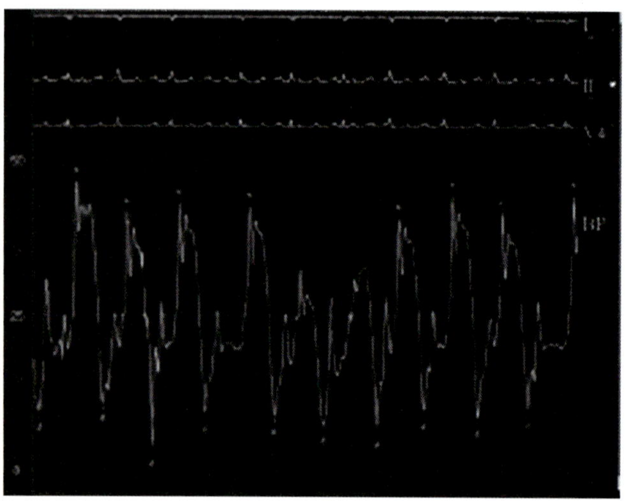

Figure Q34-1

(A) Pulsus paradoxus is likely to be present
(B) Presence of right ventricular collapse lasting more than one-third of diastole is a more sensitive echo finding in this condition than right atrial collapse
(C) Blunt or absent Y descent on the right atrial pressure tracing is typically described in this condition
(D) Ventricular interdependence may be accentuated

34.2 Pericardial tamponade in the absence of pulsus paradoxus is described with all of the following, EXCEPT:

(A) Aortic regurgitation
(B) Severe rheumatoid spondylitis
(C) Constrictive pericarditis
(D) Large atrial septal defect (ASD)

34.3 Consider the percutaneous pericardial intervention depicted in Figure Q34-3. Which of the following statements is INCORRECT?

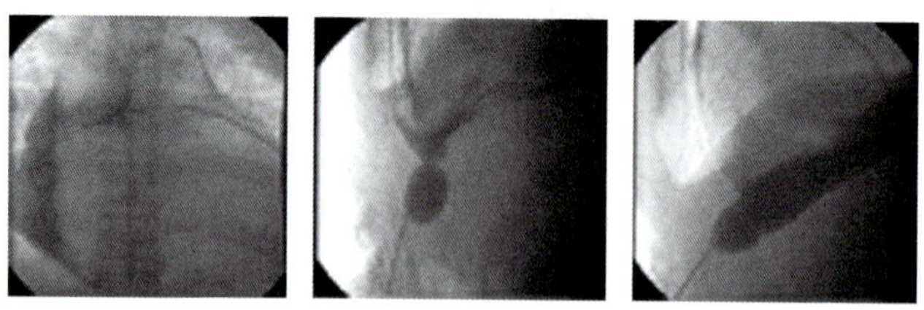

Figure Q34-3

(A) Left pleural effusion occurs in 1% to 2% of cases
(B) A pericardiocutaneous fistula is a potential complication
(C) It is recommended that the balloon be inflated until the waist disappears
(D) Biplane fluoroscopy is recommended

34.4 All of the following are relative contraindications to percutaneous balloon pericardiotomy, EXCEPT:

(A) Marginal respiratory reserve
(B) Presence of a large pleural effusion
(C) Thrombocytopenia
(D) Malignant pericardial effusion

34.5 Which of the following catheterization findings most reliably supports a diagnosis of pericardial constriction over restrictive cardiomyopathy?

(A) Pulmonary artery systolic pressure <50 mm Hg
(B) A prominent Y descent
(C) Equalization of right and left heart late diastolic pressures
(D) Ventricular interdependence

34.6 Regarding pericardiocentesis, which of the following statements is MOST accurate?

(A) It is advisable to drain <500 mL at a time to avoid acute right ventricular dilatation
(B) Recurrence rate with drainage of large idiopathic pericardial effusions is no better than with conservative management
(C) Major complications occur in 1.3% to 1.6% of pericardiocentesis
(D) Effusions measured by echo tend to be larger than those measured by computed tomography (CT) or magnetic resonance imaging (MRI)

34.7 In the setting of aortic dissection, which of the following statements is INCORRECT?

(A) Pericardial effusion coincides with 17% to 45% of cases
(B) Pericardial tamponade occurs most frequently with a DeBakey type I dissection
(C) Pericardiocentesis may cause extension of the dissection
(D) Surgery should be performed as soon as possible

34.8 In patients with large malignancy-related pericardial effusion treated with percutaneous balloon pericardiotomy, which of the following is INCORRECT?

(A) Fever occurs in approximately one-third of patients post-procedure
(B) Recurrence rate at 4 months is approximately 50%
(C) Results with immediate and deferred procedures are similar
(D) Lung and breast cancer-associated effusions are most common

34.9 A 64-year-old man with a history of alcohol dependency presented to the emergency room with increasing dyspnea, chronic cough, hemoptysis, and persistent fever. Echocardiography confirms the presence of a large pericardial effusion. Simultaneous right atrial pressure and pericardial opening pressure are shown in Figure Q34-9. Regarding this hemodynamic tracing, which of the following statements is INCORRECT?

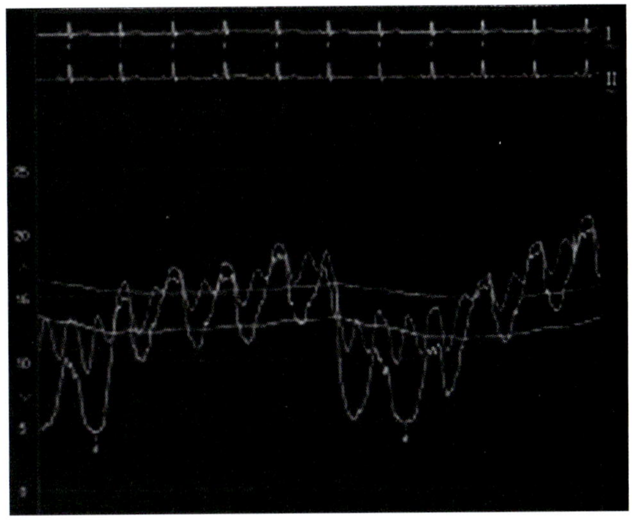

Figure Q34-9

(A) The X descent during ventricular systole is the dominant waveform
(B) The right atrial and pericardial pressures fall during inspiration
(C) With increased pericardial fluid accumulation, the X descent will become less prominent and the Y decent more pronounced
(D) RV mid-diastolic pressure may be elevated and equal to the right atrial and pericardial pressure

34.10 The patient discussed in Question 34.9 had a cardiac CT (short axis shown in Fig. Q34-10) on admission. He had a reasonable symptomatic response to pericardiocentesis and his pericardial pressure returned to zero post-tap; however, his right atrial pressure remained elevated. On the basis of his findings on cardiac CT scan and his hemodynamic parameters, a presumptive diagnosis of effusive-constrictive pericarditis was made. Which of the following findings does NOT support this diagnosis?

(A) Equalization of the right and left ventricular end diastolic pressures
(B) A prominent dip and plateau waveform in the right ventricular tracing

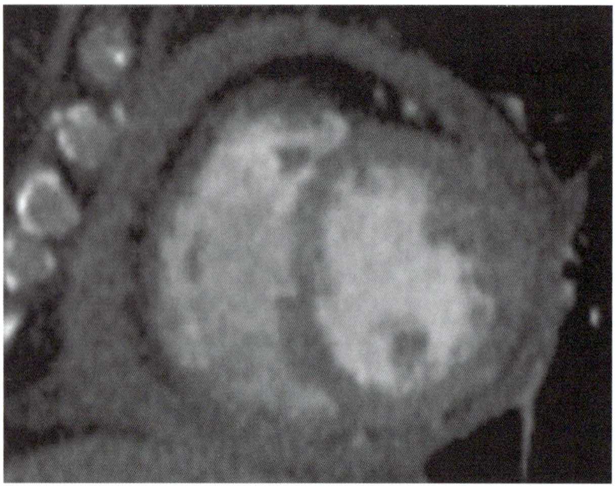

Figure Q34-10

(C) Concordance between the left and the right ventricular systolic pressures
(D) Right ventricular end systolic pressure <50 mm Hg

34.11 *Mycobacterium tuberculosis* was found in the same patient's (discussed in Questions 34.9 and 34.10) pericardial fluid. Which of the following statements regarding tuberculous pericarditis is INCORRECT?

(A) Pericardial constriction occurs in 10% to 15% of cases
(B) The mortality rate approaches 85% in untreated cases
(C) A rapid diagnosis can be made from a small volume fluid sample by polymerase chain reaction (PCR)
(D) The tuberculin skin test is falsely negative in 25% to 30% of cases

34.12 A patient with a history of tuberculous pericarditis presents with progressively increasing dyspnea and undergoes the noninvasive study depicted in Figure Q34-12. Regarding this investigative study, which of the following statements is CORRECT?

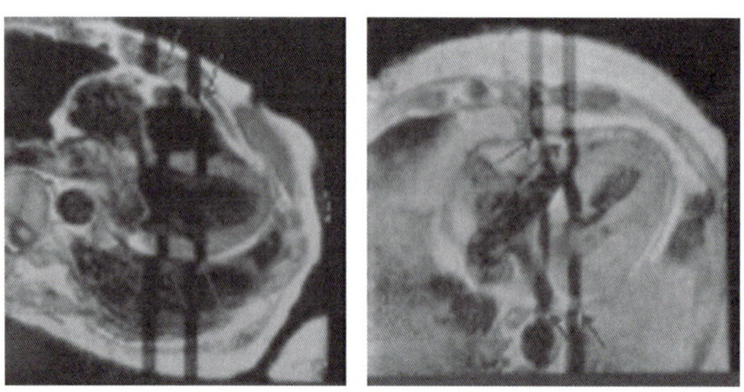

Figure Q34-12

(A) The image on the left represents evidence of pericardial constriction and tethered movement of the heart
(B) The images represent CT scan tagging, which can be used to diagnose pericardial constriction
(C) Pericardial thickening is absent in approximately 18% of cases of constrictive pericarditis
(D) Pericardiectomy for constrictive pericarditis has a mortality rate of 1% to 2%

34.13 Which of the following statements regarding endomyocardial biopsy or temporary pacemaker lead placement is FALSE?

(A) The rate of perforation during right ventricular biopsy is 0.3% to 5%
(B) Tamponade and circulatory collapse follow right ventricular perforation 75% of the time
(C) Pericardial hemorrhage complicates 0.1% to 3.3% of left ventricular biopsies
(D) Presence of right rather than left bundle-branch block (LBBB) configuration suggests pacemaker lead penetration of the RV

34.14 During insertion of an implantable cardioverter defibrillator (ICD), the patient becomes acutely hypotensive and an echo confirms the presence of an effusion. Which finding in the hemodynamic tracing in Figure Q34-14 does NOT support a diagnosis of pericardial tamponade?

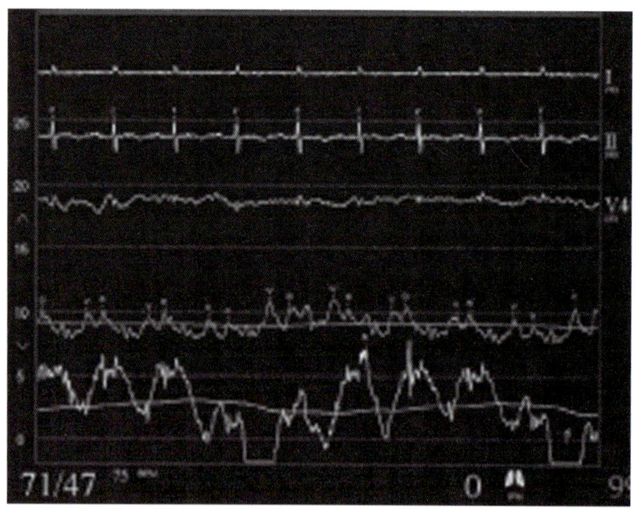

Figure Q34-14

(A) Presence of an elevated right atrial pressure
(B) Blunting of the Y descent in expiration
(C) Absence of respiratory variation in the right atrial tracing
(D) Pericardial pressure approaching right atrial diastolic pressure in expiration

34.15 A 43-year-old male presents with chest pain. He reports mild, flulike symptoms 2 weeks ago. You are considering a provisional diagnosis of pericarditis. Which of the following is most specific for pericarditis?

(A) Sharp nature of the chest pain
(B) Elevated C-reactive protein (CRP)
(C) A triphasic rub on auscultation
(D) Transthoracic echocardiogram (TTE)

34.16 A patient with a significant medical history of lung cancer treated with surgical resection and radiotherapy presents with a 3-week history of progressive dyspnea, anorexia, malaise, and dark-colored urine. Physical examination shows a temperature of 36.5°C, heart rate (HR) 116/min, respiratory rate (RR) 19/min, blood pressure (BP) 103/70 mm Hg, oxygen saturation (SaO_2) 90%, prominent neck veins, mild bilateral pedal edema, and sensitivity on palpating the right hypochondrium. All of the following are appropriate to be performed, EXCEPT:

(A) TTE
(B) CT scan
(C) 12-lead electrocardiogram (ECG)
(D) Intravenous (IV) furosemide to relieve congestion

34.17 A 27-year-old woman presents with sharp retrosternal pain aggravated by inspiration and supine position. A review of her past medical history revealed two episodes of acute pericarditis. Prior laboratory findings were largely unremarkable, including serology for antinuclear antibodies (ANA) and rheumatoid factor. She was treated with standard dose nonsteroidal, anti-inflammatory, and colchicine but had minimal relief of symptoms. All of the following are appropriate in her management, EXCEPT:

(A) Higher dose and longer duration of nonsteroidal
(B) Higher dose and longer duration of colchicine
(C) Steroids
(D) Etanercept

34.18 All of the following statements about constrictive pericarditis are TRUE, EXCEPT:

(A) Invasive right heart catheterization is essential prior to pericardiectomy
(B) Chest CT scan has highest sensitivity to detect pericardial calcification
(C) TTE is a good early test
(D) Constrictive pericarditis is a progressive disease and requires early pericardiectomy

34.19 Regarding percutaneous approach to pericardiocentesis, which of the following statements is FALSE?

(A) A right xiphocostal approach is associated with right atrium (RA) and inferior vena cava (IVC) injury
(B) Puncture of the left pleura and lingual is more frequent with an apical approach
(C) Puncture of the left anterior descending (LAD) coronary artery and left internal mammary artery (LIMA) is more common with the parasternal approach
(D) Left chest wall approach should not be used when performed with echo-guided procedures

34.20 Regarding percutaneous balloon pericardiotomy, which of the following is INCORRECT?

(A) Thoracocentesis is required following balloon pericardiotomy in 30% to 40% of cases
(B) Drainage of >100 mL fluid per 24 hours, 3 days after standard catheter drainage indicates the need for more definitive intervention
(C) Surgical window may be preferred if a loculated fibrinous effusion is present
(D) Reaccumulation of pericardial fluid with recurrent tamponade is considered a strong indication for performing percutaneous balloon pericardiotomy

34.21 Which of the following statements regarding pericardial effusion following cardiac surgery is FALSE?

(A) Postoperative pericardial effusion occurs in 50% to 85% of cases
(B) Cardiac tamponade occurs in 1% to 2% of patients who undergo cardiac surgery
(C) Cardiac tamponade occurs most frequently within 48 hours of surgery
(D) Nonsteroidal anti-inflammatory drugs (NSAIDs) do not reduce the risk of pericardial tamponade

34.22 Which of the following statements with regard to perforation by an implanted lead of a cardiac perforation electronic device is TRUE?

(A) The incidence is approximately <1%
(B) Late perforation is defined as perforation of the lead through the myocardium more than 1 week after implantation
(C) A fall in lead impedance is typical of lead perforation
(D) All of the above

34.23 A 77-year-old male with known coronary artery disease (CAD), prior aortic valve replacement and three-vessel bypass grafting presents with chronic stable angina. Cardiovascular risk factors include treated hypertension, diabetes, and elevated cholesterol. Based on a myocardial perfusion (MIBI) scan showing a large area of reversibility in the lateral wall, the patient was referred for a coronary angiogram. Approximately 8 hours after percutaneous coronary intervention (PCI) to a complex lesion in the left circumflex (LCx) artery, the patient complained of pleuritic chest pain, dyspnea, and became hypotensive. ECG was unchanged. All of the following are true EXCEPT:

(A) Unremarkable TTE can exclude pericardial tamponade with good confidence
(B) Coronary perforation from guidewires should be considered here
(C) CT scan can be good diagnostic aid
(D) Cardiothoracic consult is appropriate

34.24 Which of the following statement with regards to pericardial effusion in patients with systemic autoimmune disease is FALSE?

(A) The pericardium may be involved in different systemic autoimmune diseases (i.e., systemic lupus erythematosus, rheumatoid arthritis, progressive systemic sclerosis, mixed connective tissue disease, Sjögren's syndrome, polyarteritis, giant cell arteritis, and other systemic vasculitides)
(B) The pericardial involvement may occur either in a symptomatic form (usually during the active phase of the disease) or as asymptomatic pericardial effusion
(C) Pericardial effusion is a common manifestation of rheumatoid arthritis
(D) Pericarditis is frequent in patients with rheumatoid arthritis. It is usually asymptomatic, but cases of constrictive pericarditis or, more rarely, tamponade have been reported. In such cases, the study of pericardial fluid is of special interest for the etiologic diagnosis
(E) Elevated rheumatoid factor is present in rheumatoid pericardial effusion
(F) A low glucose concentration is typically present in patients with rheumatoid pericardial effusion

34.25 Which of the following is least likely to cause constrictive pericarditis?

(A) Tuberculous pericardial effusion
(B) Radiotherapy for esophageal cancer
(C) Postcardiac surgery
(D) Systemic lupus erythematosus

ANSWERS AND EXPLANATIONS

34.1 Answer B. The hemodynamic tracing depicts an elevated RV pressure with exaggerated respiratory variation consistent with pericardial tamponade. Echocardiographic evidence of right ventricular collapse lasting more than one-third of diastole is a more specific but less sensitive sign of cardiac tamponade than right atrial collapse (Singh S, et al. *Circulation* 1984;70(6):966–971). Pulsus paradoxus, which is an exaggeration of the normal respiratory variation in blood pressure and is defined as a >10-mm Hg drop in the systolic arterial pressure during inspiration, is likely to be present. In pericardial tamponade due to high intrapericardial pressures, there is loss of pressure difference between the RA and RV, hence the blunted Y descent that corresponds to the tricuspid valve opening and RA emptying. The X descent is preserved or may be exaggerated in some cases. Enhanced ventricular interdependence is also a well-described finding in pericardial tamponade.

34.2 Answer C. Constrictive pericarditis is a well-described cause of pulsus paradoxus. Pericardial tamponade in the presence of the other three conditions may occur in the absence of pulsus paradoxus. In the presence of aortic incompetence, which may accompany aortic dissection, the LV fills from the aorta during inspiration. The increase in systemic venous return during inspiration is balanced by a decrease in left-to-right shunting by a large ASD, which results in minimal change in the right ventricular volume and thereby a minimal displacement of the interventricular septum. Severe thoracic skeletal disease prevents wide changes in intrathoracic pressure (Khasnis A, et al. *J Postgrad Med* 2002;48(1):46–49).

34.3 Answer A. Left pleural effusion occurring within 24 to 48 hours of percutaneous balloon pericardiotomy is a common occurrence, which occurs in up to 50% of patients. Thoracentesis or chest tube placement is required in up to 16% of cases (Ziskind AA, et al. *J Am Coll Cardiol* 1993;21(1):1–5). When carrying out the procedure, care must be taken to advance the balloon so that it straddles the parietal pericardium (Fig. A34-3); however, its proximal end needs to be clear of the skin and subcutaneous tissue to avoid pericardiocutaneous fistula formation. Biplane fluoroscopy is recommended to confirm the position of the balloon in two planes before inflation. Two to three balloon inflations are ideally performed, resulting in complete obliteration of the waist caused by the parietal pericardium.

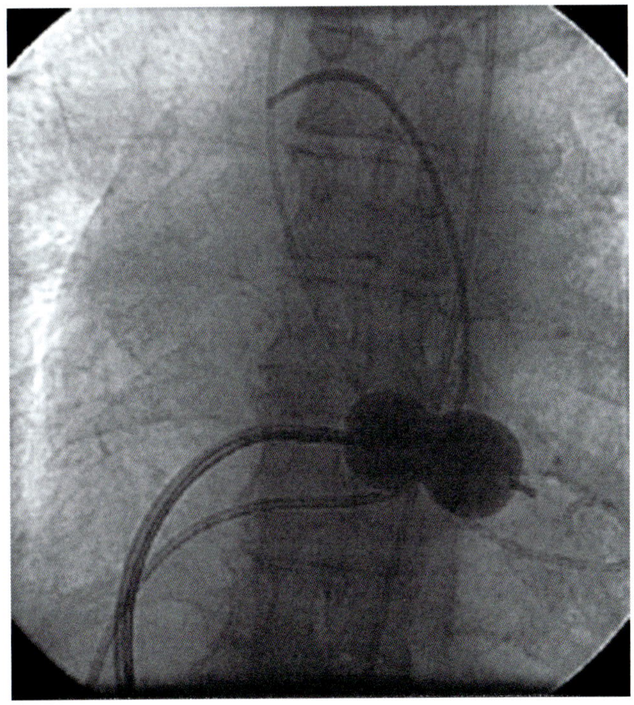

Figure A34-3

34.4 Answer D. If a large pleural effusion precedes percutaneous balloon pericardiotomy, then the chances of requiring thoracocentesis are high and procedure benefit must outweigh this risk. It is ill-advised to perform the procedure in patients with marginal pulmonary reserve, such as in those postpneumonectomy, owing to the risk of further compromise by a pleural effusion. Platelet or coagulation abnormalities are relative contraindications for the procedure because excessive bleeding from trauma to pericardial vessels may require surgical intervention (Ziskind AA, et al. *J Am Coll Cardiol* 1993;21(1):1–5). The procedure is of particular benefit in patients with recurrent malignant pericardial effusions (Palacios IF, et al. *Cathet Cardiovasc Diagn* 1991;22(4):244–249). In the presence of a pyopericardium due to bacterial or fungal infection, percutaneous balloon pericardiotomy should not be performed.

34.5 Answer D. Dynamic respiratory variation consistent with ventricular interdependence is the best hemodynamic parameter for distinguishing pericardial constriction from a restrictive cardiomyopathy. During inspiration, the right ventricular systolic pressure increases, and the left ventricular systolic pressure decreases, and the inverse occurs during expiration. This finding is >90% sensitive and specific in distinguishing the two conditions (Hurrell DG, et al. *Circulation* 1996;93(11):2007–2013). A prominent Y descent in the right atrial pressure tracing is described with constriction along with equalization of right and left heart diastolic pressures; however, these are less reliable distinguishing parameters. In the presence of a restrictive cardiomyopathy, the left ventricular end diastolic pressure generally exceeds that of the RV. Pulmonary hypertension with a pulmonary artery systolic pressure >50 mm Hg is more typical of a restrictive process (Little WC, et al. *Circulation* 2006;113(12):1622–1632).

34.6 Answer C. Major complications are reported in 1.3% to 1.6% of cases of pericardiocentesis (Maisch B, et al. *Eur Heart J* 2004;25(7):587–610). Drainage of more than 1 L of pericardial fluid at a time may be associated with right ventricular dilatation (Armstrong WF, et al. *Am Heart J* 1984;107(6):1266–1270). Pericardial catheter drainage on large idiopathic effusions is associated with lower recurrence rate than with conservative treatment (Fernandes V, et al. *Am J Cardiol* 2002;89(6):704–710). Effusions measured by CT or MRI tend to be larger than when studied by echocardiography.

34.7 Answer B. Tamponade is more common with DeBakey type II (18% to 45%) than type I (17% to 33%) or type III (6%) aortic dissections (Hausmann D, et al. *N Engl J Med* 1992;327(7):500–501). Pericardial effusions are confirmed in 17% to 45% of patients presenting with aortic dissection and in 48% at autopsy (Erbel R. *Heart* 2001;86:227–234). Pericardiocentesis is contraindicated in these patients due to the risk of further hemorrhage and extension of the dissection (Erbel R, et al. *Eur Heart J* 2001;22(18):1642–1681).

34.8 Answer B. Percutaneous balloon pericardiotomy in patients with large malignancy-related pericardial effusions is highly successful with approximately 88% freedom from recurrence at 4 months. Malignancy-related effusions are most commonly associated with lung and breast cancer. Results with immediate or deferred intervention are comparable and the procedure is associated with fever in approximately one-third of patients (Wang HJ, et al. *Chest* 2002;122(3):893–899).

34.9 Answer C. The patient has elevated right atrial and pericardial pressures. The pericardial pressure approaches right atrial pressure in expiration and thereby represents early pericardial tamponade. The X descent, which occurs after the A wave and before and after the C wave, represents systolic decline in atrial pressure. It is well preserved during cardiac tamponade unlike the Y descent. The Y descent follows the V wave (venous filling of atrium in late systole) and represents diastolic decline in atrial pressure. The Y descent is initially blunted and then obliterated as pericardial pressure rises with increasing pericardial fluid accumulation. Both pericardial and right atrial pressures fall during inspiration and increase during expiration. Right ventricular middiastolic pressures are elevated and may equal the right atrial and pericardial pressures. Ultimately, diastolic equalization of pressures occurs and interventricular dependence becomes more apparent.

34.10 Answer C. Effusive-constrictive pericarditis exists when constrictive pericardial hemodynamic findings result after a pericardial effusion is treated. Pericardial constriction results in increased ventricular interdependence and discordance between the right and the left ventricular pressures. This is the best hemodynamic parameter for distinguishing constriction from a restrictive cardiomyopathy. The right and left ventricular end diastolic pressures usually differ by <5 mm Hg and a classic dip and plateau pattern is seen in diastole. Right ventricular end systolic pressure is usually <50 mm Hg, unlike in restrictive cardiomyopathy where it can often be higher (Ignacio Inglessis, et al. *Curr Treat Options Cardiovasc Med* 1999;1:63–71).

34.11 Answer A. Pericardial constriction occurs in 30% to 50% of patients with tuberculous pericarditis. Mortality rate can be as high as 85% if untreated and the disease follows a relapsing and remitting course. Use of PCR to identify *M. tuberculosis* deoxyribonucleic acid is rapid and highly sensitive and can be performed on very limited samples. The tuberculin skin test is falsely negative in 25% to 33% of patients (Sagristà-Sauleda J, et al. *J Am Coll Cardiol* 1988;11(4):724–728).

34.12 Answer C. Pericardial thickening (>2 mm) was found to be absent in 18% of operatively proven cases of constrictive pericarditis (Talreja DR, et al.

Circulation 2003;108(15):1852-1857). The mortality rate for pericardiectomy to treat constrictive pericarditis is approximately 6% to 12% (Ling LH, et al. *Circulation* 1999;100(13):1380-1386). The images represent MRI tagging and show a normal heart on the left and an example of pericardial constriction on the right. The arrows accompanying the image on the left indicate normal pericardial sliding and those on the right indicated tethered pericardium in the presence of constriction. The ventricles on the right are classically tubular in appearance supporting the diagnosis.

34.13 Answer B. Tamponade and circulatory collapse follow right ventricular perforation in <50% of cases. Endomyocardial biopsy is complicated by right ventricular perforation in 0.3% to 5% of cases and left ventricular perforation in 0.1% to 3.3% of cases. Perforation of the RV by a pacemaker lead results in a right rather than LBBB pattern (Maisch B, et al. *Eur Heart J* 2004;25(7):587-610).

34.14 Answer C. Exaggerated respiratory variation in the right heart pressure trace is expected in the setting of pericardial tamponade. Elevated right atrial pressure, blunted Y descent, and gradual narrowing in the difference between the pericardial and the right atrial pressures are all consistent with early evidence of pericardial tamponade.

34.15 Answer C. Pericardial friction rub is caused by contact between two layers of inflamed pericardium. It typically consists of three phases during diastolic filling, corresponding to ventricular systole, early diastole, and atrial contraction. When present, pericardial rub is a pathognomonic sign of pericardial inflammation. The sensitivity of this physical finding is low since it is often evanescent and may recur and hence the need for repeated auscultation. Elevated CRP or white cell count is nonspecific. TTE early in the course of disease is usually normal.

34.16 Answer D. The differential diagnosis of the clinical syndrome consistent with right heart failure in a patient with prior malignancy should include pericardial metastasis, pulmonary embolism, and chemotherapy-induced cardiomyotoxicity. Metastatic pericardial effusion in these patients evolves gradually and presents with state of fluid overload. Reduced left ventricular preload is reflected as lower cardiac output and poor perfusion to kidneys, as often reflected by concentrated urine and modest reduction in glomerular filtration rate (GFR). Volume expansion may be appropriate for early resuscitation. Forced diuresis can be associated with further reduction in preload, declining cardiac output, and hypotension and hence is not recommended.

34.17 Answer B. Six percent of idiopathic recurrent pericarditis may be due to TRAPS (tumor necrosis factor recurrent acute pericarditis syndrome). TRAPS is caused by mutations in the TNFRSF1A gene. Patients with TRAPS report recurrent fever (1 to 3 weeks), skin rash, arthralgia, myalgia, and polyserositis with involvement of pericardium and pleura in up to 27% of subjects. Patients with TRAPS are typically poorly responsive to colchicine but are responsive to corticosteroids. A family history of pericarditis or periodic fever syndrome, poor response to colchicine, recurrence on colchicine treatment, or after the first year from the index attack are clues to possible presence of TNFRSF1A gene mutations (Cantarini L, et al. *Clin Res Cardiol* 2012;101(7):525-531).

34.18 Answer D. Traditionally, constrictive pericarditis was considered to be progressive and irreversible. Pericardiectomy is usually required to definitively relieve heart failure symptoms. A definitive diagnosis must be established before referring patients with constrictive pericarditis for pericardiectomy, since mortality is high even in the most experienced medical centers (4% to 6%). A subset of patients had been reported in the literature in whom the constrictive physiology was transient and resolved completely with medical therapy at a mean of 8 weeks. This was more often noticed in patients with constrictive physiology developing after cardiac surgery (Haley JH, et al. *J Am Coll Cardiol* 2004;43(2):271-275). Recently, late gadolinium enhancement on cardiac MRI and elevated inflammatory markers have been suggested as predictive markers for reversibility (Feng D, et al. *Circulation* 2011;124(17):1830-1837).

34.19 Answer D. Multiple approaches to pericardiocentesis can be taken and include subxiphisternal, right xiphocostal, apical, and parasternal approaches. The left chest wall approach is often favored with echo-guided pericardiocentesis. Trauma to the RA and IVC is more with right xiphocostal approach, trauma to the left pleura and lingual with the apical approach, and puncture of the LAD coronary artery and LIMA with the parasternal approach.

34.20 Answer A. Thoracocentesis is required following approximately 10% to 15% of cases of percutaneous balloon pericardiotomy. Continuous drainage of >100 mL in 24 hours, 3 days postprocedure, and reaccumulation of an effusion with tamponade both indicate the need for a more definitive percutaneous or surgical procedure. A primary surgical approach may be preferred if a loculated fibrinous effusion is present (Palacios IF, et al. *Cathet Cardiovasc Diagn* 1991;22(4):244–249).

34.21 Answer C. Pericardial effusion occurs commonly after coronary artery bypass surgery and has an incidence of 50% to 85% (Weitzman LB, et al. *Circulation* 1984;69(3):506–511). Cardiac tamponade occurs in approximately 1% to 2% of cases. It is typically insidious in onset and occurs most frequently more than a week postoperatively (Tsang TSM, et al. *Chest* 1999;116(2):322–331). Evidence would indicate that NSAIDs use neither reduces the size of the effusion nor reduces the risk of tamponade (Meurin P, et al. *Ann Intern Med* 2010;152(3):137–143).

34.22 Answer A. The incidence of cardiac perforation by an implanted lead of a cardiac implantable electronic device is <1%. Late perforation is defined as perforation of the lead through the myocardium more than 1 month after implantation. Although early perforation is more common, late perforation is increasingly recognized (Khan MN, et al. *Pacing Clin Electrophysiol* 2005;28(3):251–253). Typically, lead impedance will increase, and there may be a failure to pace and sense or an increase in the pacing threshold. Lead perforation is commonly associated with a pericardial effusion and is a recognized cause of pericardial tamponade.

34.23 Answer A. A variety of causes should be considered for chest pain and hypotension following PCI: stent thrombosis, pericardial effusion, and severe hemorrhagic shock. This patient complained of pleuritic pain, which is highly suspicious for pericardial irritation from pericardial effusion. In patients with prior cardiac surgery, adhesions are fairly common, thus limiting free spread of blood through the pericardial sac. Localized effusions are not uncommon and can still result in tamponade physiology from intense pressure on single chamber of heart (Aggarwal C, et al. *Catheter Cardiovasc Interv* 2013;82(5):770–775). TTE often fails to detect localized effusion in the posterior location, behind the LA, and in the atrioventricular (AV) grove. In situations where clinical suspicion is high, a cardiac CT with contrast can clarify diagnosis with certainty, particularly in patients with prior cardiac surgery and pericardial adhesions (Floerchinger B, et al. *J Cardiothorac Surg* 2013;8:158).

34.24 Answer C. Pericardial effusion is a rare manifestation in patients afflicted with rheumatoid arthritis. Typically, the pericardial fluid of patients with rheumatoid effusion has a low glucose concentration and elevated rheumatoid factor titer. The pericardial involvement may occur either in a symptomatic form (usually during the active phase of the disease) or as asymptomatic pericardial effusion. Pericardial involvement in rheumatoid arthritis can present as pericardial effusion with tamponade, constrictive-effusive, or constrictive disease.

34.25 Answer D. Etiology for constrictive pericarditis is varied. Tuberculosis remains the most common cause in developing countries and early treatment with antituberculous therapy and adjunctive steroids is recommended. Mediastinal radiotherapy for malignancies like esophageal cancer or lymphoma can be associated with pericardial scarring. Systemic lupus erythematosus and other autoimmune conditions are rarely associated with extensive pericardial scarring and constriction.

35 Percutaneous Alcohol Septal Ablation for Hypertrophic Cardiomyopathy and Left Atrial Appendage Closure for Prevention of Stroke

Srihari S. Naidu, Sei Iwai, and Ryan Kaple

QUESTIONS

35.1 A 43-year-old man with hypertrophic cardiomyopathy (HCM) and a resting left ventricular outflow tract (LVOT) gradient of 60 mm Hg is referred to you for consideration of alcohol septal ablation. He has dyspnea when walking rapidly up a flight of stairs or more than two blocks on level ground. His blood pressure is 140/80 mm Hg, and his heart rate is 85 beats per minute (bpm) with normal intervals. His exam is consistent with dynamic LVOT obstruction; however, there are no signs of congestive heart failure. He is taking 12.5 mg of metoprolol ER daily. You should:

(A) Arrange for left heart catheterization followed by alcohol ablation if severe coronary artery disease (CAD) is not present
(B) Increase his metoprolol to 25 mg twice daily (BID) and have him follow-up with his cardiologist for further uptitration of beta-blockers as tolerated and then reevaluate the symptoms
(C) Refer him for surgical consultation because he is too young for alcohol ablation
(D) Tell him that he should not be considered for alcohol ablation unless he develops New York Heart Association (NYHA) Class IV symptoms

35.2 A 57-year-old patient with HCM presents to your office because she is short of breath upon minimal exertion. Echocardiography demonstrates mild systolic anterior motion (SAM) of the mitral valve leaflet tips, mild mitral regurgitation, and a resting LVOT gradient of 10 mm Hg. What should you do next?

(A) Perform alcohol septal ablation
(B) Refer her for myectomy
(C) Arrange for a stress echocardiogram or other testing to evoke provocable gradient in order to determine if the LVOT gradient increases
(D) Tell her that her symptoms are unlikely related to LVOT obstruction

35.3 A 70-year-old HCM patient with resting and provokable LVOT gradients of 30 and 160 mm Hg, respectively, comes to you for alcohol septal ablation. She has NYHA functional Class IV symptoms in spite of maximal medical therapy. Her echocardiogram demonstrates normal left ventricular function, severe asymmetric left ventricular hypertrophy with an upper septal diameter of 2.0 cm, and SAM of the anterior mitral valve leaflet. The anterior mitral valve leaflet is excessively long, and there is posterior mitral valve leaflet override as a result. There is moderate to severe mitral regurgitation at rest, which is both posteriorly and centrally directed. Left heart catheterization shows mild, nonobstructive CAD. What would you recommend?

(A) Refer her for myectomy and possible repair of the mitral valve
(B) Proceed with alcohol septal ablation because you feel that her septal and valvular anatomy is ideal for this form of therapy
(C) Proceed with alcohol septal ablation because she does not have significant obstructive CAD that requires coronary artery bypass (CABG) surgery, and she is over the age of 60

35.4 Mortality following myectomy in experienced centers is higher than that following alcohol septal ablation in experienced centers.

(A) True
(B) False

35.5 Current credentialing statements and guidelines for alcohol septal ablation include each of the following, EXCEPT:

(A) An experienced operator is one who has performed over 20 successful procedures
(B) To maintain skills, an operator should perform 10 procedures per year
(C) An operator's first procedure should be proctored by an experienced operator

35.6 A 75-year-old man with HCM and severe LVOT obstruction comes to you because he wants alcohol septal ablation. He heard that it was a noninvasive procedure that will provide him with complete and immediate relief of his symptoms. He is NYHA functional Class III on maximum tolerated doses of verapamil and disopyramide, has SAM of the anterior mitral valve leaflet that is responsible for his LVOT obstruction, and has no unfavorable anatomical features to suggest that he would be better served by myectomy. How would you proceed?

(A) Schedule him for alcohol septal ablation because you feel confident that it will result in an immediate reduction in his LVOT gradient and therefore immediate resolution of his current symptoms
(B) Explain to him that while alcohol septal ablation is less invasive than myectomy, the reduction in LVOT gradient is not as complete immediately after alcohol ablation as that following myectomy. As a result, he initially may not experience a dramatic decrease in his symptoms
(C) Tell him that LVOT gradients are reduced significantly following alcohol septal ablation; however, the gradients gradually increase to preprocedure levels within a year's time

35.7 The most common conduction abnormality following percutaneous transluminal septal myocardial ablation (PTSMA) is:

(A) Complete heart block
(B) Left bundle branch block (LBBB)
(C) Right bundle branch block (RBBB)
(D) Alternating RBBB and LBBB

35.8 All of the following patients should have a temporary transvenous pacemaker placed prior to performing alcohol septal ablation, EXCEPT:

(A) Patients without preexisting conduction abnormalities on electrocardiogram (ECG)
(B) Patients in whom you feel you may need to ablate more than one septal perforator
(C) Patients with a preexisting LBBB on ECG
(D) Patients with a permanent pacemaker positioned at the apical septum

35.9 What imaging modality has become standard practice to help with identification of the most appropriate septal branch targets for alcohol septal ablation?

(A) Intracardiac echocardiography (ICE)
(B) Cardiac computed tomography (CT)
(C) Myocardial contrast echocardiography (MCE)
(D) Cardiac magnetic resonance imaging (MRI)

35.10 What step is necessary prior to instillation of alcohol into the targeted septal branch?

(A) No steps are necessary once the targeted branch is identified
(B) Iodinated contrast must be injected into the central lumen of the balloon to make sure that alcohol will only go to the intended target
(C) A second flexible guidewire must be placed into the distal left anterior descending (LAD) artery and a balloon inflated over that wire just distal to the origin of the targeted septal artery. This will prevent extravasation of alcohol into the mid and distal portions of the LAD beyond the targeted branch
(D) None of the above

35.11 Approximately 5 mL of ethanol is necessary for successful ablation of a single septal perforator.

(A) True
(B) False

35.12 Once the procedure is complete, the operator must do all of the following, EXCEPT:

(A) Place the patient in the intensive care unit for at least 48 hours
(B) Remove the temporary pacemaker wire if complete heart block did not occur during the course of the procedure
(C) Cycle cardiac biomarkers until they have peaked
(D) Review ECG and telemetry daily for the occurrence of high-grade conduction disease

35.13 What features of this hemodynamic tracing distinguish it as HCM with LVOT obstruction rather than aortic stenosis (Fig. Q35-13)?

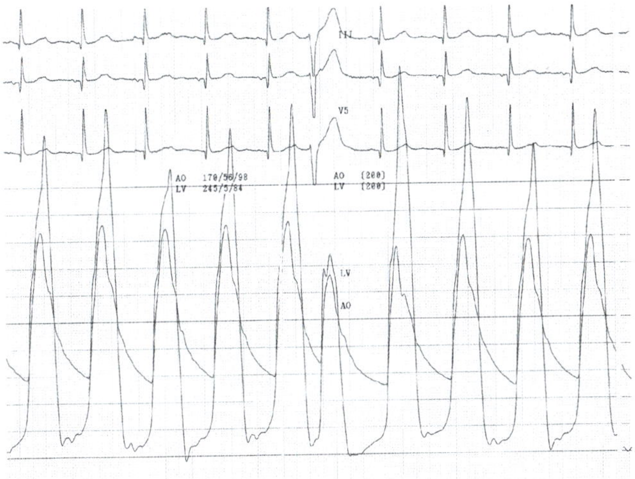

Figure Q35-13

(A) There is a decrease in aortic pulse pressure following a premature ventricular contraction
(B) There is an increase in the gradient between the left ventricle and aorta following a premature ventricular contraction
(C) There is a significant reduction in the gradient between the aorta and left ventricle in the beat of the premature ventricular contraction (PVC)
(D) (A) and (B)

35.14 A 24-year-old female with HCM and a resting LVOT gradient of 70 mm Hg comes to you for alcohol septal ablation. She is otherwise healthy and has NYHA Class III symptoms in spite of maximal medical therapy. There are no anatomic reasons to suggest that she would be better served by a myectomy. You should:

(A) Schedule her for alcohol septal ablation and explain that her risk of developing a lethal ventricular arrhythmia is equivalent to that following myectomy
(B) Schedule her for a myectomy because there is a much higher risk of developing lethal ventricular arrhythmias following alcohol septal ablation
(C) Discuss with her that we do not yet know the true risk of lethal ventricular arrhythmias following alcohol septal ablation. Long-term data about the myectomy are more robust. She is young and at a surgical center that has extensive experience and excellent outcomes following myectomy; therefore, you would recommend at this point in time that she has a myectomy
(D) Schedule her for alcohol septal ablation because the risk of lethal ventricular arrhythmias following myectomy is much higher in young patients

35.15 The following angiograms (Fig. Q35-15) were taken to document the key steps used during alcohol septal ablation in a 60-year-old patient with HCM and severe LVOT obstruction. A long 0.014-in. flexible guidewire followed by an over-the-wire balloon (2 × 10 mm) was introduced into the first major septal perforator prior to documenting the angiograms below. Before alcohol injection, the operator used MCE to confirm septal perfusion at the appropriate locations. The patient developed severe chest pain and an anterior ST elevation in multiple anterior leads following alcohol injection. Based on the information above and the angiograms below, what was the most likely cause?

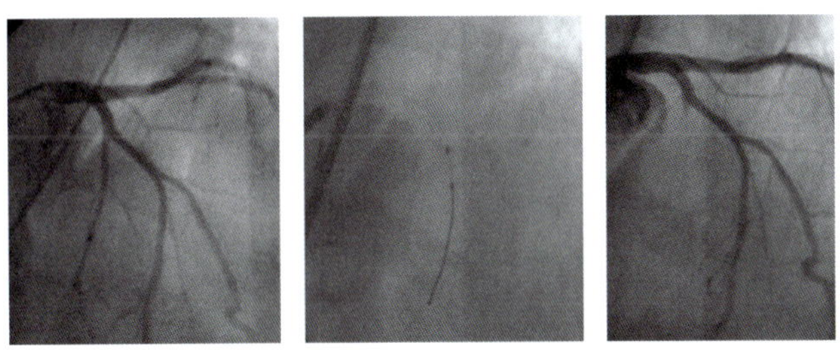
Figure Q35-15

(A) Plaque in the proximal LAD was disrupted by the guidewire during initial wiring of the septal perforator
(B) The guidewire caused dissection of the proximal LAD
(C) There was spillover of alcohol into the LAD beyond the septal perforator
(D) The septal perforator supplied portions of the anterior wall of the left ventricle

35.16 In looking at the following angiograms, which patient will likely have the best result in terms of LVOT gradient reduction following alcohol septal ablation?

(A) Figure Q35-16A

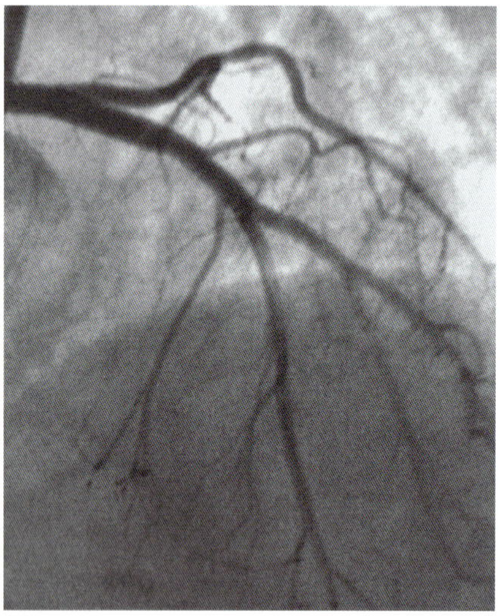

A

(B) Figure Q35-16B

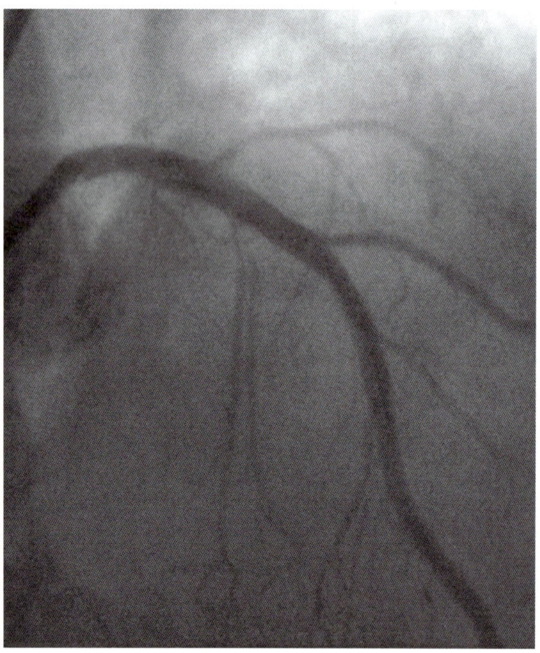

B

(C) Figure Q35-16C

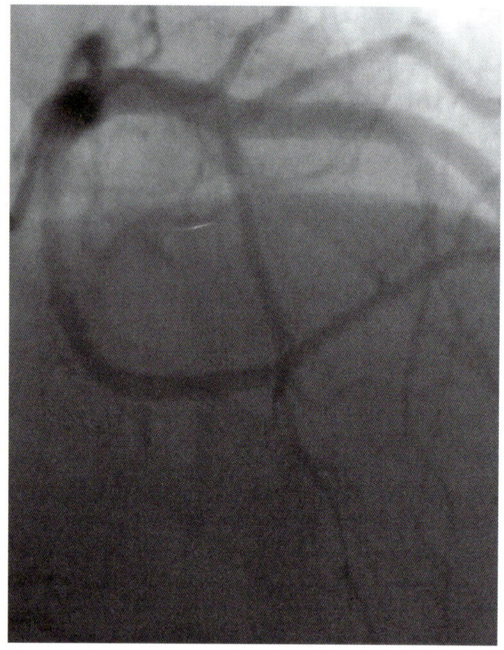

C

(D) Unable to determine

35.17 Alcohol septal ablation has surpassed myectomy as the gold standard mechanical intervention (septal reduction therapy) for treatment of HCM with LVOT gradient obstruction.

(A) True
(B) False

35.18 A combination of anatomic and hemodynamic criteria exist to suggest when the procedure is complete.

(A) True
(B) False

35.19 If a patient experiences chest pain and ST elevation in V1 and V2 during alcohol infusion, what should you do?

(A) Immediately stop the infusion of alcohol
(B) Immediately deflate the balloon
(C) Evaluate for wall motion abnormalities by echo and administer an intravenous (IV) analgesic agent like fentanyl
(D) Administer sublingual nitroglycerin

35.20 How should alcohol be administered into the central lumen of the balloon?

(A) As a rapid bolus injection
(B) At a rate of 1 mL/60 to 120 seconds
(C) At a rate of 1 mL/30 seconds
(D) At a rate of 1 mL/10 seconds

35.21 You are referred a 61-year-old patient with HCM and an LVOT gradient of 65 mm Hg. He has NYHA Class III symptoms despite optimal beta-blocker therapy. You determine that he has anatomy suitable for both alcohol septal ablation and surgical septal myectomy. After discussing the patient's options, he chooses to go forward with alcohol septal ablation. Compared to septal myectomy, this patient undergoing alcohol septal ablation is more likely to have which of the following?

(A) Improved short-term mortality
(B) Improved long-term mortality
(C) Increased risk for ventricular tachyarrhythmia
(D) Increased risk for pacemaker implantation

35.22 A patient has successful alcohol septal ablation and is transferred to the intensive care unit. He is 58 years old and has a family history of hypertrophic cardiomyopathy and a maximal wall thickness of 2.4 cm. Upon transferring from the stretcher to the bed, his eyes roll back and he is found to be in sustained ventricular tachycardia. He is successfully cardioverted and does not require intubation. Appropriate care may include each of the following, EXCEPT:

(A) Resumption of his preprocedure beta-blockers
(B) Monitoring of telemetry for recurrence
(C) Electrophysiology consultation
(D) Implantable cardioverter–defibrillator (ICD) placement

35.23 Long-term clinical benefits of alcohol septal ablation are attributed to each of the following anatomic findings, EXCEPT:

(A) Reduction in resting and/or dynamic left ventricle outflow tract gradients
(B) Reduction in mitral regurgitation
(C) Improved diastolic function
(D) Regression of left ventricular hypertrophy
(E) Improved right ventricular function

35.24 You are referred a 70-year-old male with prior lobectomy for lung cancer who has HCM and NYHA Class III heart failure symptoms despite optimal medical therapy, including beta-blockers and mild diuretics for lower extremity edema. On echocardiogram, he has a 2.1-cm septum, systolic anterior motion (SAM), a 60-mm Hg resting gradient, and mild aortic regurgitation. The most appropriate next step in management is:

(A) Cardiac catheterization to determine suitability for alcohol septal ablation
(B) Stress testing to determine if CAD is present
(C) Transesophageal echocardiogram (TEE) to determine if a subaortic membrane is present
(D) Alcohol septal ablation given his age and comorbidities

35.25 Relative contraindications to alcohol septal ablation include all of the following, EXCEPT:

(A) Age < 40
(B) Septal thickness > 30 mm
(C) Moderate to severe mitral regurgitation
(D) Midventricular obstruction

35.26 The rationale for left atrial appendage (LAA) occlusion is based on the theory that most left atrial thrombi originate from the LAA. What percentage of thrombi occur in the LAA?

(A) 60%
(B) 70%
(C) 80%
(D) >90%

35.27 Which of the following is a known complication of surgical LAA closure?

(A) LAA tear
(B) Residual communication between the appendage and the left atrium
(C) Residual stump of the appendage
(D) All of the above

35.28 A 73-year-old man has just undergone placement of a Watchman (Boston Scientific, Marlborough, MA) LAA occlusion device. TEE performed 6 weeks after device implantation shows a leak around the device with a maximum width of 2 mm. What is the appropriate antithrombotic strategy going forward?

(A) Aspirin 325 mg daily and clopidogrel 75 mg daily for 6 months, followed by aspirin indefinitely
(B) Warfarin, with a goal international normalized ratio (INR) of 2.0 to 3.0 for 45 days, followed by aspirin and clopidogrel up to 6 months, followed by aspirin indefinitely
(C) Warfarin, with a goal INR 2.0 to 3.0 for 6 months, followed by aspirin indefinitely
(D) Warfarin, with a goal INR of 1.5 to 2.0 for 6 months, followed by aspirin indefinitely

35.29 Which of the following was the most common adverse event in the device intervention arm of the PROTECT AF trial?

(A) Vascular complication
(B) Bleeding, requiring transfusion of >2 units
(C) Pericardial effusion
(D) Stroke
(E) (A) and (B)

35.30 The Centers for Medicare and Medicaid (CMS) require that all institutions in the United States performing LAA occlusion with Watchman need to participate in a national registry.

(A) True
(B) False

35.31 Which of the following are considered to be contraindications to LAA occlusion with the Watchman (Boston Scientific, Marlborough, MA) device?

(A) An inability to take therapeutic warfarin therapy
(B) The maximum LAA ostium measures <17 mm
(C) The patient has an inferior vena cava (IVC) thromboembolic filter in place
(D) Both (A) and (B)

35.32 You evaluate a 72-year-old man for potential LAA occlusion with the Watchman device (Boston Scientific, Marlborough, MA). Preprocedural TEE demonstrates a maximum LAA ostium of 22.5 mm. A 24-mm device was subsequently deployed in the LAA, and the maximum device diameter prior to detachment of the device delivery cable was 24 mm. There is a leak around the device of 6 mm in width. Which of the following statements are TRUE?

(A) The patient should have undergone LAA assessment by a CT scan with contrast to assess the size and morphology of the LAA
(B) Once positioned in the LAA, the device was able to recoil to its original diameter, which is imaging confirmation that the correct-sized device was implanted
(C) A residual leak 6 mm demonstrates an adequate seal of the LAA
(D) Both (B) and (C)
(E) The device is too small and does not adequately occlude the LAA in this patient

35.33 You are asked to evaluate an 82-year-old woman with a history of hypertension, peripheral vascular disease, and nonvalvular atrial fibrillation for LAA occlusion. Which of the statements is FALSE regarding the potential long-term benefit of LAA occlusion as compared to warfarin therapy?

(A) There is a reduced risk of hemorrhagic stroke
(B) There is a reduced risk of ischemic stroke
(C) There is a reduced risk of cardiovascular death

35.34 The LARIAT system (SentreHeart, Redwood City, CA) remains under investigation regarding its safety and efficacy when utilized to exclude LAA. Potential benefits of this device over LAA occlusive devices delivered via the transseptal approach include:

(A) Electrical isolation of the LAA tissue
(B) Anticoagulation with warfarin is not required after device implantation
(C) It has fewer procedure-related complications
(D) Both (A) and (B)

35.35 TEE is performed in this 74-year-old woman with a history of hypertension, hyperlipidemia, and prior stroke 6 weeks following implantation of the LAA occlusion device. She has been taking warfarin for the prior 6 weeks with a therapeutic INR ranging from 2 to 3. Imaging demonstrates a leak around the device of 7 mm in diameter. What is the appropriate strategy for anticoagulation going forward?

(A) Warfarin should be continued, with a goal INR 2.0 to 3.0, until subsequent imaging demonstrates the leak has decreased to ≤5 mm
(B) Aspirin 325 mg daily and clopidogrel 75 mg daily for 6 months, followed by aspirin indefinitely
(C) Warfarin, with a goal INR of 2.0 to 3.0 for 45 days, followed by aspirin and clopidogrel up to 6 months, followed by aspirin indefinitely
(D) Warfarin, with a goal INR 2.0 to 3.0 for 6 months, followed by aspirin indefinitely

35.36 A 66-year-old male with hypertension and paroxysmal atrial fibrillation diagnosed 2 years ago, but with no otherwise past medical history, had prior bleeding due to peptic ulcers treated endoscopically 4 years ago. There has been no recent bleeding. He has been on apixaban (5 mg bid) since his diagnosis but is concerned about the chance of recurrent gastrointestinal bleeding. Which of the following are reasonable options?

(A) Switch to warfarin and aim for INR of 1.5
(B) Switch back to aspirin 325 mg once daily
(C) Implant a Watchman device
(D) Continue apixaban
(E) (C) and (D)

35.37 According to pooled data from the PROTECT AF and PREVAIL trials, which of the following statements is TRUE when comparing bleeding rates of the Watchman device to warfarin therapy?

(A) The overall rate of major bleeding is similar between the two groups over 3 years of follow-up
(B) The Watchman device significantly reduced bleeding, when excluding the periprocedural period (i.e., first 7 days)
(C) (A) and (B)

35.38 In the PROTECT AF trial, which of the following statement(s) was TRUE regarding Watchman device?

(A) Patients required a CHADS2 score of at least two to be eligible for randomization
(B) Watchman was demonstrated to be superior to warfarin therapy in the primary efficacy end point (stroke, cardiovascular death, systemic embolism)
(C) There was a higher incidence of primary safety events (i.e., major bleeding, pericardial effusion, and device embolization) in the Watchman group compared to the warfarin therapy group
(D) The rate of ischemic stroke was lower in the Watchman group compared to the warfarin therapy group
(E) The Watchman device was implanted successfully in over 97% of patients in the intervention group

35.39 Which patient(s) would be an appropriate candidate for LAA occlusion with a Watchman device?

(A) 65-year-old female with diabetes mellitus, mechanical mitral valve replacement, and persistent atrial fibrillation
(B) 80-year-old male with hypertension, nonvalvular atrial fibrillation, and frequent falls
(C) 68-year-old male with CAD and paroxysmal atrial fibrillation
(D) (B) and (C)

35.40 Regarding the LARIAT system (SentreHeart, Redwood City, CA) for LAA closure, which of the following statements are FALSE?

(A) Preprocedural screening includes CT angiography to assess the LAA
(B) LARIAT has been shown to be noninferior to warfarin in terms of reduction of stroke and systemic embolism
(C) Presence of LAA thrombus is a contraindication to LARIAT procedure
(D) Prior cardiac surgery is a contraindication to LARIAT procedure
(E) (B) and (C)

ANSWERS AND EXPLANATIONS

35.1 Answer B. PTSMA for the relief of LVOT obstruction in HCM should not be considered until a patient develops drug refractory severe symptoms, defined as NYHA Class III or IV. This patient is currently NYHA functional Class II without optimal medical therapy, which makes him an inappropriate candidate for septal reduction. Uptitration of beta-blockers would be the next step in this patient with heart rate of 85 with normal intervals. This is important because drug refractory symptoms, a criteria for mechanical intervention, implies that the patient is on maximum tolerated doses of negative inotropic agents used to reduce the degree of LVOT obstruction (Kimmelstiel CD, et al. *Circulation* 2004;109(4):452–456; Maron BJ. *JAMA* 2002;287(10):1308–1320; Maron BJ, et al. *J Am Coll Cardiol* 2003;42(9):1687–1713). These medications include beta-blockers, nondihydropyridine calcium channel blockers, and in some cases, the antiarrhythmic disopyramide.

35.2 Answer C. For many years, it was felt that LVOT obstruction occurred in only 25% of the HCM population. However, recent literature and expert opinion suggests that it is much more common and occurs in up to 70% of HCM patients when both resting and provokable gradients are considered (Rozner MA, et al. *J Am Coll Cardiol* 2005;45(1):161–162). It is therefore always important to assess for provokable LVOT gradient obstruction, especially when patients report symptoms primarily on exertion. This can be done with provocative maneuvers designed to decrease preload, decrease afterload, or increase cardiac contractility. While a resting echo with Valsalva maneuver is the most typical form of provocation in the cooperative patient, amyl nitrite, which decreases afterload, can also be used with echocardiography. Stress echocardiography is helpful because changes in the degree of LVOT obstruction and mitral regurgitation at peak stress can be correlated with a patient's symptoms. Finally, invasive hemodynamics with intraprocedural provocative maneuvers, such as Valsalva and Brockenbrough, can also be performed if the diagnosis remains in doubt. Alcohol septal ablation should only be considered when there is a resting or provokable LVOT gradient of 50 mm Hg or more documented (Maron BJ. *JAMA* 2002;287(10):1308–1320).

35.3 Answer A. In spite of maximal medical therapy, 15% of HCM patients with LVOT obstruction will develop debilitating heart failure and should be considered for mechanical intervention designed to relieve outflow tract obstruction (Cohn LH, et al. *Am J Cardiol* 1992;70:657–660). Several factors must be considered in order to determine the most appropriate form of mechanical intervention. For PTSMA to be effective, the mechanism of LVOT obstruction must be SAM of the anterior mitral valve leaflet with leaflet to ventricular septal contact (Maron BJ, et al. *J Am Coll Cardiol* 2003;42(9):1687–1713). In addition, there should be no intrinsic structural abnormalities of the mitral valve and/or its apparatus, severe CAD amenable to CABG, or atypical patterns or excessive degrees of septal hypertrophy (Kimmelstiel CD, et al. *Circulation* 2004;109(4):452–456; Maron BJ, et al. *J Am Coll Cardiol* 2003;42(9):1687–1713). While this patient does have LVOT obstruction secondary to SAM of the anterior mitral valve leaflet, the leaflet is excessively long and allows for posterior mitral valve leaflet override. While this in and of itself may not be a contraindication to alcohol ablation, the centrally directed mitral regurgitation implies intrinsic abnormality of the mitral valve, which would not be responsive to alcohol ablation or myectomy alone. Thus, this patient would be better served with myectomy and valvular repair or replacement if, after myectomy, the mitral regurgitation persists.

35.4 Answer B. While mortality associated with both myectomy and alcohol septal ablation is center dependent, both are similar at experienced centers at <1% in the modern era (Maron BJ, et al. *J Am Coll Cardiol* 2015;66(11):1307–1308; Nagueh SF, et al. *J Am Coll Cardiol* 2011;58(22):2322–2328). In the real world, both mortality rates decline by tertile of increasing procedural volume, although myectomy mortality appears higher at all tertiles than alcohol septal ablation, indicating that alcohol septal ablation outcomes may be more generalizable than surgery and thereby prompting a recent push to perform both procedures only within the confines of designated high-volume HCM centers (Kim LK, et al. *JAMA Cardiol* 2016;1(3):324–332).

35.5 Answer C. A 2013 clinical competency statement included criteria for training and proficiency in alcohol septal ablation. Operators should perform the first 5 procedures under the proctorship of an experienced operator, defined as an operator who has performed at least 20 successful procedures. To maintain proficiency, an operator should perform at least 10 procedures per year (Harold JG, et al. *J Am Coll Cardiol* 2013;62(4):357–396).

35.6 Answer B. Since the start of alcohol septal ablation in 1995, several observational studies have shown that both resting and provokable gradients following the procedure are reduced immediately by more than 50%, with a majority being reduced by 90% or more (Faber L, et al. *Heart* 2000;83:326–331; Faber L, et al. *Circulation* 1999;98(22):2415–2421; Gietzen FH, et al. *Eur Heart J* 1999;20(18):1342–1354; Knight C, et al. *Circulation* 1997;95(8):2075–2081; Lakkis NM, et al. *J Am Coll Cardiol* 2000;36(3):852–855; Lakkis NM, et al. *Circulation* 1998;98(17):1750–1755; Mazur W, et al. *Circulation* 2001;103(11):1492–1496; Seggewiss H, et al. *J Thorac Cardiovasc Surg* 1999;47(2):94–100; *Lancet* 1995;346(8969):211–214). However, the decrease in LVOT gradient following myectomy is more complete and immediate than that following alcohol septal ablation (Qin JX, et al. *J Am Coll Cardiol* 2001;38(7):1994–2000). Three meta-analyses have compared outcomes in patients following alcohol septal ablation and surgical myectomy (Agarwal S, et al. *J Am Coll Cardiol* 2010;55(8):823–834; Alam M, et al. *Eur Heart J* 2009;30(9):1080–1087; Leonardi RA, et al. *Circ Cardiovasc Interv* 2010;3(2):97–104). Although short- and long-term mortality has been consistently shown to be equivalent in patients undergoing alcohol septal ablation and surgical myectomy, it does appear that in patients undergoing surgical myectomy, the reduction in LVOT gradient is more robust. The clinician must also consider the time course of LVOT obstruction as well. For patients undergoing alcohol septal ablation, infarction and remodeling of the septum require some time to mature; thus, the permanent result of the procedure is not determined until approximately 3 to 6 months (Yoerger DM, et al. *Am J Cardiol* 2006;97(10):1511–1514). Alternatively, in surgical myectomy, the LVOT obstruction is relieved immediately following the procedure.

35.7 Answer C. The most common conduction abnormality following alcohol septal ablation is RBBB. Its high incidence of approximately 60% can be explained by the location of the right bundle branch in relation to the myocardial infarction (MI) created by alcohol septal ablation (Qin JX, et al. *Am J Cardiol* 2004;93(2):171–175; Talreja DR, et al. *J Am Coll Cardiol* 2004;44(12):2329–2332). Unlike the left bundle, when the right bundle enters the muscular portion of the interventricular septum, it remains as a discrete, cord-like structure located deep within its mid-portion and does not begin to branch until it reaches the level of the papillary muscles. This is unlike the left bundle branch, which enters the muscular portion of the interventricular septum as multiple branches in a sheetlike array that are located much closer to the septum's endocardial surface throughout its anterior, mid-, and inferior portions (Talreja DR, et al. *J Am Coll Cardiol* 2004;44:2329–2332). During alcohol septal ablation, a transmural infarction is created in the mid-portion of the septum, which often contains the right bundle branch and spares the more subendocardially located left bundle branch. It is important to keep in mind, however, that individual septal perfusion patterns do vary and a variety of conduction abnormalities can occur. In contrast, in patients undergoing myectomy, LBBB is commonplace due to the subendocardial resection that occurs in all patients (Gersh BJ, et al. *J Am Coll Cardiol* 2011;58(25):2703–2738).

35.8 Answer D. A temporary pacemaker wire must be placed in the right ventricle prior to alcohol septal ablation in all patients without an apically placed permanent pacemaker or implantable defibrillator, regardless of whether there is preexisting conduction disease and/or the operator feels that it may be necessary to ablate additional septal perforators. This is because complete heart block can occur transiently in up to 50% of patients undergoing the procedure (Chang SM, et al. *J Am Coll Cardiol* 2003;42(2):296–300). Stable and reliable pacing thresholds are of utmost importance, and some operators will utilize screw-in leads for this purpose. While all patients can develop this complication, there are risk factors for its development. Pre-existing conduction disease, particularly pre-existing LBBB, appears to place patients at greatest risk (Chang SM, et al. *J Am Coll Cardiol* 2003;42(2):296–300; Qin JX, et al. *Am J Cardiol* 2004;93(2):171–175). In addition, female gender, rapid injection of ethanol, and ablation of more than one septal perforator have been associated with higher incidences of complete heart block (Chang SM, et al. *J Am Coll Cardiol* 2003;42(2):296–300).

35.9 Answer C. Prior to the use of MCE, operators determined the most appropriate septal branches by either always assuming the first perforator was the likely target or assessing the impact that temporary balloon occlusion had on the LVOT gradient. If balloon occlusion caused an acute and significant reduction in the LVOT gradient, typically ≥50%, the branch was selected if unwanted areas of myocardium were not at risk (Gietzen FH, et al. *Eur Heart J* 1999;20(18):1342–1354). MCE has now become standard to aid in selecting the most appropriate target branches. After the septal branch has been wired and a balloon placed over the wire in the septal perforator's most proximal portion, the guidewire is removed and the balloon inflated. One milliliter of an agitated angiographic contrast agent is then injected into the balloon's central lumen, and TTE images are obtained (Faber L, et al. *Circulation* 1999;98(22):2415–2421; Nagueh SF, et al. *J Am Coll Cardiol* 1998;32(1):225–229). The contrast defines the myocardial territory supplied by the branch and delineates the area of planned infarction. The branch is chosen if the area of SAM-septal contact is opacified at the area of maximal flow acceleration and remote regions of the left and right ventricle are not involved (Faber L, et al. *Circulation* 1999;98(22):2415–2421). When compared to routine probatory balloon occlusion, ablations utilizing MCE result in smaller infarcts, greater LVOT gradient reductions, faster atrioventricular (AV) nodal recovery times, more significant reductions in NYHA functional class, and reduced incidences of recurrent LVOT obstruction.

35.10 Answer B. If retrograde spillover of alcohol occurs during infusion, an MI secondary to abrupt closure of the LAD distal to the targeted branch can occur (Knight C, et al. *Circulation* 1997;95(8):2075–2081; Wigle ED, et al. *J Am Coll Cardiol* 2001;38(6):1707–1710). There is no known treatment for when this happens, and a patient may develop large anterior wall MI and/or ventricular tachycardia. This highlights the need to confirm precise balloon positioning in the proximal portion of the branch and exclude reflux of dye into the LAD through contrast injection while the balloon is inflated, prior to alcohol infusion. If reflux of contrast is seen, the balloon should be replaced with a larger diameter balloon and contrast infusion reattempted prior to alcohol infusion. In addition to retrograde spillover, antegrade contrast perfusion to distant myocardium via collateral vessels should also be ruled out prior to alcohol infusion. These can be visualized both angiographically and by way of MCE utilizing multiple views. MCE should pay particular attention to the midseptum at the point of papillary muscles, the moderator band, the RV free wall, and both the anterior and inferior walls of the LV to confirm no opacification prior to alcohol infusion. These views should be repeated during alcohol infusion to confirm lack of alcohol ablation to these distant segments in addition to confirming opacification of the basal septum at the SAM contact point (Khouzam RN, et al. *Curr Cardiol Rep* 2014;16(5):478).

35.11 Answer B. Although not uncommon in the early era, 5 mL of ethanol is excessive for alcohol ablation. There is a higher incidence of complete heart block and permanent pacemaker implantation when large volumes are used, and typically, 1 to 2 mL is adequate as long as the appropriate target septal perforator branch is chosen (Chang SM, et al. *J Am Coll Cardiol* 2003;42(2):296–300; Maron BJ, et al. *J Am Coll Cardiol* 2003;42(9):1687–1713). Current recommendations are to infuse roughly the same volume in milliliters as the thickness of the septum at the point of SAM contact point or roughly the same volume in milliliters as the diameter of the septal perforator. In the modern era, it is not uncommon to infuse as little as 0.5 mL of alcohol if the target area opacifies fully. Despite lower volumes of alcohol infusion in the modern era, clinical efficacy has remained high while safety has improved, including pacemaker rates, which are now roughly 6% to 7% (Nagueh SF, et al. *J Am Coll Cardiol* 2011;58(22):2322–2328).

35.12 Answer B. Following completion of the procedure, the temporary pacemaker wire must remain in place due to the high incidence of complete heart block that can occur during or following the procedure. Although complete heart block can occur during the procedure, the incidence has decreased with reduced amounts of alcohol and slower infusion rates in the modern era. Heart block occurring for the first time 24 to 48 hours after the procedure, although rare, can occur up to 6 days afterward (Chang SM, et al. *J Am Coll Cardiol* 2003;42(2):296–300; Faber L, et al. *Circulation* 1999;98(22):2415–2421; Lakkis NM, et al. *Circulation* 1998;98(17):1750–1755; Lakkis NM, et al. *J Am Coll Cardiol* 2000;36(3):852–855). If the patient remains free of any concerning AV conduction abnormalities for up to 48 hours, the temporary wire can be removed. Monitoring should occur in an intensive care unit for the first 48 hours, and telemetry continued for the duration of the patient's stay, usually 4 to 5 days, to detect subacute heart block. An ECG should be performed daily to track any progression of conduction disease that could require prolonged monitoring or permanent pacemaker (PPM) placement. Cardiac biomarkers should be cycled and follow a pattern similar to that seen following an acute MI, with peak creatine kinase (CK) targets of 800 to 1,500, depending on septum thickness and amount of alcohol infused.

35.13 Answer D. This hemodynamic tracing demonstrates many of the features characteristic of the dynamic LVOT obstruction that occurs with HCM. What distinguishes it from aortic stenosis, which is a fixed obstruction to left ventricular outflow, is the decrease in the aortic pulse pressure and increase in LVOT gradient in the beat following the PVC. The former is referred to as the Brockenbrough-Braunwald-Morrow sign and signifies the decreased stroke volume due to dynamic obstruction. When a PVC occurs, there is an increase in cardiac contractility and typically, although not present in this tracing, a compensatory pause that allows for an increase in left ventricular end diastolic volume. In a patient without a dynamic LVOT obstruction or in a patient with a fixed obstruction at the level of the aortic valve, the increase in contractility and increased end diastolic volume will lead to an increase in aortic pulse pressure. In HCM with LVOT obstruction, the increase in cardiac contractility following a PVC increases the degree of LVOT obstruction and the aortic pulse pressure consequently decreases while the gradient increases. This will occur even in situations where a compensatory pause allows for increased left ventricle filling.

35.14 Answer C. Alcohol septal ablation carries with it the concern that scar tissue, as a result of the infarction, may serve as a substrate for the development of lethal ventricular arrhythmias, which would be an undesirable complication in a group of patients already prone to their occurrence (Kimmelstiel CD, et al. *Circulation* 2004;109(4):452-456; Maron BJ. *JAMA* 2002;287(10):1308-1320; Maron BJ, et al. *J Am Coll Cardiol* 2003;42(9):1687-1713). Nonetheless, studies examining the risk of sudden death and ventricular tachyarrhythmia following alcohol septal ablation have shown that there is no increase in the attributable risk of sudden death (Agarwal S, et al. *J Am Coll Cardiol* 2010;55(8):823-834; Cuoco FA, et al. *J Am Coll Cardiol* 2008;52(21):1718-1723). The most recent data continue to support equipoise in long-term mortality and sudden cardiac death, although follow-up is limited in patients after alcohol septal ablation due to the fact that myectomy has been around twice as long. Accordingly, long-term data in most observational series have looked at 8 to 10 years. While these data are reassuring for middle and later age groups of patients, it may not be sufficient for children and young adults. Accordingly, guidelines recommend myectomy in healthy, young patients (Gersh BJ, et al. *J Am Coll Cardiol* 2011;58(25):2703-2738).

35.15 Answer C. While not frequently reported, MI, most commonly involving the LAD territory, can occur at sites beyond the intended septal region (Wigle ED, et al. *J Am Coll Cardiol* 2001;38(6):1707-1710). The operator in this scenario failed to ensure proper balloon positioning within the proximal portion of the septal artery and did not ensure that there was no spillover of contrast into the LAD prior to injecting alcohol. A short balloon was used, and this is important because these are easier to position solely within septal branches, which will decrease the risk of LAD dissection upon balloon inflation. Positioning of the balloon can then be confirmed by inflating the balloon within the septal branch and injecting contrast into the left main. It is also important to confirm that the diameter of the balloon is adequate to completely occlude the proximal portion of the septal branch during alcohol injection. This is done by injecting contrast into the central lumen of the balloon while it is inflated. This step, which was not performed during this procedure, will exclude the reflux of contrast into the LAD, which would necessitate upsizing the balloon diameter.

35.16 Answer D. Not only is it impossible to determine the degree of LVOT gradient reduction one will achieve with alcohol septal ablation by looking at an angiogram alone, it is impossible to determine which vessel(s) are appropriate for ablation. Individual septal perfusion patterns vary widely, as do the anatomical features related to LVOT obstruction. This is why it is important to assess the physiologic impact that temporary balloon occlusion has on the LVOT gradient, in addition to employing MCE, which will confirm that the septal artery(ies) supply the region where the mitral valve leaflets contact the septum and maximal flow acceleration occurs.

35.17 Answer B. The 2011 guidelines state that the current gold standard mechanical intervention remains surgical myectomy and gave it a Class IIa indication in acceptable surgical candidates. It involves excision of approximately 5 g of muscle from the basal anterior portion of the interventricular septum to just beyond the distal margins of the mitral valve leaflets (Gersh BJ, et al. *J Am Coll Cardiol* 2011;58(25):2703-2738; Kimmelstiel CD, et al. *Circulation* 2004;109(4):452-456; Maron BJ. *JAMA* 2002;287(10):1308-1320; Maron BJ, et al. *J Am Coll Cardiol* 2003;42(9):1687-1713). Removal of the hypertrophied tissue decreases the degree of outflow tract obstruction and frequently improves the severity of mitral regurgitation secondary to SAM. Surgical treatment also allows for concomitant correction of intrinsic mitral valve and papillary muscle abnormalities. Mortality is 0% to 3% and patients experience long-lasting symptomatic improvement that often includes an enhanced exercise capacity (Cohn LH, et al. *Am J Cardiol* 1992;70:657–660; *JAMA* 2002;287:1308–1320; Maron BJ, et al. *J Am Coll Cardiol* 2003;42(9):1687–1713; Ommen SR, et al. *J Am Coll Cardiol* 2005;46(3):470–476; ten Berg JM, et al. *Circulation* 1994;90(4):1781–1785; Woo A, et al. *Circulation* 2005;111(16):2033–2041). Alcohol septal ablation was developed as a less invasive alternative because elderly patients and those with multiple comorbidities are not always optimal candidates for surgery. The 2011 guidelines state that alcohol ablation is a Class IIa recommendation in patients who are not acceptable surgical candidates for myectomy, and a Class IIb in patients who are candidates for myectomy but who choose the minimally invasive option after a balanced discussion (Gersh BJ, et al. *J Am Coll Cardiol* 2011;58(25):2703–2738). More recently, the 2014 European Society of Cardiology (ESC) guidelines stated there is no gold standard therapy, giving both alcohol septal ablation and myectomy the same Class I indication in patients with acceptable clinical, anatomic, and hemodynamic indications for septal reduction therapy, with myectomy preferred only in those with concomitant surgical indications (Authors/Task Force Members, et al. *Eur Heart J* 2014;35(39):2733–2779). There is significant regional variation in the utilization of one therapy over the other, with myectomy and alcohol septal ablation evenly split in volumes in the United States. Alcohol septal ablation is significantly preferred throughout Europe and Asia. The differences within the United States and European guidelines may partly explain these differences.

35.18 Answer A. Although there are no absolute criteria to determine when to end the procedure, and practice patterns differ, there are anatomic and hemodynamic criteria that suggest a successful outcome. In general, success is defined hemodynamically by at least a 50% reduction in resting and/or provokable gradient, and ideally <10 to 20 mm residual gradients (Kimmelstiel C, et al. *Circulation* 2004;109:452–456; Lakkis NM, et al. *J Am Coll Cardiol* 2000;36(3):852–855). Anatomically, it is reasonable to complete the procedure when MCE shows opacification of the basal septum at the area of SAM–septal contact and maximal flow acceleration. Both criteria are utilized in all procedures, with the MCE anatomic criteria being absolutely essential, regardless of acute hemodynamic outcome. If the target myocardium is not opacified by MCE, or hemodynamic criteria are not met, additional septal perforators selected on the basis of MCE should be identified for repeat alcohol infusion, with the combined alcohol dosage remaining preferably <3 mL.

35.19 Answer C. Almost all awake patients experience chest pain during and several hours following alcohol infusion. The pain is maximal during alcohol infusion and reduces significantly as soon as infusion ceases. This typically responds to IV analgesic agents (i.e., morphine and fentanyl), not sublingual nitroglycerin. If the ECG shows ST elevation in the septal leads, as in this case, then this is consistent with the desired ablation. If, however, the EKG shows ST elevations in V3 to V6 or the lateral leads, then this would indicate alcohol spillage into the mid and distal LAD and its branches. Alcohol infusion should only be stopped if there is evidence of acute infarction in territories other than the septum. Accordingly, MCE during the procedure should evaluate the mid-distal anterior wall in the apical two-chamber view to document normal wall motion in real time. The balloon should not be deflated in response to chest pain because alcohol in the septal perforator can spill into the LAD and can cause abrupt occlusion of this vessel.

35.20 Answer B. Alcohol is not given as a rapid bolus injection as this leads to higher incidences of complete heart block (Chang SM, et al. *J Am Coll Cardiol* 2003;42(2):296–300). Indeed, bolus injection can result in complete heart block in the majority of patients. Rather, alcohol is infused into the central lumen of the balloon at a rate of 1 mL per 60 to 120 seconds (1 mL/min minimum) and the balloon should remain inflated for 5 to 10 minutes after infusion. Operators should remember that the balloon lumen can hold 0.3 mL of fluid, and thus, alcohol infusion should be chased with 0.3 mL of saline in order to assure delivery of the total desired dose of alcohol (Khouzam RN, et al. *Curr Cardiol Rep* 2014;16(5):478).

35.21 Answer D. To date, there are no randomized controlled trials comparing alcohol septal ablation and septal myectomy. One published meta-analysis (Agarwal S, et al. *J Am Coll Cardiol* 2010;55(8):823–834) examines outcomes from nonrandomized studies. In this pooled analysis, there was no statistically significant difference in short-term or long-term mortality. There has been a theoretic concern for increased ventricular tachyarrhythmia risk following alcohol septal ablation because of the scar created by infarction. To date, the studies examining this have not corroborated this hypothesis (Agarwal S, et al. *J Am Coll Cardiol* 2010;55(8):823–834; Cuoco FA, et al. *J Am Coll Cardiol* 2008;52(21):1718–1723; Noseworthy PA, et al. *Am J Cardiol* 2009;104:128–132). Similar long-term sudden cardiac death and mortality have been demonstrated in a more recent contemporary meta-analysis (Liebregts M, et al. *JACC Heart Fail* 2015;3(11):896–905). There has been an established difference in risk for postprocedural need for PPM implantation, with those undergoing alcohol septal ablation demonstrating somewhat higher rates for this complication (Agarwal S, et al. *J Am Coll Cardiol* 2010;55(8):823–834).

35.22 **Answer D.** Ventricular arrhythmias, although rare in the modern era of alcohol septal ablation, continue to occur at a rate of 1% to 2%. They are more frequent with higher doses of alcohol infusion. When they occur, the patient should be monitored more frequently on telemetry, and beta-blockers continued. Antiarrhythmic therapy is not routinely required. Although it is not unreasonable to obtain an electrophysiology consultation, placement of an implantable cardioverter–defibrillator (ICD) for ventricular arrhythmias that occur within the first 48 hours of ablation are not warranted. If the patient subsequently requires a PPM for subacute heart block, there remains no indication for ICD placement (Gersh BJ, et al. *J Am Coll Cardiol* 2011;58(25):2703–2738).

35.23 **Answer E.** Alcohol septal ablation's immediate benefit is a reduction in resting and/or provoked gradients, leading to improved stroke volume and cardiac output. In addition, the relief of obstruction decreases SAM-related mitral regurgitation, which has been shown to further improve clinical outcome and reduce left atrium pressure and size, which might reduce the incidence of atrial fibrillation, although this latter benefit has not been shown definitively. Interestingly, relief of obstruction appears to improve diastolic function and also produce a global regression of left ventricular hypertrophy not only in the basal septum but in remote regions, likely due to the unloading of the left ventricle once outflow tract obstruction is resolved. These benefits as a whole contribute to improved functional status and likely also to continued clinical benefits that evolve out to 1 to 3 years from the procedure (Gersh BJ, et al. *J Am Coll Cardiol* 2011;58(25):2703–2738; van Dockum WG, et al. *Circulation* 2005;111:2503).

35.24 **Answer C.** This patient meets clinical, hemodynamic, and anatomic indications for septal reduction therapy. He is already on beta-blockers and has evidence of congestion, which occurs late in the HCM disease process. While cardiac catheterization leading to either septal reduction therapy is appropriate, the mild aortic regurgitation should prompt TEE first in order to evaluate for subaortic membrane. Aortic regurgitation is common with subaortic membranes, which would indicate the patient requires myectomy as opposed to alcohol ablation despite his comorbidities and older age. If no membrane is found, then cardiac catheterization can be performed, and alcohol septal ablation preferred in this patient with advanced age and prior lung surgery, if acceptable septal perforators are found (Gersh BJ, et al. *J Am Coll Cardiol* 2011;58(25):2703–2738).

35.25 **Answer C.** The long-term efficacy past 10 years has not been studied, and thus, alcohol septal ablation is contraindicated in children <21 and discouraged in adults <40, according to national guidelines. In addition, the efficacy appears reduced in the setting of midventricular obstruction and/or septal thickness >30 mm, and surgery is preferred in these settings. In contrast, moderate to severe mitral regurgitation is not a contraindication if the etiology is SAM, resulting in posteriorly directed mitral regurgitation. Alcohol septal ablation in this setting should eliminate both outflow tract obstruction and mitral regurgitation in such patients. If the mitral regurgitation is centrally or anteriorly directed, then this degree of mitral regurgitation would warrant surgical myectomy and mitral repair, due to intrinsic mitral valve pathology (Gersh BJ, et al. *J Am Coll Cardiol* 2011;58(25):2703–2738; Khouzam RN, et al. *Curr Cardiol Rep* 2014;16(5):478).

35.26 **Answer D.** In one series of 229 patients with atrial fibrillation undergoing TEE, surgery was used as the gold standard for identification of LAA thrombus (Manning WJ, et al. *Ann Intern Med* 1995;123(11):817–822). In this cohort, 14 patients with LAA thrombus were identified; 13 of the 14 patients had thrombus that involved the LAA (92%). In most patients (12 of 14), the thrombus was confined completely in the appendage. A second TEE series of 272 patients with atrial fibrillation identified 19 patients with LAA thrombus, all of which were either entirely situated within the LAA or involved the LAA orifice (Leung DY, et al. *J Am Coll Cardiol* 1994;24(3):755–762).

35.27 **Answer D.** The LAAOS trial was the first randomized trial of surgical closure of the LAA in patients at risk for atrial fibrillation (Healey JS, et al. *Am Heart J* 2005;150(2):288–293). This was a small trial of 77 patients looking at early, postoperative outcomes. During the procedure, 17% of patients suffered an atrial tear; most of these were related to a stapling device and were repaired intraoperatively. Eight weeks following surgical closure, patients underwent follow-up TEE. This demonstrated that 44% of patients had inadequate closure, defined as residual blood flow into the appendage, or a >1 cm residual stump of the appendage. Failure due to ongoing communication was more common with suture-based closure, while failure associated with the stapling device was related to distal deployment of the staples and a large residual stump at the base of the appendage. An observational study performed at the Cleveland Clinic showed that up to 60% of surgical appendage closures were a failure (Kanderian AS, et al. *J Am Coll Cardiol* 2008;52(11):924–929). New surgical techniques and devices are being developed, including the AtriClip (AtriCure, Inc., West Chester, OH), which was approved for use by the U.S. Food and Drug Administration (FDA) in June 2010.

35.28 Answer B. PROTECT AF (Holmes DR, et al. *Lancet* 2009;374(9689):534–542) is the first randomized trial examining the use of the Watchman LAA occluder vs. conventional warfarin therapy in patients with a CHADS2 scores of 1 or more. Following placement of the device, patients were placed on warfarin for 45 days, at which point they were examined with TEE. If TEE demonstrated complete appendage closure or only a small peridevice leak (≤5 mm), the patient was taken off of warfarin and started on aspirin (81 to 325 mg) and Plavix 75 mg up to the 6-month follow-up. Following that, the patient was placed on aspirin 300 to 325 mg indefinitely. The safety of placing the Watchman device without postprocedural use of warfarin is unknown.

35.29 Answer C. The incidence of serious pericardial effusion, defined as the need for drainage, was 4.8% in the intervention arm of the PROTECT AF trial (Holmes DR, et al. *Lancet* 2009;374(9689): 534–542), making it the most common serious adverse event. This is related, in part, to operator experience. In the subsequent PROTECT CAP registry (Reddy VY, et al. *Circulation* 2011;123(4): 417–424), the rates of serious pericardial effusion decreased to 2.2%. Major bleeding (3.5%) and ischemic stroke (1.1%) are also listed as important adverse events. The rate of ischemic stroke is thought to be related to air embolism through the transseptal sheath. This is also thought to be related to operator experience, as subsequent registry data show a 0% incidence in 460 patients.

35.30 Answer A. The CMS requires that all institutions in the United States performing LAA occlusion (LAAO) procedures participate in the National Cardiovascular Data Registry (NCDR). This registry began in August 2016 and is designed to analyze procedural safety and device effectiveness (https://cvquality.acc.org/NCDR-Home/Registries.aspx).

35.31 Answer D. The clinical trials that led to the FDA approval of Watchman for the prevention of thromboembolic strokes due to nonvalvular atrial fibrillation include PROTECT AF and PREVAIL (Holmes DR, et al. *Lancet* 2009;374(9689):534–542; Holmes DR Jr, et al. *J Am Coll Cardiol* 2014;64(1):1–12). These studies compared Watchman implantation to long-term warfarin therapy. Therefore, this device has been approved in patients who are able to take warfarin in the perioperative period. The safety and efficacy of Watchman in patients not concurrently taking warfarin are under investigation. There are five different sizes of the Watchman device available, allowing closure of the LAA when the maximum diameter ranges from 17 to 31 mm. Patients with IVC filters can still be considered for device implantation, but care must be taken when crossing the filter with wires and sheaths.

35.32 Answer E. At the present time, CT scanning with contrast is not recommended as the primary imaging modality to size LAAO devices. TEE sizing was used in the landmark trials and appears to provide accurate measurements for sizing. In this case, the correct-sized device was chosen based on the manufacturer's guidelines (a 24-mm device is intended for LAA ostia ranging from 20 to 22.9 mm). However, when the device is positioned, there is no imaging evidence by TEE that the device is compressed. A properly sized device will expand to a diameter ranging between 80% and 92% of its original diameter when positioned in the LAA. Thus, a 24-mm device should measure between 19.2 and 22.1 mm at its maximum diameter when deployed in the LAA. Also, a residual jet of 6 mm shows there is an inadequate seal of the LAA. Any jet >3 mm at the time of device implantation demonstrates an inadequate seal. Thus, the answer is E, this device should be removed and a larger device should be implanted.

35.33 Answer B. In the long-term data from PROTECT AF (Reddy VY, et al. *JAMA* 2014;312(19): 1988–1998), reporting results after a mean follow-up time of 3.8 years, LAAO with the Watchman (Boston Scientific, Marlborough, MA) was associated with reduced rates of cardiovascular death (3.7% in the device arm vs. 9.0% in the warfarin arm, RR 0.40; 95% CI 0.23 to 0.82) and hemorrhagic stroke (0.6% in the device arm vs. 4.0% in the warfarin arm, RR 0.15; 95% CI 0.03 to 0.49). The rates of ischemic stroke were equivalent between the two groups (5.2% for the device arm, and 4.1% for the warfarin arm, RR 1.26; 95% CI 0.72 to 3.28).

35.34 Answer D. The LARIAT system utilizes both transseptal and epicardial access to deliver and tighten a snare around the LAA ostium. Successful ligation of the LAA with the LARIAT results in a permanent transmural lesion at the level of the appendage ostium. This lesion excludes the LAA from the left atrium, both anatomically and electrically. Because of the anatomic isolation of the LAA, warfarin therapy is not needed after device deployment. However, there is a higher risk of pericardial effusion related to epicardial access and trauma to the LAA and surrounding tissue (16% in a series of 154 consecutive patients (Price MJ. *Interv Cardiol Clin* 2014;3(2):301–311). There is also a risk of LAA laceration or perforation when the snare is tightened. Late pericardial effusions have been reported due to inflammation related to LAA necrosis.

35.35 Answer A. The available data on the management of anticoagulation in the setting of incomplete LAA closure are limited. Recommendations by the manufacturer of the only currently FDA-approved device, Watchman (Boston Scientific, Marlborough, MA), provide some guidance. When a residual leak >5 mm is present 6 weeks after device implantation, they recommend that warfarin therapy be continued until such time that the leak is ≤5 mm on subsequent imaging. However, analysis of the PROTECT AF study did not demonstrate an increased risk of stroke in patients with residual peridevice leak, regardless of ongoing warfarin therapy or the size of the leak (Viles-Gonzalez JF, et al. *J Am Coll Cardiol* 2012;59(10):923–929). However, the authors conclude that the low rates of events make it difficult to base therapeutic decisions from this study; ongoing investigation is required.

35.36 Answer D. There are no data to support stroke risk reduction with an INR target of 1.5. The patient described has a CHA2DS2-VASc score of 2 (hypertension and age), and thus, aspirin therapy alone would be insufficient. He has tolerated anticoagulation with apixaban (for 2 years) and thus is not unable to take long-term oral anticoagulation. This would preclude consideration for Watchman per the CMS decision memo (https://www.cms.gov/medicare-coverage-database/details/nca-decision-memo.aspx?NCAId=281) along with his CHA2DS2-VASc score of 2 (and CHADS2 score of 1).

35.37 Answer C. In a pooled, patient-level analysis of the PROTECT AF and PREVAIL trials (Price MJ, et al. *J Am Coll Cardiol Interv* 2015;8(15):1925–1932; Holmes DR Jr, et al. *J Am Coll Cardiol* 2014;64(1):1–12), there was no difference in the overall rate of major bleeding between the two groups over a median follow-up of 3.1 years. However, LAA closure significantly reduced bleeding beyond the procedural period, with the difference emerging 6 months after randomization.

35.38 Answer C. In the PROTECT AF trial (Holmes DR, et al. *Lancet* 2009;374(9689):534–542), patients were required to have at least one of the CHADS2 risk factors, not two. The Watchman device was found to be *noninferior*, but not superior, to warfarin therapy. Probability of noninferiority was >99.9%. There was, indeed, a higher incidence of primary safety events in the Watchman group compared to the warfarin therapy group (RR 1.69; 95% CI 1.01 to 3.19). The Watchman group had a *higher* incidence of ischemic stroke compared to warfarin. The Watchman was successfully implanted in 88% of patients assigned to this intervention, and in 91% of those in whom implantation was attempted.

35.39 Answer B. Patients with another indication for ongoing systemic anticoagulation (e.g., a mechanical valve) are not appropriate candidates for Watchman. In addition, the CMS decision memo (https://www.cms.gov/medicare-coverage-database/details/nca-decision-memo.aspx?NCAId=281) requires a CHADS2 score of at least 2 or a CHA2DS2-VASc score of at least 3. Patient C has a CHADS2 score of 0 and a CHA2DS2-VASc score of only 2 and thus would not be eligible. Patient B has nonvalvular atrial fibrillation with a CHADS2 score of 2 (age and hypertension) and a CHA2DS2-VASc score of 3 (age over 74 and hypertension) and is suitable for short-term warfarin but at high risk for long-term anticoagulation given his history of falls.

35.40 Answer B. In the initial clinical experience (Bartus K, et al. *J Am Coll Cardiol* 2013;62(2):108–118) and in subsequent studies, CT angiography was utilized to assess the characteristics of the LAA, including size, orientation of the LAA apex, presence and orientation LAA lobes (if more than one was present), and rotation of the heart. There have been no randomized clinical trials comparing LARIAT procedure to warfarin in terms of reduction of stroke and systemic embolism. Presence of LAA thrombus and prior cardiac surgery preclude safe deployment of the LARIAT system.

36 Chronic Stable Angina: American College of Cardiology/American Heart Association Guidelines

Karen Segerson and Stephan D. Fihn

QUESTIONS

36.1 A 63-year-old woman is evaluated in clinic for a 2-month history of dyspnea on exertion. History is notable for prior anginal symptoms and percutaneous coronary intervention (PCI) to the mid-right coronary artery (RCA) 18 months ago. She was diagnosed with diabetes 3 years ago, but has no other significant past medical history. Her blood pressure (BP) is 142/82 and ejection fraction (EF) is 55%. Her hemoglobin A1C is noted to be 8.0% and creatinine is 0.9. She is not taking any medications for management of diabetes. Which of the following is FALSE regarding her diabetes management?

(A) Therapy with rosiglitazone is contraindicated
(B) A goal hemoglobin A1C of 7% or less is reasonable
(C) An angiotensin-converting enzyme (ACE) inhibitor should be prescribed
(D) Empagliflozin should be prescribed as a first-line glucose-lowering agent

36.2 Which of the following is a FALSE statement regarding the use of angiography for the diagnosis of coronary artery disease (CAD)?

(A) Angiography may underestimate lesion severity in diffusely diseased coronary arteries
(B) There is minimal intraobserver variability in the grading of coronary artery stenosis with conventional coronary angiography
(C) Angiography remains the "gold standard" for diagnosis of CAD
(D) Intravascular ultrasound (IVUS) and optical coherence tomography (OCT) provide more precise information about the severity of stenosis and plaque morphology than does coronary angiography

36.3 Which of the following would NOT be an indication for hybrid coronary revascularization (planned combination of left internal mammary artery [LIMA]-to-left anterior descending [LAD] artery grafting and PCI of ≥1 non-LAD coronary arteries)?

(A) Limitations to traditional coronary artery bypass grafting (CABG), such as heavily calcified proximal aorta or poor target vessels
(B) Multivessel CAD and diabetes mellitus
(C) Lack of suitable graft conduits
(D) Unfavorable LAD artery for PCI

36.4 Which of the following is NOT considered a "significant coronary stenosis" when assessing clinical scenarios for clinical guidelines in stable ischemic heart disease?

(A) ≥70% mid-LAD stenosis as seen in "worst view" angiographic projection
(B) ≥50% left main stenosis as seen in "worst view" angiographic projection
(C) ≥60% bifurcation stenosis affecting both the mid-LAD and the ostium of the first diagonal branch
(D) ≥45% proximal circumflex stenosis as seen in "worst view" angiographic projection, with a fraction flow reserve (FFR) of 0.70

36.5 A 71-year-old female is referred for angiography with history of atypical chest pain, no previous medical therapy, and intermediate-risk myocardial perfusion scan (MPS). Angiography reveals 70% mid-circumflex and 65% mid-LAD stenoses. FFR of these stenoses were 0.85 and 0.75, respectively. Which statement would not be consistent with guideline support for PCI in this patient?

(A) PCI may be appropriate for two-vessel disease
(B) PCI is appropriate for symptom-based indication for single-vessel PCI
(C) PCI may be appropriate for symptom-based indication for single-vessel PCI
(D) PCI would rarely be appropriate

36.6 A 64-year-old male with diabetes mellitus, chronic obstructive pulmonary disease (COPD), and s/p two-vessel CABG remotely presents with intermediate-risk MPS and progressing stable angina despite beta-blocker therapy. Angiography demonstrates patent LIMA-proximal LAD, 75% left main stenosis, patent saphenous vein graft (SVG)-distal RCA, and minimally diseased circumflex and posterior descending artery (PDA) systems. The SYNTAX score is 25. Which of the following statements best describes revascularization appropriateness?

(A) Given redo sternotomy and intermediate complexity score, mortality benefit is expected for percutaneous intervention to left main stenosis
(B) Redo CABG is indicated given left main disease and increased PCI complexity score
(C) Left main PCI is indicated for symptom reduction
(D) Medical management is preferred and no revascularization is indicated

36.7 Which is not part of the SYNTAX score?

(A) Tortuosity
(B) Poststenotic dilatation
(C) Length of stenosis
(D) Calcification
(E) Presence thrombus/filling defect

36.8 Which statement is true regarding the SYNTAX trial?

(A) The majority of the patients deemed low complexity for PCI had single- or two-vessel disease
(B) PCI appeared to reduce mortality relative to CABG for low and intermediate complexity patients at 3 years follow-up
(C) CABG was superior to PCI for major adverse cardiac and cerebrovascular events (MACCE) at 1 year when all patient groups were included
(D) For low and intermediate complexity patients at 5 years follow-up, PCI was superior to CABG for MACCE

36.9 Which of the following statements is false regarding evaluation of stable ischemic heart disease (SIHD) in patients with prior CABG?

(A) Assessment of ischemia due to a stenosis may be complicated by the potential for competing flow from both the native and conduit vessels
(B) The FFR across an SVG stenosis could be normal if the native and collateral supply are sufficiently large
(C) The data supporting use of FFR in vein grafts and native vessels are equally well validated
(D) The presence of collaterals from long-standing native coronary occlusion may complicate the assessment of ischemia

36.10 A 40-year-old female airline pilot presents with a 2-month history of intermittent chest pain. Her symptoms arise in her left inframammary region. They can be reproduced with physical exertion but can also occur spontaneously and in the postprandial state. The symptoms do not reliably dissipate with rest. She inquires about whether she should have a coronary angiogram. Select the BEST management:

(A) Calcium channel antagonists
(B) Invasive coronary angiography
(C) Reassurance that her symptoms are not typical for angina pectoris
(D) Noninvasive risk stratification

36.11 A 74-year-old man with type II diabetes and a 3-month history of stable angina undergoes coronary angiography (Fig. Q36-11). Select the correct statement in regard to this patient's case:

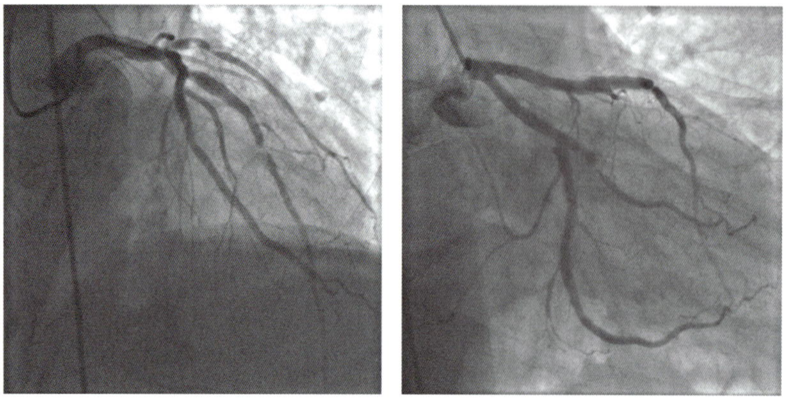

Figure Q36-11

(A) A heart team approach to revascularization is recommended
(B) An initial strategy of balloon angioplasty results in similar survival in comparison to CABG
(C) A drug-eluting stent (DES) results in superior long-term survival in comparison to bypass grafting
(D) An insulin-sensitization program is preferred over insulin provision

36.12 A 55-year-old woman is referred to your office with mild dyspnea. Six weeks ago, she suffered a myocardial infarction (MI) and did not undergo reperfusion therapy. Her referring physician had obtained a viability study with positron emission tomography (PET), and those images are shown in Figure Q36-12. The study is interpreted as showing a large area of nonviable myocardium involving the anterior, apical, septal, and inferior regions. There was also severe left ventricular and moderate right ventricular enlargement. No myocardial ischemia is found. Her EF is calculated to be 22%. Select the BEST management:

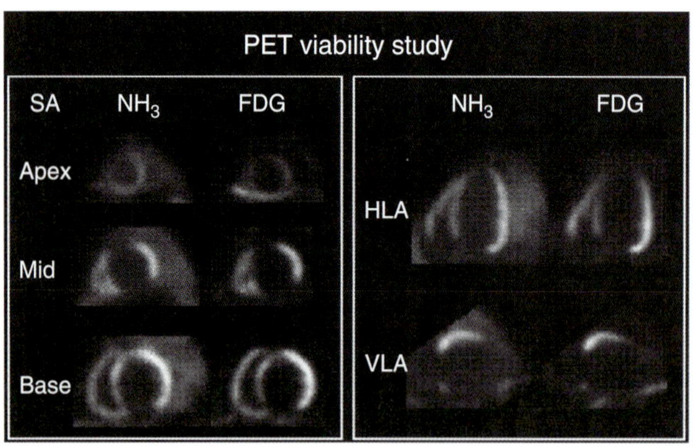

Figure Q36-12

(A) Coronary angiography and percutaneous revascularization
(B) Coronary angiography and CABG
(C) Medical therapy only
(D) Dobutamine stress echocardiogram

36.13 A 69-year-old man is referred for evaluation of chest pain. He exercises frequently, and his symptoms of angina occur near the completion of his regular three-mile run. On a treadmill study with the Bruce protocol, he exercises for 7 minutes with no electrocardiographic evidence of ischemia or precipitation of angina. The patient takes no medications. He undergoes coronary angiography (Fig. Q36-13). Select the BEST management for this patient:

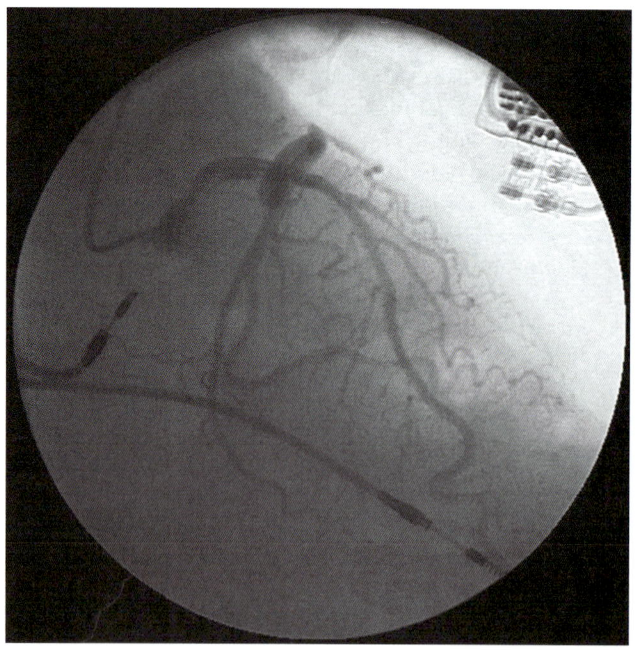

Figure Q36-13

(A) Initiation of guideline-directed medical therapy including a statin drug
(B) Referral to a cardiac surgeon
(C) PCI
(D) Stress echocardiography

36.14 A 60-year-old man is referred for angina. His symptoms began 3 months ago and progressed to where they have interfered with his job as a construction worker for the past 3 weeks. Apart from nicotine dependence, he has no other health problems. A recent echocardiogram showed his EF to be 50%. His coronary angiogram is shown in Figure Q36-14. Select the true statement in regard to this patient:

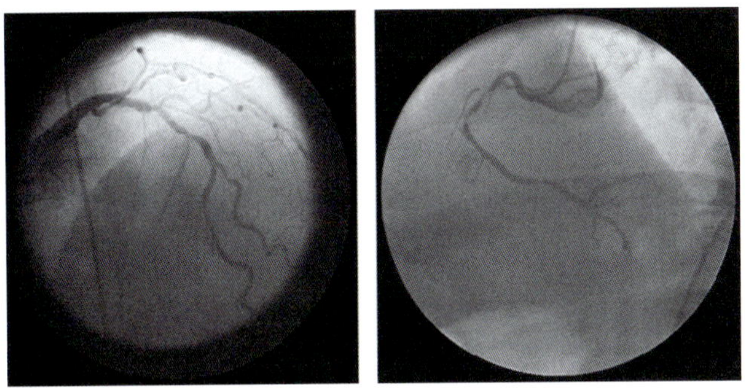

Figure Q36-14

(A) Randomized trials have shown equivalent long-term survival for CABG as compared to the initial strategy of PCI with stenting for similar patients
(B) Randomized trials of PCI vs. CABG frequently enrolled much older and severely symptomatic patients with abnormal ventricular function
(C) Balloon angioplasty alone results in reduced cumulative costs compared with an initial strategy of bypass grafting

36.15 A 78-year-old man is referred for evaluation of 3 months of progressive angina. During an exercise treadmill study, the patient developed angina with an ischemic electrocardiogram (ECG) with 2 mm horizontal ST-segment depression during stage 2 of the Bruce protocol. His comorbidities include hypertension, hyperlipidemia, and COPD, which has been stable with steroid inhalers. His coronary angiogram is shown in Figure Q36-15. Select the CORRECT statement:

(A) CABG is the preferred mode of revascularization in patients with significant left main disease
(B) The absence of distal left main disease indicates that the outcomes after revascularization with PCI or CABG would be comparable

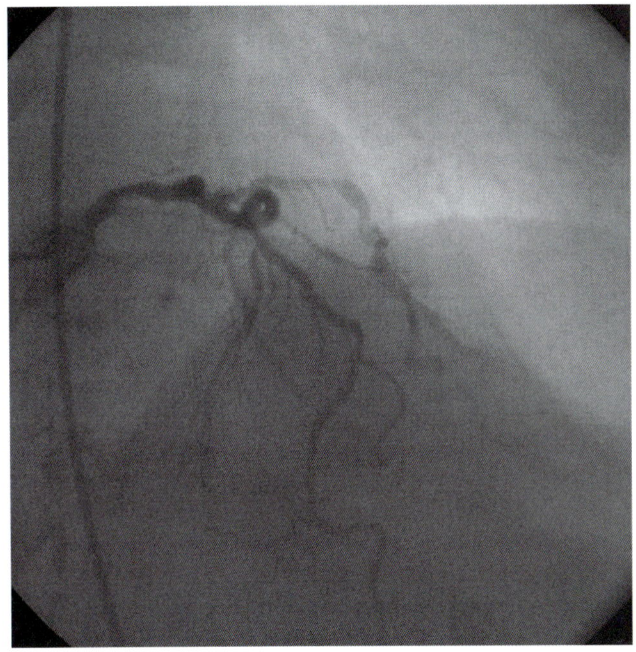

Figure Q36-15

(C) PCI is contraindicated
(D) IVUS or FFR should be performed to determine the need for revascularization

36.16 Which of the following is a TRUE statement with regard to periprocedural rise in cardiac biomarkers among patients undergoing elective PCI?

(A) Positive linear relationship exists between the risk of cardiac mortality and peak creatinine kinase (or CK-MB) for intermediate (1.5 to 3.0 times normal) and higher (>3 times normal) levels of rise
(B) A positive linear relationship exists between the risk of cardiac mortality and elevation of troponin isoforms (I or T) at intermediate levels of elevation (<5 times normal)
(C) Elevation of troponin isoforms is common and not of prognostic value
(D) In comparisons of CABG to PCI, studies have utilized the same levels of cardiac biomarker rise in defining the rates of periprocedural MI for both procedures

36.17 A 57-year-old man is referred for angina. His symptoms began 2 months ago when he was shoveling heavy snow. He is able to clear his driveway without stopping, but he is worried that he could "drop dead." On a treadmill exercise study with the Bruce protocol, he exercised for 12 minutes and developed 1 mm horizontal ST-segment depression without chest pain. His only medication is atenolol, which he takes for hypertension. His angiogram is shown in Figure Q36-17. Which of the following would not be appropriate management?

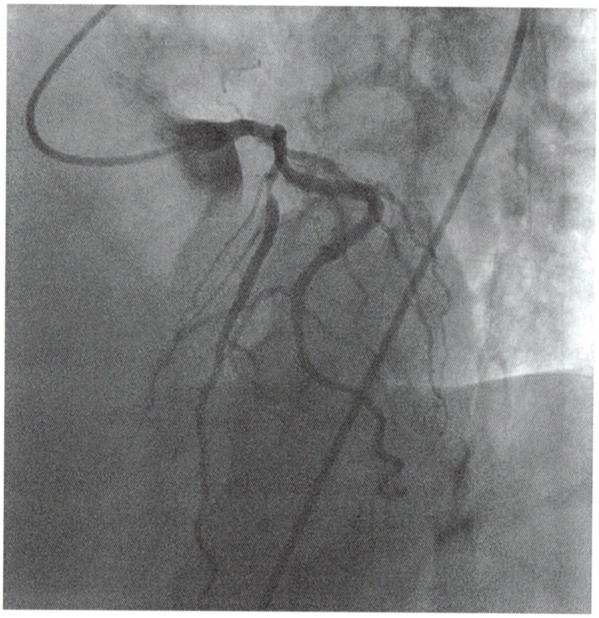

Figure Q36-17

(A) Intensification of medical therapy and lifestyle modification
(B) Bypass surgery with placement of an internal mammary graft to his LAD artery
(C) Percutaneous coronary revascularization
(D) External extracorporeal counterpulsation

36.18 A 45-year-old male executive undergoes a treadmill study with nuclear perfusion imaging as part of an annual exam. He recently began exercising for health maintenance and has no cardiovascular symptoms. He exercises for 4 minutes and develops 1.5-mm horizontal ST-segment depression that returns to normal after 5 minutes of recovery. He has no chest pain during the study. His nuclear imaging demonstrates impaired coronary flow reserve in the anterior and anterolateral walls of his left ventricle with mild dilatation on the poststress images. Select the BEST management:

(A) Medical therapy alone with additional primary prevention measures
(B) Stress echocardiography
(C) Coronary angiography and revascularization warranted by anatomic findings
(D) Cardiac MRI with gadolinium for delayed hyperenhancement

36.19 Which of the following is an indication for invasive coronary angiography?

(A) A 67-year-old asymptomatic man with a prior history of bypass grafting, mildly positive stress test, and metastatic lung adenocarcinoma
(B) A 42-year-old woman who desires a definitive diagnosis of CAD in the presence of noncardiac chest pain
(C) A 55-year-old man who was successfully resuscitated from ventricular fibrillation
(D) A 74-year-old asymptomatic woman with hypertension, hyperlipidemia, and peripheral vascular disease

36.20 A 56-year-old woman returns 6 months after having elective PCI of a proximal left circumflex (LCx) lesion. She had entered a cardiovascular health program near her home after the procedure and reports no symptoms with good functional capacity. Before the intervention, she had inquired about the possibility of restenosis during follow-up. She now wants to have a stress test to evaluate the status of the intervention. Select the BEST next step:

(A) Exercise ECG
(B) Stress echocardiography
(C) Invasive coronary angiography
(D) Cardiac computed tomography angiogram
(E) Reassurance

36.21 Which of the following is a TRUE statement?

(A) Approximately 40% of SVGs become occluded within 1 year after surgery
(B) Perioperative and long-term treatment with platelet inhibitors does not significantly improve the patency rate of SVGs
(C) Use of the internal thoracic artery in place of a saphenous vein significantly improves long-term graft patency
(D) Aggressive lipid-lowering therapy does not significantly decrease vein graft atherosclerosis

36.22 A 66-year-old man recently underwent successful balloon angioplasty of a mid-LAD lesion after having a 2-month history of severe angina. His past medical history consisted of hyperlipidemia, but there was no history of diabetes or heart failure. Currently he is asymptomatic with an excellent functional capacity. The physical examination is normal. He undergoes electrocardiography (Fig. Q36-22). Select the most appropriate method for evaluating left ventricular function:

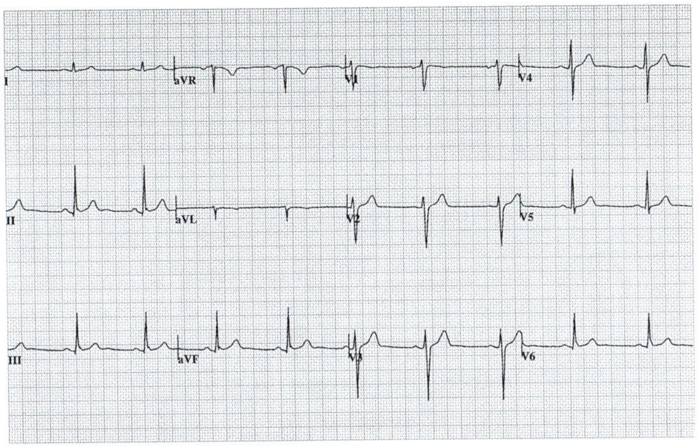

Figure Q36-22

(A) Transthoracic echocardiography (TTE)
(B) Radionuclide angiography
(C) Cardiac magnetic resonance imaging (MRI) with gadolinium hyperenhancement
(D) Left ventriculography
(E) No further evaluation

36.23 A 72-year-old asymptomatic man presents for a second opinion regarding his CAD. As part of a general medical evaluation, he performed a treadmill study with the Bruce protocol where he exercised for 11 minutes. His ECG became positive for ischemia at 10 minutes of exercise with 1 mm, horizontal ST-segment depression. There was no accompanying chest pain. The patient subsequently underwent coronary angiography (Fig. Q36-23). He was advised to undergo PCI of this lesion but was reluctant because he felt that the interventionalist was being "pushy." Select the CORRECT statement:

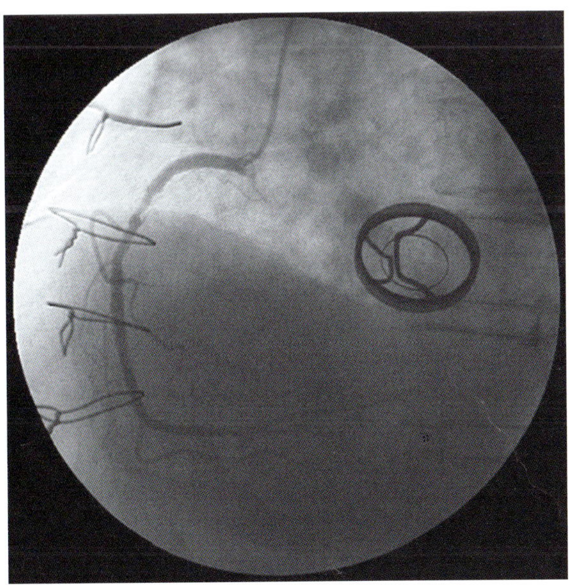

Figure Q36-23

(A) Revascularization of this lesion will reduce the risk of nonfatal infarction
(B) Surgery is preferred due to the complexity of the lesion
(C) Intensive medical therapy will result in similar long-term outcome compared to PCI

36.24 Which of the following findings on noninvasive testing is consistent with a high rate of annual cardiovascular events (>3% per year)?

(A) Left ventricular ejection fraction (LVEF) < 35% not readily explained by noncoronary causes
(B) Single moderate-sized, lateral wall defect on stress thallium imaging
(C) New apical and inferior hypokinesis occurring at a heart rate of 130 beats per minute (bpm) during dobutamine echocardiography
(D) A Duke treadmill score of −8

36.25 A 43-year-old man is referred for coronary angiography. He recently underwent an exercise echocardiogram. During exercise, he had developed mild pain in his right lower chest after 8 minutes of exercise on the Bruce protocol. Both the exercise ECG and stress echocardiographic images showed no evidence of ischemia. The exercise test is interpreted as equivocal, and he undergoes angiography. This demonstrates a 40% left main lesion. Using IVUS, the minimal lumen area is determined to 8.9 mm^2. Select the BEST management:

(A) CABG
(B) Balloon angioplasty only
(C) PCI with DES
(D) Reassurance and no revascularization

36.26 Which of the following is a FALSE statement concerning the randomized trials of CABG vs. medical therapy?

(A) The majority of patients had severe symptoms and left ventricular dysfunction
(B) The survival advantage of the patients initially treated with surgery persisted to 10 postoperative years
(C) There was a 40% crossover rate to surgery by the medical therapy patients during follow-up
(D) The benefit of surgery was greater in high-risk patients

36.27 A 58-year-old healthy man is referred for treatment of his CAD. The patient states that he exercises regularly and reports no cardiovascular symptoms. He has a remote history of smoking but no other comorbidities. As part of a general medical evaluation, he underwent a CT scan of his chest, which suggested significant coronary atherosclerosis. Subsequently, an angiogram demonstrates a 50% lesion in the distal left main with good distal targets. IVUS of the left main lesion demonstrates the minimal lumen area to be 5.0 mm^2. Select the BEST management:

(A) CABG
(B) PCI with DES
(C) Stress echocardiography
(D) Medical therapy only

36.28 A 62-year-old woman is referred with a 3-month history of worsening angina. Two years ago, she underwent PCI of a diagonal lesion with placement of a 3.0 × 13 mm sirolimus-eluting stent (SES). Presently, walking a distance of 15 feet from her front door to the mailbox reliably precipitates her symptoms, but there are no unstable features. She has been faithfully taking her previously prescribed medications, including metoprolol (75 mg twice daily), isosorbide dinitrate (40 mg twice daily), aspirin (81 mg daily), atorvastatin (20 mg daily), and clopidogrel (75 mg daily). Which of the following would be the appropriate next step?

(A) Treadmill study
(B) Stress radionuclide imaging
(C) Stress echocardiography
(D) Coronary angiography
(E) B, C, or D

36.29 A 77-year-old man with a 4-year history of stable angina is admitted to your hospital with dyspnea. On examination, crackles are auscultated in the lower halves of both lung fields. The first heart sound is slightly diminished, and a third heart sound is heard. His chest x-ray shows a cardiothoracic ratio of 0.6 with mild bilateral pulmonary infiltrates. Select the most appropriate next step:

(A) Intravenous (IV) diuresis
(B) IV diuresis and ACE inhibitor therapy
(C) IV diuresis, ACE inhibitor therapy, and coronary angiography

36.30 A 60-year-old woman undergoes placement of a 3.0 × 23 mm everolimus-eluting stent (EES) in her mid-RCA. She had received 300 mg clopidogrel and aspirin prior to the procedure. There are no postprocedural complications. Which of the following is indicated (more than one answer may be correct)?

(A) Clopidogrel (75 mg daily) and aspirin (81 to 325 mg daily)
(B) Oral hormone replacement therapy
(C) Vitamin E (400 IU daily)
(D) Lipid-lowering therapy with a statin
(E) A and D

ANSWERS AND EXPLANATIONS

36.1 Answer D. Therapy with rosiglitazone should not be initiated in patients with SIHD (Level of Evidence: C). In patients with a short duration of diabetes mellitus and a long life expectancy, a goal A1C of 7% or less is reasonable (Level of Evidence B). The HOPE and EUROPA studies showed that high-risk patients with SIHD who have diabetes mellitus should be prescribed an ACE inhibitor (Yusuf S, et al. *N Engl J Med* 2000;342(3):145-153; Fox KM. *Lancet* 2003;362(9386):782-788). This patient is hypertensive and treatment with an ACE inhibitor is recommended (Level of Evidence A). Although empagliflozin has been demonstrated to reduce blood pressure, hyperglycemia, and major adverse cardiac events (MACE), it is not considered to be a first-line treatment for hyperglycemia (Loke YK, et al. BMJ 2011;342:d1309; Woodcock J. Center for Drug Evaluation and Research. *Decision on continued marketing of rosiglitazone (Avandia, Avandamet, Avandaryl)* [Report NDA 021071]. 2010; The Diabetes Control and Complications Trial Research Group. *N Engl J Med* 1993;329(14):977-986; UK Prospective Diabetes Study Group. *Lancet* 1998; 352(9131):837-853; Patel A, et al. *N Engl J Med* 2008;358(24):2560-2572; Braunwald E, et al. *N Engl J Med* 2004;351(20):2058-2068; Zinman B, et al. *N Engl J Med* 2015;373(22):2117-2128; Dormandy JA, et al. *Lancet* 2005;366(9493):1279-1289; UKPDS Study Group. *Lancet* 1998;352(9131):854-865).

36.2 Answer B. Studies have documented significant intraobserver variability in grading of coronary artery stenosis (Zir LM, et al. *Circulation* 1976;53(4):627-632). Lack of a normal reference segment may lead to underestimation of lesion severity as angiography assessment of stenosis severity relies on comparison to an adjacent, nondiseased reference segment. IVUS and OCT provide more precise information about the severity of stenosis and plaque morphology than angiography. Nonetheless, coronary angiography remains the "gold standard" for diagnosis of CAD (Leape LL, et al. *Am Heart J* 2000;139(1 Pt 1):106-113; Fleming RM, et al. *J Am Coll Cardiol* 1991;18(4):945-951).

36.3 Answer B. Limitations to traditional CABG, lack of suitable graft conduits, and an unfavorable LAD artery for PCI are all Class IIa indications for hybrid coronary revascularization. Hybrid revascularization may also be considered in an attempt to improve the overall risk-benefit ratio of the procedures (Class IIb indication). While hybrid revascularization could be considered in a patient with multivessel CAD and diabetes mellitus for the reasons mentioned above, these conditions alone are not indications for hybrid revascularization (Bonatti J, et al. *Cardiology* 2008;110(2):92-95; Gilard M, et al. *Cardiology* 2007;108(4):363-367; Holzhey DM, et al. *Ann Thorac Surg* 2008;86(6):1856-1860; Kon ZN, et al. *J Thorac Cardiovasc Surg* 2008;135(2):367-375; Reicher B, et al. *Am Heart J* 2008;155(4):661-667; Vassiliades TA Jr, et al. *J Thorac Cardiovasc Surg* 2006;131(5):956-962; Zhao DX, et al. *J Am Coll Cardiol* 2009;53(3):232-241; *Circulation* 1997;96(6):1761-1769; Hoffman SN, et al. *J Am Coll Cardiol* 2003;41(8):1293-1304; Serruys PW, et al. *N Engl J Med* 2009;360(10):961-972; Farkouh ME, et al. *N Engl J Med* 2012;367(25):2375-2384; Hannan EL, et al. *N Engl J Med* 2005;352(21):2174-2183; Hlatky MA, et al. *Lancet* 2009;373(9670):1190-1197; Kapur A, et al. *J Am Coll Cardiol* 2010;55(5):432-440).

36.4 Answer C. The phrase "significant clinical stenosis" is used throughout SIHD guidelines in various clinical scenarios. When assessed in the "worst view" angiographic projection, left main stenoses are considered significant if ≥50% luminal diameter narrowing, and in all other locations, stenoses are significant if ≥70%. Intermediate lesions from 40% to 70% are deemed significant with FFR ≤ 0.80. Bifurcation or sequential lesions ≤70% are not considered significant without further functional information (Fihn SD, et al. *J Am Coll Cardiol* 2012;60(24):e44-e164; Patel MR, et al. *J Am Coll Cardiol* 2017;69(17):2212-2241).

36.5 Answer A. The LAD lesion is intermediate by fluoroscopy, but FFR reveals this stenosis is, in fact, functionally significant. This anatomy describes two-vessel disease, but without left-main or proximal LAD disease (Fihn SD, et al. *J Am Coll Cardiol* 2012;60(24):e44-e164; Patel MR, et al. *J Am Coll Cardiol* 2017;69(17):2212-2241).

36.6 Answer C. With *unprotected* left main disease, there is mortality benefit from revascularization, and evidence for improved mortality with PCI relative to CABG for unprotected left main disease when there is low or intermediate predicted complexity (SYNTAX < 33) and increased surgical risk (STS > 2% mortality). However, the anatomy here describes *protected* left main disease, where the mortality benefit would be attenuated. As for single-vessel proximal circumflex vessel disease, PCI is indicated to improve symptoms (Morice MC, et al. *Circulation* 2010;21(24):2645–2653; Chakravarty T, et al. *Am J Cardiol* 2011;107(3):360–366; Kim YH, et al. *J Am Coll Cardiol Interv* 2010;3(6):612–623; Buszman PE, et al. *J Am Coll Cardiol* 2008;51(5):538–545; Capodanno D, et al. *J Am Coll Cardiol Interv* 2011;4(3):287–297; Hannan EL, et al. *N Engl J Med* 2008;358(4):331–341; Ellis SG, et al. *Circulation* 1997;96(11):3867–3872; Biondi-Zoccai CG, et al. *Am Heart J* 2008;155(2):274–283; Boudriot E, et al. *J Am Coll Cardiol* 2011;57(5):538–545; Brener SJ, et al. *Am J Cardiol* 2008;101(2):169–172; Chieffo A, et al. *J Am Coll Cardiol Interv* 2010;3(6):595–560; Chieffo A, et al. *Circulation* 2006;113(21):2542–2547; Lee MS, et al. *J Am Coll Cardiol* 2006;47(4):864–870; Makikallio TH, et al. *Ann Med* 2008;40(6):437–443; Naik H, et al. *J Am Coll Cardiol Interv* 2009;2(8):739–747; Palmerini T, et al. *Am J Cardiol* 2006;98(1):54–59; Park DW, et al. *J Am Coll Cardiol* 2010;56(2):117–124; Rodes-Cabau J, et al. *Circulation* 2008;118(23):2374–2381; Sanmartin M, et al. *Am J Cardiol* 2007;100(6):970–973; Seung KB, et al. *N Engl J Med* 2008;358(17):1781–1792; White A, et al. *J Am Coll Cardiol Card Interv* 2008;1(3):236–245; Kappetein AP, et al. *Eur Heart J* 2011;32(17):2125–2134; Park SJ, et al. *N Engl J Med* 2011;364(18):1718–1727; Gurfinkel EP, et al. *Int J Cardiol* 2007;119(1):65–72; Subramanian S, et al. *Ann Thorac Surg* 2009;87(5):1392–1398).

36.7 Answer B. All others are comprised in the SYNTAX score (Morice MC, et al. *Circulation* 2010;121(24):2645–2653).

36.8 Answer B. All patients had left main disease. Low complexity scores tend to be seen with isolated left main or adjunctive single vessel disease. Patients with adjunctive two-vessel disease were associated with moderate complexity scores. MACCE (composite of death, stroke, MI, or repeat revascularization) was equivalent across all groups at 1 year. Despite suggestion of improved mortality for PCI in low- and intermediate-risk patients at 3 years, a benefit in MACCE was not demonstrated in 5-year data (Morice MC, et al. *Circulation* 2010;121(24):2645–2653; Mohr FW, et al. *Lancet* 2013;381(9867):629–638).

36.9 Answer C. FFR measurements are well validated in native vessels, but data on the use of FFR in vein grafts are limited (Patel MR, et al. *J Am Coll Cardiol* 2017;69(17):2212–2241; Aqel R, et al. *Catheter Cardiovasc Interv* 2008;72(4):479–485).

36.10 Answer D. The patient's symptoms do not meet criteria for typical angina, and thus, noninvasive stress testing may be considered as the next appropriate step. The patient's symptoms would be characterized as nonanginal pain. Given her age and gender, the Diamond and Forrester pretest probability of CAD is very low. Therefore, exercise ECG would be the recommended study (Wolk MJ, et al. *J Am Coll Cardiol* 2014;63(4):380–406; Fihn SD, et al. *J Am Coll Cardiol* 2012;60(24):e44–e164; Fihn SD, et al. *J Am Coll Cardiol* 2014;64(18):1929–1949).

36.11 Answer A. The randomized Bypass vs. Angioplasty Revascularization Investigation (BARI) study demonstrated equivalent long-term survival for angioplasty or bypass grafting among patients with multivessel disease (Bypass Angioplasty Revascularization Investigation (BARI) Investigators. *N Engl J Med* 1996;335(4):217–225). However, superior survival was observed in diabetic patients who received an internal mammary graft to their LAD artery. Several additional studies have supported the American College of Cardiology (ACC) and American Heart Association (AHA) guideline recommendation that CABG generally is preferred over balloon angioplasty or PCI for diabetics with multivessel disease for which revascularization is likely to improve survival (Class I recommendation). The efficacy of DES vs. bypass grafting in diabetic patients is the subject of ongoing investigation as therapeutic options advance. The CARDia, SYNTAX, and FREEDOM trials (Kapur A, et al. *J Am Coll Cardiol* 2010;55(5):432–440; Groot MW, et al. *Herz* 2012;37(3):281–286; Kappetein AP, et al. *Eur J Cardiothorac Surg* 2013;43(5):1006–1013; Farkough ME, et al. *N Engl J Med* 2012;367(25):2375–2384) suggest that CABG is superior to PCI in patients with diabetes. Other studies have had a mixed picture, but no studies have demonstrated long-term mortality benefit with PCI (Hlatky MA, et al. *Lancet* 2009;373(9670):1190–1197; Alserius T, et al. *J Thorac Cardiovasc Surg* 2009;138(5):1115–1122; Hillis LD, et al. *Circulation* 2011;124(23):2610–2642; Serruys PW, et al. *N Engl J Med* 2009;360(10):961–972; Daemen J, et al. *Circulation* 2008;118(11):1146–1154; Verma S, et al. *Lancet Diabetes Endocrinol* 2013;1(4):317–328; Bangalore S, et al. *N Engl J Med* 2015; 372(13):1213–1222; Bangalore S, et al. *Circ Cardiovasc Interv* 2015;8(7):e002626; Fihn, SD, et al. *J Am Coll Cardiol* 2014;64(18):1929–1949).

36.12 **Answer C.** The patient is unlikely to derive clinical benefit from revascularization due to the large areas of nonviable myocardium in the absence of ischemia. There are limited studies on the use of viability data in determining appropriateness for revascularization. In the OAT study, where 91% of patients with occluded arteries had mild or no ischemia 3 to 28 hours after infarction, there was no benefit of percutaneous revascularization over medical therapy. A meta-analysis demonstrated that patients with viable myocardium had better clinical outcomes when revascularized, while patients with nonviable myocardium had superior outcomes when not revascularized (Patel MR, et al. *J Am Coll Cardiol* 2017;69(17):2212–2241; Patel MR, et al. *J Am Coll Cardiol* 2012;59(22):1995–2027; Allman KC, et al. *J Am Coll Cardiol* 2002;39(7):1151–1158).

36.13 **Answer A.** Revascularization is harmful in patients with one-vessel disease without proximal LAD involvement (ACC/AHA Class III) and of uncertain benefit for patients with two-vessel disease without proximal LAD involvement or extensive ischemia (ACC/AHA Class IIb). It would not be indicated in a patient who has not received an adequate trial of medical therapy and has no demonstrable evidence of ischemia. Guideline directed medical therapy with a statin would be appropriate (Patel MR, et al. *J Am Coll Cardiol* 2017;69(17):2212–2241).

36.14 **Answer A.** Equivalent long-term survival has been observed in randomized trials of stenting or CABG in patients with multivessel disease and low-risk anatomy. Patients enrolled in such randomized trials characteristically were relatively young (age 60 years), and most frequently had two-vessel disease, preserved ventricular function, and stable symptoms, although some studies enrolled patients with unstable angina. A cost-effectiveness analysis of the BARI trial demonstrated cost-effectiveness of CABG compared to angioplasty, principally due to the need for repeat procedures in the angioplasty group (Hlatky MA, et al. *N Engl J Med* 1997;336(2):92–99). The FREEDOM and SYNTAX trials (Magnuson EA, et al. *Circulation* 2013;12(7):820–831; Cohen DJ, et al. *Catheter Cardiovasc Interv* 2012;79(2):198–209) similarly demonstrated long-term cost-effectiveness of CABG in this population.

36.15 **Answer A.** The left main lesion is approachable by PCI because of its distance from the bifurcation of the LAD and circumflex. The current guidelines favor CABG over PCI in patients who are suitable for surgery (Patel MR, et al. *J Am Coll Cardiol* 2017;69(17):2212–2241). In the SYNTAX study (Mohr FW, et al. *Lancet* 2013;381(867):629–638), complexity of disease, with or without distal left main involvement, was a major determinant of outcome in comparing CABG to PCI. The ACC/AHA guidelines upgraded the recommendation for revascularization of left main disease with PCI from a Class III to Class IIb when anatomy is suitable and clinical characteristics predict an increased risk of adverse surgical outcomes. This patient does not have clinical characteristics predicting increased operative mortality. Further assessment with IVUS or FFR would only be indicated in the presence of equivocal angiographic findings (Morice MC, et al. *Circulation* 2010;21(24):2645–2653; Buszman PE, et al. *JACC Cardiovasc Interv* 2016;9(4):318–327).

36.16 **Answer A.** A linear relationship between adverse outcomes and all levels of creatine kinase (CK) rise has been demonstrated, but not for mild elevations of troponin isoforms. However, marked troponin elevations (>5 times normal) have been associated with increased mortality. In comparison studies, definitions of periprocedural infarction typically use higher levels of biomarker rise (5 to 10 times normal) for CABG procedures than for PCI (Pervaiz MH, et al. *Circ Cardiovasc Interv* 2012;5:150–156).

36.17 **Answer D.** The MASS study demonstrated comparable survival for patients with LAD disease, irrespective of whether they received medical therapy, PCI, or CABG. However, revascularization was associated with superior relief of angina and reduced need for antianginal medications. The COURAGE study (Sedlis SP, et al. *N Engl J Med* 2015;373(20):1937–1946) showed comparable outcomes for PCI vs. intense medical therapy in stable patients over 15 years of follow-up. The patient's symptoms are mild. In addition, the Duke treadmill score is +7, which suggests a low annual risk of cardiovascular events (<1% per year). The updated 2017 guidelines state that revascularization with PCI or LIMA to LAD may be appropriate in patient with symptoms and proximal LAD or proximal left-dominant circumflex. External extracorporeal counterpulsation should be considered only in patients with angina refractory to medical therapy (Patel MR, et al. *J Am Coll Cardiol* 2017;69(17):2212–2241; Fletcher GF, et al. *Circulation* 2013;128(8):873–934; Pijls NH, et al. *J Am Coll Cardiol* 2007;49(21):2105–2111; Zimmermann FM, et al.

Eur Heart J 2015;36(45):3182–3188; Boden WE, et al. *N Engl J Med* 2007;356(15):1503–1516; Hannan EL, et al. *Circulation* 2012;125(15):1870–1879).

36.18 Answer C. Although the patient is asymptomatic, there are high-risk features on his nuclear stress study that suggest significant left main or multivessel disease. The ACC/AHA guidelines recommend coronary angiography for risk stratification with high-risk criteria on noninvasive testing irrespective of anginal severity. As in symptomatic patients, revascularization is indicated for asymptomatic patients when a large ischemic burden is present.

36.19 Answer C. Patients with possible or known history of angina and who have survived sudden cardiac death should undergo coronary angiography to establish diagnosis of CAD (Class I recommendation). Coronary angiography would be contraindicated in all of the remaining cases (Class III recommendations).

36.20 Answer E. Although restenosis may be clinically silent, the prognostic benefit of controlling silent ischemia remains unproven. Thus, stress testing after revascularization should only be performed in patients with a significant change in their angina symptoms (Class I recommendation). For patients with an indication for stress testing, adjunctive imaging is recommended to improve the sensitivity of the test and to help localize the site of ischemia.

36.21 Answer C. Angiographic follow-up studies have demonstrated that up to 22% of SVGs become occluded within the first year after surgery. Greater patency has been observed in patients treated with platelet inhibition and aggressive lipid-lowering therapy. Use of the internal thoracic artery has greatly improved graft patency with 90% of grafts still functioning >10 years after surgery. Over the same time, SVGs have an occlusion rate of 40%, with significant atherosclerosis being present in 50% of those that are still patent (Barner HB, et al. *Ann Thorac Surg* 1994;57(6):1526–1528; Sabik JF III, et al. *Ann Thorac Surg* 2005;79(2):544–551).

36.22 Answer E. In patients with a normal ECG, no prior MI, and no heart failure, routine assessment of left ventricular function is not recommended (Class III recommendation). Of note, several large studies of CAD patients have shown that >90% of patients with a normal ECG have normal left ventricular function.

36.23 Answer C. Based on his performance on the treadmill, the patient's prognosis is excellent (Duke score = 6; annual cardiac mortality < 1%) and cannot be improved with revascularization by any means. Revascularization has not been shown to decrease rates of nonfatal infarction (Pursnani S, et al. *Circ Cardiovasc Interv* 2012;5(4):476–490; Stergiopoulos K, et al. *Arch Intern Med* 2012;172(4):312–319; De Bruyne B, et al. *N Engl J Med* 2012;367(11):991–1001).

36.24 Answer A. Table A36-24 lists noninvasive findings for prognosis in patients with CAD.

Table A36-24 Noninvasive risk stratification

High Risk (>3% annual mortality rate)
1. Severe resting left ventricular dysfunction (LVEF < 35%)
2. High-risk treadmill score (score ≤ −11)
3. Severe exercise left ventricular dysfunction (exercise LVEF < 35%)
4. Stress-induced large perfusion defect (particularly if anterior)
5. Stress-induced multiple perfusion defects of moderate size
6. Large, fixed perfusion defect with left ventricular dilation or increased lung uptake (thallium-201)
7. Stress-induced moderate perfusion defect with left ventricular dilation or increased lung uptake (thallium-201)
8. Echocardiographic wall motion abnormality (involving greater than two segments) developing at low dose of dobutamine (≤10 mcg/kg/min) or at a low heart rate (<120 bpm)
9. Stress echocardiographic evidence of extensive ischemia
Intermediate Risk (1%–3% annual mortality rate)
1. Mild/moderate resting left ventricular dysfunction (LVEF = 35%–49%)
2. Intermediate-risk treadmill score (−11 < score < 5)
3. Stress-induced moderate perfusion defect without LV dilation or increased lung intake (thallium-201)
4. Limited stress echocardiographic ischemia with a wall motion abnormality involving less than or equal to two segments only at higher doses of dobutamine
Low Risk (<1% annual mortality rate)
1. Low-risk treadmill score (score ≥ 5)
2. Normal or small myocardial perfusion defect at rest or with stress[a]
3. Normal stress echocardiographic wall motion or no change of limited resting wall motion abnormalities during stress[a]

[a]Although the published data are limited, patients with these findings will probably not be at low risk in the presence of either a high-risk treadmill score or severe resting left ventricular dysfunction (LVEF < 35%).
LV, left ventricular; LVEF, left ventricular ejection fraction.

36.25 **Answer D.** This lesion does not meet criteria for a significant left main lesion (≥50% left main stenosis as seen in "worst view" angiographic projection). Revascularization may be deferred in lesions with minimal lumen area of >7.5 mm^2. In this patient, revascularization with either CABG or PCI is contraindicated in the absence of demonstrable ischemia on noninvasive testing (ACC/AHA III recommendation) (Patel MR, et al. *J Am Coll Cardiol* 2017;69(17):2212–2241).

36.26 **Answer A.** The majority of enrolled patients in these trials had mild or no symptoms and had preserved left ventricular function. The survival advantage of surgery persisted at 10 years. Patients who were in the highest risk categories received the greatest benefit with CABG, particularly those with left main disease (Takaro T, et al. *Circulation* 1976;54(6 Suppl):III107–III117; Caracciolo EA, et al. *Circulation* 1995;91(9):2335–2344; Yusuf S, et al. *Lancet* 1994;344(8922):563–570).

36.27 **Answer A.** The lesion is suggestive of functional significance as it has ≥50% luminal diameter narrowing and the lumen area is <5 mm^2. Even in the absence of symptoms, CABG is recommended for patients with significant left main disease (Class I recommendation). PCI may be appropriate for a patient with left main disease depending on the anatomy, particularly in the absence of bifurcation involvement and disease burden in other areas. However, in this healthy patient without surgical comorbidities, CABG would be most appropriate (Patel MR, et al. *J Am Coll Cardiol* 2017;69(17):2212–2241).

36.28 **Answer E.** Stress testing with adjunctive imaging is recommended over treadmill study alone in patients with prior revascularization who have had a change in clinical status (Class I recommendation). Ideally, the imaging modality selected would be the same as prior studies to facilitate comparison. Coronary angiography also may be performed as the initial step in patients with CCS Class III angina despite maximal medical therapy (Class I recommendation).

36.29 **Answer C.** Coronary angiography, in addition to appropriate medical therapy, is indicated for patients with angina and symptoms and signs of congestive heart failure (Class I recommendation).

36.30 **Answer E.** Both dual antiplatelet agents and lipid-lowering strategies are established therapies for patients undergoing PCI. Despite early promising studies, hormone replacement therapy for postmenopausal women has not been found to be beneficial and may result in harm. In one randomized investigation, hormone replacement therapy resulted in higher rates of MI and thromboembolism. Thus, hormone replacement therapy is not recommended in postmenopausal patients for reduction of cardiovascular events (Class IV recommendation). Vitamin E was examined in a large study (>20,000 patients) and also not found to be beneficial (Class III recommendation).

37 Non–ST-Elevation Acute Coronary Syndromes: Insights from the AHA/ACC Guidelines

Waleed Kayani, Ali Denktas, and Hani Jneid

QUESTIONS

37.1 A 59-year-old man presents with non–ST-segment myocardial infarction (NSTEMI) and undergoes percutaneous coronary intervention (PCI) to the left anterior descending (LAD) and D1 with two everolimus-eluting stents (EES). He has no procedural complications, and clinical success is achieved with complete resolution of anginal symptoms. He has a history of hypertension, diabetes, and transient ischemic attack (TIA). His hemoglobin A1c = 7.6%. His blood pressure (BP) is 137/89 mm Hg. His LDL = 50 mg/dL. He has severe left ventricular (LV) dysfunction with a left ventricular ejection fraction (LVEF) of 25%. His inpatient medical regimen consists of aspirin 81 mg, prasugrel 10 mg, metformin 500 mg twice daily, lisinopril 20 mg, atorvastatin 40 mg, metoprolol XL 25 mg, and a multivitamin. Which of the following adjustment to his medical regimen is recommended?

(A) Add ranolazine
(B) Add ticagrelor and stop prasugrel
(C) Add insulin to lower HbA1c
(D) Add short-acting nifedipine to lower his blood pressure
(E) Increase atorvastatin dose to lower LDL

37.2 An 84-year-old man is admitted at midnight with a NSTEMI (initial troponin I = 4 ng/mL). He is angina-free and hemodynamically stable (except for borderline low blood pressure, systolic blood pressure [SBP] 100 mm Hg). He has ST-segment depression in leads II, III, and aVF. He reports excellent quality of life prior to his hospitalization. He has longstanding diabetic nephropathy, and his creatinine is 1.6 mg/dL (which reflects his known baseline stage chronic kidney disease [CKD]). When should he undergo coronary angiography?

(A) He should never undergo coronary angiography because of his age and CKD
(B) He should undergo an early invasive strategy within 72 hours
(C) He should undergo immediate invasive strategy within 2 hours
(D) He should undergo an early invasive strategy within 12 to 24 hours
(E) He should undergo an ischemia-guided strategy

37.3 An 80-year-old diabetic woman presents with 8 hours of chest heaviness. Her blood work shows elevated troponin. Electrocardiogram (ECG) reveals sinus rhythm with deep T-wave inversion in leads V1 to V4. Aspirin 325 mg, ticagrelor 180 mg, and two doses of sublingual nitroglycerin are administered. Twenty minutes later, she continues to feel 3/10 chest pressure. Repeat examination shows a BP of 100/62 mm Hg and a heart rate of (HR) 112 beats per minute (bpm); she appears anxious, but the rest of the examination is unremarkable. She underwent urgent coronary angiography, which reveals critical stenosis (95%) of the proximal LAD with moderate angiographic stenoses in the left circumflex (LCx) and right coronary arteries (RCAs) (40% to 50%). Decision is made to proceed with PCI to the LAD with a drug-eluting stent (DES). Which of the following is a CORRECT statement regarding this patient's management?

(A) Bivalirudin is a safe adjunctive therapy during PCI
(B) Heparin and tirofiban should be added during PCI
(C) Heparin and eptifibatide should be added during PCI
(D) Fondaparinux alone is safer in this patient
(E) An ischemia-guided strategy is preferred in this older patient

37.4 Which of the following is INCORRECT regarding late hospital or posthospital care of patients with non–ST-elevation acute coronary syndrome (NSTE-ACS)?

(A) Aspirin should be continued indefinitely in all NSTE-ACS patients at a daily dose of 325 mg
(B) All eligible patients with NSTE-ACS should be referred to a cardiac rehabilitation program
(C) A $P2Y_{12}$ receptor inhibitor should be continued for at least 12 months
(D) Folic acid should not be used for secondary prevention in NSTE-ACS patients
(E) An annual influenza vaccine is recommended in NSTE-ACS patients

37.5 Of the following medications, which does NOT have an American College of Cardiology (ACC) and American Heart Association (AHA) Class I recommendation for use in NSTE-ACS patients?

(A) Angiotensin-converting enzyme (ACE) inhibitors
(B) Beta-adrenergic antagonists
(C) Immediate-release nifedipine
(D) Non–dihydropyridine calcium channel blockers
(E) Sublingual nitroglycerin

37.6 A 67-year-old woman presents with 5 hours of chest heaviness. Her initial blood work included an elevated troponin T level. ECG reveals sinus rhythm with anterolateral ST-segment depression. She is diagnosed with NSTEMI. Aspirin 325 mg and two doses of sublingual nitroglycerin are administered. Twenty minutes later, she continues to feel 3/10 chest pressure. Decision is made to proceed with urgent coronary angiography. What is the best oral antiplatelet therapy to be added to this patient?

(A) A repeat dose of aspirin 81 mg
(B) Clopidogrel 600 mg
(C) Ticagrelor 180 mg
(D) Prasugrel 60 mg
(E) Clopidogrel 150 mg

37.7 A 66-year-old woman with no prior history of bleeding presents with a NSTEMI. A coronary angiography shows a spontaneously recanalized RCA with only mild residual stenosis identified. No PCI is performed. She is prescribed aspirin and atorvastatin. Should she also be prescribed clopidogrel on discharge?

(A) Yes, for 6 months
(B) Yes, for 12 months
(C) Yes, for 2 years
(D) Yes, indefinitely
(E) No

37.8 A 71-year-old man with mild dementia (vascular in nature, following earlier ischemic stroke) and a history of prior coronary artery bypass grafting (CABG) surgery is admitted to the hospital with several hours of anginal symptoms. His HR is 63 bpm and his BP is 111/54 mm Hg. His troponin I level is 0.06 ng/mL. His ECG reveals sinus rhythm and no dynamic ECG changes. He and his family refuse coronary angiography. He is administered heparin, enoxaparin, simvastatin, intravenous (IV) nitroglycerin, and metoprolol. What is the best way to improve his medical regimen?

(A) Add abciximab
(B) Add clopidogrel and switch him to atorvastatin 40 mg
(C) Add prasugrel and switch him to rosuvastatin 20 mg
(D) Add clopidogrel and switch him to atorvastatin 20 mg
(E) Substitute unfractionated heparin (UFH) for enoxaparin

37.9 A 60-year-old man presents to the emergency department with 10 hours of severe ongoing chest heaviness. He has a history of type II diabetes mellitus, hyperlipidemia, hypertension, obesity, obstructive sleep apnea, and renal insufficiency. His Tn I measurement is 1.87 ng/mL and creatinine is 1.5 mg/dL (baseline renal function). His ECG reveals sinus rhythm without ischemic changes. His ischemic symptoms are relieved after receiving aspirin, heparin, and nitroglycerin in the emergency department. What is the most appropriate next step in management?

(A) Coronary angiography (and PCI, if needed) within 24 hours
(B) An ischemia-guided strategy, given the absence of chest discomfort and a normal ECG
(C) Resting nuclear sestamibi scan to evaluate for a perfusion abnormality at rest
(D) Continue monitoring his renal function with plans for coronary angiography if his renal function improves
(E) Immediate coronary angiography within 2 hours

37.10 A 68-year-old woman presents with unstable angina. She has prior CABG surgery (left internal mammary artery [LIMA]-LAD, saphenous vein graft [SVG]-obtuse marginal [OM] 2, SVG-right posterior descending artery [RPDA]). Her ECG reveals 2-mm ST-segment depressions in leads I and aVL during chest discomfort. Troponin level is 0.07 ng/mL. Coronary and graft angiography reveals severely diseased and calcified left main trunk disease, occluded mid-LAD, severe proximal circumflex stenosis (also heavily calcified and tortuous), and an occluded dominant RCA. The LAD and RCA grafts are patent. The proximal portion of the vein graft to the OM branch has a severe ulcerated stenosis with thrombolysis in myocardial infarction (TIMI) 2 flow. The best treatment strategy for this patient is:

(A) Medical therapy because the LAD and RCA grafts are patent
(B) Redo CABG to the OM
(C) PCI to the SVG to OM with distal embolic protection
(D) PCI to SVG with adjunctive glycoprotein (GP) IIb/IIIa inhibitor
(E) PCI to left main trunk and proximal circumflex

37.11 A 56-year-old diabetic woman presents with NSTEMI and undergoes a successful PCI with a zotarolimus-eluting stent (ZES) deployed in the LAD. Post-PCI echocardiogram reveals mild mitral regurgitation and normal ventricular function. What should her discharge medications include?

(A) Aspirin 325 mg daily, clopidogrel 75 mg daily, simvastatin 40 mg daily, a beta-adrenergic blocker, and an ACE inhibitor
(B) Aspirin 325 mg daily indefinitely, clopidogrel 75 mg daily, atorvastatin 20 mg daily, and a beta-adrenergic blocker
(C) Aspirin 325 mg daily for at least 3 months, clopidogrel 75 mg daily, and atorvastatin 10 mg daily
(D) Aspirin 81 mg, clopidogrel 75 mg daily, atorvastatin 40 mg daily, a beta-adrenergic blocker, and an ACE inhibitor
(E) Aspirin 325 mg daily, clopidogrel 75 mg daily, rosuvastatin 10 mg daily, and an ACE inhibitor

37.12 A 53-year-old man is diagnosed with NSTE-ACS at an outside hospital. He is transferred and undergoes PCI with implantation of two bare metal stents (BMS) to the RCA. His bleeding risk is normal. He is prescribed a low-dose aspirin. What is the appropriate clopidogrel regimen for this patient?

(A) 150 mg daily for at least 12 months
(B) 150 mg daily for 2 years
(C) 150 mg daily for 9 to 12 months
(D) 75 mg daily for at least 12 months
(E) 75 mg daily for 2 years

37.13 A 63-year-old woman presents with crescendo angina over the last 8 weeks. She has hypertension and hyperlipidemia. She has been taking atorvastatin and aspirin. Her discomfort was not relieved after two sublingual nitroglycerin tablets. Cardiac biomarkers are elevated, and her ECG shows nonspecific ST changes. She is referred for urgent coronary angiography shortly after receiving aspirin 325 mg and atorvastatin 80 mg. Angiography reveals a large OM2 branch with 90% tubular thrombotic lesion. She is to undergo PCI with stenting. The optimal adjunctive medical therapy for this patient is:

(A) Bivalirudin only
(B) Heparin only
(C) Heparin and eptifibatide
(D) Fondaparinux only
(E) Subcutaneous enoxaparin

37.14 A 59-year-old man undergoes PCI to the LAD and D1 with an everolimus-eluting cobalt-chromium (CoCr) stent. He is diabetic with a hemoglobin A1c of 7.6%. His BP is 137/89 mm Hg and his LDL is 105 mg/dL. His LVEF is 30%. His daily inpatient medical regimen consists of aspirin 81 mg, clopidogrel 75 mg, atorvastatin 20 mg, metoprolol, and a multivitamin. Which of the following adjustment to his discharge medications is NOT recommended?

(A) Add an ACE inhibitor to lower his blood pressure and to afford benefits given his diabetes and depressed LVEF
(B) Sublingual nitroglycerin as needed for angina
(C) Add metformin to lower HbA1c
(D) Add short-acting nifedipine to lower his blood pressure
(E) Increase atorvastatin dose to 40 mg

37.15 A 73-year-old woman with prior CABG presents to the emergency room with 6 hours of chest discomfort. Her ECG reveals anterolateral ST-segment depression, and her initial troponin I is elevated. She is diagnosed with a NSTEMI, and coronary angiography is scheduled within 12 hours of presentation. Her only medication is metformin. Which antiplatelet agents should be immediately initiated?

(A) Aspirin and abciximab
(B) Aspirin only
(C) Aspirin and clopidogrel
(D) Aspirin and prasugrel
(E) Aspirin, clopidogrel, and eptifibatide

37.16 A 43-year-old woman presents to the emergency department with new atypical chest pain. The pain is mild, continuous, and sharp in nature, worsens with inspiration and lying supine, and improves with sitting upright. She received one EES 3 years earlier following a NSTEMI presentation. She is scheduled to undergo surgical laminectomy in 3 weeks. A recent coronary angiography at an outside facility demonstrates a patent RCA stent and mild left coronary artery (LCA) disease. Her cardiac medications are aspirin and clopidogrel. Recommendations include perioperative beta-blockade. What other perioperative recommendations are appropriate?

(A) Continuous ST-segment monitoring following the operation
(B) Pharmacologic stress test with either echocardiographic or nuclear imaging
(C) In-hospital GP IIb/IIIa inhibitor therapy during the period of aspirin and clopidogrel discontinuation
(D) Intraoperative monitoring with Swan-Ganz catheter
(E) Discontinuation of clopidogrel at least 5 days before surgery. There is no need to resume it afterward

37.17 A 37-year-old woman presents to the emergency department with 30 minutes of new-onset non-radiating chest tightness at rest. Her symptoms started 1 hour after snorting cocaine. Cardiac biomarkers are negative. Her ECG reveals sinus tachycardia with upsloping 2-mm inferolateral ST-segment depression. Her blood pressure is 200/110 mm Hg (equal in both arms), and her lungs are clear. Her chest x-ray is normal. What is the most appropriate management?

(A) IV esmolol
(B) IV labetalol
(C) IV metoprolol
(D) IV amiodarone
(E) IV nitroglycerin and IV midazolam, followed by coronary angiography if the chest discomfort and ECG changes persist

37.18 A 46-year-old obese man is hospitalized with a diagnosis of unstable angina. He recently underwent a resection for colorectal cancer, and he is scheduled for an ileostomy reversal. His left heart catheterization reveals a 90% focal stenosis (8 mm length) in a large RCA. The reference vessel diameter is estimated at 4.5 mm. His other coronary arteries have only mild disease. What is the most appropriate strategy for this patient?

(A) PCI with balloon angioplasty with no stenting
(B) PCI with BMS
(C) PCI with a ZES
(D) PCI with an EES
(E) Single-vessel CABG surgery

37.19 A 49-year-old woman with a family history of coronary artery disease (CAD) presents to the emergency room with 12 hours of chest heaviness. Her initial blood work and physical examination are unremarkable. Her ECG reveals sinus rhythm with deep lateral ST-segment depression. She is diagnosed with NSTEMI, and coronary angiography is scheduled within the next few hours. Her weight is 65 kg. What antiplatelet agents should be administered?

(A) Clopidogrel 150 mg
(B) Prasugrel 10 mg
(C) Prasugrel 60 mg
(D) Ticagrelor 180 mg

37.20 The GRACE risk score includes all of the following, EXCEPT:

(A) More than three cardiovascular risk factors
(B) Heart rate
(C) SBP
(D) Serum Creatinine level
(E) ST-segment deviation

37.21 A 57-year-old man with diabetes mellitus was diagnosed with NSTEMI at an outside facility and is now being transferred to undergo urgent coronary angiography and possible PCI. He arrives in the catheterization laboratory with no signs of heart failure and no ongoing chest pain. The onset of ischemic symptoms was 9 hours earlier, and the cardiac troponin T biomarkers from the outside facility are elevated. He received non-enteric-coated aspirin 325 mg and enoxaparin 1 mg/kg SQ at the outside hospital 8 hours earlier. Serum creatinine is normal. Coronary angiography reveals a mid-LAD culprit lesion with a large amount of thrombus. Which of the following anticoagulant regimen is not recommended at this point?

(A) IV UFH
(B) Eptifibatide
(C) Enoxaparin 0.3 mg/kg IV
(D) Cangrelor
(E) Bivalirudin

37.22 A 48-year-old woman with a history of chronic renal insufficiency and severe knee osteoarthritis presents with exertional chest heaviness over the past 3 weeks. The chest heaviness is not consistently reproducible on exertion and sometimes lasts >1 hour at a time. She is admitted to the hospital. Her creatine kinase (CK), CK-MB, and troponin T are within normal limits. Her ECG reveals sinus rhythm and borderline nondynamic and nonspecific ST changes. At rest, she is asymptomatic. Her HR is 75 bpm, her BP is 150/90 mm Hg, and her cardiac examination is normal. Which is an appropriate risk stratification strategy in this patient?

(A) Proceed with coronary angiography immediately given high-risk features
(B) Obtain serial CK-MB levels and proceed with coronary angiography when CK-MB levels are elevated
(C) Obtain a symptom-limited exercise stress test, without an echocardiogram or nuclear imaging, 1 to 2 days after admission or shortly after discharge
(D) Obtain a symptom-limited exercise stress test, with an echocardiogram or nuclear imaging, 1 to 2 days after admission or shortly after discharge
(E) None of the above

37.23 A 56-year-old diabetic man presents to the emergency room with chest heaviness radiating to both arms and diaphoresis for the past 45 minutes. He has known CAD and his symptoms are similar to his prior cardiac presentation with unstable angina 2 years earlier. His clinical exam is normal. Recommendations that should be followed or considered (ACC/AHA Class I or II) for early risk stratification for this patient include all of the following, EXCEPT:

(A) 12-lead ECG within 10 minutes of emergency department arrival
(B) Serial cardiac troponin measurements
(C) Continuous 12-lead ECG monitoring
(D) Assessment of CK-MB or myoglobin, for patients who present within 6 hours of symptom onset
(E) Serial ECGs during the initial hour of presentation when the initial ECG is nondiagnostic

37.24 A 75-year-old woman with a history of remote CABG surgery presents with 4 hours of chest heaviness and dyspnea. Her blood pressure is 96/56 mm Hg, and heart rate is 112 bpm. Her ECG reveals sinus tachycardia with anterolateral ST-segment depression. Pulse oximetry is 86% on room air. The patient is diaphoretic. She has a cough productive of pink sputum. She has elevated jugular venous pulsations and bilateral wet crackles midway up the lung fields. Outpatient medications are aspirin and simvastatin. Which constitute the HIGHEST-risk clinical feature in this patient?

(A) Prior obstructive coronary artery disease requiring CABG
(B) ST-segment depression on the ECG
(C) Evidence of pulmonary edema on physical examination
(D) History of aspirin use
(E) Age ≥65 years

37.25 A 77-year-old woman with a history of hypertension and diabetes presents to the emergency room. Twenty-four hours prior to her arrival, she experienced 2 hours of chest pressure radiating to her left arm and jaw. Her ECG reveals sinus rhythm with 3-mm ST-segment depression in leads V1 to V4 and an elevated troponin I. Her physical examination is unremarkable. Blood oxygen saturation is 98%. Her heart rate is 75 bpm. Currently, she is asymptomatic and her estimated LVEF by echocardiography is 40%. Which of the following steps is recommended for her initial therapy?

(A) IV beta-blocker within the first 24 hours
(B) IV morphine within the first 24 hours
(C) Supplemental oxygen during the first 6 hours
(D) Sublingual nitroglycerin
(E) Bed or chair rest with continuing ECG monitoring in the emergency room

37.26 A 75-year-old woman with advanced rheumatoid arthritis is brought to the emergency room by her husband who is her primary caregiver. Twenty-four hours prior to her arrival, she experienced 2 hours of chest pain radiating to her left arm and jaw. Her ECG reveals sinus rhythm with deep T-wave inversions in leads V1 to V4 and an elevated troponin I level. Her cardiovascular exam is normal. Blood oxygen saturation is 98%. Her heart rate is 75 bpm. Currently, she is chest pain-free and her estimated LVEF by echocardiography is 45%. Despite understanding the need for coronary angiography and benefit with possible revascularization, she decides not to undergo any invasive procedures. Her husband, who lives with her, is present during the meeting and agrees with her decision. She receives 48 hours of heparin infusion, along with aspirin 81 mg daily, ticagrelor 90 mg twice daily, atorvastatin 40 mg, lisinopril 5 mg, and metoprolol XL 12.5 mg daily. Which of the following is the next best course of action?

(A) Add ranolazine
(B) Stop ticagrelor; start clopidogrel 75 mg daily
(C) Stop ticagrelor; start prasugrel 10 mg daily
(D) Arrange another family meeting to convince them about the need for coronary angiography and possible revascularization
(E) Administer pneumococcal vaccine prior to discharge

37.27 The TIMI risk score components for unstable angina/NSTEMI patients include all of the following, EXCEPT:

(A) Positive cardiac marker
(B) Aspirin used within the last month
(C) Known coronary artery disease >50% stenosis in a major epicardial artery
(D) Age ≥65
(E) ST changes ≥0.5 mm

37.28 A 67-year-old patient presents to the emergency room with severe shortness of breath and diaphoresis. The patient is producing pink frothy sputum and is obtunded. His blood pressure is 92/55 mm Hg, heart rate is 115 bpm, and oxygen saturation on room air is 84%. Initial ECG shows anterolateral ST-segment depression and initial troponin of 14 ng/mL. What is an inappropriate course of action in this patient?

(A) Endotracheal intubation and mechanical ventilation
(B) Proceed with immediate invasive angiography and possibly complete revascularization
(C) Obtain a bedside transthoracic echocardiogram (TTE) immediately
(D) Immediate placement of an intra-aortic balloon pump (IABP)
(E) Start norepinephrine infusion to maintain a SBP > 60 mm Hg and a mean arterial pressure (MAP) > 65 mm Hg

37.29 Which of the following statements is FALSE in the setting of NSTE-ACS?

(A) Nitroglycerin is contraindicated in patients who have received vardenafil within the past 48 hours
(B) Abciximab is contraindicated in patients in whom PCI is not planned
(C) IV beta-blockers are contraindicated in patients with a low-output state
(D) Angiotensin receptor blockers are contraindicated in pregnant women

37.30 Which of the following is useful to provoke coronary artery spasm in variant angina when clinical criteria and noninvasive testing fail to establish the diagnosis?

(A) Epinephrine
(B) Norepinephrine
(C) Adenosine
(D) Vasopressin
(E) Acetylcholine

ANSWERS AND EXPLANATIONS

37.1 Answer B. The 2014 AHA/ACC NSTE-ACS guideline gives a Class I recommendation for the use of either clopidogrel, ticagrelor, or prasugrel in patients with NSTE-ACS (on top of aspirin). There is, however, a Class IIa indication for the preferential use of ticagrelor or prasugrel (over clopidogrel) in patients undergoing PCI and in the absence of contraindications. Prasugrel is contraindicated in patients with a history of cerebrovascular accident or TIA (because of harm) and is best avoided in patients older than 75 years or <60 kg in weight (given no net clinical benefit in the latter two groups). Adding ranolazine is of no benefit given the absence of anginal symptoms. Adding insulin is the wrong choice, as the patient's metformin can be further uptitrated (maximal clinical effectiveness is obtained with a total of 2,000 mg of metformin total dose daily). The patient is already receiving a high-intensity HMG-CoA reductase inhibitor (atorvastatin 40 mg) and has achieved an acceptable LDL level indicating compliance to his lipid-lowering therapy. Use of short-acting nifedipine is contraindicated in patients with NSTE-ACS.

37.2 Answer D. This elderly patient has excellent quality of life and is presenting with NSTEMI that appears to be initially stabilized. Ischemia-guided strategy (previously called initial conservative management) is a poor choice given he is NOT a low-risk patient. In fact, despite the absence of all components that enable one to calculate his GRACE risk score, he is most likely to be at high risk with a GRACE risk score > 140. The eight variables used in the GRACE risk model are age, Killip class, systolic blood pressure, serum creatinine level, heart rate, ST-segment deviation, cardiac arrest at admission, and positive cardiac biomarkers level. A patient's GRACE risk score is calculated by adding points corresponding to all these variables and helps stratify patients into low, intermediate, and high risk of in-hospital and postdischarge 6-month mortality. Therefore, an early invasive strategy (within 12 to 24 hours) with intention to revascularize is the best option in this patient (as supported by the TIMACS clinical trial). A delayed invasive strategy (defined by a time period between 24- and 72-hour of presentation) is an acceptable strategy in those with intermediate-risk features. Overall, an invasive strategy is not contraindicated in elderly patients and in those with stable kidney function. Elderly patients with acute myocardial infarction (MI) are undertreated with evidence-based therapies (including invasive therapies), despite the fact they are usually at higher risk and derive higher benefits compared with their younger counterparts. A routine invasive strategy is, in general, superior, to an ischemia-guided strategy (in most patients, except low-risk patients) and will help rapidly diagnose, risk stratify and dictate therapy, and expedite discharge. An immediate or urgent invasive strategy (within 2 hours) for NSTE-ACS patients is reserved to those with hemodynamic instability, heart failure, refractory ischemia, or cardiogenic shock (i.e., in those who are not initially stabilized). This patient has only borderline low blood pressure and does not qualify as having hemodynamic instability. (See Tables A37-2A and A37-2B.)

Table A37-2A Selection of initial treatment strategy: invasive vs. conservative strategy

Strategy	Patient Characteristic
Immediate invasive (within 2 h)	Refractory angina Signs or symptoms of HF or new or worsening mitral regurgitation Hemodynamic instability Recurrent angina or ischemia at rest or with low-level activities despite intensive medical therapy Sustained VT or VF
Early invasive (within 24 h)	None of the above, but GRACE risk score > 140 temporal change in Tn New or presumably new ST depression
Delayed invasive (within 25–72 h)	None of the above but diabetes mellitus, renal dysfunction GFR < 60 mL/min/1.73 m^2) PCI within 6 mo Prior CABG Reduced left ventricular function (LVEF < 40%) GRACE risk score 109–140; TIMI score ≥ 2 Early postinfarction angina
Ischemia-guided strategy	Low-risk score (e.g., TIMI 0–1, GRACE < 109) Patient or physician preference in the absence of high-risk features Low-risk Tn-negative female patients

CABG, coronary artery bypass graft; GRACE, Global Registry of Acute Coronary Events; h, hours; HF, heart failure; LVEF, left ventricular ejection fraction; PCI, percutaneous coronary intervention; TIMI, thrombolysis in myocardial infarction; Tn, troponin; VF, ventricular fibrillation; VT, ventricular tachycardia.
Modified from Amsterdam EA, et al. *Circulation* 2014;130(25):e344–e426.

Table A37-2B Mortality in hospital and at 6 months in low-, intermediate-, and high-risk categories in registry populations, according to the GRACE risk score

Risk Category (Tertile)	**GRACE Risk Score**	**In-Hospital Death (%)**
Low	<109	<1
Intermediate	109–140	1–3
High	>140	>3
Risk Category (Tertile)	**GRACE Risk Score**	**Postdischarge 6 months (%)**
Low	≤88	<3
Intermediate	89–118	3–8
High	>118	>8

GRACE risk model uses patient's age, Killip class, SBP, serum creatinine level, heart rate, ST-segment deviation, cardiac arrest at admission, and positive cardiac biomarkers level to predict in-hospital and postdischarge mortality in patients presenting with NSTE-ACS.

37.3 Answer A. Bivalirudin is a safer regimen in patients with NSTE-ACS undergoing PCI when compared with heparin plus GP IIb/IIIa inhibitors (lesser bleeding and similar efficacy). Older patients with NSTE-ACS, who are initially stabilized, benefit as much or more than younger patients from an early invasive strategy compared with an ischemia-guided strategy. In one meta-analysis of randomized controlled trials with 5-year follow-up, an early invasive strategy vs. an ischemia-guided strategy was associated with a significant reduction in death/MI in patients ≥75 years of age. Although the highest risk reduction in death/MI with an early invasive strategy occurred in those ≥75 years of age, this strategy was associated with a threefold bleeding risk; hence, strategies to minimize bleeding in this population must be considered. In this particular clinical scenario, the patient requires an urgent/immediate invasive strategy (within 2 hours) given she has refractory ischemic symptoms and appears unstable. Fondaparinux should never be used alone during PCI, as it is associated with catheter thrombosis; an additional anticoagulant with anti-IIa activity should be administered when fondaparinux is used during PCI. (See Table A37-3.)

Table A37-3 Medications used for stabilized NSTE-ACS patients

Anti-Ischemic and Antithrombotic/ Antiplatelet Agents	Drug Action	Class/Level of Evidence
Aspirin	Antiplatelet	I/A
Clopidogrel	Antiplatelet	I/B
Ticagrelor[a]	Antiplatelet	I/B
Prasugrel[b]	Antiplatelet	I/B
Beta-blockers	Anti-ischemic	I/A—use in the absence of HF, low-output state, risk for cardiogenic shock
ACEI	Inhibitor of the renin–angiotenin–aldosterone system	I/A, EF < 0.40 and HTN, DM, and CKD
ARBs	Inhibitor of the renin–angiotenin–aldosterone system	I/A, EF < 0.40, if ACE intolerant
Aldosterone antagonists	Inhibitor of the renin–angiotenin–aldosterone system	I/A, If EF < 0.40, DM or HF
Nitrates	Antianginal	I/C for ischemic symptoms
Nitrates—if phosphodiesterase inhibitors recently used	Antianginal	III
Calcium channel blockers (nondihydropyridine)	Antianginal	I—for ischemic symptoms; when beta-blockers are not successful (B) or contraindicated or cause unacceptable side effects and in coronary spasm (C)
Calcium channel blockers (short-acting dihydropyridines)		III B
GP IIb/IIIa inhibitors	Antiplatelet	I—at the time of PCI in patients NOT adequately pretreated with dual antiplatelet therapy
GP IIb/IIIa inhibitors	Antiplatelet	IIB—routine use in patients with NSTE-ACS
Enoxaparin	Anticoagulant	I A—till discharge or PCI
Unfractionated heparin	Anticoagulant	I B—till PCI or 48 hours
Bivalirudin[c]	Anticoagulant	I B—till angiography or PCI ONLY in patients undergoing early invasive therapy
Subcutaneous fondaparinux	Anticoagulant	I B—till discharge or PCI along with another anticoagulant
Additional Agents for Secondary Prevention and Other Indications	**Risk Factor**	**Class/Level of Evidence**
High-intensity statin therapy	Hyperlipidemia	I/SA
Pneumococcal vaccine	Patients >65 y of age or immunocompromised	I/B
Hormone therapy (initiation)[d]	Postmenopausal state	III/A
Hormone therapy (continuation)[d]	Postmenopausal state	III/B
NSAIDs except aspirin	Chronic pain	III/B
Vitamins C, E, beta-carotene; folic acid, B_6, B_{12}	Antioxidant effect; homocysteine lowering	III/A

[a]Preferred to clopidogrel either an early invasive or initial ischemia-guided strategy (IIa).
[b]Preferred to clopidogrel in patients treated with stents (IIa).
[c]Especially useful in patients with higher bleeding risk or those >75 y of age.
[d]For risk reduction of coronary artery disease.
ACEI, angiotensin-converting enzyme inhibitor; ARBs, angiotensin II receptor blockers; CHF, congestive heart failure; CKD, chronic kidney disease; COX-2, cyclooxygenase 2; DM, diabetes mellitus; EF, ejection fraction; GP, glycoprotein; HF, heart failure; HDL, high-density lipoprotein; HTN, hypertension; NSAID, nonsteroidal anti-inflammatory drug; NSTE-ACS, non–ST-segment elevation acute coronary syndrome.

37.4 Answer A. The 2016 ACC/AHA Guideline Focused Update on Duration of Antiplatelet Therapy (Levine, et al. *JACC* 2016;68(10):1082–1115) clearly specifies that the recommended long-term aspirin dose is 81 mg daily. A higher dose does not confer added ischemic benefits and rather increased the bleeding hazards. Antioxidant vitamins and folic acid (with or without vitamins B_6 or B_{12}) have no role in secondary prevention after NSTE-ACS. Referral to a cardiovascular rehabilitation program, especially a comprehensive program (e.g., exercise, nutrition and activity counseling, and medications compliance), is recommended to all eligible NSTE-ACS patients either before or shortly after hospital discharge. An annual influenza vaccine, as well as a pneumococcal vaccine (for those 65 years old and high-risk patients), are also recommended. A $P2Y_{12}$ receptor inhibitor should be continued in all NSTE-ACS patients, irrespective of the stent choice (whether a DES or BMS). (See Table A37-3.)

37.5 Answer C. Immediate-release nifedipine can cause precipitous drop in blood pressure and is contraindicated in patients with NSTE-ACS (Class III recommendation because of harm). Oral non-dihydropyridine calcium antagonists (verapamil and diltiazem) are recommended in patients with NSTE-ACS who have recurrent ischemia in the absence of contraindications after appropriate use of beta-blockers and nitrates or if beta-blockers are contraindicated. ACE inhibitors have a Class I recommendation and should be started and continued indefinitely in all ACS patients with LVEF < 40% and in those with hypertension, diabetes mellitus, or stable CKD, unless contraindicated.

37.6 Answer C. Although both ticagrelor 180 mg and clopidogrel 600 mg have a Class I indication for use in patients with acute NSTEMI regardless of the treatment strategy (invasive or medical treatment), ticagrelor is more potent and a faster acting antiplatelet agent than clopidogrel (there is a Class IIA-LOE B-indication for using ticagrelor preferentially over clopidogrel). Compared with clopidogrel, ticagrelor is associated with a reduction in vascular and total mortality and in recurrent MI (findings from the head-to-head PLATO trial comparing both agents on the background of aspirin therapy). Prasugrel use is only recommended in patients with NSTEMI after delineation of the coronary anatomy and PCI is planned. Clopidogrel loading dose is 600 mg before PCI and not 150 mg.

37.7 Answer B. In the CURE study, the benefit of dual antiplatelet therapy (DAPT) with aspirin and clopidogrel was observed compared with aspirin alone in patients with ACS following three to 12 months of therapy. The majority of subjects in the CURE study had medically treated NSTE-ACS. In terms of the recommended duration of clopidogrel or ticagrelor (or prasugrel, if PCI is performed) treatment, the current 2014 ACC/AHA NSTE-ACS guidelines and the 2016 focused update of the guideline on the duration of antiplatelet therapy recommend a period of 12 months of antiplatelet therapy whether treated medically or with PCI/stenting (and irrespective of the type of stent). However, in patients with ACS treated with DAPT after DES implantation who develop a high risk of bleeding, are at high risk of severe bleeding complication, or develop significant overt bleeding, discontinuation of $P2Y_{12}$ inhibitor therapy after 6 months may be reasonable (Class IIb recommendation).

37.8 Answer B. The CURE trial demonstrated that, compared to aspirin alone in patients with ACS, the addition of clopidogrel on top of aspirin was associated with a lower incidence of adverse ischemic events. In this case of medically treated ACS, clopidogrel should be started and continued for up to 12 months. The GUSTO IV trial demonstrated harm with the strategy of administering abciximab to ACS patients with no planned PCI. Prasugrel is contraindicated in patients with prior TIA or stroke. All patients <75 years of age that have atherosclerotic cerebrovascular disease should receive a high-intensity statin (20/40 mg rosuvastatin or 40/80 mg atorvastatin), unless intolerance or drug-drug interaction exists. Enoxaparin is slightly superior to UFH among medically treated ACS patients.

37.9 Answer A. The 2014 ACC/AHA NSTE-ACS guideline recommends early invasive therapy (within 24 hours) in this high-risk patient. Immediate or urgent invasive therapy (within 2 hours) is recommended in patients with refractory angina, signs of heart failure or worsening mitral regurgitation, hemodynamic instability, ventricular tachycardia, or ventricular fibrillation. Ischemia-guided strategy is recommended for patients at low risk (especially low-risk women and those without elevated biomarkers and no active ischemia) and involves a noninvasive stress test for risk stratification before or shortly after discharge. (See Tables A37-2A and A37-2B.)

37.10 Answer C. Since the graft is on the verge of occlusion, it is reasonable to expect PCI to provide superior preservation of myocardial function.

The risk/benefit ratio for reoperation for a single circumflex territory target is unfavorable. In this particular case, PCI to native left main and proximal circumflex is more difficult (given severe calcification and tortuosity), and it is best to hold this strategy in reserve as an option for the future (if needed, and if technically feasible then). Distal embolic protection devices are beneficial (they usually reduce periprocedural MI) in vein graft PCI and should be used when technically feasible, as in this patient with proximal lesion location in the graft (Class I recommendation, LOE B according to the 2011 ACCF, AHA, and Society for Cardiovascular Angiography and Interventions [SCAI] Guidelines for PCI). GP IIb/IIIa inhibitors are not indicated in patients undergoing PCI for vein graft disease.

37.11 Answer D. After PCI with implantation of a DES, DAPT with aspirin and a $P2Y_{12}$ receptor inhibitor (clopidogrel, ticagrelor or prasugrel) is recommended for at least 12 months. For NSTEMI patients treated with DES, aspirin 81 mg (range 75 to 100 mg) per day should be continued indefinitely, and there is no need for higher doses of aspirin (no added antiplatelet efficacy and increased hazards of gastrointestinal bleeding). Of note, the recommended dose of aspirin to be used with ticagrelor is <100 mg as the efficacy of ticagrelor seems to be decreased in patients treated with higher aspirin doses (the US Food and Drug Administration [FDA] issued a boxed warning on this regard). Because this patient has established atherosclerotic CAD (NSTEMI presentation), she should receive a high-intensity statin daily at bedtime (e.g., rosuvastatin 20 or 40 mg; atorvastatin 40 or 80 mg). Following MI, all patients should be treated with a beta-adrenergic blocker, unless contraindicated. This patient should also receive an ACE inhibitor, which is a Class I recommendation for NSTE-ACS patients with ventricular systolic dysfunction (LVEF < 40%), hypertension, diabetes mellitus, or stable CKD.

37.12 Answer D. A $P2Y_{12}$ inhibitor (clopidogrel, prasugrel or ticagrelor) in addition to aspirin should be administered for at least 12 months in all patients with NSTE-ACS undergoing PCI with stenting (irrespective of whether they received a DES or BMS).

37.13 Answer C. In a patient with NSTE-ACS who is not adequately pretreated with a $P2Y_{12}$ inhibitor, a GP IIb/IIIa receptor inhibitor (abciximab, double-bolus eptifibatide, or high-dose bolus tirofiban) should be used during PCI to reduce the incidence of ischemic events. A loading dose with a $P2Y_{12}$ inhibitor as soon as feasible is also advised. Even among adequately pretreated patients (with DAPT), a GP IIb/IIIa inhibitor may be reasonable to use during PCI selectively (e.g., large thrombus burden, side-branch occlusion, or distal embolization).

37.14 Answer D. Short-acting nifedipine is contraindicated after NSTE-ACS (Class III recommendation for harm). Adding SL nitroglycerin for use as needed is a reasonable option. Adding metformin is likely to help him achieve a target Hb A1c of <7%, although newer agents are also available than can potentially reduce recurrent cardiovascular agents. ACE inhibitors are particularly beneficial for diabetics, especially in the context of elevated blood pressure or depressed LV systolic function. The patient is on moderate-intensity statin, which needs to be further advanced (especially given suboptimally controlled LDL level).

37.15 Answer C. Except for patients known to be intolerant of aspirin, all patients with an ACS should be loaded with a non–enteric-coated aspirin 162 to 325 mg (followed by 81 mg once daily). Patients should also receive an oral loading dose of clopidogrel 300 to 600 mg (a pre-PCI loading dose is 600 mg) and ticagrelor 180 mg (whether medically managed or treated with PCI). A loading of prasugrel 60 mg should be given only in patients undergoing PCI and once the coronary anatomy is delineated. The likelihood that this 73-year-old patient with prior CABG undergoes an emergent or urgent redo CABG is very small, and thus a loading with a $P2Y_{12}$ receptor inhibitor is reasonable. Platelet GP IIb/IIIa receptor antagonists (preferably the small molecules eptifibatide or tirofiban) may be selectively used as part of an initial antiplatelet regimen in patients with an ACS undergoing an early invasive strategy and who have been pretreated with DAPT (Class IIb recommendation, LOE B). However, the routine upfront use of GP IIb/IIIa receptor inhibitors in patients with intermediate-/high-risk ACS who are pretreated with DAPT and undergoing early invasive strategy is no longer recommended (following the findings from the EARY-ACS trial).

37.16 Answer E. The patient received more than 12 months of DAPT following NSTEMI and DES implantation. Therefore, it is appropriate to stop clopidogrel with no need to resume it after surgery. She needs lifelong aspirin 81 mg daily (which should be maintained perioperatively). For patients receiving a $P2Y_{12}$ receptor inhibitor and undergoing elective surgery, clopidogrel and ticagrelor should be withheld 5 days before the procedure, while prasugrel should be withheld 7 days before. The patient's discomfort does not indicate myocardial ischemia due to coronary disease, but is likely a mild episode of pericarditis. Stress testing is not indicated in this patient with noncardiac pain and who has no obstructive CAD on coronary angiography (which was not clinically warranted in the first place). In addition, if there was angiographic suspicion of stenotic lesions significantly affecting the patient's coronary flow reserve, the interventional cardiologist would likely have performed an invasive coronary physiologic assessment (e.g., fractional flow reserve [FFR]) during the invasive procedure. Bridging with antiplatelet therapy, such as a GP IIb/IIIa inhibitor, is not indicated in this patient with remote ACS and DES implantation. Notably, bridging strategies in patients with recent DES remain controversial and are supported by a paucity of data.

37.17 Answer E. Cocaine use is associated with several cardiac conditions, including accelerated atherosclerosis (with chronic abuse), coronary vasospasm, elevated blood pressure and heart rate, and in situ thrombosis. Cocaine use therefore results in increased incidence of MI, aortic dissection, stroke, and other cardiovascular complications. Overall, ACS in patients with a history of cocaine use should be treated in the same manner as patients without cocaine use. The exception is in patients with ACS in the presence of acute cocaine intoxication. For patients with acute cocaine intoxication, cautious lowering of blood pressure is the most important next step. In addition, patients with signs of acute cocaine intoxication (e.g., euphoria, tachycardia, and hypertension), beta-blockers should be avoided unless patients are receiving coronary vasodilator therapy. In these patients, it is reasonable to use benzodiazepines alone or in combination with IV nitroglycerin to manage hypertension and tachycardia and signs of acute cocaine intoxication. In the absence of acute intoxication and when beta-blockers are likely to be safe to use, labetalol may be preferable due to its concomitant α-blocking action. In this case, the patient has acute intoxication and the concern is more for myocardial ischemia, especially vasospasm, and less for aortic dissection (different pain characteristics—no radiation to back; not worse pain of lifetime; not sudden in onset—also, no mediastinal widening on chest x-ray and equal BP in both arms). If the patient has persistent tachycardia and has normal LVEF by bedside echocardiogram, non-dihydropyridine calcium channel blockers can also be added to nitroglycerin and benzodiazepine, if needed. Coronary angiography is advisable if the discomfort and the ECG changes persist after optimization of the blood pressure.

37.18 Answer B. The patient will require interruption in clopidogrel therapy with his upcoming surgery. Although contemporary DES have much lower rates of late stent thrombosis, they still require at least 12 months of DAPT after ACS. The requirement for at least 12 months of DAPT after ACS applies for both DES and BMS. The risk of stent thrombosis in patients treated with any stent is greatest in the first days to weeks after implantation. Cessation of DAPT during this period, particularly for patients undergoing surgery, is associated with increased rate of stent thrombosis. Therefore, a BMS is best reserved for patients who cannot receive DAPT for more than ≈1 month for reasons of active bleeding, nonadherence to medical therapy, or planned surgery (whereas a minimum of 3 months may be reasonable with DES). This patient has fortunately a low risk for restenosis with a BMS, given he has a very large reference vessel diameter, a short lesion length, and no diabetes (all three are major predictors of restenosis).

37.19 Answer D. For patients with NSTEMI, ticagrelor 180 mg loading dose followed by 90 mg twice daily or clopidogrel 300 mg or 600 mg loading dose followed by 75 mg daily are indicated (Class I recommendation). In patients who are planned for an invasive or an ischemia-guided strategy, ticagrelor use is preferred over clopidogrel because it has incremental benefits and further reduces ischemic complications (namely the composite end-point of vascular death, MI, or—driven by a significant reduction in vascular death and MI). An overall mortality benefit was also observed with ticagrelor compared to clopidogrel in the PLATO trial. Prasugrel use (60 mg followed by 10 mg daily) is reserved for patients in whom the coronary anatomy is delineated and for those who are undergoing PCI (as per the design of the TRITON-TIMI 38 trial). Prasugrel was superior to clopidogrel in the head-to-head TRITON-TIMI 38 trial and reduced the composite end-point significantly, which was driven solely by a reduction in MI (no mortality benefit). Prasugrel, on the other hand, increased the primary safety end-point of major bleeding, is contraindicated in patients with prior TIA/stroke and had no net clinical benefit in elderly (>75 years of age) or underweight (<60 kg) patients. Prasugrel benefits appear more pronounced in acute MI patients with diabetes. Both prasugrel and ticagrelor are FDA approved for acute MI patients (and not for elective PCI, for which their use is off-label).

37.20 Answer A. Criterion A is a component of the TIMI risk score. The GRACE (Global Registry of Acute Coronary Events) risk score for ACS patients was derived and from over 11,000 patients in the GRACE registry and was validated in two additional datasets encompassing more than 16,000 ACS patients in general clinical practice. The eight variables used in the GRACE risk model are age, Killip class, SBP, serum creatinine level, heart rate (defined as continuous outcomes); ST-segment deviation, cardiac arrest at admission, and positive cardiac biomarkers level (defined as binary outcomes) (Granger CB, et al. *Arch Intern Med* 2003;163(19):2345–2353). A patient's GRACE risk score is calculated by adding points corresponding to all these variables (https://www.mdcalc.com/grace-acs-risk-mortality-calculator). Other common risk assessment tools include the TIMI risk score, the PURSUIT (Platelet Glycoprotein IIb/IIIa in Unstable Angina: Receptor Suppression Using Integrilin Therapy) risk score, the GRACE risk score, and the NCDR-ACTION (National Cardiovascular Data Registry-Acute Coronary Treatment and Intervention Outcomes Network) registry risk score. The 2014 AHA/ACC NSTE-ACS Guideline emphasizes that risk scores should be used to assess prognosis in patients with NSTE-ACS (Class I recommendation, LOE A).

37.21 Answer A. It is ill-advised to switch to UFH in patients who already received enoxaparin. The SYNERGY (Superior Yield of the New Strategy of Enoxaparin, Revascularization and Glycoprotein IIb/IIIa Inhibitors) trial compared enoxaparin to UFH in patients with NSTE-ACS undergoing PCI. Although there were no significant differences in the ischemic efficacy endpoint, more bleeding was noted in the enoxaparin group. A post hoc analysis suggested that this increase in bleeding may be attributed to the higher rate of bleeding among patients who were switched from enoxaparin to heparin during the PCI. The ACUITY (Acute Catheterization and Urgent Intervention Triage Strategy) trial demonstrated that bivalirudin may be safer (lesser TIMI major bleeding) than, but equally efficacious to, heparin/enoxaparin with a GP IIb/IIIa inhibitor among moderate- to high-risk patients undergoing PCI for NSTE-ACS. Also of note, in patients who have received fewer than two doses of therapeutic enoxaparin or received the last dose more than 8 to 12 hours before PCI, additional 0.3 mg/kg IV of enoxaparin is recommended. Cangrelor and eptifibatide are parenteral antiplatelet and not anticoagulant therapies (adenosine diphosphate [ADP] and glycoprotein IIb/IIIa antagonists, respectively).

37.22 Answer E. This patient's clinical presentation has overall low-risk features. She even has some attributes that make her symptoms atypical or noncardiac (i.e., prolonged duration of symptoms without evidence of myonecrosis). Therefore, she does not need an invasive strategy (coronary angiography with intent to revascularize) and certainly not an immediate/urgent invasive strategy (within 2 hours). The latter strategy is indicated in patients with definite NSTE-ACS who have hemodynamic instability, refractory ischemia, heart failure, etc. (representing, in general, <5% to 10% of all NSTE-ACS patients). Troponin levels, when available, should be the biomarkers of choice to rule out and diagnose MI (please refer to the third Universal Definition of Myocardial Infarction released in 2012). CK-MB levels can be used only when troponin measurements are not available; otherwise, they should not be used routinely. The 2014 AHA/ACC NSTE-ACS Guideline clearly states that with contemporary troponin assays, CK myocardial isoenzyme (CK-MB) and myoglobin are not useful for diagnosis of ACS. In 2017 (3 years after the release of the 2014 NSTE-ACS guidelines), the fourth-generation troponin assays became approved by the FDA for clinical use, and these are very highly sensitive compared to the existing assays and will likely enable rapid emergency department triage of patients suspected with NSTE-ACS. CK is a very nonspecific marker to diagnose myonecrosis and should be completely abandoned (same for myoglobin). A noninvasive stress test is appropriate, but she is unlikely to be able to exercise adequately (to achieve 85% of her maximally predicted heart rate) given her severe knee osteoarthritis. Therefore, she likely will need pharmacologic stress testing (e.g., adenosine vasodilator or dobutamine). Finally, an imaging modality added to the stress ECG test appears to be needed given abnormalities in her baseline ECG tracing (and likely presence of left ventricular hypertrophy, given suboptimal blood pressure control and CKD—even if not manifest on ECG).

37.23 Answer D. The patient presents to the emergency room with symptoms consistent with an ACS. Rapid assessment and monitoring are needed.

Current ACC/AHA guidelines recommend against the use of CK-MB and myoglobin for the diagnosis of ACS (Class III recommendation). This is concordant with the recommendation of the Writing Committee of the Third Universal Definition of MI, which support the use of the highly sensitive and highly specific cardiac troponin levels as the biomarkers of choice to diagnose MI. The other recommendations are either Class I or Class II for early risk stratification in this patient. In addition to obtaining (and evaluating) an ECG within 10 minutes of presentation, and subsequently obtaining serial ECG or continuous ECG monitoring when the initial ECG is nondiagnostic, the 2014 AHA/ACC NSTE-ACS Guideline state that it is reasonable to obtain supplemental ECG leads V7 to V9 in patients whose initial ECG is nondiagnostic and who are at intermediate/high risk of ACS. Leads V7-V9 may help diagnose lateral ischemia—usually involving the left circumflex artery, which can be sometimes electrically silent on a standard 12-lead ECG.

37.24 Answer C. In an ACS patient, pulmonary edema is associated with a very high short-term risk, as it indicates the ACS is complicated with heart failure. Complications of ACS (predominantly MI) include hemodynamic complications (isolated left or right heart failure, biventricular failure, cardiogenic shock, and mechanical complications), arrhythmias (e.g., ventricular tachycardia or fibrillation, atrial fibrillation, and atrioventricular [AV] nodal block), pericardial complication, and other miscellaneous complications. The other features listed are components of the TIMI risk score and certainly denote increased risk. However, pulmonary edema indicative of CHF likely represents the highest risk clinical feature. Examples of low-risk features include normal levels of cardiac biomarkers and a normal ECG with ongoing chest discomfort.

37.25 Answer E. Sublingual nitroglycerin is indicated for ongoing ischemic symptoms. Nitroglycerin is excellent antianginal/anti-ischemic medications. They reduce myocardial oxygen demand by reducing preload and wall stress, but they do not confer survival benefit and are not indicated in this asymptomatic patient. Supplemental oxygen should be administered to patients with NSTE-ACS with arterial oxygen saturation <90%, respiratory distress, or other high-risk features of hypoxemia. Data indicate that supplemental oxygen may be even deleterious in normoxemic patients. IV morphine should be used cautiously and may be reasonable for continued ischemi chest pain despite maximally tolerated anti-ischemic medications. IV beta-blockers are ill-advised in patients with ACS; they are associated with increased complications and especially a small but existent risk of cardiogenic shock (particularly in those with large MI and low-output state). Oral beta-blockers maybe started within the first 24 hours in the absence of heart failure, low-output state, risk for cardiogenic shock, or other contraindications.

37.26 Answer E. In this older patient with NSTEMI who chooses medical management after fully understanding its risks and benefits, optimizing medical therapy is the best course of action. The 2014 ACC/AHA NSTE-ACS Guideline gives a Class I recommendation to pneumococcal vaccine in patients 65 years or older and in high-risk patients (smokers, asthmatics) with CAD. Immunocompromised adults should receive the 13-valent conjugate vaccine in addition to the 23-valent vaccine. Treatment decisions after NSTE-ACS should be patient-centered and consider patient preferences, comorbidities, functional and cognitive status, and life expectancy. Adding ranolazine or switching to clopidogrel or prasugrel is not the next best course of action. Ranolazine is an antianginal medication that is usually added for symptom relief, on top of conventional anti-anginal agents (or when intolerant to antianginal medications); it confers no hard-outcome benefit and it is therefore not indicated in the absence of anginal symptoms. Ticagrelor is the preferred antiplatelet agent (along with aspirin 81 mg) in patients with medically treated NSTE-ACS, as it was shown to be superior to clopidogrel in the PLATO trial (with significant reduction in vascular and overall mortality and in nonfatal MI). On the other hand, prasugrel is not indicated in this medically managed NSTE-ACS patient.

37.27 Answer B. The TIMI risk score is developed as a simple tool to assess the prognosis of patients presenting with unstable angina/NSTEMI. It is therefore a risk stratification tool—not a diagnostic tool. It is a simple tool, nowadays available as an electronic calculator, composed of seven risk indicators that help predict the risk of cardiac events (Table A37-27). The rates of all-cause mortality, MI, and severe recurrent ischemia prompting urgent revascularization through 14 days increase as TIMI risk score increases. Aspirin used within the last *7 days* is one of the risk indicators (Antman EM, et al. *JAMA* 2000;284(7):835-842).

Table A37-27 TIMI risk score for unstable angina/non–ST-elevation MI

TIMI Risk Score	All-Cause Mortality, New or Recurrent MI, or Severe Recurrent Ischemia Requiring Urgent Revascularization Through 14 d After Randomization, %
0–1	4.7
2	8.3
3	13.2
4	19.9
5	26.2
6–7	40.9

The TIMI risk score is determined by the sum of the presence of seven variables at admission. One point is given for each of the following variables: age 65 y or older, at least three risk factors for CAD, prior coronary stenosis of 50% or more, ST-segment deviation on ECG presentation, at least two anginal events in the prior 24 h, use of aspirin in the prior 7 days, and elevated serum cardiac biomarkers. Prior coronary stenosis of 50% or more remained relatively insensitive to missing information and remained a significant predictor of events.

CAD, coronary artery disease; ECG, electrocardiogram; h, hours; MI, myocardial infarction; y, year.

Modified from Antman EM, et al. *JAMA* 2000;284(7):835–842.

37.28 Answer D. Acute MI with pump failure is the most common etiology of cardiogenic shock (around 80% of cases). An IABP insertion is no longer recommended routinely in patients with cardiogenic shock. In the SHOCK II trial, IABP did not confer a survival benefit at 30 days or 1 year in acute MI-related cardiogenic shock who underwent PCI. Given the patient is obtunded (unable to protect his airways) and hypoxemic, urgent endotracheal intubation and mechanical ventilation are reasonable. A 2-D echocardiogram should be obtained at the bedside to assess the left and right ventricular function, rule out mechanical complications (e.g., ventricular septal defect, mitral regurgitation, free wall rupture), and basically confirm the clinically suspected diagnosis of cardiogenic shock. All cardiogenic shock patients should undergo immediate angiography and revascularization (preferably complete, although definitive data on the merits of complete revascularization in shock patients are not yet available). Beta-blockers (IV or oral) are contraindicated in patients with cardiogenic shock, and the elevated heart rate in a patient with cardiogenic shock is physiologic and helps maintain the patient's cardiac output (in the presence of diminished stroke volume).

37.29 Answer A. The vasodilator effect of phosphodiesterase inhibitors and nitroglycerin is mediated by the release of nitric oxide. The combination can cause severe hazardous hypotension and is thus contraindicated—especially in patients with ACS. Because of sildenafil half-life of 4 hours and vardenafil half-life of 4 to 6 hours, nitroglycerin is contraindicated (Class III recommendation) after the use of sildenafil or vardenafil within the previous 24 hours (or within 48 hours of tadalafil use).

37.30 Answer E. Vasospastic angina (Prinzmetal angina) typically occurs spontaneously at rest and is associated with transient ST elevation. It often occurs in clusters with long periods of no attacks. Variant angina is caused by coronary spasm that occurs in either normal or diseased vessels. Coronary spasm leads to myocardial ischemia and chest discomfort. Long-acting calcium channel blockers alone or in combination with long acting nitrates are useful to treat and reduce the frequency of vasospastic angina. Statins and cessation of tobacco use and additional atherosclerosis risk factor modification are also useful in these patients.

Provocative testing during invasive coronary angiography may be considered for suspected vasospastic angina when clinical criteria and noninvasive assessment fail to determine the diagnosis. Provocative testing during invasive coronary angiography (e.g., using ergonovine, acetylcholine, or methylergonovine) is relatively safe, especially when performed in a controlled manner by experienced operators. However, sustained spasm, serious arrhythmias, and even death can also occur but very infrequently. Therefore, provocative tests should be avoided in patients at risk (e.g., significant left main disease, advanced three-vessel disease, presence of high-grade obstructive lesions, significant valvular stenosis, significant LV systolic dysfunction, and advanced heart failure).

38 Percutaneous Coronary Intervention Guidelines*

Glenn N. Levine

QUESTIONS

38.1 A 54-year-old physically fit female that does not smoke complains of 6 months of progressive exertional dyspnea. She has hyperlipidemia (LDL cholesterol 221 mg/dL before treatment initiated 5 years ago) and a strong family history of premature coronary artery disease (CAD). You refer her for nuclear stress testing, which reveals transient left ventricular (LV) dilation and decreased LV ejection fraction (EF) with exercise. You perform diagnostic angiography and find a 40% to 50% mid-left main coronary artery narrowing, an 80% mid-right coronary artery (RCA) lesion, and diffuse but noncritical disease in the left anterior descending (LAD) and left circumflex (LCx) arteries. Her calculated SYNTAX score is 34. You perform an intravascular ultrasound (IVUS) on the left main lesion, and the findings are shown in Figure Q38-1. What is the recommended way to proceed?

(A) Medical management only
(B) Repeat angiography and IVUS in 6 months to assess for left main lesion progression
(C) Percutaneous coronary intervention (PCI) of left main and RCA lesions
(D) Coronary artery bypass graft (CABG) surgery

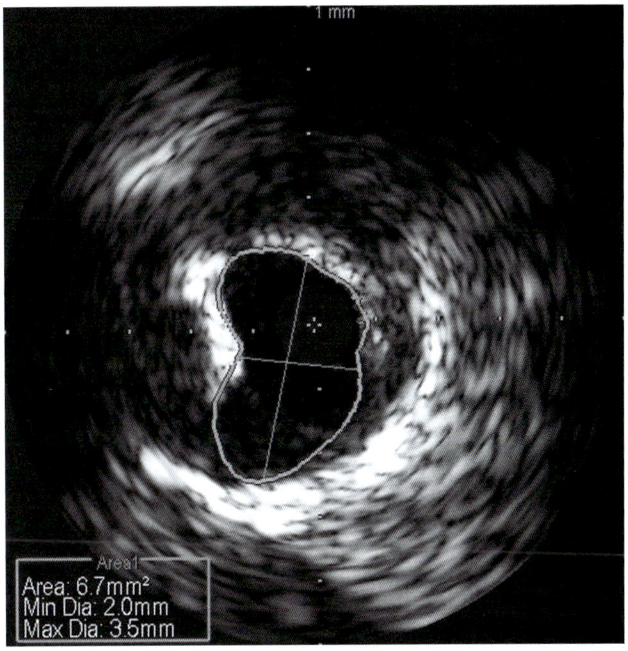

Figure Q38-1 Intravascular ultrasound of the left main coronary artery.

*Questions based on the 2011 ACC/AHA/SCAI PCI Guideline, the 2013 ACC/AHA STEMI Guideline, the 2014 ACC/AHA NSTE-ACS Guideline, the 2014 ACC/AHA/AATS/PCNA/SCAI/STS SIHD Focused Update, the 2015 ACC/AHA/SCAI Primary PCI Focused Update, and the 2016 ACC/AHA Duration of DAPT Focused Update.

38.2 A 57-year-old woman with a history of hypertension and hyperlipidemia presents to your office for a second opinion. She underwent LAD stenting with a second-generation drug-eluting stent (DES) 3 years ago for chronic stable angina. She has been on atenolol, amlodipine, atorvastatin, aspirin, and nitrates and is angina-free. Her primary care physician (PCP) ordered an exercise stress test, in which she exercised for 11 minutes on a Bruce protocol and achieved 12 METS and 94% maximum predicted heart rate with no evidence of ischemia. She underwent cardiac computed tomography (CT) at her own request and was found to have a significant stenosis in her LCx artery. She then underwent catheterization that showed minimal (30%) restenosis in the LAD, a large dominant RCA with a 40% distal stenosis, and 80% proximal stenosis in a moderate-sized LCx artery. She wants your opinion regarding her management and how best to decrease her future risk of myocardial infarction (MI) or death. You would advise:

(A) Continue current medication regimen but no revascularization
(B) Fractional flow reserve (FFR) of the LCx artery; if <0.80, proceed to PCI
(C) PCI of the LCx artery
(D) Add clopidogrel therapy but no revascularization

38.3 She is not satisfied with your answer and goes to another cardiologist who evaluates the LCx artery lesion with IVUS and FFR. Studies show an FFR of 0.86, and 70% cross-sectional area stenosis by IVUS, with minimal lumen diameter of 2.1 mm^2 and minimal lumen area of 4.2 mm^2. She is still asymptomatic and returns to your office wanting your opinion regarding revascularization.

(A) The IVUS data demonstrate a clear indication for PCI
(B) FFR indicates a benefit for proceeding with PCI
(C) Both the IVUS data and the FFR data indicate a benefit with PCI
(D) Both the IVUS and FFR data indicate a likely good prognosis with continued medical therapy

38.4 A 46-year-old male with a history of hyperlipidemia and tobacco use presents with stable exertional chest pain for 3 months. On a stress thallium test, he exercises to 11 METS and has a large anterior wall ischemic defect and LVEF of 60%. He undergoes cardiac catheterization, which shows a 75% mid-LAD stenosis that is treated with a 21-mm everolimus-eluting stent. He is not on chronic nonsteroidal anti-inflammatory drugs (NSAID) or oral anticoagulation, consumes 2 to 3 beers per week, and has normal hemoglobin and platelet counts. According to the 2016 American College of Cardiology (ACC)/American Heart Association (AHA) Duration of Dual Antiplatelet Therapy (DAPT) focused update, what should you recommend regarding duration of clopidogrel therapy?

(A) Three months of DAPT is appropriate for him to minimize the risk of bleeding
(B) At least 6 months of DAPT is recommended and >6 months of therapy may be reasonable
(C) At least 12 months of DAPT is recommended and >12 months of therapy may be reasonable
(D) Prolonged (>12 months) of DAPT is recommended

38.5 You are at a tertiary care institute with PCI capabilities and are called on for management advice of a 44-year-old female who presents to a rural ER with 1 hour of chest pain. She has a history of uterine fibroids, hypertension, and heavy cigarette use. On presentation, she is in significant distress with a heart rate of 110 beats per minute (bpm) and a blood pressure of 110/60 mm Hg. Electrocardiography (ECG) shows 3-mm ST-segment elevation in the anterior leads. It will take approximately 150 minutes to transfer her to your tertiary care facility. What should you advise the rural ER physician?

(A) Administer aspirin and heparin and transfer the patient for primary PCI
(B) Administer aspirin, heparin, and thrombolytic therapy, and then transfer the patient
(C) Administer aspirin, heparin, and half-dose thrombolytic therapy, and then transfer the patient
(D) Perform a diagnostic catheterization there, and then transfer the patient if she has thrombotic occlusion of the LAD

38.6 A 79-year-old male presented to a hospital 3 days ago with chest pain for 10 hours. At that time, he had ST-segment elevation in the inferior ECG leads and received fibrinolytic therapy because the hospital was not PCI-capable. With fibrinolytic therapy, there was no resolution of ST-segment changes, and he continued to have chest pain, which only gradually decreased and then resolved after 6 hours. His peak troponin was 46 ng/mL. He did well clinically over the next 2 days. His children urged him to undergo catheterization, which showed a 100% posterior descending artery (PDA) lesion and a diffuse 60% lesion in the LAD. No left-to-right collateral artery flow was visualized. The patient's cardiologist and family asked that he be transferred to your hospital for PCI of the occluded PDA. What would you advise?

(A) On the basis of observational and experimental data, infarct artery patency favorably influences LV remodeling and electrical stability; therefore, PCI to the PDA is recommended
(B) PCI of the occluded PDA and the 60% LAD stenosis will improve his prognosis and should be done in one procedure
(C) PCI of the occluded PDA, and the 60% LAD stenosis will improve his prognosis but should be done as a staged procedure
(D) PCI of the occluded PDA at this time is not of benefit and should not be performed

38.7 You have recently been appointed to the quality review board of your hospital. They are reviewing a protocol of cardiac biomarker (creatine-kinase-MB [CK-MB], troponin I or T) measurement after every PCI. Which of the following is NOT true?

(A) Per the 2011 ACC/AHA guidelines, in patients who have signs or symptoms suggestive of MI during or after PCI, or in asymptomatic patients with significant persistent angiographic complications (e.g., large side-branch occlusion, flow-limiting dissection, no-reflow phenomenon, or coronary thrombosis), CK-MB and troponin I or T should be measured (Class I)
(B) Routine measurement of cardiac biomarkers (CK-MB and/or troponin I or T) in all patients after PCI may be reasonable (Class IIb)
(C) The benefit of routinely measuring cardiac biomarkers in patients undergoing PCI has been demonstrated in multiple observational and randomized studies
(D) Recommendations regarding measurements of cardiac biomarkers after PCI are essentially "expert opinion" recommendations (i.e., without supporting studies demonstrating benefit)

38.8 A 76-year-old retired acupuncturist presents to your office with increasing shortness of breath. The patient's history is only remarkable for hyperlipidemia for which he takes red rice yeast. He is referred for cardiac catheterization after a stress test that shows anterior ischemia and is found to have a 90% mid-LAD lesion and a normal EF. He states that he is willing to take medicine but does not want PCI or CABG. His concerned wife wants to know which treatment is best for his long-term survival? What do you tell her?

(A) This lesion is called the "widow maker" and should be expeditiously treated with PCI to improve long-term survival
(B) Head-to-head trials of PCI vs. CABG for such lesions show a mortality benefit with CABG, so her husband should undergo CABG
(C) Minimally invasive surgery with placement of a left internal mammary artery (LIMA) graft to the LAD is the best option to improve survival
(D) Neither PCI nor CABG is recommended to improve survival

38.9 A 76-year-old woman with diabetes and chronic kidney disease (CKD) (creatinine = 1.9 mg/dL; estimated GFR = 43 mL/min) comes to your clinic. She has exertional chest pain consistent with angina. She gets this several times a week when walking up a hill. Her heart rate is 78 bpm and her blood pressure is 140/80 mm Hg. Her current medications include insulin, aspirin, and terazosin. She desires to have better exercise capacity so she can take her dog on longer walks in the hilly area where she lives. You consider the options of a trial of medical therapy vs. catheterization and possible stent implantation, as well as the risk of contrast nephropathy. Regarding contrast nephropathy, which of the following is NOT correct?

(A) Both the patient's diabetes and CKD place her at increased risk of contrast nephropathy
(B) Administration of *N*-acetylcysteine is useful to reduce the risk of contrast nephropathy
(C) Preprocedural hydration is useful to reduce the risk of contrast nephropathy
(D) Minimization of contrast reduces the risk of contrast nephropathy

38.10 In the precath clinic, you see a 58-year-old woman with Class III angina despite treatment with metoprolol, amlodipine, and isosorbide. She does not remember having any adverse reaction to past studies, but she does recall feeling ill and flushed after eating shellfish several years ago. A 73-year-old man also with Class III angina despite good medical therapy underwent a contrast CT study several years ago and remembers developing urticarial and mild bronchospasm afterward. What is the best way to manage these two patients?

(A) Neither patient requires anaphylactoid prophylaxis (steroid and antihistamine)
(B) Both patients require anaphylactoid prophylaxis (steroid and antihistamine)
(C) The 58-year-old woman does not require anaphylactoid prophylaxis, but the 73-year-old man does require anaphylactoid prophylaxis (steroid and antihistamine)
(D) The 58-year-old woman can safely undergo catheterization with anaphylactoid prophylaxis, but the 73-year-old man should not be exposed to the risk of anaphylaxis and should not undergo the catheterization

38.11 A 48-year-old malpractice lawyer recently underwent implantation of a single DES to the mid-LAD for stable angina and was placed on clopidogrel. He is concerned that he was prescribed clopidogrel and seeks your opinion on his management. He has heard of "clopidogrel resistance" but was never sent for platelet function testing or genetic testing (for CYP2C19). The best response to him is:

(A) Since this was an LAD lesion, he should have undergone both platelet function testing and genetic testing
(B) He should have undergone platelet function testing but not genetic testing
(C) Genetic testing is more predictive of clopidogrel efficacy, so he should have undergone this, but not platelet function testing
(D) Neither routine platelet function testing nor genetic testing is recommended

38.12 A 46-year-old woman who underwent placement of two DES to the proximal RCA several years ago for worsening chronic stable angina moved to your town and makes an appointment with you for cardiology follow-up. As best she remembers, she was told her other arteries had only "mild blockage." She is now able to engage in daily moderate exercise without chest pains or dyspnea on exertion (DOE). She is concerned that she has had no follow-up testing to make sure the other blockages have not progressed or that the stent has not "blocked up again." The most appropriate advice you can give to her is:

(A) She is right to be concerned about silent restenosis or progression of disease and a nuclear stress test should be performed
(B) She is right to be concerned about silent restenosis or progression of disease and a cardiac catheterization should be performed
(C) She is right to be concerned about silent restenosis or progression of disease and a coronary CT scan should be performed
(D) Routine periodic stress testing of asymptomatic patients after PCI without specific clinical indications is of no benefit and is not recommended

38.13 A 73-year-old man admitted for several days of rest angina has a 20-year history of non–insulin-dependent diabetes, hypertension, and hyperlipidemia. His troponin was mildly elevated, and his ECG showed left ventricular hypertrophy with repolarization abnormalities that were similar to prior ECGs. Echocardiogram revealed LVEF 45% with anterior wall and mid/distal inferior wall hypokinesis. You perform diagnostic catheterization that reveals an 80% proximal LAD lesion and three sequential proximal RCA lesions. The left circumflex has diffuse but noncritical disease. The calculated SYNTAX score is 27. The LAD and RCA can be treated with either PCI or CABG. Based on recent studies and the guidelines, what is the best advice you can give the patient?

(A) Now that we have DES, your outcome with stents is as good as CABG
(B) Treatment with DES will lead to a better long-term outcome than CABG
(C) Given your diabetes, you are best treated with CABG
(D) Randomized trial data do not apply to you, so either treatment option is fine

38.14 A 55-year-old literature professor is brought by ambulance to the emergency room with 3 hours of crushing chest pain. ECG shows 3 mm of inferior ST-segment elevation. You rapidly bring the patient to the catheterization laboratory and demonstrate occlusion of the distal RCA. A wire is easily passed across the occlusion. You consider manual aspiration thrombectomy. You should:

(A) Routinely perform manual aspiration thrombectomy in ST-elevation myocardial infarction (STEMI) based on the benefit shown in the TAPAS study
(B) Not routinely perform manual aspiration thrombectomy in primary PCI
(C) Perform rheolytic thrombectomy, which yields greater thrombus removal
(D) Manually aspirate the blood proximal to the thrombus to prevent further thrombus formation

38.15 You are referred a 67-year-old man for PCI before knee surgery. He had not experienced angina with modest activity (4 to 5 METS), but because of his limited exercise capacity, his PCP ordered a nuclear stress test before his scheduled knee replacement. The stress test revealed inferior wall ischemia, and the patient underwent diagnostic angiography that revealed a 70% to 80% mid-RCA lesion. Echocardiogram reveals normal EF without focal wall motion abnormalities. The knee surgery is scheduled for 5 weeks from now. You recommend to the patient:

(A) He should proceed to knee replacement without revascularization
(B) He should have balloon angioplasty but not stent implantation
(C) He should have a bare metal stent (BMS) and treatment with DAPT for 4 weeks

(D) He should have a bioabsorbable scaffold DES and treatment with DAPT for 4 weeks
(E) He should have a second-generation DES and delay knee replacement for 3 to 6 months

38.16 An 87-year-old man is admitted to the coronary care unit (CCU) with non-ST-elevation acute coronary syndrome (NSTE-ACS). The peak troponin is 1.3 ng/mL, and the ECG shows a prior known left bundle-branch block (LBBB). The patient experienced 2 days of stuttering chest pain, with the last pain occurring sometime yesterday. He has a history of several strokes, metastatic prostate cancer treated with antiandrogen therapy, CKD stage II, and a below-the-knee amputation. He tells you that several friends and relatives have had bad experiences with stents and bypass surgery. He is willing to undergo diagnostic catheterization if you think he should, but will not agree to either PCI or CABG. The most appropriate plan of action for you is to:

(A) Perform diagnostic catheterization for risk stratification within 24 to 48 hours of admission
(B) Perform urgent diagnostic catheterization for risk stratification that day
(C) Request a psychiatry evaluation of his competence
(D) Not perform catheterization and treat medically

38.17 A 49-year-old woman is admitted to the step-down unit with NSTE-ACS. ECG shows 0.5-mm inferior ST depression, and peak troponin is 2.7 ng/mL. She is treated with aspirin, ticagrelor, and fondaparinux. The next day you perform diagnostic catheterization that shows a 90% mid-RCA lesion. How should you manage her anticoagulation during PCI?

(A) Proceed with PCI without additional anticoagulation, as she recently received fondaparinux
(B) Check activated clotting time (ACT) and proceed based on that result (i.e., administer additional fondaparinux if ACT < 180 seconds).
(C) Give an additional dose of 0.3 mg/kg of intravenous (IV) fondaparinux
(D) Administer full-dose unfractionated heparin and proceed with PCI

38.18 You are emergently called to perform angiography on a 69-year-old woman who presented to the emergency room with 4 hours of left arm heaviness and shortness of breath. ECG shows 2-mm lateral ST-segment elevation. She has no prior cardiac history and is on hydrochlorothiazide for hypertension and Naprosyn for osteoarthritis. Catheterization reveals a totally occluded mid-LCx artery, a 70% mid-LAD stenosis, and diffuse but mild disease of the RCA. Primary PCI of the occluded LCx proceeds expeditiously and without complication. Which of the following is a reasonable approach for the mid-LAD lesion?

(A) Stick to a strategy of culprit vessel-only PCI
(B) Perform PCI now
(C) Perform PCI several days later during the hospitalization
(D) Perform FFR of the LAD lesion in several days and stent only if the FFR is <0.8
(E) Any of the above

38.19 You are managing a 79-year-old patient with a history of several significant gastrointestinal (GI) bleeds for which the etiology is unknown, despite extensive workup. He also has diabetes, CKD, and chronic mild anemia. Despite treatment with metoprolol, isosorbide, amlodipine, and ranolazine, the patient has an unacceptable quality of life and desires to undergo catheterization and stent implantation, if appropriate. Catheterization demonstrates a long (40 mm), tight mid-RCA lesion. The artery is only 2.5 mm in diameter. You are reluctant to place a BMS, out of concern about a high risk of restenosis, so you proceed with second-generation DES implantation. What is the most appropriate antiplatelet therapy?

(A) Clopidogrel only for 3 months
(B) Acetylsalicylic acid (ASA) 81 mg only indefinitely
(C) ASA 81 mg indefinitely and clopidogrel for 3 months
(D) ASA 81 mg indefinitely and clopidogrel for 6 months
(E) ASA 81 mg indefinitely and clopidogrel for 30 months based on the DAPT study

38.20 A very anxious 78-year-old man with Class IV angina comes to your office for consultation. He has had progressive angina for the last several years but is worried about the complications of angiography and coronary stenting. He has CKD stage III, diabetes, and hypertension. You inform him that there are many things you can do to decrease the risk of procedural complications. All of the following are associated with a decreased risk of complications, EXCEPT:

(A) Preprocedure hydration
(B) Pre- and postprocedure administration of *N*-acetylcysteine
(C) Pre-PCI high-dose statin administration
(D) Perform catheterization via the radial artery
(E) Minimize dose of contrast agent

38.21 A 54-year-old woman presents to a community hospital with 1 hour of chest discomfort and nausea. ECG shows 3-mm ST-segment elevation in the inferior leads, and she is treated with fibrinolytic therapy. Her chest discomfort and ST elevations resolve shortly afterward. She is then transferred to your hospital. On arrival 1 hour later, she is comfortable. On exam, her heart rate is 80 bpm, blood pressure is 120/80 mm Hg, and she is not in heart failure. The most reasonable next step in her management is:

(A) Immediate catheterization and PCI (if appropriate)
(B) Angiography 3 to 24 hours after fibrinolysis and PCI (if appropriate)
(C) Coronary angiography before hospital discharge
(D) Coronary angiography 2 to 4 weeks after discharge

38.22 You have placed a DES in the proximal LCx artery of a 73-year-old patient admitted with NSTE-ACS. The patient has a history of diabetes, a cerebrovascular accident (CVA) 3 years ago, irritable bowel syndrome, and vitiligo. He has been on aspirin, 81 mg daily, and clopidogrel, 75 mg daily, for the last 2 years since implantation of a DES in the proximal LAD. Platelet function testing reveals a platelet reactivity unit (PRU) of 247 (high platelet reactivity). Reasonable management options would include all the following, EXCEPT:

(A) Continue him on aspirin and clopidogrel
(B) Treat him with aspirin and ticagrelor
(C) Treat him with aspirin and prasugrel

38.23 You are planning to perform PCI in a patient who underwent diagnostic angiography one week ago and was found to have sequential mid-LAD lesions. The patient has a recent history of heparin-induced thrombocytopenia. His current platelet count is 110. The most appropriate anticoagulant to use during PCI is:

(A) Unfractionated heparin (UFH)
(B) Low molecular weight heparin (enoxaparin)
(C) Anti-Xa inhibitor, such as fondaparinux
(D) Bivalirudin

38.24 An 87-year-old gentleman with history of CABG 11 years ago now presents with NSTE-ACS. As you contemplate the potential of PCI of an old saphenous vein graft (SVG), you review the guidelines on SVG PCI. Which of the following is INCORRECT?

(A) Adverse cardiac events rates are doubled after SVG PCI compared with native-artery PCI
(B) Embolic protection devices should be used during SVG PCI when technically feasible
(C) Platelet glycoprotein IIb/IIIa inhibitors should be used during SVG PCI
(D) PCI of a chronic SVG occlusion is not recommended

38.25 A 43-year-old man was admitted from the ER after complaining of 1 week of stuttering, angina-quality chest pain. High-sensitivity serum troponin was mildly elevated, and ECG showed 1 mm anterior ST depression. He was given 1 mg/kg subcutaneous enoxaparin. Six hours later, he develops diaphoresis and heavy chest pressure. Repeat ECG shows 4-mm ST elevation and emergent angiography demonstrates an occluded mid-LAD. According to published studies and the 2014 ACC/AHA NSTE-ACS guideline, how should you manage his anticoagulation therapy as you proceed with PCI?

(A) No further anticoagulation is required as he received enoxaparin 6 hours prior
(B) An additional 1 mg/kg subcutaneous enoxaparin should be administered
(C) An additional 0.3 mg/kg IV should be administered
(D) Full-dose UFH should be administered

38.26 One year ago, you placed two second-generation DES in a complex LAD/diagonal bifurcation lesion of a 61-year-old patient with long-standing diabetes and heavy smoking history who experienced acute coronary syndrome (ACS). The stent in the LAD was 30 mm long and 2.75 mm in diameter; the stent in the diagonal was 18 mm long and 2.25 mm in diameter. He has done well since. His medications include insulin, metoprolol, lisinopril, aspirin, and prasugrel. Based on study data and current guidelines, the best management of his antiplatelet therapy at this time is probably:

(A) Stop the aspirin and continue prasugrel
(B) Stop the prasugrel and continue aspirin
(C) Continue the aspirin and continue the prasugrel at least 18 to 30 months more
(D) Continue the aspirin and change the prasugrel to rivaroxaban 2.5 mg daily

38.27 A 93-year-old patient with chronic stable angina comes to your clinic. The patient has a history of hypertension, CKD stage III, upper GI bleed, osteoarthritis, and gout. Despite intensive antianginal therapy, his angina has progressed and he now has chest pain with minimal activity. You reluctantly proceed with catheterization. A distal RCA lesion is present and you place a 16-mm DES. To decrease bleeding risk in this patient while on DAPT, you should:

(A) Have him take aspirin in the morning and clopidogrel in the evening, both with meals
(B) Prescribe Tums be taken 3 times daily
(C) Prescribe a histamine 2 (H2) blocker
(D) Prescribe a proton pump inhibitor (PPI)

38.28 You are called at 3 AM for a STEMI. The patient presented with 1 hour of epigastric pain and nausea. ECG shows 2-mm ST-segment elevation in the inferior leads. Angiography reveals a complex 70% distal left main stenosis, an 80% proximal LCx artery lesion, and a totally occluded proximal RCA that appears to be a freshly occluded vessel (Fig. Q38-28). You perform primary PCI on the RCA with placement of a DES. Two weeks later, the patient undergoes CABG. What would you recommend to the patient with respect to further DAPT therapy?

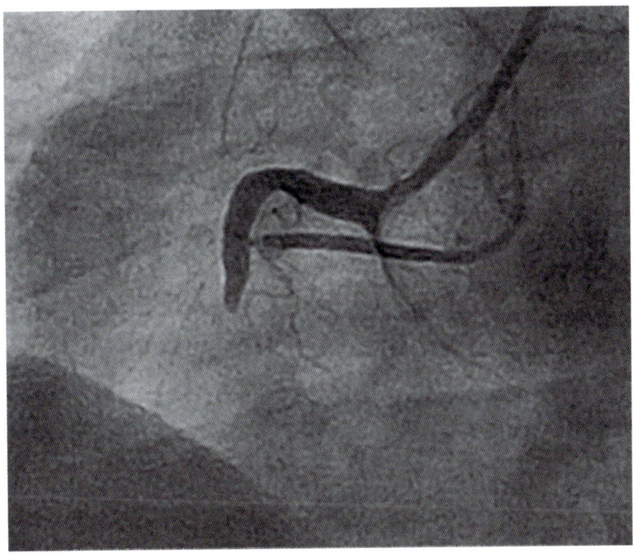

Figure Q38-28 Angiogram of the right coronary artery in a patient presenting with inferior ST-segment elevation. (Courtesy of Glenn Levine.)

(A) Continue aspirin, but stop clopidogrel now that CABG has been performed
(B) Continue aspirin; stop clopidogrel after a total of 3 months of therapy
(C) Continue aspirin; continue clopidogrel for a total of 12 months (or more) of DAPT
(D) Stop aspirin; continue clopidogrel indefinitely

38.29 You perform angiography on a 67-year-old admitted for NSTE-ACS. The patient has diabetes; CKD stage II; hypertension; a history of CVA 7 years ago with some residual left-sided weakness; a poorly healing foot ulcer; right leg cellulitis, for which he is receiving antibiotics; a history of GI bleed 4 years ago due to a gastric ulcer that has since been treated; and an EF of 44% with anterior and inferior hypokinesis. Angiography reveals a 40% to 50% ostial left main lesion, a discrete 70% proximal LAD lesion, a 50% mid-LCx lesion, and an 80% discrete proximal RCA lesion. All lesions and vessels are amenable to PCI and to bypass. The calculated Society of Thoracic Surgeons (STS) score for mortality is 4.2; the SYNTAX score is 24. The best treatment strategy is for you to recommend is:

(A) Multivessel PCI in one procedure
(B) Staged multivessel PCI
(C) CABG
(D) Hybrid PCI and CABG with minimally invasive bypass to the LAD and stenting of the RCA
(E) Discuss as a heart team

38.30 You are helping in the management of a 79-year-old patient with 70% distal left main disease and a 90% mid-RCA stenosis. Her EF is 35%. Because of multiple comorbidities, the patient is felt to be a prohibitively high-risk patient for CABG. You recommend:

(A) PCI with intra-aortic balloon pump (IABP) support, as this has been shown to improve outcome
(B) PCI with Impella, as this has been shown in a randomized trial to improve the risk of procedure-related death
(C) PCI with TandemHeart, as this has been shown in a randomized trial to improve the risk of procedure-related death
(D) PCI with hemodynamic support, although this has never been shown in a randomized trial to improve the risk of procedure-related death

ANSWERS AND EXPLANATIONS

38.1 Answer D. The IVUS of the left main coronary artery shows a minimal lumen area of 6.7 mm^2. The 2011 PCI guidelines state that for the left main coronary artery, a finding of a minimal lumen area >7.5 mm^2 by IVUS suggests that revascularization may be deferred (Levine GN, et al. *J Am Coll Cardiol* 2011;58(24):e44–e122). A minimal lumen area between 6 and 7.5 mm^2 requires further physiologic assessment. The patient has already had physiologic assessment with the nuclear stress test suggesting stress-induced global ischemia. Thus, the patient should be considered to have significant left main disease. CABG for significant left main disease is a Class I indication. PCI for left main disease is a Class IIa or Class IIb indication, depending on left main anatomy, likelihood of good long-term outcome, and the predicted risk of adverse surgical outcomes. One of the criteria for predicting this is the SYNTAX score. This patient has a high (≥33) SYNTAX score. As described, the patient is at low surgical risk. Thus, although stenting may be a reasonable approach, CABG is the recommended preferred approach in this patient, with revascularization of both the left main and RCA.

38.2 Answer A. The 2011 PCI guidelines give a Class III harm recommendation for PCI of non-LAD single-vessel disease for improvement of survival (Levine GN, et al. *J Am Coll Cardiol* 2011;58(24): e44–e122). The COURAGE trial (Boden WE, et al. *N Engl J Med* 2007;356(15):1503–1516) and other studies of such patients show that PCI does not decrease the future risk of MI or death. Although the FAME 2 trial (De Bruyne B, et al. *N Engl J Med* 2012;367(11):991–1001), published after the 2011 PCI guidelines, showed that FFR-guided PCI reduced the composite ischemic end point, the study did not show an overall reduction in the risk of either MI or death (only the landmark analysis after 8 days showed this). In addition, this patient would not have been enrolled in FAME 2, as patients needed to have either angina or documented ischemia on noninvasive testing to be enrolled in the study (see the study supplement), and this patient has neither. The patient does not have angina and thus PCI cannot improve her symptoms. The addition of clopidogrel to a patient with stable ischemic heart disease, and without prior MI, has not been shown to be of benefit. It would be extremely unlikely that the addition of clopidogrel now, 3 years after implantation of a second-generation DES in the LAD, would decrease the risk of very late stent thrombosis. Therefore, the best management option is continued current medical therapy.

38.3 Answer D. Per the 2011 PCI guidelines for non-left main stenoses, a minimal lumen diameter of >2.0 mm^2 and minimal lumen area of >4.0 mm^2 correlate with low rates of ischemic events (Levine GN, et al. *J Am Coll Cardiol* 2011;58(24): e44–e122). Furthermore, the FAME study found low clinical event rates at 2 years in patients with a FFR ≥ 0.8 (Tonino PA, et al. *N Engl J Med* 2009;360(3): 213–224). Thus, the best management option is continued current medical therapy.

38.4 Answer B. Recommendations for the duration of DAPT were updated in 2016 (Levine GN, et al. *J Am Coll Cardiol* 2016;68(10):1082–1115) based on the analysis of 11 studies. The recommendation also considered post-MI studies, such as PEGASUS (Bonaca MP, et al. *N Engl J Med* 2015;372(19): 1791–1800). In patients with stable ischemic heart disease undergoing second-generation DES implantation, the Class I recommendations is at least 6 months of DAPT (decreased from 12 months of treatment in the 2011 PCI guidelines); >6 months of DAPT may be reasonable and is a Class IIb recommendation. Treatment duration of at least 12 months applies to ACS patients undergoing coronary stent implantation; this patient has stable ischemic heart disease (SIHD). The patient is not at high bleeding risk, so he would not fall into the Class IIb recommendation that only 3 months of therapy may be reasonable in high bleeding-risk patients.

38.5 Answer B. Per the 2013 ACC/AHA STEMI guidelines, in the absence of contraindications, fibrinolytic therapy should be given to patients with STEMI and the onset of ischemic symptoms within the previous 12 hours when it is anticipated that primary PCI cannot be performed within 120 minutes of first medical contact (FMC) (O'Gara PT, et al. *J Am Coll Cardiol* 2013;61(4):e78–e140). Half-dose lytic therapy and a strategy of facilitated PCI have generally not been shown to be of benefit compared to more standard therapy and are not recommended in the guidelines. If this patient had an absolute contraindication to fibrinolytic therapy (which she does not), then immediate transfer for primary PCI (regardless of the transfer time) would be appropriate.

38.6 Answer D. Per the 2011 ACC/AHA PCI guidelines, PCI of a totally occluded infarct artery more than 24 hours after STEMI should not be performed in asymptomatic patients with one- or two-vessel disease, if patients are hemodynamically and electrically stable and do not have evidence of severe ischemia (Class III—no benefit) (Levine GN, et al. *J Am Coll Cardiol* 2011;58(24):e44–e122). The OAT (Open Artery Trial) study demonstrated no benefit for the routine PCI of a totally occluded infarct artery >24 hours after STEMI (Hochman JS, et al. *N Engl J Med* 2006;355(23):2395–2407). This patient is hemodynamically and electrically stable and has no symptoms to suggest ischemia or viable myocardium.

38.7 Answer C. Recommendations regarding the measurement of serum cardiac biomarkers are Level of Evidence C, with no studies cited to support this practice. While some analyses have shown that serum troponin elevations post-PCI are associated with worse in-hospital and long-term outcome, there is no study that has actually shown that the measurement of serum cardiac biomarkers (as opposed to not measuring serum cardiac biomarkers) improves patient management or prognosis. This is not to state that such measurements should not be done—but merely to point out that this practice is based on "expert opinion" rather than confirmatory studies.

38.8 Answer D. For single-vessel disease with a proximal LAD lesion, revascularization to improve survival is a Class IIa (can be beneficial) recommendation for CABG (with use of a LIMA) and a Class IIb (uncertain benefit) recommendation for PCI (Hillis LD, et al. *J Am Coll Cardiol* 2011;58(24):e123–e210). However, for single-vessel disease without proximal LAD involvement, neither PCI nor CABG is recommended for the purpose of improving survival (and, in fact, are Class III—harm—recommendations). No study has demonstrated mortality benefit with revascularization of mid-LAD lesions alone. Conversely, if the patient has unacceptable symptoms despite guideline-directed medical therapy, either PCI or CABG is useful (Class I) to improve symptoms.

38.9 Answer B. Diabetes and pre-existing renal disease both increase the risk of contrast nephropathy. Preprocedural hydration and minimization of contrast are both recommended (Class I) to decrease the risk of contrast nephropathy. Although the first trial of *N*-acetylcysteine in patients undergoing radiologic procedures suggested it was beneficial in reducing the risk of contrast nephropathy, subsequent studies—including ACT (Acetylcysteine for Contrast-Induced Nephropathy Trial)—and meta-analyses found no overall benefit with *N*-acetylcysteine. Per the 2011 ACC/AHA/SCAI PCI guidelines, it is considered Class III—no benefit (Levine GN, et al. *J Am Coll Cardiol* 2011;58(24):e44–e122). Despite these numerous, more recent trials and meta-analyses, some remain unconvinced that there is no benefit. As of this writing, a large U.S. Department of Veterans Affairs (VA) trial of *N*-acetylcysteine will provide additional information.

38.10 Answer C. Patients with prior anaphylactoid reactions to contrast media should receive appropriate prophylaxis with a steroid and antihistamine (Class I), which reduces the risk of recurrent reaction to <1%. There are no data that suggest that patients with seafood or shellfish allergies are at risk for an anaphylactoid reaction from exposure to contrast media; iodine does not mediate seafood, shellfish, or contrast media reactions. The 2011 ACC/AHA PCI guidelines state that in patients with a prior history of allergic reactions to shellfish or seafood, anaphylactoid prophylaxis for contrast reaction is not beneficial (Class III—no benefit) (Levine GN, et al. *J Am Coll Cardiol* 2011;58(24):e44–e122).

38.11 Answer D. Although high platelet reactivity during clopidogrel treatment is associated with worse outcome post-PCI, no study (i.e., GRAVITAS [Price MJ, et al. *JAMA* 2011;305:1097–1105] or ARCTIC [Collet JP, et al. *Lancet* 2014;384(9954):1577–1585]) of tailored therapy based on routine platelet function testing has shown benefit. Similarly, routine genetic testing has not been shown to improve outcome. For these reasons, routine platelet function and genetic testing to screen patients treated with clopidogrel are both Class III—no benefit—recommendations in the 2011 ACC/AHA PCI guidelines (Levine GN, et al. *J Am Coll Cardiol* 2011;58(24):e44–e122). Although there is a Class IIb recommendation that platelet function testing may be considered in patients at high risk for poor clinical outcomes, placement of a single DES in the mid-LAD of a patient with stable angina does not fall into this category, and this recommendation does not imply that testing, even in such cases, should be done.

38.12 Answer D. Even if there is some restenosis and "silent ischemia," there is no evidence that the detection of silent restenosis leads to improved outcome. Routine periodic stress testing of asymptomatic patients after PCI without specific clinical indications has never been shown to be of benefit and thus should not be performed (Class III—no benefit). Note also that all three diagnostic procedures will expose this relatively young patient to additional radiation.

38.13 Answer C. Based on studies, including BARI, FREEDOM, and SYNTAX, the 2014 SIHD guideline focused update (Fihn SD, et al. *J Thorac Cardiovasc Surg* 2015;149(3):e5–e23) states that CABG is generally recommended instead of PCI to improve survival in patients with diabetes mellitus and multivessel CAD for which revascularization is likely to improve survival (i.e., three-vessel CAD or complex two-vessel CAD involving the proximal LAD). This is particularly endorsed if a LIMA graft can be anastomosed to the LAD artery. DES was used in the most recent PCI vs. CABG trials, and this patient would have met study enrollment criteria for most trials. So, the results of these most recent studies apply to a patient such as this.

38.14 Answer B. Although the relatively small TAPAS study did show benefit with routine manual aspiration thrombectomy, three subsequent and larger studies (i.e., INFUSE-AMI, TASTE, and TOTAL) failed to show benefit with such a strategy. Even subgroup analysis of patients with anterior MI or large thrombus burden did not show benefit with such a strategy. For these reasons, in the 2015 ACC/AHA/SCAI PCI guideline focused update, the recommendation regarding routine aspiration thrombectomy was "downgraded" to Class III—no benefit. Routine aspiration thrombectomy before primary PCI is not useful (Levine GN, et al. *Circulation* 2017;136(7)).

38.15 Answer A. Routine coronary revascularization before noncardiac surgery has not been shown to improve outcome. The patient has no angina with moderate exercise, and ischemia was demonstrated only with stress testing. The 2011 ACC/AHA/SCAI PCI guidelines state that "routine prophylactic coronary revascularization should not be performed in patients with stable CAD before noncardiac surgery" and gives this a Class III, or harm Class recommendation (Levine GN, et al. *J Am Coll Cardiol* 2011;58(24):e44–e122).

38.16 Answer D. An early invasive strategy is not recommended for patients with extensive comorbidities who will not grant consent for revascularization.

38.17 Answer D. As discussed in the 2014 ACC/AHA NSTE-ACS guideline, fondaparinux as the sole anticoagulant during PCI has been associated with catheter thrombosis, and use of an anticoagulant with anti-IIa activity is recommended (Class I) when patients treated with fondaparinux undergo PCI (Amsterdam EA, et al. *J Am Coll Cardiol* 2014;64(24):e139–e228). Performance of PCI with fondaparinux as the anticoagulant is not recommended (Class III—harm).

38.18 Answer E. PCI of a noninfarct artery at the time of primary PCI was previously a Class III harm recommendation based on the findings of numerous observational studies and meta-analyses. However, PRAMI, CvLPRIT, and DANAMI-3 PRIMULTI demonstrated safety and the potential benefit of nonculprit artery PCI at the time of primary PCI as a staged procedure or based on an FFR assessment several days after primary PCI. The 2015 ACC/AHA primary PCI focused update revised the recommendation regarding nonculprit artery PCI; it now states that PCI of a noninfarct artery may be considered either at the time of primary PCI or as a planned staged procedure in selected patients with STEMI and multivessel disease who are hemodynamically stable (Levine GN, et al. *Circulation* 2017;136(7)). Therefore, choices A to D are all acceptable ways to proceed.

38.19 Answer C. According to the 2016 ACC/AHA Duration of DAPT focused update, standard DAPT duration for patients with SIHD treated with DES is at least 6 months, but a treatment period of 3 months may be reasonable in patients at high bleeding risk (Levine GN, et al. *J Am Coll Cardiol* 2016;68(10):1082–1115). The patient's history of GI bleeding, older age, CKD, and anemia all put him at higher bleeding risk. No study that did not involve concomitant oral anticoagulant therapy has shown efficacy of antiplatelet monotherapy. This patient would not have qualified for enrollment in the DAPT study (Fig. A38-19).

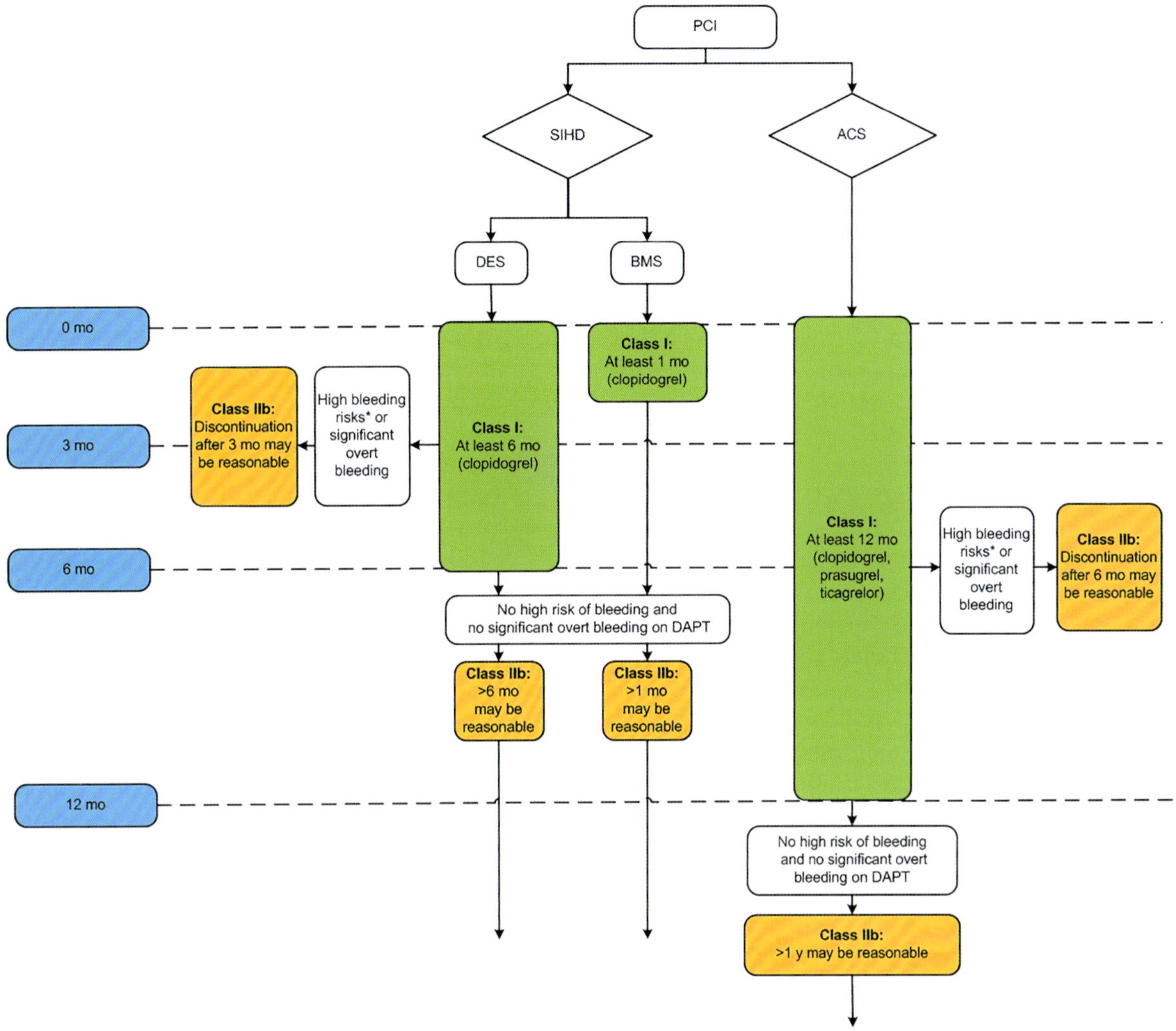

Figure A38-19 Algorithm for the duration of $P2Y_{12}$ inhibitor therapy in patients undergoing coronary stent implantation. (From Levine GN, et al. *Circulation* 2016;134(10):e123–e155.)

38.20 Answer B. Preprocedural hydration and minimization of the dose of contrast agent decrease the risk of contrast nephropathy. *N*-acetylcysteine has not been shown to have a meaningful or consistent benefit with regard to the incidence of contrast nephropathy or renal failure. High-dose statin therapy started 7 days before PCI is associated with a reduction in periprocedural MI. Use of the radial access can decrease access site complications (Levine GN, et al. *J Am Coll Cardiol* 2011;58(24):e44–e122).

38.21 Answer B. The 2011 ACC/AHA/SCAI PCI guideline (Levine GN, et al. *J Am Coll Cardiol* 2011;58(24):e44–e122) and the 2013 ACC/AHA STEMI guideline (O'Gara PT, et al. *J Am Coll Cardiol* 2013;61(4):e78–e140) give several options and recommendations regarding the timing of angiography and PCI following fibrinolytic therapy. Patients in severe heart failure or cardiogenic shock should undergo immediate angiography. In patients with suspected failed reperfusion, immediate angiography is also reasonable. Due to concerns about bleeding risk in the first several hours after fibrinolytic therapy, coronary angiography 3 to 24 hours after fibrinolytic therapy is considered reasonable in hemodynamically stable patients with evidence for successful reperfusion (Class IIa). In this same patient, coronary angiography performed at a point "before hospital discharge" is given a Class IIb recommendation. Thus, in this patient, angiography 3 to 24 hours after fibrinolysis is likely the best strategy.

38.22 Answer C. Since "tailored therapy" based on platelet function testing has not been shown to be of benefit, continuing the clopidogrel is not unreasonable. Since the patient was treated for ACS, using ticagrelor—per the PLATO study—would be a reasonable strategy. Because the patient had a prior history of stroke, per findings in TRITON, the patient should not be treated with prasugrel.

38.23 Answer D. UFH should not be used because of the history of heparin-induced thrombocytopenia. Enoxaparin is essentially shorter polysaccharide chains of UFH and can have cross-reactivity, so it should not be used. PCI should not be performed on patients treated with fondaparinux alone, as it is associated with catheter thrombosis. Bivalirudin, as a direct thrombin inhibitor, is recommended (Class I) for patients with heparin-induced thrombocytopenia (HIT) undergoing PCI (Levine GN, et al. *J Am Coll Cardiol* 2011;58(24):e44–e122).

38.24 Answer C. The 2011 ACC/AHA/SCAI guidelines (Levine GN, et al. *J Am Coll Cardiol* 2011;58(24):e44–e122) give three specific recommendations regarding SVG PCI. First, platelet GP IIb/IIIa inhibitors are not beneficial in SVG PCI. Second, embolic protection devices decrease ischemic adverse events and thus should be used when possible. Third, PCI in chronic SVG occlusion is associated with low success rates, high complication rates, and poor long-term patency rates and thus is not recommended.

38.25 Answer C. Studies have shown that PCI can safely be performed in patients treated with enoxaparin, including subcutaneous administration. However, in the 2014 ACC/AHA NSTE-ACS guideline, it is recommended that an additional dose of 0.3 mg/kg of IV enoxaparin should be administered at the time of PCI to patients with NSTE-ACS who have received fewer than two therapeutic subcutaneous doses (e.g., 1 mg/kg SC) or received the last subcutaneous enoxaparin dose 8 to 12 hours before PCI (Amsterdam EA, et al. *J Am Coll Cardiol* 2014;64(24):e139–e228). Administration of full-dose UFH to patients treated with enoxaparin was associated in the SYNERGY study with an increased risk of bleeding and is not recommended. It is Class III—harm—in the 2011 PCI guidelines (Ferguson JJ, et al. *JAMA* 2004;292(1):45–54).

38.26 Answer C. The patient has a plethora of factors associated with increased risk of stent thrombosis and recurrent spontaneous MI, including diabetes, continued smoking, complex bifurcation stenting, and small stent diameter. The patient's "DAPT score" would be 4. He has tolerated DAPT without bleeding and, other than diabetes, has no factors that put him at increased bleeding risk. Therefore, it would be reasonable to continue him on DAPT at least for a few more years. Both the PEGASUS (Bonaca MP, et al. *N Engl J Med* 2015;372(19):1791–1800) and DAPT study (Mauri L, et al. *N Engl J Med* 2014;371(23):2155–2166) suggest that such prolonged DAPT will decrease the risk of future ischemic events.

38.27 Answer D. Patients with a history of GI bleeding should be prescribed a PPI while on DAPT, per the 2011 ACC/AHA PCI guidelines (Levine GN, et al. *J Am Coll Cardiol* 2011;58(24):e44–e122), the 2016 ACC/AHA Duration of DAPT guideline focused update (Levine GN, et al. *J Am Coll Cardiol* 2016;68(10):1082–1115), and ACC/AGA expert documents (Bhatt DL, et al. *J Am Coll Cardiol* 2008;52(18):1502–1517). There are no data to support the strategies suggested in the other answer options.

38.28 Answer C. The 2016 ACC/AHA Duration of DAPT focused update gives recommendations on DAPT after CABG (Levine GN, et al. *J Am Coll Cardiol* 2016;68(10):1082–1115). In patients treated with coronary stent implantation before CABG, DAPT should be resumed or continued for the recommended duration of DAPT with respect to the stent itself. Since the stent was placed for ACS, at least 1 year of therapy is recommended. Additionally, and irrespective of the stent, since the patient had recent ACS, at least a year of DAPT is recommended. The former recommendation is admittedly based only on expert opinion, and the latter recommendation is based only on a subgroup analysis of the patients in the CURE study who underwent CABG.

38.29 Answer E. The first recommendation in the 2011 ACC/AHA/SCAI PCI guideline is a Class I recommendation for a heart team approach in cases of revascularization in patients with unprotected left main or complex CAD (Levine GN, et al. *J Am Coll Cardiol* 2011;58(24):e44–e122). This is a complex patient with complex anatomy, and there are reasons to consider either CABG or PCI.

38.30 Answer D. In BCIS-1 (Perera D, et al. *Circulation* 2013;127(2):207–212), there was no difference in the primary composite end point between routine and provisional use of IABP with PCI in high-risk patients. In similar patients, neither PROTECT I nor PROTECT II demonstrated benefit in hard end points with the use of Impella (O'Neill WW, et al. *Circulation* 2012;126(14):1717–1727). No randomized trial of PCI has been conducted showing benefit in hard end point with the TandemHeart. The 2011 ACC/AHA/SCAI PCI guidelines state that the elective insertion of an appropriate hemodynamic support device as an adjunct to PCI may be reasonable in carefully selected high-risk patients (C IIb), but this recommendation is based on level C evidence (Levine GN, et al. *J Am Coll Cardiol* 2011;58(24):e44–e122).

39 ST-Elevation Myocardial Infarction: ACC/AHA Guidelines

Hussein Othman and Rajendra H. Mehta

QUESTIONS

39.1 The emergency department calls you about a 54-year-old woman with interscapular pain radiating to the left shoulder that began 6 hours ago. She has a history of diabetes, hypertension, hyperlipidemia, and tobacco smoking. Per report, her physical exam reveals blood pressure (BP) 155/70 mm Hg, pulse 71, respiratory rate 18, 98% oxygen saturation on 2-L nasal cannula, normal jugular venous pressure, clear lungs, and normal first and second heart sounds. Her electrocardiogram (ECG) is shown in Figure Q39-1. Which of the following treatment goals is optimal in this patient:

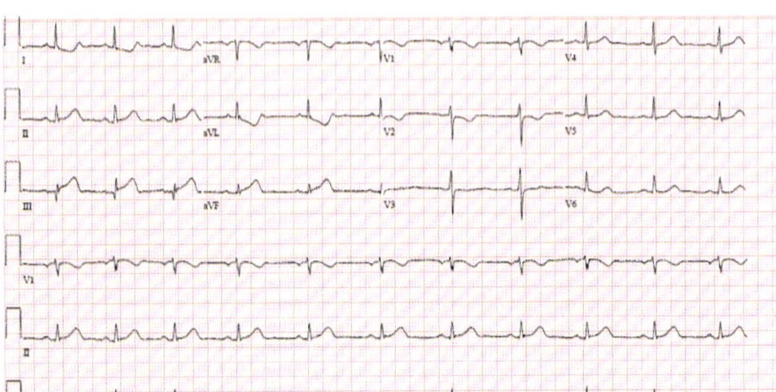

Figure Q39-1

(A) Emergency department arrival-to-femoral arterial puncture time of <60 minutes
(B) Total ischemic time of <150 minutes
(C) Total ischemic time of <180 minutes
(D) Less than 60 minutes from first medical contact to intravenous bolus of alteplase
(E) Less than 90 minutes from first medical contact to balloon dilation

39.2 An 87-year-old man with hypertension who is a tobacco user presented to the emergency department with substernal chest pain. The chest pain started 90 minutes ago and is associated with nausea and diaphoresis. A prior ECG from 1 year ago and his current ECG on presentation are shown in Figures Q39-2A and Q39-2B. On physical examination, his blood pressure (BP) is 146/84 mm Hg with a pulse of 84 beats per minute (bpm). His lungs are clear to auscultation. His neck veins are flat. He has a regular rate and rhythm with no murmurs, rubs, or gallops. He has 2+ pulses in his distal extremities. He is placed on telemetry and is given oral (PO) aspirin 325 mg and nitroglycerin 0.4 mg sublingual (SL) and started on an intravenous (IV) unfractionated heparin (UFH) drip. He has some relief in his chest pain. The most appropriate next step in this patient's management should include:

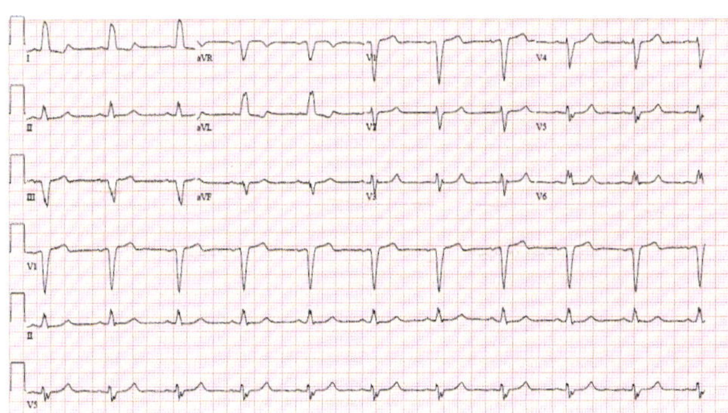

Figure Q39-2A

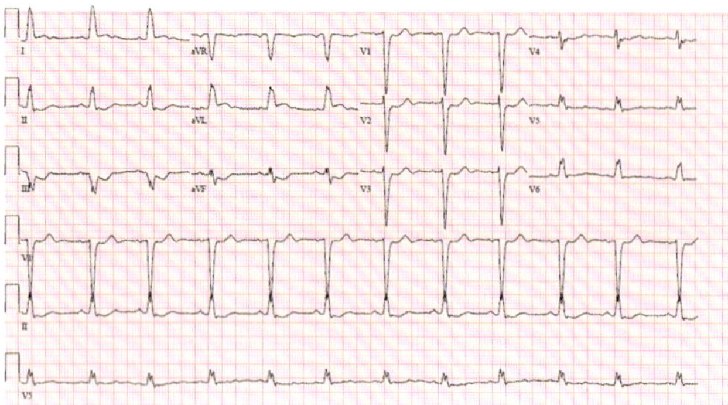

Figure Q39-2B

(A) Initiation of eptifibatide: 180 μg/kg IV bolus, followed by an infusion at 2 μg/kg/min IV and admittance to the cardiac care unit
(B) Admission to the cardiac care unit for further monitoring while awaiting results of serial cardiac biomarkers
(C) Order a single-photon emission computerized tomography (SPECT) radionuclide imaging stress test
(D) Activate the catheterization laboratory for possible primary angioplasty

39.3 A 55-year-old male with history of hypertension and type II diabetes was brought to the emergency department following cardiac arrest. The patient was having lunch with his family when he complained of chest pain, showed diaphoresis, and then suddenly collapsed. Chest compressions were immediately initiated by his family. He received two shocks by the emergency medical service and was intubated in the field. On arrival, his BP was 106/70 and heart rate (HR) was 56. He was unresponsive on arrival and initial ECG showed 2-mm ST elevation in leads I, aVL, and V2 to V6, with ST depressions in leads II, III, and aVF. The catheterization lab was activated. Aspirin, ticagrelor, and heparin were administered. While awaiting arrival of the catheterization team, you should:

(A) Start hypothermia protocol
(B) Administer a single bolus of eptifibatide
(C) Request a computed tomography (CT) head scan to assess for stroke or intracranial bleed
(D) Request echocardiography to evaluate for wall motion abnormalities

39.4 A 76-year-old patient with medical history of hypertension and hyperlipidemia presented to a local hospital with 2 hours of crushing substernal chest pain. The pain radiates to the left arm and is associated with diaphoresis, nausea, and mild shortness of breath. Physical examination revealed a BP of 154/85 mm Hg, a pulse of 105, a respiratory rate of 22, and 96% on 2-L nasal cannula. S4 was heard over the apex. ECG showed inferior ST elevation of 2 mm with ST depression in the lateral leads. The nearest hospital with percutaneous coronary intervention (PCI) capability is 130 minutes away. You decide to administer IV alteplase alongside with 325 mg of aspirin. Which of the following $P2Y_{12}$ inhibitors is indicated?

(A) Clopidogrel 300 mg
(B) Clopidogrel 75 mg
(C) Ticagrelor 180 mg
(D) Prasugrel 60 mg

39.5 A 70-year-old male with medical history of end-stage renal disease (ESRD) on hemodialysis, hypertension, type II diabetes, coronary artery disease (CAD) with a stent to left anterior descending (LAD) artery 8 years ago, smoking, and hyperlipidemia presented to the hospital for chest pain for 2 days. The pain was substernal with radiation to the neck and left shoulder. The patient appeared sweaty, anxious, and in mild distress. His BP was 170/102 mm Hg, heart rate was 120, and oxygen saturation was 92% on 2 L of oxygen. He had S3 on physical examination with mild crackles in the bases of his lungs. ECG showed 2-mm ST elevations in leads I, aVL, and V4 to V6. He was taken emergently to the catheterization lab. 325 mg of aspirin, 600 mg of clopidogrel, and weight-based heparin were administrated. Attempts to access his right radial were unsuccessful and the operator decided to proceed with right femoral arterial access. Cardiac catheterization showed stent thrombosis in the mid-LAD artery, but no significant disease in other vessels. Attempts to wire the lesion were unsuccessful and result in dissection proximal to the stent. Despite nitroglycerine and morphine, the patient is still complaining of 7/10 chest pain. Your next best step in the management of this patient is to:

(A) Page the surgeon on call for emergent coronary artery bypass grafting (CABG)
(B) Place an intra-aortic balloon pump (IABP) for hemodynamic support
(C) Change your wire to a stiff coronary wire
(D) Administer a fibrinolytic

39.6 After primary PCI, which of the following findings is associated with the worst mortality?

(A) Thrombolysis in myocardial infarction (TIMI) 2 flow grade
(B) Transient no-reflow
(C) Persistent ST-segment elevation
(D) TIMI 1 myocardial perfusion grade

39.7 Immediate β-blockers should NOT be used in which of the following situations?

(A) First-degree atrioventricular (AV) block
(B) HR < 70 bpm
(C) Systolic blood pressure (SBP) <100 mm Hg
(D) Patients undergoing primary PCI

39.8 Which of the following strategies has NOT been shown to reduce door-to-device time in the management of ST-segment elevation myocardial infarction (STEMI)?

(A) Catheterization laboratory activation by the emergency department physician
(B) Prehospital ECG to diagnose STEMI is used to activate the PCI team while the patient is en route to the hospital
(C) Catheterization team arrival in <20 minutes from alert
(D) Biannual feedback between catheterization laboratory and emergency department
(E) The emergency department makes a single contact to all members of the catheterization team

39.9 You receive a call from an intensive care unit physician at a community hospital without PCI capability (but a catheterization laboratory is available 20 minutes away) where a 53-year-old woman with a family history of premature CAD was admitted with 6 hours of chest pain. Her initial ECG revealed anterolateral ST elevations. She received IV alteplase, heparin, nitroglycerine, and fentanyl, as well as clopidogrel, aspirin, and metoprolol. Her initial troponin I was 20 times the upper limit of normal. Her chest pain subsided in the first hour after thrombolysis and her ST-segment elevations resolved. Thereafter, her chest pain returns despite increasing doses of nitrates, and she has 0.5-mm reelevations of the anterolateral ST segments on ECG. BP is 100/60 mm Hg and pulse is 110 bpm. She appears cold and clammy. Which of the following should be done next?

(A) Repeat bolus and infusion of alteplase
(B) Metoprolol 5 mg IV
(C) Immediate transfer to a catheterization laboratory for emergency cardiac catheterization
(D) IV dobutamine 5 μg/kg/h

39.10 A 57-year-old female with a medical history of hypertension, diabetes, and chronic obstructive pulmonary disease (COPD) presented with chest pain, shortness of breath, nausea, and sweating for 1 hour. Her vitals were BP 95/55 mm Hg, HR 110, and respiratory rate 24 with 92% on 4-L nasal cannula. Her neck veins were distended, lungs sounds were clear without crackles, and heart sounds were normal. Her right-sided ECG is shown on the image below (Fig. Q39-10). Which of the following medications should be avoided?

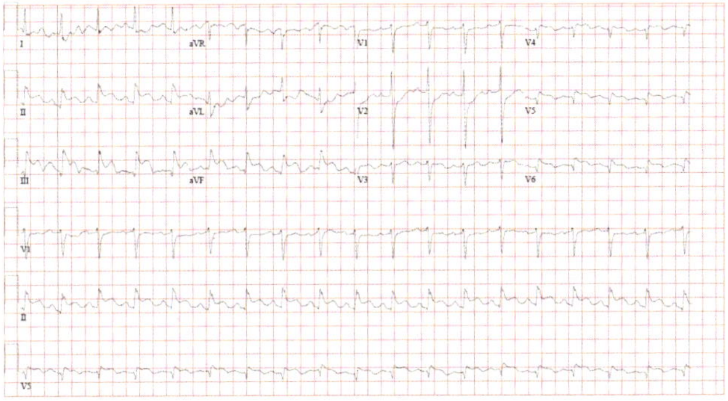

Figure Q39-10

(A) Morphine sulfate
(B) Heparin
(C) Aspirin
(D) Ticagrelor
(E) Nitroglycerine

39.11 The abovementioned patient was taken emergently to cardiac catheterization lab. Coronary catheterization through left radial access showed 100% thrombotic occlusion of the proximal right coronary artery (RCA). The lesion was successfully wired with a hydrophobic wire. Flow was restored partially and the patient reported improvement in her pain. All of the following are appropriate steps in management of this patient, EXCEPT:

(A) Dilation using semicompliance balloon
(B) Direct stenting with a bare metal stent (BMS)
(C) Direct stenting with a drug-eluting stent (DES)
(D) Manual aspiration catheter

39.12 Which of the following statements is TRUE regarding facilitated PCI compared to primary PCI?

(A) TIMI flow grade is worse
(B) Major bleeding risk is higher
(C) Mortality risk is lower
(D) Urgent target vessel revascularization (TVR) rates are lower
(E) Stroke risk is equal

39.13 Which of the following statements about heparin plus a glycoprotein (GP) IIb/IIIa inhibitor vs. bivalirudin in STEMI is supported by findings from the HORIZONS-AMI trial?

(A) Stroke risk was lower
(B) Major adverse cardiac event (MACE) rates are similar
(C) Major bleeding risk is similar
(D) Thrombocytopenia is less common
(E) Revascularization rates were significantly lower for bivalirudin

39.14 An 86-year-old very active female patient with type II diabetes, hypertension, and previous myocardial (MI) with PCI of the left circumflex (LCx) and RCA arteries presented to the emergency room with shortness of breath and fatigue for 3 days. Upon arrival to emergency department, she was dyspneic on physical exam and had a BP of 85/45 mm Hg and a heart rate of 116 bpm. Jugular vein distention (JVD) was present up to the angle of the jaw. Lung exam revealed bibasilar crackles up to the lower one-third of lung fields. CVS examination revealed a right ventricular lift. A grade 4/6 holosystolic murmur was heard at the left sternal border over the precordium. ECG on arrival showed 1.5-mm ST elevation and Q wave in the leads I, aVL, and V3 to V6, with ST depressions in leads II, III, and aVF. A stat echocardiogram was ordered, and the patient was rushed for cardiac catheterization that was performed emergently. It revealed a completely occluded LAD artery in proximal portion with patent stents in the LCx and RCA. Your next best step in management of this patient is to:

(A) Proceed with insertion of a IABP and revascularize the LAD while awaiting echocardiogram
(B) Obtain immediate echocardiogram and request emergent cardiac surgical consultation
(C) Proceed with right heart catheterization
(D) Given the patient's advanced age and comorbidities, along with late presentation, manage the patient medically

39.15 A 61-year-old man with history of hypertension, obesity, and tobacco smoking presents to an emergency department of a community hospital without PCI capability with jaw and bilateral arm pain, shortness of breath, and diaphoresis of 5 hours duration. An ECG obtained within 5 minutes of arrival reveals 2-mm anterior ST-segment elevations. On physical examination, he is diaphoretic, has a BP of 105/85 and a pulse of 104, is 91% on room air, and has a respiratory rate of 21. He has JVD to 8 cm, bibasilar crackles, a normal first and second heart sound, a third heart sound heard best at the apex, no murmurs or rubs, and diminished pedal pulses. He receives aspirin 325 mg, clopidogrel 600 mg, heparin, and tenecteplase. Which of the following outcomes is more likely if the patient is transferred immediately for PCI to a PCI-capable hospital?

(A) A higher risk of death
(B) A lower risk of cardiogenic shock
(C) A lower risk of reinfarction
(D) A lower risk of new congestive heart failure

39.16 Which of the following patients should be transferred urgently to a PCI-capable hospital after thrombolysis based upon the American College of Cardiology and American Heart Association (AHA) STEMI guidelines?

(A) All patients
(B) Only high-risk patients
(C) Patients at high risk of reinfarction
(D) Patients with new right bundle-branch block (RBBB) and left anterior hemiblock

39.17 Which of the following contrast agents is recommended for patients with chronic renal insufficiency undergoing coronary angiography?

(A) Iodixanol
(B) Iohexol
(C) Ioxaglate
(D) All of the above

39.18 A 60-year-old man with hyperlipidemia, hypertension, and diabetes presents with substernal chest pain for 1 hour. His ECG is shown in Figure Q39-18A. On exam, his BP is 130/70, pulse is 105, and he is breathing at 24/min. His oxygen saturation is 98% on 2 L. He is anxious, his lungs are clear, he has a normal first and second heart sound with no rubs, murmurs, or gallops, his jugular venous pressure is not elevated, and his extremities are warm. Coronary angiography is shown in Figure Q39-18B. Which of the following interventions would you recommend for this patient?

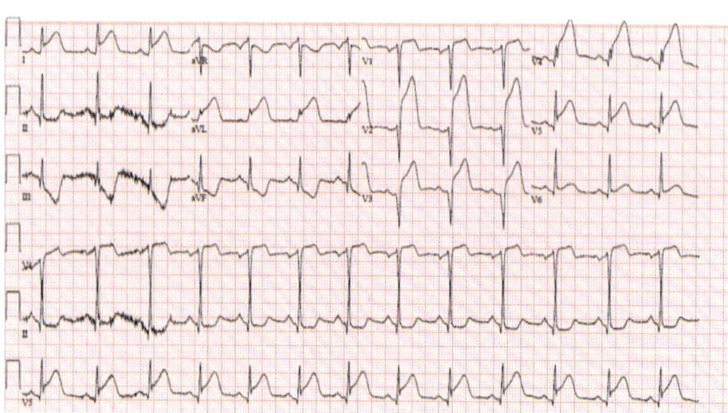

Figure Q39-18A

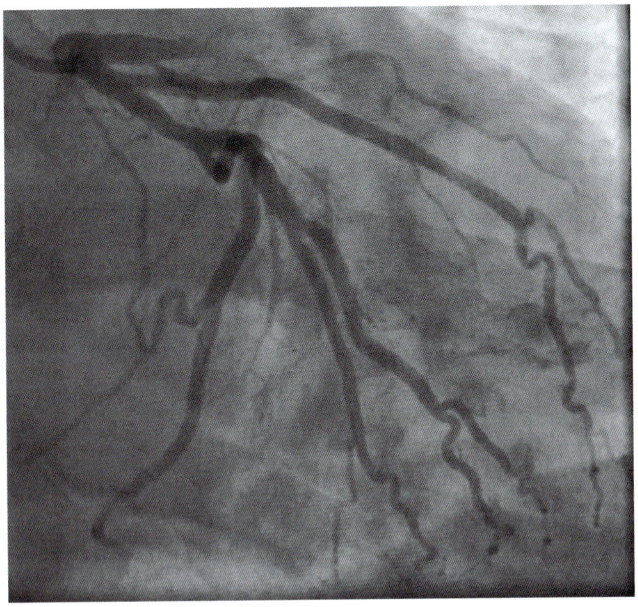

Figure Q39-18B

(A) A BMS
(B) A DES
(C) Either a DES or BMS
(D) Balloon angioplasty only

39.19 Which of the following outcomes occurred in the HORIZONS-AMI trial?

(A) The 1-year stent thrombosis rate was higher for paclitaxel stents
(B) The 1-year MACE (i.e., death, MI, and stroke) rate was similar for BMS and paclitaxel stents
(C) The rate of ischemic TVR was higher in the BMS group
(D) All of the above
(E) B and C

39.20 A 61-year-old male with hypertension and hyperlipidemia presents to the emergency department with 2 hours of substernal chest pain radiating to his jaw that began during an argument with his wife. His ECG reveals 3-mm ST-segment elevations in leads II, III, aVF, and V5 to V6. On exam, he is diaphoretic and anxious with a pulse of 61 bpm, a BP of 105/70 mm Hg in the left arm and 118/76 mm Hg in the right arm, breathing at 16/min, and 98% on 3-L nasal cannula. He has JVD to 6 mm above the sternal angle. His lungs are clear to auscultation. His point of maximal impulse is nondisplaced; he has a normal S1 and S2 with no rubs, murmurs, or gallops. His distal pulses are 2+ and his extremities are warm without cyanosis, clubbing, or edema. In the emergency department, he is loaded with prasugrel 60 mg before primary PCI. The findings of the TRITON-TIMI 38 trial suggest which of the following relative risks for patients such as this one treated with prasugrel instead of clopidogrel?

(A) Stent thrombosis is lower
(B) Death from a cardiovascular cause is similar
(C) Urgent TVR is lower
(D) All of the above

39.21 A 65-year-old female patient with history of type II diabetes, hypertension, and anemia presented to your hospital with 10-hour chest pressure. Her BP was 145/65 mm Hg and HR was 120 with 97% saturation on room air. Physical exam showed flat neck veins, clear lung sounds, and no murmur, gallop, or rub. An initial 12-lead ECG showed a 2-mm ST elevation in leads I, aVL, and V5 and V6, with depressions in leads V1 to V3. The patient was taken to the catheterization lab emergently. Attempts to access the left and then also the right radial arteries were unsuccessful, and you had to switch to right femoral access. Radial access compared to femoral access is associated with all of the following, EXCEPT:

(A) Decreased mortality
(B) Decreased bleeding complications
(C) Decreased vascular complications
(D) Higher risk of stroke

39.22 You are called to the emergency department to evaluate a 71-year-old man with history of a pacemaker, hypertension, diabetes, and 6 hours of upper back and neck pain. An ECG obtained within 5 minutes of arrival reveals an ectopic atrial rhythm at 86 BPM with a left bundle-branch block (LBBB). You confirm this by placing a magnet over the implanted device. He has received aspirin 162 mg and morphine 2 mg IV. His daughter has stated that the patient has a slow heart rate, but she is unaware of the LBBB through his primary care physician, and that for 2 weeks, her father has been complaining of increasing fatigue. On exam, he appears uncomfortable, with a BP of 100/85 mm Hg on the right and 95/80 mm Hg on the left, a pulse of 105, and a regular respiratory rate of 20 on 3-L nasal cannula with a 97% oxygen saturation. His neck veins are distended to 6 cm above the sternal angle. Auscultation reveals trace bibasilar rales, and his cardiac exam reveals a laterally displaced point of maximal impulse, a paradoxically split second heart sound, and a II/VI holosystolic murmur loudest at the apex. His feet are cool with 2+ edema to his ankles. Chest x-rays are shown in Figures Q39-22A and Q39-22B. Which of the following should be done next?

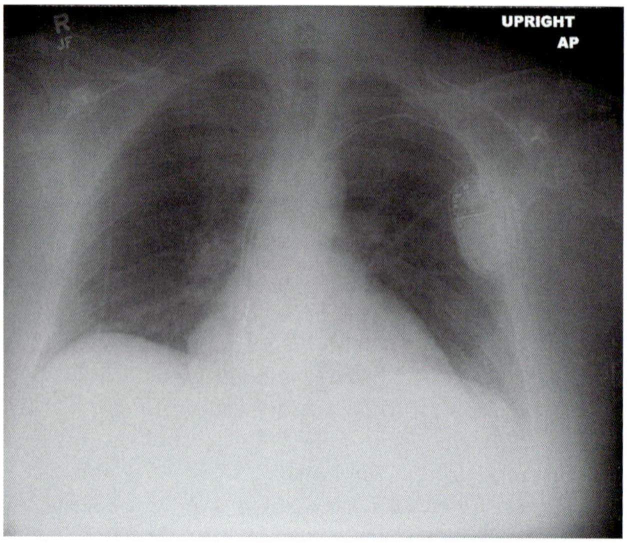

Figure Q39-22A (Courtesy of Hussein Othman.)

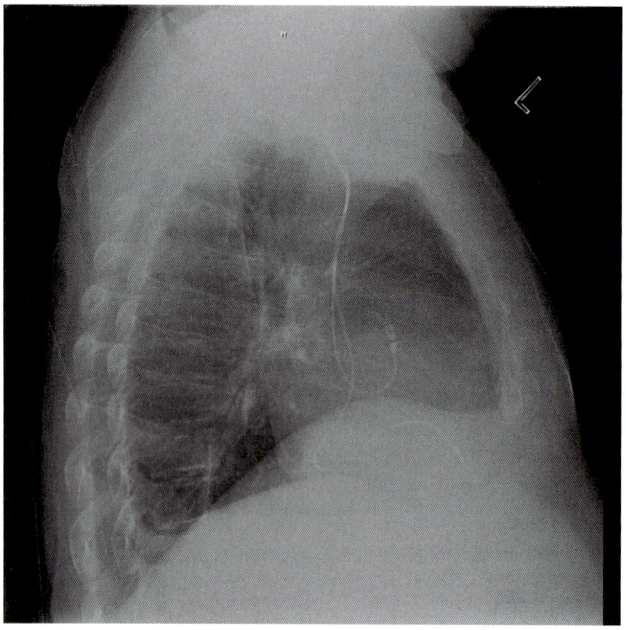

Figure Q39-22B (Courtesy of Hussein Othman.)

(A) Chest CT with contrast
(B) Coronary angiography
(C) Thrombolysis
(D) Myocardial perfusion imaging
(E) Medical therapy with serial cardiac enzymes

39.23 A 67-year-old female with past medical history of hemorrhagic stroke 4 years ago, hypertension, and hyperlipidemia presented with chest pain and shortness of breath that started 4 hours ago. She was also diaphoretic and nauseated. Examination revealed a BP of 158/94 mm Hg, a heart rate of 108, and oxygen saturation of 95% on 4-L nasal cannula. She had bibasilar crackles, S3 gallop, and a +3 pulse in all extremities. Initial ECG showed ST elevation in the anterior leads I, aVL, and V2 to V6, with ST depression in leads II and aVF. She was given 325 mg aspirin and weight-based heparin. The operator preferred to load with $P2Y_{12}$ upon knowing the anatomy. Cardiac catheterization showed a small RCA with no obstruction, a patent left main and LCx, and a proximal 100% occlusion in LAD artery. Plans to proceed with PCI were made. Which of the following medications should be given?

(A) 600 mg clopidogrel
(B) 60 mg prasugrel
(C) 180 mg ticagrelor
(D) IV cangrelor

39.24 Which of the following time delays in primary PCI is associated with the highest mortality?

(A) Door-to-balloon time
(B) Door-to-balloon time minus door-to-needle time
(C) Symptoms-to-balloon time
(D) Symptoms-to-door time

39.25 Which of the following interventions to reduce reperfusion injury have been shown to reduce infarct size in humans?

(A) Superoxide dismutase
(B) Glucose-insulin-potassium (GIK) infusion
(C) Pexelizumab (complement inhibitor)
(D) Ischemic preconditioning

39.26 Which of the following patients is most likely to have acute shortness of breath with no chest pain as their presenting symptoms of a STEMI?

(A) A 75-year-old white woman
(B) A 49-year-old white man
(C) A 49-year-old white woman
(D) A 75-year-old African American man

39.27 A 49-year-old man with hypertension presents to the emergency department with 16 hours of severe substernal chest pain. The initial ECG shows Q waves and 1-mm ST-segment elevation in leads V1 to V4. He continues to have 3/10 chest discomfort despite nitroglycerine (NTG) and morphine. On physical examination, his BP is 110/60 with a pulse of 95 bpm. An S3 is present with rales halfway up both lung fields. The monitor shows two 10-beat runs of nonsustained ventricular tachycardia (VT) at 160 bpm. The patient is started on lidocaine. What would be the next step in the management of this patient?

(A) Immediate catheterization and possible PCI
(B) IV β-blocker and IV Lasix with medical management
(C) IABP insertion with medical management
(D) Pulmonary artery (PA) catheter insertion with medical management

39.28 A 67-year-old woman presents to the emergency department with 4 hours of substernal chest pain and shortness of breath. ECG shows 4-mm ST-segment elevation in leads II, III, and aVF. Physical examination shows a BP of 140/70 with a pulse of 80 bpm. An S4 is audible. The patient is given aspirin, heparin, SL nitroglycerin, and clopidogrel and is taken to the catheterization laboratory. She is found to have a 99% lesion of the proximal RCA with large clot burden and TIMI 2 flow. The LAD has a 50% midlesion, and first obtuse marginal (OM) branch has an ostial 70% lesion. The patient had ventricular ectopy during the contrast injections. The patient is started on abciximab. What additional therapy is indicated prior to primary angioplasty?

(A) IV β-blocker
(B) IV lidocaine
(C) Intracoronary (IC) tissue plasminogen activator t-PA
(D) IC adenosine

39.29 According to PRAMI trial, multivessel PCI vs. culprit-only PCI was associated with all of the following, EXCEPT:

(A) Reduced all-cause mortality
(B) Reduced nonfatal MI
(C) Contrast-induced nephropathy requiring dialysis
(D) Reduced refractory angina

39.30 Primary angioplasty with stenting compared with primary angioplasty with balloon angioplasty alone has been shown to:

(A) Reduce restenosis and TVR
(B) Reduce restenosis and reinfarction
(C) Reduce restenosis and mortality
(D) Reduce restenosis, mortality, and CHF

39.31 A 59-year-old previously healthy woman presented with fatigue and a 4-hour history of chest discomfort. Her ECG demonstrated ST-segment elevations in V3 to V6. She was started on aspirin, heparin, nitroglycerin, and metoprolol. Primary PCI was chosen as the strategy for reperfusion. En route to the catheterization laboratory, she became unresponsive. The monitor showed ventricular fibrillation. She was successfully defibrillated with 150 J of biphasic energy. At catheterization, she had a total occlusion of the proximal- to mid-LAD. The lesion was stented with an excellent angiographic result with restoration of TIMI 3 flow. A transthoracic echo done 1 day after presentation showed an ejection fraction of 30% with hypokinesis of the anterior and lateral walls and apical akinesis. She has had no evidence of recurrent ischemia and no further ventricular arrhythmias. She has no evidence of CHF. Her medical regimen now includes aspirin, clopidogrel, metoprolol, lisinopril, and atorvastatin. What additional step should be taken in regard to the patient's episode of ventricular fibrillation?

(A) Implantable cardioverter defibrillator (ICD) placement before discharge
(B) Electrophysiologic study before discharge
(C) ICD placement 1 month post discharge
(D) Reassessment of left ventricular (LV) function 40 days post infarct

39.32 A 73-year-old male with a medical history of hypertension, type II diabetes, and CABG surgery presented to the hospital with chest pain. Initial EKG showed ST elevations in leads II, III, and aVF of 2 mm with ST depressions of 1 mm in V1 to V3. Emergent cardiac catheterization showed 100% occlusion of proximal saphenous vein graft (SVG) to RCA. Percutaneous transluminal coronary angioplasty (PTCA) was performed with a 2.0 × 15-mm semicompliant balloon followed by placement of FilterWire across the lesion. A repeat PTCA using a 3.0 × 15-mm semicompliant balloon was performed with resolution of the ST elevation with 80% residual stenosis in the proximal occluded segment. Following stenting with a 4 × 23-mm DES, ST-segment elevation was noted in inferior leads with sluggish flow. Which of the medications have shown no benefit in treating this patient?

(A) Nitroprusside
(B) Verapamil
(C) Adenosine
(D) Nitroglycerin

39.33 A 67-year-old woman presents with confusion and shortness of breath that started 8 hours ago. Her ECG shows 3-mm ST-segment elevation and Q waves in II, III, aVF, and V4 to V6. On physical examination, she has no focal neurologic signs. Her BP is 120/80 and pulse is 90 bpm. She has minimal crackles at the base of the lung fields. She is given aspirin, IV heparin, SL nitroglycerin, and IV reteplase. Within 30 minutes, the ST elevations have decreased. At 60 minutes, she becomes unresponsive. Her BP is 130/90 and pulse 100 bpm. What should you do now?

(A) Obtain transesophageal echocardiogram (TEE)
(B) Obtain a head CT
(C) Take the patient to the catheterization laboratory emergently
(D) Stop heparin and obtain a head CT

39.34 A 57-year-old female with no significant past medical history presented with ST elevation in leads II, III and aVF to a local hospital without catheterization lab. She was a smoker for 15 years. The nearest PCI facility is 2-hour away. The emergency physician administrated alteplase and heparin. The patient ECG changes and chest pain resolved completely within 34 minutes. She remained asymptomatic for the next 3 days with no recurrent chest pain, hemodynamic instability, or arrhythmias. Echocardiogram revealed a normal left ventricular ejection fraction without any wall motion abnormalities, normal RV systolic function, and no other significant abnormalities. All of the following should be part of the discharge planning, EXCEPT:

(A) Exercise stress test prior to discharge
(B) Referral to cardiac rehabilitation
(C) Smoking cessation counseling
(D) Pharmacologic stress testing

39.35 A 41-year-old obese man with no known past medical history presents with chest pain while shoveling snow. ECG obtained on arrival reveals inferolateral STEMI. He remains hemodynamically stable and primary PCI is planned. A point-of-care glucose measurement obtained in the ambulance was "out of range high," and repeat serum glucose available to you during post dilation of the stent placed to a large first OM artery is reported to you as 620 mg/dL (normal 70 to 100 mg/dL). Which of the following statements is supported by the ACC/AHA guidelines?

(A) Insulin should be given to all STEMI patients with glucose >200 mg/dL to achieve a serum glucose of 70 to 140 mg/dL
(B) An insulin infusion to normalize blood glucose is recommended for patients with STEMI and complicated courses
(C) It is reasonable to use an insulin-based regimen to achieve and maintain glucose levels <180 mg/dL while avoiding hypoglycemia for patients with STEMI with either a complicated or uncomplicated course

39.36 A 64-year-old female with a medical history of hypertension, type II diabetes, and smoking presents to the emergency room with shortness of breath for 3 hours. Her medications include 50 mg of metoprolol succinate, 20 mg of lisinopril, and a baby aspirin daily. Her blood pressure is 139/56 mm Hg, heart rate is 123, and oxygen saturation is 99% on 3-L nasal cannula. Physical examination showed flat neck veins, S3 gallop was heard, and her lungs revealed bilateral basal crepitations to auscultation. ECG showed ST elevation in I aVL and V6 with depression in V1 to V3. She was taken to the catheterization lab. She had 100% occlusion in her first OM artery. She was loaded with 325 mg acetylsalicylic acid, 60 mg prasugrel, and bivalirudin. A DES was placed with good results. Her left ventriculogram showed an ejection fraction of 35% with mild anterolateral hypokinesis. Atorvastatin 80 mg daily was added on the day of admission. She remained stable and was being discharged on day 3. Which one of the following medications should be added to her discharge medications besides those listed above?

(A) Long-acting nitrate
(B) Eplerenone
(C) Acetylsalicylic acid 325 mg
(D) Ranolazine

39.37 A 65-year-old male presented to your hospital with chest pain for 45 minutes. The patient has history of hypertension, diabetes, and atrial fibrillation on warfarin. Vitals showed BP of 145/88 mm Hg and a heart rate of 130. His heart sounds were irregular but no murmur or gallop was heard. ECG showed atrial fibrillation with an inferior ST-segment elevation of 1.5 mm. He was taken emergently to the catheterization lab. His angiography showed a 100% occluded RCA. Which of the following $P2Y_{12}$ inhibitors is indicated?

(A) Clopidogrel
(B) Ticagrelor
(C) Prasugrel
(D) Cangrelor

39.38 A 57-year-old patient with a medical history of hypertension and rheumatoid arthritis presented to a local facility with chest discomfort for 2 hours. Examination showed a BP of 160/94 mm Hg, a heart rate of 98, clear lung sounds, and normal first and second heart sounds without a murmur. His initial ECG showed inferior ST-segment elevation. The nearest facility with PCI capability is 1 hour away by airplane. However, due to weather conditions, the patient could not be airlifted. Fibrinolytics were administrated with resolution of ST-segment elevation. His dual antiplatelet therapy should include aspirin and:

(A) Clopidogrel for 1 month
(B) Ticagrelor for 1 year
(C) Clopidogrel for 1 year
(D) Prasugrel for 1 month

ANSWERS AND EXPLANATIONS

39.1 Answer E. When thrombolysis is the strategy for the management of STEMI, the "door-to-needle" time should be <30 minutes. When primary PCI is the revascularization strategy, the first medical contact-to-primary device time should be <90 minutes (ACC/AHA 2013). This period is commonly referred to as "door-to-balloon" time but would also include the first deployment of a manual thrombectomy device or direct deployment of a stent. Total ischemic time of <2 hours, and ideally <1 hour, is the overall goal of system's based management of STEMI and is defined as the onset of symptoms to needle or balloon time (ACC/AHA 2007).

39.2 Answer D. Diagnosis of STEMI in the setting of an old LBBB is a challenge. The 2013 ACC/AHA guidelines suggest the use of the Sgarbossa criteria in patients with an old LBBB. A score ≥3 has a specificity of 90% for diagnosing MI. The criteria are:

- Concordant ST elevation ≥1 mm in leads with a positive QRS complex (score 5)
- Concordant ST depression ≥1 mm in V1 to V3 (score 3)
- Discordant ST elevation ≥5 mm in leads with a negative QRS complex (score 2)

This patient has concordant ST elevation in the lateral leads I and aVL and concordant ST depression in leads III and aVF. Thus, STEMI is highly suspected. In addition to standard medical treatment for acute STEMI (aspirin, $P2Y_{12}$ inhibitors, etc.), a strategy for early reperfusion should be implemented in a timely fashion.

The 2013 ACC/AHA guidelines define STEMI as a new ST elevation at the J point in at least two contiguous leads of ≥2 mm (0.2 mV) in men or ≥1.5 mm (0.15 mV) in women in leads V2 to V3 and/or of ≥1 mm (0.1 mV) in other contiguous chest leads or the limb leads. Besides, a new LBBB is considered STEMI-equivalent. Other STEMI equivalents are

- ST depression in precordial leads (V1 to V4) indicating transmural posterior injury.
- Multilead ST depression with coexistent ST elevation in lead aVR has been described in patients with left main or proximal LAD artery occlusion.
- Hyperacute T-wave changes may be observed in the very early phase of STEMI, before the development of ST elevation.

Cardiac catheterization should be considered in these cases, and an echocardiogram can be very helpful to establish the diagnosis if in doubt.

39.3 Answer A. Therapeutic hypothermia should be started as soon as possible in comatose patients with STEMI and out-of-hospital cardiac arrest caused by ventricular fibrillation or pulseless ventricular tachycardia, including patients who undergo primary PCI (Class I, Level of Evidence B). This is based on two randomized studies showing improved neurologic outcomes when using hypothermia (cooling to 32°C to 34°C for 12 or 24 hours) in comatose patients following ventricular fibrillation/pulseless VT cardiac arrest (Bernard SA, et al. *N Engl J Med* 2002;346(8):557–563; *N Engl J Med* 2002;346(22):1756). Given that ticagrelor was given as a load, the role of eptifibatide is not well defined. Also if used, eptifibatide should be given as a continuous drip rather than just a bolus. CT head scan is less useful when the patient had chest pain and had a witnessed arrest. Echo is not useful given STEMI and stable hemodynamics.

39.4 Answer B. STEMI patients treated with fibrinolytics should be loaded with clopidogrel 300 mg if the patient is 75 years old or less and with clopidogrel 75 mg if the patient is older than 75. Newer-generation $P2Y_{12}$ receptor inhibitors (prasugrel and ticagrelor) have not been studied with fibrinolytics.

39.5 Answer A. The role of CABG in the treatment of STEMI has decreased since the introduction of modern PCI techniques. However, emergent CABG is indicated in failed PCI, especially in those at high risk (the current patient is high risk given age, diabetes, ESRD, tachycardia, and CHF at presentation) if coronary anatomy is not amenable to PCI and in cases of mechanical complications (Class I, Level of Evidence B). Using stiff coronary wire is associated with high complication rate including coronary perforation and dissection. IABP can be placed while awaiting surgical evaluation. Fibrinolytic therapy has not been studied in those with failed PCI and perhaps has no role in those with failed PCI.

39.6 Answer D. Despite TIMI 3 flow in an epicardial vessel after reperfusion, impaired myocardial perfusion may still be present and is associated with worse outcomes. The TIMI myocardial perfusion grading (TMPG) system or myocardial blush grade is a marker of myocardial perfusion and corresponds to higher mortality rates independent of epicardial flow (Gibson CM, et al. *Circulation* 2000;101(2):125–130). TMPG grade 0 is defined as no apparent tissue-level perfusion (no ground-glass appearance of blush or opacification of the myocardium) in the distribution of the culprit artery. TMPG grade 1 indicates presence of myocardial blush, but no clearance from the microvasculature (blush or a stain is present on the next injection). TMPG grade 2 is when blush clears slowly (blush is strongly persistent and diminishes minimally or not at all during three cardiac cycles of the washout phase). TMPG grade 3 indicates that blush begins to clear during washout (blush is minimally persistent after three cardiac cycles of washout). No-reflow is defined as a profound reduction in antegrade coronary blood flow despite vessel patency and the absence of dissection, spasm, or distal macroembolus. It is presumed to reflect microvascular dysfunction and appears to be more common in diabetic patients. The TMPG system is a stronger independent predictor of mortality outcomes in STEMI patients after reperfusion therapy than persistent ST-segment elevations, TIMI flow grade, or the presence of no-reflow. Patients with a TIMI grade 2 flow may have a normal TMPG secondary to collateral circulation. Patients with both normal epicardial flow (TIMI grade 3 flow) and normal tissue-level perfusion (TMPG grade 3) have an extremely low risk of mortality (Gibson CM, et al. *Circulation* 2002;105(16):1909–1913).

39.7 Answer C. Systolic BP < 100 mm Hg. The current ACC/AHA guidelines in regard to immediate administration of β-blockers are:

- Class I: Oral β-blocker therapy should be initiated in 24 hours in those patients without a contraindication (Level of Evidence B).
- Class I: Patients with initial contraindications to β-blockers in the first 24 hours of STEMI should be reevaluated for their use (Level of Evidence C).
- Class I: β-blockers should be continued during and after hospitalization for all patients with STEMI and with no contraindications to their use (Level of Evidence B).
- Class IIa: It is reasonable to administer IV β-blockers promptly to STEMI patients without contraindications who are hypertensive or have ongoing ischemia (Level of Evidence B).

The following are relative contraindications to β-blocker therapy: HR < 60 bpm, systolic arterial pressure <100 mm Hg, moderate or severe LV failure, signs of peripheral hypoperfusion, shock, PR interval >0.24 seconds, second- or third-degree AV block, active asthma, or reactive airway disease. The Clopidogrel and Metoprolol in Myocardial Infarction Trial/Second Chinese Cardiac Study (COMMIT/CCS-2) enrolled 45,852 patients at 1,250 centers (Chen ZM, et al. *Lancet* 2005;366(9497):1622–1632). COMMIT/CCS-2 was a randomized, parallel-controlled trial that used a 2 × 2 factorial design to assess the effects of adding 75 mg of clopidogrel (vs. placebo) and the effects of adding the β-blocker metoprolol (vs. placebo) in patients with acute MI on aspirin therapy (162 mg daily). The study enrolled patients with suspected acute MI (ST change or new LBBB) within 24 hours of symptom onset. Patients with shock, systolic BP >100 mm Hg, HR > 50 bpm, or second- or third-degree AV block were excluded. The findings on metoprolol showed that giving three IV doses of 5 mg metoprolol followed by daily oral doses of 200 mg reduced the relative risks of reinfarction and vascular events by 15% to 20%, but increased the relative risk of cardiac shock by 30%, especially during the first day of treatment. This finding emphasizes that β-blocker therapy in the setting of acute STEMI should be tailored to the individual patient. In patients at high risk of cardiogenic shock (i.e., patients >70 years of age, systolic BP 120 mm Hg, presenting heart rate 110 bpm, or increased time since onset of symptoms of STEMI), β-blockers should either be delayed until such patients are hemodynamically stable or they should be slowly up titrated.

39.8 Answer D. Feedback between the emergency department and catheterization laboratory regarding the efficiency of STEMI care and door-to-device times should happen on a real-time basis, within hours or days of the event so that swift system improvements to PCI management are possible. In a multicenter study of 365 acute care hospitals with PCI capability that performed 25 or more PCIs for STEMI annually, the following six factors were associated with reduced door-to-device times: real-time feedback, single call to the catheterization team, emergency department activation of the catheterization team, an in-house interventionalist, arrival of the catheterization team in <20 minutes from the STEMI alert, and having the emergency department physician activate the catheterization laboratory while the patient is en route (Bradley EH, et al. *N Engl J Med* 2006;355(22):2308–2320).

39.9 **Answer C.** This patient is unstable after thrombolysis for STEMI. Transfer directly to a catheterization laboratory with acute care capability for PCI is indicated with persistent ST elevations 90 minutes after thrombolysis or with clinical instability (Gershlick AH, et al. *N Engl J Med* 2005;353(26):2758–2768; ACC/AHA Class I). Based on the SHOCK registry, approximately 5% of patients with STEMI develop cardiogenic shock (Goldberg RJ, et al. *N Engl J Med* 1999;340(15):1162–1168). STEMI patients with cardiogenic shock should be managed with a primary PCI strategy (ACC/AHA Class I). IV β-blockers should be avoided in patients at risk of cardiogenic shock (ACC/AHA Class I).

39.10 **Answer E.** This patient has inferior STEMI with evidence of right ventricle (RV) infarction upon exam. Right-sided ECG shows ST elevation in V4 to V6, which is consistent with RV infarction. Nitrates should be avoided in this case as they may cause profound hypotension. Other contraindications to nitrates include hypotension, marked bradycardia or tachycardia, or phosphodiesterase 5 inhibitor use within the previous 24 to 48 hours.

39.11 **Answer D.** In the previous 2013 ACC/AHA STEMI guidelines, aspiration thrombectomy had a Class IIa recommendation. This was based on a single-center TAPAS trial (Vlaar PJ, et al. *Lancet* 2008;371(9628):1915–1920) that showed improved outcomes at 1 year when aspiration thrombectomy was used prior to stenting. However, three recent multicenter studies found no significant reduction in death, reinfarction, or stent thrombosis with routine aspiration thrombectomy (Fröbert O, et al. *N Engl J Med* 2013;369(17):1587–1597; Stone GW, et al. *JAMA* 2012;307(17):1817–1826; Jolly SS, et al. *N Engl J Med* 2015;372(15):1389–1398). Aspiration thrombectomy was associated with a small but nonsignificant increase in the risk of stroke (Elgendy IY, et al. *Circ Cardiovasc Interv* 2015;8:e002258). Accordingly, the new ACC/AHA 2015 guidelines give routine use of aspiration thrombectomy a Class III recommendation. Direct stenting using a BMS or DES and preparing the lesion with a semi-compliant balloon are all acceptable approaches in this patient.

39.12 **Answer B.** The term "facilitated PCI" was used previously to describe a strategy of full- or half-dose fibrinolysis with or without administration of a GP IIb/IIIa receptor antagonist, with immediate transfer for planned PCI within 90 to 120 minutes. Half-dose reteplase with or without abciximab before PCI was associated with more major bleeding than abciximab at the time of PCI and no improvement in MACE rates (Ellis SG, et al. *N Engl J Med* 2008;358(21):2205–2217). A large meta-analysis showed that facilitated PCI was associated with higher rates of death, stroke, urgent revascularization, reinfarction, and major bleeding, although TIMI flow grade on initial angiography was better in the pharmacologically pretreated patients (Keeley EC, et al. *Lancet* 2006;367(9510):579–588). Facilitated PCI is currently not recommended.

39.13 **Answer B.** The results of the HORIZONS-AMI trial suggest that bivalirudin vs. heparin plus a IIb/IIIa inhibitor in STEMI show no significant difference for MACE or stroke (Stone GW, et al. *N Engl J Med* 2008;358(21):2218–2230). While thrombocytopenia was significantly more common in the IIb/IIIa inhibitor group, bleeding risk was significantly lower in the bivalirudin group. There was a numerically higher rate of TVR in the bivalirudin group, which did not reach statistical significance. There was an increased risk of acute stent thrombosis within 24 hours in the bivalirudin group, but no significant increase was present by 30 days. Supportive use of either heparin with or without a IIb/IIIa inhibitor or bivalirudin at the time of PCI is an ACC/AHA Class I recommendation.

39.14 **Answer B.** This patient is a late presenter (as evident by the 3-day symptoms of shortness of breath and anterior Q wave) and she is at high risk for mechanical complications. Holosystolic murmur can be seen in ventricular septal rupture (VSR) or acute mitral regurgitation, but the presence of RV dysfunction signs (RV lift, increased JVD) makes the diagnosis of VSR more likely. VSR should be confirmed immediately with an echocardiogram that will also provide information on other prognostic markers (i.e., LV and RV systolic function). VSR is an indication for emergent CABG. IABP, inotropes, and vasodilators can be used as bridge to surgery. PCI should not be performed in presence of VSR, and while right heart catheterization is reasonable, it is not therapeutic. As the patient was very active before this incidence, a more aggressive approach is justified.

39.15 **Answer C.** TRANSFER AMI was a multicenter randomized trial of high-risk STEMI patients undergoing thrombolysis at hospitals without PCI capability (Cantor WJ, et al. *N Engl J Med* 2009;360(26):2705–2718). After the initiation of tenecteplase, patients were randomized to transfer for PCI as follows: (1) immediate transfer for PCI within 6 hours of thrombolysis; (2) delayed transfer in patients with persistent ST elevations, hemodynamic instability, or chest pain; and (3) delayed transfer for angiography >24 hours after thrombolysis in patients with successful reperfusion. This study showed that the immediate and delayed transfer strategies were equivalent with respect to mortality, but reinfarction and recurrent ischemia were significantly less common in the immediate transfer group (Fig. A39-15). Immediate transfer to a PCI-capable hospital for coronary angiography is recommended for suitable patients with STEMI who develop cardiogenic shock or acute severe heart failure, irrespective of the time delay from MI onset (Level of Evidence B).

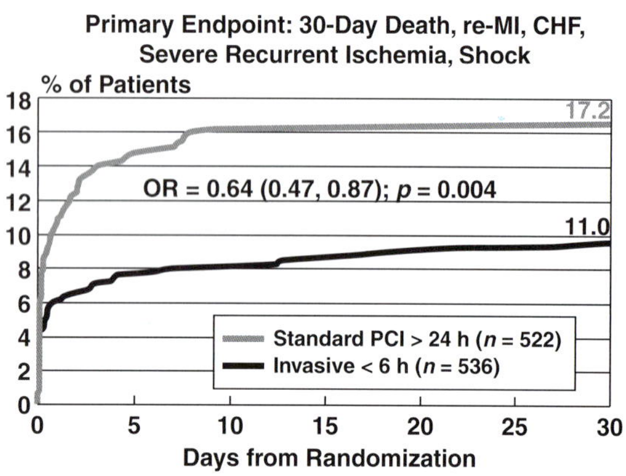

Figure A39-15

39.16 Answer A. The following recommendations are for patients who receive fibrinolytics:

- Class I indication for immediate transfer to a PCI-capable hospital for coronary angiography is recommended for suitable patients with STEMI who develop cardiogenic shock or acute severe heart failure.
- Class IIa recommendation for urgent transfer to a PCI-capable facility for rescue PCI after failed fibrinolytics.
- Class IIa recommendation to transfer to a PCI-capable hospital for coronary angiography in patients with STEMI who have received fibrinolytic therapy even when hemodynamically stable and with clinical evidence of successful reperfusion. Angiography should be performed ideally within 24 hours, but should not be performed within the first 2 to 3 hours after administration of fibrinolytic therapy.

39.17 Answer A. Isosmolar and lower molecular weight contrast agents have a Class I recommendation for angiography in patients with chronic kidney disease (CKD) not undergoing dialysis. Iodixanol is a low molecular weight agent associated with less contrast-induced nephropathy than iohexol and ioxaglate (Solomon RJ, et al. *Circulation* 2007;115(25):3189–3196; Jo SH, et al. *J Am Coll Cardiol* 2006;48(5):924–930).

39.18 Answer C. This ECG reveals a marked anterolateral injury with reciprocal inferior ST depressions consistent with evolving acute anterolateral MI. This patient's angiogram reveals a thrombotic 90% lesion in the proximal LAD. Compared with balloon angioplasty, BMS reduces revascularization and reinfarction rates but not mortality (Nordmann AJ, et al. *Am J Med* 2004;116(4):253–262). Compared with BMS, DES decreases restenosis rates without an effect on mortality. Due to risk of stent thrombosis, DES should be avoided in patients who cannot comply with or afford dual antiplatelet therapy (DAPT) or who have bleeding disorders (Class III). Either a BMS or DES would be reasonable in this patient based on his ability to comply with prolonged DAPT (Class I, Level of Evidence C).

39.19 Answer E. In addition to comparing bivalirudin with heparin and a GP IIb/IIIa inhibitor for STEMI, the HORIZONS-AMI trial compared paclitaxel-eluting stents with BMS in a 3:1 randomization (Stone GW, et al. *N Engl J Med* 2009;360(19):1946–1959). The paclitaxel stent arm had less TVR and a similar rate of death or recurrent MI compared to the BMS arm. Stent thrombosis was similar (Fig. A39-19).

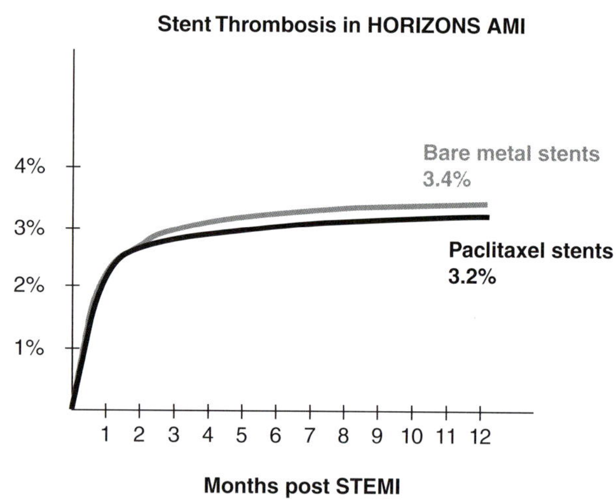

Figure A39-19 (Adapted from Stone GW, et al. *N Engl J Med* 2009;360(19):1946–1959.)

39.20 Answer D. Use of prasugrel vs. clopidogrel in STEMI is associated with a lower risk of the combined primary end point of death from cardiovascular causes, nonfatal MI, or nonfatal stroke (Wiviott SD, et al. *N Engl J Med* 2007;357(20):2001–2015). Prasugrel is also associated with a lower risk of stent thrombosis and urgent TVR. There is a higher rate of major non-CABG-associated bleeding with prasugrel. The number needed to treat for benefit over clopidogrel was 46. The number needed to harm was 167 (Fig. A39-20). Prasugrel 60 mg should be given as early as possible for STEMI patients (ACC/AHA 2009 Class Ib).

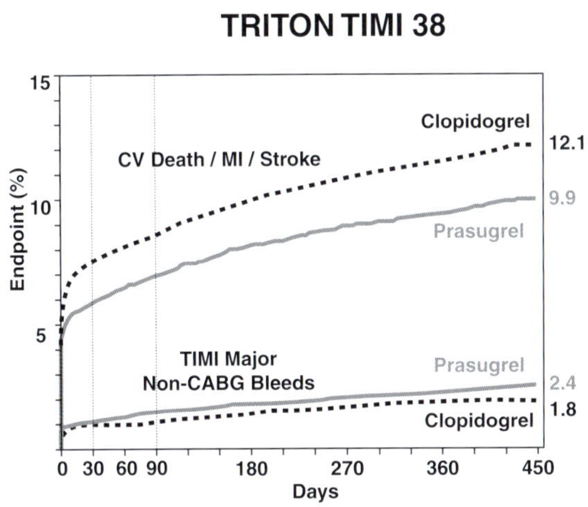

Figure A39-20 (Adapted from Wiviott SD, et al. *N Engl J Med* 2007;357(20):2001–2015.)

39.21 Answer D. Radial access compared with femoral access improves survival and decreases bleeding and vascular complications without an increase in stroke rates (Ferrante G, et al. *JACC Cardiovasc Interv* 2016;9(14):1419–1434). If performed by an experienced radial operator, radial access should be preferred over femoral access in STEMI patients as recommended by European Society of Cardiology (Steg PG, et al. *Eur Heart J* 2012;33(20):2569–2619).

39.22 Answer B. Given his advanced age and risk factors for CAD, the pretest likelihood of obstructive CAD in this man is high. A new LBBB is a STEMI equivalent and an ACC/AHA Class I indication for primary PCI or thrombolysis. This chest x-ray reveals cardiomegaly and increased pulmonary vascularity, as well as a subclavian permanent pacemaker. The chronicity of the LBBB in this case is in doubt so immediate thrombolysis would be inappropriate. Further testing with emergent diagnostic angiography is the best answer.

39.23 Answer A. Both prasugrel and ticagrelor are contraindicated in patients with a prior history of intracranial hemorrhage. Besides, prasugrel is contraindicated in patients with prior transient ischemic attack (TIA) or stroke. IV cangrelor has not been studied or approved for this indication.

39.24 Answer C. Symptoms-to-balloon time. Symptom onset to balloon inflation represents the true ischemic time in patients undergoing primary PCI. De Luca et al. demonstrated that for every 30-minute delay from the onset of symptoms to balloon inflation, the risk of 1-year mortality is increased by 7.5% (De Luca G, et al. *Circulation* 2004;109(10):1223–1225). Figure A39-24 depicts this relationship between ischemic time and 1-year mortality; the dotted line represents 95% confidence intervals of predicted mortality.

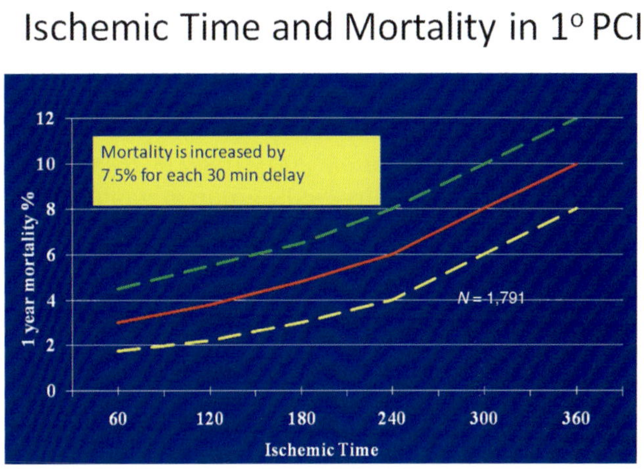

Figure A39-24 (From De Luca G, et al. *Circulation* 2004;109(10): 1223–1225, with permission.)

39.25 Answer D. Ischemic preconditioning is the phenomenon in which brief nonlethal episodes of ischemia protect the myocardium before a subsequent prolonged ischemic event through a variety of adaptive physiologic measures. This concept was initially described in animal models, but it has subsequently been described in humans and shown to decrease infarct size. It likely accounts for some of the cardiovascular benefit seen in individuals who exercise. Superoxide dismutase is an endogenous free radical scavenger that has been studied in a variety of animal models of reperfusion injury. To date, no human studies have shown a reduction in infarct size. The effects of GIK therapy were studied in the CREATE-ECLA trial (Cobb LA, et al. *JAMA* 2005;293(21):437–446). Patients presenting with STEMI within 12 hours of symptom onset were randomized to GIK infusion or placebo. There was no difference in all-cause mortality, cardiac arrest, cardiogenic shock, or reinfarction. Pexelizumab is a monoclonal antibody against C5 complement and functions to inhibit the activation of the complement system. Complement activation is a mediator of inflammatory damage seen with reperfusion injury. In the COMMA trial (Granger CB, et al. *Circulation* 2003;108(10):1184–1190), pexelizumab was administered (bolus alone or bolus plus infusion) to patients with STEMI undergoing mechanical reperfusion. Administration of this monoclonal antibody failed to show a reduction in infarct size, but patients receiving the bolus plus infusion showed a significant reduction in 90-day mortality. Other agents have also been unsuccessful in clinical trials. This includes monoclonal antibodies against white cell CD11/18 integrin receptors, calcium channel blockers, the Na/H exchange inhibitor, cariporide, the K_{ATP} channel opener, nicorandil, and adenosine. Whereas adenosine showed benefit following thrombolysis in initial trials, subsequent trials in patients undergoing primary PCI have been negative.

39.26 Answer A. McSweeney et al. (McSweeney JC, et al. *Circulation* 2003;108(21):2619–2623) retrospectively surveyed a group of women diagnosed with acute MI to determine the symptoms at presentation. In this cohort of predominantly white women, the most frequent presenting symptoms were shortness of breath (58%), weakness (55%), and fatigue (43%). Acute chest pain was absent in 43% of patients. In general, women and the elderly present with more atypical symptoms leading to delays in presentation and diagnosis.

39.27 Answer A. This patient is presenting >12 hours after his initial symptoms. However, he has evidence of heart failure, electric instability, and persistent symptoms. An emergent cardiac catheterization should be performed. The pertinent ACC/AHA guidelines are:

- Class I (Level of Evidence B): To perform primary PCI if there is evidence of cardiogenic shock or acute severe heart failure irrespective of time delay from MI onset
- Class IIa (Level of Evidence B): To perform PCI if there is evidence of ongoing ischemia 12 to 24 hours after symptom onset

39.28 Answer A. Administration of β-blockers in the acute phase of STEMI diminishes myocardial oxygen demand, reduces systemic arterial pressure, and reduces myocardial contractility. β-Blockers are part of the standard of care for STEMI management except for the scenarios reviewed in Question 39.7. Through a reduction in HR and prolongation of diastole, β-blockers are thought to augment myocardial perfusion. β-Blockers have been shown to decrease the size of infarction, decrease the rate of reinfarction, and decrease the frequency of life-threatening ventricular arrhythmias regardless of the reperfusion strategy. Several nonrandomized trials (e.g., PAMI and CADILLAC) have shown improved short- and long-term mortality with pretreatment with β-blockers in patients undergoing primary PCI.

39.29 Answer C. The Preventive Angioplasty in Acute Myocardial Infarction (PRAMI) trial (Wald DS, et al. *N Engl J Med* 2013;369(12):1115–1123) was a multicenter randomized trial where patients with STEMI were assigned to infarct-only PCI or multivessel PCI. After 23 months of follow-up, multivessel PCI was associated with a reduction in the primary outcome (a composite of death from cardiac causes, nonfatal MI, or refractory angina) compared with culprit-only PCI. There was no increase in adverse events, including procedure-related stroke, bleeding requiring transfusion or surgery, and contrast-induced nephropathy requiring dialysis. Current ACC/AHA 2015 guidelines state PCI of a noninfarct artery may be considered in selected patients with STEMI and multivessel disease who are hemodynamically stable, either at the time of primary PCI or as a planned staged procedure (Class IIb, Level of Evidence B).

39.30 Answer A. Compared with PTCA, several studies show that intracoronary stents achieve better immediate angiographic results with a larger arterial lumen. No significant differences in mortality or reinfarction have been observed, but with primary stenting, there is less vessel reocclusion and restenosis, leading to less TVR (Antoniucci D, et al. *J Am Coll Cardiol* 1998;31(6):1234–1239).

39.31 Answer D. This patient has ventricular fibrillation in the setting of acute MI. With prompt reperfusion therapy for STEMI and medical optimization in the ensuing weeks, it is likely that her LV function will improve and that her risk of a recurrent lethal arrhythmia is very low. The relevant guidelines come from the ACC/AHA/HRS 2012 consensus document (Epstein AE, et al. *Circulation* 2013;127(3):e283–e352).

- Class I: ICD therapy is indicated in patients who are survivors of cardiac arrest due to ventricular fibrillation or hemodynamically unstable sustained VT after evaluation to define the cause of the event and to exclude any completely reversible causes (Level of Evidence A).
- Class I: ICD therapy is indicated in patients with LV ejection fraction ≤35% due to prior MI who are at least 40 days post-MI and are in New York Heart Association (NYHA) functional Class II or III (Level of Evidence A).

- Class I: ICD therapy is indicated in patients with LV dysfunction due to prior MI who are at least 40 days post-MI, have an LV ejection fraction ≤ 30%, and are in NYHA Functional Class I (Level of Evidence A).

39.32 Answer D. The "no-reflow" phenomenon refers to suboptimal myocardial perfusion despite restoration of epicardial flow in the infarct artery and has been attributed to the combined effects of inflammation, endothelial injury, edema, atheroembolization, vasospasm, and myocyte reperfusion injury (Niccoli G, et al. *J Am Coll Cardiol* 2009;54(4):281–292). It is associated with reduced survival and is more common in STEMI and SVG PCI. Vasodilators including nitroprusside, adenosine, and verapamil have been used for treatment of no-reflow with variable success (Rezkalla SH, et al. *JACC Cardiovasc Interv* 2017;10(3):215–223). Aspiration thrombectomy and intracoronary GP IIb/IIIa inhibitors have also been used.

39.33 Answer D. An abrupt decline in consciousness or other new central nervous system deficit in a patient undergoing thrombolysis is an immediate indication to stop further fibrinolysis, anticoagulation, and antiplatelet agents. PT, aPTT, platelets, and fibrinogen should be drawn. STAT brain imaging and consultation with neurology should be obtained. Protamine, cryoprecipitate, fresh frozen plasma, or platelets should be given where clinically indicated. This is based on the algorithm for evaluation of intracranial hemorrhage complicating fibrinolytic therapy for STEMI (ACC/AHA, 2004).

39.34 Answer D. The ACC/AHA 2013 guidelines recommend (Class I) that noninvasive testing for ischemia should be performed before discharge to assess the presence and extent of inducible ischemia in patients with STEMI who have not had coronary angiography and do not have high-risk clinical features for which coronary angiography would be warranted. Exercise stress testing is preferred over pharmacologic stress testing unless the patient cannot exercise. In addition to the prescription of medications shown to improve subsequent events, referral to cardiac rehabilitation and smoking and diet counseling should be discussed with all STEMI patients.

39.35 Answer C. There is a U-shaped relationship between mortality and glucose level in critically ill patients as evident from the NICE-SUGAR trial (*N Engl J Med* 2009;360(13):1283–1297). In medical and intensive care unit patients, tight glucose control (81 to 108 mg/dL) compared to modest control (180 mg/dL) was associated with increased mortality rate (primarily from cardiovascular causes) and more episodes of hypoglycemia. Thus, it is reasonable to use an insulin-based regimen to achieve and maintain glucose levels <180 mg/dL while avoiding hypoglycemia for patients with STEMI with either a complicated or uncomplicated course (ACC/AHA guidelines, 2013).

39.36 Answer B. The EPHESUS trial (Pitt B, et al. *N Engl J Med* 2003;348(14):1309–1321) showed reduced mortality in patients with heart failure and MI when aldosterone antagonist is added to a beta-blocker and angiotensin inhibitor blocker. An aldosterone antagonist should be given to patients with STEMI and with no contraindications who are already receiving an angiotensin-converting enzyme (ACE) inhibitor and beta-blocker and who have an ejection fraction less than or equal to 0.40 and either symptomatic heart failure or diabetes mellitus (Class I, Level of Evidence B).

39.37 Answer A. This patient has an indication for triple therapy with warfarin, aspirin, and a $P2Y_{12}$ inhibitor. Ticagrelor and prasugrel are both more potent newer-generation inhibitors that were associated with improved outcomes compared with clopidogrel. However, they are associated with higher risk of bleeding. Thus, clopidogrel is recommended when triple therapy is indicated as explained in the ACC/AHA 2016 guidelines on duration of DAPT (Levine GN, et al. *Circulation* 2016;134(10):e123–e155). Lower target of the international normalized ratio (INR) (2 to 2.5) is also appropriate. Cangrelor is an IV form of $P2Y_{12}$ inhibitor that is used if oral agents are contraindicated. However, it has not been studied with triple therapy, nor is available in oral form for long-term use.

39.38 Answer C. In patients with STEMI, DAPT is indicated for 1 year regardless of reperfusion strategy (i.e., PCI, fibrinolytics, or surgical) (Class I). Clopidogrel is the only $P2Y_{12}$ inhibitor that has been studied in association with fibrinolytics.

40 Ethical Issues and Risks Associated with Catheterization and Interventional Procedures

Debabrata Mukherjee

QUESTIONS

40.1 A 73-year-old man with diabetes, hypertension, and dyslipidemia presents to your office with exertional chest pain. A stress test is performed, which reveals moderate-size inferolateral ischemia. You recommend cardiac catheterization with coronary angiography and possible percutaneous coronary intervention (PCI). The patient and daughter ask you about the type of stent you will implant if he needs PCI. You are on the advisory board of a stent manufacturer, which makes a bioresorbable scaffold. The appropriate course of action regarding using this particular device in this patient would be:

(A) Treat the patient based on your personal preference
(B) You should inform the patient of any conflicts of interest arising from your relationships with, or investments in, companies that manufacture or supply medications, devices, or therapies to be used for the patient. Any conflict of interest must be resolved in the best interest of the patient
(C) When caring for patients, physicians must hold the hospital's interest paramount
(D) You need not disclose your own or, your institution's, financial relationship with the manufacturer of a drug or device whenever clinical research or experience with a particular procedure or device is presented by you at a meeting or is published

40.2 All of the following are suggested by the Society for Cardiovascular Angiography and Intervention (SCAI)'s Code of Ethics, EXCEPT:

(A) The patient's welfare and best interest will always be first and foremost in the member's clinical decision-making
(B) Procedures will be performed with the expectation that the patient's quality of life will be improved and/or the risk of postprocedure adverse outcomes will be reduced
(C) A member has no obligation to accept periodic peer review and cooperate with this as a component of continuous quality improvement and appropriateness review
(D) Prior to the member performing a procedure, the patient will be given an explanation regarding details of the procedure, potential risks and benefits, and all reasonable alternatives to the procedure, so the patient can make as fully an informed decision as possible

40.3 A 45-year-old man with a history of hypertension and cigarette smoking presents to the office of a board-certified interventional cardiologist with coronary and peripheral artery expertise, with recent-onset exertional chest discomfort as well as pain in the right calf with walking. The cardiac exam and resting electrocardiogram (ECG) are normal. Exercise echocardiography results are consistent with inferior ischemia. Coronary arteriography is subsequently performed and demonstrates important two-vessel involvement amenable to PCI, with a 90% unstable-appearing proximal right coronary artery (RCA) stenosis and a 75% left anterior descending (LAD) stenosis, but no significant left main or circumflex disease. There is difficulty noted in guidewire passage into the central aorta from the right iliac. Left ventriculography demonstrates normal wall motion. After completion of the diagnostic portion of the procedure, the patient reports he has been experiencing chest discomfort and discomfort in the right thigh that has worsened as the procedure has progressed. Right iliac and femoral angiography demonstrates a 90% right common iliac stenosis. On the basis of these findings, how best should the interventional cardiologist proceed?

(A) End the procedure and schedule the patient for LAD and RCA PCIs and right iliac intervention at three separate procedures
(B) Carry out PCI only for right iliac stenosis and have the patient return for coronary intervention at a later date
(C) Perform PCI for both coronary lesions and have the patient return at a later date for iliac intervention
(D) Carry out RCA and right common iliac interventions and have the patient return for the LAD intervention

40.4 An 84-year-old woman with a history of chronic obstructive pulmonary disease (COPD) who is 2 days status post total arthroplasty following right hip fracture develops respiratory distress that responds to continuous positive airway pressure with a mask, but from which the patient subsequently cannot be weaned. Cardiac markers include a troponin I of 6.25. Coronary arteriography demonstrates serial severe LAD lesions. The circumflex is dominant and free of hemodynamically significant-appearing disease. The patient is restive from the beginning of the procedure and then becomes agitated and combative—twice contaminating the catheterization fields. The interventional cardiologist does not have privileges for deep conscious sedation—defined at the institution as bolus or brief continuous administration of general anesthetic agents such as propofol—but feels that deeper sedation is the optimum means of managing the patient's combativeness. Which of the following is the optimal approach for managing the patient's sedation and airway during the procedure?

(A) Stop the procedure and refer the patient for emergency surgical revascularization
(B) Administer increasing doses of fentanyl and midazolam in an effort to sedate the patient
(C) Contact anesthesiology for appropriate deep sedation
(D) Use forcible restraints to prevent the patient from contaminating the field
(E) The interventional cardiologist should break scrub and administer a propofol 50 mg intravenous (IV) bolus and initiate 0.1 to 0.2 mg/kg/min continuous infusion, and then rescrub and perform PCI for the LAD

40.5 An interventional cardiologist in a highly competitive environment is considering strategies to increase market share. Of the following options, which would constitute an ethical way of garnering more patient referrals?

(A) Contract with an advertising firm for an Internet and billboard campaign that describes the physician as "World Class Heart Care in Our Area" and "Advanced Experienced, Exceptional Cardiac Care in our Community"
(B) Have in practice a seasonal gift-giving plan in which physicians who refer five or more patients are sent a minimum of $1,000 for professional development purposes, and monies for these payments are derived from the collections from the respective patients
(C) Initiate a system whereby in return for patient referrals, the interventional cardiologist will send the patient back to the referring physician for nonindicated procedures, such as surveillance radionuclide stress testing
(D) Have in place a system whereby in return for referring friends and acquaintances, patients will be charged "insurance only"

40.6 An 80-year-old woman with a history of age-related cognitive decline who resides in an assisted living facility has been admitted to hospital with a non–ST-segment elevation myocardial infarction (NSTEMI). The patient's husband is deceased. There are five children, all of whom frequently visit the patient. The eldest daughter has power of attorney. There is a valid living will. An interventional cardiologist has been following the patient and discusses treatment options with the siblings, who agree on an initial course of conservative management with aspirin, clopidogrel, β-blockade, and statin therapy; they reiterate the patient's request in the living will to not be resuscitated. The patient had been admitted to the coronary care unit (CCU) and has now been transferred to a nontelemetry floor bed. On the floor, the patient has experienced two episodes of prolonged chest discomfort associated with ST-segment depression on the ECG. The children have met, and four out of the five, including the daughter with power of attorney, wish to continue conservative management. The youngest son has demanded that the patient be taken for coronary arteriography and percutaneous coronary revascularization and that the patient be resuscitated in the event of an arrest. What is the CORRECT approach in this situation?

(A) The interventional cardiologist is supremely confident in his ability to see patients safely through complex, high-risk interventional procedures. The youngest son tells the physician that he has spoken with the rest of the family and that they now agree with him. Using an informed consent signed by the youngest son, the interventional cardiologist takes the patient to the cardiac catheterization laboratory
(B) The interventional cardiologist realizes the legal significance of power of attorney and recommends a joint meeting with all five siblings
(C) Discuss the situation with the telemetry floor nursing staff, who have dealt with many such situations
(D) Because of the family strife, the interventional cardiologist notifies the family of his withdrawal from management of the patient

40.7 What, if any, federal regulation exists concerning self-referral?

(A) The Belmont Statute
(B) The Stark Law
(C) The Medicare–Medicaid Anti-Kickback Statute
(D) The Proxmire Designated Health Services Law, also referred to as the Golden Fleece Law
(E) There is no federal regulation regarding self-referral in medicine

40.8 You are actively enrolling patients at your institution in an ongoing clinical trial and have provided scientific, privacy-protected information to the study sponsor while at the same time ensuring that patient care is not negatively impacted by your financial relationship to the study. In addition to the study, you have begun to do continuing medical education (CME) presentations that are underwritten by the study. To date, you have received approximately $7,500 in compensation for your participation in the CME activities. What level of compensation is considered significant?

(A) Any compensation is considered significant for CME activities
(B) Any compensation >$500
(C) Any compensation >$5,000
(D) Any compensation >$10,000

40.9 You are the medical director of a catheterization laboratory, which has just hired a female radiology technologist to assist with the increasing volume of cases. She is well trained and eager to help. The catheterization laboratory nurse manager reports to you that a catheterization laboratory employee has recounted overhearing another male employee speak in overt sexual contexts both around and directly to the new female technician. The new female staff member confirms that these conversations took place, but she assures you that she is not affected by this environment. However, you feel that she is simply trying to protect her new job and that such coworker behavior is inappropriate and unprofessional. What is the most appropriate way to handle this situation?

(A) Refer to the policy of your institution regarding sexual harassment in the workplace and then instruct the catheterization laboratory nurse or technical manager to address this issue directly with the coworker at the earliest opportunity, enforcing the principles of professionalism and the consequences (both legal and professional) of sexual harassment either real or perceived
(B) Reassure the employee that this conduct is likely due to the predominance of men in the workplace and that this behavior is a benign part of male-dominated workplaces
(C) Because the female technician stated that such conduct did not bother her, take no further action at this point
(D) See that the particular offending male staff members and physicians avoid working with the new female technician

40.10 You are carrying out a coronary interventional procedure in a live-demonstration course and will be using an investigational device as part of the procedure. A standard informed consent for the procedure includes consent for participation in the live demonstration that was electronically signed and is in the electronic record. The intervention is complex but proceeds smoothly and successfully until near the conclusion of the procedure when the patient acutely develops diaphoresis and asks for the live demonstration to be terminated.

A guidewire perforation is noted on arteriography. Despite efforts, a covered stent cannot be delivered to remedy the perforation. Attempts at coil embolization of the artery at the perforation are successful, and the patient stabilizes. Which of the answers best summarizes the conduct of the case?

(A) Rather than agreeing to the patient's request to terminate the live demonstration, efforts should be directed at identification of the problem and stabilization of the patient
(B) The informed process for the live demonstration and use of an investigational device were appropriate
(C) The informed consent process was appropriate, but the live demonstration should have been terminated at the instant of the patient's request
(D) There are ethical problems with the standard informed consent process, and the patient may terminate the live demonstration at any time

40.11 Accepted criteria for not starting CPR include all of the following, EXCEPT:

(A) The patient has a valid "do not resuscitate" (DNR) order
(B) The patient has signs of irreversible death: rigor mortis, decapitation, or dependent lividity
(C) Attending physician discretion
(D) No physiologic benefit can be expected because the vital functions have deteriorated despite maximal therapy for such conditions as progressive cardiogenic shock

40.12 Regarding management of a patient with ischemic syndromes, which of the following is TRUE?

(A) Either PCI or coronary artery bypass grafting (CABG) is not to be pursued if a competent patient or power of attorney refuses informed consent or expresses irrevocable DNR/do not intubate (DNI) orders
(B) Medical therapy should not be provided if there are DNR/DNI orders
(C) Primary PCI should not be performed in hospitals without on-site cardiac surgery capabilities
(D) DNR orders cannot be rescinded by patients

40.13 The primary ethical principles that are operational in the allocation of scarce resources, such as heart transplantation, include all of the following, EXCEPT:

(A) Equity
(B) Beneficence
(C) Justice
(D) Utility

40.14 You were notified of a 78-year-old woman now 45 minutes status post percutaneous circumflex coronary intervention, with flank pain, diaphoresis, and suspected retroperitoneal hemorrhage. The patient has a body surface area (BSA) of 1.6 m^2 and a history of systolic hypertension, and in spite of 2,000 mL of crystalloid administered, the systolic blood pressure in the catheterization laboratory recovery area remains 90 to 100 mm Hg. The IIb/IIIa glycoprotein (GP) inhibitor was stopped. The ECG remains normal. The physician now responsible has seen the patient and is moving her to the computed tomography (CT) scanner for imaging. On the way to the scanner, her systolic blood pressure falls to 70 mm Hg, necessitating return of the patient post haste to the catheterization laboratory recovery area for further resuscitation. What of the options below is NOT part of the optimal treatment approach in this case?

(A) Sufficient volume expansion to stabilize the blood pressure before imaging to confirm retroperitoneal hemorrhage
(B) Type and cross-match for blood transfusion
(C) Rather than return to the recovery area, continue on to the radiology suite for CT scanning to confirm the diagnosis of retroperitoneal hemorrhage
(D) Obtain immediate consultation from vascular surgery and/or a peripheral interventional cardiologist in order to prepare for possible catheter-based closure of a retroperitoneal leak
(E) Ascertain the availability in the catheterization laboratory inventory of embolization coils and covered stents of sufficient size to repair an iliac perforation

40.15 Regarding deactivation of an implantable cardioverter–defibrillator (ICD) in an end-of-life patient, all of the following are reasonable discussion points, EXCEPT:

(A) Leaving the defibrillation function on could potentially cause the patient to experience pain if the device delivers shocks near the end of life
(B) Turning off the ICD will not cause death
(C) Turning off the ICD will not be painful, nor will a patient's death be more painful if it is turned off
(D) Turning off the ICD function will also turn off the pacemaker

40.16 A 73-year-old man with known coronary artery disease (CAD), severe left ventricular systolic dysfunction, and New York Heart Association (NYHA) Class III heart failure symptoms presents by emergency medical transport to the emergency department with an unequivocal anterior STEMI. The patient has altered mental status, a blood pressure of 90 mm Hg palpable systolic, and a heart rate of 100 beats per minute (bpm) and is unable to give informed consent. He is well known to you from follow-up in your clinic and has no living relatives. Recently, although in a better state of health, the patient told you that it is his desire to have no further cardiac interventions in the future, and he indicated that he had completed appropriate "DNR" orders with his primary care provider. Which of the following offers the most optimal and appropriate cardiovascular care for this patient?

(A) In addition to standard medical therapy, consider inserting an intra-aortic balloon pump (IABP)
(B) Quickly confer with other medical professionals in the emergency room and proceed to the catheterization laboratory under an emergency informed consent signed by you
(C) Tell the patient that you feel he needs to go directly to the catheterization laboratory or he will likely die
(D) Consider thrombolytic therapy along with aspirin, oxygen, nitroglycerin, and heparin, and move the patient to the CCU for further management and observation

40.17 A colleague consults you regarding a patient who has undergone diagnostic coronary angiography. Your colleague has identified a single lesion that he feels would benefit from PCI. Informed consent for possible PCI had been obtained before the procedure, and the patient is aware that you would be performing the procedure. You initially agree to perform the procedure, but as the equipment for the intervention is being pulled from electronic cabinets, your earlier doubt that the procedure is indicated intensifies because you, in fact, believe the stenosis is not hemodynamically significant. How do you proceed?

(A) Tell the patient you are uncertain of the potential benefit of the planned procedure, and ask if he chooses to proceed
(B) Tell the patient that your assessment is that the procedure is not indicated, should be canceled, and that you will review his records further and discuss your findings with him
(C) Advise the patient that although you are unsure of the ultimate outcome, the potential risks of the procedure are low and proceed
(D) Proceed without expressing your opinion to the patient in deference to both your colleague's opinion and the catheterization laboratory schedule

40.18 Before proceeding with a planned percutaneous mitral valvotomy, you explain the procedure to the patient, along with the risks, benefits, and alternatives. The patient is 75 years of age and has a history of "a touch of Alzheimer disease," according to a daughter who accompanies him. He is otherwise independent, and no separate provision, such as a health care power of attorney, has been established. What is the proper way to proceed with ensuring that informed consent is obtained?

(A) Ask your nurse to spend extra time assessing the patient's understanding of the procedure and to let you know if the patient seems to understand the plan
(B) Ask the daughter if she understands the procedure and if she is agreeable to proceeding
(C) Have the daughter convince the patient to proceed and sign the consent form despite his reluctance
(D) Ensure that the patient displays competence, understanding, and autonomy in providing consent free of undue influence or coercion

40.19 You are carrying out a coronary intervention that has immediately followed the diagnostic procedure. The patient is a 68-year-old woman with no history of drug allergies who underwent an uncomplicated renal arteriogram several years ago and since that procedure has been taking lisinopril for control of hypertension. Within the past week, a lung nodule was found on chest x-ray, and coincidentally, the patient has experienced several episodes of chest discomfort radiating to the left arm lasting for 10 to 15 minutes. Because her son was in town for the procedure, they went out for soft-shell crabs at the local French restaurant the night before the procedure. The precatheterization ECG is normal. For the procedure, the patient has received aspirin, clopidogrel, IV β-blocker, heparin, small doses of fentanyl and midazolam, and 150 mL of low-osmolality nonionic contrast material. The procedure has been going smoothly, but you have just encountered difficulty advancing a drug-eluting stent (DES) across a target lesion that was predilated with an appropriately sized balloon when the patient first says, "I feel funny," and then a minute later complains of intense itching, queasy stomach, and a feeling of being unable to clear her throat; her blood pressure drops to 80 mm Hg systolic. On examination, the patient is found to have diffusely raised urticaria, including a 10-cm diameter right neck lesion extending from dorsal of the right ear lobe to the sternal notch. What is the most likely explanation for the patient's findings?

(A) The patient is having an immune-mediated reaction to contrast material
(B) The patient is having a delayed hypersensitivity reaction to the soft-shell crab she had for dinner the night before the procedure
(C) The patient is experiencing an anaphylactoid reaction to iodinated contrast material
(D) The episode constitutes evidence that the patient has a paraneoplastic syndrome in which a tumor is producing histamine
(E) The cutaneous findings are angioedema due to lisinopril

40.20 Several months after an acute coronary event, you are seeing a 40-year-old male in follow-up in the clinic. In the course of left leg trauma from a motor vehicular accident, the patient sustained an inferior myocardial infarction (MI), for which you performed PCI of the RCA, including placement of a stent. You noted during the catheterization that the coronary arteries appeared smooth and normal, with the exception of the right coronary occlusion, which had the appearance of a meniscus convex in the direction of vessel origin (retrograde), suggesting an embolic coronary occlusion, which could have occurred as a result of the leg trauma rather than a primary plaque rupture. Following the interventional procedure, you had ordered an echocardiogram including contrast study, which was performed in the catheterization laboratory holding area. However, it was a busy day in the laboratory, and the patient was transferred to the care of trauma surgery without disposition on the echocardiographic findings. In fact, the echocardiographic contrast study had demonstrated passage of contrast from the right atrium into the left atrium, consistent with a patent foramen ovale (PFO). As a result of the leg trauma, the patient underwent left below-the-knee amputation and now will require reconstructive knee surgery. In the clinic now several weeks later, your adept midlevel associate has uncovered the echocardiographic contrast result. What is the best approach to convey this overlooked result to the patient?

(A) The echocardiographic contrast result should be conveyed to the patient as having been an incidental finding on the echocardiogram during the hospitalization
(B) A personal policy of full disclosure should be held by the physician, and in this case, the physician should explicitly relate to the patient that the echocardiographic contrast result was overlooked, followed by a discussion of the test's potential significance
(C) The echocardiographic result need not be discussed with the patient, because the findings are not germane to the present illness
(D) The interventional cardiologist should disclose the echocardiographic findings to the patient and tell him that it was the responsibility of the trauma surgeon to notify the patient of the echocardiographic findings

ANSWERS AND EXPLANATIONS

40.1 Answer B. The ethical standards for physicians relating to industry recommend that when caring for patients, members must hold the patient's welfare paramount. Physicians must prescribe drugs, devices, and treatment based solely on medical considerations and patients' preferences, regardless of any direct or indirect inducements by industry. Furthermore, physicians should inform a patient of any conflicts of interest arising from their relationships with or investments in companies that manufacture or supply medications, devices, or therapies to be used for the patient. Any conflict of interest must be resolved in the best interest of the patient. When faced with a conflict of interest that cannot be easily resolved, a physician should consult with disinterested colleagues or an institutional ethics committee to determine if an actual or potential conflict of interest is present and, if so, how to address it.

Physicians must accept no direct or indirect financial inducements from industry for utilizing one particular device or drug over another or for switching from one manufacturer's product to another. Unacceptable inducements include payment over and above the actual cost of completing postmarketing surveys of drug or device use. Physicians should disclose their own or their institution's financial relationship with the manufacturer of a drug or device whenever clinical research or experience with a particular procedure or device is presented at a meeting or is published. Clinicians who serve as the principal investigator of any research project should report fully any influence from funding sources on designing the project, controlling access to the data, preparing a presentation or paper, or controlling timing of presentation or publication.

40.2 Answer C. SCAI recognizes that ethical issues surrounding medical practice are more complex and critical than ever. The society also recognizes its responsibility to promote the highest possible ethical behavior by its members. The society recommends that the patient's welfare and best interest will always be first and foremost in the member's clinical decision-making. A member will be dedicated to providing competent, appropriate, evidence-based medical care with compassion and respect for human dignity and welfare, and a member's interactions with patients will occur without inappropriate external influence. Procedures will be performed with the expectation that the patient's quality of life will be improved and/or the risk of postprocedure adverse outcomes will be reduced. Prior to the member performing a procedure, the patient will be given an explanation regarding details of the procedure, potential risks and benefits, and all reasonable alternatives to the procedure, so the patient can make as fully an informed decision as possible. Maximizing a patient's safety and comfort will be a priority before, during, and after the procedure. A member's decision to perform an invasive/interventional procedure will be based upon what is in the best interest of the individual patient. A member will accept the importance of independent, impartial, and periodic peer review and cooperate fully with this as a critical component of continuous quality improvement and appropriateness review. Finally, performing inappropriate procedures on patients is profoundly unethical and any member doing so will suffer permanent loss of membership in the society.

40.3 Answer D. The ethical choice for managing the patient is to ameliorate the unstable coronary lesion, and as long as the coronary intervention is uncomplicated, carry out right iliac intervention as well because the patient has experienced leg pain at rest during the procedure. Schedule the patient to return at a later date for the LAD intervention. Had not the right iliac lesion been present and produced symptoms during the procedure, consideration of two-vessel coronary intervention at the same setting would also have been reasonable. Detailing options for treatment is part of the informed consent process, and therefore, it is appropriate before catheterization to discuss surgical revascularization as an option for managing selected subsets of coronary anatomy. In some instances, reimbursement may be influenced by whether multiple coronary interventions are carried out at the same or in different settings. In these cases, it is essential for the well-being of the patient that the interventional cardiologist's efforts be directed solely toward what is most appropriate for the patient without consideration of reimbursement. In the absence of the peripheral artery situation described in this case, a reasonable approach in multivessel cases is to take into account the complexity of the lesions to be intervened and endeavor to complete all the interventions in no more than two separate procedures; however, the approach should be guided by lesion complexity.

40.4 Answer C. Further narcotics and benzodiazepines in this patient may not result in the desired level of sedation, and apnea could result. The lack of deep conscious sedation privileges presents the interventional cardiologist with an ethical dilemma. Lacking these, the interventional cardiologist does not have the authority to administer propofol, although this may be the most medically optimal approach. Forcible restraints may keep the patient from contaminating the field, but they will not stop the patient's movement. A valid advanced cardiac life support (ACLS) card may not constitute sufficient expertise in airway management to afford the interventional cardiologist deep conscious sedation privileges. Although deep sedation during interventional procedures is very rarely necessary, in our experience, most such patients can safely be administered propofol without resorting to elective intubation of the patient, utilizing the deep conscious sedation monitoring protocol of the catheterization laboratory; however, it is incumbent upon the interventional cardiologist to have the appropriate hospital privilege, as otherwise, to administer a drug that has the potential to result in apnea would be unethical. If the cardiac catheterization laboratory is staffed by a full-time certified nurse anesthetist, this individual may administer drugs such as propofol, but under current nurse professional guidelines, as well as Joint Accreditation of Hospital Organization assessments, nurses with critical care qualifications are not authorized to administer deep sedation unless the patient is already intubated. Therefore, if only he or she had the appropriate privilege in the present case, the interventional cardiologist could break scrub and personally administer therapy of deep sedation. The most appropriate course would be to have an anesthesiologist administer deep sedation safely.

40.5 Answer A. It is ethical for physicians to market their practices on a billboard or on the Internet provided that the communication is truthful and not misleading, deceptive, or discriminatory. The remaining options are unethical, illegal, or both. Option B constitutes payola, a kickback to the primary physician in return for the referral of a patient and is a prosecutable offense under the Medicare-Medicaid Anti-Kickback provision in 42 U.S.C.; 1320a-7b of the United States Code. Similarly, charging "insurance only" is considered Medicare fraud and is a practice that is prohibited by the Commission for Medicare and Medicaid Services. Any such *quid pro quo* arrangements are unethical. Similarly, the practice of referring patients for any procedure that is not indicated is to be decried. For a Medicare patient, it would constitute fraud.

40.6 Answer B. Continued communication with the youngest son is essential to the well-being of this grief-stricken individual and the well-being of the family unit. Regarding clinical decisions, the physician is legally obligated to follow the instructions of the power of attorney, and the law is clear in this situation that only the power of attorney's signature constitutes valid informed consent. Therefore, whether the procedure was successful, Option A would result in legal action by the family. Option D is unsavory and comes close to an abdication of the physician's covenant to care for the patient, who should never be abandoned in time of medical need. Open, inclusive, and compassionate communication by engaged care providers virtually never fails to aid bereaved relatives, such as the youngest son, and an approach by the physician in concert with other providers, such as the patient's nurse, can gently move the process forward. Palliative care services are now available in many inpatient health facilities and can provide significant benefit in the management of bereavement and comfort to the patient (Goodlin SJ. *J Am Coll Cardiol* 1999;54(5):386-396; Mularski RA, et al. *Chest* 2009;135(5):1360-1369).

40.7 Answer B. The Federal Physician Self-Referral Law, also known as the Stark Law (United States Code Section 1395nn), prohibits referrals by a physician for "designated health services" covered by Medicare or Medicaid to entities in which the physician has a financial relationship (broadly defined as an ownership interest or compensation agreement). There has been dramatic growth in the volume of both invasive and noninvasive procedures over the past decade. The impact of this law in cardiology practice is ACCF/AHA Consensus Conference Report on Professionalism and Ethics (Ritchie JL, et al. *J Am Coll Cardiol* 2004;44(8):1740-1746). The Stark Law was conceived to curtail unnecessary usage of limited resources. The Medicare-Medicaid Anti-Kickback Statute (Chapter 42, United States Code Section 1320a-7b[b]) prohibits individuals or entities from knowingly and willfully offering, paying, soliciting, or receiving remuneration to induce referrals of items or services covered by Medicare or Medicaid. The Stark legislation is complex but, in essence, is an attempt to control self-referrals motivated by personal or financial gain, hence creating overutilization of resources. The Stark Laws are distinct from the Anti-Kickback Statute in that Stark focuses on the financial aspects of referral relationships and is a civil rather than criminal statute. Regarding Answer D, there is no such statute as the Proxmire Designated Health Services Law. The late Senator William Proxmire, Wisconsin, was a force against overcharging of the federal government by private industry and for many years recognized egregious examples of bilking with the Golden Fleece Award. He is perhaps better known as the senate sponsor of legislation in 1987, ratifying the International Convention on the Prevention and Punishment of the Crime of Genocide approved by the United Nations General Assembly in 1948.

40.8 Answer C. Transparency is the key to ensuring that the public and individual patients feel confident that we as cardiovascular clinician-researchers are keeping the public's best interests at the forefront of our activities. The Pharmaceutical Research and Manufacturers of America developed guidelines for the pharmaceutical industry's relationship with health care professionals. These voluntary guidelines took effect in 2009. Similarly, in 2009, the Advanced Medical Technology Association adopted a code of ethics to guide its members (medical technology companies) in interacting with health care professionals. This code of ethics generally addressed the same issues as the Pharmaceutical Research and Manufacturers of America guidelines but also addressed grants to institutions to subsidize fellows. Significant financial interests for investigators at this time include a minimal value of $5,000 for payments and equity interests, including any equity interest in nonpublicly traded entities.

40.9 Answer A. Given your concerns regarding this conduct, you should personally review your established policies regarding sexual harassment and promptly address the issue with the employee who is making the inappropriate comments, and review the sexual harassment policy with the entire catheterization laboratory staff. Stated succinctly, there should be zero tolerance for sexual harassment in the workplace. As the laboratory director, you have the obligation to ensure that all policies are current, available, and in practice on a daily basis in the catheterization laboratory. It is the supervisor's responsibility to provide a professional atmosphere and a safe, nonhostile working environment (Bashore TM, et al. *J Am Coll Cardiol* 2001;37(8):2170–2214). Employees should participate in regular sexual harassment training and understand that harassment is a violation of federal, state, and local laws. The first federal guidelines regarding sexual harassment in the workplace were published by the Equal Employment Opportunity Commission (EEOC) in 1980. The EEOC is the federal organization that is responsible for enforcing and interpreting federal discrimination laws. The EEOC defines sexual harassment as:

- Unwelcome sexual advances, requests for sexual favors, and other verbal or physical conduct of a sexual nature, where,
  - Submission to such conduct is made either implicitly or explicitly a term or condition of employment; or
  - Submission to or rejection of such conduct by an individual is used as a basis for employment decisions affecting the individual.
- Unwelcome sexual advances, requests for sexual favors, and other verbal or physical conduct of a sexual nature, where such conduct has the purpose or effect of unreasonably interfering with the individual's work performance or creating an intimidating, hostile, or offensive working environment.

In this case, it is reasonable to conclude that the explicit and suggestive behavior of the male colleague could interfere substantially with the ability of the female technician to carry out her work because the environment is offensive, hostile, and intimidating. Therefore, such behavior must be considered inappropriate and a potential violation of federal antiharassment laws. If a "zero tolerance" policy is to be effective, there must be strict enforcement of the antiharassment policies and bylaws that are in place. While the female technician suggests that such explicit language and behavior does not excessively bother her, it is incumbent upon you as laboratory director to take the necessary actions to ensure that all staff members are free to work in a nonoffensive, nonhostile environment free of harassment.

40.10 Answer D. A work group of the SCAI, ACCF, the Heart Rhythm Society, the European Society of Cardiology (ESC), the Sociedad Latinoamericana de Cardiología Intervencionista, and the Asian Pacific Society of Interventional Cardiology has recently published a consensus document on the use of live case demonstrations at cardiology meetings (Dehmer GJ, et al. *J Am Coll Cardiol* 2010;56(15):1267–1282). It is worthwhile to keep in mind the Belmont principles: beneficence, respect for persons, and justice. These guiding tenets can serve not only as the ethical basis for best clinical practice in the conduct of human research but also as the model for activities involving patients such as live demonstrations, even the basis for how to provide care to patients. The consensus document notes that a potential conflict of interest will exist when using investigational devices in a live demonstration, and the well-being of the patient takes precedence. In the case presented, there, of course, should have been a signed informed consent approved by the human investigations and studies committee (IRB) to participate in an IRB-approved study involving an investigational device. In addition, the writers of the consensus document recommend an IRB-approved informed consent be utilized for live-demonstration participation. As with consent to participate in a human investigation, so, too, the patient may withdraw consent to participate in a live demonstration at any time and the request should be honored. Beneficence, respect for persons, and justice should prevail.

40.11 Answer C. The ethical aspects of the cardiopulmonary resuscitation (CPR) and emergency cardiovascular care (ECC) guidelines state that scientific evaluation has shown that there are no clearly defined criteria to predict the futility of CPR (AHA, et al. *Circulation* 2000;102(8 Suppl):I-12–I-21). Therefore, it is recommended that all patients in cardiac arrest receive resuscitation unless:

- The patient has a valid DNR order.
- The patient has signs of irreversible death: rigor mortis, decapitation, or dependent lividity.
- No physiologic benefit can be expected because the vital functions have deteriorated, despite maximal therapy for such conditions as progressive septic or cardiogenic shock.
- Withholding attempts to resuscitate in the delivery room is appropriate for newly born infants with confirmed gestation <23 weeks or birth weight <400 g, or anencephaly—confirmed trisomy 13 or 18.

40.12 Answer A. Current guidelines (Fihn SD, et al. *Circulation* 2012;126(25):e354–e471) recommend that other than when prompted by a decision for comfort care, there is no contraindication to medical therapies in those with DNR/DNI orders. However, PCI or CABG is not to be pursued if a competent patient or power of attorney refuses informed consent or expresses irrevocable DNR/DNI orders. The 2011 ACCF/AHA/SCAI Guideline for PCI (Levine GN, et al. *Circulation* 2011;124(23):e574–e651) stipulated new classification ratings for both primary and elective PCI at hospitals without on-site cardiac surgery. Primary PCI was assigned a Class IIa recommendation (Level of Evidence B) stating that primary PCI is "reasonable," provided appropriate planning for program development has been accomplished. Elective PCI was given a Class IIb recommendation (Level of Evidence B) stating it "might be considered in hospitals without on-site cardiac surgery, provided that appropriate planning for program development has been accomplished and rigorous clinical and angiographic criteria are used for proper patient selection."

40.13 Answer B. The primary ethical principles that are operational in the allocation of scarce resources problem are equity, justice, and utility (Freeman RB, et al. *Prog Cardiovasc Dis* 2012;55(3):282–289). Justice is the lawful and moral maintenance of what is right for a person or what is due to a person. This principle includes both distributive justice, distributing a resource fairly to a given population, and compensatory justice, which is the belief that an injured person should receive a benefit proportional to their loss. Utility is the principle that directs policymakers to achieve the maximal benefits from a limited resource (e.g., supply of donor organs) for the population under consideration. Equity in medical practice is achieved when patients with similar expected degrees of illness and similar expected outcomes have comparable access to treatment.

40.14 Answer C. The management of acute hypotension in patients postcatheterization is fundamentally the same as in any other setting. At times, we in cardiology may err in overthinking cardiac etiologies for hypotension. A 12-lead ECG is appropriate. The presence of bradycardia and vagal symptoms should alert the clinician to the possibility of vasovagal (autonomic) hypotension, as well as anaphylactoid reaction, the latter especially if there is stridor, wheezing, or dyspnea. For postintervention patients with hypotension, in whom heparin, low molecular weight heparin, GP IIb/IIIa inhibitors, or a direct thrombin inhibitor will have been used, retroperitoneal hemorrhage or abdominal rectus hematoma should be given high priority in the differential. It is to be emphasized that key management is like a trauma alert, with all the effort directed at normalization and stabilization of the blood pressure (Trimarchi S, et al. *JACC Cardiovasc Interv* 2010;3(8):845–850) before considering diagnostic testing. The need for IV pressors for blood pressure support is an indication for consideration of catheter or surgical intervention. Combined covered stent placement and coil embolization are emerging as an effective strategy in the management of retroperitoneal hemorrhage with hemodynamic instability (Boufi M, et al. *Ann Vasc Surg* 2010;25(3):352–358).

40.15 Answer D. After an ICD has been identified, the physician should engage in an informed consent discussion with the end-of-life terminally ill patient or legally authorized surrogate about the potential benefits and burdens of the device at this point in the patient's illness. The physician should emphasize the following points during the discussion:

- Leaving the defibrillation function on could potentially cause the patient to experience pain if the device delivers shocks near the end of life.
- Leaving the shocking function active does not guarantee, however, that the heart will return to a normal pattern of beating after an arrhythmia.
- Turning off the ICD will not cause death.
- Turning off the ICD will not be painful, nor will a patient's death be more painful if it is turned off.
- The ICD has a built-in pacemaker, which is separate from the shocking function, and the pacemaker function is not turned off when shock is turned off.
- Decisions about deactivating a pacemaker are often made separately from the decision to turn off an ICD, and they depend on the indication for the pacemaker and the patient's underlying intrinsic cardiac rhythm.

40.16 Answer D. Advanced directive dilemmas are relatively common for the interventional cardiologist. The issue of advance directives (ADs), advanced care plans (ACPs), living wills, and DNR orders will become increasingly prominent in cardiovascular medicine practice as the patient population continues to age and with the presentation of patients who have higher morbidity. Individuals have the right to forgo potentially life-sustaining treatment based on the principle of patient autonomy, which is the ethical centerpiece of the doctor–patient relationship. In this case, a competent patient has expressed directly, and in writing, that he desires to have no further invasive procedures, even in an emergency. In patients who cannot make competent decisions, the issue of substitute decision-making arises. The "substitute" decision-maker must approximate the patient's wishes. Who can legally assume the role of substitute decision-maker and act as a proxy for the patient, as well as manage legal aspects of ADs, ACPs, living wills, and DNR orders, varies by jurisdiction. However, the underlying ethical principles that guide therapy in this situation should not vary, and it is paramount to respect patient autonomy and decision-making, recognizing that patients do have the right to refuse potentially lifesaving therapies. The surrogate decision-maker must consider in decreasing order of priority the patient's wishes, the patient's values and beliefs, and then patient's best interests (Parmley WW, et al. *J Am Coll Cardiol* 1998;31(5):917–925). In the case presented, the patient's wishes are clear: no further invasive procedures, and he does not wish to be resuscitated in the event of an emergency. A key responsibility in the physician's job description is to inform, counsel, and guide patients and families through this process. The choice of IABP is not appealing because this is an invasive treatment typically precluded in the setting of a DNR order. Physicians should familiarize themselves with state law and advance directive policies in their practice settings. In the present scenario, there is ample information about the patient's prior wishes to proceed with palliative therapy, though one may feel that PCI is the best option. This approach respects the patient's autonomy and protects his trust.

40.17 Answer B. In this scenario, in which the first interaction with the patient is in the catheterization laboratory itself, the interventional cardiologist has a duty to advise the patient of his/her assessment of the findings and either evaluate the hemodynamic significance of the stenosis or cancel the procedure. It is unethical for the interventional cardiologist to perform a procedure that he/she in fact judges to not be indicated, and in the present scenario would amount to a failure to take part in the clinical decision-making process, and would violate all three Belmont principles. It would be better that the interventional physician does what he or she judges to be the right thing for the patient than to later have to reconcile a complication during a nonindicated procedure. In our experience, a true colleague will virtually always understand such a change in management when the physician's best judgment is the basis for taking the alternate approach. Like all physicians, the interventional cardiologist's first responsibility is to be an advocate for the patient, be free of avoidable conflicts of interest in decision-making, and use ethical judgment in providing patient care. The interventional physician is responsible for determining the appropriateness and timing of a procedure and ensuring that the patient is informed of the various options, risks, and benefits of any planned procedures (Cameron AA, et al. *Catheter Cardiovasc Interv* 2004;61(2):157–162). Another way out of the present case that both protects the patient's interests and addresses the physiologic significance of the lesion in question, of course, is fractional flow reserve (FFR), as used in the FAME study (Tonino PA, et al. *N Engl J Med* 2009;360(3):213–224).

40.18 **Answer D.** Neglect of ensuring proper informed consent can occur. The concept of informed consent is integral to the good clinical practice of any physician. Appropriate informed consent procedures must be maintained and constitute the main method of demonstrating respect for patient autonomy and protecting the patient's trust in the physician. In the present scenario, the interventional cardiologist must spend adequate time to ensure that the patient possesses competence to understand the risks, benefits, and alternatives to the procedure and does so with autonomy, that is, free of undue influence or coercion. Generally accepted essential elements of informed consent include:

- Documentation of full disclosure of the risks and benefits of the planned procedure;
- Demonstration that the patient possesses the proper understanding of the planned procedure;
- Demonstration of patient competence to understand the procedure, as well as the risks and benefits it entails;
- Demonstration of autonomy to make decisions regarding care without undo influence or coercion;
- And documentation that the patient, after having displayed competence, understanding, and autonomy, has authorized the operator to proceed with the planned procedure (Albarran JW, et al. *Nurs Crit Care* 1996;1(3):127–133).

The patient was mentally capable of presenting a cogent history of exertional dyspnea, which signifies a level competency sufficient to consent to a procedure intended to relieve symptoms. As a general rule, the patient should be considered competent to provide informed consent unless there is a legally authorized health care power of attorney. However, in the course of the informed consent process, if the physician performing the anticipated procedure and an independent health provider, such as a catheterization laboratory holding area nurse, agree an informed consent problem exists, the process should continue until such time as acceptable informed consent is obtained, if necessary involving next of kin in the consent, and documenting the process in the progress notes. Proceeding when there is a lack of agreement about the quality of consent among providers is a recipe for problems for the patient and practitioners.

40.19 **Answer C.** When a patient undergoing a catheterization procedure says, "I feel funny," in the next minute, the patient may be incommunicative (procedural stroke) or, as in the case presented, have an anaphylactoid reaction. Although an anaphylactic reaction, an IgE-mediated immune response such as to a beesting, is possible, the incidence of immunoglobulin E (IgE) antibodies in patients who have sustained immediate hypersensitivity reactions in the catheterization laboratory is vanishingly low, and the likelihood is that the patient is experiencing an anaphylactoid reaction, most probably to iodinated contrast material. Angioedema due to lisinopril would be in the differential but is unlikely because the patient has been taking this drug for several years. So-called anaphylactoid reactions to contrast material are uncommon, especially in the era of the newer contrast agents, but such reactions do occur and have manifestations similar to the classic anaphylactic reaction. Anaphylactoid reactions, as can be judged by the name, resemble anaphylactic reactions but are nonimmune mediated. These reactions are characterized by the release of vasoactive substances, such as histamine and serotonin, presumably through a cytokine mechanism that is triggered by contrast administration, leading to the development of urticaria, indigestion, hypotension, and respiratory distress that are usually manageable by appropriate medical interventions. Iodine contained in the contrast material is not necessarily the only anaphylactoid trigger. The "queasy stomach" is a clinical sign of endogenous histamine release giving rise to secretion of stomach acid. If the patient in fact had IgE antibody to contrast material, an anaphylactic reaction would have been likely to occur immediately upon the initial administration of contrast and would have been associated with laryngeal edema and stridor, which, in this patient, did not occur. There is some delay in the development of a contrast reaction, as described in the scenario. Treatment consists of volume expansion, IV diphenhydramine and H2 receptor blocker, and IV glucocorticoid and, if necessary, administration of a pressor such as phenylephrine. Epinephrine 0.1 to 0.3 mL should be administered intramuscularly (1:1,000 dilution) for moderate reactions (Nayak KR, et al. *J Invasive Cardiol* 2009;21(10):548–551). In the event of a severe reaction, such as severe bronchospasm, laryngeal edema, or cardiopulmonary arrest, IV epinephrine may be given in a diluted form (1:10,000) at a dose of 1 to 3 mL, recognizing that nearly all adverse outcomes caused by epinephrine result when given intravenously. Completion of the patient's interventional procedure should be delayed until the patient has been stabilized.

Rarely, the hypotension of an anaphylactoid event can be sustained and sluggishly responsive to volume expansion and phenylephrine, and it is in these cases that postponement of the process becomes an option. An ounce of prevention for patients who give any history of contrast reaction, pretreatment with the preventive agents above beginning 24 hours before and again at the time of the procedure is the best practice. It is possible that the patient is experiencing a delayed hypersensitivity reaction to the soft-shell crab, but such a reaction would most probably have awakened the patient in the middle of the night before the procedure.

40.20 **Answer B.** Full and honest disclosure is always the best policy when disclosing medical errors. The physician has only to fully disclose the echocardiographic contrast findings to the patient, explicitly take responsibility that the oversight was his/her error alone, and the patient, although perhaps briefly dismayed about this health history development, will see that the physician has the patient's best interest as the first priority. Any approach other than full disclosure constitutes dissembling, and there could be no other conclusion by the patient in that event other than the physician wishes to hide something. In the present scenario, nothing untoward has occurred as a result of the patient's PFO, but the possibility of paradoxic embolism as a cause of MI must be introduced to the patient. For errors of commission or omission, an approach of full disclosure allows the patient and physician to proceed without emotional encumbrances, and for the physician, precludes feelings of guilt for not having been forthcoming to the patient. In the present case, full disclosure allows the physician to proceed with a positive discussion regarding management of the PFO, including the possibility that the patient's left leg trauma resulted in either a thromboembolism or fat embolism that could have passed paradoxically to the RCA causing the heart attack. Breach of the physician–patient relationship as result of dishonesty may also result in litigation (Gallagher TH, et al. *Arch Intern Med* 2005;165(16):1819–1824).

41 Statistics Related to Interventional Cardiology Procedures

Harsh Agrawal

QUESTIONS

41.1 A recent journal article reported the results of a randomized clinical trial (RCT) comparing two medical therapies used in conjunction with transcatheter aortic valve implantation. The primary end point was 30-day mortality. In addition to the results for the overall study population, results of a subgroup analysis by gender were also reported (Fig. Q41-1). Based upon these results, you conclude the following:

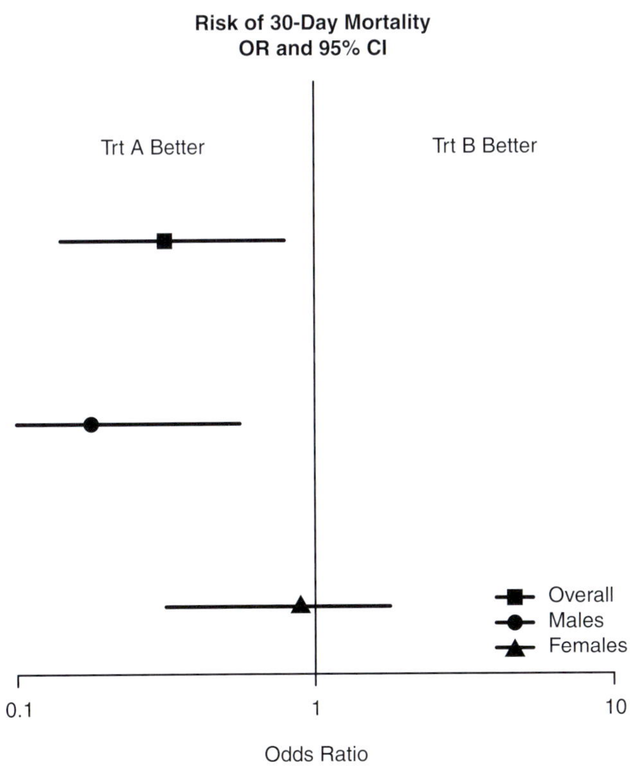

Figure Q41-1

(A) Females can be treated with either treatment
(B) Females should be treated with treatment B
(C) Neither treatment is effective at reducing 30-day mortality
(D) The results for the overall study population contain the most information

41.2 A catheterization laboratory colleague practicing at a hospital in North Carolina is preparing to treat a patient who has a very long lesion (>25 mm) in the right coronary artery. She is considering two approaches: overlapping two drug-eluting stents (DES–DES) or overlapping a drug-eluting stent and bare-metal stent (DES–BMS). She brings you two articles to review and asks for advice on how to proceed. The first reports the results of a large, well-powered RCT in South African patients. The trial found DES–DES to be a safer and more effective means of treatment than the alternative approach. The second article reports the results of a large observational study in the United States that found no significant advantage to either treatment over the other. What do you recommend?

(A) She should proceed with DES–DES because randomized trials are more reliable than observational studies
(B) She can treat with either because observational studies are more reliable than randomized clinical studies
(C) She should broaden her literature review to include RCTs conducted in the United States before making her decision
(D) She should broaden her literature review to include observational studies conducted in South Africa before making her decision

41.3 You are given access to data collected from a large randomized trial designed to assess the effectiveness of a new intracoronary stent (Stent A) in reducing mortality compared with Stent B. While the primary end point of the original study was mortality, patients were also followed to determine if repeat revascularization was required following the index procedure. Demographic data, such as a patient's diabetic status, age, race, etc., were also recorded. You would like to use this dataset to determine if Stent A is effective in diabetic patients. After removing nondiabetic patients, 1,000 patients remain, 500 randomized to Stent A, and 500 to Stent B. You are considering the composite end point of mortality or revascularization. The statistician on the project summarizes the data in Figure Q41-3. Based on the figure, the composite end point is a reasonable end point to consider since there will be so many more events with the inclusion of revascularization, which will in turn increase statistical power.

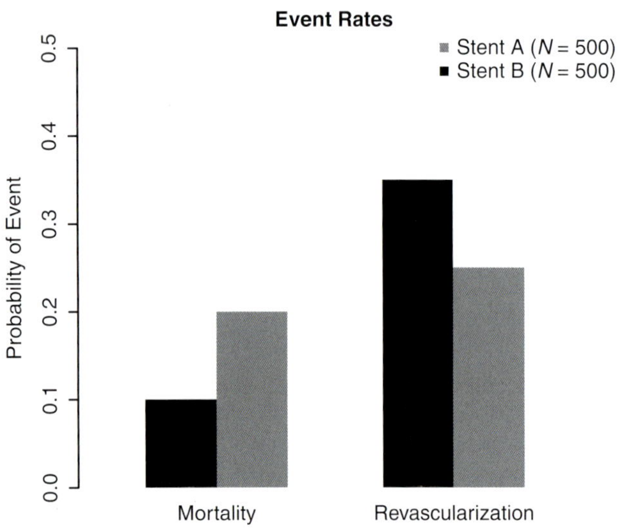

Figure Q41-3

(A) True
(B) False

41.4 What is not a potential benefit of a registry-based randomized controlled trial (RRCT) over a conventional randomized control trial (RCT)?

(A) Cost of trial is less than an RCT
(B) Relatively large number of patients can be enrolled in a shorter time frame
(C) Patients are more representative of the real-world population
(D) Both the patients and physicians can be blinded to prevent potential bias

41.5 Table Q41-5 reports the baseline characteristics of patients with de novo left main disease from two different studies. Both studies compared the efficacy of percutaneous coronary intervention (PCI) using paclitaxel-eluting stents and coronary artery bypass graft treatment. Based on these characteristics, which study most likely corresponds to the randomized Synergy Between PCI with TAXUS and Cardiac Surgery (SYNTAX) trial and which belongs to an observational study?

Table Q41-5

	Study A		Study B	
	CABG	PCI	CABG	PCI
Age, y	65.6	65.4	61.3	58.6
Men, %	75.6	72.0	73.9	70.1
Left main only	14.1	11.8	10.0	41.8
Diabetes mellitus, %	25.6	23.8	31.0	23.9
Prior myocardial infarction (MI), %	24.0	17.9	12.7	8.2

All continuous covariates are presented as the mean value, and categorical measures are presented as percents. Table reused from the second edition.

(A) Study A most likely corresponds to the SYNTAX trial
(B) Study B most likely corresponds to the SYNTAX trial
(C) There is not enough information to decide

41.6 In a registry comparing PCI of the unprotected left main coronary artery to coronary artery bypass surgery, traditional trial designs have used a single composite end point as primary outcome, with the assumption that each component of the composite end point carries similar weight and treatment and is the same for each component. However, this is seldom true as death is not equivalent to a nonfatal myocardial infarction (MI). Multiple statistical approaches have been introduced to overcome this issue. Which of the following is the new statistical method?

(A) Andersen–Gill Counting Process
(B) WIN ratio (WR)
(C) Competing Risk Method
(D) Weighted composite end point (WCE)
(E) All of the above

41.7 A pharmaceutical sales representative is presenting his company's literature on the use of a medical treatment for coronary artery disease (CAD). The medical treatment, if beneficial, would reduce the need for PCI when treating CAD. He describes a large randomized trial investigating the superiority of the medical treatment when compared with PCI. The primary end point of the study was periprocedural or spontaneous MI. The sales representative presents the Kaplan–Meier estimates of the survival curves over the first 48 hours following treatment for both treatment groups (Fig. Q41-7). Which of the following is a possible explanation for the results seen in the figure?

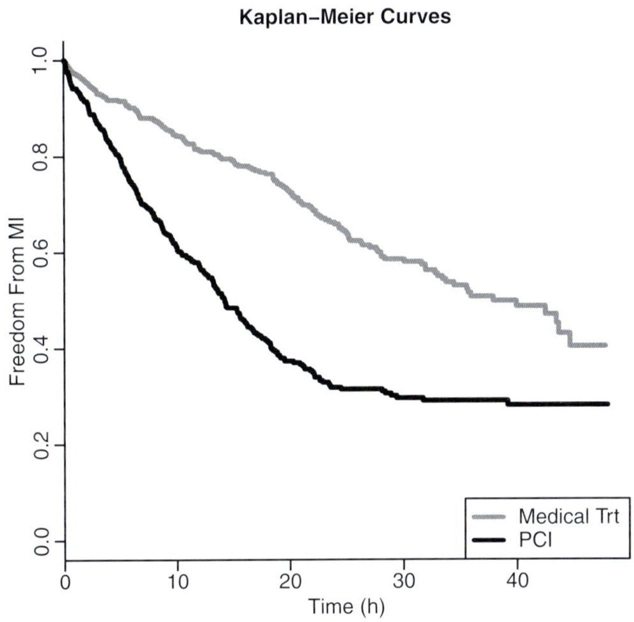

Figure Q41-7

(A) Medical treatment is superior to PCI
(B) The inclusion of periprocedural MI in the endpoint definition is biasing the results in favor of medical treatment
(C) Both A and B
(D) Neither A nor B

41.8 You are part of a proposed study's steering committee, which has been charged with designing a clinical trial to test whether new Stent A is better than old Stent B. The new stent has many attractive design features and your research group would like to be sure that the study is large enough to definitively conclude that Stent A is truly superior to Stent B if the rates hypothesized are seen. Which component of sample size calculation does this refer to?

(A) Type I error
(B) Type II error
(C) Number needed to treat (NNT)
(D) Study *p*-value

41.9 A recently published journal article reported the results of an RCT comparing two invasive techniques, fractional flow reserve (FFR), and instantaneous wave-free ratio (iFR), for determining the severity of coronary artery disease to guide revascularization. The authors concluded that iFR is noninferior to FFR in terms of major cardiovascular outcomes. Which option on the forest plot Figure Q41-9 best demonstrates this finding?

(A) A
(B) B
(C) C
(D) D

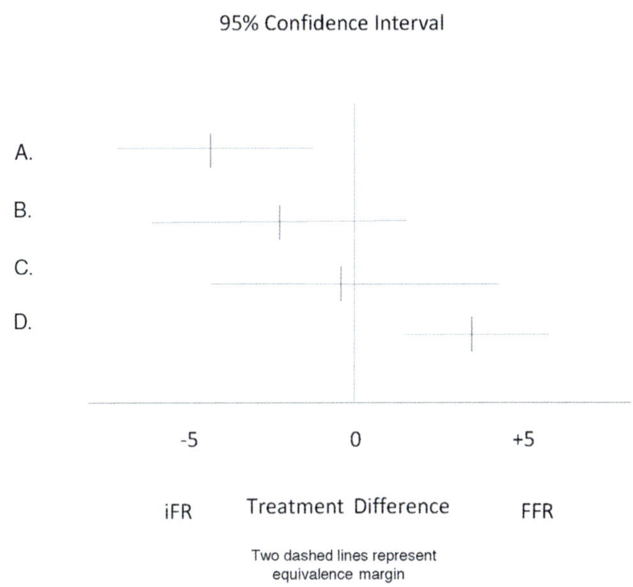

Figure Q41-9 (Courtesy of Harsh Agrawal.)

41.10 Two years ago, a new DES was introduced to a practice within a community-based catheterization laboratory that performs approximately 500 PCIs per year. It quickly became popular and was used in 45% of procedures. The laboratory collects information at the time of procedure and over the first year following discharge. You have noticed that there have been several recent cases of subacute stent thrombosis and wonder if these events are related to the new stent. You are preparing a proposal to investigate this relationship for the director of the laboratory. What is the most appropriate study design to get information quickly in this setting that might be useful in addressing your concerns?

(A) Case–control study
(B) Nonrandomized observational registry
(C) Cohort study
(D) Randomized clinical trial

41.11 Regardless of your answer to Question Q41.10, suppose you decide to perform a cohort study. You divide patients into two groups (those whose interventions included the new DESs and those whose interventions did not), and you follow them for the next year. You calculate the rate of subacute stent thrombosis in each group and determine the odds ratio (OR). You conduct your study at a 0.05 nominal level. What do you conclude?

(A) Due to the randomization in a cohort study, you can easily conclude that the stent is harmful
(B) Due to the lack of randomization in a cohort study, you cannot conclude the stent is harmful without first adjusting for other possible confounders
(C) Regardless of the randomization, the stent is harmful
(D) Regardless of the randomization, the stent is beneficial

41.12 For which of the following reason(s) is blinding (or "masking") in a clinical trial important?

(A) It helps prevent introduction of treatment-specific biases
(B) It helps maintain objectivity in assessment of clinical events
(C) It preserves Type I error rate
(D) A and B

41.13 A new treatment is being considered as a low-cost alternative to the current standard of care. As the primary benefit of this new treatment is the lower cost, a large noninferiority trial was conducted to investigate the performance of the new treatment; see Figure Q41-13 for a summary of the findings.

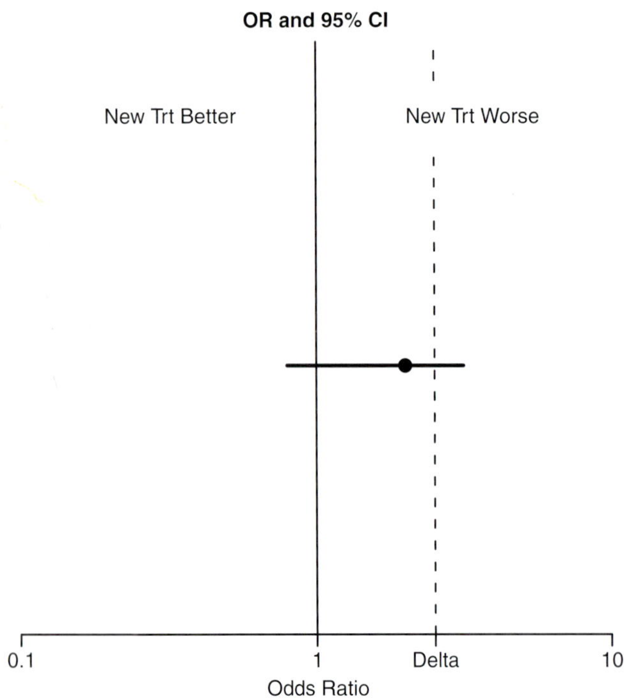

Figure Q41-13

Some patients randomized to receive the new low-cost treatment were inadvertently given the old treatment. The decision was made to analyze the data with an intention-to-treat protocol (ITT). The study reported the findings to be inconclusive. Which of the following statements is the best possible explanation of the results?

(A) The study was underpowered to correctly determine noninferiority, resulting in a wide confidence interval
(B) The ITT analysis favored the inferiority hypothesis, resulting in a wide confidence interval
(C) Both A and B
(D) Neither A nor B

41.14 You are interpreting the results of a clinical trial that compared fibrinolysis with primary angioplasty for ST-segment elevation acute MI. There were 6,600 patients randomly assigned to one of two treatments, with 3,300 patients in each group. If there were 300 deaths in the fibrinolysis group and 200 deaths in the PCI group, what is the OR that most appropriately compares the two groups?

(A) 0.065
(B) 0.10
(C) 0.65
(D) 9.1%

41.15 The results of a clinical study are provided in Table Q41-15. Your local formulary committee asks you to put this into clinical context and provide them with an absolute risk reduction by using this drug. What is it?

Table Q41-15

	Placebo	Treatment	Total
MI	10	8	18
No MI	90	92	182
Total	100	100	200

Table reused from the second edition.

(A) 8%
(B) 10%
(C) 2%
(D) 15%

41.16 The committee also wants to know the number needed to treat (NNT) one patient with the new drug to prevent one MI. The NNT is:

(A) 0.02
(B) 0.50
(C) 42
(D) 50

41.17 You are conducting a case-control study to compare the long-term efficacy of BMS and DES in your local catheterization laboratory. Looking through the database available, you find that patients are categorized based on the type of stent implanted. All patients had a follow-up exam 12 months following their index procedure, and the amount of restenosis in the artery was recorded. In conducting this case-control study, you use propensity scores to match each DES patient with a similar BMS patient. The matching is done to account for possible confounders, such as age, gender, body mass index (BMI), etc. (Fig. Q41-17). Is this figure an appropriate way to visually compare these data?

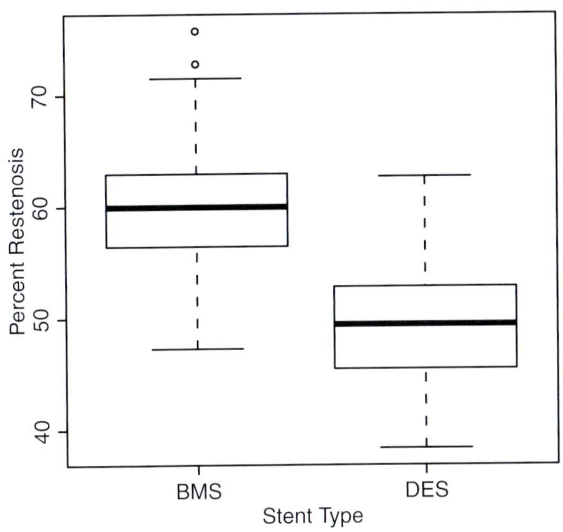

Figure Q41-17

(A) Yes
(B) No

41.18 Your colleague hypothesizes that the amount of restenosis 10 years following the implantation of a stent is associated with the BMI of the patient at the time of the PCI. Using a pre-existing database from a clinical trial comparing two stents that measured a patient's BMI and other risk factors, he divides patients into two groups: those with a BMI > 20 at the time of PCI and those with a BMI no more than 20 at the time of PCI. His analysis, summarized in Figure Q41-18, found little relationship between BMI and the amount of restenosis 10 years following PCI. He submits the article for publication. Which of the following is a possible response from a reviewer?

(A) BMI should not be broken up into two arbitrarily defined categories, as this might mask the effect of BMI on restenosis
(B) The amount of restenosis is a categorical variable, and therefore, a box plot is not an appropriate method of displaying the data

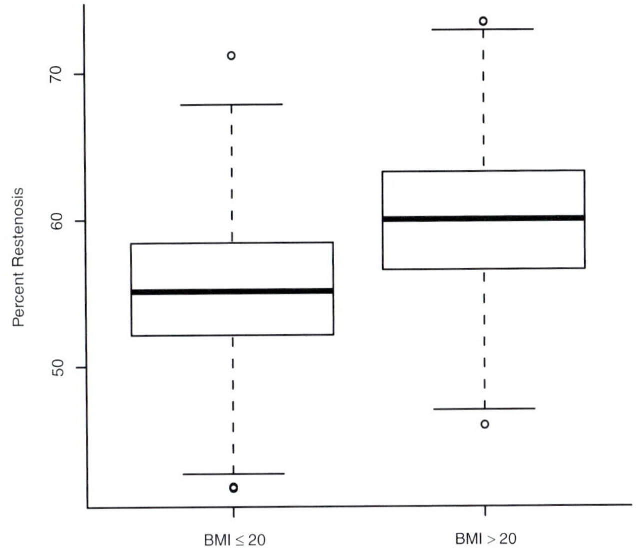

Figure Q41-18

(C) When considering various groups based on a variable, you should consider at least 10 groups
(D) None of the above

41.19 Three hundred and seventy-eight patients in a prospective study presented to the cardiac catheterization laboratory for a coronary angiogram and were found to have intermediate stenosis (50% to 70%). The researchers sought to evaluate the accuracy of the visual estimation of the stenosis as significant enough for PCI vs. gold standard for assessing the significance of the lesion by FFR and subsequent PCI. Table Q41-19 shows a 4 × 4 design of the study. What is the sensitivity of visual estimation for PCI as compared to FFR-guided PCI?

Table Q41-19

Visual Assessment of Stenosis and Subsequent PCI	FFR Positive	FFR Negative	Total
Yes	105	171	276
No	15	87	102
Total	120	258	378

Table courtesy of Harsh Agrawal.

(A) 88%
(B) 34%
(C) 38%
(D) 85%

41.20 In the above question, what is the diagnostic effectiveness of visual estimation for PCI vs. FFR-guided PCI?

(A) 88%
(B) 34%
(C) 38%
(D) 50.8%

ANSWERS AND EXPLANATIONS

41.1 Answer D. Clinical trials are typically designed and powered to answer one question, represented by the primary end point. Subgroups of patients, defined by patient characteristics (such as gender or age) or disease characteristics (such as the presence or absence of diabetes or other risk factors), are best viewed for consistency. If there is a positive treatment effect in favor of one therapy over another, there may well be *quantitative* differences (differences in the absolute treatment effect) in the magnitude of the observed treatment effect that favor certain subgroups, but it is unlikely that there will be important *qualitative* differences (treatment effect that is truly directionally different from the main result) among subgroups. The most appropriate way to view RCT results is from the perspective of the overall trial results.

41.2 Answer C. While RCTs are generally preferred to observational studies, the results of the trial should be generalizable to the patient of interest before making treatment decisions. In this case, the randomized trial was conducted solely in South Africa while the patient of interest is from the United States. Because of differences in patient characteristics, the result seen in the trial may not generalize to the patient of interest. If randomized trials including US patients are available, these results should be considered prior to making a treatment decision. If such trials are not available, the results of the South African trial are likely more useful and reliable than the US-based observational study.

41.3 Answer B. The figure illustrates that Stent A appears to be associated with a lower revascularization rate, but it also appears to be associated with an increased mortality rate. Since Stent A has a different effect on each of the components of the composite, considering a composite end point with these two events would be inappropriate.

41.4 Answer D. Randomized clinical trials are the strongest type of clinical trials that can be performed. They are the cornerstones for establishing the effectiveness or harm of any therapy or drug by accounting for the effects of the confounders. However, RCTs are very costly to perform; take years to perform, in which time the standard of care may change; and might not be completely representative of the real-world population. However, RCTs are blinded, which makes them potentially free of selection and treatment bias. RRCTs are a new kind of randomized clinical trial; they use registry data to randomize patients to measure the effect of a therapy. This has several benefits as mentioned above except that there is no way to blind the physician or the patient. In addition, long-term follow-up, measurement of composite outcomes, generalizability, data quality, and missing data are some of the challenges faced by this kind of trial design.

41.5 Answer A. The primary benefit of randomizing patients into treatment groups is that the groups are then "balanced" across other covariate information. This ensures that any associations we observe are due to the treatment under study and not to extraneous covariate differences (confounding). In the table, the data related to Study A appear to be balanced (similar between the two treatment groups), while in Study B, the characteristics differ between the groups. Notice that without knowing if the sample sizes are similar for the two studies, the balance only refers to the additional covariate information. Since the SYNTAX trial is a randomized study, it most likely corresponds to Study A.

41.6 Answer E. All of the abovementioned methods can be used for statistical analysis over and above the traditional time-to-event analysis (TTE). The Andersen–Gill method uses first event as well as subsequent events as long as the subject is still being observed with equal probability. It does not give different weight to different events. WR is a rank-based method, which first ranks and then pairs the patients to different treatment methods according to a risk score to test for treatment superiority. Competing risk is an event than can modify the chances of occurrence of an event of interest or hinder its occurrence. Competing risk methodology takes this into account and can help quantify the effect of an intervention on each composite endpoint components individually. The WCE method is an extension of the TTE method where each of the nonfatal events carries a weight. Patients start with a weight of 1 and their contribution to the cohort reduces in weight with each nonfatal event (which is assigned a weight with value of <1) and full or all remaining weight is lost in the event of death.

41.7 Answer C. The survival curve for medically treated patients is shifted upward from that corresponding to patients undergoing PCI. Therefore, it is possible that the medical treatment is indeed reducing the risk of MI. However, the inclusion of periprocedural MI in the endpoint definition will bias the results in favor of medical treatment. That is, since those patients undergoing medical treatment do not undergo a procedure, by definition, they cannot experience a periprocedural MI, and the survival probability for the PCI group will look worse at first (carry an early hazard). If periprocedural MI is not included in the end point, PCI might actually appear similar or even superior to the medical treatment. It is important to carefully consider the definition of an end point and the definition of the treatment under study when examining study results.

41.8 Answer B. Type II error (β) occurs when no effect is seen between the studied treatments when, in fact, a treatment effect truly exists. One minus the Type II error ($1 - \beta$) is also known as the *trial's power*. By understanding the risk of a tType II error, or conversely, the importance of power in examining clinical trial results, one can appreciate whether a study actually had adequate power or was truly large enough in size to answer the desired question. Many studies that fail to show a statistical difference between therapies suffer from a lack of power; that is, the study design accepted a large potential Type II error (Yusuf S, et al. *Prog Cardiovasc Disc* 1985;27(5):335-371). By convention, a well-powered clinical trial accepts a potential β error of <10% to no more than 20%. In the example given, one would want to be sure that the planned trial had a minimum of 80% power (but preferably ≥90%) to definitively conclude that Stent A was truly superior to Stent B.

41.9 Answer C. Figure A41-9 depicts four different results. Plot A depicts that iFR is superior to FFR as the line of unity (0) is not crossed. Plot B depicts noninferiority of iFR as compared to FFR. Here, we are interested in whether the confidence interval (CI) falls below the bound (the minimally important difference or MID). Plot C depicts equivalence of the two treatments given the wide confidence interval and not crossing the MID on both sides, and plot depicts that FFR is superior to iFR. Noninferiority trials are designed to test if a new treatment is as efficacious as the current standard of care. With significant advancement in health care technology, patient safety, and clinical outcomes, demonstrating significant benefit of new therapies over existing treatments may not be possible and assigning such patients to a placebo may be unethical. No two drugs can have exactly the same effects or are equivalent. Hence, clinical equivalence means that their effects differ by no more than a prespecified amount, known as equivalence margin. Noninferiority trials, on the contrary, are geared to demonstrate that an experimental treatment is not less effective than an active control by more than the equivalence margin.

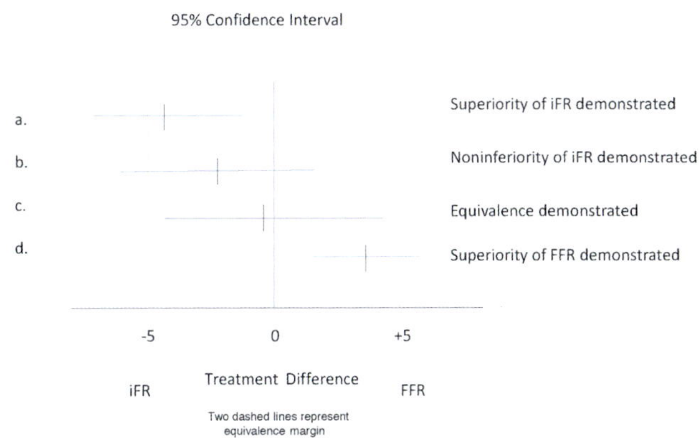

Figure A41-9 (Courtesy of Harsh Agrawal.)

41.10 Answer A. The case-control study is well suited for providing preliminary information on a question using previously collected data (Narins CR, et al. *Circulation* 1996;93(4):667-671). Since you can identify patients who have experienced stent thrombosis and a matched group who have not, you should be able to get some preliminary information regarding the factors that are associated with the outcome. There are problems with the case-control study, most notably bias that arises from the data already collected before occurrence of the event. Randomized trials prove the overall best method of evaluating and comparing treatments, but such studies are much larger and take longer than is practical to provide preliminary insight into your concerns.

41.11 Answer B. Observational studies do not randomize patients. As no attempts were made to account for the effect of possible confounders, we cannot make a strong causal interpretation of the results. It is possible that the difference observed is due to differences in the age of the patients receiving the different types of stent. For example, suppose all patients who received the new stent are older than those patients who did not; then, it is not possible to determine if the observed effect is due to the stent or the age of the patient. This is a limitation of observational studies. The use of analytical methods such as propensity scores to match patients is an example of how one might attempt to overcome this drawback by accounting for the effects of other confounders, such as age. This example demonstrates why RCTs are seen as the gold standard in the evaluation of new therapies. The randomization allows us to make causal links based on the results as the treatment groups are balanced (i.e., the same) except for the randomly assigned treatment.

41.12 Answer D. Blinding in a clinical trial can reduce the likelihood of biased behavior on the part of investigators, patients, or other study personnel. For example, knowledge of the treatment assignment might cause an investigator to look harder for certain drug effects, both expected and unexpected. For trials that include an independent assessment of the study's endpoint events, such as review by a clinical events committee, blinding is essential to maintain the integrity of a process that relies on a completely objective determination of suspected endpoint events (Mahaffey KW, et al. *Curr Control Trials Cardiovasc Med* 2001;2(4):180–186).

41.13 Answer C. When a study is underpowered, the resulting confidence intervals for an estimate are very wide. That is, it is difficult to detect whether a treatment is noninferior (or superior, depending on the context). In addition, ITT analyses are conservative in a superiority trial but are not so in a noninferiority trial. Suppose that the new treatment is superior; the patients who incorrectly took the standard treatment will bias the estimated treatment effect in favor of the standard treatment. This will result in a wider confidence interval and can lead to inconclusive or even incorrect conclusions. In most trials that are testing first for superiority, the ITT analysis is the appropriate one; in a noninferiority test, it is frequently preferred to use a treatment received or even an on-treatment comparison for the most informative assessment.

41.14 Answer C. ORs and risk ratios are two of the more common ways to display comparative data in the medical literature. To calculate the odds of having an event in any one group, we divide the number of events in that group by the number of patients in that group who did not have an event. The OR is the ratio of those two odds. Risk is calculated by dividing the number of events by the total number of patients in a group. Risk ratios are then calculated by dividing the risks of the individual groups. In the example given, the odds of dying in the fibrinolysis group are 0.10 (300/3,000) and in the PCI group are 0.065 (200/3,100). This provides an OR of 0.65 (0.065/0.10).

41.15 Answer C. Absolute risk reduction (ARR) is also called the risk difference. It answers the question: As a result of using the treatment, is the risk of an event reduced by a clinically meaningful amount? The calculation is just the difference between the risk of an event in the placebo group and the risk of an event in the treated group. The risk under placebo is 10% (10/100), and the risk under the treatment is 8% (8/100), giving a risk difference, or ARR, of 2%.

41.16 Answer D. The NNT is defined as 1/(risk difference or ARR), as we already calculated the ARR or the risk difference of 2%. To calculate NNT, we take 1/0.02 = 50.

41.17 Answer B. No, we cannot use the box plots to compare the data. The existence of confounders has been accounted for by matching each DES patient to a similar BMS patient. However, this creates a correlation structure in the data. That is, each matched pair is more similar to one another than to other patients in the sample. For example, suppose we recorded blood pressure in 10 individuals before and after a stress test. The two measurements taken on patient 1 will be more similar to one another than the measurements of patient 1 and patient 2. So the data are not independent. When the data are correlated, other visual and statistical methods must be considered that account for this correlation.

41.18 Answer A. Continuous variables, such as age, BMI, and creatinine clearance, typically should not be broken into categories (called discretizing). This process discards potentially valuable information and can actually mask the effect. For example, suppose the relationship between BMI and the amount of restenosis was curved; then, by grouping patients based on an arbitrary cutpoint of BMI, it is possible to miss the underlying effect in the analysis.

41.19 Answer A and 41.20 Answer D. The sensitivity of the test is the proportion of patients with disease who have a positive test. Thus, sensitivity is (True Positives [TP]/TP + False Negatives [FN]). In this case, that's 105/105 + 15 = 0.88 or 88%. The high sensitivity test is useful to rule out a disease with confidence; chances of missing a disease are low.

The specificity of a test is the proportion of patients without the disease who test negative. High specificity is helpful in classifying a patient with the disease if positive. Specificity is TN/TN + FP. Negative predictive value is the proportion of the patients correctly classified as negative among all the negative patients. NPV = TN/TN + FN. Positive predictive value is proportion of correctly diagnosed positives among all positive tests. PPV = TP/TP + FP. Unlike sensitivity and specificity, predictive values are largely dependent on disease prevalence in the population. Accuracy or diagnostic effectiveness of a test is the proportion of correctly diagnosed patients among all the patients tested. Thus, in this case, diagnostic effectiveness or accuracy is TP + TN/TP + FP + FN + TN or (105 + 87)/378 = 0.508 or 50.8%.

42 Approach to Interventional Boards and Test-Taking Strategies

Debabrata Mukherjee

QUESTIONS

42.1 What identification will you need to take the American Board of Internal Medicine (ABIM) interventional exam?

(A) A valid credit card
(B) Social security card
(C) A primary and secondary identification. Candidates without a valid primary and secondary ID may not be admitted to the exam. Primary ID can be a current government-issued form of ID that contains both your signature and a recent photograph. A valid driver's license, passport, or state identification card is acceptable. Secondary ID can be a form of ID that includes either your signature or a photograph. For example, a social security card, valid credit card, or ATM card is acceptable
(D) Workplace ID
(E) A copy of your examination confirmation email

42.2 Once you gather all the material you need to study for the interventional board exam, you are ready to start your preparation. After acquiring your study material for the board exam, you should organize your study plan to:

(A) Begin with the subject matter you know best to build your confidence
(B) Focus on doing practice questions
(C) Focus on the content you have heard is most important for the exam
(D) Map out how many pages of material you will cover each day
(E) Start by focusing on the content area where you are least confident

42.3 You have just finished reading through all of your study materials for the board exam and you have some additional time before you are scheduled to take the test. To make the best use of this remaining preparation time you should:

(A) Do as many practice questions from the *1133 Questions: An Interventional Cardiology Board Review* book as possible in the time you have left
(B) Do practice questions from the *1133 Questions: An Interventional Cardiology Board Review book* and let the ones you get wrong tell you what to go back and study again
(C) Find and review new study material to give you an alternative perspective on the core concepts for the exam
(D) Read over your study materials again
(E) Take a break from studying so that you will be fresh for the exam itself

42.4 There is a lot of information to commit to memory for the board exam. The most efficient way to commit critical study material to memory is to:

(A) Copy the details from your study material into a personal study notebook
(B) Do a lot of practice questions
(C) Organize the material into clusters
(D) Read over it repeatedly
(E) Talk it over with a friend or colleague

42.5 There is a lot of material to study to prepare for the board exam and people often feel some frustration during the study process. When you feel frustrated in the middle of your study process, the best thing to do is:

(A) Find a different source to study from
(B) Shift to a different topic area
(C) Stop studying for the day and come back to look at the material the next day
(D) Take a 30-minute break from study
(E) Take a deep breath and focus your attention on the material before you

42.6 When answering questions during the board exam, if you are able to eliminate all but two of the presented options but cannot come up with a reason to select one or the other, the best strategy is to:

(A) Go back and reread the questions to check for important details you might have missed
(B) Make an argument to yourself about why one option, then the other, must be right
(C) Read each option again and think about what it reminds you of
(D) Read each option again and think carefully about the exact wording
(E) Take a guess

42.7 Taking time to do practice questions is an important part of preparation for the board exam. The best strategy for getting the most benefit out of practice questions is to:

(A) Do as many practice questions as you can from as many different sources as you can
(B) Focus on a particular set of questions and do them repeatedly until you get them all correct
(C) Save your practice questions until you have completed your study of content material
(D) Take your time when doing practice questions to give yourself a chance to think clearly about each one
(E) Use questions you get wrong to guide you on what you need to go back and review again

42.8 In medical practice, experts often disagree on the proper course of action in a given circumstance. When confronting a presented situation in an exam question where you know there may be some difference of opinion among practitioners in the field, the best way to decide on an answer is:

(A) Become familiar with clinical findings and research published in the last year
(B) Consider what you think most of the colleagues you know would do in a similar situation
(C) Select an answer based on existing practice guidelines
(D) Think about how you would handle the situation in your own practice
(E) Think back to the direction you received in handling similar situations when you were in residency and fellowship training

42.9 People have a lot of different advice as to how to best prepare for the board exam. Some of this advice is good and some is not. Most people find that the best way to understand and remember important information for the board exam is to:

(A) Focus on linking the material you study to real-life patients you have encountered
(B) Rearrange study materials to focus on differences among concepts
(C) Reread the details to reinforce their importance
(D) Try hard to remember the material exactly as it was presented
(E) Write everything out longhand in parallel with your study material

42.10 For the exam usually does not occur all at once, but in a series of study sessions across several weeks or months, the best thing to do at the end of each of these study sessions is to:

(A) Chart your progress in covering the material you will need to master for the exam
(B) Look ahead at the study material you have left for the specific topic you are studying
(C) Map out what you will study next
(D) Summarize the key concepts covered during your study session
(E) Think about something besides the study material to give yourself a mental break

42.11 To do well on the board exam, you must apply the knowledge you have learned to the questions presented. During the actual exam, the first thing you should do is:

(A) Read and focus on the questions at the end of the clinical case
(B) Read the presented case content and check on relevant details
(C) Read over the presented options/answers to see what comes to mind
(D) Take a moment and think about the issues that the presentation brings to mind
(E) Try to connect what you have read to a real-life patient you have encountered

42.12 Practice questions are usually a part of everyone's preparation for the board exam. The best way to integrate practice questions into the weeks and months of your study is to:

(A) Begin doing a few questions early and increase the number as the exam gets closer
(B) Don't limit practice questions to study time, but do them whenever you have a spare moment in your day
(C) Spend most of your study time on practice questions and reading the annotated answers
(D) Begin studying by doing a lot of questions as guidance as to what to study

42.13 Different people need to take different amounts of time to prepare for the board exam depending on their general familiarity with the material. The best way to decide how much time you need to take to prepare for your board exam is to:

(A) Assume that you will need about 2 weeks of preparation for every year that you are out of fellowship
(B) Begin preparation early to get a sense of what is familiar and your comfort with the material
(C) Check with people who recently took the exam and see how long they studied
(D) Decide how many pages of study material you can cover in a week and project the time needed to complete the material
(E) Take a practice exam and see how well you do

42.14 The way we learn should be different for different types of material and different kinds of tests. The best way to get ready for a multiple-choice exam is to:

(A) Focus on memorizing important details just as they are presented in study materials
(B) Organize material in modules, and modules in clusters, that emphasize differentiation
(C) Read your study material aloud to make sure you cover it all and to help with memorization
(D) Talk to colleagues who have taken the exam in the past and focus your study on the things that were prominently featured in their exam
(E) Write or type out explanations of important concepts in sentence form to get familiar with the essential details

42.15 Some of the material you have to learn for the board exam will be relatively easy and simple memorization will suffice. Other material is more complex and will require more sophisticated techniques to master. When trying to master difficult or complex material for the board exam, the best strategy is to:

(A) Block out time and sit studying the material until you have mastered it
(B) Focus on practice questions so you will know how it will appear on the exam
(C) Gather all the reference material you can on the subject and work your way through all of it
(D) Look at it for a little bit of time every day until you feel comfortable with it
(E) Skip it completely and hope that it will not account for much of the exam

42.16 For people who have recently completed a relevant fellowship prior to taking the board, the best suggestion for planning how to spend study time would be:

(A) Feel confident that your fellowship has given you exposure to the best and most recent information and work on maintaining confidence and getting well rested
(B) Organize a study group of colleagues who you know from your fellowship program
(C) Plan an extensive review based on notes and materials collected from the recently completed fellowship
(D) Select study material that is independent of your fellowship and organize your time for a complete review of all of it
(E) Wait to study until right before the exam so that your knowledge will be as fresh as possible

42.17 The best strategy for helping yourself remember and understand the material at the level you will need for the board exam is:

(A) Be consistent: Doing the same study procedures every day is the key to success
(B) Follow your nose: Trust your instincts as to what is important and what you need to learn
(C) Nose to the grindstone: Keep at it and do not stop until you have completed the task
(D) Repetition is best: Reading over material again is always a good use of time
(E) Variety is the spice of life: Doing different things with the material will give better results than getting stuck on one approach

42.18 In the week immediately leading up to the exam, the best strategy to maximize performance on the exam would be to:

(A) Maintain my clinical schedule, but do as many practice questions as possible in the evening
(B) Maintain my clinical schedule, but meet with colleagues in the evening to have them grill me on essential concepts
(C) Stick with my regular professional routine to maintain the appropriate clinical perspective
(D) Take time off from clinical work and spend all the time possible in intensive reading and study
(E) Take time off from clinical work and spend the day alternating between practice questions and reviewing material as you deem best

42.19 Because the board exam is a timed test, it is important to have a strategy for managing time over the course of the exam. For this exam, the best strategy to manage your time would be:

(A) Answer easy questions and very hard questions quickly so you will have the time to think about questions when you need it
(B) Go slow and concentrate at the beginning of the exam and pick up the pace if you find you run short of time
(C) Practice allocating time evenly and spending the same amount of time on each question
(D) Relax and proceed at a measured pace without focusing on the time issue
(E) Work as quickly as possible from the very beginning to be sure that there is enough time

42.20 If you feel short of time during the board exam, the best strategy to pick up speed would be to read:

(A) The first line and the last line of the question stem and then move to the options
(B) The last line of the stem—the actual question—and take your best guess at an answer after looking at the options
(C) The presented options first so you will know what the key issues are as you read though the question stem
(D) The question (lead-in or last line) first, then the case content and spend just enough time on the presented options/answers to make a decision
(E) Through the question stem quickly so you will have time to think about the answer options

42.21 Some people are concerned that the makeup of the board examination is unknown and obscure and that this makes it difficult for them to study for the examination correctly. This concern is often heightened as they discover that few of their colleagues who have previously taken the examination have been helpful in telling them what questions were asked and what types of material was covered other than to say "everything." In the face of this uncertainty, the best strategy for getting a clear sense of what is tested on the board exam is to:

(A) Buy a couple of large textbooks on interventional cardiology and read each one cover-to-cover, focusing on memorizing as much as possible
(B) Contact the college of education at a local university for insight and advice on how to prepare for these examinations
(C) Hire an educational/testing consultant to assist you in preparation
(D) Rely on your developed clinical instincts as to what is most important and most likely to be tested
(E) Visit the ABIM Web site for guidance

42.22 The ABIM Web site states that "the examination will assess the candidate's knowledge and clinical judgment in aspects of interventional cardiology required to perform at a high level of competence." Since performing at a high level of competence demands current knowledge, and good clinical judgment demands that you be aware of the latest thinking and trends, your best sources of information for studying will be:

(A) Controversies and debates at the most recent appropriate annual professional meetings
(B) Recent media releases from the American College of Cardiology Extended Learning (ACCEL) and other cardiology organizations
(C) Recent issues in major cardiovascular journals dealing with interventional cardiology
(D) Textbooks and practice guideline documents published at least 6 months before the exam and material from recent board review courses

42.23 Sometimes, what physicians do in practice and what the research suggests is best may be different. On the ABIM exam, the CORRECT answer will most likely be defined by:

(A) The consensus of actual practice by the physicians in the specialty
(B) What the leading physicians in the specialty are doing
(C) Standards set by the national guidelines of the American College of Cardiology Foundation (ACCF) and the American Heart Association (AHA)
(D) Historical standards for practice in the specialty
(E) The most recent peer-reviewed publications

42.24 When taking your exam, you read the question and are about to select an answer choice. At that moment, you remember something from your recent studies that suggests that the answer is different than that you are about to select. At this point, your best course of action would be to:

(A) Reread the question again to gain a fresh perspective
(B) Mark the answer you had selected first
(C) Move on to the next question and come back to sort it out later
(D) Mark the second answer as suggested by your studies
(E) Make a random choice between the two options you are considering

42.25 As you are studying for your exam, you find that you have a hard time remembering the names of some of the newer pharmacology options. The best way to help you remember these new options would be to:

(A) Think about the drug as one set of options along with other similar drugs and focus on what sets it apart from the others
(B) Read the details about the drug over and over and over again until you can remember it
(C) Associate the drug with a patient you can remember from your own practice
(D) Associate the drug with the representative from the company who markets the drug
(E) Look up the fact sheet provided by the company that makes the drug and spend time reading over the provided material

42.26 Finding time to study for your exam in the middle of a busy professional practice and personal life can be difficult. The best way to organize your study time would be to:

(A) Block out one full day a week to study until you take the exam
(B) Keep study material with you and study every chance that you get
(C) Set aside the same time each day and commit yourself to using it for study
(D) Just focus on doing questions whenever you have a chance
(E) Focus on your practice and take a week off before the exam to do whatever studying you need

42.27 On previous exams, you sometimes have felt yourself to be nervous and jumpy and to have a hard time concentrating. For this exam, the best way to deal with these feelings would be to:

(A) Tell yourself that these reactions are not helpful and they need to stop
(B) Consider taking a 1-week course of bupropion just before the exam
(C) Stop thinking about what might happen during the exam and focus on your study and preparation
(D) Do several practice exams before the actual exam to become more accustomed to the exam situation
(E) Consider psychotherapy to address your exam reactions

42.28 Of all the material that you have to review for your exam, there is one topic that you just cannot stand. You do not deal with it during your clinical practice and really do not feel comfortable with the material. The best way to deal with this topic as you prepare for your exam would be to:

(A) Begin your studies with the topic
(B) Ignore the topic completely and study what makes more sense
(C) Find a colleague who can explain the details of the topic to you
(D) Focus on the topic right before the exam so it will be fresh in your mind
(E) Find as many questions as you can on the topic and do them all

42.29 In general, which of the following statements is TRUE about ABIM answers?

(A) The examination tests the ability to recite facts and figures
(B) It is important to know all late-breaking clinical studies
(C) The obvious answer is usually incorrect
(D) Absolutes, such as ALWAYS, NEVER, and ONLY, are typically incorrect answers

ANSWERS AND EXPLANATIONS

42.1 **Answer C.** Arrive 30 minutes prior to the appointment time specified on your confirmation email. If you arrive after your appointment time, you may not be admitted to the exam. When you arrive at the test center, you will need to present primary and secondary identification. Candidates without both valid primary and secondary ID may not be admitted to the exam. A primary ID is a current government-issued form of ID that contains both your signature and a recent photograph. A valid driver's license, passport, or state identification card is acceptable. Note: Any form of ID issued by the Syrian government cannot be used as a primary ID, per US government regulations. A secondary ID is a form of ID that includes either your signature or a photograph. For example, a social security card, valid credit card, or ATM card is acceptable.

42.2 **Answer E.** It is best to start by focusing on the content area where you are least confident. Most people are likely to spend the most time on the things that they already know fairly well. Although this might make you feel good, it does little to identify and correct deficits that should be the main goal of your exam preparation. Starting with the weakest subject assures that you will give it the time and attention it deserves. It is easier to bring your worst subject area to average than to try to make your best subject areas even better. Doing practice questions too early is like hunting without ammunition. You have to have a good sense of the material already before practice questions can really guide you further. Focusing on what others have told you can be dangerous. First, memory of exam takers is selective and what people remember is often not a good representation of what was really on the exam. In addition, what was on the exam last year may not be your best guide as to what will be on the exam that you take this year. Trying to cover a set number of pages each day misses the fact that some content will be easy and some will be hard for you. You need to spend enough time on a subject until you understand it, but not waste time on content you already know fairly well. Covering a set number of pages per day means you are not tailoring your study time to your specific needs.

42.3 **Answer B.** Do some practice questions and let the ones you get wrong tell you what to go back and study again. Questions benefit you in two ways. First, they give you experience in the behaviors and thought processes you need for the exam. Second, they can uncover weaknesses in your knowledge and understanding before the real exam. Your task is to take the information provided by questions you miss and do something about it. If you find you do not understand a concept, go back and look at it again—and don't just look at the exact issue you missed. If you missed one issue in a subject area, the odds are you have other weaknesses there as well. Just doing a lot of questions provides no real benefit. All you are doing is retesting yourself, but doing nothing to improve and increase your chances of success. Looking at brand-new study material will simply expand the amount of material you have to master and will likely result in you feeling confused or overloaded. Rereading repetitiously increases boredom but does little to give you a better grasp or increased understanding of material. Replowing the same field over and over again does not give you a better crop. The issue now is to move from simple repetition to something that will help direct your study efforts; question-guided study will do that.

42.4 **Answer C.** Organize the material into clusters. Our minds are not wired to learn lists, but classes of things. You must organize study to take advantage of this fact. Group like content together. What are key differentials? How will you decide when to choose among a select set of procedures or techniques? These are the questions you will be called upon to address on the exam. Organize your study to anticipate this. Copying details from your study material takes quite a bit of time and does not provide much return. Keeping things in the format of your study material does not render it in a form that has the most resonance with you and focusing on all the details risks having you overwhelmed by the weight of the particulars. Questions test what you know, but do not help you with the process of memorization. Rereading gets boring and eventually results in diminishing returns. Mechanically rereading means that you must cover a lot of material you already know just to uncover a few nuggets of new insight. Talking with a friend can really help you sort out and learn to articulate your understanding of difficult concepts, but memorization is an individual process done in private.

42.5 Answer D. Take a break from study. Nothing fuels frustration as much as to pushing on the thing that is frustrating you. You need to walk away briefly and take a mental break. When you return to the material, you will find you have a different perspective and what was obscure before now makes sense. Changing to a different source risks increasing the volume of material you have to study and can result in overload. There is no reason that our break should be 24 hours. A short time away from the content is usually all it takes. Shifting topics can make your study schedule choppy, makes it hard to track what you have and have not studied, and often means that you never return to the point of frustration to clarify and achieve resolution.

42.6 Answer E. If you are able to eliminate all but two options and you do not know which one to select, you have taken the questions as far as you can. You now have a 50% shot. Take it and run. It is time to guess and move on to the next question. Most people get <½ of these questions correct because they do one of several bad strategies. They reread the questions, which takes time and usually does not clarify. Making an argument usually means inventing a different question and losing track of exactly what it is you are supposed to answer. Reading each option again and reflecting usually causes you to think about things not anticipated by the question's writer. And looking carefully at the wording of options may cause you to overinterpret simple wording and talk yourself out of a right answer. When you get to two and you are through, it is time to guess.

42.7 Answer E. Use questions you get wrong to guide you as to what to go back and review again. Questions test you, but do not teach you. The learning occurs when you respond to the deficit uncovered by the questions by fixing it. Usually, this means returning to your primary study materials and reexamining the sections relevant to the question you just got incorrect. Doing a lot of questions from a lot of different sources will have you spend your time getting comfortable doing questions but will not help you improve your score. Doing more questions without additional review simply gives a more reliable assessment of your current level of expertise. Doing the same questions over and over will help you to memorize those questions but will not help you to learn the material in the way you will need for the new questions you will face on the board exam. Saving practice questions until the end of studying means you will not have the benefit of a reminder of what it is you are preparing for. You need to be reminded of the task at hand to help you focus on what is essential rather than what is simply interesting. And because the exam is timed, you should do your practice questions under timed conditions to get used to the pressures of the exam. Doing well on the exam means not just being able to answer the questions, but being able to answer them within the given timeframe.

42.8 Answer C. Select an answer based on existing practice guidelines. Established practice guidelines represent the consensus of the best minds in the field. When question writers are constructing questions, they are very likely to use existing guidelines as templates for writing questions and as arbiters for what makes the best answer. The most recently published clinical work is likely to be too new and was not available when the questions for your exam were written. What everyone thinks is right is not always what objective research tells us is correct. Consider that questions writers are especially likely to write a question about a topic where what many practitioners actually do is not supported by the empirical research. When everyone knows the right thing to do, it simply does not make a very good question. And keep in mind that the field is constantly undergoing changes. What was state-of-the-art several years ago may not be so today. In residency, the right answer is whatever your current attending physician says it is. On the board exam, the right answer is what the committee of experts relying on empirical research says that it is.

42.9 Answer B. Rearrange study materials to focus on differences among concepts. This is one of the most important issues for efficient study. Your task on a multiple-choice exam is to select among the presented options. To do your best, you need to study the same way. Focus on learning sets options and then how to choose among those options. Learning all the details of something will not be nearly as useful as knowing what clinical detail makes one option better than another. Differential diagnosis should be your template. You need to be able to do more than recognize a patient with a certain condition. You need to be able to tell yourself why it is that condition and not something similar. The same logic holds for choosing among procedures, techniques, and patient management options. Real-life cases may not offer the type of choices you will be given on the actual exam. Rereading and remembering something exactly as they are presented helps memorize the text but does not give you an understanding of the material in your own words and on your own terms. Material memorized does not help you decide. Material you have organized in your head for that purpose does. And writing everything out longhand just takes too much time given the amount of material you have to master for the exam.

42.10 **Answer D.** Summarize for yourself the key concepts covered during your study session. A quick mental review of what you have covered is the best way to get closure for your study session, to facilitate remembering key concepts, and it forces you to think about things on your own terms rather than just mimicking the words you have studied. Focusing on where you are in your progress tends to make the task seem longer. Each time you focus on looking ahead, you risk your inner child asking, "Are we there yet?" Before you look ahead, be sure of what you have just covered. Looking ahead to the next topic can make it hard to concentrate on and retain the current issues under study. At the end of your study session, you will have a mental break as you move on to other things in your life. Just be sure to summarize and reinforce what you have done before moving on.

42.11 **Answer A.** First, focus on the question at the end (called lead-in) of the clinical case. One of the most common, and avoidable, mistakes on a multiple-choice exam is to answer the questions you wanted or expected rather than the one you were actually asked. This error costs otherwise well-prepared people valuable points they deserve to have. The best strategy is to read and understand what the focus of the question is and then scan the answer options to see what types of answers are being sought. Following that, read the case vignette carefully and reread the question at the end of the clinical case and choose your answer. Without the guidance of the questions, options tend to only confuse you. Thinking in general or about a real-life patient takes you away from that matter at hand. Focus on the questions asked and let your thinking be about that!

42.12 **Answer A.** Begin doing a few questions early and increase the number as the exam gets closer. Questions are the target that you are in training to hit. You need to be reminded of why you are studying. Start doing practice questions, just a few, early in your study. As you progress through the material, day by day, you can increase the number of questions you do and the time you spend reviewing them. Do not do questions haphazardly in spare moments, but keep your practice as close as you can to the real exam situation. This means questions should be done in clusters and with a clock. Do a set of questions before looking up the answer to any one question. But also remember that questions themselves will not get you where you need to be. The hard work of studying is how you learn what you need to learn. Questions just help you refine your knowledge and gain perspective on how an issue might be approached on an exam. Study is first; questions are second. Do not leave them until the end.

42.13 **Answer B.** Begin preparation early to get a sense of what is familiar and your comfort with the material. One size does not fit all. There is no magic number of days, weeks, or months required to prepare for the exam. You simply need to make sure that you have the time that *you* need, which may be different than that of other people. By starting early, you will ensure that you have the time, if you need it, and will be able to get a real concrete sense of how familiar or unfamiliar the material might be. The key is not to adopt some formula, like a set number of weeks or a certain number of pages per day, but to select a solution and study schedule that meet your particular needs. A practice exam is always a nice idea, if possible, and can pinpoint areas of weakness, but it cannot tell you how long you, personally, need to prepare. When are you ready to take the exam? When you get it! You should be at the level of being able to argue and explain the material to others. Most people have pretty good gut instinct as to when they have reached this level.

42.14 **Answer B.** Organize material in modules and modules in clusters that emphasize differentiation. The two most important issues in studying are to organize the material in a way that makes sense to you and to make sure that you focus on being able to make choices among the presented options. If you can lay out everything that is known about a procedure or a technique, this will not help you. You will not be asked to lay out everything you know. Instead, you will have to be able to say why "this" and not "that." Details that help you make these kinds of decisions are essential. Details that do not are mere knowledge ornamentation with no value for improving your exam performance. Not all the details matter. Everything in your study material is not important. Make choices and focus on what matters. Review courses help you with this, but you can also give yourself guidance by remembering the type of decisions the exam will ask you to make. Reading aloud is a good way to reinforce memory regarding difficult concepts, but simply takes too long given the body of material you have to master, nor does reading someone else's words help to get concepts framed in the way that makes the most sense to you. Studying what was on the exam last year can be a recipe for disaster. Board exams tend to shift content year to year. Study for *this* exam, not for the one last year. Outlines and tales showing similarities and differences among concepts are much better choices than writing out content in full sentences.

42.15 Answer D. Look at it for a little bit of time every day until you feel comfortable with it. Sequential study sessions over a period of days are by far the most effective and efficient way to master complex materials. Learning theory tells us that "spaced practice is better than massed practice," which means that sitting and trying to grasp content all at once is not nearly as effective as looking at it repeatedly over time. Trying to get it all in one day is a residual of the days when you had to cram for an exam in only a day or two. Preparing for the board exam is different. You will be studying over weeks and months and have the time to take the time when you need it. Practice questions are an excellent vehicle to get you to think about the exam and to break you from the monotony of rote rereading of material, but they will likely not show you the material just as you will encounter it on the exam. Most people walk out of the exam surprised that although practice questions do cover much of the same information as on the exam, they do so in a different, and sometimes, surprising way. You cannot anticipate all the questions, but you can arm yourself with the information you need and train yourself to be able to think with it and solve whatever problem you are presented with. Gathering all the reference material available is a sure way to end up overloaded and overwhelmed. Do not skip over complex material. Complex material is more likely than easier material to be the source of questions. Take the time you need, look at it repeatedly, and you will find you are able to master what you could not master before.

42.16 Answer D. No matter how well-known and structured the program and how compulsive the fellow, it is unlikely that any program will impart all of the possible testable knowledge in an ABIM examination. In each program or curriculum, there is an intended curriculum (objectives, examination blueprint, etc.) and an informal curriculum (content emphasized during lectures and small group discussions, etc.) (McLaughlin K, et al. *BMC Med Educ* 2005;5:39). Frequently, it is the informal curriculum that flavors a trainee's data retention and clinical practice patterns. The examiners for the ABIM-sponsored examinations, however, are focused on assessing core knowledge of generally accepted practice standards. Therefore, it is important to recognize that the examiners' perception of core knowledge may not be consistent with the exam taker's experience with an informal curriculum. All programs have strengths and weaknesses, and it is the latter components in which it is particularly important to study and increase one's knowledge. A casual attitude of preparation is likely to lead to disappointing results in testing.

42.17 Answer E. Variety is the spice of life: Doing different things with the material will give better results than getting stuck on one approach. Effective study requires a series of steps in which you do different things with the material as your familiarity with it changes. Step one is to decide what you will study. Step two requires repetition and reading over the essential material. Step three requires fostering recollection by doing something active with the material, such as making outlines, drawing pictures, talking to yourself about it, or talking with others. Step four moves on to practice using the material as you focus on practice questions. Doing the exact same things every day does not make sense as your understanding changes and improves. Following your instincts will likely have you study what you like but avoid what you hate. You need guidance as to what to study beyond your personal preferences. Pushing on for weeks at a time without a break is emotionally damaging and cognitively ineffective. Schedule some pauses in your study. You will come back to it fresher, with more insight and more motivation. Rereading helps to get content into your head but does not help you get it out when you need it. At some point, you need to change from repetition to active processes that promote recollection.

42.18 Answer E. Take time off from clinical work and spend the day alternating between doing practice questions and reviewing material as you decide you need to. The board exam will require different mental processes and a different perspective than daily clinical work. Taking a break from your clinical duties will aid you in making this transition. It will also help to ensure that you do not walk into the exam sleep deprived by giving up sleep in order to try to do your job and your exam preparation at the same time. When you take time off, do not spend every waking moment in preparation. Instead, set up each day like a job; put in the time you planned and then stop and allow yourself some downtime to relax.

42.19 Answer A. Answer easy questions and very hard questions quickly so you will have the time to think about questions when you need it. The essential notion here is to have the time when you need it by not wasting it on difficult questions you do not know or lingering over easy questions when the answer is obvious to you. Going slow and focusing on concentration will result in you having too little time at the end. Not all questions take the same amount of time. Spend just what is needed on each one and then move on. If you do not think about time at all, you will be ambushed by a shortage of time at the end of the exam period. The trick is to track the time without being panicked by the ticking of the clock. Working as quickly as possible makes most people feel rushed and unable to have that moment of reflection that makes the difference. Questions will require you to think. You need to move efficiently through the exam. But not at the expense of giving up applying your intelligence and thinking through to the best answer.

42.20 Answer D. First focus on the question at the end (called lead-in) of the clinical case. The best strategy when pressed for time is to read and understand what the focus of the question is and then scan the answer options to see what types of answers are being sought. After that, read the case vignette for clues and choose your answer. Getting to the options/answers before reading and processing the clues given in the question is essentially hunting in the dark. You are unlikely to get the right option that gives you the point and improves your chances of passing.

42.21 Answer E. To get specific information about the exam you are preparing for, go right to the source. An educational consultant or the local college of education at the university will provide useful information about a broad field of study techniques, improving data retention, and the like. They will not be knowledgeable, however, about the structure of the ABIM content in interventional cardiology. Knowing that structure and content makeup can help you target your preparation better. It is available at the ABIM Web site (www.abim.org) and currently has a Web address of www.abim.org/cert/aqic.shtm. The primary content areas and their relative proportions on the examination as of July 2017 are shown in Table A42-21:

Table A42-21

Medical Content Category	% of Exam
Case Selection and Management	20%
Procedural Techniques	20%
Complications of Coronary Intervention	8%
Catheter-Based Management of Noncoronary Disease	13%
Basic Science	6%
Anatomy, Anatomic Variants, Anatomic Pathology	6%
Pharmacology	12%
Cardiac Imaging and Assessment	9%
Miscellaneous	6%
	100%

Source: http://www.abim.org/~/media/ABIM%20Public/Files/pdf/exam-blueprints/certification/interventional-cardiology.pdf

The Web site provides additional information as to specific content within each of these broad areas. Merging this information with your own awareness of strengths and weaknesses in your own knowledge base allows you to tailor your studying, spending more time on relatively weaker areas of knowledge and slightly less in areas of greater proficiency.

42.22 Answer D. Board questions are focused on core knowledge required to support excellent clinical judgment. As such, the boards do not examine the latest and greatest theories, ideas, and personal opinions of interventional thought leaders. Guidelines documents are a rich source of information as they are robust, amply referenced, and based on levels of evidence. Since they are evidence based, they provide a rich source of potential examination material with "single best answers." Textbooks are also excellent sources of information, but this information is often a bit more dated. Nonetheless, such information is often highly relevant and "testable." Remember that the board questions are written, vetted, and "put to bed" several months before the actual examination. The ABIM has never given an exact cutoff date for inclusion of information in the examination, but a general time frame of 6 to 9 months pre-examination has been suggested as reasonable. Data more recent than that are not felt to be widely enough known, disseminated, and incorporated to stand as valid test material. Also, the controversies or debates at large annual meetings, recent reports and opinions from interventional cardiology leaders, and other such opinion-based material are not the core information used for ABIM testing. Board review courses are rich sources of information for preparation as they are focused on core knowledge and not the latest, hottest new topics.

42.23 Answer C. One of the aims of this certification exam is to be sure you are abreast of current evidence-based medical knowledge. The medical specialty societies (ACC and AHA) set forth practice guidelines from time to time based on robust clinical evidence. These guidelines are based on the best knowledge available, which means concrete evidence as presented in publications that were able to stand the test of peer review. The best answer on your exam is not what everyone does, but what everyone ought to do based on the most current evidence-based knowledge.

42.24 Answer D. In spite of what has become common wisdom, your first impulse is not necessarily your best answer. Research has shown us that changing your mind when new information occurs increases your score when compared to always sticking to the first answer that occurs to you. This is different from second guessing yourself or simply having doubts. In those instances, your first instinct is likely your best. But when you are thinking about a problem and new information occurs to you, that new information is likely useful and your response should change accordingly. Note that moving away from the question and coming back later interrupts the thought process in which you were engaged. When you come back, you must re-engage the question and repeat the thought process all over again.

42.25 Answer A. Comparing the drugs with other options creates an anchor for the new information and fosters retention. Remember that our brains are basically lazy and retain information only if we are going to use it or if it connected to other information of value. By thinking about how these new drugs are similar to and different than the pharmacology you already know, you have placed the drugs in a content from that's easier to recall. Reading about the drugs over and over again is an exercise in brute memory. This type of memory is short term, and the information is easily forgotten when you move on to something else. Linking the drug to a patient is only useful if the exam presents to you the same type of patient and you have some actual experience using the drug. Thinking about the pharmacy representative removes you from the clinical thought process the exam question will require of you.

42.26 Answer C. Learning is most efficient when it occurs regularly over time. Having study time as a part of your routine makes it less likely that you will forget to put the time in or be distracted by something else. Blocking out one day a week can be difficult in the face of clinical practice demands and can create a feeling that too much has to be accomplished on this day. Trying to study every spare moment can be fatiguing and can distract you from clinical and personal life demands. Questions are a great way to self-evaluate and get guidance for future study but do not, by themselves, give you the overview and content you need to make sense of material. Waiting until the last week before the exam to study may mean that you do not have enough time to really prepare and is unlikely to allow you to reflect on and think about the material as you study.

42.27 Answer D. Familiarity tends to lessen anxiety. Spending time in practice situations will help you have more emotional control during the exam when it matters. This process has the added benefit of providing the questions that you get wrong to give you guidance as to what you should study as your exam preparation moves forward. Telling yourself to not have your emotional reactions is rarely effective. Our cognitive processes can influence but often have little control over our emotional reactions. Self-medication is never a good idea, and when the trigger for anxiety is situational rather than systemic, general antianxiety medications are not the answer. Trying not to think about something that is a worry for you often enhances, rather than suppresses, our emotional reaction. The reaction you have is real and cannot simply be ignored. Finally, having some nervousness during exams is relatively normal and does not suggest the need for psychotherapy. Remember that getting nervous during exams is normal. The issue is to get used to the situation so anxiety does not rise to the level of becoming a problem.

42.28 Answer A. We all have material we do not like and do not want to study. The best way to tackle this material is to get it out of the way early. If you put it off, you will likely find that you never really have time to get to it and your score will suffer correspondingly. If you are going to run the race, tackle the big hill at the start of the race; do not wait and let it defeat you at the end of the process. Getting a colleague to talk to you about the topic may prove difficult. If you do not deal with these issues in your own practice, you may not know who to approach. Even if you do find someone, just because they can explain it to you does not mean that you will gain the understanding you need. You need to make the content yours, which means getting an understanding in ways that make sense to you. Doing questions will confirm that you do not know the topic but will not teach it to you. Start with the hardest stuff first in your study. This will give you the time you need to master it. And once you have mastered the hard stuff, the rest is (literally) easy.

42.29 Answer D. The board examination does not test the ability to recite facts and figures. It is, in fact, designed to test the breadth and depth of interventional cardiology knowledge. The board questions are set at least a year or so in advance, and while it may be important to know late-breaking clinical studies that were reported last month for practice, it is not going to be tested in the boards. The board examination is not trying to trick you, and the obvious answer is usually correct. Absolutes, such as ALWAYS, NEVER, and ONLY, are typically incorrect answers since very few things in medicine are absolute.

INDEX

(Note: Page numbers followed by *t* indicate table and those followed by *f* indicate figure.)

E

M

N

O

P

Q

R

T